DeGowin's

DIAGNOSTIC EXAMINATION

NOTICE

Medicine is an ever-changing science. As research and clinical experience broaden our knowledge, changes in treatment and drug therapy are required. In their efforts to provide information that is complete and generally in accord with the standards accepted at the time of publication, the editor and the publisher of this work have checked with sources believed to be reliable. However, human error and changes in medical science are unavoidable. Neither the editor nor the publisher nor any other party who has been involved in the preparation or publication of this work warrants that the information contained herein is in every respect accurate or complete, and they are not responsible for any errors or omissions or the results obtained from the use of such information. Readers are encouraged to confirm the information contained herein with other sources. For example and in particular, readers are advised to check the product information sheet included in the package of each drug they plan to administer to be certain that the information contained in this book is accurate and that changes have not been made in the recommended dose or in the contraindications for administration. This recommendation is of particular importance in connection with new or infrequently used drugs.

DeGowin's
DIAGNOSTIC EXAMINATION

Eighth Edition

Richard F. LeBlond, M.D., F.A.C.P.

Professor of Internal Medicine (Clinical)
The University of Iowa College of Medicine
Iowa City, Iowa

Richard L. DeGowin, M.D., F.A.C.P.

Professor Emeritus of Internal Medicine
The University of Iowa College of Medicine
Iowa City, Iowa

Donald D. Brown, M.D., F.A.C.P.

Professor of Internal Medicine
The University of Iowa College of Medicine
Iowa City, Iowa

Illustrated by

**Elmer DeGowin, M.D.,
Jim Abel,
and Shawn Roach**

McGraw-Hill
Medical Publishing Division

*New York   St. Louis   San Francisco   Auckland   Bogotá   Caracas
Lisbon   London   Madrid   Mexico City   Milan   Montreal
New Delhi   San Juan   Singapore   Sydney   Tokyo   Toronto*

The **McGraw·Hill** *Companies*

DeGowin's Diagnostic Examination, Eighth Edition

1234567890   DOC DOC 0987654

ISBN 0-07-140923-8

This book was set in Palatino by Matrix Publishing Services.
The editors were Jim Shanahan and Karen Edmonson.
The production supervisor was Rick Ruzycka.
The text designer was Marsha Cohen/Parallelogram
The cover designer was Aimee Nordin.
The index was prepared by Nancy Newman.
RR Donnelley Crawfordsville, was printer and binder.

This book is printed on acid-free paper.

Library of Congress Cataloging-in-Publication Data
DeGowin's diagnostic examination.—8th ed. / edited by Richard F.
  LeBlond, Richard L. DeGowin, Donald D. Brown
      p. ; cm.
   Includes bibliographical references and index.
   ISBN 0-07-140923-8
   1. Physical diagnosis. 2. Diagnosis. I. Title: Diagnostic
examination. II. DeGowin, Richard L. III. LeBlond, Richard F.
IV. Brown, Donald D., 1940–
   [DNLM: 1. Physical Examination. 2. Diagnosis. 3. Signs and
Symptoms. WB 200 D3194 2004]
   RC76.D45 2004
   616.07'54—dc22   2003061420

Dedication

To my wife, Annie,
and children, Sueño and Ned,
for your patience,
understanding, and encouragement.
Richard F. LeBlond

It is not easy to give exact and complete details of an operation in writing; but the reader should form an outline of it from the description.

HIPPOCRATES
"On Joints"

[Studies] perfect Nature, and are perfected by Experience: For Natural Abilities, are like Natural Plants, that need proyning by study: And Studies themselves, due give forth Directions too much at Large, except they be bounded in by experience. Crafty Men Contemne Studies; Simple Men Admire them; And Wise Men Use them; For they teach not their owne Use; But that is a Wisdome without them, and above them, won by Observation. Reade not to Contradict, and Confute; Nor to Beleeve and Take for granted; Nor to Finde Talke and Disourse; But to weigh and Consider.

FRANCIS BACON
"Of Studies"

It is only by persistent intelligent study of disease upon a methodical plan of examination that a man gradually learns to correlate his daily lessons with the facts of his previous experience and that of his fellows, and so acquires clinical wisdom.

SIR WILLIAM OSLER

Sources for Quotations:

Brecht quotation from: Bertolt Brecht. *Poems 1913–1956*. London, Methuen London Ltd., 1979.

Eliot quotation from: T.S. Eliot. *The Complete Poems and Plays, 1909–1950*. New York, Harcourt, Brace & World, Inc., 1971.

Frazer quotation from: Sir James George Frazer. *The Golden Bough, A Study in Magic and Religion*, abridged edition. New York, MacMillan Publishing Company, 1922.

Hippocrates quotation from: Jacques Jouanna (M.B. DeBevoise translator). *Hippocrates*. Baltimore, The Johns Hopkins University Press, 1999.

Osler quotation from: Sir William Osler. *Aequanimitas, with other Addresses to Medical Students, Nurses and Practictioners of Medicine*. Philadelphia, P. Blakiston's Son and Co., 1928

Roethke quotations from: Theodore Roethke. *On Poetry and Craft*. Port Townsend, Washington Copper Canyon Press, 2001.

Contents

Part I

THE DIAGNOSTIC FRAMEWORK

Part II

THE DIAGNOSTIC EXAMINATION

Part III

PREOPERATIVE EVALUATION

Part IV

USE OF THE LABORATORY AND DIAGNOSTIC IMAGING

Quick-Find Guide

Part 1

THE DIAGNOSTIC FRAMEWORK

Chapter 1

DIAGNOSIS / 1

Chapter 2

HISTORY TAKING AND THE MEDICAL RECORD / 17

Chapter 3

THE SCREENING PHYSICAL EXAMINATION: METHODS AND PROCEDURE / 39

Part II

THE DIAGNOSTIC EXAM

Chapter 4

VITAL SIGNS, ANTHROPOMETRIC DATA AND PAIN / 59

Chapter 5

NON-REGIONAL SYSTEMS AND DISEASES / 99

Chapter 6
_____

THE SKIN AND NAILS / 129

Chapter 7

THE HEAD AND NECK / 197

Edema-Papillitis, Anterior Optic Neuritis,
Papilledema; Pseudopapilledema, Venous
Engorgement, Hemorrhages, CMV Retinitis,
Arterial Occlusion, Venous Occlusion, Arteriolar
Sclerosis, Retinal Spots-Cotton Wool Spots, Hard
Exudates, Pigmented Spots; Refractile Spots in
Retinal Arteries, White or Yellow Spots in Retinal
Arteries, Macular Degeneration, Diabetic
Retinopathy, White Macular Region, Retinitis
Pigmentosa, Angioid Streaks, Retinal Detachment

Protuberance, Palatine Mass-Carcinoma, Mixed
Tumor of Ectopic Salivary Gland; Arched Palate,
Cleft Palate, Palatine Perforation

Chapter 8

THE CHEST: CHEST WALL, PULMONARY, AND CARDIOVASCULAR SYSTEMS; THE BREASTS / 339

Chapter 9

THE ABDOMEN, PERINEUM, ANUS, AND RECTOSIGMOID / 509

Chapter 12

MALE GENITALIA AND REPRODUCTIVE TRACT / 649

Chapter 13
_____

THE SPINE AND EXTREMITIES: THE MUSCULOSKELETAL AND SOFT TISSUE EXAM / 675

Chapter 14

THE NEUROLOGIC EXAMINATION / 797

Chapter 15

THE MENTAL STATUS, PSYCHIATRIC, AND SOCIAL EVALUATIONS / 881

Part III

THE PREOPERATIVE EVALUATION

Chapter 16

THE PREOPERATIVE EVALUATION / 903

Part IV

USE OF THE LABORATORY AND DIAGNOSTIC IMAGING

Chapter 17

PRINCIPLES OF DIAGNOSTIC TESTING / 915

Chapter 18

COMMON LABORATORY TESTS / 933

Preface

The clinician's goal in performing a history and physical examination is to generate diagnostic hypotheses. This was true for Hippocrates and Olser and remains true today. The practice of medicine would be simple if each symptom or sign could be matched to a single disease, but this is not the case. There are a large number of symptoms and signs; we cover several hundred in this book, and they can occur in a nearly infinite number of combinations and temporal patterns. The clinician's diagnostic task has four parts:

(1) To become familiar with the symptoms and signs of common and unusual diseases;
(2) To elicit the pattern of the symptoms and signs from each patient;
(3) To generate a differential diagnosis, a list of those diseases or conditions most likely to be causes of the patient's illness; and
(4) To test those hypotheses with appropriate laboratory tests or clinical interventions.

DeGowin's Diagnostic Examination has been used by students and clinicians for nearly forty years precisely because of its usefulness in this diagnostic process:

(1) It describes the techniques for obtaining a complete history and performing a thorough physical examination;
(2) It links symptoms and signs with the pathophysiology of disease;
(3) It presents an approach to differential diagnosis, based upon the pathophysiology of disease, which can be efficiently tested in the laboratory.
(4) It does all of this in a format that can be used as a quick reference at the "point of care" and as a text to study the principles and practice of history taking and physical examination.

When Dr. Richard DeGowin asked me to undertake revision of the seventh edition, I was honored, and not a little intimidated. My goal was to preserve the unique strengths of previous editions, while making organizational changes for greater ease of use. The second edition was one of the few books I have retained from medical school, thirty years ago. The reason is that *DeGowin's Diagnostic Examination* emphasizes the unchanging aspects of clinical medicine: the symptoms and signs of disease as related by the patient and discovered by physical examination.

Pathophysiology links the patient's story of their illness (the history), the physical signs of disease, and the changes in biologic structure and function revealed by imaging studies and laboratory testing. Patients describe symptoms, we need to *hear* pathophysiology; we observe signs, we need to *see* pathophysiology; the radiologist and laboratories report findings, we need to *think* pathophysiology. Understanding pathophysiology gives us the tools to understand *disease* as alterations in physiology and anatomy and *illness* as the patient's experience of these changes.

In keeping with this theme, I have placed a discussion of the *Pathophysiology* of many of the signs and symptoms immediately following the heading, highlighted in blue. The discussions are brief and the reader is encouraged to consult physiology texts to develop a full understanding of normal and abnormal physiology [Guyton AC, Hall JE. *Textbook of Medical Physiology,* 10th edition. Philadelphia, W.B. Saunders Company, 2000 and Lingappa VR, Farey K. *Physiological Medicine: A Clinical Approach to Basic Medical Physiology.* New York, McGraw-Hill, 2000].

I should emphasize that *DeGowin's Diagnostic Examination* is not just a descriptive text on how to do a history and physical exam. It is, uniquely, a text to assist the clinician in *thinking* about symptoms and physical signs to facilitate generation of reasonable, testable diagnostic hypotheses. This subject is covered in detail in Chapters 1 through 3 and 17.

The chapters in the body of the book, Part II, continue to be organized around the regions of the body examined sequentially during the physical examination. I have added two chapters that bring together and expand material previously scattered in several chapters: Chapter 4 discusses the vital signs, and Chapter 5 discusses major physiologic systems that do not have a primary representation in a single body region or unique set of examination methods.

In reorganizing the text, I have introduced a common structure to the body-region chapters in Part II, Chapters 6 through 14. See the Introduction for an outline of this structure. To avoid duplication, the text is heavily cross-referenced. I hope the reader will find this useful and not too cumbersome.

A detailed outline of the contents (Quick-Find Guide) of each chapter follows the Contents. This allows the reader to quickly scan the organization and content of each chapter.

References to articles from the medical literature are included in the body of the text. We have chosen articles which provide useful clinical information including excellent descriptions of diseases and syndromes and, in some cases, photographs illustrating key findings. Evidence-based articles on the utility of the physical exam are included, mostly from the *Rational Clinical Examination* series published over the last decade in the Journal of the American Medical Association. *They are included with the caveat that they evaluate the physical exam as a hypothesis-testing tool, <u>not</u> as a hypothesis generating task.* Some references may be dated in their recommendations for laboratory testing and treatment; they are included because they give thorough descriptions of the relevant clinical syndromes, often with excellent discussions of the approach to differential diagnosis. Tests and treatments come and go, but good thinking has staying power. *The reader must always check current resources before initiating a laboratory evaluation or therapeutic program.*

Each chapter was reviewed and revised by my co-authors and independently reviewed by faculty members of the University of Iowa, Roy J. and Lucille A. Carver College of Medicine. Their feedback and assistance is gratefully acknowledged. Reviewers for this edition are: Caroline Carney-Doebbling M.D., M.Sc., Associate Professor of Psychiatry and Internal Medicine, Indiana University School of Medicine (Chapter 15); Jane Engeldinger, M.D., Professor, Clinical Obstetrics and Gynecology (Chapters 10 and 11); Bruce J. Gantz, M.D., F.A.C.S., Professor and Head, Brian F. McCabe Distinguished Chair in Otolaryngology, Department of Otolaryngology (Chapter 7); Christopher J. Goerdt, M.D., M.P.H., Associate Professor, Clinical Internal Medicine, Division of General Internal Medicine (Chapters 1–3, 9, 16 and 17); George V. Lawry III, M.D., Professor, Clinical Internal Medicine, Division of Rheumatology (Chapter 13); Warren W. Piette, M.D., Professor and Vice-Chair, Department of Dermatology (Chapter 6); Gary Rosenthal, M.D., M.P.H., Professor of Internal Medicine and Division Director for General Internal Medicine (Chapter 17); Jay Sandlow, M.D., Associate Professor and Vice Chair, Department of Urology, Medical College of Wisconsin (Chapters 10 and 12); William B. Silverman, M.D., Professor, Clinical Internal Medicine, Division of Gastroenterology and Hepatobiliary Diseases (Chapter 9); Haraldine A. Stafford, M.D., Ph.D., Associate Professor, Clinical Internal Medicine, Divisions of Rheumatology (Chapter 13); and Michael Wall, M.D., Professor of Neurology and Ophthalmology (Chapters 7 and 14). As noted above, Drs. Carney-Doebbling and Sandlow have been recruited to other institutions; they will be missed.

Once again, Mr. Shawn Roach has done an excellent job of revising many of the illustrations for this edition. I greatly appreciate his patience and cooperation. Mrs. Denise Floerchinger was instrumental in coordinating the many details of manuscript preparation and reviews. Her assistance is gratefully acknowledged.

My co-authors for this edition, Donald D. Brown, MD, and Richard L. DeGowin, MD, have been instrumental in seeing that the eighth edition maintains the strengths of previous editions. Dr. Brown directed the history taking and physical examination course at the University of Iowa for over 25 years. He is annually nominated for best teacher awards by the students in recognition of his knowledge and enthusiasm for teaching these essential skills. Dr. Brown has reviewed the entire text and made many corrections and additions to the initial drafts. In addition, as a practicing cardiologist, he is the primary reviewer for Chapters 8 and 16.

I am especially appreciative of the encouragement and support of Dr. Richard DeGowin during the extensive revisions for this edition. He has carefully read each chapter and made many suggestions and corrections to my drafts. He is a wonderful collaborator and I appreciate the opportunity he has given me to guide the eighth edition of *DeGowin's Diagnostic Examination.*

Mr. James Shanahan, our editor at McGraw-Hill, has been actively involved from the beginning in the planning and execution of the eighth edition. His encouragement and support are deeply appreciated. The McGraw-Hill editorial and publishing staff under his direction, especially Ms. Michelle Watt, have been prompt and professional throughout manuscript preparation, editing, and production. The continued success of *DeGowin's Diagnostic Examination* is due in large measure to the support and enthusiasm of Mr. Martin Wonsiewicz of McGraw-Hill. We could not have asked for a more professional and supportive publisher.

I wish to thank my colleagues who have encouraged me throughout the course of this project. I have incorporated many suggestions from my co-authors and each of the reviewers; any remaining deficiencies are mine. Ultimately, you, the reader, will determine the strengths and weaknesses of this edition. I welcome your feedback and suggestions. Email your comments to richard-leblond@uiowa.edu (please include "DeGowin's" on the subject line).

Richard F. LeBlond, M.D., F.A.C.P.
Iowa City, Iowa

Introduction and User's Guide

> Read with two objectives: first to acquaint yourself with the current knowledge on the subject and the steps by which it has been reached; and secondly, and more important, read to understand and analyze your cases.
>
> SIR WILLIAM OSLER
> *"The Student Life"*

Despite recent advances in testing and imaging, the clinician's skills in taking a history and performing a physical examination are needed now more than ever. Proper use of the laboratory and imaging are based upon accurate diagnostic hypotheses derived from the history and physical examination. The history is the patient's story of their illness related as the time course of their symptoms; the physical examination reveals the signs of disordered anatomy and physiology. The symptoms and signs of disease form temporal patterns which the clinician recognizes from his experience and knowledge of diseases. From the history and physical examination the clinician generates a set of testable pathophysiologic and diagnostic hypotheses, the differential diagnosis. It is this differential diagnosis which is subjected to laboratory testing.

Members of the American Board of Internal Medicine have expressed concern about the atrophy of diagnostic skills among trainees and have recommended improvements in training programs [Schechter GP, Blank LL, Godwin HA, Jr., LaCombe MA, Novack DH, and Rosse WF. Refocusing of history-taking skills during internal medicine training. *Am J Med* 1996;101:210–216]. They point out that reliance on technological testing has contributed to this deficiency. *DeGowin's Diagnostic Examination* is intended to assist the student and clinician in practice in making reasonable diagnostic hypotheses from the history and physical examination. Part I, Chapters 1–3, discuss the diagnostic framework in detail. Chapter 1 discusses the importance of diagnosis and the process of forming a differential diagnosis specific to each patient. Chapter 2 discusses the process of history taking and documentation of your findings in the medical record. Chapter 3 presents an outline of the screening physical examination.

The heart of *DeGowin's Diagnostic Examination* is Part II, Chapters 4–15. It is organized in the sequence in which the clinician traditionally performs the examination. Chapter 4 discusses the vital signs. Chapter 5 introduces some systems to keep in mind throughout the examination since they present with symptoms and signs not easily referable to a specific body region. Chapters 6–13 discuss the diagnostic examination by body region: the skin (Chapter 6), the head and neck (Chapter 7), the chest and breasts (Chapter 8), the abdomen (Chapter 9), the urinary system (Chapter 10), the female genitalia and reproductive system (Chapter 11), the male genitalia and reproductive system (Chapter 12), the spine and extremities (Chapter 13), the neurologic examination (Chapter 14), and the psychiatric and social evaluations (Chapter 15).

Parts III and IV provide supplemental information. Chapter 16 discusses the preoperative examination. The intent is to give the reader a framework for evaluating the medical risks of surgical procedures and an approach to communicating those risks to the patient and surgeon. Chapter 17 introduces the principles of laboratory testing and imaging. These principles are critical to an efficient use of the laboratory and radiology. Chapter 18 lists many common (not "routine") laboratory tests which provide important information about the patient's condition not accessible from the history or physical examination. More specialized tests used to evaluate specific diagnostic hypotheses are not discussed.

Chapters 6–14 have a uniform organization: (A) each chapter begins with a brief overview of the major organ systems to be considered; (B) following is a discussion of the superficial and deep anatomy of the body region; (C) the physical examination of the region or system is described in detail in the usual order of performance; (D) the symptoms particularly relevant to the body region and systems are presented; (E) the physical signs in the region or system exams are listed (some findings can be both symptoms and signs; discussion of a finding is in the section where it is most likely to be encountered, then cross referenced in the other section); and (F) discusses some diseases and syndromes commonly in the differential diagnosis of symptoms and signs in the body region and systems under discussion. To avoid duplication, the text is heavily cross-referenced.

Brief discussions of many diseases and clinical syndromes are included so the reader can appreciate the patterns of symptoms and signs they commonly manifest. This will help the clinician determine whether that disease or syndrome should be included in the differential diagnosis of the symptoms and signs *in their specific patient*. Particularly useful points of differentiation are listed after the DDX symbol. This is not a textbook of medicine. The reader must use *DeGowin's Diagnostic Examination* with a comprehensive textbook of medicine to fully understand the diseases and syndromes. We strongly recommend *Harrison's Principles of Internal Medicine* as a companion text [Kaspar DL, Braunwald E, Fauci AS, et al (editors). *Harrison's Principles of Internal Medicine,* 16th edition. New York, McGraw-Hill, 2004].

We emphasize the characteristics of diseases because a clinician who knows the manifestations of many diseases will ask the right questions, obtain the key history, and elicit the pertinent signs to differentiate one disease from another. Instructions on how to elicit the specific signs are included in the physical examination section for each region; if the maneuver is not generally part of the routine exam, it is discussed with the sign itself. Following the descriptions of many symptoms and signs is a highlighted *CLINICAL OCCURRENCE* section. This is a list of diseases from which to begin a differential diagnosis. The organization of the *CLINICAL OCCURRENCE* section is based upon the approach to the differential diagnosis of the symptom or sign felt to be most useful clinically.

Where a broad differential exists, we have introduced an organizational scheme for the **CLINICAL OCCURRENCE** based upon the pathophysiologic mechanisms of disease. The clinician can often narrow their differential diagnosis to one or a few of the basic mechanisms of disease: congenital, endocrine, idiopathic, infectious, inflammatory/immune, mechanical/traumatic, metabolic/toxic, neoplastic, neurologic, psychosocial, or vascular. This facilitates the creation of a reasonable differential diagnosis. The categories in this scheme are not mutually exclusive; a congenital syndrome may be metabolic, infections are usually accompanied by inflammation, and a neoplastic process may cause mechanical obstruction. Though not rigid, this is a useful conceptual construct for *thinking* about the patient's problems.

Key symptoms, signs, syndromes, and diseases are highlighted. These are important in understanding common disease processes. Critical symptoms, signs, syndromes, and diseases are noted by the ▶ marginal symbol. These are symptoms, signs, syndromes, and diseases which may indicate an emergent condition requiring immediate and complete evaluation.

By using our understanding of normal and abnormal anatomy and physiology as the basis for thinking within clinical medicine, it is possible to avoid the trap of "word space." This is the term one of us (RFL) has given to the common practice of using lists and word association as a means of thinking (or, rather not thinking) about diagnosis: associating a word (for instance, cough) with a memorized list of other words (pneumonia, bronchitis, asthma, post-nasal drip, gastroesophageal reflux, etc.). The emphasis on memorization inherent in this scheme is the bane of all medical students; fortunately, it is not only unnecessary, it is counter-productive. Cough is a protective reflex arising from sensory phenomena in the upper airway, bronchi, lungs, and esophagus mediated through peripheral and central nervous system pathways and executed by coordinated contraction of the diaphragm, chest wall, and laryngeal muscles. With this physiologic context, and our understanding of the mechanisms of disease, we can hypothesize the irritants most likely to be relevant *in each specific patient*.

New diseases are being encountered with surprising frequency. They present not with new symptoms and signs but with new combinations of the old symptoms and signs. It is our hope that the reader will learn to recognize the patterns of known diseases and to be alert for patterns that are unfamiliar (those not yet in their knowledge base) or previously unrecognized (the new diseases). HIV/AIDS was recognized as an unprecedented clinical syndrome with a new pattern of familiar symptoms (weight loss, fever, fatigue, dyspnea, cough) and signs (wasting, generalized lymphadenopathy, mucocutaneous lesions, Kaposi's sarcoma, opportunistic infections) in a unique population (homosexual males and IV drug users). Continuously expanding our personal knowledge of the known while welcoming the unfamiliar and unknown is the excitement of clinical practice.

The proper testing of diagnostic hypotheses is beyond the scope of this book. It is a subject of constant change as new tests are developed and their usefulness evaluated in clinical trials. Part IV discusses the principles of laboratory testing (Chapter 17) and some common laboratory tests (Chapter 18). The reader should consult *Harrison's Principles of Internal Medicine,* 16th edition, and the current literature when selecting specific tests to evaluate their diagnostic hypotheses [Guyatt G, Rennie D. (editors). *Users' Guides to the Medical Literature: A Manual for Evidence-based Clinical Practice.* Chicago, AMA Press, 2002].

User's Guide:

DeGowin's Diagnostic Examination can be read cover to cover with benefit to the student or practitioner; however, most will not, and should not, choose this strategy. As Osler said, read to understand your patients and to answer your questions.

We strongly suggest that all readers start with Chapters 1–3 and 17 which outline the conceptual basis for the diagnostic examination, including the approach to laboratory testing and imaging. This context is critical to an efficient use of time and resources.

If you have questions about the systems being examined in a given body region consult part A of the relevant chapter and *Harrison's Principles of Internal Medicine,* 16th edition. If your question concerns anatomy, consult part B and an anatomy textbook [Agur AMR, Lee MJ. *Grant's Atlas of Anatomy,* 10th edition. Philadelphia, Lippincott Williams & Wilkins, 1999]. If you are uncertain of the techniques of the physical examination, see Chapter 3 and part C of the body region chapters. If you are uncertain what to make of a symptom see part D of the relevant chapter. If you are wondering how to elicit or interpret a particular sign, see part E of the relevant chapter. To find out more about the diseases mentioned in the section, consult part F of that chapter or look in the index for the page where it is discussed. Remember, the disease and syndrome discussions in this book are brief and must be complemented with reading in a textbook of medicine, e.g., *Harrison's Principles of Internal Medicine,* 16th edition.

You can always consult the index to find the location of any of the material in the text.

There is no right way to use a book. The key is to use the information to inform your thinking about your patients and the problems they present. No text is definitive and the reader is encouraged to consult other texts and the current and historic literature to develop a full understanding of your patients and their illnesses. The acquisition of clinical skills is a journey without end; this is an intimidating thought for the student, but is the source of lifelong stimulation for the practitioner.

After all, what we call truth is only the hypotheses which is found to work best.

SIR JAMES GEORGE FRAZER
The Golden Bough, Abridged edition. New York, Collier Books, Macmillan Publishing Company, 1922, pg. 307.

DeGowin's

DIAGNOSTIC
EXAMINATION

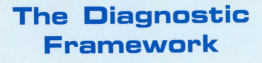

Part

1

The Diagnostic Framework

To carefully observe the phenomena of life in all its phases, normal and perverted, to make perfect that most difficult of all arts, the art of observation, to call to aid the science of experimentation, to cultivate the reasoning faculty, so as to be able to know the true from the false—these are our methods.

Sir William Osler

Don't strain for arrangement. Look and put down and let your sensibility be the sieve.

Theodore Roethke
"Poetry and Craft"

. . . the framing of hypotheses is the most difficult part of scientific work, and the part where great ability is indispensable. So far, no method has been found which would make it possible to invent hypotheses by rule. Usually some hypothesis is a necessary preliminary to the collection of facts, since the selection of facts demands some way of determining relevance. Without something of this kind, the multiplicity of facts is baffling.

Bertrand Russell
"A History of Western Philosophy"

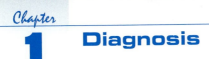

Chapter

1

Diagnosis

Varieties of Medical Examinations

There are at least seven varieties of medical examinations that differ from one another in their purposes, their stereotyped procedures, and their diagnostic tests.

The first six examinations involve special, stereotyped routines for persons having no symptoms and who are presumed to be well. Recommendations based on yield and cost are periodically revised by various professional groups. The absence of symptoms makes the performance and interpretation of these examinations different from that of a diagnostic examination.

1. *Examination of Young Schoolchildren*: The examination usually emphasizes tests of vision and hearing, physical and social development, coordination, and language skills.
2. *Examination of Athletes*: The examiner stresses tests of cardiopulmonary function, muscle performance, flexibility, and injury prevention.
3. *Examination for Military Service*: This resembles the examination for athletes but adds testing of the special senses and psyche.
4. *Examination for Life Insurance*: The routine is generally established by the insurance company; it usually consists of a history form, an abbreviated physical examination, and a few laboratory tests to exclude the presence of chronic diseases that affect longevity, substance abuse, and HIV infection.
5. *Periodic Health Examination*: For infants, follow the recommendations of the American Academy of Pediatrics for well-child examinations and immunizations. The clinician especially searches for birth defects and measures growth and social development. Annual examinations of sexually active adults with new sexual partners should be performed with Pap testing of women and screening for sexually transmitted diseases in women, and possibly men. In persons older than age 45 years, annual examinations seek to detect the early onset of cardiovascular disease, diabetes mellitus, hypercholesterolemia, hypertension, and cancer. In addition, the clinician provides counseling about age-related life changes, diet and exercise,

3

and appropriate immunizations. The visits may foster optimal patient–physician relationships. See the current recommendations of the US Public Health Service Task Force [Han PKJ. Historical changes in the objectives of the periodic health examination. *Ann Intern Med* 1997;127:910–917].

6. *Industrial Examinations*: Specialized procedures detect the hazards of particular industries: testing for lead and carbon monoxide in the blood, seeking signs of pneumoconiosis or tuberculosis in radiographs of the chest, measuring the radiation exposure of those who work with x-rays or radioisotopes.

7. *Preoperative Screening*: See Part III, Chapter 16.

8. *Diagnostic Examination*: This procedure is not restricted in its approach, but is more searching. It starts with the patient's chief complaint and, using symptoms and signs as clues, seeks to find an explanation for the discomfort or dysfunction, a diagnosis. The urgency of the situation dictates the form the examination will take. For example, in a patient with chronic complaints and an exam that reveals no urgent problems, the diagnostic evaluation might span several clinic visits over a month or two. In contrast, the trauma patient requires an expedited primary survey of the airway, breathing, circulation, and neurologic functions to determine the need for resuscitation. This is followed by a secondary survey: the history, a physical examination, and selection of laboratory and radiologic studies to permit formulation of a definitive care plan.

A conceptual approach to the diagnostic exam is the focus of this chapter.

The Diagnostic Examination

Appropriate medical care depends upon the physician's recognizing the abnormalities of the patient's physiologic functions, structure, and mentation. Each recognizable disease possesses clinical and/or laboratory features that serve as clues to differentiate it from similar conditions. During the diagnostic examination, the clinician is performing two parallel tasks: (a) a search for symptoms and signs to develop a list of problems, and from this, (b) the generation and selection of physiologic and diagnostic hypotheses aimed at establishing one or more diagnoses.

Why is Diagnosis Important?

The purpose of performing a history and physical examination is to assist in making the diagnosis. Accurate diagnosis allows the clinician to perform the three tasks that are central to the healing professions: explanation, prognostication, and therapy. These three tasks have been consistently performed by physicians throughout time and across cultures, regardless of the belief system or theory underpinning the practice: magic, faith, rationalism, or science. They provide answers to the patient's three fundamental questions: (a) What is happening to me and why? (b) What does this mean for my future? (c) What can be done about it and how will that change my future? [Cohen JJ. Remembering the real questions. *Ann Intern Med* 1998;128:563–566; Kravitz RL, Callahan EJ. Patients' perceptions of omitted examinations and tests: A qualitative analysis. *J Gen Intern Med* 2000;15:38–45].

Failure to pursue a diagnosis may permit your patient's disease to progress from a stage that responds to treatment to one that does not. Paradoxically, for many acute complaints, in otherwise healthy people with no alarm symptoms or signs, an accurate and good prognosis can be ascertained without knowing the exact cause of the complaint, for instance, an upper respiratory infection or back pain. In this situation, the experienced clinician can reassure the patient that further testing to establish the exact cause is unnecessary and will not change the prognosis or treatment. It takes experience, knowledge of the medical literature, good judgment, and an understanding of the fundamentals of clinical epidemiology and decision making to determine when pursuit of a specific diagnosis is warranted. For an excellent review of the principles of epidemiology in a highly readable format, see Fletcher et al. [Fletcher RH, Fletcher SW, Wagner EH. *Clinical Epidemiology, the Essentials.* 3rd ed. Baltimore: Williams & Wilkins, 1996].

Diseases and Syndromes: An Entry to the Medical Literature

For thousands of years physicians have recorded recurring patterns of disordered bodily structure, function, and mentation that suggest a common cause. Each pattern receives a specific name. When a common etiology and pathophysiology are confirmed, we designate the condition a *disease*. Other clusters of attributes, known by a combination of features not clearly related to a single cause, are called *syndromes*. Diseases and syndromes are intellectual constructs allowing the physicians to study groups of patients with relatively homogeneous physiologic disorders; they do not exist independently of the patients who manifest them. The diagnosis of a disease or syndrome provides an entry to the medical literature to obtain information about etiology, diagnostic findings, treatment, and prognosis.

An accurate diagnosis is indispensable to offering your patients evidence-based therapy, that is, therapy validated in clinical trials based upon accurate diagnosis of participating subjects.

Finding Clues to the Diagnosis

The diagnostic examination has four components: (a) history taking, where clues are *symptoms* (abnormalities perceived by the patient's own senses); (b) physical examination, where the physical *signs* are clues (abnormalities perceived by the examiner's senses); (c) laboratory examination, where the clues are findings from cytologic, chemical and immunologic tests of tissues, body fluids, and excreta; and (d) special anatomic and physiologic examinations, where the clues appear on x-ray films, computed tomography (CT) or magnetic resonance imaging

(MRI) scans, ultrasonograms, intravascular pressure recordings and electrical measurements such as electrocardiograms (ECGs), cardiac electrophysiologic studies, electromyograms (EMGs), nerve conduction velocity studies (NCV), electroencephalograms (EEGs), or polysomnography. Our focus is on the history and physical examination and the process of hypothesis generation [Boland BJ, Wollan PC, Silverstein MD. Review of systems, physical examination, and routine tests for case-finding in ambulatory patients. *Am J Med Sci* 1995;309:194–200; Boland BJ, Wollan PC, Silverstein MD. Yield of laboratory tests for case-finding in the ambulatory general medical examination. *Am J Med* 1996;101:142–152]. Current evidence suggests that most diagnoses result from findings in the history, and to a lesser extent, the physical examination and laboratory testing [Peterson MC, Holbrook JH, Von Hales D, et al. Contributions of the history, physical examination, and laboratory investigation in making medical diagnoses. *West J Med* 1992;156:163–165; Reilly BM. Physical examination in the care of medical inpatients: an observational study. *Lancet* 2003, 362:1100–1105].

The clinician uses a recursive process to work his way toward the final diagnosis. First, from the history and physical examination, a *differential diagnosis* is constructed of the most probable pathophysiologic abnormalities and/or specific disease states. Second, choosing tests with appropriate likelihood ratios, these hypotheses are tested. The results of the testing changes the probability of each hypothesis; some are now more probable, while others are less probable. The clinician returns to the patient, reviews the history, and repeats specific parts of the examination to reach a new, refined differential diagnosis to be tested more specifically. This process repeats, *each time returning to the patient* for the patient's ongoing history and to search for new or changing physical findings, until one or more specific diagnoses are established that fully explain the patient's illness.

The diagnostic exam begins with the first patient contact. The patient's age is a surrogate for diseases more or less common in that age group. The duration of illness is important; for example, a disease lasting more than 3 years is unlikely to be aggressive cancer. Ethnicity is important for diagnosing some diseases; for example, sickle cell anemia rarely occurs in northern European whites. Sex-linked diseases such as hemophilia are rarely encountered in females. Males don't get pregnant. Although obvious, it is important to make each of these categorical probability decisions explicit. Sometimes it is a disease that was excluded by using one of these criteria (usually without consciously recognizing it) that turns out to be the diagnosis, such as appendicitis in the 80-year-old with abdominal pain.

While searching, each emerging clue is examined closely before it is accepted. If it is a symptom, assess the reliability of the observer: Are the observer's perceptions accurate and consistent or are they colored by emotion or secondary considerations? Is the observer's memory adequate? What importance does the patient attach to the symptom? Does the patient regard it fearfully or with relative unconcern? Obtain history from collateral observers, family, and friends whenever possible. Do they corroborate the patient's history?

If the clue is a *sign*, is it within the range of normal, has it changed from previous exams or is it clearly abnormal? Is it constantly present or does it vary with position or motion? With laboratory findings, one must constantly suspect the mixing of specimens and laboratory error. Do the reports accord with what you expected? Was there opportunity for the adulteration of specimens? What is the laboratory's reputation for accuracy? If the clue was found in the x-ray films, was it present in previous films? Was there proper identification of the patient in obtaining the images? Were the images interpreted by competent persons?

Select Hypotheses: The Differential Diagnosis

Physiologic and Diagnostic Hypotheses

Clues are sought by taking a history, performing a physical examination, and obtaining laboratory tests and imaging. The specific findings suggest a list of problems from which is generated *physiologic hypotheses* to explain the mechanism of disease and *diagnostic hypotheses*, diseases that are known to cause the specific symptoms, signs, and pathophysiology. A list of all possible diagnoses is rarely of much benefit, and does not provide a guide for efficient evaluation. Rather, from this list we use the specific findings from the history and exam *of this patient* to *differentiate* the relative probabilities of the potential conditions to create a short list of the most likely conditions, the *differential diagnosis*. Further history and exam and specific laboratory tests are used to support or refute each condition in the differential diagnosis to finally arrive at a diagnosis. Problem-based learning prepares the student to embrace this diagnostic process.

Because the clues that allow us to differentiate between disease of high and low probability *for this patient* are unique to this patient, a differential diagnosis is only possible for an individual patient, not a problem. For an isolated symptom or sign we can generate a list of potential diagnoses, but have no means to differentiate their probabilities. In this book, under many symptoms and signs, we have placed a list of such **Clinical Occurrences**. It is up to the clinician, perhaps using this list as a organizational tool, to generate a meaningful differential diagnosis for her patient. When specific clues will help in generating the differential diagnosis, we have listed them after the DDX: symbol in the text.

The differential diagnoses are a list of the diseases that are considered as hypotheses for further evaluation. Each disease or condition is more or less probable based upon how well it explains the full range of the patient's problems. Studies show that the average clinician carries coincidentally 4 or 5 diseases on the clinician's differential list; but often a total of 13 to 15 diseases will have appeared on the differential list at some time during the examination.

Hypothesis Generation

The process by which skilled clinicians arrive at hypotheses has attracted attention from physicians, mathematicians, and psychologists. Much of this literature is found in writings on medical decision making, medical logic, or clinical problem solving. Although several methods of problem solving have been considered, branching and matching are most commonly used when pattern recognition has not occurred.

PATTERN RECOGNITION. The whole of the patient's illness is greater than the sum of its parts and a simple mathematical summing of the sensitivity and specificity of each finding is probably far less accurate than the pattern formed in the mind of the skilled examiner by the totality of the observations. For example, it is unlikely that we could accurately identify a person by looking singly at each ear, each eye, the hair, the forehead, the cheeks, the nose, the lips, or the chin. Each exam would lack the sensitivity and specificity we desire for identification. But with just a glance at the pattern of the whole, we can identify with great accuracy literally hundreds of distinct faces. We even recognize our friends after injuries or when much of the face is covered (i.e., many of the parts are different or distorted) because of the persisting unity of the whole. We use this powerful cognitive ability in everyday life and in medical practice. It is not an exercise in reductionism: the whole is greater than the sum of the parts. This ability to recognize patterns is one of the most powerful properties of the human brain, which no computer or algorithm can match.

Most clinicians believe that composite pictures of disease, although comprising many signs, strike them at a glance. The Germans recognize this concept when they refer to Augenblick diagnoses (literally, "a blink of the eye"). Pattern recognition is the current English term describing this concept.

BRANCHING HYPOTHESES. Clinicians follow a search for clues that leads from one hypothesis to another. A clue calls to mind a disease with similar attributes and the other attributes of the disease are considered. The hypotheses are entered on the examiner's imaginary slate, revised, and reviewed, and each new clue may hint at other diseases for consideration.

MATCHING HYPOTHESES. The patient's symptoms and signs are matched with those of the hypothesized diseases. The best match is selected as the diagnosis of the patient. For example, suppose the examination of the patient (pt) yields attributes, or clues, a, d, e, k, and n; we may designate the patient as (pt) adekn. From memory, or references in this book under the head "Clinical Occurrence," the examiner enters on the imaginary slate a list of diseases having the same attribute a. The diseases on the list can be designated as V, W, X, Y, and Z. In matching, the examiner finds that the diseases have the following attributes in common with the patient: (V) abcde has ade in common; (W) acefg has ae in common; (X) adfij has ad in common; (Y) afhkl has ak in common; and (Z) aekgn has aekn in common. Without any other considerations, this last would be eligible as the diagnosis.

DECISIONS BASED ON PROBABILITY. As far as we know, the mathematics applied to decision making in medicine has been focused on determining the most probable diagnosis. If the examiner followed this principle rigidly, a rare disease would never be diagnosed.

Nevertheless, using statistical methods to evaluate the sensitivity and specificity of clinical findings and tests and the positive and negative likelihood ratios for various test results helps us to understand the usefulness of each individual part of the diagnostic examination. A very useful book that summarizes most of what is currently known about the sensitivity, specificity, and positive and negative likelihood ratios for specific physical findings is *Evidence-Based Physical Diagnosis* [McGee S. *Evidence-Based Physical Diagnosis.* Philadelphia: WB Saunders, 2001].

Soft Focus and Hard Focus

Pattern recognition results from a soft focus, taking in the observations without undue emphasis on any one; the observer lets the pattern emerge as their systematic observations are filtered through the lens of their knowledge and experience. Performance of the screening physical exam in a structured and relatively stereotypic sequence allows the examiner to observe each patient in a similar manner so that the repetitive patterns between patients become more evident. When the examination process becomes a routine, little or no thought is required to perform or sequence the physical acts of the exam, so the mind is free to observe.

When the focus of attention is sharp, as is often the case with beginners, one thing may be seen, while much is missed. This is demonstrated by a classic example from psychology. In the days when pocket watches were common and often had the 6 on the dial replaced by a second hand, a lecturing professor pointed out to his students that they had looked at their watches thousands of times, but many probably could not recall if they had a 6 on their dials. Many in the audience took surreptitious glances at their timepieces. After the watches had been pocketed, the professor asked if they knew what time it was; many had not noted the time. They had seen what they were looking for, but not all that was to be seen. The time for sharp focus is when testing your hypotheses by searching for specific signs.

One of the most important observations made by the experienced clinician using pattern recognition with a soft focus is the overall assessment of severity of illness: How sick is the patient? Although one could list many attributes of severe illness, for example, abnormal vital signs, pallor, diaphoresis, anxious or frightened expression, the global assessment of severity made by the experienced clinician also includes many intangibles, often based upon prior knowledge and experience with the patient. Severity of illness scores, such as APACHE (Acute Physiology and Chronic Health Evaluation) II scores, are attempts to systematize this global assessment. Your experience-based emotional cues are an important part of this assessment.

Use of Computers

There are several areas in which computers have proven valuable in the diagnostic examination. One of these is in the rapid communication of laboratory results and radiologic images and interpretations to clinicians. Another is in the comprehensive search of the medical literature to evaluate clues and hypotheses generated during an examination. Computer literature searches should be available on the clinical floors of every hospital and in the offices and homes of physicians.

A computer output listing the rank order of disease probability based upon a simple list of symptoms and signs may reassure physicians who fear they will forget a disease for inclusion in the differential diagnosis. Such a list might be valuable in solving complex problems of differential diagnosis, or identifying rare diseases, but its utility for an experienced clinician is probably too low to encourage its use for most problems. Moreover, you still must have the experience and judgment to evaluate the list and determine which items to pursue and how. If you have those skills, you probably do not need the computer-generated list.

Undoubtedly, technologic progress will provide physicians with new opportunities for computer assistance in the diagnostic examination. Satisfactory answers to a few basic questions should precede the adoption of a computer-assisted diagnostic system: Who developed the program and with which data? How frequently will the program be updated and by whom? [Miller RA, Gardner RM. Summary recommendations for responsible monitoring and regulation of clinical software systems. *Ann Intern Med* 1997;127:842–845]. Will it save time? Is it portable? How will access to confidential information be controlled? How expensive is it?

Tests of the Diagnosis

In choosing a diagnosis from several hypotheses, the matching of the patient's attributes with those of the hypothetical disease may not be entirely conclusive. Several additional criteria may be used to help elucidate the most likely diagnosis.

Parsimony

The diagnosis has a higher probability of being correct if one disease can explain the entire cluster of clues, rather than attempting to account for the findings by a coincidence of several diseases. This is known as Occam's razor: the simplest solution is likely to be correct. When one diagnosis does not explain all the findings, those that are able to account for the greatest proportion of the patient's signs and symptoms are most likely to be correct. Older persons more often have two or more coincident disorders.

Chronology

It is possible to have a perfect match of attributes between patient and disease, but if the epidemiology, onset, and course are not appropriate to the disease, the hypothesis is probably wrong.

Severity of Illness

Not infrequently, an inexperienced clinician will diagnose the patient's condition as, for instance, an upper respiratory infection, whereas a more experienced clinician will look at the patient and suggest the diagnosis of pneumonia, explaining that the patient looks "too sick" for the first condition. The severity of illness is valid and diagnostically useful, but it is difficult to explain or describe.

Prognosis

If two hypotheses seem equally probable and neither can be proved immediately, the patient should be informed of the diagnostic and prognostic possibilities and encouraged to discuss this with his family. In these situations, we have found it best to help the patient prepare for the worst and hope for the best. Regular follow-up and frequent reevaluation are required. Often, referral to a specialist will help both the patient and the physician deal with the uncertainty.

Therapeutic Trials

If there is uncertainty between an untreatable morbid disease and one with potentially successful therapy, try a therapeutic trial. Although experience shows that such trials are often inconclusive or difficult to interpret, they may save a life; for example, when appendicitis cannot be excluded, perform an appendectomy accepting that some normal appendices will be removed.

Selection of Diagnostic Tests

Experienced clinicians select diagnostic tests indicated by clues from the history and the physical examination. They have repeatedly learned that routine testing or uncritical testing for remote diagnostic possibilities frequently yield results that require explanation by more testing, all without answering the primary diagnostic question. This "cascade effect" heightens the patient's anxiety, is hazardous and expensive, and delays treatment. See Chapter 17 for a discussion of the appropriate selection of diagnostic tests.

Rare Diseases

Some physicians, especially the inexpert, have a tendency to diagnose rare diseases with uncommon frequency. It is well to recall that rare diseases occur rarely. The old saying is, "when you hear hoofbeats think of horses, not zebras." Just remember, this works in America, not Africa, so you need to know the epidemiology and demographics of your patient and patient population before you really know what is common and what is rare.

Certainty and Diagnosis

When a diagnosis is established for the patient, how certain should the examiner be that it is correct? Unfortunately, there is no accepted scale of degrees of certainty whereby the examiner can express the extent to which the diagnosis has been established. On the one hand, the diagnosis is defined by the image, the laboratory test, the culture, or the biopsy result. For instance, a fracture of the tibia is diagnosed when the fracture can be seen on the x-ray film with absolute assurance. Many types of neoplasia and inflammatory diseases are diagnosed by biopsy. Culture, serology or polymerase chain reaction (PCR) identification of specific organisms establishes the diagnosis of specific infectious diseases. Laboratory tests are specific for endocrine and metabolic diseases. On the other hand, we speak of a diagnosis of rheumatoid arthritis, where often there is much less certainty, and no definitive diagnostic tests. The diagnosis is supported by the clinical picture, and by such nonspecific tests as x-ray examinations and tests for rheumatoid factor.

In each clinical situation, the clinician must consciously establish a "stopping rule." That is, the clinician must decide how much certainty is required, and stop further investigation when that point is reached. This decision is based upon the severity of the illness, an estimate of the prognosis (based upon the severity of illness and the patient's comorbidities), and whether a specific diagnosis is needed to guide a decision between mutually exclusive interventions which would harm the patient if applied to the wrong disease; for example, antibiotics or corticosteroids.

Deferred Diagnoses

When a satisfactory diagnosis cannot be identified, the physician can proceed with the following five supplementary steps.

Repeat the History and the Physical Examination

This tests the patient's memory; it may prove to have been faulty, or recall may have been stimulated by the first inquiry. Talk to more relatives and attendants to confirm or deny the original story and to add details. Carefully repeat the physical examination to confirm your previous evaluation and to search for signs that were overlooked the first time.

Repeat Laboratory Tests

Specimens may have been mixed on the initial occasion, or an error in the first test may be uncovered.

Make a Provisional Diagnosis

Although a meticulous physician may qualify the diagnosis by the word probable or a question mark, these modifiers often get dropped when the record has passed through several transcriptions. Unfortunately, these important adjectives and adverbs may be impatiently discarded by lawyers, insurance adjustors, and medical chart coders. Other statements of uncertainty are preliminary diagnosis, diagnostic impression, tentative diagnosis, working diagnosis, provisional diagnosis, and probable diagnosis.

Defer Diagnosis

Carefully explain the situation to secure the patient's confidence so that a return examination may be made when new symptoms or signs have appeared or time has given more perspective to the case. Retain the problem list, but mark the record "Diagnosis Deferred"; do not let the medical record rules or the insurance company force a premature diagnosis.

Seek Wise Consultation

Often presenting the case to colleagues as an unknown and asking for their input, or seeking consultation with an excellent generalist or appropriate subspecialist will assist in making the diagnosis, and, even if not, may reassure the patient and physician. It is better to offer this option to the patient than to wait for the patient to insist out of frustration. However, avoid excessive consultation or visits to multiple physicians. Like excessive laboratory testing, this is more likely to add confusion than clarity.

A Summary of the Diagnostic Process

Step 1: Take a History

Elicit symptoms and the pattern of the illness to begin a problem list.

Step 2: Develop Hypotheses

Generate a mental list of pathophysiologic processes and diseases that might produce the symptoms.

Step 3: Perform a Physical Examination

Look for signs of the physiologic processes and diseases suggested by the history, and identify new findings for the problem list.

Step 4: Generate a Differential Diagnoses

List the most probable hypotheses in the order of their probability.

Step 5: Test the Hypotheses

Select laboratory tests, imaging studies, and other procedures with appropriate likelihood ratios to evaluate your hypotheses.

Step 6: Modify your Differential Diagnosis

Use the results of all of the tests to evaluate your hypotheses, perhaps eliminating some and adding others and adjusting the probabilities.

Step 7: Repeat Steps 1 to 6

Reiterate your process until you have reached a diagnosis or decided that a definite diagnosis is neither likely or necessary.

Step 8: Make the Diagnosis or Diagnoses

When the tests of your hypotheses are of sufficient certainty that they meet your stopping rule, you have reached a diagnosis.

Step 9: If Uncertain, Consider a Provisional Diagnosis or Watchful Waiting

Decide whether more investigation (return to step 1), consultation, treatment, or watchful observation is the best course based upon the severity of illness, the prognosis, and comorbidities. If the diagnosis remains obscure, retain a problem list of the unexplained symptoms and signs, as well as laboratory and imaging findings, assess the urgency for further evaluation and schedule regular follow-up visits.

Caveat

The complex process we have discussed is primarily suited to the problems of chronic and relatively obscure diseases commonly encountered in the fields of internal medicine and pediatrics. A majority of patients seen by most physicians do not require such a comprehensive process. Although the principles of diagnosis hold for all patients, variations from the described process may be appropriate for a given patient's condition and the medical or surgical specialty involved. Many conditions requiring minor surgery need few or no symptoms to make a diagnosis; the situation is obvious by noting the anatomic derangement or by taking x-ray films. The dermatologist can make many diagnoses without hearing about any symptoms. On the other hand, the psychiatrist leans heavily on the history given by friends, relatives, and attendants, and on dialogue with the patient. It follows that the scope and length of the history vary greatly among medical specialties.

An Example of the Diagnostic Process

The objective of the diagnostic examination is to discover the physiologic cause of the patient's complaint, identify the specific disease, and determine the severity and prognosis of the disease. You need these data to counsel your patient regarding the indications for treatment.

A 21-year-old woman consults you about a painless lump in her neck (symptom). You consider her age and select hypotheses that include lymphoma, infection, and collagen vascular disease, which lead to questions about fever, itching, weight loss, exposure to pets, tuberculosis, arthralgias, and Raynaud phenomenon. Your examination reveals a single, firm, 3-cm nontender lymph node in the right cervical chain (sign), but the spleen is not palpable and there are no other signs of disease. The patient's blood counts are normal (lab), and a biopsy of the enlarged node (supplemental test) discloses Hodgkin disease. Bone marrow biopsy and imaging studies of the chest and abdomen fail to reveal more disease (prognosis and staging tests).

You make a diagnosis of stage I Hodgkin disease and discuss the diagnosis with your patient, informing her of the prognosis without treatment, and the risks and benefits of radiotherapy at this stage of the disease.

The Autopsy

The gold standard since the mid-nineteenth century for diagnostic accuracy has been the autopsy, and it remains so. Unfortunately, autopsy rates have declined in recent decades, and with them valuable learning experiences for physicians to validate or correct their diagnostic impressions. In the current climate many physicians have not learned the value of an autopsy and many families have not received a full explanation of the diseases of their loved ones. Despite the current abundance of laboratory tests and imaging technologies, there is considerable evidence that clinical diagnoses in difficult cases are not uncommonly wrong, that significant disease is missed, and that the addition of technology has not substantially altered these facts [Kirch W, Schafi C. Misdiagnosis at a university hospital in 4 medical eras. *Medicine (Baltimore)* 1996;75:29–40].

Physicians should work closely with patients and their families to encourage autopsies in most in-hospital deaths. This is a critical part of our professional development and the continuous struggle to improve our clinical skills [McPhee SJ. The autopsy. An antidote to misdiagnosis. *Medicine (Baltimore)* 1996;75:41–43]. The issue is not one of assigning blame or responsibility, it is one of improving our diagnostic and therapeutic strategies.

2 History Taking and the Medical Record

> *. . . [T]here is no more difficult art to acquire than the art of observation, and for some men it is quite as difficult to record an observation in brief and plain language.*

Sir William Osler

Proper care of a patient over time requires that a complete medical record be kept at the site of care. The record should record, preferably on standardized forms, basic patient data, such as their demographics, list of active and past medical problems, surgical history, injury history, medication history, allergies and drug intolerances, sexual history, family history, social history, personal habits, prostheses used, preventive care services, and specific counseling provided. Using standardized forms enables the information to be recorded in a uniform way for each patient, allowing rapid review of the pertinent information at each visit. When recording information on these forms, it is important to enter information in such a way that it is always current; for example, in the family history record, the first names of children and siblings with their year of birth (rather than age).

Outline of the Medical Record

The parts of the medical history follow a standardized sequence, differing only in small details from one institution to another. The following sequence is used for adult patients in the Department of Internal Medicine at the University of Iowa. A different order is usually preferred by pediatricians, who set the birth history and the past history ahead of the present illness.

    I.   Identification
   II.   Informant
  III.   Chief Complaints (CC)
  IV.   History of Present Illness (HPI)
   V.   Past Medical and Surgical History (PH)
       A.   General health
       B.   Chronic and episodic illnesses

Procedure for Taking the History

Definition of the Medical History

The medical history is an account of the events in the patient's life that have relevance to the patient's mental and physical health. Much more than the patient's unprompted narrative, it is a specialized literary form in which the physician writes an account of the perceptions and events supplied by the patient or other informants. The history may be offered spontaneously or secured by skillful probing. Often, additional history is revealed by repeated questioning over time, as the patient is encouraged to reflect on her experience. In taking the history, the clinician should record key statements in the patient's words. *The history is the patient's history of their illness, not the physician's interpretation of the patient's history.* The clinician should take particular care to establish the sequence of events. *The clinician's task at this time is to try to understand the patient's experience and interpretation of her illness.*

Scope of the History

When patients consult their physicians for dermatitis, the necessary diagnostic history is very brief, possibly only a few sentences. For a person brought into the hospital with a fractured tibia, a long diagnostic history is unnecessary and even inhumane. In contrast, a chronic, obscure disease may require a long, careful history, perhaps repeated and expanded, with supplements from time to time as the results of further studies open new diagnostic possibilities. Writings on history taking always discuss the extended history, which is complicated and demands maximal skill. However, it would be folly to insist on an extended history for every patient; in many conditions, it would be unnecessary, and by insisting on it the physician would be able to care for only a few patients in a day. The experienced physician adjusts to the patient's problems. To test if the history is sufficient for the individual case, ask yourself if you can picture the patient's lifestyle and how the patient's illness affects it and is affected by it.

Methods in History Taking

The best history is obtained by the clinician who is empathetic with the patient, knows the manifestations of disease, and understands how patients describe the symptoms of various diseases. Your skill in history taking will continue to improve the more you learn of people, life, and disease. The face-to-face interaction of taking a good history permits you to see the emphasis your patient puts on his or her symptoms, allows you to learn about your patient's personality, and provides an opportunity to develop a supportive physician–patient relationship. Use of medical intake questionnaires to assist in obtaining a complete medical, family, and social history within the time constraints of practice is encouraged [Ramsey PG, Curtis JR, Paauw DS, et al. History-taking and preventive medicine skills among primary care physicians: An assessment using standardized patients. *Am J Med* 1998;104:152–158].

We believe that extensive written instructions about interrogation of the patient are unrewarding; you can only become proficient at history taking by actually interviewing patients. A few guidelines are useful: (a) listen actively; (b) don't interrupt the patient; (c) ask open-ended questions; and (d) be patient, give the patient time to think and speak.

Clinical experience, and reflection upon your experience, is necessary to link your knowledge of diseases with the history being obtained from the patient without conscious thought. When a disease or syndrome thus comes to mind, it should recall a cluster of symptoms and signs and chronologic data about which to ask the patient. When you have acquired this knowledge and experience, you can face the patient confidently and readily improvise methods of interrogation.

Taking a diagnostic history has four objectives: (a) discovering symptoms, (b) obtaining accurate quantitative descriptions, (c) securing a precise chronology of events, and (d) determining how the illness has changed the patient's life.

Conducting the Interview

Arrangement

This description deals with the taking of an extended history in the physician's clinic in the following circumstances: the patient is in no acute distress; time limitations are not urgent; and the disease is relatively obscure. Circumstances often vary greatly from these stipulations.

Address patients formally, do not use their first name unless they request it. The conversation should not be overhead by others, although the presence of the patient's spouse or a relative is often helpful in confirming the narrative and supplementing the patient's observations. Limit the interview to the patient and one other informant; more informants waste time in their disagreements on details that outweigh the slight extra yield of information.

Physician's Manner

To obtain the patient's confidence and rapport, present yourself as unhurried, interested, and sympathetic. Sit at eye level without a desk between you. In no way should you express a moral judgment on the patient's actions or beliefs. Permit patients to begin their story in their own way; listen for several minutes before gradually injecting questions to guide the interview. Gently, but firmly, keep the discussion centered on the patient's problems. By all means, avoid discussing your own health, even when a patient invites you to do so.

Note Taking

Write sparingly while the patient talks. After you have recorded some routine data, sit back and *listen* to the narrative for a while, interjecting only a few questions. Avoid writing the patient's narrative verbatim; it is usually too lengthy and poorly organized. Use of standardized forms for recording the past medical history, family history, and social history (which can be filled out by the patient before the interview) will greatly decrease the need for making notes. Remember that the patient is telling you a story; you should try to understand their story and remember key words and phrases. These can be jotted down to assist recall.

Language

From the beginning, gauge the patient's meaning of the words they use; words may have different meanings for different people. Put your questions in simple, nontechnical words. Even lay words may be misunderstood. The English vocabulary is vast and formidable, even to the scholar. Excluding your scientific and medical vocabulary, you may be able to use 100,000 words, while the adult with average education gets along with 30,000 to 60,000. So the patient may not know half the words you use in English. Patients may leave the interview with the fear that they have presented their symptoms poorly because they have answered questions they did not understand.

Belief Systems

Physicians are trained in the scientific method and in science-based rules of evidence. For many patients, if not most, this is not the structure of their belief system. Other belief systems include magic, religion, and rationalism. It is essential to understand how the patient views cause and effect, to what sources they attribute disease and illness. The clinician's task is to understand the patient; it is not, primarily, the patient's task to understand the clinician. Education of patients becomes an important part of providing proper care for many chronic diseases.

Patient's Motivation

The usefulness of the history for diagnosis depends on the assumption, frequently forgotten, that the patient's sole motive is to assist the physician in diagnosis and treatment, and, therefore, the descriptions of the patient's symptoms are truthful. As far as possible, this assumption must be confirmed by excluding other motives that might prompt misrepresentation. Some patients, entirely truthful, present symptoms that are baffling until the physician learns of their resemblance to those of a friend or relative who has died of cancer, and the patient fears the same fate. The physician must ascertain whether the patient is contemplating a lawsuit for damages, claiming worker's compensation, or applying for veteran's benefits. The narcotic addict may present symptoms calculated to obtain drugs. Lacking discernible motives, a few patients fabricate medical histories that may lead to extensive diagnostic examinations [Asher R. Munchausen's syndrome. *Lancet* 1951;1:339–341].

Procedure

After introducing yourself and confirming the identifying data for the patient, start the patient's narrative by saying, "Tell me about your problem," or "Give me your story." Don't ask, "What is the matter with you?" or "What is troubling you?" because the patient is likely to respond, "That's what I came here to find out." Listen to the story without interruption for several minutes; use open-ended questions to encourage the patient to speak. After the general outline becomes apparent, you may need to ask specific directed questions to establish the nature of the symptoms, the medication, the chronology, and the disability. Also ask about symptoms not mentioned that are prompted by your search for diagnostic clues. Then pause and write down notes to assist your recall, including key words and phrases.

Next, record any remaining information to complete the past medical history; surgical history; injury history; review of medications and allergies; family history; social history; sexual, obstetrical, and gynecologic history; review of systems and preventive care history, including procedures (e.g., mammography, colonoscopy); tests (e.g. Pap smears, purified protein derivative [PPD]); and immunizations.

Completion of the Medical Record

It is the clinician's responsibility to see that the medical record is complete and accurate. Your signature attests to the accuracy of the information and that you have verified it to your satisfaction. *Once entered and signed, the information in the medical record cannot be altered,* though addendums and corrections can be *added.*

Identification

Data under this heading are frequently recorded by the physician's receptionist or the hospital registration clerk. During the history taking, the physician should check the accuracy of all previously recorded items.

Patient's Name

Insist on recording the complete name, including the family name and all given names. The family name should be placed first, followed by a comma and all given names. Be careful to obtain the correct spelling. Any medical records department of considerable size contains the records of several patients with identical or closely similar names. Because fatal errors have occurred when two patients with the same name have been under treatment in the hospital simultaneously, each patient is given a unique hospital number, which should be used for identification before a treatment is instituted.

For a married woman who has taken her husband's name, use her own given names after the family name of her husband; after these, place her husband's given names in parentheses, as Brown, Mary Elizabeth (Mrs. Edward Charles). This arrangement is necessary because she may sign her name as Mrs. Edward C. Brown in correspondence about her case. She can be distinguished from other Mary Browns with differing middle names. Determine whether she wishes to be addressed as Ms. or Mrs.

Sex

Usually, this is obvious. In cases of intersex, the problem of sex may be difficult to establish accurately, but it is sufficient to give the sex the patient has assumed.

Residence

The address should be confirmed and recorded as completely as possible to facilitate efficient mailing of correspondence. Occasionally, the address is used to distinguish the identity of two patients with the same name.

Birth Date and Age

The patient's statement of the birth date should be recorded, in addition to the stated age. The birth date is required for most insurance claims. Comparison of it with the stated age on subsequent hospital visits may disclose discrepancies, reflecting on the patient's veracity or memory. The birth date may help distinguish between patients with the same name.

Source of Referral

If your patient was referred by another physician, confirm the name, address, telephone number, and reason for referral.

The Informant

The Sources of the History

The history may be obtained from the patient or others. In either case, record your judgment of the accuracy and credibility of the informant's answers. Errors are frequent when orientation is judged from a casual conversation. A person who converses normally may, on direct questioning, be unable to tell the day of the week, the month, the year, or even the name of the city where you are meeting.

Interpreters

When the patient does not speak your language, be cautious about interpreters who are not medically trained. A frequent experience with a lay interpreter resembles the following. You ask, "Does the patient have any pain?" The interpreter engages the patient in animated conversation in language incomprehensible to you. After 3 or 4 minutes, much longer than a simple question should take, you think surely the interpreter will provide you with a detailed story. Finally, the interpreter turns back to you and says, "No, she doesn't have any pain." If you could have followed this mysterious exchange, you would have found that the interpreter had embraced the opportunity to apply his or her concepts of medicine to history taking and had stated all sorts of questions that you did not propose. You cannot evaluate the answers unless you know what questions were asked. Your only recourse is to ask short questions and firmly insist that the resulting conversation is not longer than you judge necessary for your question.

Chief Complaints

The history of symptoms begins with the chief complaints, abbreviated CC. These should consist of a list of one or more symptoms that caused the patient to seek attention. The complaints are usually tabulated, each on a separate line, followed by the approximate duration in time units; they are written as words or phrases, not as complete sentences. Complaints are not diagnoses by the physician or the patient. It is customary to advise the patient to state the chief complaints in the patient's own words so that interpretation does not alter them. The patient's words may be so ambiguous as to be useless without further interrogation. The chief complaints should be expressed as the problems of most concern to the patient.

There are two purposes for isolating certain symptoms as chief complaints. First, they often serve as important clues with which to begin making a differential diagnosis; the details of these symptoms should always be sought out. Second is to remind you that these are the symptoms that brought the patient to seek treatment; they require therapy or an explanation of why therapy is not given. The patient's chief complaint should be the first problem on your problem list. This would seem obvious, but occasionally the physician finds an interesting disease, entirely unrelated to the chief complaints; the medically attractive condition receives all the attention, and the chief complaints are ignored.

In eliciting the chief complaints, do not press patients for them too early in the interview. Patients will be better able to select them after they have told some of their story; you may have to help identify them. Occasionally, when patients are asked for their symptoms, they produce a piece of paper containing a list of notes. The French label this *la maladie de petit papier.* Formerly, this practice was considered a sign of neurosis. Many doctors now encourage their patients to keep track of symptoms, signs, temperature, blood pressure, weight, blood sugars, blood counts, and the like, so as to obtain a more accurate evaluation of their progress.

History of Present Illness (HPI)

Symptoms

The word symptom is derived from a Greek word meaning "something that has befallen one." A symptom is usually considered to be an abnormal sensation that is perceived by the patient, in contrast to a physical sign that can be seen, felt, or heard by the examiner. The elements of the medical history can be classified as (a) sensations that can never be observed by the examiner; (b) abnormalities noted by the patient at some past time so they cannot be confirmed by the physical examination; (c) events in the past, not readily verifiable, such as former diagnoses or treatments; and (d) the patient's understanding of their family history and description of their social situation. Diagnostic evaluation of a symptom is simple when the patient says, "I've found a lump in my neck" (symptom), and the examiner can palpate a mass (physical sign). But when the patient complains of pain in the chest and no physical signs can be detected, much more information about the nature of the pain is required before the symptom can serve as a diagnostic clue. You can obtain more diagnostic information by further questioning the patient about the attributes of his symptoms. Specifically ask about *P*rovocative or *P*alliative maneuvers, *Q*uality of the symptom, the *R*egion involved, the *S*everity and *T*emporal pattern of the symptom. Use the initials *PQRST* as a mnemonic to remember to ask these questions. See the discussion of pain (Chapter 4, page 95) as an example.

The history of present illness is the heart of the diagnostic history. It should be written as a lucid, succinct, chronologic narrative with complete sentences in good English. The patient's symptoms should be accurately recorded in their own words; insist on symptoms from the patient and do not accept diagnoses or medical jargon. When a symptom is mentioned that suggests several conditions, accompany it with statements about the absence of concomitant symptoms that you have ascertained by direct questioning (pertinent negatives). For example, when the patient has had attacks of pain in the right upper abdominal quadrant, your description should include the fact that jaundice was not present, the urine was not dark-colored, no pruritus was experienced, and the pain did not radiate to the right scapula (all signs and symptoms of hepatobiliary disease).

Ideally, the HPI should be brief, so that it is easily read and digested. This objective can only be achieved if the diagnosis is relatively simple and easily made. When the condition is obscure, the author includes more details, being uncertain what is pertinent and will ultimately be useful. Because of this uncertainty, the clinician must avoid overinterpretation of the patient's history, replacement of their words with interpretive medical terminology, and elimination of seemingly irrelevant details.

Searching for Diagnostic Clues

The chief purpose of the history is to furnish clues for diagnosis. As the narrative unfolds, you should be simultaneously performing three operations: (a) the accumulation of facts (obtaining the history), (b) evaluation of the facts (testing the credibility of symptoms, seeking more details of time and quantity), and (c) preparation of hypotheses. Having formed a list of hypotheses, question the patient about other symptoms specific for diseases on the list, either to support or to discard a hypothesis. For example, when the patient complains of pain in the chest, ask if it is related to respiratory movements. A positive answer prompts questions about inflamed muscles, fractured ribs, and pleurisy. When the patient denies exacerbation of pain by thoracic movement, ask for an association with exertion and distribution of pain resembling that of angina pectoris. If the patient admits to such a distribution, then ask about onset of pain and its duration. Thus, each step in the narrative leads to another run through the sequence, resulting in frequent shifts in the list of hypotheses.

Nature of the Symptoms

The patient's description of symptoms must be clarified and quantified.

CLARIFICATION. Question the patient until sufficient details are obtained to categorize the symptom. Do not accept vague complaints such as "I don't feel well." If the patient complains of weakness, ascertain if she is weak in one or more muscle groups or if she experiences lassitude, malaise, or myalgia. When a patient says she is dizzy, inquire if she feels weak and unstable or if her surroundings seem to whirl about, as in vertigo. Determine whether dyspnea occurs at rest or with exertion.

QUANTIFICATION. Quantification is important to the evaluation of symptoms. Avoid recording a symptom without a statement of quantity. A woman may tell you that she has a "terrible pain," but her remark attains a different significance when she admits on questioning that the pain has never interfered with her work, sleep, or other activities. Although pain cannot be measured, its severity can be judged by how it affects the patient. Exertional dyspnea can be assessed by the amount of exertion required to produce it; for example, ask, "Can you climb a flight of stairs? Can you walk two blocks without stopping?" Neither you nor your reader can interpret what a "heavy smoker" means. Heavy is a value judgment whose meaning varies from one person to another; but a record of smoking 20 cigarettes a day is a measure everyone can understand. Don't label a patient as an "alcoholic"; put down the volume of alcohol the patient drinks in a stated time. The patient who had hemoptysis should be instructed to estimate the amount of blood lost in household measures, such as teaspoonfuls, cupfuls, or quarts. The amount of sputum raised should be recorded; the volume serves as an important consideration in differential diagnosis.

CHRONOLOGY. The duration of a symptom and its time of appearance in the course of disease are frequently significant for diagnosis. When the disease is chronic and the course complicated, the patient may disclaim ability to place events in chronologic sequence. A work chart may be sketched that will assist the patient in clarifying the details. On a piece of paper, the physician draws a series of steps, with their horizontal dimensions representing duration in approximate time units, such as days, weeks, months, or years. After labeling the time units, the physician indicates on the chart the few dates supplied by the patient. Seeing the chart, the patient can frequently recall further details and indicate the occurrence of symptoms on the time scale. The sequence and doses of medication can also be graphed.

CURRENT ACTIVITY.   Include this in a separate paragraph of the "Present Illness." The physician needs to determine how the disease has diminished the patient's quality of life and whether therapy has improved it. This information is also needed to substantiate the patient's claim for insurance. Obtain a detailed picture of the patient's average day to evaluate the patient's reaction to illness, the severity of the disease, and the response to therapy.

SUMMARIZATION.   Review your understanding of the history and ask the patient for corrections and confirmation. Test the completeness of your history by asking whether your summary conveys a clear picture of the patient's experience of their illness, that is, how the illness has affected them and their family, how it has interfered with their work, and how the symptoms have progressed.

Past Medical and Surgical History

Ordinarily, the items in the past history have less diagnostic value. If they provide clues for the diagnosis, the facts may be interpolated in the present illness, but they still should be recorded separately in this section. The significance of past illnesses may be appreciated after future developments in the patient's condition and as newly recognized disease associations are reported.

General Health

The patient's lifetime health, before the present illness, is sometimes revealing. Factors to consider include body weight (present, maximum, and minimum, with dates of each), previous physical examinations (dates and findings), and any periods of medical disability.

Chronic and Episodic Illnesses

CHRONIC MEDICAL ILLNESS.   List all illness for which the patient receives, or has received, chronic medical treatments. These include, but are not limited to, obesity, diabetes, hypertension, gout, rheumatoid arthritis, cancer, psychiatric illnesses, seizure disorders, and sleep disorders.

INFECTIOUS DISEASES.   Infectious diseases have had an important history in medicine. Knowledge of past infections is important to understand current and future infection risk. List dates and complications of measles, German measles, mumps, whooping cough, chickenpox, smallpox, diphtheria, typhoid fever, malaria, hepatitis, scarlet fever, rheumatic fever, chorea, pneumonia, tuberculosis, sexually transmitted diseases, and HIV. Give dates of chemotherapy and antibiotic treatment. Include reactions to antibiotics under the heading, "Allergies and Medication Intolerances."

Operations and Injuries

Give dates and nature of injuries, operations, operative diagnoses, and infection, hemorrhage or other complications.

Previous Hospitalizations

Record each hospitalization, including the dates and names of hospitals and their locations. If the hospital records are available, summarize the dates and diagnoses for each admission.

Family History (FH)

A family history is essential for all patients receiving more than the most cursory of care. This should include four generations, when available: grandparents, parents, aunts and uncles, siblings, and children. For parents and grandparents, record the birth year and current health or age at death and causes. For aunts, uncles, siblings, and children, record the birth year, first name, and current health or cause of death and age at death. Make note of any family history of hypertension, heart disease, diabetes, kidney disease, autoimmune diseases, gout, atopy, asthma, obesity, endocrine disorders, osteoporosis, cancer (particularly breast, colon, ovarian and endocrine cancers), hemophilia or other bleeding diseases, venous thromboembolism, stroke, migraine, neurologic or muscular disorders, mental or emotional disturbances, substance abuse, and epilepsy.

Social History (SH)

PLACE OF BIRTH. This information may be useful in assessing social or national incidence of disease. The examiner may gain some insight into the probability of the patient's understanding the nuances of the English language in giving a history.

NATIONALITY AND ETHNICITY. The correct classification may require considerable knowledge of geography, history, and anthropology. The patient may not be able to give a precise answer. It may be helpful to learn the nationality and ethnicity of the parents. Ethnic and genetic backgrounds are of some importance in diagnosis, for example, of diseases such as hemoglobinopathies and Familial Mediterranean Fever.

MARITAL STATUS. Under this heading, note whether the patient is single, married, divorced, or widowed, and the duration of each marriage and an explanation of its termination.

OCCUPATIONS. Precise knowledge of the patient's work history sheds light on education, social status, physical exertion, psychologic trauma, exposure to noxious agents, and a variety of conditions that may cause disease. Some diseases produce symptoms years after exposure, so tabulate past occupations as well as current work. Do not accept the patient's categorization of an occupation without detailed questioning about what is actually done at work. The manual laborer may actually engage in little heavy physical work on the job but may be exposed to heavy-metal poisons or silica dust. Ask the patient if coworkers recognize some disease connected with their surroundings. Some women may give their occupation as "housewife," neglecting to mention additional part-time or full-time employment. When a woman says she is a housewife, ascertain the number of rooms in the house, how many persons she cares for, if she has assistance with her work, and if she takes a nap during the day. If the woman lives on a farm, how much fieldwork does she perform? For both sexes on the farm, learn what contacts with poisonous chemicals they have and how much exposure? With factory workers ascertain if other workers in the same plant or department have symptoms similar to those of the patient. Determine how much anxiety and tension accompany the job, the attitudes of superiors, and the degree of fatigue from work.

MILITARY HISTORY.   Note admissions to the armed services, branch of service, geographic locations of service, discharge (honorable or dishonorable), and eligibility for veteran's benefits.

GENDER PREFERENCE.   Labels such as heterosexual, homosexual, and bisexual are often more confusing than helpful. Ask each patient if they have had sex with anyone of the same sex. For example, ask men, "Have you ever had sex with men?" If the patient answers "yes," you should ask further questions about sex with women and the patient's past and current practices and preference. Nonjudgmental inquiry about exchange of sex for drugs, money, or services can disclose high-risk behaviors.

SOCIAL AND ECONOMIC STATUS.   Record the patient's years of formal education, vocational training, current housing type, living arrangements, and any special financial problems.

HABITS.   Determine the patient's former and current use of tobacco, coffee, alcohol, sedatives, illicit drugs (especially any injection drug use), placement of tattoos, and body piercing.

VIOLENCE AND SAFETY.   Record the patient's use of vehicle restraints, helmets with bicycling or motorcycling, and the presence of smoke and carbon monoxide alarms in the home.

Domestic, child, and elder abuse are common problems that go unidentified unless they are asked about explicitly, but discreetly. In complete privacy, inquire whether the patient has ever been in a relationship in which she felt unsafe. If the answer is "yes," ask if her situation is safe at the present time. If she answers "no," ask if she wishes you to help her find a safe environment. At no time try to explicitly identify the individual whom the patient finds threatening, unless this information is volunteered by the patient [Felhaus KM, Koziol-McLain J, Amsbury HL, et al. Accuracy of 3 brief screening questions for detecting partner violence in the emergency department. *JAMA* 1997;277:1357–1361].

PROSTHESES AND IN-HOME ASSISTANCE.   Record the patient's use of eyeglasses, dentures and dental appliances, hearing aides, ambulation assistance devices (cane, walker, scooter, wheelchair), braces, prosthetic footwear, and any aide or assistance received in the home (visiting nurse, physical therapy, homemaker services).

Review of Systems (ROS)

The following outline can help you make a careful review of the history by inquiring for salient symptoms associated with each system or anatomic region. Symptoms related to the patient's current problem, discovered during your ROS inquiry, should be recorded under "Present Illness." Become familiar with these symptoms and learn their diagnostic significance. In practice, the patient's answers are not written down except when they are positive, or when a negative response is particularly pertinent to the differential diagnosis. We suggest that you ask the questions while examining the part of the body to which the questions pertain. In taking the present illness, when one of the symptoms emerges, inquire about the associated symptoms in this outline. Use of a standardized patient questionnaire will greatly facilitate identification of positive items on a thorough system review and save the clinician valuable time.

Integument

Skin: Color, pigmentation, temperature, moisture, eruptions, pruritus, scaling, bruising, bleeding. *Hair:* Color, texture, abnormal loss or growth, distribution. *Nails:* Color changes, brittleness, ridging, pitting, curvature.

Lymph Nodes

Enlargement, pain, suppuration, draining sinuses, location.

Bones, Joints, and Muscles

Fractures, dislocations, sprains, arthritis, myositis, pain, swelling, stiffness, migratory distribution, degree of disability, muscular weakness, wasting, or atrophy, night cramps.

Hemopoietic System

Anemia (type, therapy, and response), lymphadenopathy, bleeding or clotting (spontaneous, traumatic, familial).

Endocrine System

History of growth, body configuration, and weight; size of hands, feet, and head, especially changes during adulthood; hair distribution; skin pigmentation; goiter, exophthalmos, dryness of skin and hair, intolerance to heat or cold, tremor; polyphagia, polydipsia, polyuria, glycosuria; secondary sex characteristics, impotence, sterility, treatment.

Allergic and Immunologic History

Dermatitis, urticaria, angioedema, eczema, hay fever, vasomotor rhinitis, asthma, migraine, vernal conjunctivitis and seasonal occurrence of these; known sensitivity to pollens, foods, danders, x-ray contrast agents, bee stings; previous skin tests and their results; results of tuberculin tests and others; desensitization, serum injections, vaccinations, and immunizations.

Head

Headaches, migraine, trauma, vertigo, syncope, convulsive seizures.

Eyes

Loss of vision or color blindness, diplopia, hemianopsia, trauma, inflammation, glasses (date of refraction), discharge, excessive tearing.

Ears

Deafness, tinnitus, vertigo, discharge from the ears, pain, mastoiditis, operations.

Nose

Coryza, rhinitis, sinusitis, discharge, obstruction, epistaxis.

Mouth

Soreness of mouth or tongue, symptoms referable to teeth.

Throat

Hoarseness, sore throats, tonsillitis, voice changes.

Neck

Swelling, suppurative lesions, enlargement of lymph nodes, goiter, stiffness, and limitation of motion.

Breasts

Development, lactation, trauma, lumps, pains, discharge from nipples, gynecomastia, changes in nipples.

Respiratory System

Pain, shortness of breath, wheezing, dyspnea, nocturnal dyspnea, orthopnea, cough, sputum, hemoptysis, night sweats, fevers, pleurisy, bronchitis, tuberculosis (history of contacts), pneumonia, asthma, other respiratory infections.

Cardiovascular System

Palpitation, tachycardia, irregularities or rhythm, pain in the chest, exertional dyspnea, paroxysmal nocturnal dyspnea, orthopnea, cough, cyanosis, ascites, edema; intermittent claudication, cold extremities, thromboses, postural or permanent changes in skin color; hypertension, rheumatic fever, chorea, syphilis, diphtheria; drugs such as digitalis, quinidine, nitroglycerin, diuretics, anticoagulants, antiplatelet agents, and other medications.

Gastrointestinal System

Appetite, changes in weight, dysphagia, nausea, eructation, flatulence, abdominal pain or colic, vomiting, hematemesis, jaundice (pain, fever, intensity, duration, color of urine and stools), stools (color, frequency, incontinence, consistency, odor, gas, cathartics), hemorrhoids, change in bowel habits.

Genitourinary System

Color of urine, polyuria, oliguria, nocturia, dysuria, hematuria, pyuria, urinary retention, urinary frequency, incontinence, pain or colic, passage of stones or gravel. *Gynecologic History:* Age of onset, frequency of periods, regularity, duration, amount of flow, leukorrhea, dysmenorrhea, date of last normal and preceding periods, date and character of menopause, postmenopausal bleeding; pregnancies (number, abortions, miscarriages, stillbirths, chronologic sequence), complications of pregnancy; birth control practices (oral contraceptive medications, barrier methods, etc.). *Male History:* Erectile dysfunction, premature ejaculation, blood in the semen, contraceptive methods and condom use. *Venereal Disease History:* Sexual activity (sex of partners and practices), chancre, bubo, urethral discharge, treatment of venereal diseases.

Nervous System

Cranial Nerves: Disturbances of smell (cranial nerve I), visual disturbances (CN II, III, IV, VI); orofacial paresthesias and difficulty in chewing (CN V); facial weakness and taste disturbances (CN VII); disturbances in hearing and equilibrium (CN VIII); difficulties in speech, swallowing, and taste (CN IX, X, XII); limitation in motion of neck (CN XII). *Motor System:* Paralyses, atrophy, involuntary movements, convulsions, gait, incoordination. *Sensory System:* Pain, lightning pain, girdle pain, paresthesia, hypesthesia, anesthesia, allodynia. *Autonomic System:* Control of urination and defecation, sweating, erythema, cyanosis, pallor, reaction to heat and cold.

Psychiatric History

Describe difficulties with interpersonal relationships (with parents, siblings, spouse, children, friends and associates), sexual adjustments, employment success and difficulties, impulse control, sleep disorders, mood swings, difficulty with concentration, thought or the presence of hallucinations.

Medications

In a separate section, list all medications being taken: their names, doses, effects, reason for taking, and duration. Ask the patient to bring the pharmacist's containers with the specific data on the labels. If the labels are absent, identify tablets, pills, capsules, and suppositories by asking the pharmacist who issued the drug. Be sure to list all nonprescription drugs, herbal remedies, supplements, and vitamins.

Allergies and Medication Intolerances

A notation of past medications and untoward drug reactions should be as explicit as possible. Ask the patient for the type of reaction or intolerance he experienced with each medication; many patients list allergies to medications to which they experienced common side effects, not allergic reactions, for example, stomach upset with codeine or erythromycin. Identify all known or suspected causes of anaphylaxis, including drugs, stings, and foods (e.g., peanuts). This summary of allergies and medication intolerances must be consulted when any drugs are prescribed in the future.

Preventive Care Services

Here you should record the patient's history of preventive care services. List the dates and results of screening tests (e.g., mammograms, Pap smears, tuberculin tests), insurance examinations, and immunizations using age- and sex-specific national guidelines as your standard.

Advance Directives

Each adult should be asked if they have a living will and or durable power of attorney for health care and, if so, who is their surrogate decision maker. All patients should be given information about these advance directives and be given an opportunity to record their wishes concerning resuscitation, mechanical ventilation, and prolonged life support. Although these discussions are more likely to be particularly relevant to the frail elderly, you should initiate this discussion with all adults over age 50, years before the anticipated time of need.

Physical Examination

Here you should record the finding from your physical examination in a systematic fashion. The sequence of presentation below is suggested as a common and practical method:

    Vital signs
    General appearance
    Head, eyes, ears, nose, and throat (HEENT)
    Neck and spine
    Chest: breasts
    Chest: chest wall and lungs
    Chest: heart, major arteries, and neck veins
    Abdomen
    Genitourinary exam, including inguinal hernias
    Rectal exam
    Extremities
    Lymph nodes
    Neurologic exam, including the mental status exam
    Skin

Laboratory

Record the results of the initial laboratory finding which you have used to assist in the development of your differential diagnosis.

Assessment

Case Summary

After recording the history and physical examination, analyze the chronology, symptoms, signs, and laboratory findings of the illness. It is advisable to write a brief summary of your findings as an abstract of the significant observations.

The Assessment or Problem List

Write down your list of all the diagnostic and management problems the patient presents (variously labeled as initial assessment, impression, problem list, or diagnosis). A diagnostic problem may be a symptom, a sign, a laboratory finding, or a complex of several items that experience has taught are associated with disease. A previously diagnosed disease, or one under consideration for diagnosis, may be listed as a problem. When the diagnosis is obscure, beware of lumping problems together prematurely; this may serve to obscure rather than to clarify the diagnosis.

Generate a *differential diagnosis* for each medical problem. As discussed in Chapter 1, the differential diagnosis can be pathophysiologic, diagnostic, or both. It is a good practice to keep the patient's chief complaint the first problem on your problem list. Beyond that, we do not feel that attempts to number the problem list in a prioritized or numerically consistent fashion is useful, because priorities change as the evaluation and treatment proceed and problems disappear or consolidate as more information is acquired.

A **Working Problem List** should be maintained as a separate page in the hospital or clinic chart to record the numbered problems with notes and dates indicating the status of each. It is important to maintain, update, and revise this problem list. By constantly reviewing the problem list, you can see that every problem is considered. Often the key to the diagnostic puzzle is finding how the odd problem fits the pattern. Diagnostic problem solving is much like putting together a jigsaw puzzle without the picture and with only a few pieces provided at a time. To get the pieces together correctly, you have to have all the pieces on the table at the same time and keep looking at them as new pieces appear to see the pattern emerge. The problem list is your table full of pieces, your hypotheses are attempts to explain the pattern. It is often the odd piece that doesn't seem to fit anywhere that is the key to the puzzle.

The Plan

For each problem, and the patient as a whole, you need to develop a plan. The plan for each problem has three parts: (a) plans for testing your hypothesis or differential diagnosis; (b) therapy to be considered or given; and (c) education for the patient and family.

A plan is only as good as the diagnostic hypotheses that generated it. Our emphasis in this text is to help you think about the information acquired in the performance of the history and physical examination so that you can generate sound, testable hypotheses. Once you have generated a concise and thoughtful differential diagnosis, you can consult textbooks of medicine, for example, *Harrison's Principles of Internal Medicine* [Braunwald E, Fauci AS, Kasper DL, et al. (eds). *Harrison's Principles of Internal Medicine.* 15th ed. New York: McGraw-Hill, 2001], or directly search the medical literature to assist in the most economical and efficient methods for testing your hypotheses.

The Oral Presentation

The optimal oral presentation holds your listener's attention for 5 to 7 minutes while you identify your patient and briefly summarize the case. Start with a statement of the patient's problems or diagnoses so your listeners can analyze your subsequent narrative for the evidence used to support the diagnosis and therapeutic plan you propose. Then summarize the history and presentation, review the vital signs and pertinent physical findings and laboratory test results, state the diagnostic impressions or problems, and then recommend a diagnostic and therapeutic plan. Excellent presentations require that you edit and organize the information you have collected, to tell the story of the illness as it appears to you. If you regurgitate all of the extensive information that you place in the medical record, you will quickly lose your audience.

The oral presentation of the diagnostic examination is not simply an academic exercise. Brief, accurate presentations will benefit your patients by clearly communicating their problems to others who will participate in their care: your teachers, fellow house officers, sign-out partners in practice, and consultants [Lehmann LS, Brancati FL, Chen M-C, et al. The effect of bedside case presentations on patient's perceptions of their medical care. *N Engl J Med* 1997;336:1150–1155; Bergus GR, Chapman GB, Levy BT, et al. Clinical diagnosis and the order of information. *Med Decis Making* 1998;18:412–417].

Other Clinical Notes

Inpatient Progress Notes

Progress notes are made daily and whenever necessary. Each note should be dated and the time of day recorded. Each note has four subheads. Use the mnemonic SOAP to remember them: *S*ubjective data (symptoms and changes in symptoms, their appearance and disappearance, and their response to therapy); *O*bjective data (changes in or new physical signs and laboratory findings and response to therapy); *As*sessments (updates to your problem list and hypotheses); and *P*lans (diagnostic tests, therapeutic interventions and instructions to the patient and nursing staff). When a problem is resolved by inclusion in another diagnosis, or by cure or disappearance, it should be so noted in the progress note and in the Working Problem List.

The full and legible name of the writer should be appended to each progress note. The name should be followed by a slash mark and an abbreviation indicating hospital rank. Here are some examples: (junior medical student), (second-year resident), or RN (student nurse or graduate), Joan Doe/S (staff).

Off-Service Note

Write a note in the chart when you leave a service and turn over the care of the patient to your successor. Customarily, a brief résumé of the case is recorded, stating the diagnosis or problems, the treatment, and response, suggestions for continuing treatment are included. Do not include statements like, "Good luck!"

Discharge Summary

When the patient leaves the hospital, the physician should enter a final note containing an abstract of the case, with the diagnosis or problem list and the treatment given in the hospital and prescribed for home use. Note the patient's condition and functional status at discharge and any information or instructions given to the patient and attendants for home and follow-up care.

Clinic Notes

Clinic notes follow the same SOAP format described for progress notes in the hospital. If the chart contains standardized forms as part of the medical record the note may refer the reader to those forms for current information, so that it need not be repeated in the written note. All clinic notes should state the expected response to interventions, when that response is anticipated and when the patient is to be seen in follow up.

The Patient's Medical Record

The patient's medical record is a document containing (a) the medical history; (b) the findings from the physical examination; (c) the reports of laboratory tests; (d) the findings and conclusions from special examinations; (e) the findings and diagnoses of consultants; (f) the diagnoses of the responsible physician; (g) notes on treatment, including medication, surgical operations, radiation, physical therapy; and (h) progress notes by physicians, nurses, and others.

Purposes

The purposes of the patient's medical record may be classified as follows:

Medical Purposes

1. To assist the physician in making diagnoses.
2. To assist physicians, nurses, and others in the care and treatment of the patient.
3. To serve as a record for teaching medicine and for clinical research.

Legal Purposes

1. To document insurance claims for the patient.
2. To serve as legal proof in cases of malpractice, claims for injury or compensation, cases of poisoning, and cases of homicide.

Reimbursement

The federal government has developed documentation guidelines for evaluation and management (E/M) services that define the standards that Medicare carriers employ in reviewing documentation physicians must use to bill for history taking, physical examinations, and medical decision making.

Usually, the physician composes the patient's record with attention focused on the medical purposes of making diagnoses, caring for the patient, teaching medicine, and furthering research [Reiser SJ. The clinical record in medicine. *Ann Intern Med* 1991;114:902–907, 980–985]. After the illness, sometimes years later, the medical record may be consulted to fulfill the legal purposes in support of claims and the demonstration of facts in litigation. In these contingencies, the physician may belatedly discover omissions and inaccuracies. To prevent late recriminations, always completely document each patient encounter at the time of service. Addendums may be added at a later date, but the original note must never be altered.

Attempts at grading diagnoses are encountered in some hospitals and in some insurance forms that call for a primary diagnosis and a secondary diagnosis. At face value, this request seems rational, but an absurdity appears when the same records are graded by different specialists. The primary diagnosis is often different from the view of the internist, the surgeon, the orthopedist, or the otolaryngologist. Each selects the disease pertaining to his or her own specialty. The confusion is diminished when the form states that the primary diagnosis is the reason for the clinic visit or hospitalization.

The primary purposes of enabling a physician to document his or her care in the medical record are to serve the memory of the caregiver and communicate these data to other physicians caring for the patient. Uses of the record for legal and billing purposes are secondary and should not distract or interfere with good patient care. Lawyers and insurers insist on written documentation as evidence of performance, but guidelines that encourage treating charts instead of patients are bad medicine [Brett AS. New guidelines for coding physician's services—A step backward. *N Engl J Med* 1998;339:1705–1708; Kassirer JP, Angell M. Evaluation and management guidelines—Fatally flawed. *N Engl J Med* 1998;339:1697–1698].

Physician's Signature

Each sheet, brief entry, and doctor's order composed by the physician for the medical record should be accompanied by the physician's signature and the date and time of signing as proof of authorship. In the hospital record, the physician's initials are inadequate; the complete written signature should be legible. All dates should include the month, day of the month, and year. In teaching hospitals, where many persons contribute to the record, the entries of medical students and nurses should be dated and accompanied by their signatures, affixed with suitable abbreviations indicating their status in the medical organization.

Custody of the Record

The record may rest in the physician's locked office files, or it may be in the custody of the hospital where the patient received medical care. The contents of the medical record must be guarded against access by unauthorized persons. The recorded facts are privileged communications under the law; they cannot be revealed to another person without the written consent of the patient.

The medical record should be composed with the constant realization that at some future time the patient may read it or that it may become a legal document; the date and authorship of each entry may be important. The record should not contain flippant or derogatory remarks about the patient or colleagues.

Electronic Medical Records

Over the past 30 years, enthusiasts of medical informatics have continued to develop the electronic medical record. Advances in technology permit a physician to dictate findings from the diagnostic examination and the treatment plan into an electronic format that can be readily viewed on a computer screen. This allows you to recall your documentation and the patient's study results at an appropriate computer terminal. It should facilitate the transfer of the patient's record to consultants, referring physicians, and insurers. Indeed, specialists in the burgeoning field of telemedicine, who have authored programs for the transfer of electrocardiograms and radiologic images, envision enhanced development of interactive visual consultation and robotic surgery directed from a remote source.

Physicians contemplating the use of a fully computerized patient chart have had concerns regarding the ease of preparing it and the time required to do so, its accessibility to the physician, its cost and protection against system failure. Moreover, they are also concerned about the security of sensitive patient information from unauthorized persons (e.g., creditors, investigators, computer hackers). The solution of these problems should overcome the reluctance of physicians to adopt the electronic medical record.

3 The Screening Physical Examination: Methods and Procedure

In our era of high technology, the continued need for the performance of a proper physical examination may surprise the uninformed [Sackett DL. The science of the art of the clinical examination. *JAMA* 1992;267: 2650–2652; Adolph RJ. The value of bedside examination in an era of high technology. *Heart Dis Stroke* 1994;31:128–131]. The importance of a systematic history and physical exam is best understood by considering the following points: (a) Attention to the story of the patient's illness and thoughtful performance of the physical examination (the "laying on of hands") establishes a personal relationship of trust and respect between the patient and clinician necessary for good medical care. (b) Performing laboratory tests and imaging studies without diagnostic hypotheses generated from the history and physical examination is expensive and often produces false-positive results, delaying proper diagnosis. (c) Conclusions drawn from the results of blood tests, imaging procedures, and even biopsy material, are based upon the pretest probability of the various diagnoses under consideration. The pretest probability is derived from the history, physical examination, and knowledge of disease prevalence. (d) Additionally, large studies have shown that the history and physical exam are more sensitive and specific than imaging tests in most difficult diagnostic situations [Kirch W, Schafi C. Misdiagnosis at a university hospital in 4 medical eras. *Medicine (Baltimore)* 1996;75:29–40].

Each physical examination is an opportunity to train the four senses: sight, touch, hearing, and smell. With reflective practice and knowledge of anatomy, physiology, and pathology, you will perceive abnormalities in structure and function overlooked by an untrained examiner. The physiologic and disease hypotheses generated during the history and physical exam are tested in the various laboratories leading to precise diagnosis with an economical use of resources.

We use each of our four senses to elicit signs of disease: inspection (sight and smell), palpation (touch), percussion (touch and hearing), and auscultation (hearing). Only minimal manual dexterity is required for percussion and palpation. Remember to be gentle on initiation of the exam; forceful palpation and percussion are rarely necessary and will cause the patient to tense their muscles and resist your examination.

With experience you will be able to assess the severity of illness and the urgency for treatment. To become a skillful diagnostician, you must constantly reflect on the findings from your examination, the correlations between your exam and the laboratory and imaging studies, and the accuracy of your findings and hypotheses based upon the final confirmed diagnoses. In short, you must practice and study. No one started as an expert history taker, physical examiner, or diagnostician. The experts are those who have learned from their experience and refined their senses and skills through repetition, reflection and correlation of their physical findings with the results of imaging and laboratory tests.

Methods for Physical Examination

Inspection

Inspection is the search for physical signs by observing the patient with your eyes and sense of smell. Of the examination methods, inspection is the least mechanical and the hardest to learn, but it yields many important physical signs. Because we tend to see things that have meaning for us, inspection depends entirely on the knowledge and expectations of the observer. This is epitomized in maxims such as "We see what's behind the eyes" (Wintrobe), "The examination does not wait the removal of the shirt" (Waring), and "Was Man Weiss, Man sieht" (Goethe: "What one knows, one sees"). The layperson looks at a person and concludes that there is something "peculiar" about that person; the physician sees acromegaly. The expert observer can dissect the "peculiarity" and recognize the diagnostic components, such as the enlarged supraorbital ridges, the widely spaced teeth, the macroglossia, the buffalo hump, the huge hands and feet. Practice is required to learn inspection: remember that sight is a faculty, whereas seeing is an art.

Smells are impossible to describe, only experience with similar sensations will give you a context for interpretation. The body odors of poor hygiene, the fetor of advanced liver disease, the putrid smell of anaerobic infections, the smell of alcohol or acetone on the breath, and many others are useful diagnostic clues apparent to the trained observer.

General Visual Inspection

The initial step in physical examination is inspection of the person as a whole. It begins at your first encounter with the patient. Note how the patient is dressed and groomed; whether eye contact is established; the tone and pattern of speech; how the patient moves and changes position; facial expression; skin type; overall body form and proportions; deformities or asymmetry of face, limbs, or trunk; nutrition; specific behaviors; signs of pain or tremor. You should also bear in mind that the patient will be inspecting you at the same time.

Close Visual Inspection

Close or focused inspection concentrates on a single anatomic region; the closer you look, the more you see. The art is in seeing what is important and distinguishing it from what is not.

Visual inspection usually refers to observation with the unaided eyes. Obviously, the dermatologist relies heavily on the appearance of skin lesions to make a diagnosis. Actually, however, visual signs are the principal findings in the use of the ophthalmoscope, slit lamp, otoscope, laryngoscope, bronchoscope, gastroscope, thoracoscope, laparoscope, cystoscope, anoscope, colonoscope, and sigmoidoscope. The pathologist uses the microscope; the radiologist inspects images generated in any number of ways. All are using visual inspection to elicit information.

Proper visual inspection of the body surface requires a uniform white light source to avoid color distortion. A hand-held lens or an otoscope or ophthalmoscope can be used for magnification. Oblique lighting is often very useful to detect subtle changes in surface contours and to detect motion that may be invisible with direct lighting; for example, looking for an apical impulse on the chest. As with all parts of the physical examination it is important not just to see an abnormality, you must learn to accurately describe what you see without using language that draws a conclusion or presumes a diagnosis.

Olfactory Inspection—Smell

Although some physicians seem to regard the use of the nose for diagnosis as indelicate, odors may provide valuable and immediate clues.

BREATH. Odors on the breath from acetone, alcohol, and some poisons may lead quickly to a diagnosis.

SPUTUM. Foul-smelling sputum suggests bronchiectasis or lung abscess.

VOMITUS. The gastric contents may emit the odors of alcohol, phenol, or other poisons, or the sour smell of fermenting food retained overlong. A fecal odor from the vomitus may indicate intestinal obstruction.

FECES. Particularly foul-smelling stools are common in pancreatic insufficiency.

URINE. An ammoniacal odor in the urine may result from fermentation within the bladder.

PUS. A nauseatingly sweet odor, like the smell of rotting apples, is evidence that pus is coming from a region of gas gangrene. A fecal odor is imparted by anaerobic bacteria. Some anaerobic bacteria in abscesses produce an odor like that of overripe Camembert cheese.

Palpation

The usual definition of palpation is the act of feeling using the sense of touch; but this is too limited. When you lay your hands on the patient, you perceive physical signs by tactile sense, temperature sense, and the kinesthetic senses of position and vibration. As with the other forms of observation, all normal persons possess these senses, but training and practice will enable you to identify findings that escape the layperson. If you doubt the influence of practice on palpation, observe a blind person reading a book printed in braille, then close your eyes and attempt to distinguish between two braille letters by touching them.

Sensitive Parts of the Hand

TACTILE SENSE.   The tips of the fingers are most sensitive for fine tactile discrimination.

TEMPERATURE SENSE.   Use the dorsa of the hands or fingers; the skin is much thinner than elsewhere on the hand.

VIBRATORY SENSE.   Palpate with the palmar aspects of the metacarpophalangeal joints or the ulnar side of the hand (fifth metacarpal and fifth phalanges) rather than with the fingertips to perceive vibrations such as thrills. Prove the superiority for yourself by touching first the fingertip and then the palmar base of your finger with a vibrating tuning fork.

SENSE OF POSITION AND CONSISTENCY.   Use the grasping fingers so you perceive with sensations from your joints and muscles.

Structures Examined by Palpation

Palpation is employed on every part of the body accessible to the examining fingers: all external structures, all structures accessible through the body orifices, the bones, joints, muscles, tendon sheaths, ligaments, superficial arteries, thrombosed or thickened veins, superficial nerves, salivary ducts, spermatic cord, solid abdominal viscera, solid contents of hollow viscera, and accumulations of body fluids, pus, or blood.

Specific Qualities Elicited by Palpation

TEXTURE.   The surface characteristics of the skin and hair are noted. Is each dry, brittle, coarse, thick, thin, roughened or smooth?

MOISTURE.   Assess the moisture content of the skin, hair, and mucous membranes. Are they moist and supple or dry and cracked?

SKIN TEMPERATURE.   Palpate the head, face, trunk, arms, hands, legs, and feet to assess the local skin temperature and the distribution of heat.

CHARACTERISTICS OF MASSES.   When a mass or enlarged organ is discovered, record its size, shape, consistency, motility, surface regularity and the presence or absence of expansile or transmitted pulsation.

PRECORDIAL CARDIAC THRUST.   Palpate the precordium for signs of heart action (see Chapter 8, page 361).

CREPITUS.   During examination of the bones, joints, tendon sheaths, pleura, and subcutaneous tissue note crepitation.

TENDERNESS.   Elicitation of discomfort or pain on palpation of accessible tissues and over major organs should be noted. How much pressure is required to induce the uncomfortable sensation?

THRILLS.   Palpate the precordium for thrills. If bruits are heard in the major arteries, palpate them for thrills.

VOCAL FREMITUS.   Palpation of vocal vibrations through the chest wall provides important information about the underlying pleura and lung (see Chapter 8, page 354).

Methods of Palpation

LIGHT PALPATION.   Always begin palpation with a light touch. Your sense of touch is most acute when lightly applied and the patient will be put at ease. Gently sliding your fingertips over the skin surface will often detect subtle or mobile masses that are undetected by forceful palpation. You will also locate areas of particular tenderness, which should be examined last.

DEEP PALPATION.   Firm pressure is applied to displace the superficial tissues allowing palpation for deeper lesions. This is especially useful in the abdomen, but is also useful in the neck, breasts, and large muscle masses. Avoid firm palpation over nerves or other tender structures whenever possible.

BIMANUAL PALPATION.   In this technique, the tissue is examined between the fingers of the two hands. It is useful for soft tissue such as the breasts, intraoral, abdominal and pelvic examinations, and examination of the muscles and joints.

Percussion

Percussion is the act of striking the surface of the body to elicit a sound. When the body surface is struck, the underlying tissues vibrate to produce percussion notes having mixed frequencies that vary with the density of the organ and the composition overlying tissue.

Bimanual, Mediate, or Indirect Method of Percussion

Striking the percussion blow on an inanimate object or your finger is indirect or mediate percussion. This is the form of percussion most commonly used. The palmar surface of the left long finger is firmly pressed onto the body surface, as a *pleximeter,* only the distal phalanx should touch the wall. As a *plexor,* the tip of the right long finger strikes a sharp blow on the distal interphalangeal joint of the pleximeter finger (Fig. 3-1). The examiner holds the plexor finger partly flexed and rigid and delivers the blow by bending only the wrist, so the weight of the hand lends momentum ensuring repetitive blows of equal force. The wrist must be relaxed and neither the elbow nor the shoulder should be moved. After the stroke, the plexor should rebound quickly from the pleximeter to avoid damping the vibrations. Usually, two or three staccato blows are struck in one place, and then the pleximeter is moved elsewhere for a second series of blows to compare the sounds. Most physicians employ this bimanual method for percussion of both the thorax and abdomen.

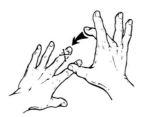

Fig. 3-1   Method of indirect (bimanual) percussion. *The terminal digit of the left long finger is firmly applied to an interspace, or other body surface, as a pleximeter. The distal interphalangeal joint of that finger is struck a sharp blow with the tip of the flexed right long finger. To furnish blows of equal intensity, the fingers of the right hand are held partly flexed and the wrist is loose so that the striking hand pivots exclusively at the relaxed wrist. To avoid dampening the vibrations after striking the blow, withdraw the plexor hand rapidly from the pleximeter.*

Direct Percussion

When you elicit sound by striking the body surface directly with your fingers, hand, or reflex hammer, the procedure is called *direct or immediate percussion*. This method is not commonly used, but can be very rewarding. Since your finger is not receiving the blow, be careful to not strike the patient too firmly.

Sonorous Percussion

Sonorous percussion is used to detect alterations in the density of an organ. For example, striking an air-filled lung produces one sound; a lung filled with fluid produces quite another. The change in sounds is determined by the change in tissue densities. The different sounds are given special names. Percussing the gastric air bubble yields a sound called *tympany;* the word is derived from the Greek for "drum," and the sound vaguely resembles a drumbeat. The percussion note from the air-filled lung is of quite different pitch and timbre, termed *resonance.* Absent in the normal body, *hyperresonance* is emitted by the emphysematous lung; it is intermediate between resonance from the lung, filled with small air sacs and septa, and tympany from the large undivided bubble in the stomach. *Dullness* is a distinctive noise elicited by percussion over the heart when it is not covered by inflated lung. Percussion of the thigh muscles yields *flatness.*

In a nontechnical sense, the percussion sounds may be regarded as the notes of a scale, which progresses from tissues of high density to tissues of low density in the following sequence: flatness, dullness, resonance, hyperresonance, and tympany. The duration of emitted sound correlates inversely with the density producing it: flatness is a very short sound and, as the density lessens, each succeeding note in the scale is longer than its predecessor.

The pitch and timbre of the sounds must be learned by listening. Language is inadequate for description of sounds, and attempts to describe these notes are futile and confusing. Proper recognition of these distinctions must be gained by listening. Some clinicians have trained themselves to feel changes in resonance, using vibration sense, as well as to perceive them as sound.

Sonorous percussion is employed to ascertain the density of the lungs, the pleural space, the pleural layers, and the hollow viscera of the abdomen. It requires a strong blow, estimated to vibrate tissue for a radius of 6 cm in the chest, 3 cm in the thoracic wall, and 3 cm in the lung parenchyma.

Definitive Percussion

When the density of an organ is invariable and contrasts with that of the surrounding tissue, the borders of the organ can be identified as the transition site of one sound quality to the other; this is *definitive percussion*. For example, percussion of the heart is employed only to locate its boundaries with the lung; the density of neither tissue is in question. A lighter blow should be struck by for definitive percussion than for sonorous percussion. Mapping of the area of greater density gives an idea of the size of the structure or the extent of its border.

Definitive percussion is commonly used to determine the location of the lung bases, the height of fluid in the pleural cavity, the width of the mediastinum, the size of the heart, the outline of dense masses in the lungs, the size and shape of the liver and spleen, the size of a distended gallbladder and urinary bladder, and the level of ascitic fluid.

Auscultation

Although auscultation literally means using hearing to obtain physical signs, it has come to mean hearing through the stethoscope. There is no technical term for hearing the patient speak, cough, groan, or shriek, although all these sounds furnish diagnostic clues; this just emphasizes the importance of *listening* to the patient, not just the patient's words.

The uses of auscultation have expanded as the correlation of auscultatory findings to physiologic and pathophysiologic processes has been revealed by ultrasonography, echocardiography, and other diagnostic studies. As every musician knows, the ear can be trained to recognize sounds more accurately. Each person learns to recognize the voices of many associates by patterns of pitch and overtones.

Use of the Stethoscope

The stethoscope contains a vibrating air column connecting the body wall to the ears. Because stethoscopes invariably modify sound to some extent, you should use a single instrument whenever possible. The usual stethoscope does not amplify sound; it merely assists in excluding extraneous noises. Electronic stethoscopes, which amplify and/or project the sound through a speaker, are particularly useful for teaching purposes.

Binaural instruments consist of a chest piece, plastic tubes, and two earpieces connected by a spring. Two chest pieces are needed to better detect the full range of frequencies. The *bell* is a hollow cone with a rim

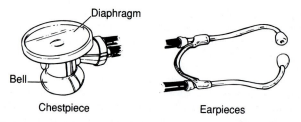

Fig. 3-2 The Sprague stethoscope. *The chest piece combines the bell and diaphragm, with a valve to direct the air through either. The earpieces are connected by a spring that holds them in place.*

of hard rubber or plastic. The bell transmits all sounds from the chest; the low-pitched sounds come through particularly well. The low-pitched murmur of mitral stenosis and the fetal heart sounds may be audible only with the bell. A wide bell can transmit sounds of lower pitch than a narrow diameter bell. The *diaphragm* is a flat cup covered with a semi-rigid diaphragm that serves as a filter to exclude low-pitched sounds, so the isolated high-pitched sounds seem louder. The diaphragm is best suited for high-pitched sounds from the heart (e.g., regurgitant aortic murmurs) and breath sounds. Cracks in the diaphragm impair its properties. The chest piece shown in Fig. 3-2 is a popular and convenient configuration of the bell and diaphragm with a valve to direct the air column from one to the other. The tubing should be thick-walled; the inside diameter should not be smaller than the caliber of the connecting tubes. For optimal acoustics, the length of the rubber tubing should not exceed 30 cm, although many physicians accept a longer, more convenient length.

The stethoscope should fit the user's ears. The plastic or rubber earpiece should impinge on the external auditory meatus without discomfort or pain, yet fit tightly without air leakage. The spring, size, and design of the earpiece determine the tightness of the fit.

More art than meets the eye is required to use the stethoscope. The diaphragm should be pressed tightly against the chest wall; in contrast, the rim of the bell should touch the chest wall lightly, but seal completely. Heavy pressure with the bell stretches the underlying skin over the bell's circumference so the skin becomes a diaphragm excluding low-pitched sounds. The entire rim of the bell must touch the skin; a roaring sound from extraneous noise warns the examiner of a leak. At first, the listener may be distracted by extraneous noises coming through the walls of the tubing, but soon learns to ignore these completely. The breath of the examiner on the tubing produces noise; try this, so the sound may be recognized and eliminated. Skin or hair rubbing on the chest piece produces sounds like crackles, which can be eliminated by wetting the hair or by placing a soft rubber rim on the bell. Movements of muscles, joints, or tendons sound like friction rubs; be certain that you can recognize them so they can be eliminated. If you do not hear the expected sounds with your first attempt, do not discredit your instrument or your ears; they are probably normal, but you need practice. Use the bell for narrow spaces such as the supraclavicular fossae. Thin-walled chests present difficulties in fitting the chest piece into the interspaces without leakage. Examine the instrument occasionally to ensure that it has no leaks or plugs of cerumen or other debris.

Auscultation is used to examine the heart and lungs. From the lungs the stethoscope conveys breath sounds, whispers, and voice sounds, as well as crackles and friction rubs. The heart generates the normal heart sounds, gallops, murmurs, rhythm disturbances, and pericardial rubs and knocks. The vessels of the neck are examined for murmurs in the thyroid, carotid, and subclavian arteries and for venous hums. Auscultation of the abdomen reveals bowel sounds and murmurs from aneurysms and stenotic arteries. The skull can be auscultated for the bruit of an arteriovenous fistula. Crepitus can be heard in joints, tendon sheaths, muscles, and fractured bones, as well as in subcutaneous emphysema.

Procedure for the Screening Physical Examination

Within practical limits, there is no such thing as a routine physical examination. Like history taking, the physical examination is a structured method for eliciting observations of the patient using multiple techniques. The emphasis of each exam varies as prompted by the symptoms, physical signs, and laboratory findings of each patient; for example, the heart and circulation will be examined more carefully and thoroughly in a patient with exertional dyspnea than in a patient who has just sustained a fractured ankle.

Either unconsciously or, preferably, after careful consideration, every physician adopts a sequence of examination. The physician develops a routine or *basic screening examination* that is periodically performed with most patients. If significant abnormalities are encountered that focus attention on an anatomic site or some physiologic problem, a more detailed examination of that area or system should be performed. The screening examination should vary very little from patient to patient of the same gender and age. The *diagnostic examination* following up on problems identified in the history or abnormalities elicited on the screening examination, is unique to each patient and problem.

Hillman et al. studied the components of screening examinations employed by various family physicians and internists in Seattle. They found that the examinations varied from 2 to 45 minutes, with wide variation in the components emphasized. We are indebted to them for making their findings available [Hillman RS, Goodall BW, Grundy SM, et al: The basic or routine physical examination of the adult, in *Clinical Skills*. New York: McGraw-Hill, 1981:97–115]. Such variation in the screening examination reflects both examinations that are too cursory and examinations that are probably too detailed for efficient screening. The clinician must master a structured, efficient screening exam, which, when combined with the history, is likely to identify most serious abnormalities.

For convenience, and for the patient's comfort, we examine the body by regions. In contrast, we recognize illness and disease by the physiologic systems involved. Consequently, *examine by regions, but think by systems.* This requires practice, reflection, and experience. The beginner sees all the regions and may identify many or most of the findings, but has trouble integrating those findings into a complete picture of the anatomy and physiology he has observed. This integration of findings is critical for generating unifying diagnostic hypotheses (see *Problem Lists,* page 33, and *Hypothesis Generation,* page 7).

A single routine that everyone should follow exactly is impractical. There are many possible sequences of examination, each with its advantages and disadvantages; none is perfect. We have based our recommendation on several observations:

1. Many physical signs are recognized and evaluated during history taking.
2. A well-organized exam room with easily accessible instruments familiar to the examiner enhances efficiency.
3. Examining each patient from head to foot in the same sequence avoids missing signs and develops an appreciation of normal variation.
4. Excessive changes of position by the examiner or patient take time and are uncomfortable for both.
5. This screening examination can be performed in 15 minutes.

Always keep the following points in mind:

1. Respecting your patient's modesty and retaining a professional approach encourages the patient's cooperation and diminishes the chances for misinterpretation of your intent to examine emotionally sensitive anatomy.
2. A screening examination not only discovers diagnostic signs but also reassures the patient.
3. Examining the problem area first responds to the patient's anxiety but should not distract from completing a complete examination.
4. Detailed evaluation of specific signs requires additional time.
5. In some circumstances, a full screening examination is inappropriate; a regional or special examination may be all that is indicated. This is particularly true for the patient returning for follow up after a short interval or an otherwise healthy patient with an acute limited problem.

Preparing for the Screening Examination

This example of a multisystem screening examination is designed to be performed with the patient in only four or five positions. It takes approximately 15 minutes (Fig. 3-3). In the following sections, we give you a description of the sequence of the examination. The methods for examination of each region are detailed in their respective chapters.

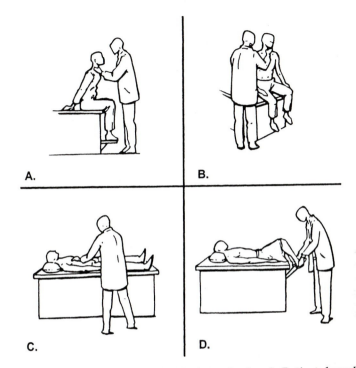

*Fig. 3-3 The office screening physical examination. A. **Patient draped and sitting** (physician facing). B. **Patient draped and sitting** (physician to right and back). C. **Patient draped and supine** (physician to right). Place the patient in the left lateral decubitus position to listen at the cardiac apex. D. **Female pelvic exam:** patient draped and supine, knees and hips flexed (physician at foot).*

Preparation: Required Equipment

A minimum list of equipment for the screening examination includes a stethoscope, sphygmomanometer, otoscope, ophthalmoscope, penlight, tongue blades, reflex hammer, tuning fork and calibrated monofilament for sensory testing, tape measure, latex or plastic gloves, lubricant for rectal and vaginal examinations, reagent for occult blood test, sterile swabs, and materials for specimen collection during the female pelvic examination. The instruments must be within easy reach. Wear gloves when examining infected skin or when you may come in contact with body fluids.

Preparation: The Patient

The patient undresses in private, puts on an examination gown, and sits on the end of the exam table with a sheet draped over the lap and legs.

Performance of the Screening Examination

Phase A: Vital Signs, General Inspection, Close Inspection, and Palpation of the Head, Ears, Eyes, Nose, and Throat

Patient and Examiner Positions: patient draped and sitting facing the examiner

To start the exam, the physician washes her hands.

VITAL SIGNS. Obtain the vital signs or, if previously obtained by a nurse, review them and confirm any abnormal findings by rechecking them yourself.

GENERAL INSPECTION. Note the general appearance of the patient. Inspect the head and face, sclera and conjunctivae, external ears, scalp, skin of the head and neck, the hands and fingernails, and the skin of the arms.

CLOSE INSPECTION. Examine the ears with the otoscope, check hearing, visual fields by confrontation, extraocular movements and pupillary size and reactions, examine the fundi, and inspect the oral cavity and oropharynx using the tongue blade.

PALPATION: Palpate any areas of head, face, or neck deformity, and use bimanual palpation of intraoral pathology. Palpate any areas of deformity of the hand, wrist, and elbow joints for synovitis or effusion. Palpate all skin rashes.

Phase B: Inspection of the Back of the Head, Neck, Back, and Shoulders; Palpation of the Neck, Shoulders, and Back; Percussion of the Spine and Lungs; Auscultation of the Lungs

Patient and Examiner Positions: patient draped and sitting; examiner on the patient's right side behind the patient

You may either stand to the patient's right side or sit on the exam table behind the patient, for part of the exam.

INSPECTION. Expose the patient's back and inspect for skin lesions, scars, rashes, and the like. Observe the neck from the side and check range of neck motion.

PALPATION. Palpate the anterior neck noting the carotid pulsations, the thyroid, and the position of the trachea. Search each lymph node bed for adenopathy. Visually and by palpation, determine the position of the thoracic and lumbar vertebral spines; note any scoliosis or excessive kyphosis or lordosis. Palpate any deformities or swelling of the neck, back, shoulders, or scapulae.

PERCUSSION. Use fist percussion to check for spinal or costovertebral angle tenderness. Percuss the chest anteriorly and posteriorly, comparing right to left and apices to bases.

AUSCULTATION. Auscultate the chest posteriorly, laterally, and anteriorly (under the gown), comparing right to left and apices to bases.

Phase C (Female Patients Only): The Sitting Breast Exam

Patient and Examiner Positions: patient draped and sitting facing the examiner

After proper explanation, lower the front of the patient's gown while the patient sits with the arms relaxed.

INSPECTION. Inspect the breasts for symmetry, skin dimpling, and nipple retraction. Have the patient press her hands to her waist, and then raise her hands over her head, each time repeating the inspection.

PALPATION. Pendulous breasts may be most easily examined in this position by using a bimanual technique.

Phase D: Examination of the Anterior Neck and Chest, Breasts, Axillae, Abdomen, Legs and Feet

Patient and Examiner Positions: patient draped and supine; examiner standing at the patient's right side

Start at the neck and work toward the feet exposing one area for examination at a time: the neck, the anterior chest and each breast separately, the abdomen, the groin, and the legs. Most left-handed clinicians are able to examine a patient from the right side.

NECK. *Inspection.* Observe the neck veins for fullness and pulsations.

CHEST AND PRECORDIUM. *Inspection.* Observe the precordium for any deformities of the sternum or ribs, and then identify the apical impulse. *Palpation.* Palpate the apical impulse and any lifts or heaves or other palpable cardiac signs. *Percussion.* Percuss the lung fields anteriorly and identify the borders of cardiac dullness. *Auscultation.* Start auscultating over the apical impulse to identify the first heart sound. Listen at the apex, the lower left and upper left sternal borders and the right second intercostal space. Auscultate the carotid arteries. Auscultate lung sounds in the anterior chest and supraclavicular fossae.

BREASTS. Expose each breast separately. *Inspection.* Inspect the breasts for symmetry, skin dimpling, or nipple retraction. *Palpation.* Palpate the breasts and nipples.

AXILLAE. *Inspection.* Lift the arms to expose the axilla for inspection. *Palpation.* Palpate the axilla and infraclavicular lymph node beds.

ABDOMEN. Reposition the drape over the chest and expose the abdomen from below the breasts to the symphysis pubis. Ask the patient to flex the hips and knees to relax the abdominal musculature. *Inspection.* Observe the symmetry and shape of the abdomen. Note any scars or skin abnormalities. Have the patient tense the abdominal muscles to reveal an abdominal wall hernia. *Percussion.* Percuss the abdomen noting any areas of tympany or pain with percussion. Use definitive percussion to identify the liver and look for splenomegaly. *Auscultation.* Auscultate over the epigastrium, both flanks, and both femoral triangles. *Palpation.* Perform superficial and deep palpation of the abdomen. Palpate deeply to identify the aorta and palpate both femoral pulses and the inguinal lymph nodes.

LEGS AND FEET.   Cover the abdomen and expose the legs and feet.   *Inspection.*   Inspect skin, muscles, and joints, and look for edema. Flex each hip to 90 degrees and perform internal and external rotation.   *Palpation.*   Palpate dorsalis pedis and posterior tibial pulses. Palpate any areas of asymmetry, deformity, or joint enlargement.

Phase E: Supplementary Neurological Exam, Sitting (*When Indicated*)

Patient and Examiner Positions: patient draped and sitting; examiner facing the patient

Return the patient to the sitting position. Now is a good time to do any remaining parts of the neurologic exam *if they are indicated* by the patient's history and examination to this point. From this position, it is easy to do precise testing of the cranial nerves, followed by testing of muscle tone and strength in the upper extremities, reflexes, and sensation (position, vibration, touch, and 10-g monofilament), followed by stance, gait, and lower extremity strength in Phase F.

Phase F: Supplemental Neurologic Examination, Standing (*When Indicated*)

Patient and Examiner Positions: patient standing facing examiner; supplementary neurologic and spine exams, when indicated

This portion of the exam is *indicated if the history or exam suggests neurologic disease or back problems.*

INSPECTION.   Have the gowned patient stand in front of you and observe the stance. Perform the Romberg maneuver. Check the range of spinal motion. Have the patient walk away from you and then toward you first on his toes, then on his heels. Have the patient hop on the balls of both feet, and then hop on one foot at a time.

Phase G: The Urogenital Exams

Patient and Examiner Positions: female patients in the lithotomy position, male patients standing; examiner at the foot of the table

FEMALE PATIENTS.   With the help of an assistant, position female patients in the lithotomy position for the female pelvic and rectal examinations (see Chapter 11, page 626 for a description of the examination).

MALE PATIENTS.   Begin the exam with the patient standing facing the examiner.   *Inspection.*   Inspect the penis, scrotum, and inguinal areas.   *Palpation.*   Palpate the testes and evaluate for inguinal hernias. Next have the patient turn and bend over the exam table, or lie on the table in the left lateral position.   *Inspection.*   Examine the perineum and anus and perform the rectal and prostate examinations. Test the stool for blood if indicated.

Provide tissues for the patient to clean themselves at the conclusion of the urogenital and rectal exams.

Phase H: Concluding the Visit

Have the patient get dressed while you are out of the exam room.

When you return and the patient is comfortable, share your synopsis of the patient's history, a summary of your physical findings, your impression of the patient's problems, and your recommendations for further diagnostic tests and/or treatment. Conclude by asking if there are any questions. Be sure to set a follow-up appointment appropriate for the patient and problems.

The preceding routine is a sequence that has served us well for many years. Remember that the purpose of the screening examination is to detect significant abnormalities in any of the body regions and systems, to establish a baseline against which future findings can be compared, and to continually hone your examination skills by experiencing the range of normal findings. Truncating the examination in the interest of excessive efficiency may lead to overlooking important findings and the loss of valuable clinical experience.

Part

2

The Diagnostic Exam

In order to observe one must learn to compare. In order to compare one must have observed. By means of observation knowledge is generated; on the other hand knowledge is needed for observation. And he observes badly who does not know how to use what he has observed. The fruit grower inspects the apple tree with a keener eye than the walker but no one can see man exactly unless he knows it is man who is the measure of man.

The art of observation applied to man is but a branch of the art of dealing with men.

Bertolt Brecht
"Speech to Danish Working Class Actors on the Art of Observation"

Early learn to appreciate the differences between the descriptions of disease and the manifestations of that disease in an individual—the difference between the composite portrait and one of the component pictures.

Sir William Osler

Not only to perceive the thing sharply, but to perceive the relationships between many things sharply perceived.

Theodore Roethke
"Poetry and Craft"

The Diagnostic Exam: Chapters 4 to 16

This section presents the classic approach to diagnosis, evolved over 2000 years, in which the diagnostic clues to diseases and syndromes are sought as *symptoms* (abnormalities perceived by the patient's own senses and conveyed to the physician during the history) and physical *signs* (abnormalities perceived by the physician's senses and found during the physical examination).

Each chapter is organized in the following sequence:

- A brief review of the **Major Systems** to be examined, including the physiology and anatomic landmarks to keep in mind during the exam.
- The **Physical Examination** of the body region.
- The **Symptoms** commonly elicited from patients which refer the clinician to this body region.
- The **Signs** the clinician may encounter during the examination of this region.
- The **Diseases and Syndromes** commonly encountered in this region.

The symptoms and signs are set in boldface type as paragraph heads, with or without preceding modifiers. To emphasize relative importance, certain symptoms and signs are distinguished as key symptoms, key signs, and key syndromes or diseases. These are the authors' choices for clues that are often most important in understanding the pathophysiology of the illness and in formulating diagnostic hypotheses. Most of the key symptoms commonly occur as chief complaints. The diseases and syndromes so marked are those that the generalist physician should be able to recognize.

Symptoms, signs, and syndromes marked with the icon ▶ are those of potentially extreme seriousness for the patient. The clinician needs to always be alert for these symptoms, signs, and conditions to avoid delayed diagnosis of life-threatening conditions.

Most of the physical signs are placed in order as they are encountered by the physician who conducts the head-to-foot physical examination of the patient.

When particular symptoms and signs are useful to help the clinician in differentiating between the various etiologies of a particular symptom or sign, they are discussed after the DDX: notation. This will help formulation of an accurate differential diagnosis.

The distinction between symptoms and signs is frequently unclear. For instance, jaundice may be a symptom that brings the patient to the physician, but it is also a sign visible to the clinician. In instances where the finding can be either a sign or a symptom, it is generally discussed where it is most likely to be found during the examination. Vomiting, although it can be witnessed, is more often a symptom, while tenderness, although it may be noted by the patient, is a sign that can be elicited by the examiner.

Diseases and syndromes in which the symptoms and signs occur are listed under *CLINICAL OCCURRENCE.*

Vital Signs, Anthropometric Data, and Pain

The vital signs are the temperature, pulse, respirations, and blood pressure; these are discussed in the first part of this chapter. In addition, we discuss measures of body size (height, weight, and body mass index) in the second part and pain assessment in the final part of the chapter. The former have direct bearing on health risk assessment, and the latter is essential in the initial evaluation and ongoing management of patients with acute or chronic illness or injury.

Vital Signs: Temperature, Pulse, Respirations, and Blood Pressure

Why are temperature, pulse, respirations, and blood pressure called *vital* signs? These are the signs of human life (L. *vitalis,* from *vita:* life); their presence confirms life and their absence confirms death. More usefully, the amount of deviation from normal is correlated, for each parameter and especially in combination, with the magnitude of threat to life. Since ancient times, practitioners have used the skin temperature, the pulse, and the respirations as prognostic signs. More recently, the blood pressure has been found to have similar predictive strength.

These signs have played a major role in the history of medicine and the evolution of our understanding of the physical examination and interpretation of physical signs. In the nineteenth century, entire texts were written on the interpretation of pulse, fever, and respiratory patterns. With the advent of modern diagnostic methods, it is now apparent that most of these signs are of insufficient specificity to be of much utility in establishing a specific diagnosis. On the other hand, they are sensitive indicators of the presence of disease and are useful in generation of pathophysiologic hypotheses and differential diagnosis. They remain strongly correlated with severity of illness and outcome.

Body Temperature

Internal body temperature is tightly regulated to maintain normal cellular function of vital organs, particularly the brain. Deviation of temperature by more than 4°C above or below normal can produce life-threatening cellular dysfunction. Regulation of internal temperature is controlled by the hypothalamus which maintains a set point for temperature. The autonomic nervous system plays a key role in maintaining body temperature by regulating blood flow conducting heat from the internal organs to the skin and innervating sweat glands. Increasing flow and dilating cutaneous capillaries radiates heat away from the body and increases conductive loss while production of sweat increases evaporative heat loss. Behavioral adaptations are also important; in hot conditions people become less active and seek shade or a cooler environment when they are able. Declines in body temperature are opposed by increased heat generation in muscles by shivering and by behavioral adaptations such as putting on clothes and seeking warmer environs. Deviations of body temperature indicate changes in the set point, increased heat production, decreased heat dissipation, failure of regulatory systems, or any combination of those.

Record the patient's temperature at each visit. Doing so establishes an individualized baseline for future reference and detects deviations from this baseline, either fever or hypothermia. Scales on clinical thermometers are either Fahrenheit or Celsius. Conveniently remembered clinical equivalents are $35°C = 95°F$, $37°C = 98.6°F$, and $40°C = 104°F$. Mercury-filled glass thermometers have been largely replaced by electronic thermometers that give rapid, accurate readings when they are well calibrated.

Normal Temperatures

DIURNAL VARIATION OF BODY TEMPERATURE.   Daytime workers who sleep at night register their minimum temperature at 3:00 to 4:00 a.m., whence it rises slowly to a maximum between 8:00 and 10:00 p.m. This pattern is reversed in nightshift workers. The transition from one pattern to the other requires several days.

SIMULTANEOUS TEMPERATURES IN VARIOUS REGIONS.   Heat is produced by the chemical reactions of cellular metabolism, so a temperature gradient extends from a maximum in the liver to a minimum on the skin surface. Customarily, the body temperature is measured in the rectum, the mouth, the ear, the axilla, or the groin. Among these sites, the rectal temperature is about 0.3°C (0.6°F) higher than that of the oral or groin reading; the axillary temperature is about 0.5°C (1.0°F) less than the oral value.

NORMAL BODY TEMPERATURE.   Internal body temperature is maintained within a narrow range, ±0.6°C (1.0°F), in each individual. However, the population range of this set point varies from 36.0–37.5°C (96.5–99.5°F) making it impossible to know an individual's normal temperature without a prior established baseline. A clinical shortcut for a patient whose normal baseline temperature is unknown is to regard as probably in the febrile range a maximum oral temperature above 37.5°C (99.5°F) and a rectal temperature exceeding 38.0°C (100.5°F). The minimum normal temperature is more difficult to define; the oral temperature often dips to 35.0°C (95.0°F) during sleep.

Elevated Temperature

Pathophysiology. Increased body temperature results from excessive production of heat or interference with heat dissipation. Each of these mechanisms may be physiologic (i.e., occurring as a normal response to a physiologic challenge), or pathologic (i.e., temperature elevation as a result of damage to the normal thermoregulatory pathways). Physiologic elevation of temperature results from an elevation of the hypothalamic physiologic set point for body temperature, a *fever.* Pathologic elevations of body temperature, *hyperthermia,* result from unregulated heat generation and/or impairment of the normal mechanisms of heat exchange with the environment.

KEY SIGN
Physiologic Elevated Temperature: Fever.
Pathophysiology. Release of endogenous pyrogens, particularly interleukin (IL)-1, triggered by tissue necrosis, infection, inflammation, and some tumors, elevates the hypothalamic set point leading to an increased body temperature. Onset of fever may be marked by a *chill* with shivering and cutaneous vasoconstriction as the body begins generating increased heat and decreasing heat loss; particularly severe chills are called *rigors.* When the new set point is reached, the skin is usually warm, moist, and flushed; but absence of these signs does not exclude fever. Occasionally, the skin temperature may be subnormal or normal while the core temperature is markedly elevated. Tachycardia usually accompanies fever, the increase in the pulse rate being proportionate to the temperature elevation. During the fever, the patient usually feels more comfortable in a warm environment. The new set point and the pattern of the fever curve depend upon the dynamics of the particular pathophysiologic process. Return of the set point to normal, either temporarily or permanently, is marked by sweat and flushing as the body dissipates the accumulated heat. *Night sweats* occur in many chronic infectious and inflammatory diseases, and some malignancies, particularly lymphomas. They represent an exaggeration of the normal diurnal variation in temperature, the sweat marking the decline of the fever at night.

Remember that some patients are unable to mount a febrile response to infection, for example, elderly patients and those with renal failure or on high doses of corticosteroids.

Fever occurring in several specific patient groups require special consideration from the clinician. These include fever in immunocompromised hosts, HIV-infected patients and nosocomial fever. Discussion of these topics is beyond the scope of this text.

Patterns of Fever. The pattern of temperature fluctuations may be a useful diagnostic clue. Many patterns have been defined.

- **Continuous Fever.** A fever with a diurnal variation of 0.5 to 1.0°C (1.0 to 1.5°F).
- **Remittent Fever.** A fever with a diurnal variation of more than 1.1°C (2.0°F) but with no normal readings.

- **Intermittent Fever.** Episodes of fever separated by days of normal temperature. Examples include *tertian fever* from *Plasmodium vivax* in which paroxysms of malaria are separated by an intervening normal day; *quartan fever* in which paroxysms from *P. malariae* occur with two intervening normal days; *intermittent hepatic fever* (Charcot hepatic fever) in which chills and fever occur at irregular intervals, marking the intermittent impaction of a gallstone and cholangitis.
- **Relapsing Fever.** Bouts of fever occurring every 5 to 7 days from infection with spirochetes of the group *Borrelia* and Colorado tick fever.
- **Episodic Fever.** Fever lasts for days or longer followed by prolonged periods (at least 2 weeks) without fever and with remission of clinical illness. This pattern is typical of the familial periodic fevers [Drenth PPH, van der Meer JWM. Hereditary periodic fever. *N Engl J Med* 2001;345:1748–1757].
- **Pel-Epstein Fever.** Occurring in Hodgkin disease, bouts of several days of continuous or remittent fever followed by afebrile remissions lasting an irregular number of days.

✓ *FEVER—CLINICAL OCCURRENCE:* *Congenital* familial Mediterranean fever, other familial periodic fevers, porphyrias; *Endocrine* hyperthyroidism, pheochromocytoma; *Infectious* bacterial, viral, rickettsial, fungal, and parasitic infections either localized or systemic (occult abscess is common); *Inflammatory* systemic lupus erythematosus, acute rheumatic fever, Still disease, vasculitis, serum sickness, any severe local or systemic inflammatory process (e.g., sarcoidosis, bullous dermatosis); *Mechanical/Traumatic* tissue necrosis (e.g., myocardial infarction, pulmonary infarction, stroke), exercise; *Metabolic/Toxic* drug reactions, gout; *Neoplastic* leukemia, lymphomas and solid tumors; *Neurologic* seizures; *Psychosocial* factitious; *Vascular* thrombophlebitis, tissue ischemia and infarction, vasculitis, subarachnoid hemorrhage.

S KEY SYNDROME

Fever of Unknown Origin (FUO): This syndrome was initially described in 1961 [Petersdorf RB, Beeson PB. Fever of unexplained origin: Report on 100 cases. *Medicine (Baltimore)* 1961;40:1–30]. To qualify as an FUO, three conditions must be met: (a) the illness must be at least 3 weeks in duration; (b) the temperature must be repeatedly >38.3°C (100.9°F); and (c) no diagnosis should have been reached after at least 1 week of hospitalization. Recent authors have suggested that the 1 week of hospitalization be replaced by at least 3 outpatient visits or at least 3 days in the hospital. The most common identified causes of FUO in immunocompetent patients in the modern era are noninfectious inflammatory diseases, infections, and malignancies, especially hematologic malignancies. Fever remains unexplained in almost 50% of patients, especially those with episodic fevers [Vanderschueren S, Knockaert D, Adriaenssens T, et al. From prolonged febrile illness to fever of unknown origin: The challenge continues. *Arch Intern Med* 2003;163:

1033–1041; Jha AK, Collard HR, Tierney LM. Diagnosis still in question. *N Engl J Med* 2002;346:1813–1816].

✓ *FUO—CLINICAL OCCURRENCE:* *Noninfectious Inflammatory Diseases* Still disease, systemic lupus erythematosus, sarcoidosis, Crohn disease, polymyalgia rheumatica, vasculitis (giant cell arteritis, Wegener disease, polyarteritis nodosa); *Infections* endocarditis, tuberculosis, urinary tract infection, cytomegalovirus, Epstein-Barr virus, HIV, subphrenic abcess, cholangitis and cholecystitis; *Neoplasms* non-Hodgkin lymphoma, Hodgkin disease, leukemia, adenocarcinoma; *Miscellaneous* habitual hyperthermia, subacute thyroiditis, Addison disease, drug fever.

D KEY DISEASE

Rheumatic Fever: *Pathophysiology:* Autoimmune carditis, polyarthritis, and chorea occur following infection with specific strains of group A streptococci. The onset is with fever, migratory pains in joints and muscles, malaise and anorexia. There may be weight loss, sweats, and precordial or abdominal pain. The arthritis is a migratory oligoarthritis of the large joints. The affected joints are red, warm, swollen, and tender. A subtle rash, erythema marginatum, may be seen. Subcutaneous nodules are often present over bony prominences. Heart exam may reveal a pericardial friction rub and valvular insufficiency murmurs; the mitral valve is most commonly affected. Chorea is a late manifestation. Symptoms and signs are markedly improved with aspirin.

KEY SIGN

▶ **Pathologic Overproduction and Impaired Dissipation of Heat: Hyperthermia:** *Pathophysiology:* Unregulated overproduction of heat or damage to the systems responsible for dissipation of heat leads to rapid and severe elevations of temperature without hypothalamic control or compensation. It is unusual for this to result from severe fever from the causes noted above, without primary failure of the normal control mechanisms. More commonly, environmental factors, behavioral events (bad judgment, impaired intellect), or toxin exposure results in loss of normal temperature control.

✓ *HYPOTHERMIA—CLINICAL OCCURRENCE:* *Impaired Heat Loss* high environmental temperature and humidity (often combined with exercise), moderately hot weather for a person with congenital absence of sweat glands, congestive heart failure, heat stroke from failure of the heat-dissipating apparatus, anticholinergic drugs and toxins. Poverty, homelessness and psychosis all inhibit the ability to adapt to environmental challenges. *Increased Heat Generation* malignant hyperthermia, neuroleptic malignant syndrome, heavy exertion in hot and humid environment.

S KEY SYNDROME

▶ **Neuroleptic Malignant Syndrome:** *Pathophysiology:* Antagonism to the central actions of dopamine is thought to play a role. One to 2 days after exposure to a neuroleptic (antipsychotic) drug, the patient develops hyperthermia, rigidity, altered mental status, labile blood pressure, tachycardia, tachypnea, and progressive metabolic acidosis. Myoglobinuria and acute renal failure can occur. It can be confused with worsening of the psychotic state leading to delayed diagnosis and administration of more neuroleptics.

D KEY DISEASE

Malignant Hyperthermia: *Pathophysiology:* This results from an inherited disorder of muscle sarcoplasmic reticulum calcium release. Exposure to inhalational anesthetics or succinylcholine precipitates sustained muscular contraction. The patient develops rigidity, hyperthermia, rhabdomyolysis, metabolic acidosis, and hemodynamic instability. Prompt recognition and treatment is lifesaving.

S KEY SYNDROME

Heat Exhaustion (Heat Prostration): *Pathophysiology:* Exertion in a hot, usually humid environment leads to loss of fluid and electrolytes and decreased ability to dissipate body heat. This is classically seen in younger individuals participating in athletic events or working in hot, humid environments. Symptoms are palpitations, faintness, lassitude, headache, nausea, vomiting, and cramps. Patients have tachycardia, diminished blood pressure, diaphoresis, ashen, cool, moist skin and dilated pupils. The core body temperature is elevated, but <40°C (104°F).

S KEY SYNDROME

Heat Stroke: *Pathophysiology:* There is failure of the thermoregulatory system producing decreased sweating and rapid increases in core body temperature. Cardiovascular disease increases the risk for heat stroke by limiting the necessary increase in cardiac output necessary to perfuse the skin. Diuretics and anticholinergic drugs also increase the risk. The typical victim is an elderly, chronically ill patient confined in a hot, humid environment during heat waves. The patient is often delirious or comatose; the diagnostic clue is the hot dry skin [Bouchama A, Knochel JP. Heat stroke. *N Engl J Med* 2002;346: 1978–1988].

S KEY SYNDROME

Factitious Fever. This is usually encountered in hospitalized patients attempting to malinger, although the motives are often obscure. The situation is suspected (a) when a series of high temperatures are recorded to form an atypical pattern of fluctuation or (b) when a recorded high temperature is unaccompanied by warm skin, tachycardia, and other signs of fever. The patient may have surreptitiously dipped the thermometer in warm water, placed it in contact with a heat source, or heated the bulb by friction with bedclothes or even the mucous membranes of the mouth. Occasionally, one thermometer is exchanged for another; the substitution may be detected by checking the serial numbers on the tubes given and returned.

Some Infections Presenting as Fever

FEVER IN TRAVELERS. In this day of global travel, this is not an un-common problem. The patient presents with a fever and history of travel to exotic, usually tropical locations. The clinician is presented with the possibility of a host of unfamiliar infectious diseases, as well as those the clinician is more used to. A clinically useful approach is presented in the references [Humar A, Keystone J. Evaluating fever in travelers re-turning from tropical countries. *BMJ* 1996;312:953–956; Ryan ET, Wilson ME, Kain KC. Illness after international travel. *N Engl J Med* 2002;347:505–516].

D KEY DISEASE

Malaria: *Pathophysiology:* Infection is with *Plasmodium vivax, P. ovale, P. malariae,* or *P. falciparum* transmitted by infected anophe-line mosquitos. Infection of the liver is followed by invasion of eryth-rocytes. Cyclical release of mature merozoites from ruptured erythrocytes produces cyclical fever. *P. fulciparum* infection can produce severe hemolysis, hypoglycemia, and obstruction of cerebral capillaries (cerebral malaria). *P. vivax* and *P. ovale* can persist in the liver causing replasing infections. Patients present with fever, headache, malaise, and myalgias. Nausea, vomiting, and abdominal pain may be present. Symp-toms may progress to delirium and coma. Establishing a history of travel to an endemic area and prompt examination fo blood smears by trained laboratory technicians are the keys to recognition. DDX: Dengue fever may present a similar clinical picture but blood smears are negative.

D KEY DISEASE

Brucellosis: *Pathophysiology:* Systemic infection with the aerobic gram-negative bacilli acquired from animals, a zoonosis. *Brucella abortus* (cattle), *suis* (pigs), *melitensis* (goats), or *canis* (dogs) are the cause. Exposure to nonpasteurized milk, contaminated meat or other animal tissues results in infection. Lassitude and weight loss accompany recurrent (undulant) fever and sweating. Pain in the back and joints is common. Physical findings include splenomegaly, lymphadenopathy, and tender bones or joints. The disease may be acute or chronic [Vogt T, Hasler P. A woman with panic attacks and double vision who liked cheese. *Lancet* 1999;354:300].

D KEY DISEASE

Tuberculosis: *Pathophysiology:* Infection with *Mycobac-terium tuberculosis* may be limited to the lung or spread via the lymph nodes or bloodstream to affect any organ. The *primary infection* is in the lung and often goes unrecognized, leaving a calcified nodule in the middle or lower lung and hilar lymph nodes (Ghon complex). *Pro-gressive primary tuberculosis* is seen more commonly in HIV-infected pa-tients and presents as progressive pulmonary infection, usually in the lower lung zones, pleural effusion, and lymphadenopathy. In immuno-suppressed hosts or dark-skinned races, there is an increased risk for early hematogenous dissemination to multiple organs, *miliary tubercu-*

losis. These patients present with fever, anorexia, and weight loss, and may have hepatomegaly, splenomegaly, or lymphadenopathy. *Reactivation tuberculosis* may be miliary or localized to one organ system, most commonly the apices of the lungs. Patients present with fever, malaise, night sweats, cough with sputum production, and findings of consolidation and/or cavity formation on pulmonary exam. Reactivation is not infrequently seen in the bones, especially the spine (Pott disease), the peritoneum, meninges, kidneys and urinary tract, lymph nodes, intestine, and pericardium [Tanoue LT, Mark EJ. Case records of the Massachusetts General Hospital. Case 1–2003. *N Engl J Med* 2003;348:151–161].

D KEY DISEASE

Typhoid Fever: *Pathophysiology:* Disseminated infection with *Salmonella typhi* or *paratyphi* following ingestion of contaminated food or water. The incubation period is 3 days to as much as 60 days. Onset begins with chills and prolonged, persistent fever, prostration, cough, epistaxis, and constipation or diarrhea. There is slowly progressing lassitude, abdominal distention and tenderness, splenomegaly, and rose spots on the trunk and chest. Delirium may occur. Complications include localized infections (gallbladder, bone, liver, spleen, endocarditis, pneumonia, meningitis, and orchitis), gastrointestinal bleeding and perforation of the bowel with peritonitis.

Lowered Body Temperature

KEY SIGN

Hypothermia: *Pathophysiology:* A decreased hypothalamic set point, insufficiency of the heat-generation systems, excessive heat loss, behaviors, and environmental conditions all can lead to sustained declines in core temperature. Core temperatures are usually lower in the elderly, and they are particularly susceptible to declines in environmental temperatures. Low body temperature impairs cellular metabolism, impairs brain function, particularly judgment, and the combination can lead to failure to take protective measures to exposure leading to fatal hypothermia. Hypothermia also protects the tissues from ischemic injury, an observation used in prolonged surgical procedures and resuscitation from cardiac arrest, so complete recovery is possible from rapid and sustained cooling even when the patient appears clinically dead. This is especially true for cold-water immersion (drowning) where the body is cooled very rapidly. Relative or absolute hypothermia in situations where fever would be expected (e.g., severe infection) is a poor prognostic sign.

✓ *HYPOTHERMIA—CLINICAL* **OCCURRENCE:** *Endocrine* hypothyroidism; *Idiopathic* advanced age; *Infectious* sepsis; *Mechanical/Traumatic* exposure and immersion, hypothalamic injury from trauma or hemorrhage, burns; *Metabolic/Toxic* antipyretics, hypoglycemia, drug overdoses; *Neoplastic* brain tumors; *Neurologic* stroke; *Psychosocial* poverty, homelessness, and psychosis all inhibit the ability to adapt to environmental challenges; *Vascular* stroke.

The Pulse: Pulse Rate, Volume, and Rhythm

The arterial pulse is generated by left ventricular systolic contraction ejecting blood into the arterial tree. The pulse wave travels along the arteries at a rate dependent upon the force of ejection and the elastic properties of the arterial wall. The regularity of the pulse wave is determined by the rhythm of cardiac electrical depolarization and subsequent contraction.

The sinoatrial (SA) node lies in the right atrial wall near the entrance of the superior vena cava (Fig. 4-1). As the normal pacemaker of the heart, it originates rhythmic waves of excitation that spread quickly through the wall of both atria until they reach the atrioventricular (AV) node near the posterior margin of the interatrial septum. Here there is a slight delay while atrial systole is completed. The excitation then passes down a specialized conducting tissue, the bundle of His, which divides into right and left branches, each passing down the corresponding side of the interventricular septum to excite the muscle of the right and left ventricles more or less simultaneously. Deviations in timing and in the pathways taken by these waves cause changes in rate and rhythm that can be analyzed with considerable accuracy in the electrocardiogram.

Examination of the Pulse

PALPATION OF THE ARTERIAL PULSE. The pulse may be palpated in any of the accessible arteries (Fig. 4-2). To the physician at the bedside, the brachial or radial pulse is usually accessible. The radial artery is pressed lightly against the radius with the examining finger; or the wrist may be encircled by the fingers and hand. The carotid pulse most accurately reflects the contour of the aortic pulse wave. The examiner ascertains the contour of the pulse wave and its volume, rate, and rhythm; the latter two are discussed under heart action (Chapter 8, page 434). Look for patterns of variability in the pulse volume.

KEY SIGN

Normal Pulse Rate and Rhythm: Sinus Rhythm: *Physiology:* In sinus rhythm, the impulse originates in the SA node and spreads throughout the walls of the atria, causing their contraction; then it reaches the AV node. The impulse then follows the two branches of the His bundle to spread into the two ventricles, causing them to contract. This is the beat of the normal heart with a rate between 55 and 100 beats per minute (BPM). Infants and children have higher normal heart rates; consult pediatric references for the normal ranges. Well-conditioned athletes may have resting pulses into the forties, while deconditioned adults may have rates approaching 100. With heart rates lower than 100 BPM, diastole is longer than systole; the two intervals become equal at about 100 BPM; above 100, systole is the longer. Heart rates lower than 55 BPM are called *bradycardias* and those above 100 BPM, *tachycardias.* Exertion may cause acceleration to rates close to 200 BPM in young, healthy adults; the maximum achievable heart rate declines predictably with age. The pulse rhythm is normally

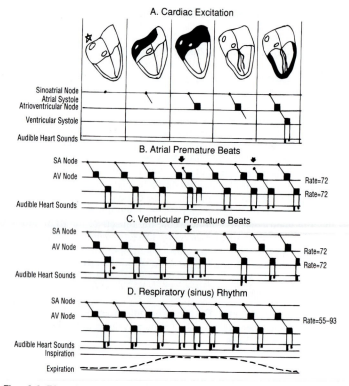

Fig. 4-1 Disturbances of Cardiac Rate and Rhythm I. A. Diagram illustrating the spread of excitation over the heart. The stimulus starts in the sinoatrial node and spreads throughout the walls of the atria, finally reaching the atrioventricular node, where there is a short delay. The stimulus then proceeds down the His bundle by its two branches along the right and left wall of the interventricular septum to the apex, spreading from there to the muscle of the right and left ventricles. The atria contract before the impulse has left the AV node; ventricular systole occurs when the impulse has spread over the walls of the lower chambers. Note that the heart sounds that result from ventricular systole are the only perceptible physical signs of this process. B. Atrial premature beat is represented as originating outside the SA node, an ectopic beat. This is followed by a short compensatory pause that cannot ordinarily be detected. C. An ectopic ventricular beat with a detectable compensatory pause. D. Respiratory or sinus arrhythmia. There is acceleration of the heart rate near the height of inspiration; this acceleration originates in the SA node. In any dysrhythmia the heart sounds of a beat following a shortened interval are often fainter than normal; beats following an abnormally long pause are louder than normal.

(continued)

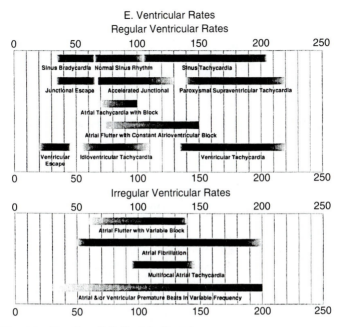

E. Ventricular Rates
Regular Ventricular Rates

Irregular Ventricular Rates

Fig. 4-1 (Continued) E. Ventricular rates.

regular with slight variation caused by respirations. Vagus stimulation by holding the breath or massage of the carotid sinus produces slowing of the rate.

Abnormal Pulse Contour

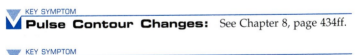

KEY SYMPTOM

Pulse Contour Changes: See Chapter 8, page 434ff.

KEY SYMPTOM

Pulse Volume Changes: See Chapter 8, page 436ff.

Variations in Ventricular Rate and Rhythm

The emphasis is deliberately placed on ventricular phenomena. Initially, many experience difficulty in appreciating the physical signs associated with cardiac dysrhythmias because they fail to realize that the signs of the heart's action are practically all ventricular (see Fig. 4-1E). The atria usually function silently, contributing no important diagnostic signs to auscultation of the precordium except for their role in generation of the fourth heart sound, the variations in loudness of the first heart sound that accompany atrioventricular (AV) dissociation, and the ventricular filling sounds associated with atrial contraction sometimes heard in AV heart block (see Chapter 8, page 413).

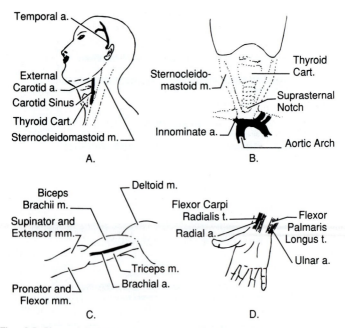

Fig. 4-2 Sites of Palpable Arteries. *A. The temporal artery is anterior to the ear and overlies the temporal bone, one of the few normally tortuous arteries. The common carotid is deep in the neck near the anterior border of the sternocleidomastoid muscle. The bifurcation of this artery is opposite the superior border of the thyroid cartilage. The carotid sinus is at the bifurcation.* **B. Elongation or dilation of the ascending aorta and arch** *makes this vessel accessible to palpation in the suprasternal notch. With slight shifting to the right or left, the innominate or left carotid arteries may also be felt in the notch.* **C. The brachial artery** *lies deep in the biceps–triceps furrow on the medial side of the arm near the elbow. It courses toward the midline of the antecubital fossa, where it is usually just medial to the biceps tendon.* **D. The radial artery** *is just medial to the outer border of the radius and lateral to the tendon of the flexor carpi radialis, where the finger can press it against the bone. The ulnar artery is in a similar position to the ulna, but it is buried deeper, so it often cannot be felt.*

(continued)

While a rhythm abnormality may be suspected on physical examination, *none can be diagnosed with the certainty required in good clinical practice without an electrocardiogram (ECG).* Nevertheless, general groupings of disorders is possible by noting the overall heart rate and whether it is regular, irregular in a rather chaotic manner, or irregular but in a reproducible manner [Mangrum JM, DiMarco JP. The evaluation and management of bradycardia. *N Engl J Med* 2000;342:703–709].

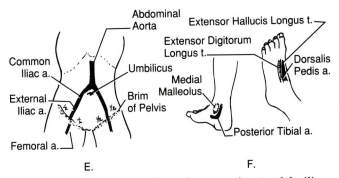

Fig. 4-2 *(Continued) E. The abdominal aorta and parts of the iliac arteries can usually be felt as generalized pulsations through the abdominal wall. The femoral artery is palpable at the inguinal ligament midway between the anterior superior iliac spine and the pubic tubercle.* **F. The posterior tibial artery** *is palpable as it curves forward below and around the medial malleolus of the tibia.* **The dorsalis pedis artery** *is felt usually in the groove between the first two tendons on the medial side of the dorsum of the foot.*

KEY SIGN

Slow Regular Rhythms: Rates below about 55 BPM, suggest sinus bradycardia, second-degree AV block (Fig. 4-3A), and third-degree AV block with junctional or ventricular escape rhythms (Fig. 4-3B).

KEY SIGN

Regular Rhythms with Rates of 60 to 120 bpm: These include sinus rhythm, accelerated junctional rhythm (also known as nonparoxysmal junctional tachycardia), atrial tachycardia with block, idioventricular tachycardia (also known as accelerated ventricular rhythm and slow or benign ventricular tachycardia), and atrial flutter (see Fig. 4-3D) with 3:1 or 4:1 atrioventricular block.

KEY SIGN

Regular Rhythms with Rates Greater than 120 bpm: Rhythms include sinus tachycardia, atrial flutter with 2:1 AV block, paroxysmal supraventricular tachycardia (see Fig. 4-3C), and ventricular tachycardia. Especially with rates of more than 140, sinus tachycardia must be distinguished from atrial flutter with 2:1 block, paroxysmal supraventricular tachycardia and ventricular tachycardia. DDX: The response to vagus stimulation may give an indication of which rhythm is present. In flutter, the rate slows in a jerky fashion. Paroxysmal atrial tachycardia does not slow, but may convert to normal rhythm and rate. Sinus rhythm may gradually slow and ventricular tachycardia does not change.

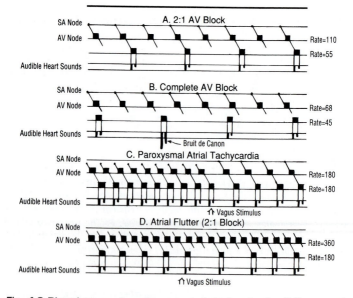

Fig. 4-3 Disturbances of cardiac rate and rhythm II. *In all diagrams, the audible heart sounds are the only physical signs to indicate the presence and operation of the mechanisms. **A. Second-degree AV block** is depicted with a 2:1 ratio. Alternate stimuli from the atria are blocked in the AV node, so the ventricles beat only half as fast as the atria. The only physical sign is a slow regular heartbeat with first sounds of equal intensity. **B. Complete AV block** is depicted, in which the ventricles beat independently of the atria and usually assume a slow rate, below 50 per minute, that accelerates little with exertion. A louder-than-common first sound occurs when ventricular filling is augmented by an atrial contraction occurring by chance at the optimal time; this is called by the French the "bruit de canon." **C** and **D**. When ventricular beats are regular with rates between 160 and 220 per minute, two conditions must be distinguished. **C. Paroxysmal atrial tachycardia**. **D. Atrial flutter.** Vagal stimulation may convert paroxysmal atrial tachycardia to normal rhythm, but there is no temporary slowing. In contrast, the only response of flutter to vagus stimulus is slowing for a few beats.*

KEY SIGN

Rhythms That Are Irregular in No Particular Repetitive Manner: Atrial flutter with variable atrioventricular block, atrial fibrillation, multifocal atrial tachycardia, and frequent atrial or ventricular premature beats that occur with no consistent pattern all need to be considered. The overall rates of such rhythms may vary from as slow as approximately 50 up to 200 BPM. However, atrial flutter with variable AV block rarely exceeds 150 BPM and the range for multifocal atrial tachycardia is usually between about 100 and 150 BPM.

KEY SIGN

Irregular Rhythms with "Reproducible Ir-regularity:" This pattern suggests either atrial or ventricular premature beats occurring at regular intervals (i.e., bigeminal, trigeminal, and quadrigeminal premature beats) or Mobitz I (Wenckebach) AV block producing grouped beats. Given the great overlap of the rhythms in these three categories, it is necessary to obtain an ECG to reach a definitive diagnosis.

Common Dysrhythmias

KEY SIGN

Respiratory (Sinus) Arrhythmia: *Pathophysiology:* The depolarizations originate in the SA node and are conducted normally through the heart. The ventricular rate accelerates as inspiration approaches its maximum and decelerates during expiration (see Fig. 4-1D). When the overall ventricular rate is slow, the association may not be as evident as expected. At rates less than 60 BPM, the rhythm may at first appear to be a series of premature beats, until the examiner remembers to check the respirations. DDX: The relation to respirations is diagnostic.

✓ *SINUS ARRHYTHMIA—CLINICAL OCCURRENCE:* Normal in children, persisting throughout life in some; occurs in many disorders but is not diagnostic of any.

KEY SIGN

Sinus Tachycardia: *Pathophysiology:* Exertion and increased sympathetic tone increase the rate of SA node depolarizations which are transmitted normally throughout the conducting system. The rate is between 100 and 160 BPM with a perfectly regular rhythm. Vagus stimulation produces smooth deceleration. DDX: Especially with rates higher than 140, sinus tachycardia must be distinguished from atrial flutter with 2:1 block. In flutter, vagus stimulation slows the rate in jerky fashion; paroxysmal atrial tachycardia does not slow, but may convert to normal rhythm and rate.

✓ *SINUS TACHYCARDIA—CLINICAL OCCURRENCE:* Exercise, anxiety, hyperthyroidism, anemia, fever, pregnancy, deconditioning, beta-adrenergic medications, and any chronic illness.

KEY SIGN

Orthostatic Tachycardia: See page 87, Orthostatic Hypotension. A pulse rise of more than 15 BPM on sitting or standing from the supine position suggests intravascular volume depletion.

KEY SIGN

Sinus Bradycardia: *Pathophysiology:* The excitation follows the normal pathways from the SA node. The slowness of the rate is attributed to vagus influence on the node. This is the natural rate for a few persons. Rates usually range from 50 to 60 BPM, rarely as low as 40 BPM. The rhythm is regular. DDX: The rate accelerates smoothly with exertion.

✓ *SINUS BRADYCARDIA—CLINICAL OCCURRENCE:*   Some normal persons, especially well-conditioned athletes; occasionally in severe infections.

S KEY SYNDROME

Sinus Rhythm with Second-Degree Block: *Pathophysiology:*   In Mobitz I (Wenckebach) AV block, there is decremental conduction in the AV node so that, after a series of conducted beats, one beat is dropped. This produces grouped beats with a P to QRS ratio of n:n-1 (e.g., 3:2, 5:4). In Mobitz II block, sinus impulses from the atria are regularly blocked below the AV node, so the atrial rate is multiple of the ventricular rate, 2:1, 3:1, 4:1, or higher. For instance, 3:1 block occurs when every third beat from the atrium is transmitted through the AV node. Mobitz I block is the most common type of AV block. The ventricular complexes appear in groups followed by a pause. The interval between beats shortens until a beat is dropped with a longer pause and the cycle recurs. The shortening of the R-R interval is usually only apparent on the ECG. In Mobitz II block, ventricular systoles occur at regular intervals with rates dependent upon the sinus rate and degree of block (see Fig. 4-3A). Each beat has the same intensity. The only distinctive physical sign may be faintly audible atrial contractions in the cycles not resulting in ventricular beats. In 2:1 block, two A-waves may be seen in the jugular vein for each ventricular contraction. Although 2:1 block is relatively common, 3:1 block is much less so. DDX: In both sinus bradycardia and second-degree heart block, the rate is accelerated with exertion, but complete heart block exhibits little response.

✓ *SECOND-DEGREE AV BLOCK—CLINICAL OCCURRENCE:*   Acute infections (especially rheumatic fever, Lyme disease, and diphtheria), valvular heart disease, digitalis intoxication, hyperkalemia, drugs (diltiazem, verapamil, beta-blockers), coronary artery disease.

S KEY SYNDROME

Third-Degree (Complete) AV Block: *Pathophysiology:*   The atria beat regularly and at normal rates in response to stimuli from the SA node, but there is no transmission from the atria to the ventricles. Block may occur in the AV node or ventricular conduction system (His bundle or both bundle branches). Escape pacemakers in junctional tissue near the AV node or the ventricular conduction system establish an escape rhythm with rates of 25 to 60 per minute; the higher the pacemaker, the faster the escape rate. The ventricular contractions are evenly timed, but the intensity of the heart sounds is augmented when an atrial systole happens to precede ventricular contraction (see Fig. 4-3B). With especially coincidental timing, there is a loud booming sound, *bruit de canon;* it may come infrequently, so auscultation should be prolonged for 60 seconds or more. More frequently, there are less-spectacular variations in intensity of the first sounds. DDX: This is the only bradycardia in which exertion does not accelerate the ventricular rate. The variation in intensity of the first sounds is distinctive.

✓ *COMPLETE AV BLOCK—CLINICAL OCCURRENCE:* Same as in second-degree heart block, plus nonischemic degenerative processes affecting the bundle branches.

S KEY SYNDROME

Premature Beats: *Pathophysiology:* A depolarization arises from an ectopic focus in the atrium or ventricle; if it arises from the atrium, it is transmitted to the ventricles, producing the premature contraction. Isolated or infrequent premature beats are usually recognized by palpation or auscultation. Among a series of normal beats, a premature contraction from an atrial impulse is heard as a beat coming through before its expected time (see Fig. 4-1B). It is followed by a compensatory pause shorter than that usually associated with ventricular premature beats, but differentiation is difficult, if not impossible, at the bedside. If the premature beat occurs soon after a normal emptying of the chamber, little blood has accumulated to be ejected during the premature systole; the resulting heart sounds are less intense, and the stroke volume may be insufficient to produce a palpable arterial pulse. When premature beats are very frequent, they present a diagnostic problem (Fig. 4-4A) [Wang K, Hodges M. The premature ventricular complex as a diagnostic aid. *Ann Intern Med* 1992;117:766–770].

KEY SIGN

Coupled Rhythm: Bigeminy, Trigeminy: *Pathophysiology:* One or two normal beats is followed regularly by a premature beat arising from an ectopic focus in the atrium or ventricle. The ventricular beats are grouped in pairs (bigeminy) or triplets (trigeminy), the last a premature beat; the compensatory pause after the premature beat separates one group from its successor (see Fig. 4-4C). If auscultation of the heart is performed, bigeminy will be recognized; but if only the arterial pulse is palpated, the premature beat of the couple may not be palpable, and a regular rhythm with half the ventricular rate may be diagnosed. This occurs whenever the premature beats follow the regular beats by an interval so short as not to permit adequate ventricular filling. As with other premature beats, exercise may cause the rhythm to resume a normal pattern. DDX: A similar pulse pattern is produced by Mobitz type I second-degree AV block (Wenckebach) with 3:2 Wenckebach simulating bigeminy and 4:3 simulating trigeminy.

✓ *COUPLED RHYTHMS—CLINICAL OCCURRENCE:* In normal hearts, organic disease of the heart and digitalis intoxication.

KEY SIGN

Grouped Beats and Dropped Beats: *Pathophysiology:* (a) Sinus pauses or sinoatrial block. (b) Second-degree AV block, Mobitz type I or II. In Mobitz type I second-degree AV block (*Wenckebach phenomenon*), during the series of equally spaced ventricular beats, each impulse from the atrium takes progressively longer to

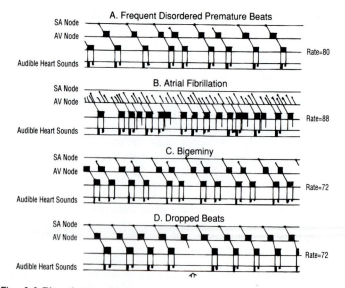

Fig. 4-4 Disturbance of cardiac rate and rhythm III. *As in previous diagrams, only the audible heart sounds are the physical signs of these disorders.* **A. Normal rhythm is interspersed with two random premature beats:** *If such beats are very frequent, the ear may not be able to distinguish them from atrial fibrillation unless some maneuvers are employed. The rhythm becomes regular as the rate accelerates to about 120 beats per minute.* **B. Atrial fibrillation:** *The ventricular rhythm is grossly irregular and continues to be irregular when the rate is accelerated by exercise to more than 120 per minute.* **C. Bigeminy:** *A normal beat is followed by a premature beat and this pattern repeats many times. The premature beats tend to fall out when exercise accelerates the rate to over 120 per minute.* **D. Dropped beats in second-degree AV block:** *Each successive impulse going through the AV node produces a longer interval until one fails to induce ventricular contraction. In contrast to premature beats, exercise tends to increase the number of dropped beats.*

pass through the AV node until one fails completely, causing a dropped ventricular beat (see Fig. 4-4D). The ratio of block is usually 3:2, 4:3, 5:4, or 6:5. In Mobitz type II there is no progressive prolongation of the conduction time through the AV node prior to the completely blocked atrial beat. The block is usually in the His bundle or below and complete heart block may occur. (c) Regularly occurring premature atrial beats in a trigeminal or quadrigeminal pattern will produce the same pattern if they occur so prematurely as to be blocked in the AV node. A series of two, three, four, or more beats is followed by a pause. The pattern may recur regularly. The rhythm is unchanged by acceleration of the heart rate. Electrocardiography is essential to distinguish between these rhythms.

✓ *GROUPED AND DROPPED BEATS—CLINICAL OCCURRENCE:* Infectious diseases, rheumatic fever, digitalis intoxication, organic heart disease.

S KEY SYNDROME

▼ **Atrial Fibrillation:** *Pathophysiology:* The atria do not contract in a synchronized fashion; different muscle segments contract separately. Stimuli arrive in complete disorder at the AV node, and a variable minority are transmitted to the ventricles at irregular intervals (see Fig. 4-4B). Accordingly, the ventricular rhythm and pulse presents no pattern. Every student can glibly recite that fibrillation is an "irregular irregularity," but experience demonstrates that the inexperienced student has great difficulty in recognizing fibrillation. Fast ventricular responses are irregularly spaced, but this cannot be recognized by the examiner. At ventricular responses of >70 BPM, the rhythm may seem regular with some premature beats. With rates >60 BPM, the irregularity of the fibrillation is very difficult to detect; one should observe longer. Because ventricular contractions occur at all stages of chamber filling, the heart sounds and pulse volume from ventricular contractions vary in intensity. The ventricular rate is accelerated by exertion. Atrial fibrillation can only be diagnosed by ECG with accurate measuring of the intervals [Falk RD. Atrial fibrillation. *N Engl J Med* 2001;344:1067–1078]. DDX: In flutter with variable AV block, exercise increases the rate by large increments.

✓ *ATRIAL FIBRILLATION—CLINICAL OCCURRENCE:* Organic heart disease (especially mitral and tricuspid valve disease or disorders causing congestive heart failure), hyperthyroidism, acute infections including rheumatic fever, postoperative (especially chest surgery), electrolyte imbalances, hypoxia and hypercarbia. "Lone atrial fibrillation" may occur in the absence of any structural heart disease or metabolic abnormalities.

S KEY SYNDROME

▼ **Atrial Flutter:** *Pathophysiology:* Regular impulses are generated in the atria at extremely high rates, causing atrial contractions from 220 to 360 times per minute (see Fig. 4-3D). The AV node cannot respond to such rapid stimuli, so block develops, for example, 2:1, 3:1, 4:1, or higher. The ventricular contractions are usually perfectly spaced, with no differences in the intensity of heart sounds from beat to beat. In some patients, there is considerable variability in the blockade of the atrial impulses. This causes variability in the ventricular response, which may be almost as irregular as in atrial fibrillation. Digitalis, verapamil, diltiazem, and beta-adrenergic blocking drugs increase the degree of block in flutter, a possibility to consider in taking the history. Vagus stimulation may produce sudden drops in ventricular rate as the degree of block is increased from 2:1 to 3:1, while the atrial rate remains constant. DDX: In sinus tachycardia, vagus stimulation causes smooth slowing. Paroxysmal atrial tachycardia cannot be slowed by the vagus, but vagus impulses may convert the rhythm to normal.

✔ *ATRIAL FLUTTER—CLINICAL OCCURRENCE:* Rheumatic heart disease, diphtheria, coronary artery disease, hyperthyroidism, and other forms of heart disease (see atrial fibrillation, page 77).

S KEY SYNDROME

Paroxysmal Atrial (Supraventricular) Tachycardia (SVT, PSVT): *Pathophysiology:* The arrhythmia is most often a reentrant or reciprocating form of tachycardia involving the AV node. True ectopic atrial tachycardia does occur. The attack begins and ends suddenly, lasting for a few minutes to many days. The ventricular rate is usually between 150 and 225 BPM. All ventricular beats have the same intensity and are equally spaced. Vagus stimulation (by massage of the carotid sinus, or a Valsalva maneuver), or the intravenous administration of adenosine does not produce temporary slowing; either there is no response, or the attack is terminated abruptly and normal rhythm resumes within a single cycle (see Fig. 4-3C). DDX: PSVT must be distinguished from sinus tachycardia, which exhibits smooth vagus slowing, and from atrial flutter, in which vagus slowing is often associated with varying AV block.

✔ *PSVT—CLINICAL OCCURRENCE:* In otherwise normal hearts, the Wolff-Parkinson-White syndrome, in various types of heart disease.

S KEY SYNDROME

Ventricular Tachycardia (VT): *Pathophysiology:* VT is usually a reentry dysrhythmia triggered by a premature ventricular contraction (PVC) and sustained by the dispersion of conduction and repolarization in damaged ventricular muscle. Diagnosis is urgently needed because this condition may induce ventricular fibrillation and death. There is usually complete AV dissociation, with the ventricles beating faster than the atria. The onset and, when self-limited, the ending are abrupt. The ventricular rate usually is between 150 and 250 BPM. The rhythm is regular, but it is not influenced by vagal stimulation, so the condition must be distinguished from atrial flutter and paroxysmal atrial tachycardia. The variable relationship of atrial to ventricular systole furnishes the most distinctive sign: variation in the intensity of the first sounds. Some sounds are especially loud cannon sounds resulting from superimposition of atrial systole with rapid passive ventricular filling. The cannon sounds are absent when the atria are fibrillating. Only the first heart sound may be audible, so mistakes in counting result in half the actual value. Occasionally, the ventricular rate is slower than 150 BPM.

✔ *VT—CLINICAL OCCURRENCE:* Acute myocardial infarction, coronary artery disease, overdoses of drugs (digitalis, quinidine, procaine amide). Trauma to the heart from surgery or catheterization.

S KEY SYNDROME

Ventricular Fibrillation (VF): *Pathophysiology:* Ventricular muscle fibers depolarize and contract in a chaotic fashion which cannot produce effective ventricular contraction. No ventricular

emptying occurs, so no heart sounds are produced. The diagnosis is made by ECG. Unless the dysrhythmia is interrupted by prompt electrical defibrillation, death follows rapidly.

Respirations: Respiratory Rate and Pattern

Respiratory Rate

KEY SIGN
Normal Respirations: At rest, the normal respiratory rate in adults is between 14 and 18 cycles per minute; in the newborn, the rate is about 44; gradually the rate diminishes until maturity. Women have slightly higher rates than men. In alert patients, the respiratory rate should be counted unobtrusively, such as pretending to count the pulse, because many persons tend to breathe faster when their attention is directed to their breathing.

KEY SIGN
▶ **Increased Respiratory Rate: Tachypnea:** *Pathophysiology:* Increased respiratory rate occurs with central nervous system stimulation and as compensation for problems in respiration. Hypoxia, increased oxygen demands, and increased CO_2 generation each lead to an increase in respiratory rate and tidal volume. Minute ventilation is maintained in restrictive disease of the lung or chest wall by increasing the respiratory rate to compensate for the reduced tidal volume. Tachypnea occurs with exertion, fear, fever, cardiac insufficiency, pain, pulmonary embolism, acute respiratory distress from infections, pleurisy, anemia, and hyperthyroidism. Breathing is faster when restricted by weakness of the respiratory muscles, emphysema, pneumothorax, or obesity.

KEY SIGN
▶ **Decreased Respiratory Rate: Bradypnea:** *Pathophysiology:* Minute ventilation is preserved when slow rates are accompanied by an increased tidal volume (*hyperpnea*). Slow rates without an increase in tidal volume produce alveolar hypoventilation indicating an abnormality of the medullary respiratory center. A slower than usual respiratory rate is not abnormal if gas exchange is preserved as demonstrated by arterial blood gas determination. When alveolar hypoventilation occurs ($PaCO_2 > 45$ mmHg), metabolic encephalopathy as a result of CNS-depressant drugs (e.g., opiates, benzodiazepines, barbiturates, alcohol) or uremia, or structural intracranial lesions (especially conditions with increased intracranial pressure) are most likely.

Respiratory Pattern

KEY SIGN
▶ **Deep Breathing: Hyperpnea (Kussmaul Breathing):** *Pathophysiology:* An increased tidal volume produces increased alveolar ventilation, which increases excretion of CO_2.

This is an appropriate compensatory response to metabolic acidosis of any cause and is a direct toxic effect of salicylates. It is also seen with hypoxia. The term Kussmaul breathing is applied to deep, regular sighing respirations, whether the rate be normal, slow, or fast. Common examples of precipitating metabolic acidoses are diabetic ketoacidosis and uremia. Hypoxemia (e.g., pneumonia, pulmonary embolism) and decreased oxygen delivery as a result of severe anemia or hemorrhage also lead to hyperpnea.

KEY SIGN
Shallow Breathing: Hypopnea: *Pathophysiology:* Decreased depth of breathing results from decreased medullary respiratory center drive, weakness of the respiratory muscles, or loss of alveolar volume from any cause. Depression of the medullary respiratory center occurs as in bradypnea. Muscular weakness can result from myasthenia gravis, amyotrophic lateral sclerosis, Guillain-Barré syndrome, drugs (e.g., paralyzing agents, rarely aminoglycosides) and exhaustion when the work of breathing is increased due to decreased chest wall and/or lung compliance as in severe asthma. Decreased lung volumes can result from alveolar filling disorders (congestive heart failure with pulmonary edema, acute lung injury, alveolar hemorrhage, pneumonia, etc.), severe restrictive disease of the lung or chest wall or severe airways obstruction (asthma, emphysema).

KEY SIGN
Periodic Breathing: Cheyne-Stokes Respiration: *Pathophysiology:* The pattern results from cyclic hyperventilation followed by compensatory apnea caused by phase delay in the normal feedback controls, which maintain a more constant PCO_2. This is the most common periodic breathing pattern. Respirations are interrupted by periods of apnea. In each cycle, the rate and amplitude of successive breaths increase to a maximum, then progressively diminish into the next apneic period. Pallor may accompany the apnea. The patient is frequently unaware of the irregular breathing. Patients may be somnolent during the apneic periods and then arouse and become restless during the hyperpneic phase.

✓ *CHEYNE-STOKES RESPIRATIONS—CLINICAL OCCURRENCE:* It may be seen during the sleep of normal children and the aged. *Disorders of the Cerebral Circulation* stroke, atherosclerosis; *Heart Failure* low cardiac output of any cause; *Increased Intracranial Pressure* meningitis, hydrocephalus, brain tumor, subarachnoid hemorrhage, intracerebral hemorrhage; *Brain Injury* syphilis, head injury; *Drugs* opiates, barbiturates, alcohol; *High Altitude* during sleep, before acclimatization.

KEY SIGN
Irregular Breathing: Biot Breathing: An uncommon variant of Cheyne-Stokes respiration, periods of apnea alternate irregularly with series of breaths of equal depth that terminate abruptly. It is most often seen in meningitis.

KEY SIGN

Irregular Breathing: Painful Respiration: Otherwise normal respirations are interrupted by the pain of thoracic movement from pleurisy, traumatized or inflamed muscles, fractured ribs or cartilage, or subphrenic inflammation, such as liver or subdiaphragmatic abscess, acute cholecystitis, or peritonitis.

S KEY SYNDROME

▶ **Irregular Breathing: Sleep Apnea (Pickwickian Syndrome):** *Pathophysiology: Obstructive sleep apnea* results from obstruction of the extrathoracic airway caused by relaxation of the pharyngeal muscles and tongue with persistence of ineffective inspiratory efforts often terminating with a loud snort or snore. *Central apnea* occurs when respiratory effort ceases because of absence of medullary respiratory drive. The periods of apnea are accompanied by hypoxia, acidosis, and cardiac dysrhythmias (bradycardia, tachycardia, especially ventricular) that sometimes cause sudden death. The original description (1965) used the term pickwickian syndrome after the obese boy in the writings of Charles Dickens. The classic patient is a morbidly obese male with daytime somnolence, polycythemia, alveolar hypoventilation, and pulmonary hypertension producing right ventricular failure; this is the picture of advanced disease. The daytime somnolence is the result of nocturnal interruptions of sleep by many arousals resulting from intervals of apnea lasting more than 10 seconds. Symptoms of early disease include early morning headaches, depression or irritability from chronic sleep deprivation, and systemic hypertension [Strollo PJ, Rogers RM. Obstructive sleep apnea. *N Engl J Med* 1996;334:99–104; Netzer MC, Stoohs RA, Netzer CM, et al. Using the Berlin questionnaire to identify patients at risk for the sleep apnea syndrome. *Ann Intern Med* 1999;131:485–491].

Irregular Breathing: Sighing Respirations: The normal respiratory rhythm at rest is occasionally interrupted by a long, deep sigh. The patient briefly senses shortness of breath without limitations of exertion when active. This is commonly encountered in anxious individuals.

Blood Pressure and Pulse Pressure

Each patient's blood pressure should be checked at each visit, both to detect hypertension and to establish a benchmark for future comparison. The blood pressure should be taken in both arms at the first office visit and again in both arms when the patient has new cardiovascular or neurologic complaints. The finding of elevated arm pressures in young persons should lead you to check the pressures in both legs. Many circumstances temporarily raise blood pressure in the absence of disease, for example, anxiety, the "white-coat syndrome," rushing to make the appointment on time, bladder distention, chronic alcoholism, and recent cigarette smoking. Under certain circumstances, you will wish to repeat it after the patient rests [Bailey RH, Bauer JH. A review of common errors in the direct measurement of blood pressure: sphygmomanometry. *Arch Intern Med* 1993;153:2741–2748].

Automated blood pressure measuring instruments record the pulse rate as well as the blood pressure, but you should count the apical heart rate during your examination of the precordium. For an apparently normal rate and rhythm, count heartbeats for 15 seconds and multiply by 4. Listen and count for longer periods if there are symptoms or signs of abnormalities.

Measurement of Arterial Blood Pressure

The intraarterial blood pressure can be measured directly by inserting a needle into the lumen of the artery, but this method is impractical and is only employed in intensive care units. Clinically, the indirect method is used, in which external pressure is applied to the overlying tissues and the compression necessary to occlude the artery is assumed equal to the intraarterial pressure. The sphygmomanometer is employed for this procedure. It consists of a flat rubber bag enclosed in a cuff of indistensible fabric or plastic. A rubber pump inflates the bag with air and tubing connects the pump to the bag and also to a manometer, either mercury or aneroid, to measure the applied air pressure in millimeters of mercury. The arm cuff should be at least 10 cm wide; for the thigh, a width of 18 cm is preferable. The tension to compress the overlying tissues is usually regarded as negligible, but a thick arm will yield readings 10 to 15 mmHg higher than the actual pressure unless a wide cuff is used [Reeves RA. The rational clinical examination. Does this patient have hypertension? How to measure blood pressure. *JAMA* 1995;273:1211–1218].

> *In hypotensive states with coincident intense peripheral vasoconstriction, the sphygmomanometric method may seriously underestimate the true intraarterial pressure. This often occurs in shock. With smaller degrees of vasoconstriction the Korotkoff sounds underestimate the systolic pressure and overestimate diastolic values.*

MEASUREMENTS OF THE BRACHIAL ARTERY PRESSURE.   The patient may be either sitting or lying in the supine position. In some cases, the pressure may be quite different with changes in posture. The patient should have been resting for some time. Bare the arm and affix the collapsed cuff snugly and smoothly, so the distal margin of the cuff is at least 3 cm proximal to the antecubital fossa. Rest the supinated arm on the table or bed with the antecubital fossa approximately at the level of the heart. Palpate for the exact location of the brachial arterial pulse; it is usually medial, but occasionally lateral, to the insertion of the biceps brachii tendon. Inflate the cuff to a pressure about 30 mmHg above the point where the palpable pulse disappears. Open the valve slightly so the pressure drops gradually (no more than 2 mmHg per second) while making observations by auscultation, or by palpation if auscultation is not possible.

Vibrations from the artery under pressure, called *Korotkoff sounds*, are used as pressure indicators. With the bell of the stethoscope pressed lightly over the brachial artery, note the pressure at which sounds first become audible: this reading is taken as the *systolic pressure*. As deflation proceeds, the sounds become louder and maintain a maximum for a considerable range before becoming muffled. Note the pressure at the point of muffling. Finally, note the point where the sounds disappear. Record these three readings, for example, 130/80/75, where the first pressure is where sounds appeared, the second pressure is where muffling occurs, and the third is where the sounds disappear completely. The highest value is the systolic pressure; but disagreement exists as to whether the second or third value represents the closest approximation to the intraarterial *diastolic pressure*. With all three values recorded, readers can draw their own conclusions, and they are not forced to guess at the criterion employed by the examiner for the diastolic pressure. The American Heart Association now recommends the point of disappearance for the diastolic pressure in most instances. Occasionally, as in hyperthyroidism and aortic regurgitation, the sounds persist to zero pressure. In such cases, accept the second value, because a diastolic pressure of zero is impossible. Palpation is an alternate method, employed to check the results by auscultation or when Korotkoff sounds are imperceptible. Palpate the brachial or radial artery distal to the cuff, and record as the systolic pressure; the pressure at which pulse waves first appear. Alternatively, a hand-held Doppler ultrasound device can be used to identify the pulse and the systolic pressure.

The *pulse pressure* is the difference between the arterial systolic and diastolic pressures. The normal mean value is 50 mmHg in men and women.

WRIST BLOOD PRESSURE.   When the blood pressure has been taken in a very fat arm, it is advisable to check the value by measuring the pressure at the wrist. The cuff is wrapped around the forearm and the stethoscope bell is placed over the radial artery.

FEMORAL ARTERY BLOOD PRESSURE.   When taking the arterial pressure in the femoral artery, have the patient lie prone on a table or bed. Wrap a wide cuff (18 cm or more) around the thigh so that the lower margin of the cuff is several centimeters proximal to the popliteal fossa. Inflate the cuff and auscultate the popliteal artery in its fossa. Considerable difficulty may be encountered in holding the cuff on the conical thigh to get even compression.

ANKLE BLOOD PRESSURE.   This may be obtained more conveniently than at the popliteal fossae. Have the patient lie supine and apply the cuff just above the malleolus. Place the chest piece of the stethoscope distal to the cuff and behind the medial malleolus on the posterior tibial artery or on the dorsal extensor retinaculum of the ankle over the dorsalis pedis artery. Pressure values by this method have been found comparable to those from the brachial artery in patients with unobstructed arteries.

MANOMETRIC DETECTION OF PULSE WAVE DISTURBANCES.   During measurement of the blood pressure, changes in the volume of individual pulse waves may be detected that are too subtle to be detected by palpation. Conditions where this is found include atrial fibrillation, pulsus

TABLE 4–1   JNC-7 Blood Pressure Classification

Classification	Systolic Pressure mmHg	Diastolic Pressure mmHg
Normal	<120	<80
Prehypertension	120–139	80–89
Hypertension		
Stage 1	140–159	90–99
Stage 2	>159	>100

paradoxus (tamponade, chronic obstructive pulmonary disease), and pulsus alternans. They are described under the appropriate headings.

KEY SIGN

Inequality of Blood Pressure in Arms.   Blood pressures normally should not differ by more than 10 mmHg between the arms, with the right arm usually greater than the left. Inequality is frequently encountered and sometimes cannot be explained. Causes to be considered are occlusion of the subclavian artery, scalenus anticus syndrome, cervical rib, superior thoracic aperture syndrome, and dissection of the aorta.

Normal Arterial Pressure

The precise bounds of the normal blood pressure are difficult to define and definitions of normal and hypertension continue to evolve (Table 4-1). The risk for cardiovascular disease begins to increase with pressures >115/75 and doubles for each 20/10 mmHg thereafter. Statistical data show an increase in the average systolic pressure with age. Normal adults exhibit a circadian variation in the blood pressure; it is highest at midmorning, falls progressively during the day, and reaches its lowest point at about 3 a.m. The Seventh Report of the Joint National Committee on Prevention, Detection, Evaluation, and Treatment of High Blood Pressure has defined the ranges for the description of blood pressure [Chobanian AV, Bakris GL, Black HR, et al. The seventh report of the joint national committee on prevention, detection, evaluation, and treatment of high blood pressure. *JAMA* 2003;289:2560–2572].

High Blood Pressure

KEY SYNDROME

Hypertension: *Pathophysiology:*   Increased diastolic pressure results from increased peripheral resistance, either by vasoconstriction or intimal thickening. Increased systolic pressure can result from increased stroke volume or decreased compliance of the aorta (in which case the pulse pressure is widened) and with increased diastolic pressure (with a normal or increased pulse pressure). The systolic pressure may be elevated with a normal diastolic pressure: isolated systolic hypertension. More commonly, both the systolic and diastolic pressures are elevated. If only the diastolic pressure is elevated, the pulse pressure is narrowed and you should suspect impaired cardiac output. The diastolic pressure represents the minimal continuous load to which the vascular tree is subjected and makes the greatest contribution to the mean arterial pressure. Both isolated systolic and systolic combined with diastolic hypertension are strongly correlated with stroke, heart failure, left ventricular hypertrophy, and chronic kidney failure. In patients older than 50 years of age, elevated systolic blood pressure is more important than diastolic blood pressure as a risk factor for cardiovascular disease. Discovery of sustained hypertension should lead you to search for hypertensive retinopathy, left ventricular hypertrophy and ischemia, and renal insufficiency.

✓ *HYPERTENSION—CLINICAL OCCURRENCE:* Most hypertension is of unknown cause and is termed "essential hypertension." The primary lesion is suspected to be in the kidney. Essential hypertension is a diagnosis of exclusion, so alternative explanations need to always be borne in mind. *Congenital* coarctation of the aorta, congenital adrenal hyperplasia (early or late onset), polycystic kidney disease; *Endocrine* pheochromocytoma, aldosteronoma, adrenal hyperplasia, hypercortisolism (Cushing disease and syndrome), hyperthyroidism, hypothyroidism, hyperparathyroidism, acromegaly; *Idiopathic* essential hypertension, toxemia of pregnancy; *Inflammatory/Immune* atherosclerosis, vasculitis; *Metabolic/Toxic* renal insufficiency, medications (estrogens, oral contraceptives, cyclosporine), drug abuse (cocaine, amphetamines, etc.), porphyria, lead poisoning, hypercalcemia; *Mechanical/Trauma* obstructive sleep apnea; *Neoplastic* adrenal adenoma, pheochromocytoma, pituitary adenoma, brain tumors; *Neurologic* stroke, diencephalic syndrome, increased intracranial pressure, acute spinal cord injury; *Psychosocial* substance abuse (cocaine, amphetamines, alcohol); *Vascular* renal artery stenosis (atherosclerosis, fibromuscular dysplasia).

S KEY SYNDROME

Isolated Systolic Hypertension: *Pathophysiology:* The increased systolic pressure is the result of either increased stroke volume of the ventricles or increased rigidity of the aorta and other large arteries. In this condition, the systolic pressure is elevated but the diastolic pressure is normal. It is correlated with an increased risk for stroke, left ventricular hypertrophy, and heart failure.

✓ *ISOLATED SYSTOLIC HYPERTENSION—CLINICAL OCCURRENCE:* Systolic hypertension is seen with increased cardiac output (hyperthyroidism, anemia, arteriovenous fistulas, aortic regurgitation, anxiety), a rigid aorta as a result of atherosclerosis, and is particularly common in the elderly.

S KEY SYNDROME

► **Malignant Hypertension:** *Pathophysiology:* Elevated blood pressure leads to end-organ dysfunction with positive feedback loops as a result of ischemia, which further aggravates the pressure. Patients present with headache, confusion, dyspnea, seizures, angina or rapidly progressive renal insufficiency, and diastolic pressures of >120 mmHg. Rapid restoration of reduced or normal pressures is required to prevent irreversible damage to the brain, heart, eyes and kidneys.

S   KEY SYNDROME

Paroxysmal Hypertension: Pheochromocytoma: *Pathophysiology:* A benign tumor of the adrenal or sympathetic chain secretes epinephrine or norepinephrine. In one-third of the patients, the tumor secretes intermittently. The patient's blood pressure may be normal except for episodes of hypertension associated with pallor, anxiety, sweating, palpitation, nausea, and vomiting. However, most patients have sustained hypertension. Orthostatic hypotension is common due to intravascular volume depletion. The condition must be distinguished from panic attacks and the "white-coat syndrome" in which some anxious patients register hypertensive readings only when their blood pressure is taken by a physician or nurse [Lenders JWM, Pacak K, Walther MM. Biochemical diagnosis of pheochromocytoma: Which test is best? *JAMA* 2002;287:1427–1434].

S   KEY SYNDROME

Paroxysmal Hypertension: Neuroleptic Malignant Syndrome: See page 63.

Low Blood Pressure

KEY SIGN

Hypotension: *Pathophysiology:* Hypotension results from a loss of blood volume, loss of vascular tone, or decreased cardiac output. Both the systolic and diastolic pressures are diminished below the usual level for the patient: values within the normal range are hypotensive for the patient who has previously had sustained hypertension. Signs of hypoperfusion (cool skin, decreased urine output, decreased mental alertness) and compensatory cardiovascular responses (peripheral vasoconstriction, tachycardia) indicate that low blood pressure is pathologic [McGee S, Abernethy WB III, Simel DL. The rational clinical examination. Is this patient hypovolemic? *JAMA* 1999;281:1022–1028].

✓ *HYPOTENSION—CLINICAL OCCURRENCE: Loss of Blood Volume* bleeding, capillary leak syndrome (anaphylaxis, sepsis, IL-2, idiopathic capillary leak syndrome), third-spacing (ascites, burns, secretory diarrheas), polyuria (diabetes mellitus, diabetes insipidus, diuretics), inadequate fluid intake, excessive sweating (heat prostration and heat stroke), adrenal insufficiency; *Loss of Vascular Tone* sepsis, drugs (vasodilators, tricyclic antidepressants, ganglionic blockers), fever, autonomic insufficiency (multisystem atrophy), acute spinal cord injury (spinal shock), arteriovenous malformations; *Decreased Cardiac Output* acute myocardial infarction, ischemic cardiomyopathy, idiopathic dilated cardiomyopathy, aortic stenosis, pulmonary embolism, pericardial tamponade.

KEY SIGN

► **Orthostatic (Postural) Hypotension:** *Pathophysiology:* The patient is hypovolemic, or normal sympathetic discharges to the heart and blood vessels are diminished, or blood is pooled, usually in the lower extremities, so that venous return to the heart is deficient. The blood pressure is normal in the recumbent position, but when the patient stands there is a fall, within 3 minutes of ≥20 mmHg in the systolic or ≥10 mmHg in the diastolic blood pressure. This is an early sign of loss of intravascular volume. When the drop in blood pressure is *not* accompanied by a rise in pulse rate, autonomic insufficiency is suggested [Robertson D, Hollister AS, Biaggioni, et al. The diagnosis and treatment of baroreflex failure. N Engl J Med 1993;329:1449–1455].

✓*ORTHOSTATIC HYPOTENSION—CLINICAL OCCURRENCE:* *Loss of Blood Volume* see Hypotension above; *Loss of Vascular Tone* deconditioning after long illnesses in bed and weightlessness of space flight, autonomic insufficiency (multisystem atrophy), peripheral neuropathies (diabetes, tabes dorsalis, alcoholic), drugs (vasodilators, tricyclic antidepressants, ganglionic blockers); *Impaired Venous Return* ascites, pregnancy, venous insufficiency, inferior vena cava obstruction or hemangiomas of the legs.

KEY SYNDROME

► **Anaphylactic Shock:** *Pathophysiology:* Immunoglobulin (Ig) E-mediated mast cell degranulation leads to release of histamine and other vasoactive substances, producing vasodilatation and opening of endothelial tight junctions with loss of plasma volume. This is a fulminant and life-threatening hypersensitivity reaction occurring on exposure to a specific allergen. Sudden vascular collapse is preceded or accompanied by malaise, pruritus, pallor, stridor, cyanosis, syncope, vomiting, diarrhea, tachypnea, tachycardia, and distant heart sounds. Angioedema and urticaria may be present, but are often absent.

✓*ANAPHYLAXIS—CLINICAL OCCURRENCE:* Hymenoptera stings, drugs (e.g., penicillin and other antibiotics), peanut ingestion, and many others. Anaphylaxis may occur with exercise, cold exposure, heat exposure or without evident cause (idiopathic anaphylaxis). Clinically identical reactions occur when mast cell release is stimulated by non-IgE–mediated mechanisms such as radiographic contrast agents.

KEY SYNDROME

► **Septic Shock:** *Pathophysiology:* This is a complex physiologic reaction to endotoxin release into the systemic circulation with activation of inflammatory and thrombotic pathways [Landry DW, Oliver JA. The pathogenesis of vasodilatory shock. N Engl J Med 2001;345:588–595]. Patients present with hypotension, often, but not always, accompanied by high fever and prostration. Initially, the skin is warm and flushed, despite the low blood pressure. As the condition worsens, peripheral vasoconstriction, decreased urine output, mental confusion, and progressive hypotension and acidosis ensue. Prompt recognition, location, and appropriate treatment of the source of infection are essential [Wheeler AP, Bernard GR. Treating patients with severe sepsis. *N Engl J Med* 1999;340:207–214].

S | KEY SYNDROME

▼**Toxic Shock Syndrome:** *Pathophysiology:* A toxin produced by certain strains of *Staphylococcus aureus* produces hypotension with high cardiac output and generalized erythroderma. This was originally described when highly absorbent vaginal tampons became infected with the organism. Now, surgical wounds containing infected foreign bodies (sutures) and sinusitis are the most common identified sources of infection. The patient, who is usually unaware of the site of infection, suddenly experiences high fever, myalgia, nausea, vomiting, and diarrhea. Within a few days, a diffuse erythematous rash (like sunburn) appears, followed by altered mentation, acute respiratory distress syndrome (ARDS), hypotension, and shock. Exfoliation of skin from the palms and soles may occur in convalescence.

Pulse Pressure

● KEY SIGN

▼**Widened Pulse Pressure:** *Pathophysiology:* Pulse pressure increases when the peak systolic pressure is increased (increased stroke volume, increased rate of ventricular contraction, decreased aortic elasticity) and there is a decreased diastolic pressure (decreased peripheral resistance, arteriovenous shunts, aortic insufficiency). A pulse pressure of ≥65 mmHg is abnormal. With a large stroke volume, the pulse is often described as bounding or, in the case of aortic regurgitation, collapsing. The head may bob with each heart beat. Thrills may be palpable and murmurs audible over AV shunts, either congenital, traumatic, or iatrogenic. With decreased peripheral resistance from vasodilation, the skin is usually warm and pink. Widened pulse pressure is associated with increased cardiovascular morbidity and mortality [Asmar R, Vol S, Vrisac A-M, Tichet J, Topouchian J. Reference values for clinical pulse pressure in a nonselected population. *Am J Hyperens* 2001;14:415–418].

✓ *WIDE PULSE PRESSURE—CLINICAL OCCURRENCE:* *Increased Systolic Pressure* systolic hypertension, atherosclerosis, increased stroke volume (aortic regurgitation, hyperthyroidism, anxiety, bradycardia, heart block, postpremature ventricular contraction, after a long pause in atrial fibrillation, pregnancy, fever, systemic arteriovenous fistulas); *Increased Diastolic Runoff* aortic regurgitation, sepsis, vasodilators, patent ductus arteriosus, hyperthyroidism, arteriovenous fistulas, beriberi.

● KEY SIGN

▼**Narrowed Pulse Pressure:** *Pathophysiology:* Pulse pressure narrows with decreased stroke volume and decreased rate of ventricular ejection. Pulse pressures less than 30 mmHg may occur in tachycardia, severe aortic stenosis, constrictive pericarditis, pericardial tamponade, and many other conditions associated with low cardiac stroke volumes.

✓ *NARROW PULSE PRESSURE—CLINICAL OCCURRENCE:* *Decreased Stroke Volume* severe aortic stenosis, dilated cardiomyopathy, restrictive heart disease, constrictive pericarditis, pericardial tamponade, intravascular volume depletion, venous vasodilatation; *Decreased Rate of Ventricular Contraction* ischemic and dilated cardiomyopathy, aortic stenosis, myocarditis.

Anthropometric Data: Height, Weight, and Body-Mass Index

Height

Linear growth occurs throughout infancy, childhood and adolescence, ending with closure of the epiphyses of the long bones of the extremities. Mature height is determined by both genetic and environmental factors, especially nutrition. Linear growth requires the presence of growth hormone, adequate nutrition (protein, calories, vitamin D, calcium, and phosphorus) and a skeleton able to respond to these signals. After achieving mature height, height should not change throughout the years of maturity into old age. With aging, there is a hormone-independent loss of bone mineral density, particularly of trabecular bone, leading to a slow and gradual loss of height. The latter is aggravated in many cases by loss of muscle tone and strength affecting posture. Addition of pathologic states such as osteoporosis and spinal compression fractures produce sometimes dramatic loss of height.

Height should be measured and recorded regularly as part of well-child examinations throughout infancy and childhood. Growth is plotted on standardized growth charts, which give a rapid, visual indication of current stature and growth trends over time. Once stable mature height is reached, it need not be measured more than once a year, or less, until the person reaches age 60. At this time, yearly measurement should be done.

MEASUREMENT OF HEIGHT. Height is measured standing with bare feet. The patient should be erect (e.g., heels, buttocks, and scapulae touching a wall) and the head in a neutral position (normally, the occiput will not touch the wall). The height is recorded by the vertical distance between the floor and a point horizontal with the highest point of the scalp. Compress the hair, or separate especially thick hair, to eliminate overestimating height. The height is recorded in inches (to the ¼ inch) or in centimeters (to 0.5 cm).

KEY SIGN
■ **Short Stature:** *Pathophysiology:* Short stature indicates a failure of growth hormone production, decreased tissue receptivity, or impaired nutrition. Expected stature can be estimated from standard

scales or by adding 6.5 cm (2.6 in) for boys and subtracting 6.5 cm (2.6 in) for girls from the mid-parental height. Consult textbooks of pediatrics for discussions of the evaluation of short stature in children.

✓ *SHORT STATURE—CLINICAL OCCURRENCE:* *Congenital* intrauterine growth retardation, pseudohypoparathyroidism, vitamin D-resistant rickets, familial short stature, Turner syndrome, achondroplasia, Noonan syndrome, Prader-Willi syndrome; *Endocrine* growth hormone deficiency, hypothyroidism, hyperthyroidism, diabetes mellitus, Cushing disease, hypogonadism; *Idiopathic* constitutional delay in growth; *Infectious* any chronic debilitating infection; *Inflammatory/Immune* juvenile rheumatoid arthritis, systemic lupus erythematosus, chronic glomerulonephritis; *Mechanical/Traumatic* brain injury; *Metabolic/Toxic* chronic glucocorticoid use, malnutrition; *Neoplastic* cancer treatment during childhood, including brain irradiation; *Neurologic* suprasellar masses; *Psychosocial* chronic emotional deprivation, misassigned paternity; *Vascular* pituitary infarction.

KEY SIGN

Accelerated Linear Growth: *Pathophysiology:* This can only occur before the epiphyses are closed in late adolescence and is a result of increased growth hormone from a pituitary tumor. Linear growth normally goes through an early and a late growth acceleration. Deviations from the expected growth rate are detected by the routine use of growth charts during childhood. Significant deviations from the expected rate of linear growth should initiate a search for a growth hormone-producing pituitary adenoma.

S KEY SYNDROME

Excessive Height: Gigantism: *Pathophysiology:* Growth hormone accelerates linear bone growth at open epiphyses. Linear growth in excess of that predicted by parental height, especially if a significant deviation from the previous record, suggests an overproduction of growth hormone from a pituitary tumor, *gigantism.* Note that excessive growth hormone production after epiphyseal closure results in acromegaly (enlarged hands, feet, skull, mandible, and soft-tissue thickening) without increase in height.

S KEY SYNDROME

Abnormal Body Proportions: Marfan Syndrome (Arachnodactyly): *Pathophysiology:* This is an autosomal dominant disorder of connective tissue. See page 774. Affected individuals are tall, of extremely slender build, and with an arm span that exceeds their height. Other features are long and slender fingers; pigeon breast or funnel breast; hyperextensibility of joints and ligaments; kyphoscoliosis; hammer toes; long, narrow skull; high palate; lenticular subluxations; myopia; and cataracts. Frequently, death occurs from dissecting aortic aneurysm.

KEY SIGN

Loss of Height: *Pathophysiology:* Decreased height after reaching skeletal maturity can only result from loss of long bone length, loss of cartilage in lower extremity joints (especially the hip and knee), loss of vertebral height, loss of intervertebral disc spaces (especially lumbar), or excessive spinal curvatures. A careful history and physical examination, combined with a minimum of radiographic investigation, can quickly identify the specific conditions affecting each individual patient. Unfortunately, unless height is measured regularly, the slow progression of height loss may go undetected until changes are severe and significant disability brings the patient to the physician's attention.

✓ *LOSS OF HEIGHT—CLINICAL OCCURRENCE: Long Bones* trauma, surgery, osteomalacia; *Cartilage* osteoarthritis, rheumatoid arthritis; *Intervertebral Discs* herniated discs, desiccated disks, disk infection; *Vertebrae* osteoporosis, osteomalacia, Paget disease, traumatic compression fracture, multiple myeloma; *Spinal Curvature* scoliosis, pregnancy, abdominal muscle weakness, myositis, polio.

Weight

Total body weight is usually thought of as a series of compartments. Gain or loss of weight should be thought of in terms of how much is added to or lost from each compartment.

One scheme is to think of the body as water and everything else: water makes up approximately 60% of the total body mass in men, slightly less in women, and it decreases with age in both sexes. The higher the proportion of body fat, the lower the proportion of water. Body water is divided into two large compartments, the intracellular water (66%) and the extracellular water (34%); it is important to note that the extracellular water is essentially saline with a sodium concentration of about 140 mEq/L, while the intracellular water is rich in potassium and relatively low in sodium. The extracellular compartment is further divided into the extravascular fluid (75%) and the intravascular fluid (25%, most of which is in the capacitance veins).

Another scheme is to visualize the body as a series of tissue compartments. There is a relatively stable component forming the visceral organs and skeleton, which vary little in mass, and a variable component made up largely of extracellular fluid, skeletal muscle and fat. Therefore, when faced with inappropriate or unexpected changes in weight, the clinician should try to determine which combinations of changes in body water and tissue compartments have occurred. This will help in determining the specific etiology of the change observed.

Weight should be measured at each visit to establish a baseline range and to detect any significant changes. Weight is measured on a scale, the most accurate being a calibrated balance scale. Properly calibrated electronic scales are quite accurate. Weight is recorded in pounds or kilograms, preferably without heavy clothing or shoes.

S KEY SYNDROME

▼ **Growth Retardation: Cystic Fibrosis:** *Pathophysiology:* Any of several autosomal recessive mutations of the epithelial chloride channel gene leads to production of viscous mucus by the exocrine glands. This results in chronic progressive disfunction of the pancreas and lungs. Patients are usually diagnosed in childhood, although some, with more mild mutations, escape detection until adulthood. Symptoms include bulky, foul-smelling stools, cough, and dyspnea. Pancreatic obstruction leads to maldigestion and growth retardation. Lung involvement produces cough and recurrent pulmonary infections, often leading to chronic infection with *Pseudomonas aeruginosa* and bronchiectasis. Involvement of the sweat glands makes affected individuals very susceptible to salt and water losses in warm environments. Complications include fecal impactions, intussusception, volvulus, and chronic bronchitis. With advanced pulmonary disease, cardiomegaly and clubbing of the fingers are present.

KEY SIGN

Weight Loss: *Pathophysiology:* Weight loss occurs when energy (calorie) utilization or loss exceeds intake. It can arise from problems of decreased effective intake (net of ingestion emesis and stool losses), maldigestion, malabsorption, increased metabolic utilization, or increased losses of calories. Remember that failure to gain weight and grow appropriately in childhood and adolescence has the same significance as weight loss in the adult. The history is most useful in formulating a probable pathophysiology. Ask the patient's estimate of the weight lost over a specific time and obtain records of weight to validate the history. Ask whether the patient's clothes fit differently or if family or friends have noted a change in appearance. Review the patient's daily intake of food and drink, and determine if there has been a change in activities. Look at the patient's belt to see if there is a change in the pattern of wear. Look for striae and loose skin over the abdomen and arms. Often more than one mechanism is at work, for example, decreased intake and increased utilization [Detsky AS, Smalley PS, Chang J. The rational clinical examination. Is this patient malnourished? *JAMA* 1994;271:54–58]. DDX: Weight loss without a decrease in intake suggests impaired nutrient assimilation (maldigestion, malabsorption), glucosuria (diabetes mellitus), or increased metabolic rate (hyperthyroidism, pheochromocytoma).

✓ *WEIGHT LOSS—CLINICAL OCCURRENCE:* *Endocrine* hyperthyroidism, adrenal insufficiency, diabetes (especially type 1); *Idiopathic* advanced age (normal adults lose weight gradually after age 60 years), any debilitating disease; *Inflammatory* any systemic inflammatory disease, for example, systemic lupus erythematosus, rheumatoid arthritis, vasculitis; *Infectious* chronic disseminated infection or advanced local infection, for example, tuberculosis, chronic active hepatitis, AIDS, intestinal parasites; *Metabolic/Toxic* organ failure (uremia, advanced liver disease, emphysema, congestive heart failure), increased physical activity, maldigestion and malabsorption, dieting, decreased intake and starvation; *Mechanical/Traumatic* bowel obstruction, dysphagia, odynophagia, dental and chewing problems, decreased mobility, paralysis, apraxia; *Neoplastic* cancers decrease appetite and increase utilization, especially when disseminated or involving viscera; *Neurologic* hypothalamic disorders; *Psychosocial* dieting, dementia, depression, anorexia nervosa, bulimia, isolation, poverty; *Vascular* vasculitis, multiinfarct dementia.

KEY SIGN
Weight Gain: *Pathophysiology:* Weight increases whenever the intake of calories exceeds the metabolic demands, or when calorie-free salt and water are retained. Therefore, weight gain can occur from increased intake, decreased metabolic demands, and/or renal retention of salt and water. Weight gain is a part of normal growth and failure to gain weight appropriately during childhood and adolescence is abnormal. Once skeletal maturity is reached, weight gain continues for a variable length of time as skeletal muscle mass increases to adult size; this is especially true in men. After reaching adult mass in the early twenties, any further increase in weight may indicate a pathologic condition, a decrease in physical exercise, or an increase in caloric intake because of increases in the quantity of food eaten or changes in the type of food ingested. Fats and alcohol have the highest energy content, 9 and 7.5 kcal/g respectively, whereas the energy content of carbohydrates and protein is 4.5 kcal/g. A careful dietary and exercise history should be obtained. Also inquire about changes in appetite, libido, skin, hair, and bowel habits. Note the pattern of weight gain during the physical exam and any evidence of retention of extracellular fluid, that is, edema.

✓ *WEIGHT GAIN—CLINICAL OCCURRENCE:* *Increased Intake* overeating, mild hyperthyroidism, insulinoma, hypothalamic injury, treatment of diabetes, anabolic steroids; *Decreased Metabolic Demands* hypothyroidism, hypogonadism, inactivity, confinement; *Salt and Water Retention* congestive heart failure, kidney failure, nephrotic syndrome, hepatic insufficiency, portal hypertension with ascites, idiopathic edema, diuretic rebound, venous insufficiency with dependent edema.

Body-Mass Index (BMI)

The body-mass index is a standardized measure of the relationship of body mass to height. It has allowed for the calculation of the risk for adverse events of populations with different BMIs. The BMI is calculated by dividing the weight in kilograms by the (height in meters)^2; the units are thus kg ÷ m^2. The upper limit of normal was identified as the point at which the risk for adverse health outcomes began to rise; the lower limit was similarly determined (Table 4–2).

TABLE 4–2 Interpretation of BMI

Body-Mass Index	Description
<18.5	Underweight
18.5–25	Normal
>25–30	Overweight
>30–35	Obese
>35	Very Obese
>40	Extremely Obese

Growth charts using the body-mass index have been developed and are being used increasingly in well-child care. Calculation of BMI and setting weight loss goals based on the BMI are clinically useful; it allows patients to compare themselves with other individuals and the population risks associated with their current and target BMI.

S KEY SYNDROME

Obesity: *Pathophysiology:* Genetics and lifestyle play very important roles in the development of obesity. Caloric intake in excess of expenditures will lead to weight gain, but obesity requires a failure of a feedback loop to control intake; the cause(s) of this failure are unknown [Leibel RL, Rosenbaum M, Hirsch J. Changes in energy expenditure resulting from altered body weight. N Engl J Med 1995;332:621–628]. Obesity is an epidemic in the United States; fully a third or more of the adult population is obese. There is a strong correlation of obesity with insulin resistance and the development of hypertension, diabetes, heart disease, cancer, and overall mortality [Peeters A, Barendregt JJ, Willekens F, et al. Obesity in adulthood and its consequences for life expectancy: A life-table analysis. *Ann Intern Med* 2003;138:24–32]. Obesity is readily recognized and diagnosed, but is very difficult to treat, especially if onset is in childhood or adolescence. Obesity can result from the causes of weight gain (see above, page 93), but more commonly the exact factors leading to the marked gain in body weight, beyond dietary and exercise habits, are obscure [Yanovski SZ, Yanovski JA. Obesity. *N Engl J Med* 2002:346:591–602].

Normal women have more subcutaneous fat than men, and with weight gain they tend to distribute the adipose tissue more diffusely, but predominately in the subcutaneous fat. Men, especially those who gain weight in mid-life, tend to develop visceral adiposity in the internal organs and omentum; this adipose tissue is metabolically different from the subcutaneous fat and appears to play a pathophysiologic role in the increased incidence of hyperlipidemia and insulin resistance in these individuals. The *waist:hip ratio* (the ratio of the body circumference at the hip and waist) has been used to quantify this type of fat distribution. An increased waist-hip ratio or a waist circumference >40 inches for men or 35 inches for women correlate with risks of adverse health events.

The *distribution of adipose tissue* can serve as a clue in diagnosis. Truncal obesity with thin limbs, round ("moon") facies and a prominent hump of fat over the upper back ("buffalo hump") are characteristic of Cushing disease, iatrogenic steroid use and, more recently, the use of protease inhibitors in the treatment of HIV-AIDS. Localized accumulations of fat are seen at sites of repetitive insulin injection (*lipodystrophy*). As noted above, *abdominal obesity* tends to seen in men with mid-life weight gain ("beer belly").

S KEY SYNDROME

Metabolic Syndrome: *Pathophysiology:* Insulin resistance underlies these disorders. The presence of three or more of these five abnormalities defines the metabolic syndrome: obesity, hypertension, low HDL cholesterol, elevated triglycerides, and elevated fasting glucose.

Pain Assessment

Pain is a complex subject and the reader is encouraged to read pain texts to gain a more complete understanding of pain pathways and the pathophysiology of acute and chronic pain, which are beyond the scope of this text.

Pain can be roughly classified as *acute* or *chronic.* Acute pain is an event, chronic pain is a persistent experience. The mechanism of most acute pain is related to direct tissue injury, ischemia or release of inflammatory mediators. Adequate treatment of acute pain not only makes the patient more comfortable, but decreases the likelihood of progression to chronic pain. Unremitting pain leads to remodeling of the central pain pathways and facilitates the persistence of pain as a chronic pain syndrome. Chronic pain is frequently accompanied by functional impairment and depression [Bennett RM. Emerging concepts in the neurobiology of chronic pain: Evidence of abnormal sensory processing in fibromyalgia. *Mayo Clin Proc* 1999:74:385–398].

The quality and localization of pain also assist the clinician in reaching a diagnosis. *Somatic pain,* arising from the skin, skeletal muscles, bones, ligaments, tendons, and soft tissues, is usually described as sharp or stabbing and is well localized (the patient can point with one finger to the site of maximal pain). *Visceral pain* arising from ischemia, inflammation, or other injury to the viscera in the body cavities, is poorly localized (the patient can only indicate a general area or areas of the pain, often described as deep or inside), is aching, pressing, or squeezing in quality, and is often accompanied by autonomic symptoms such as nausea, vomiting, diaphoresis, and intestinal ileus. *Neuropathic pain* arises from damage to the nerve cells themselves, rather than to other tissues; it is usually described as a burning or hot pain in the distribution of the affected nerve or nerves. These distinctions are far from exact, but have been found to be clinically useful.

Diagnostic Attributes of Pain

Pain is a common symptom which often prompts the patient to seek medical care. It directs attention to a specific anatomic region and often, though not always, indicates tissue injury. You can obtain diagnostic clues by further questioning the patient about the attributes of his pain (use the initials ***PQRST*** as a mnemonic as follows). Use the same questioning for other symptoms.

P: Provocative-Palliative Factors

An association of pain with bodily movement often localizes inflammation of a specific tissue known to be displaced by such a motion. If the point is sufficiently accessible, the location may be confirmed by pressure to elicit tenderness. Pain associated with respiratory motions may indicate a lesion in the thoracic wall or the parietal pleura. Flexion of the spine may cause pain in the region of an injured intervertebral joint. The relief of chest pain by nitroglycerin suggests angina pectoris. Ingestion of antacids may relieve the pain of acid-peptic disease.

Q: Quality

The patient is asked to liken the quality of the pain to some common experience such as a toothache, menstrual cramps, labor pains, or a sore throat. Three qualities of pain are recognized: (a) bright, pricking, often described as sharp, cutting, knife-like, lightning-like; (b) burning, also reported as hot or stinging; and (c) deep, aching, variously called boring, pounding, sore, heavy, constricting, gnawing. Physiologically, superficial pain includes types 1 and 2 (pricking and burning); the origin is accurately localized and the pain may be associated with paresthesias, itching, tickling, or hyperalgesia. Type 3, deep pain, is more diffuse and difficult to localize; it persists longer and includes the qualities of throbbing and cramping, depending on the cause. This is more likely to be visceral pain.

R: Region

Pain is usually confined to one or more anatomic regions to which the patient can point. Because each region comprises a separate group of tissues and organs, the diagnostic significance of pain is conveniently discussed in this book in the chapters dealing with the examination of each region.

S: Severity

Assessment of each patient's level of pain should be performed at each visit, and is mandated by Medicare for its beneficiaries. Pain is a subjective sensation so the patient's statement of her perception should be taken at face value without debate. It is useful to ask the patient to describe her pain on a 0 to 10 scale: with 0 being no pain and 10 being the worst pain she can imagine; the pain score is expressed as, for example, 7/10. This technique has proved reliable and useful. The pain scores can be used to follow a patient's pain progression and the response to its management, and it is useful to communicate the caregiver's goals for pain relief: "We should be able to reduce your pain to a 3 after this type of injury."

Intense pain is usually accompanied by physiologic signs perceptible to the examiner and often noted by the patient, such as facial expressions (a grimace), bodily postures (protecting a limb by holding it, flexion of the thighs on the belly for severe abdominal pain), reduced activity, sweating, pallor, dilatation of the pupils, elevation of the blood pressure and acceleration of the heart rate, retching, and vomiting.

Tests with a stimulus of measured intensity indicate that individuals have remarkably similar thresholds for pain. But clinical observation teaches that persons vary greatly in their reactions to pain, depending on their emotional and social backgrounds. Fear may aggravate the pain.

Persons who have never endured sickness seem more sensitive to pain than those who are more accustomed to it.

T: Temporal Characteristics

The duration of the pain often indicates the course of the disease. The duration of a single sensation may be short or prolonged, steady or worsening, and relenting in waves. Shooting pain usually results from irritation of a nerve trunk. Displacement of inflamed tissues surrounding a pulsating artery causes throbbing pain. Daytime pain is common to many conditions in which motions or muscle spasm intensifies it; daytime relief suggests muscle or joint stiffening, which improves with motion. Nighttime pain is likely to result when muscle spasm relaxes its protection of tender tissues.

Pain Syndromes

Site-specific pain is discussed in each of the chapters dealing with a specific region of the body.

S KEY SYNDROME

Complex Regional Pain Syndrome (CRPS): Reflex Sympathetic Dystrophy, Causalgia: This syndrome is characterized by burning pain, autonomic instability, and tissue changes that typically occur after surgery or injury to an extremity, especially of the hands and feet. There is poor correlation between the extent of the injury and the severity of CRPS. The pain may involve an entire anatomic region and can occur days to weeks after the event. The patient usually describes the pain as constant, burning, aching, and/or throbbing. Early skin changes include warmth, dryness, and erythema. Later, the skin becomes cool, moist, and cyanotic. Bone and muscle atrophy and flexor tendon contractures may occur. Two forms are recognized, CRPS type 1 occurs without nerve injury and CRPS type 2 (causalgia) is associated with major nerve injury. Early recognition and treatment is necessary [Kaplan PE. Complex regional pain syndrome. *Lancet* 2001;358:1552; Stanton-Hicks M, Janig W, Hassenbusch S, et al. Reflex sympathetic dystrophy: Changing concepts and taxonomy. *Pain* 1995;63:127–133].

S KEY SYNDROME

Postherpetic Neuralgia: *Pathophysiology:* Reactivation of latent varicella-zoster virus in the dorsal root ganglia produces clinical herpes zoster and can result in a subacute or chronic painful neuropathy. Most patients with acute herpes zoster have intense pain which abates over a period of weeks to months. The pain is sometimes very severe, burning in quality, and associated with severe allodynia where the slightest disturbance of the skin induces lancinating pain. The elderly are at increased risk for persistent postherpetic neuralgia [Kost RG, Straus SE. Postherpetic neuralgia—Pathogenesis, treatment and prevention. *N Engl J Med* 1996;335:32–42].

5 Non-Regional Systems and Diseases

Several body systems are located diffusely or within multiple regions of the body. As a result, the clinician assesses these systems continuously throughout the exam to a greater extent than the more localized systems. Although disease predominately arising in any body system can present with generalized or constitutional symptoms, this is generally more true of the systems discussed here. It is important to keep these systems in mind throughout the examination process. Diseases and syndromes within these systems are exemplars of the need to integrate the findings from all parts of the diagnostic examination into your hypothesis generating process. This concept is reflected in the century-old saying that "he who knows syphilis, knows medicine." This can be applied to knowing HIV/AIDS today.

Constitutional Symptoms

Constitutional symptoms are those that relate to the body or person as a whole, generally excluding psychological symptoms. Many of these symptoms are very nonspecific, but may be clues to serious systemic illness. Because of their nonspecific nature, they must be combined with other clues from the physical exam and laboratory tests before a specific set of physiologic or diagnostic hypotheses can be generated. It may, however, be possible to posit a class or two of general physiologic processes. For instance, the middle-aged patient who presents with anorexia, weight loss, and night sweats suggests the presence of neoplastic or chronic infectious or inflammatory disease, or possibly Addison disease.

▼ KEY SYMPTOM
☑ **Fatigue:** *Pathophysiology:* Fatigue is a nonspecific symptom that can result from serious organic disease, neuropsychiatric disease, or deconditioning. Patients describe decreased energy, decreased endurance for normal activities, and a feeling of increased effort in usual tasks. It is important to distinguish fatigue from shortness of breath and excessive sleepiness; if these conditions are present, they should be evaluated. If other signs or symptoms suggest specific diseases or condi-

tions, these should be pursued. Fatigue can complicate any chronic disease or medical condition; especially common causes are anemia, hypothyroidism, and hyperthyroidism. DDX: When a complete history, physical exam, and screening laboratory evaluation do not find a specific explanation, three conditions should be considered: deconditioning, depression, and chronic fatigue syndrome.

✓ *FATIGUE—CLINICAL OCCURRENCE* These are examples only. *Congenital* muscular dystrophies, mitochondrial myopathy; *Endocrine* hypothyroidism, hyperthyroidism, Addison disease, hypopituitarism, hypoparathyroidism, hypogonadism; *Idiopathic* chronic fatigue syndrome, inclusion body myositis; *Infectious* tuberculosis, acute infectious mononucleosis, acute hepatitis, following other viral illnesses, hookworm infestation, HIV infection; *Inflammatory/Immune* systemic lupus erythematosus, rheumatoid arthritis, polymyositis, dermatomyositis, vasculitis; *Metabolic/Toxic* hypokalemia, hypocalcemia, hypomagnesemia, hyponatremia, anemia, uremia, hypoglycemia, congestive heart failure, drugs (e.g., beta-blockers, sedatives, anticholinergics), alcohol; *Neoplastic* acute and chronic leukemia, myelodysplastic syndromes, myeloproliferative syndromes, solid tumors, lymphomas; *Neurologic* myasthenia gravis, amyotrophic lateral sclerosis, multiple sclerosis, dementia; *Psychosocial* depression, deconditioning, overwork and overtraining, chronic anxiety; *Vascular* claudication, strokes.

S KEY SYNDROME

Chronic Fatigue Syndrome: *Pathophysiology:* The cause is unknown, but frequently follows a viral infection. This usually is seen in young to middle-aged adults. The case definition requires new onset of fatigue not related to exertion and not relieved by rest, which results in substantial limitation of previous occupational, educational, social, or personal activities. Four or more of the following should have started with the fatigue and recur or persist for at least 6 months: impaired short-term memory, sore throat, tender cervical or axillary nodes, muscle pain, polyarthralgias without arthritis, headaches, unrefreshing sleep, and postexertional malaise that lasts longer than 24 hours [Fukuda K, Straus SE, Hickie I, et al. The chronic fatigue syndrome. *Ann Intern Med* 1994;121:953–959].

KEY SYMPTOM

Disturbance of Appetite: *Pathophysiology:* Appetite is controlled by the hypothalamus under the influence of hormones (insulin, cortisol, leptin), metabolites, neural afferents (especially from the viscera via the vagus), and cortical inputs reflecting emotional and cognitive state. Change in appetite can result from a disturbance in any of these systems.

ANOREXIA. A lack of appetite for food is anorexia. Although anorexia lacks specificity, it is sensitive to the presence and severity of many diseases; few patients with significant illness have normal appetites. When the caloric expenditure is unchanged, anorexia results in weight loss.

✔ *ANOREXIA—CLINICAL OCCURRENCE* *Endocrine* adrenal insufficiency, hypothyroidism, hypopituitary; *Inflammatory/Immune* inflammatory cytokines (interleukin-1, tumor necrosis factor) suppress appetite, so any systemic inflammatory process can depress appetite; *Infectious* hepatitis, any acute or chronic systemic infection; *Metabolic/Toxic* uremia, advanced liver disease, amphetamines, and the like; *Mechanical/Traumatic* gastrointestinal obstruction; *Neoplastic* malignancy, especially when metastatic to the liver or regionally advanced; *Neurologic* dementia, delirium; *Psychosocial* depression, poverty, social isolation, abuse, school problems, anorexia and bulimia nervosa; *Vascular* vasculitis, stroke.

POLYPHAGIA. Increased or insatiable appetite is uncommon and may be associated with weight gain if caloric intake exceeds losses, weight loss when losses exceed intake, or no change in weight when intake and losses remain in balance. It is important to remember that losses include caloric expenditures, ingested calories not absorbed because of vomiting, maldigestion, or malabsorption, and calories absorbed but lost to the body's economy (glucosuria, proteinuria).

✔ *POLYPHAGIA—CLINICAL OCCURRENCE* *Endocrine* diabetes, hyperthyroidism, insulinoma; *Metabolic/Toxic* malnutrition (protein, essential fatty acids) iron deficiency; *Neoplastic* insulinoma; *Neurologic* hypothalamic lesions; *Psychosocial* bulimia.

◤ KEY SYMPTOM
◢ **Abnormal Eating Behaviors:** *Pathophysiology:* Behaviors associated with the selection, acquisition, preparation, serving, and eating of food are culturally determined and socially important. Changes in food-related behaviors suggest medical, psychiatric, and social problems. See Chapter 15, page 894.

✔ *ABNORMAL EATING BEHAVIORS—CLINICAL OCCURRENCE:* *Endocrine* pregnancy; *Idiopathic* anosmia; *Infectious* hookworm infestation; *Metabolic/Toxic* iron deficiency, trace metal deficiency; *Neoplastic* food preferences and taste are frequently disturbed with malignant disease, especially with liver involvement; *Psychosocial* psychosis, delusions.

PICA. An unusual craving or appetite leading to the ingestion of unnatural foods such as clay, chips of old paint, plaster, laundry starch (with pregnancy), and ice chips (with iron deficiency). The symptoms depend upon the substance eaten: ingestion of paint may cause lead poisoning, while ingestion of laundry starch may cause obesity and hypochromic anemia.

◤ KEY SYMPTOM
◢ **Thirst:** *Pathophysiology:* Thirst is triggered by water depletion (increased osmolarity and serum sodium concentration) or moderate to severe extracellular volume depletion; normally, both produce increased release of antidiuretic hormone (ADH) leading to increased water intake and increased water absorption by the collecting ducts. A

defect in the production of ADH or the response of the renal collecting duct to ADH leads to water loss and persistent thirst. The sudden development of thirst is a reliable indication of dehydration when it appears with hemorrhage, traumatic shock, the polyuria of diabetes insipidus, and in some cases of severe electrolyte or fluid imbalance. It is important to distinguish between isolated water loss (increased osmolarity with normal extracellular volume), loss of extracellular saline alone (normal osmolarity, but decreased volume), and combined losses of saline and water (increased osmolarity and decreased volume).

✓ *THIRST—CLINICAL OCCURRENCE* Diabetes insipidus (central or nephrogenic), diabetes mellitus, hemorrhage, hypotension of any cause, overuse of diuretics, dry mouth of any cause, psychogenic polydipsia.

DIABETES INSIPIDUS. *Pathophysiology:* Decreased production of antidiuretic hormone (vasopressin) or unresponsiveness of the renal collecting duct to ADH results in an excessive, constant water diuresis. Patients present with an unquenchable thirst, polydipsia, and tremendous polyuria with a low urine specific gravity.

The Immune System

To understand the disorders of the immune system and how they will present to the clinician, it is essential to understand the normal physiology of the immune system. The reader should consult *Harrison's Principles of Internal Medicine*, 16th edition (HPIM-16), Chapters 295 and 296, for a complete discussion of the subject [Kasper DL, Braunwald E, Fauci AS, et al. (eds). *Harrison's Principles of Internal Medicine.* 16th ed. New York: McGraw-Hill, 2004]. For practical purposes, the immune system is thought of as having an innate, nonspecific component, and an adaptive component. The latter has evolved more recently. Disorders of innate immunity are often quantitative or qualitative disorders of neutrophils and macrophages. These are discussed under the hematopoietic system. Here we are concerned with disorders of adaptive immunity.

Serious congenital disorders of the immune system present in infancy or childhood and are beyond the scope of this book. See HPIM-16, Chapter 297, for a complete discussion of these topics. Acquired immunologic deficiencies can present to the clinician at any age. Immunologic disorders are conceptually divided into defects in antibody production (humoral immunity) and defects in cell-mediated immunity. Because humoral immunity requires functioning T cells for proper regulation, defects in cell-mediated immunity are often accompanied by impaired humoral immunity as well.

Patients with altered immune systems present with a variety of illnesses. Most commonly, they have infections, neoplastic diseases, or autoimmune illnesses. Combinations of these disorders are not uncommon. This can be the result of a common primary problem (e.g., immunosuppressive drugs), or the cause of the immune disturbance may be the presence of a neoplastic disease (e.g., multiple myeloma), severe autoimmune disease (e.g., systemic lupus erythematosus), or a chronic infection (e.g., HIV/AIDS, tuberculosis). Treatment of many neoplastic and autoimmune disorders is highly immunosuppressive. In practice, iatrogenic immunosuppression is the most common form of immunodeficiency encountered.

Defects in humoral immunity are most commonly manifest by infections with organisms that require opsonizing antibodies for recognition and elimination. These are the encapsulated bacteria such as *Streptococcus pneumonia*, *Haemophilus influenzae*, and *Neisseria meningitidis*. Because the spleen is the major site of clearance of opsonized bacteria from the blood, overwhelming infections with these organisms are more likely in patients with normal immune systems following splenectomy. All patients in whom splenectomy is contemplated should be immunized for these organisms before the procedure if possible.

Patients with defects in cellular immunity have an increased risk for neoplastic diseases and infections with intracellular pathogens (e.g., tuberculosis) and opportunistic bacterial, viral, and fungal organisms.

Autoimmune disorders are discussed in HPIM-16, Chapter 299. The major autoimmune diseases (systemic lupus erythematosus, rheumatoid arthritis, vasculitis syndromes, Addison disease, etc.) are discussed elsewhere in this text. It is important to recall that autoimmune endocrine deficiency is common and may present as an autoimmune polyglandular syndrome with multiple insufficiencies.

Two Common Syndromes

S KEY SYNDROME

Acquired Immunodeficiency Syndrome (AIDS): *Pathophysiology:* Infection with human immunodeficiency virus (HIV) leads to progressive destruction of CD4 cells and impaired cellular and humoral immunity. AIDS is defined by <200 CD4 cells/mm^3 or the presence of an AIDS-defining illness, either opportunistic infection or AIDS-associated neoplasm. Risk factors for infection are unprotected sexual intercourse (male homosexuals and heterosexuals of both sexes) intravenous drug use with needle sharing, contact with infected blood or body fluids, and vertical transmission from mother to newborn. Opportunistic infections include parasites (*Pneumocystis carinii* pneumonia, toxoplasmosis encephalitis, and cryptosporidium enteritis), viruses (cytomegalovirus, Epstein-Barr virus, herpes simplex, herpes zoster, and human herpes type 8, the cause of Kaposi sarcoma), fungi (candidiasis, cryptococcal meningitis, coccidioidomycosis, histoplasmosis, aspergillosis), bacteria (salmonellosis, *Streptococcus pneumoniae*, *Haemophilus influenzae*), mycobacteria (*Mycobacterium tuberculosis*, *M. avium* complex), listeriosis, *Treponema pallidum*, and nocardiosis. **Symptoms and Signs.** Acute HIV infection presents a nonspecific viral syndrome often with an exanthem; it may be mistaken for Ebstein-Barr virus infection. After a latent period of several years, the patient develops an immunosuppressive syndrome manifest as lymphadenopathy, weight loss, dermatitis, opportunistic infections, and malignancies (e.g., Kaposi sarcoma, CNS lymphoma, human papillomavirus-associated anal and cervical carcinomas) [Paauw DS, Wenrich MD, Curtis JR, et al. Ability of primary care physicians to recognize physical findings associated with HIV infection. *JAMA* 1995;274:1380–1382]. See HPIM-16, Chapter 173.

KEY SYMPTOM

Common Variable Immunodeficiency: *Pathophysiology:* An acquired defect in the maturation of B cells leads to decreased immunoglobulin production and decreased circulating levels of immunoglobulin IgG, IgM, and/or IgA. Patients are usually adults who present with chronic and recurrent infections of the upper and lower airways, especially sinusitis and pneumonia. They have an increased risk of developing non-Hodgkin lymphomas.

The Lymphatic System

The lymph channels and their nodes are part of a discontinuous circulation whose efferent loop is the arteries, arterioles, and capillaries of the vascular system, and whose afferent loop is the network of lymphatic vessels that drain centrally through the regional lymph nodes to the thoracic duct, which empties into the left subclavian vein. The lymphatic system plays a major role in the recognition and response to foreign antigens. Macrophages and Langerhans cells from the periphery (antigen-presenting cells) migrate from peripheral sites with processed antigen, which they present to T cells and B cells in the lymph nodes. T cells circulate from the capillary circulation to the lymphatics and nodes and back into the circulation until they are presented with an antigen specific to their T-cell receptor; recognition leads to activation and proliferation, generating an immune response. Disorders of the lymphatics produce only three physical signs: palpable lymph nodes, red streaks in the skin from superficial lymphangitis, and lymphedema. Palpable lymph nodes indicate *lymphadenopathy*.

Examination of the Lymph Nodes

Enlarged nodes may be visible by inspection, especially with oblique light. Examination is primarily by palpation. The following characteristics of palpable lymph nodes should be noted: number, size, consistency, mobility, tenderness, warmth, and whether they are discrete or matted together. Procedures for examining the major lymph node beds are described below, but all lymph node-bearing areas should be palpated when searching for generalized lymphadenopathy. *The spleen should always be examined as part of the examination of the lymphatic system.*

PALPATION OF THE CERVICAL LYMPH NODES. Seat the patient in a chair; stand behind the patient to palpate the neck with your fingertips. Examine, in sequence, the various lymph node sites (Fig. 5-1): (1) *submen-*

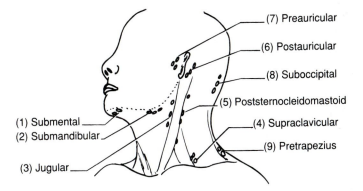

(7) Preauricular
(6) Postauricular
(8) Suboccipital
(5) Poststernocleidomastoid
(4) Supraclavicular
(9) Pretrapezius
(1) Submental
(2) Submandibular
(3) Jugular

Fig. 5-1 Superficial Lymph Nodes of the Neck.   Palpation of the neck for lymphadenopathy is accurate when the region of each group of nodes is examined in systematic fashion. The drawing contains a numbered scheme for examining nine groups of nodes in sequence.

tal, under the chin in the midline and on either side; (2) *submandibular*, under the jaw near its angle; (3) *jugular (anterior triangle)*, along the anterior border of the sternocleidomastoid; (4) *supraclavicular*, behind the midportion of the clavicle; (5) *poststernocleidomastoid (posterior triangle)*, behind the posterior border of the upper half of the sternocleidomastoid; (6) *postauricular*, behind the pinna on the mastoid process; (7) *preauricular*, slightly in front of the tragus of the pinna; (8) *suboccipital*, in the midline under the occiput and to either side; (9) *pretrapezius*, in front of the upper border of the trapezius. When an enlarged lymph node is found, carefully examine the drainage region for a primary lesion: anterior cervical triangle—the anterior third of the scalp and face; posterior cervical triangle and occiput—the posterior two-thirds of the scalp. Examine the other regional lymph node beds to determine if the lymphadenopathy is localized to the neck or generalized. Characterize the enlarged nodes by size, consistency, tenderness, and whether they are discrete or matted together, fixed or mobile.

PALPATION OF AXILLARY, INFRACLAVICULAR AND SUPRACLAVICULAR LYMPH NODES.   Examine the sitting patient palpating the left axilla with your right hand and vise versa (Fig. 5-2A). Relax the patient's left arm and axillary muscles by holding her left wrist with your left hand and elevating her upper arm toward the chest wall. Place your hand in the axilla with the extended fingers approximated and the palm toward the chest wall. Point your fingers obliquely toward the apex of the axilla. Then let her rest her left hand on your examining arm, while your released left hand is used to support her behind the shoulders. Gently, but firmly, rake the pulps of your examining fingers along the thoracic cage to feel for enlarged lymph nodes. Note the size, location, consistency, and mobility of the nodes. The central group of nodes occurs near the middle of the thoracic wall of the axilla (Fig. 5-3). The lateral axil-

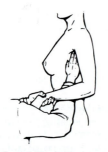 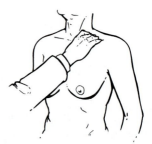

A. Search for Axillary Nodes   B. Search for Supraclavicular Nodes

Fig. 5-2 Palpation of Axillary and Supraclavicular Lymph Nodes. ***A. Axilla:*** *In palpation of the left axilla, the examiner slides his right hand toward the axillary apex, with palm toward the chest wall and approximated fingers extended so the pulps feel the structures on the thoracic cage. With his left hand, he directs the patient's upper arm close to the chest to relax the axillary muscles. He asks the patient to rest her arm on his examining arm and he supports her shoulder with his left hand. The positions are reversed to examine the right side.* ***B. Supraclavicular Fossa.***

lary group is located near the upper part of the humerus and is best demonstrated by having the patient's arm elevated so that you can feel along the axillary vein. With the patient's arm still elevated, feel along beneath the lateral edge of the pectoralis major muscle for the pectoral group. Palpate the subscapular nodes from behind the patient with the arm raised, palpating with the left hand under the anterior edge of the latissimus dorsi muscle. Palpate under the clavicle for the infraclavicular group. Enlargement in the supraclavicular group is sought by feeling the soft tissues above and behind the clavicle (Fig. 5-2B).

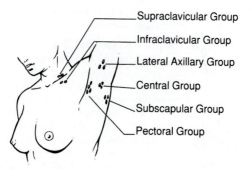

Supraclavicular Group

Infraclavicular Group

Lateral Axillary Group

Central Group

Subscapular Group

Pectoral Group

Fig. 5-3 Axillary Lymph Node Groups. *Note that the lateral axillary group is on the inner aspect of the upper arm, near the axillary vein. The subscapular group lies deep to the anterior edge of the latissimus dorsi muscle. The pectoral group is behind the lateral edge of the pectoralis major muscle.*

PALPATION OF THE INGUINAL NODES. Palpate at and just below the inguinal ligament then distally along the course of the greater saphenous vein.

Lymph Node Signs

KEY SIGN

Lymphadenopathy: *Pathophysiology:* Lymph node enlargement occurs as a result of a stimulated regional or systemic immune response, direct infection of the node, which can lead to suppuration, deposition of intracellular or extracellular material, or infiltration with neoplastic cells. Physical examination of the nodes should describe their distribution, number in each location, size, mobility, consistency (fluctuant, soft, firm, hard), surface (smooth, irregular), and the presence of tenderness, warmth, and/or sinus tracts draining to the skin. A meticulous examination of the skin and soft tissues of the involved region is mandatory when looking for signs of regional inflammation, infection, or neoplasm. Pain and tenderness suggests inflammation and/or infection, while painless lymphadenopathy is more likely to be neoplastic. Fluctuant nodes suggest suppuration from bacterial, mycobacterial, or fungal infection. Fixation of the nodes to underlying tissue is most common with metastatic carcinoma, but may occur with chronic inflammation. Matting together of nodes suggests lymphoma or chronic inflammation. Lymph node enlargement may be the presenting sign in many diseases. Lymphadenopathy which is widespread, involving several lymph node regions both above and below the diaphragm, suggests a widespread systemic disease.

Lymph Node Syndromes

KEY SIGN

Generalized Lymphadenopathy: Generalized lymphadenopathy suggests a systemic process, usually infectious, inflammatory or neoplastic.

✓ *CLINICAL OCCURRENCE* *Congenital* Niemann-Pick disease, Gaucher disease; *Idiopathic* sarcoidosis; *Inflammatory/Immune* rheumatoid arthritis, Still disease, dermatomyositis, systemic lupus erythematosus, amyloidosis, serum sickness, drug allergy; *Infectious Bacterial* scarlet fever, brucellosis, Lyme disease, secondary syphilis, tularemia, bubonic plague, cat-scratch fever, Whipple disease, African trypanosomiasis (African sleeping sickness), kala-azar, scrub typhus; *Viral* rubella (German measles), rubeola (measles), infectious mononucleosis, HIV infection; *Protozoal* African sleeping sickness, Chagas disease, kala-azar, toxoplasmosis; *Fungal* sporotrichosis; *Ectoparasites* scabies; *Metabolic/Toxic* drugs (e.g., diphenylhydantoin); *Neoplastic* Hodgkin disease, non-Hodgkin lymphoma, chronic lymphocytic leukemia.

D KEY DISEASE

Non-Hodgkin Lymphoma: *Pathophysiology:* Clonal proliferation of lymphocytes at a specific stage of maturation and with specific surface markers identifies these disorders. Patients may present with systemic symptoms of fever, weight loss, and night sweats, with abdominal pain or fullness, or with palpable lymphadenopathy. These diseases involve multiple sites and may arise in nonlymphoid tissue such as the lung, stomach, intestine, and central nervous system. Clinically, they are separated into high-grade disease that tends to be rapidly progressive, but potentially curable, and low-grade disease for which curative therapy is not generally available.

D KEY DISEASE

Hodgkin Disease: *Pathophysiology:* This is a malignant disease of lymphoid tissue of unknown etiology that spreads to contiguous lymph node beds, the spleen, liver, and bone marrow. There are two age peaks, in the third and eighth decades. Symptoms include pruritus, painless enlargement of lymph nodes, abdominal pain, and occasionally periodic or continuous fever and cachexia. Although the disease may involve any lymph nodes in the body, frequently only a single group is affected, most often in the neck (Fig. 5-4A). The lymph nodes may enlarge rapidly over 1 to 3 weeks, or slowly over a few months; the enlargement is much greater than in acute adenitis. Lymphadenopathy in non-Hodgkin lymphoma is usually generalized and rarely confined to the neck. The nodes are resilient or rubbery. The ingestion of alcohol may rarely produce severe pain in the nodes; the pain may be so severe and predictable that patients voluntarily abstain from alcohol. Hepatomegaly and splenomegaly may be present. Nephrotic syndrome may accompany or precede the diagnosis. A thorough examination of all accessible nodes by is required.

D KEY DISEASE

Chronic Lymphocytic Leukemia: *Pathophysiology:* A clonal proliferation of mature lymphocytes (90% B-cell, 10% T-cell) leads to infiltration of the lymph nodes and bone marrow with progressive cytopenias and impaired humoral immunity. Patients are often

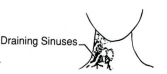

Draining Sinuses

A. Cervical Lymphadenopathy of Hodgkin Disease

B. Cervical Lymphadenopathy of Tuberculosis

Fig. 5-4 Cervical Lymphadenopathy.   *A. Hodgkin Disease: There is no specific pattern of involvement of the nodes. The neck is frequently affected first, often unilaterally. The nodes are large, firm, discrete, nontender, and nonsuppurative. B. Tuberculosis: One finds a matted mass of nontender lymph nodes. The nodes are firm, but some have suppurated and formed draining sinuses.*

asymptomatic until relatively late in the disease. They present with lymphadenopathy and progress to anemia, neutropenia and thrombocytopenia with recurrent infections. Death usually results from infection or hemorrhage.

D KEY DISEASE

▼ **HIV Infection:**   See page 103.

S KEY SYNDROME

▼ **Lymphedema:** *Pathophysiology:* Obstruction of lymphatic drainage by whatever cause leads to the accumulation of interstitial fluid with a high protein content. Massive enlargement of the part may occur and fibrosis develops over time. Patients present with progressive painless swelling of a body part. Common causes are surgical or irradiation injury to lymphatics, trauma and neoplastic invasion of the lymphatics. Longstanding lymphedema is associated with an increased risk for lymphangiosarcoma. DDX: The edema may pit at first, but characteristically is not pitting.

D KEY DISEASE

▼ **Filariasis (Wuchereriasis):** *Pathophysiology:* Infection of lymphatic system with larvae of *Wuchereria bancrofti* or *Brugia malayi* follows the bite of an infected mosquito. There is inflammation and later scarring with lymphatic obstruction, and lymphedema. Headache, photophobia, vertigo, fatigue, low-grade fever, and myalgia are common symptoms. Signs include conjunctivitis, orchitis, lymphangitis, and lymphadenopathy acutely; later, obstruction of lymphatic and venous drainage with edema, hydrocele, elephantiasis of breasts, scrotum, vulva, or legs.

Important Regional Lymph Node Syndromes

More limited, regional lymphadenopathy may be an early sign of a generalized disease, or might represent regional or local disease. Four specific syndromes involving regional lymphadenopathy are worthy of special consideration:

S KEY SYNDROME

▼ **Inoculation Lesion with Regional Lymphadenopathy:** See also, Chapter 6, Ulceroglandular syndromes, page 176ff. *Pathophysiology:* Cutaneous inoculation of infectious agents is followed by spread through the subcutaneous lymphatics, with varying degrees of inflammation and induration, to regional lymph nodes. The cutaneous inoculation site may show minimal signs, or may be marked by local inflammation, ulceration, and/or necrosis with eschar formation. A careful history, including the time of year and occupational or avocational exposures, is essential to an accurate and timely diagnosis [Kostman JR, EiNubile MJ. Nodular lymphangitis: A distinctive but often unrecognized syndrome. *Ann Intern Med* 1993;118:883–888].

✓**INOCULATION LESION WITH REGIONAL LYMPHADENOPATHY—CLINI-CAL OCCURRENCE** *Infectious Bacterial* streptococcal infections, syphilitic chancre, anthrax, erysipeloid, tularemia (ulceroglandular type), bubonic plague, rat-bite fever, cat-scratch disease, nocardia, actinomycosis, glanders; *Mycobacterial* inoculation tuberculosis, atypical mycobacteria; *Fungal* sporotrichosis; *Rickettsial* scrub typhus, boutonneuse fever, South African tick fever, Kenya typhus, rickettsialpox; *Viral* herpes simplex; *Helminths* filariasis, trypanosomiasis, leishmaniasis; *Neoplastic* melanoma, squamous cell carcinoma, lymphangioleiomyomas.

S KEY SYNDROME

▼ **Acute Cervical Lymphadenopathy: Localized Lymphadenitis:** *Pathophysiology:* Infections of the scalp, face, mouth, teeth, pharynx, or ear cause localized lymphadenitis of the neck in the particular group of nodes draining the involved region. Included in localized lesions is chancre of the face with its regional lymphadenitis. Cervical adenopathy is also common in erythema nodosum, although the subcutaneous lesions are almost always limited to the legs.

S KEY SYNDROME

▼ **Genital Lesion with Satellite Nodes:** Syphilis, gonorrhea, chancroid, herpes simplex, lymphogranuloma venereum, tuberculosis, and cancer of penis need to be considered.

S KEY SYNDROME

▼ **Suppurative Lymphadenopathy:** The following diseases commonly cause suppuration of lymph nodes: streptococcal infections, staphylococcal infections, tuberculosis (bovine type), lymphogranuloma venereum, coccidioidomycosis, anthrax, cat-scratch fever, sporotrichosis, plague, tularemia.

Syndromes of Specific Regional Lymph Nodes

Infectious, inflammatory, or neoplastic lesions within the regional drainage give rise to regional lymphadenopathy. *To avoid repetition, only singular or unusual entities specific to a given region are mentioned under CLINICAL OCCURRENCE in this section*:

The Head and Jaw

KEY SIGN

▌ **Suboccipital Nodes:** *Location:* Midway between the external occipital protuberance and the mastoid process (see Fig. 5-1), near the great occipital nerve. *Drainage:* Afferents from back of scalp and head; efferents to deep cervical nodes. *Symptoms:* Impingement of the enlarged nodes on the great occipital nerve may produce headache.

✓**CLINICAL OCCURRENCE** Ringworm of scalp, bites in pediculosis capitis, seborrheic dermatitis of scalp, secondary syphilis, cancer.

Postauricular Nodes: *Location:* On mastoid process and at insertion of sternocleidomastoid muscle, behind pinna (see Fig. 5-1). *Drainage:* Afferents from external acoustic meatus, back of pinna, temporal scalp, efferents to superior cervical nodes. *Symptoms:* Mastoid tenderness simulating mastoiditis.

✓*CLINICAL OCCURRENCE* Bacterial or herpetic infections of the acoustic meatus, rubella (but not in rubeola), leishmaniasis.

Preauricular Nodes: *Location:* In front of the tragus of the external ear (see Fig. 5-1). *Drainage:* Afferents from lateral portions of eyelids and their palpebral conjunctivae, skin of temporal region, external acoustic meatus, anterior surface of pinna.

✓*CLINICAL OCCURRENCE* Ulcerating basal cell carcinoma, epithelioma, chancre of face, erysipelas, ophthalmic herpes zoster, rubella, trachoma. *Ocular-Glandular Syndrome:* Gonorrheal ophthalmia, tuberculosis, syphilis, sporotrichosis, glanders, chancroid, epidemic keratoconjunctivitis, adenoidal-pharyngeal-conjunctival virus (APC), *Leptothrix* infection, lymphogranuloma venereum, tularemia, cat-scratch fever, Chagas disease.

Mandibular Nodes: *Location:* Under the mandible (see Fig. 5-1). *Drainage:* Afferents from tongue, submaxillary gland, submental nodes, medial conjunctivae, mucosa of lips and mouth; efferents to superficial and deep jugular nodes.

Submental Nodes: *Location:* In midline under apex of mandibular junction (see Fig. 5-1). *Drainage:* Afferents from central lower lip, floor of mouth, tip of tongue, skin of cheek; efferents to mandibular nodes, deep jugular nodes.

The Neck

Chronic Localized Cervical Lymphadenopathy: Tuberculosis (Scrofula): *Pathophysiology:* Usually the disease is caused by the bovine strain of tubercle bacilli, although human strains have been implicated. The disease has a predilection for the cervical lymph nodes. The nodes are large, multiple, and nontender. Classically, the nodes are matted together, but this is often difficult to determine by palpation (Fig. 5-4B). Frequently the nodes suppurate and form indolent sinus tracts. Extensive scarring of the neck often results.

Chronic Localized Cervical Lymphadenopathy: Kikuchi Lymphadenitis: This unusual syndrome affects young women who present with cervical lymphadenopathy. It is benign, but often confused with other entities [Dorfman RF, Berry GJ. Kikuchi's histiocytic necrotizing lymphadenitis: An analysis of 108 cases with emphasis on differential diagnosis. *Semin Diagn Pathol* 1988;5:329–345].

D KEY DISEASE

Chronic Localized Cervical Lymphadenopathy: Actinomycosis: *Pathophysiology:* Infection by bacteria of the genus *Actinomyces* from the oral flora involve the mouth, face, and cervical lymph nodes. The infection crosses tissue planes. The nodes are prone to suppurate, forming sinuses with a bright-red hue. The pus contains *sulfur granules*, 1–2 mm in diameter.

KEY SIGN

Subacute Localized Cervical Lymphadenopathy: Metastatic Carcinoma: *Pathophysiology:* Asymptomatic cancers of the head and neck frequently present as metastases in a cervical lymph node. The nodes are usually stony hard, nontender, and nonsuppurative. Epidermoid carcinoma predominates. With *anterior triangle* involvement, primary malignancies are found in the upper aerodigestive tract, including the maxillary sinus, oral cavity, tongue, tonsil, hypopharynx, and larynx. In the *submental region,* metastases occur from primary neoplasms in the lower lip, anterior tongue, and floor of the mouth. In the *posterior triangle,* the nasopharynx and scalp are common sites of origin. Carefully examine suspicious areas and the remainder of the upper aerodigestive tract. *Never surgically biopsy a solitary cervical lymph node suspicious for metastatic cancer.* Violation of the tissue planes of the neck may preclude surgical cure. Always refer such a patient for direct examination of the aerodigestive tract by an experienced observer to search for the primary tumor.

KEY SIGN

Jugular Nodes: *Location:* Along anterior border of the sternocleidomastoid, from angle of mandible to clavicle (see Fig. 5-1). *Drainage:* Afferents from tongue except apex, tonsil, pinna, parotid gland; efferents to deep jugular nodes.

✓ *CLINICAL OCCURRENCE* Infection or neoplasm of tonsil and oral cavity; thyroid cancer.

KEY SIGN

Poststernocleidomastoid Nodes: *Location:* Along the posterior border of the sternocleidomastoid muscle are the posterior cervical and inferior deep cervical nodes, not readily separated clinically (see Fig. 5-1). *Drainage:* Afferents from the scalp and neck, upper cervical nodes, axillary nodes, skin of arms and pectoral region, surface of the thorax.

✓ *CLINICAL OCCURRENCE* Bilateral enlargement in trypanosomiasis is *Winterbottom sign.*

KEY SIGN

Scalene Nodes: *Location:* These are part of the inferior deep cervical nodes that lie deep in the supraclavicular fossa behind the sternocleidomastoid muscle. *Drainage:* Afferents from the thorax. Although not palpable, they are easily biopsied.

✓ *CLINICAL OCCURRENCE* Intrathoracic granulomas and neoplasms.

KEY SIGN

► **Chronic Localized Supraclavicular Lymphadenopathy: Virchow Node (Sentinel Node):** *Pathophysiology:* The node is the site of metastasis via the thoracic duct from a primary carcinoma in the upper abdomen. This classic physical sign is an enlargement of a single lymph node, usually in the left supraclavicular group, frequently behind the clavicular head of the left sternocleidomastoid. Often it is so deep in the neck that it escapes casual examination. A purposeful search requires the patient's trunk to be erect and the examiner facing him; the fingers explore the region behind the muscle head. The node may rise to be palpated as the patient performs the Valsalva maneuver. When a primary carcinoma is found in the abdomen, demonstration of the sentinel node is proof of distant metastasis. Breast and lung cancers spread to the supraclavicular nodes, usually more laterally in the supraclavicular fossa.

The Chest, Axilla, and Arms

KEY SYMPTOM

Supraclavicular Nodes: *Location:* Part of the inferior deep cervical chain, behind the origin of the sternocleidomastoid muscle (see Fig. 5-1). *Drainage:* Afferents from head, arm, chest wall, breast.

✓ *CLINICAL OCCURRENCE* On the right side granuloma or neoplasm from lung or esophagus; on the left side neoplasm from the abdominal cavity.

KEY SIGN

Axillary Nodes: *Location:* Five groups lie on the medial aspect of the humerus, the axillary border of the scapula, and the lateral border of the pectoralis major (see Fig. 5-3). *Drainage:* Afferents from the upper limb, the thoracic wall, and the breast. In women, enlarged axillary nodes on the thoracic wall must be distinguished from axillary tail of the breast.

✓ *CLINICAL OCCURRENCE* Many normal persons have slight permanent enlargement of the axillary nodes from previous infections.

KEY SIGN

Epitrochlear Nodes: *Location:* About 3 cm proximal to the medial humeral epicondyle, in the groove between the biceps and triceps brachii. *Drainage:* Afferents from ulnar aspect of forearm and hand, and entire little and ring fingers, the ulnar half of the long finger.

✓ **CLINICAL OCCURRENCE** Acute local infections within the regional drainage, cat-scratch disease, secondary syphilis (*father-in-law sign*); commonly the inoculation site of generalized infections.

🔵 KEY SIGN
Mediastinal Nodes: *Location:* These are not accessible to palpation. Chest radiographs show widening of the mediastinum, a mass in the anterior mediastinum, and masses in the hilar regions.

✓ **CLINICAL OCCURRENCE** Tuberculosis, coccidioidomycosis, histoplasmosis, anthrax, sarcoidosis, silicosis, beryllium poisoning, erythema nodosum, Hodgkin disease, non-Hodgkin lymphoma (lymphoblastic lymphoma), chronic lymphocytic leukemia, testicular cancer.

The Abdominal and Inguinal Nodes

🔵 KEY SIGN
Abdominal Nodes: *Location:* Distinction between intraabdominal and retroperitoneal nodes cannot be made clinically. Occasionally, large nodes may be palpated as vague masses in the abdomen. Calcified nodes may be seen in the x-ray films.

✓ **CLINICAL OCCURRENCE** Malignant lymphoma and testicular carcinoma.

🔵 KEY SYMPTOM
Inguinal Nodes: *Location:* A horizontal group lies along the inguinal ligament and a vertical group is beside the great saphenous vein in the proximal thigh. *Drainage:* Afferents of the horizontal group come from the skin of the lower anterior abdominal wall, retroperitoneal region, penis, scrotum, vulva, vagina, perineum, gluteal region, and lower anal canal; afferents of the vertical group come from the lower limb, along the great saphenous vein, penis, scrotum, and gluteal region.

✓ **CLINICAL OCCURRENCE** Many persons have moderately enlarged nodes from recurrent infections or trauma. Remember that tumors of the testis metastasize directly to the paraaortic nodes and do not involve the inguinal nodes.

Disorders of B Cells

🇩 KEY DISEASE
Chronic Lymphocytic Leukemia: See page 108.

🇩 KEY DISEASE
Waldenström Macroglobulinemia: *Pathophysiology:* Proliferation and infiltration of the bone marrow, spleen, and liver by plasmacytoid lymphocytes producing excessive monoclonal IgM (macroglobulin) leads to hemolytic anemia, immune thrombocy-

topenia, and increased blood viscosity. Symptoms are insidious in onset with anorexia, malaise, and weakness, nasal and gingival bleeding,
and exertional dyspnea. Signs include any combination of pallor, petechiae, ecchymoses, retinal hemorrhages, lymphadenopathy, hepatosplenomegaly, edema, and signs of heart failure. The disease runs
a very prolonged course.

D KEY DISEASE

Multiple Myeloma: *Pathophysiology:* A clonal proliferation of plasma cells produces intact immunoglobulins and/or light
chains that are detected in the serum and urine. Humoral activation of
osteoclasts leads to bone resorption without healing, hypercalcemia, and
pathologic fractures. Symptoms include bone and muscle pain, backache, weakness, weight loss, and fatigue. There are no specific signs;
bone pain may indicate pathologic fractures.

S KEY SYNDROME

Amyloidosis: *Pathophysiology:* Deposition of the fibrillar
amyloid proteins leads to organ enlargement and dysfunction. Several
specific types exist, identified by the specific protein in the deposits. AL
amyloidosis results from deposition of immunoglobulin light chains. AA
amyloidosis occurs in chronic inflammatory diseases. The hereditary
amyloidoses have specific fibrillar proteins depending upon the specific
familial syndrome. Deposition of amyloid proteins, either generally or
locally, can be asymptomatic or can cause organ dysfunction. Symptoms
are nonspecific with constitutional complaints of weakness and fatigue;
specific complaints referable to the organ systems involve diarrhea, dysphagia, and weight loss (GI involvement); paresthesias (peripheral
nerves); and dyspnea, orthopnea, and pleural effusions (restrictive cardiomyopathy with heart involvement). The signs depend upon the organs involved: macroglossia, eyelid plaques, hypertension, lymphadenopathy, hepatomegaly, splenomegaly, purpura, nephrotic
syndrome, edema, shoulder-pad sign, joint and muscle pain, neuropathy, and fluid in serous cavities. See HPIM-15, Chapter 319.

✓*AMYLOIDOSIS—CLINICAL OCCURRENCE* *AL Amyloidosis* multiple
myeloma, monoclonal gammopathies, primary idiopathic amyloidosis;
AA Amyloidosis chronic inflammatory diseases (e.g., osteomyelitis, tuberculosis, leprosy), familial Mediterranean fever, other familial periodic fevers (see page 62, Episodic Fever).

The Hematopoietic System and Hemostasis

The *hematopoietic system* is intimately linked to the immune system
through the production of B cells and T cells and the production of cells
of the innate immune system (monocytes, macrophages, neutrophils,
eosinophils, and basophils). In practice, disorders of the hematopoietic

system are those that affect the major cellular elements of the blood (red blood cells, neutrophils and platelets). Hematopoietic disorders can be thought of as quantitative, an increase or decrease in the specific cell type, or qualitative, a disorder of function with, usually, a normal numbers of cells. It is useful to think of the presentations of the diseases by the cell type involved.

Red Blood Cell (Erythrocyte) Disorders

S KEY SYNDROME

Anemia: *Pathophysiology:* Anemia is caused by a decreased production of erythrocytes from hypoproliferation or ineffective erythropoiesis as a result of defects in normoblast maturation, increased erythrocyte destruction (hemolysis), hemorrhage, or sequestration of erythrocytes in an enlarged spleen. Patients present with nonspecific symptoms of fatigue, dyspnea, decreased exercise tolerance, and weakness. Pallor is present on examination, and is especially notable in the conjunctivae and the palmar skin creases. The examiner should look for jaundice, lymphadenopathy, enlargement of the spleen or liver, and signs of hemorrhage. DDX: Patients with dyspnea on exertion due to anemia do not have orthopnea, unlike patients with congestive heart failure.

✓ *ANEMIA—CLINICAL OCCURRENCE Hypoproliferation* iron deficiency, anemia of chronic disease, hypothyroidism, kidney failure, marrow damage (tumor infiltration, granulomatous disease, myelofibrosis); *Ineffective erythropoiesis* thalassemias, sickle cell disease, vitamin B_{12} and folate deficiency, myelodysplastic syndrome; *Hemolysis* congenital erythrocyte disorders (hereditary spherocytosis, hereditary elliptocytosis, glucose-6-phosphate dehydrogenase deficiency, pyruvate kinase deficiency), erythroblastosis foetalis, autoimmune hemolytic anemias (warm-reacting, IgG; cold-reacting, IgM), paroxysmal nocturnal hemoglobinuria (PNH), microangiopathic states (thrombotic thrombocytopenic purpura, malignant hypertension), infections, hemophagocytic syndromes, hypersplenism; *Sequestration* massive splenomegaly (chronic myelogenous leukemia, portal hypertension); *Hemorrhage* this is usually obvious, but occult gastrointestinal hemorrhage is common.

D KEY DISEASE

Sickle Cell Disease: *Pathophysiology:* This is an autosomal recessive disease with affected patients homozygous for hemoglobin S. This hemoglobin is unstable in low-oxygen tensions, leading to aggregation and "sickling" deformity of erythrocytes, which then obstruct the microcirculation and produce tissue ischemia and hemolysis. Patients of African ancestry are most commonly affected. Compound heterozygotes with other hemoglobinopathies may present with more mild symptoms. The disease becomes apparent in childhood with painful crises associated with fever, malaise, headache, epistaxis, and pains in legs and abdomen associated with hemolysis. Abnormalities of growth include tower skull, short trunk, thoracic kyphosis, and small stature. Additional physical findings are abdominal and bone tenderness, pallor, yellow-green sclerae, cardiomegaly, hepatomegaly, splenomegaly, and ulcers on shins.

D KEY DISEASE
▼ **Beta-thalassemia Major: Cooley Anemia:** *Pathophysiology:* There is a homozygous defect of hemoglobin A beta-chain synthesis leading to hemolysis and ineffective erythropoiesis. There is expansion of the marrow, extramedullary hematopoiesis, and increased production of hemoglobin F. The disease is evident in childhood with mongoloid facies, prominent frontal bosses, hepatomegaly, splenomegaly, pallor, cardiac dilatation, and failure to grow normally.

D KEY DISEASE
▼ **Beta-Thalassemia Minor: Cooley Trait:** *Pathophysiology:* There is a heterozygous defect of the beta-globulin gene leading to a mild hypochromic, microcytic anemia. The patients are generally asymptomatic or may have mild fatigue. They are often misdiagnosed as having iron deficiency on the basis of the hypochromic microcytic anemia. Iron overload can occur if iron is given inappropriately.

D KEY DISEASE
▼ **Paroxysmal Nocturnal Hemoglobinuria:** *Pathophysiology:* There is increased sensitivity of erythrocytes to complement as a result of acquired loss of a membrane anchor protein. Symptoms include abdominal, retrosternal, or lumbar pain. There is chronic anemia, superficial migratory thrombophlebitis, and hemoglobinuria at night. There is an increased risk for developing acute leukemia.

D KEY DISEASE
▼ **Pernicious Anemia and Vitamin B_{12} Deficiency:** *Pathophysiology:* In pernicious anemia, autoimmune gastritis leads to decreased production of intrinsic factor and vitamin B_{12} malabsorption. Other causes of B_{12} malabsorption from the terminal ileum are more common. Patients present with fatigue, glossitis, or proprioception deficits caused by posterior column disease or dementia. A high index of suspicion is required. Up to 5% of persons older than 75 years of age are B_{12} deficient.

✓ *VITAMIN B-12 DEFICIENCY—CLINICAL OCCURRENCE* Pernicious anemia, postgastrectomy, bacterial overgrowth of the small intestine, intestinal parasites, distal ileal resection, dietary deficiency.

S KEY SYNDROME
▼ **Erythrocytosis: Polycythemia:** *Pathophysiology:* Increased production of erythrocytes can be a result of a clonal proliferation (polycythemia vera) or secondary to either hypoxemia, abnormal hemoglobins, or renal tumors. Patients present with plethora and

dyspnea. In secondary polycythemia, there may be signs of advanced chronic lung disease. Congestive heart failure with edema occurs with hematocrits >60% and hyperviscosity of the blood can produce signs of organ dysfunction, stroke, and thrombosis. DDX: In polycythemia vera, there is splenomegaly and the plasma volume is elevated, along with the increase in red blood cell volume. Usually there is also a leukocytosis and thrombocythemia.

Neutrophil Disorders

KEY SIGN

Neutropenia: *Pathophysiology:* Decreased production of neutrophils (granulocytes, segmented polymorphonuclear leukocytes [PMNs]) can be a result of aplastic anemia, a myeloproliferative syndrome, leukemia, hypersplenism, or infection, or it can be drug induced. The patient may be asymptomatic, but when the neutrophil count falls below 500 per mm^3, the risk of infection with the patient's own flora, especially *Staphylococcus aureus, Streptococcus pyogenes,* and gram-negative flora from the gastrointestinal tract, is greatly increased. Patients may present with fever and signs of septicemia as the first indication of a problem. Fever in the neutropenic patient (febrile neutropenia) is especially common in the setting of cancer chemotherapy and presents a diagnostic and therapeutic challenge.

KEY SIGN

Leukocytosis: *Pathophysiology:* Increased production of neutrophils is a normal response to infection and hemorrhage. Early release of band forms is most consistent with infection. Epinephrine and corticosteroids cause neutrophils adherent to the vessel walls (the marginated pool) to demarginate and may increase the neutrophil count by 50–100%. Increases in mature leukocyte counts are asymptomatic, even at levels greater than 200,000 per mm^3. The keys to the diagnosis are the symptoms and signs of the underlying disease. Persistent neutrophilia without evident cause, especially with immature forms circulating suggests chronic myelogenous leukemia.

Myeloproliferative Disorders and Acute Leukemia

KEY SYMPTOM

Chronic Myelogenous Leukemia: *Pathophysiology:* An acquired balanced genetic translocation of the *bcr* gene on chromosome 9 and the *abl* gene on chromosome 22 leads to a fusion *bcr-abl* functional product associated with the disease. Unregulated granulocytic proliferation produces high neutrophil numbers in the circulating blood. Symptoms begin gradually with fatigue, malaise, loss of appetite, and abdominal fullness. There is usually palabable splenomegaly which may become massive. With progression, anemia and thrombocytopenia occur; the disease terminates in a "blast crisis" with transformation to a relatively refractory acute leukemia.

D KEY DISEASE

Polycythemia Vera: *Pathophysiology:* There is increased proliferation of erythrocytes, neutrophils and platelets. Increases in both the red cell mass and the plasma volume lead to increased blood volume, increased hematocrit, and decreased blood flow in the capillaries as a consequence of increased viscosity of the blood. Patients present with fatigue, neurologic symptoms, aquagenic pruritus, and thromboses. Physical findings are plethora and splenomegaly.

D KEY DISEASE

Essential Thrombocytosis: *Pathophysiology:* In essential thrombocytosis, there is unregulated proliferation of thrombocytes (platelets) leading to very high platelet counts (>500,000 and often >1,000,000 per mm^3). Patients are usually asymptomatic until they present with bleeding or thrombosis. They may present with headache, transient ischemic attacks, or frank hemorrhage.

D KEY DISEASE

Myelofibrosis: Myeloid Metaplasia: *Pathophysiology:* Fibrosis of the bone marrow obliterates the marrow space. There is extramedullary hemopoiesis in the spleen and liver and progressive pancytopenia. The cause is unknown. Patients complain of weakness, increased fatigability, weight loss, pallor, fullness in the left upper quadrant. Splenomegaly and hepatomegaly are usually evident, and dependent edema, bone pain, and fever may be present.

D KEY DISEASE

► **Acute Leukemias:** *Pathophysiology:* Several different forms occur, all presenting with clonal proliferation of very immature myeloid or lymphoid precursors leading to marrow replacement with neutropenia and thrombocytopenia. The onset and progression are acute and rapid. Symptoms may be fever, bleeding, or malaise. Prompt recognition and treatment are required. Acute promyelocytic leukemia is associated with a high risk for disseminated intravascular coagulation; recognition of this entity and treatment with all-*trans* retinoic acid has greatly improved survival.

Platelet Disorders

S KEY SYNDROME

Disorders of Platelet Function: See Chapter 6, page 159ff, Intradermal Hemorrhage.

S KEY SYNDROME

Thrombocytopenia: *Pathophysiology:* Decreased platelet production, increased platelet consumption, immune-mediated platelet destruction, or hypersplenism are the common causes. Patients present with a hemostatic disorder that manifests as easy bleeding from the gums, bruising, epistaxis, or bleeding following trauma or minor surgical procedures. Signs include purpura, from petechiae to large ecchymoses. The examiner should look for splenomegaly, hepatomegaly, and lymphadenopathy. Spontaneous intracranial hemorrhage is a significant risk with counts below 10,000 per mm^3.

✓ **THROMBOCYTOPENIA—CLINICAL OCCURRENCE** *Decreased Production* cytotoxic chemotherapy, other drugs (e.g., heparin, thiazides, ethanol, quinine); *Increased Consumption* massive hemorrhage, hypertransfusion syndrome, thrombotic thrombocytopenic purpura (TTP), disseminated intravascular coagulation (DIC); *Immune Destruction* immune thrombocytopenic purpura (ITP), lymphomas, monoclonal gammopathy of unknown significance (MGUS), systemic lupus erythematosus, HIV infection; *Hypersplenism* portal hypertension, lymphoma.

S KEY SYNDROME

▼ **Thrombocytosis:** *Pathophysiology:* Increased production of platelets occurs with myeloproliferative diseases, iron deficiency, chronic inflammatory disorders, and hemorrhage. This is usually asymptomatic until the platelet counts are >750,000 per mm^3. Hemorrhage is the most common complication, although thrombosis also occurs. See *Essential Thrombocytosis*, page 119.

Coagulation Disorders

Disorders of blood coagulation may be congenital or acquired. Congenital abnormalities usually are deficiencies of specific factors or decreased factor function. Acquired disorders may be factor deficiencies or functional inhibition of coagulation. In either case, patients present with delayed bleeding from sites of trauma, spontaneous hemorrhage into joints and severe hemorrhage following surgical procedures. See HPIM-15, Chapter 117, for a complete discussion.

S KEY SYNDROME

▼ **Hypoprothrombinemia:** *Pathophysiology:* Warfarin administration, vitamin K deficiency (dietary or absorptive), or hepatic insufficiency lead to loss of the vitamin K-dependent coagulation factors (II, VII, IX, X) and to loss of proteins S and C. Patients present with visceral bleeding including epistaxis, bleeding from gums, easy bruising, ecchymoses hematuria, melena, and/or menorrhagia. Ecchymoses are evident on the skin.

D KEY DISEASE

▼ **Hemophilia: Factor VIII Deficiency (Hemophilia A) and Factor IX Deficiency (Christmas Disease, Hemophilia B):** *Pathophysiology:* These X-linked disorders produce deficiency of the physiologically active coagulation factors. Clinically they are indistinguishable. Symptoms and signs begin in childhood with spontaneous bleeding or excessive hemorrhage following dental extractions and surgery. Hemarthroses lead to joint deformities and contractures.

D KEY DISEASE

▼ **von Willebrand Disease:** *Pathophysiology:* This is an autosomal dominant defect in factor VIII, von Willebrand factor, production or function. Patients present with signs of platelet dysfunction as a result of ineffective platelet adhesion. The use of aspirin by these patients greatly augments their symptoms. Many affected people are never recognized.

S KEY SYNDROME

▶ ▼ **Thrombophilia:** *Pathophysiology:* Congenital or acquired disorders of coagulation and fibrinolytic pathways lead to an increased risk for thromboembolism. Patients present with venous, and less commonly arterial, thromboembolism. Often there is no identifiable risk factor (e.g., trauma, surgery, immobility) other than a family history of thromboembolic disease. Common causes are factor V Leiden, deficiencies of antithrombin III and of proteins C and S, prothrombin gene mutations, and the antiphospholipid syndrome. DDX: Arterial thromboembolism suggests antiphospholipid syndrome, nonbacterial thrombotic endocarditis, or Trousseau syndrome associated with cancer [Levine JS, Branch DW, Rauch J. The antiphospholipid syndrome. *N Engl J Med* 2002;346:752–763; Bessis D, Sotto A, Viard JP, et al. Trousseau's syndrome with nonbacterial thrombotic endocarditis: Pathogenic role of antiphospholipid syndrome. *Am J Med* 1995;98:511–513].

The Endocrine System

Endocrine disorders are common and often present with nonspecific symptoms and signs. The clinician should always think of endocrine disorders when patients present with systemic symptoms, such as fatigue, weakness, anorexia, change in weight, and malaise, especially in the absence of fever or other localizing symptoms and signs.

Diabetes and Hypoglycemia

D KEY DISEASE

▼ **Diabetes Mellitus Type 1:** *Pathophysiology:* Destruction of beta-cells in the pancreatic islets produces an absolute deficit of insulin resulting in hyperglycemia, osmotic diuresis, and impaired energy metabolism, with reliance on oxidation of fatty acids leading to ketosis and ketoacidosis. With chronic disease, there is progressive injury to the microvasculature in the eyes, glomeruli, and nerves, and large vessel atherosclerosis. Symptoms include polydipsia, polyuria, polyphagia, weight loss and weakness. Physical findings are dryness of the skin and acetone on the breath. With chronic disease the symptoms and signs of peripheral neuropathy, atherosclerosis, renal insufficiency and retinopathy are seen. See HPIM-16, Chapter 323.

D KEY DISEASE

Diabetes Mellitus Type 2: *Pathophysiology:* Insulin resistance is the primary disorder with hyperglycemia despite elevated circulating insulin levels. Patients are usually obese adults, though increasingly children are diagnosed with the disorder. There is a strong familial predisposition, and an increase risk in some racial groups (e.g., Pima Indians). The metabolic abnormalities are similar to those of type 1 diabetes, but less acute, so many patients escape detection until complications (e.g., myocardial infarction, neuropathy, retinopathy, renal insufficiency) bring them to medical attention. Polyuria and polydipsia are gradual in onset and less pronounced than in type 1.

S KEY SYNDROME

Hypoglycemia: *Pathophysiology:* Low blood glucose results from increased insulin effects or a decreased ability of the liver to produce glucose from other substrates. Patients frequently give a history of "hypoglycemia" in themselves or relatives. Often the complaints are nonspecific and related to autonomic activity (sweating, shakiness, flushing, anxiety, or nausea). True symptoms of hypoglycemia are classified as neuroglycopenic (dizziness, confusion, tiredness, dysarthria, headache, and thinking difficulty) [Service FJ. Hypoglycemic disorders. *N Engl J Med* 1995;332:1144–1152]. Inadvertent or surreptitious use of insulin or hypoglycemia-inducing medications is the most common cause of true hypoglycemia, usually in patients with known diabetes. Insulinoma is rare and reactive hypoglycemia (alimentary hypoglycemia) is an unproven concept.

Disorders of Thyroid Function

Thyroid Disorders: Anatomic alterations of the thyroid gland are frequently associated with disturbances of function. Excesses or deficits of thyroid hormone alter the physical structure of the body to produce physical signs. Therefore, examine your patient (a) to determine the size and morbid anatomy of the thyroid gland, (b) to assess thyroid function, and (c) to judge the likelihood of cancer. Once you have assessed the gross anatomic changes in the thyroid, mostly by inspection and palpation, evaluate thyroid function by seeking symptoms and signs of two clinical entities, hypothyroidism and hyperthyroidism. Pay particular attention to the pulse, pulse pressure, appearance of the eyes and face, voice, skin and hair, neuromuscular function (especially the stretch reflexes), affect, and mood. Confirm the diagnosis by laboratory tests.

Abnormalities of Thyroid Function: Hyperthyroidism and Hypothyroidism: *Physiology:* Thyroid production of T_4 is controlled by *thyrotropin* (thyroid-stimulating hormone, TSH), which is released by the anterior pituitary under the control of the hypothalamic hormone, *thyrotropin-releasing hormone* (TRH).

l-Thyroxine (T4) and triiodothyronine (T3) are released into the circulation from the thyroid follicles in a ratio of >20:1. In peripheral tissues, T4 is converted to the active hormone, T3, at a rate determined within each tissue. T4 and T3 inhibit TRH release from the hypothalamus and TSH release by the pituitary. Thyroid hormones bind to nuclear thyroid hormone receptors, which affect transcription of multiple genes affecting cellular metabolism through binding to thyroid response elements.

S KEY SYNDROME

Hypothyroidism: *Pathophysiology:* Underproduction of thyroid hormone slows the metabolism of all tissues producing cellular, organ, and whole-body hypofunction. The most severe form is known as *myxedema,* from the soft-tissue thickening as a consequence of accumulation of interstitial mucopolysaccharides. *Symptoms:* Patients complain of fatigue, loss of energy, decreased concentration, coldness, constipation, and weight gain despite decreased food intake. The onset is often gradual and overlooked. *Signs:* The *face* of the myxedematous patient is rounded, relaxed, and indefinably puffy without frank edema. The expression is placid and good-natured. Responses are slow. The *voice* is frequently hoarse and coarse from edema of the vocal cords. The singer can no longer sing; her friends are solicitous because of her "cold." There is a paucity of unnecessary motion (hypokinesia); the motions are slow and deliberate. The *speech* is slow and distinct. The rate of alternating motions rate is slowed. There is some generalized *weakness,* but focal atrophy or disability is absent. When the knee and ankle *reflexes* are elicited, you can see and feel the slow relaxation of muscles as if the *reflex were "hung up."* The *tongue* may seem large and awkward. The *skin* feels cold, dry, and thick; often there is scaling that is difficult to distinguish from ichthyosis. The palms and circumoral skin may be yellow from carotenemia. The *hairs* on the head are dry and coarse, so that they emit a crackling sound when lightly brushed. They break easily. Looking at the profile of the forearm, one sees paucity or absence of lanugo hairs. The lateral thirds of the *eyebrows* are often thinned, but this occurs in many normal persons past middle age. The *nails* are dry and brittle; sometimes they are longitudinally ridged. The only ocular sign is *periorbital edema.* **Cardiovascular signs** include a reduced strength of *myocardial contraction,* producing a feeble precordial thrust. Angina and heart failure may occur initially or with thyroid hormone replacement. *Pericardial effusion* (with low-voltage QRS complexes on the ECG), *ascites,* and *edema* of the ankles occur without heart failure. The ventricular rate is normal or slow. Dysrhythmias are rare. The *blood pressure* is normal or there is moderate elevation of both systolic and diastolic pressure. **Constipation** is very common; the resulting tympanites may suggest ileus. **Menorrhagia** is common. There are changes in the **mental status.** The patient often complains of *thinking* more slowly, is *irritable* and emotionally labile. Most patients with long-standing hypothyroidism appear cheerful and placid, but those with recently acquired symptoms complain bitterly and are often dejected. Patients may develop *depression. Myxedema coma* is a rare but grave occurrence.

S KEY SYNDROME

Hyperthyroidism: *Pathophysiology:* Overproduction of thyroid hormone, or ingestion of excessive thyroid medication, increases the metabolic rate, producing changes in all tissues in the body. Increased stimulation of the sympathetic nervous system produces many of the symptoms and signs. See Chapter 7, page 334ff for discussion of specific thyroid disorders. *Symptoms:* Patients initially feel energetic and are often happy that they are losing weight. As the symptoms progress they develop tremor, sweaty skin, frequent defecation, and progressive weight loss despite increased food intake. *Signs:* The *face* is thin, the features are sharp, the expression is alert and vigilant; movements of the facial and neck muscles are frequent and fast. The responses to questions are quick and the emotions are labile. The *voice* is normal in hyperthyroidism. Movements are excessive (*hyperkinesia*) and their speed is faster than normal. Speech cadence is accelerated. There is often some generalized *muscle weakness*. The quadriceps femoris are most often affected, so that the patient must push with her arms to arise from a sitting position. Both shoulder girdles may be weak; symmetrical pairs of eye muscles may be paralyzed. The *reflexes* in hyperthyroidism are normal or hyperactive with unsustained clonus; in patients incidentally taking beta-blockers, this may be the only sign of hyperthyroidism. Almost always in hyperthyroidism the extended fingers and tongue exhibit a fine *tremor*. In addition, there may be a coarse tremor in a group of muscles in the calf or thigh as the result of weakness. The *tongue* is normal in hyperthyroidism. The *skin* feels softer than normal; it is thin, moist, and sweaty. The *hair* on the head is fine in texture, oily, and abundant. The *fingernail* may separate from its matrix (*onycholysis*); usually only one or two pairs of nails are involved. **Lid lag** and **lid spasm** occur in patients without Graves disease. **Cardiovascular signs** include an increased strength of *myocardial contraction*, as manifest by the accentuated precordial thrust and the sharpness of the heart sounds. Angina and congestive failure may be precipitated. *Tachycardia* is almost the rule in hyperthyroidism. The systolic blood pressure is slightly elevated, the diastolic diminished, so the *pulse pressure* is widened; thus, a pistol-shot sound is often present in the femoral arteries. There is a high incidence of **atrial fibrillation**. **Defecation** may be more frequent; the onset of true diarrhea is a grave prognostic sign. Extracellular fluid does not accumulate unless cardiac failure occurs. **Menses** are usually normal; occasionally there is oligomenorrhea. Changes in **mental status** commonly include irritability, emotional lability, and depression in hyperthyroidism; occasionally, manic states develop.

S KEY SYNDROME

Subacute Thyroiditis: Postpartum Thyroiditis: *Pathophysiology:* Painless inflammation of the thyroid gland is common following normal pregnancy. Onset is usually 3–6 months postpartum and is signaled by signs of either hyper- or hypothyroidism. The latter is often confused with the fatigue and stress of caring for a newborn. The gland is diffusely enlarged and nontender. The condition usually resolves completely over a period of months [Pearce EN, Farwell AP, Braverman LE. Thyroiditis. *N Engl J Med* 2003;348:2646–2655].

Chronic Thyroiditis: Hashimoto Thyroiditis:
Pathophysiology: Lymphocytic inflammation of the gland leads to induration and gradual loss of function. This is the most common cause of hypothyroidism; it occurs most commonly in women after the fifth decade. The gland is firm, only slightly enlarged; nontender and nodules may be present.

Disorders of Adrenal Function

Corticosteroid Excess: Cushing Syndrome:
Pathophysiology: Hypercortisolism results from adenoma or adenocarcinoma of the adrenal cortex, from stimulation by excess adrenocorticotropic hormone (ACTH) from a pituitary adenoma, or therapy with corticosteroids. Patients present with complaints of weakness, weight gain, amenorrhea, and/or back pain. Physical findings include hypertension, moon face, acne, thoracic kyphosis, supraclavicular fat pad development, hypertrichosis, purple striae on the abdomen and thighs, and peripheral edema [Raff H, Findling JW. A physiologic approach to diagnosis of the Cushing syndrome. *Ann Intern Med* 2003;138:980–991].

▶ Primary Adrenal Insufficiency: Addison Disease: *Pathophysiology:* Primary failure of adrenal glands results from destruction by tuberculosis, fungi, or other granulomatous processes, amyloidosis, hemochromatosis, tumor, or autoimmune mechanisms. This results in cortisol and mineralocorticoid (aldosterone) deficiency and increased circulating adrenocorticotropic hormone (ACTH). Symptoms include weakness, fatigue, lethargy, nausea and vomiting, diarrhea, weight loss, abdominal pain, and craving for salt. Physical exam may reveal mottled skin pigmentation, pigment in buccal mucosa (in whites), lips, vagina, rectum, reduced growth of hair, hypotension (especially orthostatic), and signs of dehydration [Oelkers W. Adrenal insufficiency. *N Engl J Med* 1996;335:1206–1212].

▶ Secondary Adrenocortical Insufficiency:
Pathophysiology: Pituitary insufficiency with decreased production of adrenocorticotropic hormone (ACTH) or adrenal suppression with inadequate recovery of ACTH responsiveness following prolonged corticosteroid administration leads to inadequate cortisol levels. Symptoms

and signs are less prominent than with primary adrenal failure because the mineralocorticoid axis remains intact. Symptoms are often precipitated by infections, trauma, and surgery, which lead to relative cortisol deficiency in a setting of increased cortisol demands.

Disorders of Parathyroid Function

S KEY SYNDROME

Hyperparathyroidism: *Pathophysiology:* An adenoma, hyperplasia, or neoplasia of the parathyroid gland leads to excessive secretion of parathyroid hormones causing bone resorption and inhibition of the renal tubular reabsorption of phosphate. Hyperparathyroidism may be *primary* or *secondary* to other disorders of calcium homeostasis, producing hypocalcemia (renal insufficiency, hypercalciuria) leading to secondary activation of the parathyroid glands. In some cases of secondary hyperparathyroidism, the gland becomes autonomous and not suppressible with correction of the underlying disorder of calcium homeostasis; this is *tertiary* hyperparathyroidism. Primary hyperparathyroidism is most common in women in the 3rd–5th decades. The onset is insidious and is often detected by abnormal calcium on serum chemistries drawn for another reason. The clinical triad that suggests the diagnosis is peptic ulcer, urinary calculi, and pancreatitis. Symptoms can include muscle weakness or stiffness, loss of appetite, nausea, constipation, polyuria, polydipsia, weight loss, deafness, paresthesias, bone pain, and renal colic. Signs include band (calcific) keratitis, hypotonia and weakness, osteopenic fractures, and skeletal deformities.

S KEY SYNDROME

Hypoparathyroidism: *Pathophysiology:* This occurs spontaneously or as a result of operative removal of the parathyroid glands at the time of thyroidectomy. Inadequate parathyroid hormone secretion leads to hypocalcemia and hyperphosphatemia. Symptoms are nervousness, weakness, paresthesias, muscle stiffness and cramps, headaches, and abdominal pain. Tetany with carpopedal spasm and positive Chvostek and Trousseau signs are characteristic. Other signs are loss of hair, cataracts, and papilledema.

Disorders of Pituitary Function

S KEY SYNDROME

Hypopituitarism: Simmonds Disease: *Pathophysiology:* The pituitary gland is destroyed by tumor, injury, infarct, or granuloma, leading to progressive pituitary insufficiency and atrophy of thyroid, adrenal cortex, and gonads. Symptoms are those of multiple endocrine failure; hypogonadal symptoms are a common early indication. Cold intolerance, weakness, nausea, vomiting, impotence, and amenorrhea are characteristic. Signs include hypothermia, bradycardia, hypotension, atrophy of skin, pallor, hypotonia, areolar depigmentation, loss of axillary and pubic hair, and atrophy of sex organs [Vance ML. Hypopituitarism. *N Engl J Med* 1994;330:1651–1662].

▼ **Hypopituitarism: Sheehan Syndrome:** *Pathophysiology:* Hemorrhage and shock during obstetrical delivery causes hypopituitarism secondary to pituitary necrosis. Symptoms include failure of lactation, amenorrhea, lethargy, sensitivity to cold, and diminished sweating. There is fine wrinkling of the skin, hair loss, depigmentation of the skin and areola, and mammary and genital atrophy.

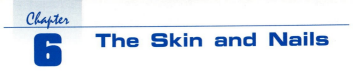

6 The Skin and Nails

This chapter presents an approach to the examination of the skin and nails to identify primary skin diseases and cutaneous signs of systemic diseases. It will help you characterize lesions sufficiently to either make a diagnosis with the assistance of atlases and textbooks or determine that referral to a dermatologist is indicated.

Physiology of the Skin and Nails

The skin forms a protective and insulating layer over the body surface protecting the underlying tissues from injury, infection, and fluid loss. It is contiguous with the mucous membranes of the body orifices at sharply demarcated borders. It supports the peripheral nerve endings. It plays an important part in the temperature regulation by dissipating heat via radiation, conduction, and convection (aided by the production of sweat), and by the insulation provided by the dermal and subcutaneous fat. Integrity of the epidermis depends upon tight intercellular adhesion to form an impermeable barrier. The dermis is rich in blood vessels that can dilate or contract to either dissipate or conserve body heat. Integrity of the dermis depends upon interlacing collagen bundles and elastic tissue.

In addition to its physical protective functions, the skin forms an immunologic barrier as well. Within the epidermis are *Langerhans cells,* antigen-presenting cells that migrate to the regional lymph nodes when activated by foreign antigens.

The skin also contains many specialized structures. Some of these are skin appendages, including the hair and glands; some are special sensory organs of the nervous system, often uniquely aggregated in certain locations. So, in addition to its protective functions, the skin and hairs also function as a sensory organ.

Functional Anatomy of the Skin and Nails

Morphologically, the three chief layers of the skin are the epidermis, the dermis, and the subcutaneous tissue.

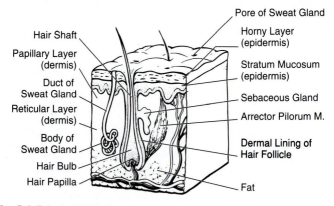

Fig. 6-1 Principal Skin Structures.

Epidermis (Cuticle)

The epidermis (cuticle) (Fig. 6-1) is the most superficial layer. It is sub-divided into two important strata. The *keratin layer* (*stratum corneum*) consists of several layers of dead keratinized cells that normally, se-quentially separate and drop off (*desquamation*). Underlying the horny layer are the *granular layer* (*stratum granulosum*), the *spinous layer* (*stratum spinosum*), and the *basal layer.* These consist of living cells deriving their nutriment from the underlying tissues, the epidermis being avas-cular. *Melanocytes* in the lower epidermis contain *melanin,* a brown or black pigment whose concentration is determined by heredity, exposure to sunlight, injury and repair, and hormonal control. The epidermis con-tains a network of furrows or rhomboid lines, visible with the unaided eye through the keratin layer; on relaxed surfaces the furrows are nar-row, while over joints they are widened.

Dermis (Cutis, Corium, True Skin)

The superficial dermis is thrown into a series of papillae into which the epidermis is molded, the *papillary dermis.* The deeper *reticular layer* con-sists of dense connective tissue containing blood vessels, lymphatics, nerves, and considerable elastic tissue. In its deeper portion are col-lagenous bundles, which are mixed with yellow elastic fibers. Between the meshes of this layer are sweat glands, sebaceous glands, hair folli-cles, and fat cells. The reticular layer merges with the deeper and looser *subcutaneous layer.* The dermis is especially thick over the palms and soles; it is extremely thin over the eyelids, scrotum, and penis. In gen-eral, the dermis is thicker over dorsal and lateral than over ventral and medial surfaces. The dermal appendages are the nails, hairs, and sweat and sebaceous glands.

The Fingernails

The astute diagnostician always examines the fingernails. With the exception of the eye, there is no region of comparable size in the body in which so many physical signs of generalized disease can be found. The nails continue to grow throughout life, providing a record of brief or prolonged disturbances of nutrition. They also serve as windows through which to view capillary changes associated with constitutional disease.

The *nail plate* is a horny, semitransparent rectangle, convex in both dimensions, with a smaller radius of curvature transversely (Fig. 6-2). The nail plate rests on and adheres to the *nail bed,* a layer of modified skin on the dorsal aspect of the terminal phalanx. The bed is studded with small longitudinal ridges containing a rich capillary network that shows through the nail plate as a pink surface. Roughly the proximal third of the nail bed is composed of partially cornified cells containing granules of *keratohyalin;* this specialized layer is the *matrix,* where new nail is made and added to the nail plate, forcing it distally. The matrix is viewed through the nail plate as the white *lunula.* The proximal part of the nail plate, buried in a dermal pouch, is the *root.* The dermal lip of the pouch is called the *mantle;* it terminates in the *cuticle,* a sharp cornified rim. The distal nail plate not adherent to the bed is the *free edge* and the *body* is the intervening portion. The sides of the nail plate are buried in lateral *nail folds* of skin and cuticle.

Throughout life, the nail plate grows continuously by elongation from the root. The average time for growing a new finger nail is about 6 months; growth is faster in youth than in old age. Most changes in the fingernails have accompanying counterparts in the toenails, but signs in the latter are not so evident.

The Toenails

The toenails undergo the same changes as the fingernails, but most of the signs are less pronounced. It takes 12–18 months for a toenail to regrow. Painful lesions are accentuated by weight bearing and by ill-fitting footwear; the fingernails have no similar irritant.

Skin Coloration

In human beings, the color of the normal skin results from a blend of four pigments: melanin (brown), carotene (yellow), oxyhemoglobin (red), and reduced hemoglobin (bluish-red). Except in albinos, the amount of melanin is the determinant of the normal skin color. In persons with dark skin, melanin may obscure colorations obvious in patients with light skin. Therefore, examine conjunctivae, buccal mucosa, nail beds, and palms to assess pallor, cyanosis, or erythema. Melanin pigment lesions lying deep in the dermis appear blue due to the change in the color spectrum of the light reflected through the overlying skin.

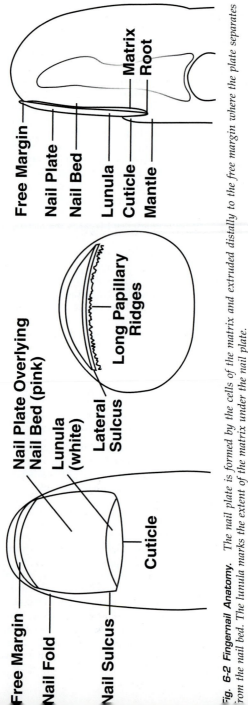

Fig. 6-2 Fingernail Anatomy. *The nail plate is formed by the cells of the matrix and extruded distally to the free margin where the plate separates from the nail bed. The lunula marks the extent of the matrix under the nail plate.*

PHYSIOLOGY OF **M**ELANIN **P**IGMENTATION. Cells in the dermis called melanocytes manufacture the enzyme tyrosinase, which converts ingested tyrosine to the pigment melanin via stages forming dopa and indoles. The melanin-containing organelles (*melanosomes*) migrate outward through the epidermis to become associated with keratinocytes in the epidermis and hair as melanin granules. Individual pigmentation is determined by two factors controlling melanin deposition: (a) hereditary factors control constitutive skin color, and (b) facultative skin color is determined by additional pigment deposition, which waxes or wanes in response to hormonal influence, ultraviolet light exposure, medications, and local stimuli such as inflammation.

Hair

The skin is covered with hairs except on the palms, soles, dorsa of the distal phalanges, glans penis, inner surface of the prepuce, and labia minora. The hair follicle is a long tubular invagination of the epidermis and dermis penetrating the dermis and often extending into the subcutaneous tissue. At its blind end, a *hair papilla* protrudes into the lumen of the follicle. The *hair shaft* is long and slender—in a straight hair, its cross section is round or oval; in a curled hair, it is flattened. The shaft consists of a *medulla,* frequently absent, and a *cortex,* whose cells contain *pigment* in colored hairs and air spaces in white hairs. On its surface is the *cuticle,* a single layer of flat scales. The proximal end of the shaft is the *root,* terminating in a hollow bulb that fits over the hair papilla; the root is softer and lighter in color than the shaft. The hair follicle penetrates the dermis obliquely forming an obtuse angle with the undersurface of the skin; in this angle is an involuntary muscle bundle, the *arrector pili,* extending from near the hair bulb to the superficial dermis. Its contraction pulls the hair to a perpendicular position.

Adults have two types of hair. Both sexes are covered in soft, colorless, short *vellus hairs. Terminal hairs* are longer, coarser, and darker than vellus hairs. Terminal hair is found on the scalp, in the pubic region, and in the axillae of both sexes. Males often exhibit terminal hair on the trunk, face, and extremities. The quantity of hair may vary.

Sebaceous Glands

A group of specialized cells in the dermal lining of the hair follicle secretes sebum through a duct that empties into the follicle near its distal end; one or more sebaceous glands are associated with each follicle.

Sweat Glands

The body of the gland is a coiled tube in the subcutaneous tissue from which a straight duct leads to the epidermis, emerging on the skin surface in a funnel-shaped opening or pore. The sweat glands receive both parasympathetic and sympathetic innervation from the autonomic nervous system. Ceruminal, ciliary, circumanal, and mammary glands are modified sweat glands.

Circulation of the Skin and Mucosa

Most lesions of the skin and mucous membranes involve the vascular system to some extent, so a comprehensive discourse on the superficial circulation would encompass the entire field of dermatology. The skin has a rich anastomotic network of vessels, so ischemia implies obstruction of the larger proximal arterioles or arteries.

Physical Examination of the Skin and Nails

The history should include (a) the symptoms attributed to the skin lesions, that is, pain, burning, and itching; (b) the site of onset and the chronology of appearance, change, and resolution of the lesions; (c) any exposure, injury, medication, or systemic disease that may have induced or altered the condition; and (d) the response to therapy.

Inspection, including use of compression and magnification, is the primary method of skin examination, supplemented by palpation to detect nodularity and induration. A systematic, sequential examination that notes (a) the anatomic distribution of the lesions, (b) the configuration of grouped lesions, if present, and (c) the morphology of the individual lesions is essential [Schwarzenberger K. The essentials of the complete skin examination. *Med Clin North Am* 1998;82:981–999].

EVALUATION OF SKIN TURGOR.   Pinch the skin over the back of the hand with the thumb and index finger, and then release it (Fig. 6-3). Normal turgid skin rapidly resumes its customary shape. Loss of turgor is indicated by persistence of the fold for a time after pinching.

EXAMINATION OF NAIL FOLD CAPILLARIES.   Examination of the nail fold capillaries is done with an ophthalmoscope. It is useful in patients with Raynaud phenomenon to look for changes in the capillaries suggestive of scleroderma. Practice is required. Select a finger without recent trauma. Place a small drop of immersion oil or lubricating jelly on the nail fold to decrease skin reflection. Use the +15–40 magnification to visualize the capillaries. Normally, the capillary arcs are fine, parallel, narrow loops extending from the base of the nail fold toward the nail and

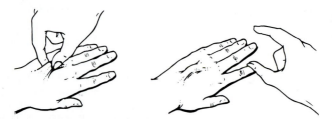

Fig. 6-3 Testing for Skin Turgor.

returning. Dilation, irregularity, and dropout of loops are abnormal [Houtman PM, Wouda AA, Kallenber CGM. The diagnostic role of nail fold capillary microscopy. *VASA* 1987;suppl 18:21–27].

TOURNIQUET TEST FOR CAPILLARY FRAGILITY.   Moderate venous stasis in normal persons produces a few petechial hemorrhages in the skin. The same degree of trauma causes many more hemorrhages when the capillaries are fragile, the *Rumpel-Leede phenomenon.* Stasis may be produced with a tourniquet or, better, with an inflatable cuff. Inscribe a circle 2.5 cm in diameter (the size of an American quarter) on the volar surface of the forearm, 4 cm distal to the antecubital fossa. Place a sphygmomanometer cuff around the arm in the usual manner and inflate to a pressure halfway between systolic and diastolic pressure. Maintain compression for 5 minutes, then release the pressure and wait 2 minutes or more before observation. Count the petechiae within the circle. Normally, the number of hemorrhages does not exceed 5 in men or 10 in women and children. Capillary fragility is commonly increased in (a) platelet disorders, for example, autoimmune thrombocytopenic purpura and platelet dysfunction, and (b) vascular disorders, such as scurvy and senile purpura.

Supplemental Aids to Dermatologic Diagnosis

DIASCOPY.   Press your magnifying glass or a glass slide on a red lesion to see if it blanches. Extravasated blood in a petechia or purpura will not blanch, but the dilated vessels in erythema or a hemangioma will.

KOH PREPARATION.   To demonstrate the hyphae of dermatophytes, the pseudohyphae and budding yeasts of *Candida,* or the spores and fragmented hyphae of tinea versicolor, make a preparation of skin scales scraped from the lesion and placed it on a glass slide. Add 2 drops of a 10–20% solution of KOH to dissolve keratin so that you can see fungal elements more easily under a microscope.

TZANCK SMEAR.   To identify lesions caused by herpes simplex or zoster, gently scrape the base of an unroofed early vesicle with a scalpel and air dry the specimen on a glass slide. Stain it with Wright or Giemsa stain. Search for multinucleated giant cells under the microscope. Culture a fresh specimen for precise identification of the virus.

WOOD LIGHT.   Shine an ultraviolet lamp (360 nm) on the lesion to demonstrate the characteristic fluorescence of infections in the scalp caused by dermatophytes such as *Microsporum canis* (yellow), or abscesses with *Pseudomonas* (pale blue), or of intertriginous infections with *Corynebacterium minutissimum* (coral red).

SKIN BIOPSY.   Biopsy of lesions suspicious for cancer or of uncertain etiology is easily performed. Techniques include using a skin punch, shaving with a scalpel or razor blade, and sharp excision. Training and experience are required.

Skin and Nail Symptoms

Itching: Pruritus: Itching is a common symptom and treatment may prove frustrating to you and your patient in the absence of a specific diagnosis. Ask what induces and relieves the itching, if it is related to a recent exposure or beginning a new medication, where it itches, whether it inhibits sleep, when it started, and whether it is constant and progressive. Look for the excoriations and lichenification that are telltale signs of scratching.

✓ *PRURITUS—CLINICAL OCCURRENCE: Local Causes:* contact dermatitis (e.g., poison ivy), insect bites, chigger bites (red larva of Trombiculidae mites), scabies, tinea, candidiasis, trichomoniasis, atopic dermatitis, neurodermatitis, seborrheic dermatitis, lichen simplex, urticaria, pruritus ani, pruritus vulvae, stasis dermatitis, dermatitis herpetiformis; *Generalized Causes:* asteatosis ("winter itch"), miliaria (heat rash), pruritus of pregnancy, pityriasis rosea, psoriasis, drug reactions, uremia, obstructive jaundice, biliary cirrhosis, myxedema, polycythemia vera (aquagenic pruritus), Hodgkin disease, cutaneous and other lymphomas, diffuse cutaneous mastocytosis, pediculosis (body lice), hook worm, onchocerciasis, filariasis.

Skin and Nail Signs

This section discusses the terminology of dermatologic diagnosis, so you can construct a description of the condition sufficient for efficient use of dermatology textbooks to assist in diagnosis. Following the description of the signs are examples of diseases that cause the lesion.

Anatomic Distribution of Lesions

Many skin diseases have characteristic anatomic patterns determined by either special regional skin features or selective exposure to noxious agents permitted by clothing, for example, sunlight, ornaments, occupational contact, and medication, amongst others. A few examples follow (Fig. 6-4).

Head and Neck: *Acne:* face, neck, and shoulders; *Actinic Keratoses:* face; *Amyloidosis:* eyelids; *Atopic Dermatitis:* face, neck; *Cancer:* face, nose, ears, lips; *Contact Dermatitis:* eyelids, face; *Discoid Lupus Erythematosus:* nose, cheeks; *Herpes Zoster:* trigeminal nerve distribution in face; *Psoriasis:* scalp; *Rosacea:* face; *Seborrhea:* scalp, eyebrows, eyelids, nasal alae; *Secondary Syphilis:* face;

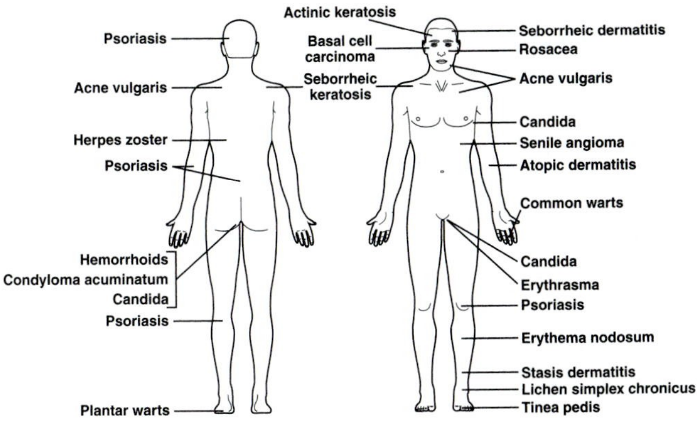

Fig. 6-4 *Distribution of Skin Lesions.*

Spider Angiomata: cheeks, neck; *Tinea Capitis:* scalp; *Xanthelasma:* eyelids; *Variola (Smallpox):* head and face > extremities > trunk.

KEY SIGN
Trunk: *Candidiasis:* under breasts, axillae, inguinal and gluteal folds; *Dermatitis Herpetiformis:* scapulae, sacrum, buttocks; *Drug Eruption:* front and back of thorax and abdomen; *Petechiae:* abdomen; *Pityriasis Rosea:* front and back of trunk; *Secondary Syphilis:* thorax and abdomen; *Spider Angiomata:* chest, shoulders, abdomen; *Varicella (Chickenpox):* trunk > extremities and face.

KEY SIGN
Extremities: *Actinic Keratoses and Cancer:* backs of the hands; *Atopic Dermatitis:* antecubital fossae; *Contact Dermatitis:* arms, hands, legs; *Erythema Multiforme:* arms, hands, legs, feet, palms, soles; *Erythema Nodosum:* legs, shins; *Granuloma Annulare:* backs of hands and fingers; *Onychomycosis:* fingernails, toenails; *Petechiae:* forearms, hands, legs, feet; *Pityriasis Rosea:* upper arms, upper legs; *Plantar Warts:* soles; *Psoriasis:* elbows, hands, fingernails; *Secondary Syphilis:* palms, soles.

Pattern of Lesions

Single lesions may have distinctive shapes and patterns, some quite large (e.g., erythema chronicum migrans of Lyme disease). In other conditions, individual, smaller lesions are grouped into more- or less-distinctive configurations (e.g., herpes zoster). Multiple single lesions often coalesce into larger less-distinctive patterns, so a careful history of the evolution of lesions is critical. Look for these *patterns* when you examine the skin.

KEY SIGN

Annular, Arciform and Polycyclic Pattern:
The individual lesions are arranged in circles, arcs, or irregular combinations of the two.

✔ *CLINICAL OCCURRENCE:* Drug eruptions, erythema multiforme, urticaria, psoriasis, granuloma annulare, tinea.

KEY SIGN

Serpiginous Pattern: The lesions occur in wavy lines (serpiginous means "creeping").

✔ *CLINICAL OCCURRENCE:* Granuloma annulare, nodular lesions of late syphilis, larva migrans.

KEY SIGN

Iris Pattern: A pattern like a bull's-eye occurs as an encircled round spot; more than one ring may be present.

✔ *CLINICAL OCCURRENCE:* Erythema multiforme.

KEY SIGN

Irregular Pattern: Groups of individual lesions with no distinct patterns except that of irregular collections.

✔ *CLINICAL OCCURRENCE:* Urticaria and insect bites.

KEY SIGN

Dermatomal Pattern: Lesions occur in bands in the pattern of the spinal root dermatome sensory distribution; they do not cross the midline.

✔ *CLINICAL OCCURRENCE:* Herpes zoster, sometimes in metastatic breast carcinoma.

KEY SIGN

Linear Pattern: These lesions follow linearly arranged cutaneous and subcutaneous structures, that is, nerves, lymphatics, or blood vessels, or they result from contact with a linear irritant.

✔ *CLINICAL OCCURRENCE:* Lymphangitis, superficial phlebitis, contact dermatitis (e.g., poison ivy), jellyfish envenomation, trauma.

KEY SIGN

Retiform Pattern: The individual lesions form a network in a pattern consistent with the cutaneous arterial or venous anatomy.

✔ *CLINICAL OCCURRENCE:* *Venous Pattern:* erythema ab igne, livedo reticularis, meningococcemia. *Arterial Pattern:* necrotizing vasculitis, cutaneous infarcts.

Extrinsic Pattern: The pattern on the skin follows no anatomic pattern and often has relatively straight borders. This suggests that the pattern is imposed from outside the patient, that is, by the wearing of clothing or other protective gear, or the pattern of exposure.

✔ *CLINICAL OCCURRENCE:* Radiation injury, including sunburn and x-ray dermatitis, contact dermatitis.

Morphology of Individual Lesions

After noting the anatomic distribution and pattern, carefully examine and characterize several individual lesions. Have the patient identify individual lesions in each stage of development: new, mature, and resolving. Palpate the lesions to identify papules, nodules, plaques, and infiltration. View the skin through a compressing magnifying glass to disclose deep lesions obscured by erythema and to determine whether red lesions blanch or persist; this will distinguish vasodilation from extravasation of blood.

Individual Lesion Types

Petechiae and Purpura: See pages 159–163.

Telangiectasia: Dilated small blood vessels blanch on pressure.

✔ *CLINICAL OCCURRENCE:* Spider angiomata, Osler-Weber-Rendu disease, rosacea.

Macules: These are localized changes in the skin color or appearance, but, by definition, they are not palpable (Fig. 6-5A). The ar-

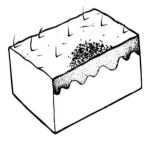

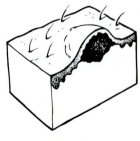

A. Macule.   **B.** Papule.

Fig. 6-5 Macules and Papules. A. Macules are visible but not palpable. B. Papules are palpable and <5mm in diameter.

eas may be small or large; they occur in many shapes and colors. There may be desquamation or scaling.

✓ *CLINICAL OCCURRENCE:* Freckles, exanthems (rubeola, rubella, secondary syphilis, rose spots of typhoid fever), drug eruptions, lichen planus, petechiae, purpura, first-degree burns, systemic lupus erythematosus, pityriasis rosea, café-au-lait spots, vitiligo.

KEY SIGN
Maculopapules: These are macules with slightly elevated portions of the lesion.

✓ *CLINICAL OCCURRENCE:* Pityriasis rosea, erythema multiforme, fixed drug eruptions, exanthems.

KEY SIGN
Papules: The lesions are solid and elevated; they are defined as less than 5 mm in diameter (see Fig. 6-5B). Their borders and tops may assume various forms.

✓ *CLINICAL OCCURRENCE: Pointed or Acuminate* bites, acne, physiologic gooseflesh; *Flat-topped* psoriasis, atopic eczema, lichen planus, molluscum contagiosum, condyloma latum; *Round or Irregular* senile angiomas, melanoma, eczematous dermatitis, papular secondary syphilis; *Filiform* condyloma acuminatum; *Pedunculate* skin tags, neurofibromas.

KEY SIGN
Plaques: Because papules have a diameter of less than 5 mm, any elevated area of greater size is a plaque, usually formed from confluent papules.

✓ *CLINICAL OCCURRENCE:* Cutaneous lymphomas (mycosis fungoides, Sézary syndrome); *Red, Scaling* psoriasis, pityriasis rosea, discoid lupus erythematosus (with atrophy); *Yellow* xanthomas; *Brown* seborrheic keratoses; *Hyperkeratotic* plantar warts; *Lichenified* atopic dermatitis.

KEY SIGN
Nodules: The lesions are solid and elevated; they are distinguished from papules by extending deeper into the dermis or even the subcutaneous tissue (Fig. 6-6A). They are usually greater than 5 mm in diameter. The depth may be inferred by palpation; when below the dermis, the skin slides over them; lesions within the dermis move with the skin.

✓ *CLINICAL OCCURRENCE:* Gummas, rheumatoid nodules, lipomas, cancer, lymphoma cutis, xanthomas, gouty tophi, erythema nodosum, bromoderma.

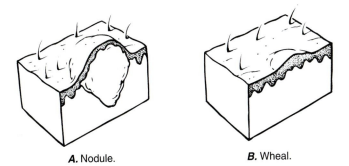

A. Nodule. *B.* Wheal.

Fig. 6-6 Nodules and Wheals. *A. Nodules are persistent, discrete and firm lesions in the skin or subcutaneous tissue. **B.** Wheals are transient, discrete areas of edema in the epidermis and dermis.*

KEY SIGN

Wheals: Caused by edema of the skin, these areas are circumscribed, irregular, and relatively transient (see Fig. 6-6B). Their color varies from red to pale, depending on the amount of fluid in the skin. Hives (*urticaria*) may itch.

✔ *CLINICAL OCCURRENCE:* Urticaria, insect bites.

KEY SIGN

Vesicles: An accumulation of fluid in the superficial layers of the skin produces an elevation covered by a translucent epithelium that is easily punctured to release the fluid (Fig. 6-7A). By definition, their diameter is limited to less than 5 mm. Umbilicated vesicles are usually the result of viral infections.

✔ *CLINICAL OCCURRENCE:* Acute contact dermatitis, second-degree burns, varicella, herpes simplex and zoster, variola.

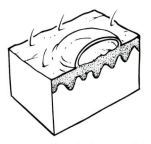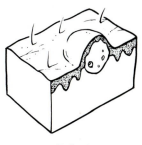

A. Vesicle, bulla, or pustule. *B.* Cyst.

Fig. 6-7 Fluctuant Skin Lesions. *A. Vesicle, bullae and pustules involve the epidermis. **B.** Cysts are subepidermal and may extend into the subcutaneous tissues.*

KEY SIGN

Bullae: Accumulations of fluid between the layers of the skin that are larger than 5 mm in diameter are bullae (Fig. 6-7A). If the layer of separation is deep to the epidermal basal layer, the bullous will be tense; if it is superficial to the basal layer, it will be flaccid and more easily ruptured.

✓ *CLINICAL OCCURRENCE:*   Contact dermatitis, second-degree burns, bullous impetigo, pemphigus, pemphigoid, dermatitis herpetiformis, erythema multiforme (rarely).

KEY SIGN

Pustules: Vesicles or bullae that become filled with pus and tiny abscesses in the skin are termed pustules (see Fig. 6-7A). Through the translucent skin covering, their contents appear milky, orange, yellow, or green, depending somewhat on the infecting organisms. Pustules frequently arise from hair follicles or sweat glands.

✓ *CLINICAL OCCURRENCE:*   Folliculitis, acne, furuncles, variola, pustular psoriasis, bromide, and iodide eruptions.

KEY SIGN

Cysts: These are lesions that contain fluid or viscous material surrounded by an epithelial layer. They appear as papules or nodules (see Fig. 6-7B). The distinction is made by removing the cyst to examine the contents and to identify the cyst wall. Similar lesions without an epithelial lining are *pseudocysts.*

✓ *CLINICAL OCCURRENCE:*   *Cysts*   sebaceous and epidermal inclusion cysts;   *Pseudocysts*   cystic acne.

KEY SIGN

Vegetations: Elevated irregular growths are called vegetations (Fig. 6-8A). When their covering is keratotic or dried, they are *verrucous;* when covered by normal epidermis, they are *papillomatous.*

✓ *CLINICAL OCCURRENCE:*   *Verrucous*   verruca vulgaris (common wart), seborrheic keratosis;   *Papilloma*   condyloma acuminatum.

KEY SIGN

Scales: Thin plates of partly separated dried cornified epithelium cling to the epidermis (see Fig. 6-8B).

✓ *CLINICAL OCCURRENCE:*   *Large Scales*   psoriasis, exfoliative dermatitis;   *Small Scales*   pityriasis rosea, seborrheic dermatitis.

KEY SIGN

Hyperkeratosis: Keratotic cells don't separate and slough normally, so they are piled up to produce elevations.

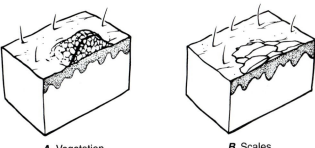

A. Vegetation.   **B.** Scales.

Fig. 6-8 Vegetations and Scales. **A.** *Vegetations are irregular growths above the skin surface.* **B.** *Scales are small or large flakes of cornified epithelium loosely adherent to the skin surface.*

✓ *CLINICAL OCCURRENCE:* Calluses, seborrheic keratoses and actinic keratoses are all common. Arsenic produces punctate keratoses of the palms and soles.

KEY SIGN
Lichenification: Repeated rubbing of the skin produces hyperplasia of all layers (Fig. 6-9A). This appears as a dry plaque in which the normal skin furrows or rhomboid lines are accentuated.

✓ *CLINICAL OCCURRENCE:* Atopic dermatitis, lichen simplex chronicus.

KEY SIGN
Crusts: A plate of dried serum, blood, pus, or sebum forms on the surface of any vesicular or pustular lesion when it ruptures (see Fig. 6-9B).

✓ *CLINICAL OCCURRENCE:* The honey-colored crusts of impetigo are typical.

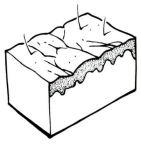
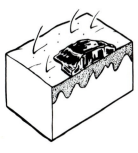

A. Lichenification.   **B.** Crust.

Fig. 6-9 Lichenification and Crusts. **A.** *Lichenification is a leathery thickening of all skin layers with prominent furrows.* **B.** *Crusts form from dried blood, serum, pus or other secretions from the skin.*

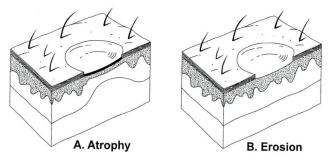

Fig. 6-10 Atrophy and Erosion. *A. With atrophy, all skin layers are present but thin. B. Erosions represent traumatic loss of the stratum corneum.*

KEY SIGN

Atrophy: The skin is thinned, as noted by the lack of resilience and loss of skin furrows or rhomboid lines (Fig. 6-10A).

✓ *CLINICAL OCCURRENCE:*   Senile atrophy, striae, discoid lupus erythematosus, prolonged application of potent topical steroids, and insulin lipodystrophy.

KEY SIGN

Sclerosis: An area of skin is indurated from collagen deposition in the cutaneous and subcutaneous tissues. It is often the result of chronic inflammation.

✓ *CLINICAL OCCURRENCE:*   Posttraumatic keloid, stasis dermatitis, scleroderma (systemic and localized), calciphylaxis.

KEY SIGN

Erosions: The moist surface uncovered by the rupture of vesicles or bullae or from rubbing is termed an erosion (see Fig. 6-10B).

KEY SIGN

Fissures: A vertical cleavage of the epidermis extending into the dermis is a fissure (Fig. 6-11A). Commonly, it occurs from trauma to thickened, dry, and inelastic skin.

✓ *CLINICAL OCCURRENCE:*   An example is chapped lips.

KEY SIGN

Ulcers: A depressed lesion results from loss of epidermis and the papillary layer of the dermis (see Fig. 6-11B).

✓ *CLINICAL OCCURRENCE:*   Trauma, pressure over bony prominences (decubitus ulcers), pyoderma gangrenosum, burns, stasis ulcers, necrotizing infections (bacterial, fungal).

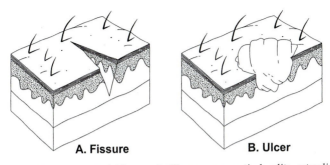

Fig. 6-11 Fissures and Ulcers. *A. Fissures are vertical splits extending through the epidermis into the dermis. B. Ulcers are actual loss of epidermal and dermal tissues that may extend into the subcutaneous tissue and muscle down to bone.*

KEY SIGN

► **Gangrene:** Ischemic necrosis of the skin and subcutaneous tissues creates a blackened, atrophic eschar. If the primary problem is arterial insufficiency the lesions are atrophic and dry (dry gangrene). If the primary lesion is a local necrotizing process, the lesion may be edematous and weeping (moist gangrene).

✓ *CLINICAL OCCURRENCE: Dry Gangrene* arterial insufficiency. *Moist Gangrene* Aspergillosis, pyoderma gangrenosum, necrotizing fasciitis.

Generalized Skin Signs

KEY SIGN

Urticaria: *Pathophysiology:* Inflammatory mediators produce local capillary dilation and leak leading to dermal and epidermal erythema and edema. The lesions are discrete raised erythematous papules and plaques, often intensely pruritic. Precipitating factors may be allergic, mechanical or physical [Greaves MW. Chronic urticaria. *N Engl J Med* 1995;332:1767–1772].

✓ *CLINICAL OCCURRENCE: These are examples only. See dermatologic texts for a complete list. Allergic:* drug eruptions, topical sensitivity; *Physical:* cold, exercise; *Mechanical: Light Trauma* dermatographia; *Systemic Diseases:* mastocytosis, systemic lupus erythematosus.

KEY SIGN

Urticaria: Dermatographia: Dermatographia is form of urticaria stimulated by stroking the skin. Normally, light scratching produces a white line limited to the skin area touched. With an urticarial response, there is a bright-red line that becomes cyanotic. In certain persons, a red, mottled flare develops by lateral extension of the red line. From this, a wheal may emerge projecting 1–2 mm above the skin level. In such cases, writing on the skin with a dull point results in embossed letters (hence the name).

S KEY SYNDROME

Urticaria: Mastocytosis: Mastocyte infiltration of the skin is associated with brown macules, which produce urticaria when stroked (*Darier sign*). Mastocytosis may be limited to the skin (urticaria pigmentosa), or systemic with organ infiltration, presenting as hepatosplenomegaly and with signs of systemic histamine release (abdominal pain, peptic ulcer, hypotension, flushing).

KEY SIGN

Angioedema: *Pathophysiology:* Localized opening of endothelial tight junctions leads to interstitial edema in the deep layer of the skin and subcutaneous tissues. The syndrome may be related to immunoglobulin (Ig) E-mediated allergy, complement activation, or nonimmunologic mast cell activation, or it may be idiopathic. Single or multiple pruritic nonpitting swellings appear on the face, tongue, larynx, hands, feet, and/or genitalia that subside with or without treatment. Nausea, vomiting, and diarrhea may be seen with gastrointestinal involvement. Laryngeal angioedema can cause fatal airway obstruction.

✓ *ANGIOEDEMA—CLINICAL OCCURRENCE:* *IgE Mediated* hymenoptera stings, drugs (e.g., penicillin and other antibiotics), food allergens (e.g., peanuts, shellfish), foreign proteins used therapeutically, many others; *Non-IgE Mediated* angiotensin-converting enzyme inhibitors, radiologic contrast agents, cold exposure; *Complement Mediated* hereditary angioedema (C1-esterase deficiency), serum sickness, vasculitis.

KEY SIGN

Dry Skin: Xerosis and Anhydrosis: *Pathophysiology:* Loss of adequate sebaceous and/or sweat gland function lead to excessive drying of the skin. The skin is dry, often cracked and leathery in texture. Paradoxically, xerotic skin is more permeable to water because it lacks the normal protective oils.

✓ *CLINICAL OCCURRENCE:* Ichthyosis, anticholinergic drugs, denervation in peripheral neuropathies such as diabetes.

KEY SIGN

Decreased Skin Turgor: Extracellular Fluid Deficit: *Pathophysiology:* Loss of extracellular fluid leads to increased viscosity of the interstitial space fluid. The turgor of the skin is decreased with losses of extracellular fluid volume. It should not be confused with a decrease in cutaneous elastic tissue (see *Decreased Skin Elasticity* below). In evaluating for dehydration, check the lying, sitting, and standing blood pressure and pulse for postural changes; check for loss of skin turgor and longitudinal furrowing of the tongue. Loss of total body water does not result in loss of skin turgor. Technically, the term *dehydration* (loss of water) is an inaccurate description of this condition.

KEY SIGN

Decreased Skin Elasticity: *Pathophysiology:* Destruction or disruption of the elastic fibers in the skin results in decreased elasticity. Decreased elasticity is evident with wrinkling and redundancy of the skin.

✓ *CLINICAL OCCURRENCE:* Sun exposure (solar elastosis), senile cutaneous atrophy, excessive stretching of the skin (e.g., pregnancy, obesity), glucocorticoid excess (Cushing syndrome), pseudoxanthoma elasticum.

KEY SIGN

Cutaneous Scars: *Pathophysiology:* Injury to the epidermis can heal without scarring, but may leave alterations in pigmentation. Injury to the elastic and collagen fibers in the dermis results in scarring. Deeper injury to the subcutaneous fat and muscle can result in visible depressions or masses. All cutaneous scars are initially raised and red; they fade through pink to a pallid hypopigmented hue over months to years as the vascularity of the fibrous tissue diminishes. Sutured wounds healing without infection produce thin scars because there is a minimum of bridging fibrosis. Wounds healing by secondary intention leave wide, inelastic scars similar to burns, but following the contour of the surgical incision. *Pattern:* The *pattern* of scarring will be indicative of the mechanism (sharp trauma, burn, excessive tension, scarification, etc.) and etiology (e.g., surgery, obesity).

KEY SIGN

Striae: *Pathophysiology:* In normal skin, stretching causes rupture of the elastic fibers in the reticular dermis. In adrenal hypercorticism, the epidermis itself becomes fragile and easily breaks under normal tension. Striae are permanent even after removal of the precipitating condition. *Pattern:* Multiple scars, 1–6 cm long, run axially under the epidermis. When recent, they are pink or blue; older scars are silvery. They occur in skin regions under chronic tension. Although striae are most common on the abdomen, deposition of adipose tissue or edema also produces them on the shoulders, thighs, and breasts. Striae should be differentiated from traumatic and therapeutic scarring, and self-inflicted injury.

✓ *CLINICAL OCCURRENCE:* Abdominal distention (pregnancy, obesity, ascites, tumors), subcutaneous edema, corticosteroid excess (Cushing syndrome usually exhibits fresh-appearing purple striae; corticosteroid therapy).

KEY SIGN

Surgical and Traumatic Scars: *Pattern:* Ask your patient to identify each scar, relating it to previous surgery or trauma. This helps to corroborate the history and provides identifying marks for the record. Without a history, the cause may only be inferred by the size, pattern, location, and contour (smooth or jagged) of the scar. The presence of suture marks indicates surgical repair of the skin, but not the depth of injury or incision. Full thickness burns cause deep, irregular, broad, inelastic scars.

Keloids: *Pathophysiology:*   In some individuals, cutaneous injury variably produces persistent raised, red, hypertrophic scars, which are called keloids. Keloids may progressively thicken over time. *Pattern:*   Keloids are more prevalent in dark-skinned persons and after complicated wounds. They can occur anywhere on the body and after seemingly minor injury.

Changes in Skin Color

Constitutive   Diffuse   Brown   Skin: Normal Melanin Pigmentation: This is the inherited constitutive skin color. The challenge is to distinguish it from acquired disorders. Persons of African descent have the greatest melanin density; lesser amounts occur, in order, from Asian Indians, Native Americans, Indonesians, Oriental Asians (Chinese and Japanese) to Western Europeans who have the least. There is also variation within anthropologic ethnic groups of related genetic background: for example, among whites, the natives of India are often very dark, while the inhabitants of the Mediterranean region are darker than the northern Europeans. Individual variation within a family is also large. DDX: The inheritance of skin color can usually be established by questioning patients or their acquaintances about the origin and appearance of their relatives.

Tattoos: Tattoos are common and indicate an increased risk for blood-borne disease if not placed using a sterile technique. Determine whether the tattoos were placed professionally or by amateurs and the degree of sterility and any sharing of instruments. Inquire about other high-risk behaviors such as intravenous drug use and high-risk sexual behaviors.

Malignant Melanoma: See page 189.

Nevi: Moles: See page 188.

Acquired   Diffuse   Brown   Skin: Melanism: *Pathophysiology:*   The mechanisms are not well known except that melanin production is stimulated by adrenocorticotropic hormone, melanocyte-stimulating hormone, and increased iron deposition in the skin. Melanism is a darkening of the skin from augmented production of melanin in the facultative pigment deposits. The brown color is diffuse, with accentuation in palmar creases, recent scars, and pressure points at elbow, knee, and knuckles. Pigmentation appears in the oral mucosa (this is abnormal when found in whites). A history of a definite onset establishes that the pigmentation was acquired. Its presence should prompt an intensive search underlying disease.

✓*MELANISM—CLINICAL OCCURRENCE:* *Congenital* hemochromato-sis, porphyria, alkaptonuria; *Endocrine* Addison disease, Nelson syndrome, Graves disease, hypothyroidism, pregnancy (melasma—primarily on the face), contraceptive hormones; *Infectious* Whipples disease; *Inflammatory/Immunologic* scleroderma; *Metabolic/Toxic* cirrhosis, pernicious anemia, B_{12} and folic acid deficiency, drugs (busulfan, arsenicals, dibromomannitol); *Neoplastic* hormone-secreting neoplasms; *Psychosocial* tanning.

KEY SIGN
Acquired Diffuse Brown Skin: Hemochromatosis: The actual color may be bronze, blue-gray, brown, or black, accentuated in the flexor folds, the nipples, recent scars, and in parts exposed to the sun. The pigment is caused by melanin, although hemosiderin is also increased. Skin color change may antedate the hepatic cirrhosis and diabetes mellitus by several years.

KEY SIGN
Skin Color Change: Blue-Grey Color: Deposition of foreign substances discolors the skin. Also, increased concentration of unsaturated or abnormal hemoglobin in the cutaneous vessels gives *cyanosis* (see page 159).

✓*CLINICAL OCCURRENCE:* Use of amiodarone or minocycline; deposition of silver (argyria), gold, or bismuth salts; hemochromatosis, cyanosis, sulfhemoglobinemia, methemoglobinemia arsenic poisoning.

Acquired Diffuse Blue-Gray Skin: Silver (Argyria): Silver salts from ingestion or intranasal absorption may be deposited in the skin to produce a blue-gray or slate color, accentuated in the areas exposed to sunlight. The mucosa and nail lunulae may be deposit sites. The pigmentation may appear years after exposure.

Acquired Spotted Blue-Gray Skin: Arsenic: The ingestion of arsenic, therapeutically or as chronic poisoning, produces a diffuse gray background with superimposed dark macules 2–10 mm in diameter. This is often accompanied by punctate hyperkeratoses of the palms and soles. The skin manifestations may appear from 1–10 years after ingestion of the chemical.

Blue-Gray Skin: Alkaptonuria (Ochronosis): *Pathophysiology:* This is an inherited metabolic error of homogentisic acid oxidase leading to appearance of black polymers of homogentisic acid in the connective tissues and in the urine. The black accumulations shine through the skin, giving a faint blue-gray color to the skin, especially over the pinnae, the tip of the nose, and in the sclerae. The blackened extensor tendons of the hands may shine through the skin. Often a dark butterfly pattern will appear on the face; the axillae and genitalia will be pigmented.

Acquired Blue-Gray Skin: Gold (Chrysoderma):
Occasionally, the parenteral administration of gold salts to treat rheumatoid arthritis causes a blue-gray pigmentation of the periocular skin and regions exposed to the sun.

KEY SIGN

Acquired Diffuse Yellow Skin: Jaundice (Icterus, Bilirubinemia):   See *Jaundice*, Chapter 9, page 539.

KEY SIGN

Acquired Diffuse Yellow Skin: Carotenemia:
Pathophysiology: The carotene surplus occurs (a) from excessive ingestion of the pigment in oranges, mangos, apricots, carrots, and all green vegetables or (b) when the liver fails to metabolize the carotene in myxedema and diabetes mellitus. Excessive deposition of carotene appears as yellowness of the skin, especially on the forehead, the nasolabial folds, behind the ears, and in the palms and soles [Mazzone A, Canton AD. Hypercarotenemia. *N Engl J Med* 2002;346:821 (picture)].

Acquired Diffuse Yellow Skin: Quinacrine (Atabrine), Dinitrophenol, Tetryl: The ingestion of quinacrine, an antimalarial suppressant and a therapeutic agent for discoid lupus erythematosus and polymorphous light eruptions, produces a greenish-yellow skin. A similar discoloration occurs from contact with dinitrophenol and tetryl, both used in the manufacture of explosives.

KEY SIGN

Skin Color Change: Erythema: Erythema is a diffuse reddening of the skin caused by dilation of the cutaneous vasculature; it is often accompanied by increased skin temperature. The borders are not discrete.

✓ *ERYTHEMA—CLINICAL OCCURRENCE:*   Local inflammatory lesions, local infection (e.g., cellulitis, lymphangitis), scarlet fever, scarlatiniform drug eruptions, polycythemia, porphyria, pellagra, lupus erythematosus, first-degree burns. Transient erythema occurs in blushing and in some cases of metastatic carcinoid.

KEY SIGN

Skin Color Change: Depigmentation: Loss of normal skin pigmentation may be patchy or diffuse, usually with discrete borders. The distribution and pattern of depigmentation is important in identification of the specific etiology.

✓ *DEPIGMENTATION—CLINICAL OCCURRENCE:*   Vitiligo, tinea versicolor, albinism, scars, stria, and sites of subcutaneous steroid injection.

KEY SIGN

Skin Color Change: Hyperpigmentation: Increased melanin deposition in the skin can result from either local or systemic factors.

✓*HYPERPIGMENTATION—CLINICAL OCCURRENCE:* Addison disease, hemochromatosis, porphyria, arsenic poisoning, progressive systemic sclerosis (scleroderma), sun exposure, chronic local irritation from burning or scratching.

KEY SIGN
Skin Color Change: Acanthosis Nigricans: Hyperpigmented lesions with a velvety texture are most commonly seen on the neck, axillae, and other body folds. They are asymptomatic.

✓*CLINICAL OCCURRENCE:* *Congenital* hereditary benign; *Endocrine* diabetes, increased androgens, acromegaly, Cushing syndrome, Addison disease, insulin resistance syndromes, hypothyroidism; *Metabolic/Toxic* obesity, drug induced, for example, nicotinic acid, glucocorticoids; *Neoplastic* paraneoplastic with adenocarcinomas or lymphoma.

Changes in the Hair

Excessive hair growth is termed *hypertrichosis* or *hirsutism.* This may occur locally over a nevus or generally. The presence of less hair than normal is *hypotrichosis,* as in some congenital ectodermal defects.

KEY SIGN
Alopecia: *Alopecia* is the loss of hair in either congenital or acquired conditions.

✓*CLINICAL OCCURRENCE:* Physiologic baldness in the male, alopecia areata, hypothyroidism, thallium intoxication, scleroderma drugs.

S KEY SYNDROME
Alopecia Areata: *Pathophysiology:* This is thought to be an autoimmune phenomenon, but the exact pathophysiology is uncertain. Sudden loss of hair may be associated with emotional disturbances or infections, but can occur without associated illness. There is painless loss of hair in patches or complete denudation of body without other visible changes to the skin.

KEY SIGN
Graying of the Hair: Canities: Loss of pigmentation in the hair is a normal event; the age of occurrence is variable and to some extent familial.

✓*CLINICAL OCCURRENCE:* Normal aging, premature aging syndromes, pernicious anemia, chloroquine therapy; localized graying occurs in vitiliginous lesions.

KEY SIGN
Hirsutism and Hypertrichosis: *Pathophysiology:* True hirsutism is excess growth of terminal hairs from androgen-sensitive pilosebaceous units. It may result from excess androgen secretion or genetically determined increased androgen sensitivity. Hirsutism is especially distressing to women, as the hair tends to grow in a masculine pattern, including hair on the face, shoulders, back, chest, abdomen,

thighs, and buttocks. The challenge is to discern normal variants from the rare, potentially morbid causes of excess androgen. *Hypertrichosis* is excess "nonsexual" hair growth. The hairs are of the vellus type and cover the body evenly.

✓ *CLINICAL OCCURRENCE: Hirsutism* androgen-secreting tumors, polycystic ovary, late-onset congenital adrenal hyperplasia, glucocorticoid excess, prolactinemia, carcinoma, drugs (e.g., certain oral contraceptives, testosterone, anabolic steroids); *Hypertrichosis* congenital, anorexia nervosa, hypothyroidism, dermatomyositis, malnutrition, drugs (minoxidil, phenytoin, hydrocortisone, cyclosporine, penicillamine, and streptomycin) [Gilchrist VJ, Hecht BR. A practical approach to hirsutism. *Am Fam Physician* 1995;52:1837–1844].

Nail Signs

Absence of Nails: As a congenital anomaly, the nails may fail to develop; sometimes this is associated with ichthyosis. A traumatized nail may be shed and damage to the matrix may prevent regrowth.

Malnourished Nails: The nails grow slowly or not at all. They are dry, brittle, and contain transverse ridges. Later, they become thickened.

KEY SIGN

Irregular, Short Nails: Bitten Nails: The free edge of the nail plate may be absent from the nervous habit of biting the nails (Fig. 6-12A).

Square, Round Nail Plates: Acromegaly and Cretinism: Disproportionate growth may produce nail plates more wide than long.

Long, Narrow Nail Plates: Eunuchoidism and Hypopituitarism: The nails are longer and narrower than usual and may resemble those in Marfan syndrome.

Brittle Nail Plates: Onychorrhexis: The cut edges of the various keratin layers may be laminated and present a step-like appearance. Borders may be frayed and torn (see Fig. 6-12B).

✓ *CLINICAL OCCURRENCE:*   Malnutrition, iron deficiency, thyrotoxicosis, or calcium deficit; many times the cause is unknown.

Friable Nail Plates: X-ray Irradiation: The edges may be frayed, the growth stunted. They are often softened (see Fig. 6-12D).

Longitudinal Ridging in Nail Plate: Reedy Nail:
An exaggeration of normal, it has been attributed to many conditions, but the diagnostic significance is meager (see Fig. 6-12C).

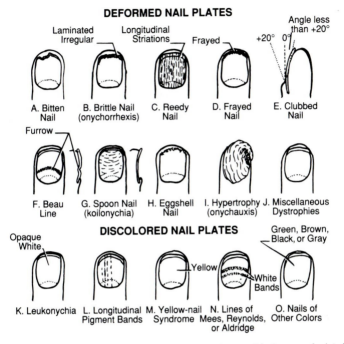

DEFORMED NAIL PLATES

A. Bitten Nail — Laminated Irregular
B. Brittle Nail (onychorrhexis) — Longitudinal Striations
C. Reedy Nail
D. Frayed Nail — Frayed
E. Clubbed Nail — Angle less than +20°, +20°, 0°

F. Beau Line — Furrow
G. Spoon Nail (koilonychia)
H. Eggshell Nail
I. Hypertrophy (onychauxis)
J. Miscellaneous Dystrophies

DISCOLORED NAIL PLATES

K. Leukonychia — Opaque White
L. Longitudinal Pigment Bands
M. Yellow-nail Syndrome — Yellow
N. Lines of Mees, Reynolds, or Aldridge — White Bands
O. Nails of Other Colors — Green, Brown, Black, or Gray

Fig. 6-12 Diagnosis of Fingernail Lesions I. *Many nail lesions are depicted here. It is necessary to know whether the lesion is in the nail plate or in the nail bed. The distinction can usually be made by noting if the abnormal color is changed by pressure on the nail plate, indicating a lesion of the nail bed. See text for descriptions.*

KEY SIGN

Transverse Furrow in Nail Plate: Beau Line: The matrix may form a transverse indentation in the nail plate during a severe illness or following chemotherapy. As the nail elongates, the furrow moves into view from beneath the mantle, progresses distally, and is finally pared off (see Fig. 6-12F).

KEY SIGN

Concave Nail Plate: Spoon Nails (Koilony-chia): The natural convexity is replaced by concave, saucer nails (see Fig. 6-12G). Often the nail plate is thinned.

✓ *CLINICAL OCCURRENCE:* Most often encountered in iron deficiency; rarely, encountered in rheumatic fever, lichen planus, and syphilis.

Concave Nail Plate: Eggshell Nails: The nail plate is thinned and its free edge is curved sharply outward from the digit (see Fig. 6-12H). The cause is obscure; it has sometimes been ascribed to a deficit in vitamin A.

Hypertrophy of the Nail Plates: Onychauxis:
The nail plate becomes greatly thickened by piling up of irregular keratin layers (see Fig. 6-12I). It may be familial or the result of chronic fungal infections.

KEY SIGN
Nail Pitting: Psoriasis: Occasional pits in the nails are normal. Large numbers of pits are seen in psoriasis, especially psoriatic arthritis; other skin signs may be absent.

Dystrophy of the Nail Plates: Under this head are grouped many ill-defined changes including opacities, furrowing, ridging, pitting, splitting, and fraying, all testaments to poor nail growth (see Fig. 6-12J).

✓ *CLINICAL OCCURRENCE:*   Chronic infections of the nails, lesions of the nerves supplying the limb, vascular deficits of the extremity, amyloidosis, and the collagen diseases.

White Nail Plates: Partial Leukonychia: Irregular white areas in the nail plates are common and are not diagnostically significant.

White Nail Plates: Total Leukonychia: The nail plates are completely chalk white (see Fig. 6-12K). The condition is inherited as a dominant character with varying penetrance.

Transverse White Banded Nail Plates: Lines of Mees, Reynolds, or Aldrich: The nail plates contain transverse white bands that are laid down during a generalized illness or poisoning. The formation ceases with recovery, producing a white band that moves distally with growth of the nail plate (see Fig. 6-12N). The bands are probably evidence of a lesser degree of injury than Beau lines.

✓ *CLINICAL OCCURRENCE:*   Poisoning (arsenic, thallium, and fluoride), chemotherapy, infectious fevers including malaria and pneumonia, and other illnesses such as renal insufficiency, cardiac failure, myocardial infarction, Hodgkin disease, and sickle cell anemia.

Yellow Nail Plates: Yellow-Nail Syndrome:
Pathophysiology: The disorder results from impeded lymphatic circulation and often antedates lymphedema elsewhere. The nail plates become yellow or yellow-green, thicken, and grow more slowly (see Fig. 6-12M) with excessive transverse curvature. Occasionally, ridging and onycholysis occur.

Discolored Nail Plates: Miscellaneous Varieties: Various drugs, infections, and stains occasionally color the

DISCOLORED NAIL BEDS

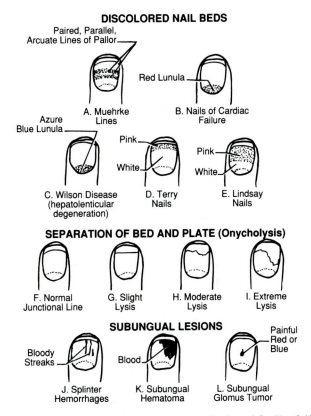

Paired, Parallel, Arcuate Lines of Pallor

A. Muehrke Lines

Red Lunula

B. Nails of Cardiac Failure

Azure Blue Lunula

C. Wilson Disease (hepatolenticular degeneration)

Pink

White

D. Terry Nails

Pink

White

E. Lindsay Nails

SEPARATION OF BED AND PLATE (Onycholysis)

F. Normal Junctional Line

G. Slight Lysis

H. Moderate Lysis

I. Extreme Lysis

SUBUNGUAL LESIONS

Bloody Streaks

J. Splinter Hemorrhages

Blood

K. Subungual Hematoma

Painful Red or Blue

L. Subungual Glomus Tumor

Fig. 6-13 Diagnosis of Fingernail Lesions II. *See legend for Fig. 6-12.*

nail plates (see Fig. 6-12O), the color giving a clue to etiology: blue-green = infection with *Pseudomonas;* brown-yellow = ingestion of phenindione; brown or black = fungal infections, fluorosis, quinacrine; and blue-gray = argyria.

White Proximal Nail Beds: Terry Nails: The mechanism is unknown. The proximal 80% or more of the nail bed is white (Fig. 6-13D), leaving a distal band of normal pink. The nail findings are associated with hepatic cirrhosis.

White Proximal Nail Beds: Half-and-Half Nail (Lindsay Nails): Somewhat similar in appearance to Terry nails, the proximal 40–80% of the nail beds is white but the distal portion is red, pink, or brown (see Fig. 6-13E). The colored portion is sharply demarcated, usually by a curved line parallel to the free edge of the nail plates. Constriction of the venous return deepens the color of the distal portion, but only a slight pink is induced in the proximal bed. Most patients have renal disease, usually advanced [Lindsay PG. The half-and-half nail. *Arch Intern Med* 1967;119:583–587].

White Banded Nail Beds: Muehrcke Lines in Hypoalbuminemia: Paired, narrow, arcuate bands of pallor, parallel to the lunulae, appear in the nail beds (see Fig. 6-13A). They occur during periods of hypoalbuminemia (less than 2.0 g/dL) and resolve when the deficit has been corrected. Because they are not in the nail plates, they do not move distally with nail growth [Muehrcke RC. The fingernails in chronic hypoalbuminaemia. *Br Med J* 1956;1:1327–1328].

Red Half-Moons in Nail Beds: Nails of Cardiac Failure: Red lunulae rather than normal white (see Fig. 6-13B) are associated with cardiac failure.

Azure Half-Moons in Nail Beds: Hepatolenticular Degeneration (Wilson Disease): The lunulae are colored light blue (see Fig. 6-13C).

KEY SIGN
Separation of the Nail: Onycholysis: Normally, the line of adhesion of plate to bed is a smooth curve (see Fig. 6-13F); in onycholysis, it separates at its free edge from the nail bed, collecting debris underneath, inaccessible to cleaning (see Fig. 6-13G-I).

✓ *CLINICAL OCCURRENCE:* Hyperthyroidism, eczematoid dermatitis, psoriasis, and mycotic diseases of the nails.

Subungual Hemorrhage: Splinter Hemorrhage: *Pathophysiology:* Bleeding from the capillaries in the nail plate is confined to the longitudinal ridges giving a longitudinal linear appearance. These lesions are asymptomatic (see Fig. 6-13J).

✓ *CLINICAL OCCURRENCE:* Trauma is most common. Local dermatologic diseases, systemic thrombotic and embolic illness can be causative (e.g., endocarditis, antiphospholipid syndrome, vasculitis).

KEY SIGN
Subungual Hemorrhage: Subungual Hematoma: This traumatic lesion is intensely painful; relief of pain is achieved either by dissection of the hemorrhage to the distal nail plate (resulting in lifting and subsequent loss of the nail) or by therapeutic drainage through the nail plate to preserve the nail.

KEY SIGN
Subungual Pigmentation: Ungual Melanoma: An unusual location for malignant melanoma (2.5% of melanomas), ungual melanoma is most frequently found under the nails of the thumb or great toe. Its characteristic sign is leaching of melanin from under the

nail to its border and into the paronychial area [Levit EK, Kagen MH, Scher RK, et al. The ABC rule for clinical detection of subungual melanoma. *J Am Acad Dermatol* 2000;42:269–274].

Painful Red or Violet Subungual Spot: Glomus Tumor: Tumors arising from sensory glomus bodies are especially common in the nail bed, where they are exquisitely painful. It is seen through the nail plate as a round red or violet spot (Fig. 6-13L). It resembles a hemangioma, but the latter is not tender.

Foot and Toenail Signs

Certain lesions of the feet and toenails need special mention.

KEY SIGN
Thickening of Skin: Callus: *Pathophysiology:*   A well circumscribed area of thickened epidermal keratin develops at locations of repeated pressure or friction. It is normal under the first and fifth metatarsal heads and the heel. Occurrence at other locations, usually with a decrease in the normal callosities, indicates unusual distributions of weight, or pressure from footwear. Calluses are infrequently painful in themselves, but pressure on underlying structures, especially periosteum, may cause pain. Hard callus transmits pressure from footwear to the underlying soft tissues impinged between the callus and the underlying bone.

KEY SIGN
Hard Corn (Heloma Durum):   Undue pressure on thin skin, especially that covering the toes, produces a conical structure of keratin pointing into the dermis, where it causes pain. It has a central core that can be seen when the top is pared away.

KEY SIGN
Soft Corn (Heloma Mollis):   This is a corn on an interdigital surface that undergoes maceration from moisture and infection. It is quite painful.

KEY SIGN
Sharply Circumscribed Thickening of the Sole: Plantar Wart (Verruca Pedis):   This wart is caused by human papilloma virus infection. The verrucous nature may not be apparent because it is overlaid with callus. The lesions are frequently multiple. Viewed through the callus, black spots of hemorrhage may appear as dark pearls. Pruritus is frequent and weight bearing causes pain. Direct pressure does not yield tenderness, but pinching from the sides is painful.

KEY SIGN
Ulcer of the Sole: Perforating Neurotrophic Ulcer: *Pathophysiology:*   Normal pressure and pain sensation are essential to protect the foot from excessive and prolonged pressure over boney prominences. In the insensitive foot (e.g., diabetic neuropathy)

this pressure can lead to painless ischemic necrosis of the soft tissue, infection, and/or ulceration. A punched-out, indolent, painless ulcer occurs under a metatarsal head, at the tip of the toe, over the proximal interphalangeal joint of a hammertoe or on the heel. Test for sensation to pressure by using graded monofilament (page 820) [Sumpio BE. Foot ulcers. *N Engl J Med* 2000;343:787–793; Caputo GM, Cavanagh PR, Ulbrecht JS, et al. Assessment and management of foot disease in patients with diabetes. *N Engl J Med* 1994;331:854–860; Grayson ML, Gibbons GW, Balogh K, et al. Probing to bone in infected pedal ulcers: A clinical sign of underlying osteomyelitis in diabetic patients. *JAMA* 1995;273:721–723; Edelman D, Hough DM, Glazebrook KN, Oddone EZ. Prognostic value of the clinical examination of the diabetic foot ulcer. *J Gen Intern Med* 1997;12:537–543].

Subungual Pain: Ingrown Toenail (Onychocryptosis): Usually the lateral nail fold of the great toe is affected. Excessive transverse growth of the nail plate causes the lateral edge to lacerate the nail fold. An ulcer is formed and maintained by repeated trauma and infection. Weight bearing is painless, but any pressure on the nail plate, as from shoe or sock, elicits tenderness. Exuberant granulation tissue may form in the nail fold.

Subungual Pain: Subungual Exostosis: The great toe is usually involved. An exostosis arises from the dorsal surface of the distal phalanx to penetrate the distal half of the nail bed and subsequently the nail plate itself. Early, a painless discoloration under the nail is visible; later, the nail is pushed upward and split. The protruding surface becomes covered with granulations that form painful ulcers.

Overgrowth of the Toenail: Ram's Horn Nail (Onychogryposis): The nail becomes thickened, conical, and curved like a ram's horn; it may assume grotesque shape and size.

Vascular Signs

Some disorders of dermal vessels furnish signs of generalized disease; these are considered together with local abnormalities, from which they must be distinguished. The selected lesions contain enough blood that their red or blue color readily identifies them as vascular disorders.

KEY SIGN

Pallor: Pallor is the lack of the normal red color imparted to the skin and mucous membranes by the blood in the superficial vessels. Skin color is modified by the thickness of the avascular epidermis and the amount of melanin and other pigments in the dermis. Inspection for generalized pallor is always supplemented by observing the color of the conjunctivae, the oral mucosa and palmar creases. In deeply pigmented persons, these may be the only reliable physical signs. Pallor can be produced by edema or myxedematous tissue surrounding the superficial blood vessels, vasoconstriction, anemia, or any combination.

✓*PALLOR—CLINICAL OCCURRENCE*: *Localized Pallor* cold exposure, vasoconstriction (e.g., Raynaud phenomenon), arterial insufficiency (narrowed lumina, thrombosis, embolism), edema; *Generalized Pallor generalized vasoconstriction*—exposure to cold, severe pain, hypoglycemia, volume depletion or low cardiac output syndrome; *chronic pallor*—normal in some persons, anemia, renal failure (anemia may contribute); *Paroxysmal Pallor* apneic periods in periodic breathing, hypertensive periods from pheochromocytoma, vertiginous periods in Ménière disease, migraine; *Obscuration of Skin Vessels* edema, myxedema (anemia may contribute), scleroderma.

KEY SIGN

Cyanosis: *Pathophysiology:* Cyanosis is the blue color seen through the skin and mucous membranes when the reduced hemoglobin concentrations in capillary blood exceed 4.0–5.0 g/dL, 0.5–1.5 g of methemoglobin, or 0.5 g of sulfhemoglobin. The amount of oxyhemoglobin does not affect the color. Local cyanosis occurs when blood is deoxygenated in the vessels in venous stasis or in the tissues from extravasation. Many normal persons have localized venous stasis in some parts of the body. Generalized cyanosis is seen in the lips, nail beds, ears, and malar regions. DDX: Central cyanosis usually becomes more prominent with exertion or exposure to a warm environment, but peripheral cyanosis does not. Because the blue color is within the venules, capillaries, and arterioles of the subpapillary plexus, it fades with superficial pressure, distinguishing it from argyria.

✓*CYANOSIS—CLINICAL OCCURRENCE*: *Local Cyanosis* localized venous stasis or arterial obstructions, Raynaud phenomenon, extravasations of blood in superficial tissues; *Central Cyanosis* hypoxemia (right-to-left shunt, impaired oxygenation as a result of lung disorders), presence of abnormal hemoglobin pigments (methemoglobin or sulfhemoglobin); *Peripheral Cyanosis* (implies normal arterial oxygen concentration but increased oxygen extraction because of sluggish flow in the capillaries of the cutaneous vessels) cutaneous vasoconstriction secondary to cold exposure, reflex response to decreased cardiac output.

KEY SIGN

Abnormal Nail Fold Capillaries: Scleroderma: Episodic digital vasospasm is common in scleroderma (Raynaud phenomena) or in otherwise normal persons (Raynaud disease). Finding abnormal nail fold capillaries is strongly associated with later appearance of scleroderma.

KEY SIGN

Intradermal Hemorrhage: *Pathophysiology:* In general, mucocutaneous bleeding occurs with platelet abnormalities (number or function) or problems of the vessel wall (e.g., scurvy); bleeding into joints or viscera is more likely related to clotting factor deficiencies or inhibitors. Extravasation of blood in the skin produces an area that is first red, then blue; in a few days, the degradation of hemoglobin changes the color to green or yellow and fades. Because the blood in the area is extravascular, the color does not blanch with pressure. A *petechia* (plural, petechiae) is a round, discrete hemorrhagic area less than 2 mm in diameter. Doubtful spots can be circled with ink; their disappearance in a few days rules out angioma. A larger spot is an *ecchymosis* (plural, ecchymoses). When hemorrhages of either size occur in groups, the condition is termed *purpura*. Purpuric lesions may become confluent and they usually do not elevate the skin or mucosa. Spontaneous purpura from platelet or vessel defects usually occurs on the lower extremities, although slight trauma to the skin may induce it elsewhere. A **hematoma** is an area in which underlying hemorrhage causes elevation of the skin or mucosa; extravasated blood frequently colors the surface and dissects along tissue planes. DDX: When the capillaries are involved by infectious disease, the resulting purpura may predominate on the thorax and abdomen. *Palpable purpura* suggests a cutaneous or systemic vasculitis; larger nodules may be palpable in polyarteritis nodosa. In subacute bacterial endocarditis, isolated petechiae from bacterial emboli may occur anywhere. In the skin, they may be distinguished from small angiomas by not blanching under pressure. Septic emboli frequently appear in the mucosa of the palate, buccal surfaces, and conjunctiva, where changes in color during resolution are not evident; in the conjunctiva, the petechiae sometimes have gray centers.

✓ **INTRADERMAL HEMORRHAGE—CLINICAL OCCURRENCE:** *Vascular Abnormalities* eroded or traumatized large vessels, hereditary hemorrhagic telangiectasia, vasculitis, infections (Rocky Mountain spotted fever), scurvy, Schamberg disease, Cushing syndrome; *Blood Abnormalities quantitative platelet defects* (e.g., autoimmune thrombocytopenic purpura, heparin-induced thrombocytopenia, hypersplenism), *qualitative platelet defects* (e.g. aspirin, von Willebrand disease, Glanzmann syndrome), thrombotic thrombocytopenic purpura, bone marrow failure (e.g., aplastic anemia, leukemia, chemotherapy), meningococcemia, cryoglobulinemia, disseminated intravascular coagulation.

S KEY SYNDROME

Purpura, Abdominal Pain and Arthralgia: Schönlein-Henoch Purpura (Anaphylactoid Purpura): See Chapter 8, page 473. This vasculitis is most commonly encountered in children, often coincident with streptococcal infections. A purpuric rash occurs in association with urticaria, arthralgias, abdominal pain, gastrointestinal blood loss, nausea and vomiting, and glomerulitis. The platelet count remains normal. The disease is self-limited in children; corticosteroids are believed helpful in severe cases.

S KEY SYNDROME

Dermal Hemorrhage: Immune Thrombocytopenic Purpura (ITP): *Pathophysiology:* Immunologic destruction of platelets leads to thrombocytopenia and increased size of circulating platelets; the bone marrow shows hyperplasia of megakaryocytes. Easy bruising, petechiae, menorrhagia, epistaxis, or other mucocutaneous bleeding signals the onset of ITP. The spleen is not palpable. Children with acute ITP frequently recover without treatment. Adults with very low platelet counts are at risk for intracranial hemorrhage and are more likely to develop chronic thrombocytopenia. DDX: The history, physical exam, and selected tests should exclude lupus erythematosus, HIV infections, cytomegalovirus, Epstein-Barr virus, drug-induced thrombocytopenia, hypersplenism, malignant lymphoma, and other hematologic disorders.

D KEY DISEASE

Dermal Hemorrhage: Scurvy: Punctate hemorrhages may occur in the skin; they are distinguishable from the usual petechiae by being perifollicular. The lesions are most common in the lower extremities. Close inspection discloses that each petechia surrounds a hair follicle. The hair is abnormal being tightly coiled. Mucous membrane bleeding and loosening of the teeth also occur.

D KEY DISEASE

▶ **Dermal Hemorrhage: Rocky Mountain Spotted Fever, Typhus:** *Pathophysiology:* Infection of the endothelium with *Rickettsia rickettsii* following the bite of an infected tick leads to loss of vessel integrity. On about the fourth day of fever, an eruption of erythematous blanching macules 2–6 mm in diameter appears on the wrists, ankles, palms, and soles. It spreads centripetally to the trunk, face, axillae, and buttocks. In 2 or 3 days, the lesions become maculopapular, assume a deep-red color, and finally become petechial hemorrhages that resolve with the usual color changes. DDX: In contrast, the eruption of **typhus fever**, with similar individual lesions, begins on the trunk and extends centrifugally, rarely involving the face, palms, or soles.

D KEY DISEASE

▶ **Dermal Hemorrhage: Meningococcemia:** Three-quarters of patients with meningococcal meningitis develop meningococcemia. The eruption involves the trunk and extremities with petechial hemorrhages, together with bright-pink, tender maculopapules 2–10 mm in diameter. Some maculopapules develop hemorrhagic centers. Large ecchymoses and hemorrhagic vesicles may form. Gangrene of soft tissues, especially fingers and toes, may occur. Livedo reticularis may be present.

S KEY SYNDROME

▶ **Dermal Hemorrhages: Disseminated Intravascular Coagulation (DIC; Consumption Coagulopathy):** *Pathophysiology:* Persistence of activated clotting factors and other procoagulants in the circulation lead to deposition of platelet-fibrin thrombi in multiple vessels with depletion of intravascular clotting factors. Simultaneous activation of the fibrinolytic system leads to dissolution of fibrin and a hemorrhagic diathesis. The onset may be sudden or gradual. It may be characterized by shock, the appearance of ecchymoses, purpura, or petechiae, fever, and bleeding from multiple sites. It usually occurs as a complication of preexisting multisystem disease.

✓ *DIC—CLINICAL OCCURRENCE:* Septicemia, malignancy (especially acute promyelocytic leukemia, certain adenocarcinomas, and sarcomas), extensive surgery, trauma, complications of pregnancy (dead fetus, amniotic fluid embolism, abruptio placenta, septic abortion, preeclampsia, and eclampsia), envenomation, hepatic failure.

S KEY SYNDROME

▼ Dermal Hemorrhages: Thrombotic Thrombocytopenic Purpura (TTP) and Hemolytic Uremic Syndrome (HUS): *Pathophysiology:* In TTP, large multimers of von Willebrand factor circulate because of a metalloprotein enzyme inhibition that appears to be immunologically mediated. Arteriolar platelet-rich thrombi produce fragmentation of circulating erythrocytes and ischemic infarcts in vital organs. The mechanism of HUS is less-well understood. Rapid diagnosis and treatment are necessary; examination of the peripheral blood smear for schistocytes is the most rapid way to establish the diagnosis. Without treatment the mortality is >90%. Most patients with **TTP** are young adults, more often women, with a history of recent viral infection. Other known risk factors are pregnancy, bee sting, AIDS, systemic lupus erythematosus (SLE), chemotherapy with mitomycin C, or recent organ transplantation. Petechiae from thrombocytopenia may be the first sign noted by the patient. The classic pentad of the syndrome is (a) thrombocytopenia, (b) microangiopathic hemolytic anemia, (c) renal insufficiency, (d) diffuse nonfocal neurologic deficits, and (e) fever, which is variably present. Headache, confusion, delirium, seizures, and other mental status changes develop in 90% of those who die. Relapses of TTP following successful treatment are common. The **hemolytic uremic syndrome (HUS)** in children produces the same arteriolar lesions and laboratory findings without signs of CNS involvement. The specific metalloprotein enzyme inhibition of TTP is not found in HUS. HUS has been reported in young children with gastroenteritis from *Escherichia coli* 0157:H7.

S KEY SYNDROME

▼ Dermal Hemorrhages: Atheroembolism: *Pathophysiology:* Embolization of cholesterol-rich contents of atherosclerotic plaques causes ischemic infarction with hemorrhage in the skin and organs distal to the site of plaque rupture. Patients frequently have had an endovascular procedure with mechanical disruption of plaques on the vessel wall. They present hours to 1–2 days later with pain and erythema followed by retiform ecchymoses and palpable purpura, which may progress to frank infarction [O'Keefe ST, Woods BO'B, Breslin DJ, Tsapatsaris NP. Blue toes syndrome: Causes and management. *Arch Intern Med* 1992;152:2197–2202].

Dermal Hemorrhages: Schamberg Disease (Progressive Pigmentary Dermatosis): A benign chronic disorder, whose cause is unknown, with repeated crops of petechiae and orange to fawn-colored macules on feet and legs.

Pink Papules: Rose Spots of Typhoid Fever: These are erythematous papules, 2–4 mm in diameter, that blanch with pressure. They appear in the second week of the fever, usually in crops, but few in number. They are commonly seen on the upper abdomen and lower thorax; each lesion persists for 2 or 3 days and then disappears, leaving a faint brown stain.

Red Macule or Papule: Cherry Angioma (Papillary Angioma): Usually less than 3 mm in diameter and often no larger than a pinhead, the cherry angioma is bright red, discrete, and irregularly round. Larger lesions may be slightly elevated; occasionally they are pedunculated. The growth is surrounded by a narrow halo of pallid skin. Pressure induces only partial blanching or none. Small lesions may be distinguished from petechiae only by their permanence when observed for several days. The angiomas occur more often on the thorax and arms than on the face and abdomen; they are less frequent on the forearms and on the lower extremities. With advancing age, some lesions become atrophic and faded. Everyone has a few; the number increases after the age of 30 years. They have no clinical significance.

Blue Papule: Venous Lakes: Thin-walled papules are filled with venous blood. Gentle pressure forces them to empty, leaving lax indentations beneath skin level. They rarely occur before the age of 35 years; their numbers increase with age. They are 10 times more common in men than in women. They are more frequent on the ears and face than on the lips and neck; they are uncommon elsewhere. Aging is the only condition with which they are associated.

Blue Papules: Scrotal Venous Angioma (Fordyce Lesion): See Fig. 6-14B and Chaper 12, page 665.

D KEY DISEASE
▼ **Punctate Macules: Hereditary Hemorrhagic Telangiectasia (Osler-Weber-Rendu Disease):** *Pathophysiology:* The disease is hereditary, transmitted as a mendelian dominant trait. It is believed that most lesions develop after puberty. The development and regression of some individual lesions has been observed, although most lesions are probably permanent. Affected children often have repeated epistaxis before diagnostic lesions appear in the skin and mucosa. The first glance at the patient often discloses a pale face, caused by anemia from continual gastrointestinal blood loss, spotted with dull red lesions. The average lesion is punctate, about 1–2 mm in diameter. Usually, it is not elevated; some appear

slightly depressed. The overlying skin may be covered with a fine silvery scale. Pressure causes fading, although blanching is incomplete in some. Through a compressing glass slide, the spots may be seen to pulsate. Occasionally, one or two fine, superficial vessels may radiate from the punctum, but the radicles in arterial spiders are more numerous and the centers smaller. The mucosa is practically always involved; lesions are almost invariably found in the Kiesselbach area on the anterior portion of the nasal septum, giving rise to frequent epistaxis, for which the disease is famous. The tip and dorsum of the tongue are favorite sites. Most frequently affected in the skin are the palmar surfaces of the hands and fingers, the skin under the nail plates, the lips, ears, face, arms, and toes. The trunk is least involved. Because any structure may be the site of these lesions, bleeding may cause epistaxis, hemoptysis, hematemesis, melena, or hematuria. There is a high incidence of pulmonary arteriovenous fistulas, which can lead to polycythemia and clubbing of the fingers [Guttmacher AE, Marchuk DA, White RI Jr. Hereditary hemorrhagic telangiectasia. *N Engl J Med* 1995;333:918–924].

Blue Nodule: Rubber-Bleb Nevi of Skin and Gastrointestinal Tract: There are three types of lesions: a large disfiguring angioma, a fluctuant thin-skinned bleb containing blood that leaves a rumpled sac when compression empties it into venous channels, and an irregular blue area that gradually merges with the surrounding skin, fading only partially with pressure. Nevi of the skin may be accompanied by similar lesions in the gastrointestinal tract that are sites of serious hemorrhage. The dermal lesions may be few, or they may be scattered throughout the body. The condition is not hereditary.

Painful Red or Blue Nodule: Glomus Tumor: *Pathophysiology:* This a benign neoplasm, thought to arise from the pericyte in the vessel walls of the glomus body. The lesions are more common in the hands and fingers, especially beneath the nail (Fig. 6-14C). The red or blue tumor is an elevated nodule, from 2–10 mm in diameter. It is exquisitely painful, completely disproportionate to its size. The pain may occur in paroxysms. The physician should learn to suspect a small spot that is very painful, because relief must be obtained by surgical excision.

S KEY SYNDROME

Irregular Spongy Tumor: Cavernous Hemangioma: *Pathophysiology:* The tumor occurs in any tissue and varies in size from microscopic to huge, where an entire extremity may be involved. Usually present at birth, it tends to enlarge with age. The tumor may involve skin, subcutaneous tissue, muscle, and even bone. The surface presents an irregular nodular mass, frequently bluish, and fluctuant. Raising the involved extremity above heart level may result in partial emptying. A patient of ours pooled enough blood in a lower-extremity tumor to cause dyspnea and tachycardia in the erect

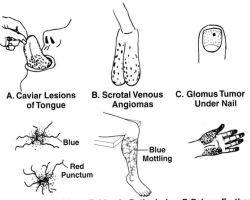

A. Caviar Lesions of Tongue

B. Scrotal Venous Angiomas

C. Glomus Tumor Under Nail

Blue

Red Punctum

D. Arterial Spider

Blue Mottling

E. Livedo Reticularis

F. Palmar Erythema

Fig. 6-14 Some Named Superficial Vascular Lesions. A. Caviar Lesions of the Tongue: Varicose veins under the tongue form bluish masses that appear as bunches of caviar. B. Scrotal Venous Angiomas: When the scrotum is spread out, multiple papules may be demonstrated, 3–4 mm in diameter, dark red or blue. C. Glomus Tumor Under the Nail: An elevated nodule, 2–10 mm in diameter, may occur any place in the skin, frequently under the nail plate. It is extremely painful. D. Venous Stars and Arterial Spiders: One form of venous star is depicted; the lesions may also appear as cascades, flares, rockets, comets, or tangles. A typical form of arterial spider, with punctum and radicles, is presented. While venous stars are bluish, spiders are fiery red. Both lesions fade with pressure. Pressing the center with a pencil tip will not blanch the branches of a star; the radicles of the spiders will fade with pressure on the punctum. The star always overlies a large vein; the spider is not associated with a visible large vessel. As seen through a pressing glass slide, the venous star does not pulsate; the arterial spider fills from the center with pulsatile spurts. E. Livedo Reticularis: Seen most often on the legs, the skin is mottled, with deeply cyanosed areas interspersed with round pale spots. In one type, the discoloration disappears with warming; in others, it does not. F. Palmar Erythema: An intense diffuse erythema occurs, which is deepest over the hypothenar eminence and less pronounced on the thenar eminence and the distal segments of the fingers. The erythema is not mottled.

position; this was relieved by a compression bandage on the tumor. The hemangioma may consume platelets and procoagulants to produce a picture of disseminated intravascular coagulation (*Kasabach-Merritt syndrome*).

Pulsating Tumor: Cirsoid Aneurysm: A cavernous angioma-eroding bone may form a congenital arteriovenous fistula. The overlying subcutaneous tissue is swollen into a visible pulsatile tumor that writhes like a nest of snakes.

Stellate Figure: Venous Star: The lesion occurs as part of the aging process or as a result of venous obstruction. Branches of small superficial veins radiate from a central point (see Fig. 6-14D). The patterns include stars, angular Vs, cascades, flares, rockets, and tangles. The entire figure may vary from a few millimeters to several centimeters in diameter. The vessels are bluish, whereas arterial spiders are bright red. When pressed upon, the color fades; the figure refills from the center when pressure is released, as do arterial spiders. In contrast to arterial spiders, pressure on the central point with a pencil does not blanch the radicles. The figure always overlies a larger vein, whereas the spider is not associated with a larger vessel. Venous stars are more common in women. The predominant sites are the dorsum of the foot, the leg, the medial aspect of the thigh above the knee, and the back of the neck. They also occur in the skin swollen from superior vena cava obstruction. Their clinical importance is to distinguish them from arterial spiders.

KEY SIGN

Stellate Figure: Arterial Spider (Spider Angioma, Spider Telangiectasis):   *Pathophysiology:* The cause of arterial spiders is unknown. Anatomic studies demonstrate that a coiled vessel arises perpendicularly from a deep artery, its distal end forming the central body from which the legs radiate in the plane of the skin, branching and rebranching. Typically, the fiery red vascular figure in the skin consists of a central body or punctum, varying from a pinpoint to a papule, 5 mm in diameter (see Fig. 6-14D). The "body" is an arteriole from which radiates arterialized capillaries forming the "legs" (radicles) of the "spider." The vessels may dip into the tissue to reappear further on, forming short, visible segments. An area of erythema surrounds the body and extends several millimeters beyond the radicular tips. The lesion feels warmer than the surrounding skin. Rarely, the body is visibly pulsatile; occasionally the pulsation may be felt. Invariably, pressure over the body with a glass slide discloses the blood emerging from the punctum in pulses. When the body is pressed with a pencil tip, the radicles fade; they fill centrifugally when pressure is released. Spiders occur commonly on the face and neck and, in diminishing order of frequency, on the shoulders, anterior chest, back, arms, forearms, and dorsa of the hands and fingers; rarely are they found below the umbilicus. DDX: Spiders are frequently accompanied by palmar erythema in liver disease and pregnancy.

✓ *CLINICAL OCCURRENCE:*   Occasionally, in normal persons, hepatic disease, hyperestrinism, pregnancy (disappearing after delivery).

Reticular Pattern: Costal Fringe: Particularly in older men, the superficial veins near the anterior rib margins and the xiphoid process form networks, sometimes in the pattern of bands with rough correspondence to the attachments of the diaphragm. The lesion is usually associated with aging, but has been seen as evidence of collateral blood flow in a patient with superior vena cava obstruction.

Reticular Pattern: Facial Telangiectasis: The vessels of the nose and face may be dilated in older persons. They are common in rosacea and in patients with hepatic disease. Frequently, but not always, they are associated with exposure to the wind and cold, as in farmers and sailors.

Reticular Pattern: Radiation Telangiectasis: Large therapeutic doses of x-rays produce changes in the skin that occur months after exposure. The chief signs of x-ray dermatitis are pigmentation, skin atrophy, and telangiectasis; the last is the most conspicuous. Fine red or blue vessels appear in the skin, forming a disordered network. The sharp border in the shape of the radiation port establishes the artificial nature of the lesion and suggests the diagnosis.

KEY SIGN

Reticular Pattern: Livedo Reticularis: The skin of the arms and legs is mottled, with a circinate bands of cyanosis surrounding patches of normal skin (see Fig. 6-14E). Three types are described. In *cutis marmorata* the mottling appears on exposure to cold and disappears with warming. The other types persist when warmed. They are *livedo reticularis idiopathica,* which is not associated with other disease, and *livedo reticularis symptomatica,* a frequent accompaniment of the antiphospholipid syndrome, cryoglobulinemia, and polyarteritis nodosa. Ulceration is sometimes a complication of the two types that persist with warming. Livedo reticularis is also seen with embolism of cholesterol from disruption of an atherosclerotic plaque.

KEY SIGN

Diffuse: Palmar Erythema: A fixed, diffuse erythema involves the hypothenar eminence and, with less intensity, the thenar prominence (see Fig. 6-14F). In severe cases, the palmar surfaces of the terminal digits and the thumb are similarly reddened. Rarely, the normal mottling of the palms becomes accentuated and fixed.

✓ *PALMAR ERYTHEMA—CLINICAL OCCURRENCE:* Hepatic disease and pregnancy (disappearing after delivery); the incidence in both conditions closely parallels that of arterial spiders, although they may not be present in the same patient.

KEY SIGN

Generalized Erythroderma: *Pathophysiology:* Diffuse dilation of the cutaneous capillaries may result from systemic inflammation, fever, or release of bacterial toxins. The patient presents with generalized cutaneous erythema, which may be asymptomatic in benign conditions, or intensely painful and burning with systemic inflammation.

✓ *ERYTHRODERMA—CLINICAL OCCURRENCE:* Fever, viral exanthems, staphylococcal or streptococcal toxic shock syndrome, staphylococcal scalded-skin syndrome, scarlet fever, drug eruptions (exfoliative dermatitis), Stevens-Johnson syndrome, toxic epidermal necrolysis, psoriasis, cutaneous T-cell lymphoma.

S KEY SYNDROME

Paroxysmal Flushing, Blanching, and Cyanosis: Metastatic Carcinoid: *Pathophysiology:* Usually a benign tumor of the ileum, carcinoid may metastasize to the liver, where it produces excessive amounts of serotonin (5-hydroxytryptamine). Circulating serotonin causes paroxysms of erythema in the skin, intermixed with areas of pallor and cyanosis. A given area of skin may exhibit all three colors in rapid succession, a bewildering display reminding the observer of the aurora borealis. The eruption is most pronounced on the face and neck, although it may extend to the chest and abdomen. The excessive serotonin also causes hypotension, cramps in the abdomen, diarrhea, and bronchospasm. Fibrosis in the right heart may result in pulmonary stenosis, tricuspid stenosis, and tricuspid insufficiency. The diagnosis is confirmed by demonstrating an increased urinary excretion of 5-hydroxyindolacetic acid.

S KEY SYNDROME

Red Burning Extremities Erythromelalgia: *Pathophysiology:* This occurs from excessive dilatation of arteries and arterioles. The patient complains of painful red skin on the extremities, especially the feet and hands, aggravated by dependency. Ambient temperatures above 31°C (87.8°F) usually initiate the attacks; they are relieved by cold exposure. During a paroxysm, the limbs are red, warm, swollen, and painful. The arterial pulses are present and normal. DDX: Similar lesions, but not true erythromelalgia, occur with atherosclerosis, hypertension, frostbite, immersion foot, trench foot, peripheral neuritis, disseminated sclerosis, hemiplegia, chronic heavy metal poisoning and gout [Kurzrock R, Cohen PR. Erythromelalgia: Review of clinical characteristics and pathophysiology. *Am J Med* 1991;91:416–422].

✓ *ERYTHROMELALGIA—CLINICAL OCCURRENCE:* Autosomal dominant and an acquired syndrome associated with drugs (e.g., nifedipine, bromocriptine) or myeloproliferative diseases (may antedate by years polycythemia vera or essential thrombocytosis).

KEY SIGN

Subungual Hemorrhages: See page 156.

Signs of Systemic Lipid Disorders

KEY SIGN

Xanthomas: *Pathophysiology:* Systemic disorders of lipid metabolism lead to deposition of lipid in cutaneous and subcutaneous structures, including tendons. The asymptomatic lesions are macules, papules, plaques, or nodules, often brown to orange in color. The distribution of the lesions is highly suggestive of the underlying disorder.

Xanthelasma: There are soft, elevated beige-colored plaques on the eyelids, usually symmetrical, and often coalescent. This is an increasingly common condition after the sixth decade. It may occur in otherwise normal people, or be a sign of elevated low-density lipoprotein (LDL) cholesterol.

Eruptive Xanthomas: Hypertriglyceridemia leads to rather sudden appearance of multiple closely packed red-to-brown cutaneous papules and nodules. They are common on the elbows and buttocks, but may occur anywhere.

Palmar Xanthomas: Infiltration of the volar creases of the hands produce yellowish ridges. This is pathognomonic for familial dysbetalipoproteinemia.

Tendinous Xanthomas: These are relatively large nodules are palpable along the tendons and ligaments particularly of the Achilles tendon and hands. They are associated with marked elevations of the serum cholesterol.

Common Skin Disorders and Syndromes

Common Skin Disorders

D KEY DISEASE
Acne Vulgaris: *Pathophysiology:* The interaction of sebaceous gland obstruction, androgens, and *Propionibacterium acnes* in the pilosebaceous unit leads to inflammation. The lesions are papular, pustular, and may progress to inflammatory pseudocysts with scarring. The distribution is in the areas with many sebaceous glands, the face, chest, and upper back. The earliest lesion are *comedones,* which are either open to the air (leading to oxidation of the sebum in the gland orifice, a blackhead) or closed (which produces a white papule). Comedones are not inflamed. Rupture of the obstructed pilosebaceous unit leads to inflammatory papules and nodules.

D KEY DISEASE
Rosacea: Patients have a history of easy flushing. After years, acneform papules and telangiectasia develop in the central face (forehead, cheeks, chin), which may progress to chronic edema and skin thickening. Women are more affected than men, although *rhinophyma,* the chronic deformity of the nose, is more common in men.

S KEY SYNDROME
Eczema: Dermatitis: Dermatitis literally means inflammation of the skin; in practice it is synonymous with eczema, a specific class of epidermal inflammation. Several types are distinguished by their etiology, pattern, and appearance. Consult dermatologic textbooks for more specific information.

S KEY SYNDROME

Atopic Dermatitis: This an inherited condition of people with an atopic, or allergic, diathesis. The exact mechanism of the skin disease is unclear. The condition begins in infancy or childhood and may be lifelong. The lesions are erythematous, intensely pruritic, papules or plaques with a predisposition for the flexor surfaces of the elbows, neck, and wrists, as well as the face, feet, and hands. Scratching temporarily relieves the itch, only to increase the inflammation and pruritus, ultimately producing lichenification [Leung DY, Bieber T. Atopic dermatitis. *Lancet* 2003;361:151–160].

S KEY SYNDROME

Lichen Simplex Chronicus: *Pathophysiology:* Chronic rubbing or scratching of the skin leads to hyperkeratotic plaques in disposed persons. The lesions are intensely pruritic plaques. Nodular lesions, *prurigo nodularis,* occur at spots of persistent picking. Atopic individuals are predisposed.

S KEY SYNDROME

Stasis Dermatitis: *Pathophysiology:* Increased venous and capillary pressures leads to inflammation, edema, subcutaneous fibrosis, and skin atrophy with hemosiderin staining. Any cause of venous insufficiency or elevated central venous pressure can produce the syndrome. There is prominent edema, erythema, and warmth, often with tenderness; it is often mistaken for cellulitis. With chronic disease, the subcutaneous tissues become fibrotic and the edema no longer pits (brawny edema). The skin becomes thin and easily injured, leading to ulceration and secondary infection.

S KEY SYNDROME

Contact Dermatitis: *Pathophysiology:* This is either a cell-mediated response to prior sensitization or an inflammatory response to skin irritants. The lesions are erythematous, intensely pruritic plaques. The distribution of the individual lesions and the history of specific exposures are critical to making a correct diagnosis. DDX: Irritant disease often forms vesicles early in the course (but so does rhus dermatitis) and evolve more rapidly than allergic disease. Irritant disease will occur in anyone given sufficient exposure to an adequate concentration of the agent (e.g., chemical burns), but allergic contact dermatitis requires prior exposure with sensitization.

✓ *CONTACT DERMATITIS—CLINICAL OCCURRENCE:* *Allergic* rhus dermatitis (poison ivy and oak), many other plant and animal sources, drugs (neomycin, sulfonamides), chromate, solvents, latex, metals, cosmetics, clothing dyes, industrial oils, and many others; *Irritants* acids and alkali, cement, solvents, cutting oils, detergents, and the like.

S KEY SYNDROME

Dyshidrotic Eczema: This is an acute condition of the hands and feet, especially the intertriginous areas, palms, and soles.

Deep pruritic vesicles form and coalesce. Scratching may produce lichenification. DDX: Consider contact allergens and autosensitization from dermatophyte infection on the feet.

S KEY SYNDROME

▼ **Nummular Eczema:** The nummular (coin-like) lesions are 1–3 cm in diameter, raised plaques with sharp borders and a raised edge. They may weep, especially with excoriation. They are most common on the legs and trunk in older men, on the hands in younger women.

S KEY SYNDROME

▼ **Autosensitization Dermatitis:** *Pathophysiology:* Sensitization to antigens at the site of a primary dermatitis, often infectious or infected, leads to distant lesions. The classic example is the "id" reaction, a vesicular eruption on the hands in patients with chronic dermatophyte infection of the feet. Characteristically, the secondary lesions only heal with treatment of the primary site of infection or inflammation.

S KEY SYNDROME

▼ **Seborrheic Dermatitis:** This very common disorder produces erythema and scaling in areas of sebaceous gland activity: the scalp (dandruff, cradle cap), eyebrows, nasolabial folds, external acoustic meatus, and chest. The skin may be mildly pruritic.

✓ *CLINICAL OCCURRENCE:* Usually of no diagnostic significance; Parkinson disease; sudden severe disease may be sign of HIV infection.

S KEY SYNDROME

▼ **Intertrigo:** The intertriginous areas, the skin folds between the buttocks, under the breasts, and in the skin creases, especially of morbidly obese persons, are common sites of superficial erythema and discomfort caused by persistent warmth, moisture, and occlusion. Secondary infections may occur with streptococci, *Pseudomonas aeruginosa, Candida albicans,* and other fungi. DDX: Psoriasis, especially inverse psoriasis, can be confused with intertrigo.

D KEY DISEASE

▼ **Psoriasis:** *Pathophysiology:* Inflammation of the dermis is associated with increased epithelial cell division leading to thickening of the skin. This is a common disorder that varies from mild to severe (the heartbreak of psoriasis). It is bilateral and symmetrical, involves the extensor surfaces (e.g., elbows, knees) more than the flexor surfaces, and frequently involves the scalp and gluteal crease. Trunk and extremities may be involved in any combination. Occasionally, the pattern is the opposite of that expected, *inverse psoriasis.* Individual lesions vary from papules to huge plaques. They have a characteristically adherent scale; the surface bleeds when the scales are removed. The nails are frequently involved with pits and dystrophy. Skin trauma from scratching may precipitate a new lesion (*Koebner phenomena*). A severe mutilating arthritis with characteristic involvement of the axial skeleton (spondy-loarthropathy) and distal interphalangeal joints may accompany or occur independently of the skin and nail disease.

Guttate Psoriasis: Following an infectious disease, often streptococcal pharyngitis, 2–10-mm pink papules appear diffusely on the trunk and extremities; the face and scalp are relatively spared and the palms and soles rarely involved. The lesions resolve spontaneously over weeks.

Pustular Psoriasis: Sudden onset of intense painful erythema is followed within 24 hours by deep pustular dermal lesions which rupture to form erosions. The patient has fever and leukocytosis. Patients may be severely ill. A localized form on the palms and soles is known as *palmoplantar pustulosis*.

S KEY SYNDROME

Infectious Exanthems: An *exanthem* is a diffuse skin eruption associated with bacterial or viral illness (See also *Erythroderma*, page 167). The viral exanthems are often accompanied by mucosal involvement, an *enanthem*. The individual lesions may take many forms: diffuse erythroderma (*scarlatiniform*), maculopapules (*morbilliform*, measles-like), or vesicles that may evolve to pustules. The diffuse erythrodermas often heal with desquamation.

✓ *EXANTHEMS—CLINICAL OCCURRENCE:* *Viral (most common)* rubella, rubeola, parvovirus B19, adenoviruses, Cytomegalovirus, Epstein-Barr virus, herpes simplex virus 6 (exanthem subitum) and 7 (roseola infantum), enteroviruses, HIV, Colorado tick fever, and many others; *Bacterial* Group A streptococcus (scarlet fever), staphylococcus (toxic shock syndrome), leptospirosis, meningococcemia; *Rickettsial* Rocky Mountain spotted fever, rickettsial pox, typhus.

D KEY DISEASE

Scarlet Fever: *Pathophysiology:* Pharyngitis from group A streptococci with toxin production causes generalized cutaneous erythema. Excruciating sore throat, often with vomiting and malaise, is accompanied by a brilliant-red edematous pharynx with gray or white exudate or membrane and cervical adenopathy. The tongue becomes denuded and beefy red and a maculopapular erythematous blanching eruption appears on the neck, axillae, and groin, and later becomes generalized. The skin may feel slightly rough, like fine sandpaper. The rash heals with desquamation beginning around the nails.

S KEY SYNDROME

Ichthyosis: *Pathophysiology:* These are hereditary diseases of the keratinocytes leading to hyperkeratosis and excessive drying of the skin. The skin is thickened and dry and, in severe forms, cracking hexagonally like dried clay. Hyperkeratosis of the hair follicles produces pointed follicular papules, *keratosis pilaris*.

D KEY DISEASE

Granuloma Annulare: Rubbery papules and plaques, often with annular or serpiginous sharply demarcated borders appear on the hands, feet, elbows, knees, and distal extremities. The lesions are pink, purple, or skin colored, and asymptomatic.

D KEY DISEASE

Lichen Planus: Pink, flat-topped, sharply demarcated macules appear on the wrists, ankles, eyelids, and shins. Mucous membrane involvement is common, appearing as white linear lesions in the mouth or genital mucosa [Case records of the Massachusetts General Hospital: Case 24–2002. *N Engl J Med* 2002;347:430–436].

D KEY DISEASE

Genital White Patches: Lichen Sclerosis Et Atrophica: White atrophic lesions with sharp borders appear most often on the vulva and penis, although other areas may be involved. The skin is thin and erosions may occur. Pruritus and dyspareunia are not uncommon.

D KEY DISEASE

Human Papilloma Virus: Warts: *Pathophysiology:* Infection of the skin or mucous membranes with human papilloma virus leads to verrucous hyperplasia; uterine cervix infection with specific strains antedates development of cervical cancer. The common wart is a well-demarcated papule with a verrucous surface, commonly on the fingers. Genital involvement is particularly troublesome. Flat confluent lesions without the verrucous surface occur, *flat warts.* Areas of particular difficulty are the sole of the foot, *plantar warts,* and around the nails, *periungual warts.*

D KEY DISEASE

Pityriasis Rosea: This common disorder affects primarily adolescents and young adults in the fall of the year. The eruption is asymptomatic, primarily involving the trunk and proximal extremities. The general eruption may be preceded by a larger single lesion, the *herald patch.* The lesions are ovate, with the long axis in the skin folds. They vary from 0.5–3 cm in diameter, and have a slightly raised border with a collar of fine superficial scales and an erythematous base. Resolution is spontaneous over weeks.

D KEY DISEASE

Actinic Keratoses: Mildly erythematous papules with an adherent hyperkeratotic scale occur in sun-exposed areas. They are premalignant lesions; squamous cell carcinoma may arise in chronic lesions.

D KEY DISEASE

Seborrheic Keratoses: These are hereditary lesions that begin to appear in midlife as brown macules. They gradually enlarge to 1–3-cm plaques with an adherent hyperkeratotic raised surface.

They give the appearance of being stuck on the skin. DDX: Pigmented lesions may be confused with malignant melanoma and macular lesions with moles or lentigos.

S KEY SYNDROME

Photodermatitis: *Pathophysiology:* Sensitization of the skin by either topical or systemic chemicals leads to a dermatitis triggered by exposure to sunlight. The rash appears within hours to a day or two of sunlight exposure and only in sun-exposed areas. It is erythematous and may have a burning quality. Blistering may occur. *Polymorphic light eruption* refers to a delayed sensitivity reaction to sunlight exposure.

✓ *PHOTODERMATITIS—CLINICAL OCCURRENCE: Only partial lists.* *Drugs* antibiotics (tetracyclines, sulfonamides), antidepressants, antihypertensives, diuretics (thiazides especially), NSAIDs, sunscreens; polymorphic light eruption; porphyria.

S KEY SYNDROME

Dermatofibroma: The lesions are 3–8 mm, variably colored papules, usually on the extremities. They are hard intradermal lesions attached to the epidermis: this is demonstrated by pinching the lesion sideways; it will retract rather than elevate, the *dimple sign*. DDX: May be confused with melanoma.

S KEY SYNDROME

Skin Tags (Acrochordons): These are dermal polyps which are more prevalent on the neck, axillary folds, and perineum. They are more common with obesity. They are of no significance but are a cosmetic concern to the patient. DDX: Large skin tags may be confused with neurofibromas.

S KEY SYNDROME

Vitiligo: *Pathophysiology:* Destruction of melanocytes (possibly immunologic or apoptotic) leads to patchy, complete loss of pigmentation. The macular lesions are symmetrical with sharp borders. They cause significant cosmetic discomfort in dark-skinned individuals. DDX: Don't confuse vitiligo with hypopigmented lesions (e.g., systemic lupus erythematosus, leprosy), depigmentation from burns or scars, or ash leaf spots of tuberous sclerosis.

✓ *VITILIGO—CLINICAL OCCURRENCE:* More common in families with other autoimmune disorders, for example, diabetes, Addison disease, Hashimoto thyroiditis.

Skin Infections and Infestations

Arthropod Bites and Stings

Mosquito and other arthropod bites are very common. They present as painful or pruritic papules with erythema and variable cutaneous edema. The central punctum marking the bite is evident with close inspection of early lesions. Most are minor and self-limited; severe local reactions with expansive erythema and edema are not uncommon with *hymenoptera* stings. Severe systemic allergic reactions occur in sensitized hosts to hymenoptera (bees, hornets, and wasps) and to certain ant species. *Black flies* leave a 1–2-mm hemorrhagic mark. Extensive bites may cause systemic toxicity.

S KEY SYNDROME

Spider Bites: Most are benign and no cause for concern. Bites of the *common aggressive house spider* cause moderate necrosis of the skin with scarring. The bites are usually on the face, hands, arms, or feet. The spider attacks the victim while sleeping. The *brown recluse spider* is common, but not aggressive. It will bite in defense when disturbed in old buildings, woodpiles, and similar habitats. The bite is intensely painful with progressive severe necrosis and scarring. The *black widow spider* bite is a minor lesion with minimal erythema; the adverse effects are caused by a systemic neurotoxin.

Bacterial Infections

D KEY DISEASE

Impetigo: Superficial erythematous erosions with crusts caused by staphylococcus and streptococcus organisms are common on the face of children. It may occur at any area of breaks in the skin. The crust is characteristically amber. Bullae may form in severe cases, *bullous impetigo*. Localized painful ulcerations, *ecthyma*, may occur with poor hygiene. Secondary infection of other skin lesions is termed *secondary impetiginization*.

S KEY SYNDROME

Folliculitis: Pustular infection of the hair follicles, commonly in the beard area of men, but also occurring on the scalp, trunk, legs, and buttocks. Organisms include *Staphylococcus aureus, Pseudomonas aeruginosa* (hot tub folliculitis), herpes simplex, and several fungi. DDX: *Pseudofolliculitis barbae* occurs in men with tightly curled hair who shave. Papules caused by retained hairs are present; pustules indicate secondary staphylococcal infection.

S KEY SYNDROME

Cellulitis: *Pathophysiology:* Infection of the dermis spreads radially within the skin and subcutaneous structures. Usually caused by streptococci or staphylococci, the lesions are warm, raised, and tender with indistinct borders. Often a break in the skin is identified at the origin. This is most common on legs and arms at sites of trauma. Fever may or may not be present. DDX: Less-common causes of cellulitis are mycobacteria, *Pseudomonas aeruginosa, Haemophilus influenzae,* and vibrios (especially in patients with liver disease). *Pasteurella multocida* is common following cat and dog bites and has a propensity to cause osteomyelitis. *Erysipeloid* is caused by *Erysipelothrix rhusiopathiae. Erythema chronicum migrans* is caused by Lyme borreliosis (see page 176). Noninfectious inflammation is often confused with cellulitis, for example, stasis dermatitis, superficial and deep thrombophlebitis, panniculitis, erythema nodosum, nephrogenic fibrosing dermopathy, tibial stress fracture.

S KEY SYNDROME

Erysipelas: *Pathophysiology:* Streptococcal infection of the dermal lymphatics produces intense dermal and epidermal edema and inflammation. The lesion is intensely erythematous with a sharp, raised border. The lesions are common on the face and often a break in the skin is not evident.

S KEY SYNDROME

Skin Abscess: Furuncle, Carbuncle: *Pathophysiology:* Skin infections with *Staphylococcus aureus* produce collections of pus. The pattern is determined by the skin structure in the area of infection. *Furuncles* (boils) are single collections that are relatively superficial. *Carbuncles* are deep collections extending into the subcutaneous tissues and involve interconnected collections arising from involvement of the deep hair follicles. Carbuncles arise in areas of especially thick fibrotic skin such as the posterior neck.

S KEY SYNDROME

Axillary and Perineal Inflammation: Hidradenitis Suppurative: This occurs most commonly in obese women and involves the axilla and perineum, rarely the scalp. It is more common in people with cystic acne. Inflammation of the apocrine gland areas leads to chronic, painful draining lesions that heal with scarring. Infection is probably not the primary problem, but occurs secondarily.

D KEY DISEASE

Erythema Migrans: Lyme Disease: *Pathophysiology:* Inoculation of *Borrelia burgdorferi* by Ixodes ticks leads to the characteristic skin lesion. At the site of inoculation an asymptomatic erythema appears, which expands progressively, often with an annular configuration. Vesiculation is uncommon. The lesions may reach several centimeters in size; more than one lesion may be present. Bell palsy, heart block, and arthritis of large joints are late manifestations of the disease.

S KEY SYNDROME

Ulceroglandular Syndromes: The inoculation site of the organism develops an ulcer that is often minimally symptomatic. Dissemination via the lymphatics leads to regional lymphadenopathy. Finding regional lymphadenopathy should always initiate a search for an inoculation lesion. The history of the type and location of exposure is key to establishing an accurate diagnosis. See also page 109.

✔ *ULCEROGLANDULAR SYNDROME—CLINICAL OCCURRENCE:* Tularemia, plague, syphilis, rat-bite fever, ricketsial pox, cat-scratch disease, anthrax, *Mycobacterium marinum*, scrub typhus, sporotrichosis, lymphogranuloma venereum, herpes simplex trypanosomiasis.

D KEY DISEASE

Ulceroglandular Syndrome: Tularemia (Rabbit Fever): *Pathophysiology:* *Francisella tularensis* is inoculated by fly or tick bites or skin contact with an infected rabbit. The incubation period is 1 to 10 days followed by lassitude, headache, chills, nausea and vomiting, and myalgia accompanied by a rather benign-looking ulcer at the inoculation site with surrounding erythema, but little pain. Regional fluctuant painful lymphadenopathy develops, which may suppurate. Splenomegaly may be present. Inoculation into the eye causes an *oculoglandular syndrome* with lacrimation, photophobia, edema of the lids, and preauricular and cervical lymphadenopathy.

D KEY DISEASE

Ulceroglandular Syndrome: Syphilis: The chancre is the primary lesion of syphilis. A painless, elevated ulcer typically appears on the finger. The underlying induration is peculiarly discoid, so it can be picked up like a small coin. Painless, nonsuppurating swelling of a regional lymph node follows.

D KEY DISEASE

▶ ### Ulceroglandular Syndrome: Anthrax: *Pathophysiology:* Infection with *Bacillus anthracis* is transmitted from infected wild or domestic animals by contact with hides or by ingestion or inhalation of the spores. Malaise and a painless pruritic pustule on the skin may be followed by dyspnea and hemoptysis during dissemination. The "malignant pustule" begins on an exposed surface as an erythematous papule which then vesiculates, ulcerates, and is surrounded by characteristic nontender brawny edema [Roche KJ, Chang MW, Lazarus H. Cutaneous anthrax infection. *N Engl J Med* 2001;345;1611 (picture)]. A black eschar may form. Regional lymphadenopathy is occasionally present. Inhalational exposure leads to a rapidly progressive pneumonia with hilar lymphadenopathy and mediastinal widening. Because anthrax has been used as a bioterrorism agent, a high index of suspicion is required and public health authorities should be contacted immediately [Swartz MN. Recognition and management of anthrax—An update. *N Engl J Med* 2001;345:1621–1626].

D KEY DISEASE

Ulceroglandular Syndrome: Cat-Scratch Disease: *Pathophysiology:* Gram-negative bacilli (*Bartonella henselae*) are inoculated by the scratch, lick, or bite of a healthy cat. The organisms travel to the regional lymph nodes and then disseminate. Symptoms are nonspecific with malaise and headache. Signs include fever, a papule or pustule at the inoculation site, followed by painful fluctuant regional lymphadenopathy with overlying reddened skin. Dissemination in immunocompromised hosts can lead to hepatitis (peliosis hepatitis), osteomyelitis or meningoencephalitis. Conjunctival infection produces preauricular lymphadenopathy (Parinaud oculoglandular syndrome).

S KEY SYNDROME

▶ ### Necrotizing Soft-Tissue Infections: *Pathophysiology:* Anaerobic or microaerophilic organisms are inoculated deep into the tissues by a puncture wound, or may ascend into the tissues via the lymphatics from an open wound on an extremity. The infection spreads longitudinally along the adipose tissue septa and the muscle fascia and vertically into the deeper structures via the neurovascular bundles that penetrate the tissue planes. The patient complains of severe pain disproportionate to the injury or the evident cutaneous erythema, which may be minimal at onset. The soft tissues are edematous, indurated, and very tender. These infections progress rapidly causing extensive tissue necrosis, edema, hypoperfusion, compartment syndromes, systemic hypotension, and death. Rapid diagnosis and extensive surgical debridement are essential to save limbs and life. If the infection extends into the fascia and muscle, compartment syndromes may develop. The most common organisms are group A or microaerophilic streptococci. Less common are gas-forming organisms, for example, *Clostridium perfringens* (*gas gangrene*).

D KEY DISEASE

Erysipeloid: *Pathophysiology:* The disease is probably caused by *Erysipelothrix rhusiopathiae* and acquired by handling infected mammals and fish. A localized dermal infection of the fingers or hands, it produces an area of swollen, slightly tender, violaceous skin defined by sharp borders, rarely extending above the wrist. The inflammation resolves in a few days, leaving pigmentation.

Mycobacterial Infections

Infection with tuberculous or nontuberculous mycobacterium may present as progressive skin infections unresponsive to antibiotics and with negative cultures on routine media. A high index of suspicion is required to make the diagnosis. Fungal infections (e.g., cryptococcus) can mimic these infections.

Digital Infection: Verruca Necrogenica (Pathologist's Wart, Butcher's Wart): A bluish-red patch appears on the skin; later it becomes papillomatous and warty; pus may exude from the tissues. The lesion results from inoculation with *Mycobacterium tuberculosis*. The pathologist is infected at the autopsy; butchers and packing-house workers handle infected meat. Usually, the lesions are indolent with no constitutional symptoms.

Fish-Tank Granuloma: Mycobacterium Marinum: A small nodule or nodules develop on the fingers after exposure to contaminated aquariums. The lesions may ulcerate or form small abscesses.

Tropical Ulcer: Buruli Ulcer: This is limited to tropical countries. A pruritic nodule breaks down to form a chronic, shallow, nonhealing ulcer. *Mycobacterium ulcerans* is the cause.

Viral Infections

Human Papilloma Virus: Warts: See page 173.

Varicella: Chickenpox: Infection with varicella virus leads to a mild systemic disease and recurrent crops of pustules. The rash and fever begin simultaneously. The initial lesion is a red papule that becomes a superficial vesicle on an erythematous base (dew drop on a rose petal). Vesicles occur in successive crops, so lesions at various stages of development and healing are present. The lesions are most common on the trunk, less so on the face and extremities. They rapidly turn to pustules that heal by crusting and leave little or no scar.

Variola: Smallpox: Infection with variola virus produces a severe systemic illness and pustular skin eruption. The rash is always preceded by 2–3 days of fever and severe myalgias and arthralgia. The skin lesions are synchronous, occurring predominately on the face and extremities. They progress from vesicles to tense deep pustules that break, crust, and heal with scarring. The mortality rate is high [Breman JG, Henderson DA. Diagnosis and management of smallpox. *N Engl J Med* 2002;346:1300–1308].

Monkeypox: *Pathophysiology:* This is a disease of African monkeys that can cross species. This infection was imported to North America in the spring of 2003. It was transmitted to humans from infected prairie dogs. The illness is acute with fever and malaise, followed by a macular rash with vesicles, which may be umbilicated. The lesions may be asynchronous.

Herpes Simplex: Herpes simples virus is common. Initial infection may be marked by a severe stomatitis with gingival involvement. Recurrent lesions occur on the lips (herpes labialis), buttocks, or elsewhere. Genital ulceration may be caused by either type 2 (genital herpes strain) or type 1.

Herpes Zoster (Shingles): *Pathophysiology:* Infection with varicella virus leads to chronic infection of the spinal sensory ganglia; reactivation of infection is associated with immunosuppression. Initially, the patient complains of severe pain and dysesthesia in a dermatomal distribution. In 1–3 days, clustered herpetic vesicles appear in the cutaneous distribution of the nerve, imparting a burning pain and erythema to the involved skin. The vesicles burst, crust, and slowly heal. The distribution is always unilateral, and it does not cross the midline unless dissemination occurs in the immunosuppressed patient. The pain may subside in a week or so, or it may persist for months as *postherpetic neuralgia.* Before the appearance of the vesicles, the clinician may be confused about the diagnosis. A Tzanck preparation or culture of varicella virus from a vesicle will confirm the diagnosis [Gnann JW Jr, Whitley RJ. Herpes zoster. *N Engl J Med* 2002;347:340–346].

D KEY DISEASE

HIV and AIDS: HIV/AIDS has many skin findings that may be clues to the diagnosis. Acute HIV infection can be associated with a morbilliform exanthem and enanthem. Herpes zoster can occur relatively early in the course of chronic HIV infection. Severe seborrheic dermatitis is common. Candida skin and vulvovaginal infections occur more frequently. Dermatophyte infections may be more common and difficult to treat. An eosinophilic folliculitis is associated with HIV infection and its treatment. Commonly, AIDS patients have a pruritic dermatitis with dry skin. Human papillomavirus-associated dysplastic changes and cervical cancer are more common in HIV-infected women than in HIV-infected men. In advanced disease, Kaposi sarcoma lesions may be present on the skin and oral and genital mucous membranes. Hairy leukoplakia is a characteristic oral lesion. Abnormalities of subcutaneous fat distribution, lipodystrophy, is associated with use of protease inhibitors in the treatment of HIV/AIDS.

Fungal Infections

D KEY DISEASE

Superficial Fungal Infections: Dermatophytosis, Tinea: *Pathophysiology:*   Dermatophytes infect the dead keratin layer of the skin, nails, and hair. The specific fungus can be cultured, but clinically the lesions are classified by their location. The clinical picture is variable, but usually involves thickening of the skin with scaling and mild erythema. In chronically moist areas, maceration and secondary bacterial infection may occur. DDX: Mycetomas (soil fungi), chromomycosis, sporotrichosis, and disseminated deep fungal infections affect the skin. Chronic non-infectious dermatitis is often confused with tinea.

TINEA PEDIS: ATHLETE'S FOOT: This occurs in the intertriginous spaces, usually between the lateral toes. Between the toes it appears as a white raised patch with fissures that may ulcerate. It may be painful or asymptomatic. It may involve the entire sole of the foot, with a sharp demarcation at edge of the sole. Vesicular forms can occur, especially on the instep.

TINEA MANUUM: This is infection of the palm of one or both hands, often occurring in association with tinea pedis.

TINEA CAPITIS: This involves of the scalp and hair. The hair is brittle. The circular areas may become inflamed and ulcerate, leading to permanent loss of hair.

TINEA BARBAE: This involves the beard area of men; the hair shafts are infected. The lesions are inflammatory papules or pustular folliculitis.

TINEA CORPORIS: RINGWORM: The erythematous lesions are usually circular or arcuate, slowly spreading with a raised scaling border and central clearing. Large plaques may form.

TINEA CRURIS: JOCK ITCH: This is often a chronic infection of the groin, scrotum, proximal thighs and pubis. The tan or reddish scaling lesion is well demarcated and may be asymptomatic.

D KEY DISEASE

Tinea Versicolor (Pityriasis Versicolor):   Infection by *Pityrosporum ovale* (*Malassezia furfur*) causes a very superficial mildly scaling rash usually on the trunk or arms. The macular lesions are hypopigmented in dark skinned individuals, but may be dark in light-skinned people. The lesions are asymptomatic but are cosmetically important.

D KEY DISEASE

Candidiasis: Skin infection is common in moist areas, especially the mouth (thrush), vagina and vulva, under pendulous breasts, and on the perineum and groin of incontinent patients. The lesions are raised, intensely erythematous, and coalesce into large plaques with smaller satellite lesions. *Candida albicans* is the most common species.

D KEY DISEASE

Sporotrichosis: *Pathophysiology:*   This is a slowly progressive infection with *Sporothrix schenckii,* a soil fungus implanted under the skin by trauma or abrasion. An ulcer at the inoculation site is followed by nodular cutaneous or subcutaneous lesions that suppurate, ulcerate, and drain through multiple sinuses. Regional lymph node enlargement is expected and dissemination to viscera or bone can occur.

Deep Fungal Infections: Fungi most commonly associated with deep tissue infections may give rise to skin disease. The lesions may be papules, nodules, ulcers, or confluent masses. Biopsy and culture based on clinical suspicion of fungi in nonhealing lesions is required for diagnosis.

✓*CLINICAL OCCURRENCE:*   Cryptococcosis, histoplasmosis, blastomycosis, aspergillosis, coccidioidomycosis.

Infestations

D KEY DISEASE

Scabies: *Pathophysiology:*   The mite, *Sarcoptes scabiei*, burrows in the epidermis, laying eggs and depositing feces, both of which incite an inflammatory reaction. The infestation is passed between persons. The lesions are linear erythematous papules that are intensely pruritic. The mite favors areas with thin skin and few hair follicles, especially the intertriginous areas of the hands, wrists, elbows, and genitalia.

D KEY DISEASE

Pediculosis: Lice: The patient complains of pruritus and close inspection or combing the hair with a fine comb reveals the lice; the egg sacs are cemented to hair shafts forming *nits*. Two species are described: *Pediculosis humanus,* which inhabits the head (pediculosis capitis) or body (pediculosis corporis), and *Phthirus pubis,* which lives in the pubic hair (pediculosis pubis).

Larval Migrations: Cutaneous Larval Migrans:
Pathophysiology: Roundworm eggs hatch in the soil into motile larvae that penetrate the skin and migrate in the skin and subcutaneous tissues to their final destinations. The lesions are linear red serpiginous and raised, migrating with time.

✓ *CLINICAL OCCURRENCE:*   *Ancylostoma braziliense* and *A. caninum,* hookworm. There are similar findings with strongyloidiasis (*larva currens*), fascioliasis, dracunculiasis, and others.

S KEY SYNDROME

Swimmer's Eruption: *Pathophysiology:*   Penetration of the skin by the larval forms of many organisms for which humans are not the primary host (bird schistosome, jellyfish, sea urchins, etc.) incite an intense cutaneous reaction. Patients present with an intensely pruritic rash hours after emerging from the water. Bathers in salt water have often showered in fresh water with their bathing suits on; freshwater exposure triggers a sting by some free-swimming larvae. The pattern of the rash may be diffuse or restricted to the area of contact with wet clothing which held the parasites next to the skin [Freudenthal AR, Joseph PR. Seabather's eruption. *N Engl J Med* 1993;329:542–544].

Bullous Skin Diseases

D KEY DISEASE

Hereditary Epidermolysis Bullosa: *Pathophysiology:*   This is a group of hereditary disorders that lead to loss of epidermal cohesion resulting in blister formation with minor trauma. Large superficial blisters develop and break leaving shallow erosions. The severity depends upon the specific genetic defect and depth of the blistering.

D KEY DISEASE

Pemphigus Vulgaris: *Pathophysiology:*   An acquired disease with immunoglobulin (Ig) G antibodies to epidermal desmosomes leading to loss of epidermal cell adhesion. The first lesions are often in the oral mucosa with cutaneous bullae appearing later. There are vesicles and flaccid bullae which rupture easily leaking serous fluid. Slight lateral pressure on the skin may cause blistering and a subsequent erosion (*Nikolsky sign*) [Nousari HC, Anhalt GJ. Pemphigus and bullous pemphigoid. *Lancet* 1999;354:667–672]. *Paraneoplastic pemphigus* has histologic findings of both pemphigus and pemphigoid.

D KEY DISEASE

Bullous Pemphigoid: *Pathophysiology:* Antibodies form against hemidesmosomes of the basal layer of the epidermis and subsequent complement activation leads to separation of the basal layer from the dermis. The lower legs, axillae, abdomen, legs, and groin are affected. Mucous membranes are involved. Early lesions may be erythematous papules or appear urticarial. Tense bullae develop that may be serous or hemorrhagic; they may rupture or heal by drying and crusting.

D KEY DISEASE

Dermatitis Herpetiformis: This is common in celiac disease (gluten sensitive enteropathy). The exact pathophysiology is uncertain. Symmetrically distributed vesicles, papules, and/or urticaria appear on the extensor surfaces of the arms and trunk. Pruritus is severe. Symptoms may precede the skin lesions by several hours. DDX: **Linear immunoglobulin (Ig) A dermatosis** appears similar but is not associated with celiac disease and is immunopathologically distinct.

Skin Manifestations of Systemic Diseases

S KEY SYNDROME

Erythema Multiforme: Target lesions appear on the palms and soles, feet, forearms, and face; mucous membranes may be involved. The lesions evolve over several days and may be painful or pruritic. They may progress to bullae (erythema multiforme bullosa). DDX: Psoriasis, secondary syphilis, urticaria.

✓ *CLINICAL OCCURRENCE:* Herpes simplex infection, drug reactions (sulfonamides, anticonvulsants, penicillin), idiopathic.

S KEY SYNDROME

Panniculitis: *Pathophysiology:* Sterile inflammation of the subcutaneous fat takes two forms: *lobular,* in which the fat lobule is primarily involved, and *septal,* in which the vascular and fibrous septa separating lobules is involved. Patients present with tender erythematous swellings of the skin and subcutaneous tissues, usually over areas of abundant subcutaneous fat. The epidermis is intact and the lesions are not fluctuant [Naschitz JE, Boss JH, Misselevich I, et al. The fasciitis-panniculitis syndromes. Clinical and pathologic features. *Medicine (Baltimore)* 1996;75:6–16]. DDX: Angioedema can give a similar appearance, but the lesions are more transient and are not restricted to adipose areas. Pyomyositis looks similar, but the lesions are within the muscle, not the fat.

✓ *PANNICULITIS—CLINICAL OCCURRENCE: Septal Panniculitis* erythema nodosum, eosinophilic fasciitis, eosinophilia myalgia syndrome, scleroderma (localized and diffuse), polyarteritis nodosa; *Lobular* trauma, cold injury, steroid induced, idiopathic lobular panniculitis (Weber-Christian syndrome), acinar pancreatic carcinoma, systemic lupus erythematosus, sarcoidosis, vasculitis.

S KEY SYNDROME

Erythema Nodosum: Tender subcutaneous nodules appear on the anterior shins. They are violaceous and slightly warm.

✓*CLINICAL   OCCURRENCE:* *Infections* mycobacteria (tuberculosis, leprosy), bacteria (cat-scratch disease, leptospirosis, tularemia, salmonellosis, yersiniosis), deep fungal infections, viruses (Epstein-Barr virus, lymphogranuloma venereum, hepatitis B); *Noninfectious* drug reactions, inflammatory bowel disease, paraneoplastic, Sweet syndrome, Behçet syndrome.

S KEY SYNDROME

Fever, Urticaria, Arthralgia After Foreign Protein Injection: Serum Sickness: *Pathophysiology:* Deposition of antigen–antibody complexes in the subendothelial space elicits a local inflammatory reaction. This belongs to the group of hypersensitivity vasculitides. *Age and Sex:* no limitations. *Antigens:* This was originally described during the therapeutic use of antiserum made from horse serum. Currently, the injection of penicillin has been the most common cause, although a variety of therapeutic agents can cause it. *Course:* A few days after administration, headache and pruritus are accompanied by wheal formation at the site of subcutaneous or intramuscular injection. The urticaria spreads, and large areas of skin may become edematous. An erythematous rash is present. Myalgias and arthralgias may be severe; nausea and vomiting may occur. Generalized lymphadenopathy is frequent. The blood counts are not significantly abnormal. *Response to Therapy and Prognosis:* the symptoms and signs promptly respond to corticosteroids and the course is self-limited.

S KEY SYNDROME

Scleroderma: *Pathophysiology:* Progressive fibrosis occurs in the dermis and subcutaneous tissues. The distribution of the lesions and the pattern of other organ involvement defines the particular syndrome.

✓*CLINICAL OCCURRENCE:* Diffuse cutaneous scleroderma, limited cutaneous scleroderma, CREST syndrome, morphea, toxic oil syndrome, arthralgia-myalgia syndrome, graft-versus-host disease, polyvinyl chloride exposure.

DIFFUSE CUTANEOUS SCLERODERMA: Tight shiny skin is present on the distal extremities and face and progresses to involve the more proximal extremities and to a lesser extent the trunk. Raynaud phenomena is common. Cutaneous sclerosis leads to joint immobility, limited mouth opening, poorly healing with minor trauma. Dysphagia, hypertension, acute renal failure, and, less commonly, pulmonary involvement occur.

LIMITED CUTANEOUS SCLERODERMA: The skin lesions are less extensive and favor the trunk. Severe pulmonary involvement with refractory pulmonary hypertension and respiratory failure are common, and kidney disease is less common.

CREST SYNDROME: CREST stands for the first letters of its cardinal features: calcinosis cutis, Raynaud phenomenon, esophageal dysfunction, sclerodactyly, and telangiectasia.

MORPHEA: Localized areas of erythema and induration progress to plaques of sclerosis on the limbs, or head. They may be linear on the extremities. Women are more affected than men. Visceral sclerosis does not occur.

S KEY SYNDROME

Dermatomyositis: *Pathophysiology:* There is atrophy, edema, or fibrosis of the skin and nonsuppurative inflammation of skin and striated muscle; the cause is unknown. Malaise, weight loss, muscle stiffness, and dysphagia are presenting symptoms. Heliotrope discoloration of the upper lids and bridge of the nose and flat-topped violaceous papules (*Gottron papules*) over the backs of the interphalangeal joints of the hands are classic signs. In addition, erythematous rashes or exfoliative dermatitis may be seen. Proximal muscle weakness and stiffness are indicative of muscle involvement. Synovial and tendon friction rubs, lymphadenopathy, and splenomegaly may be found. An increased association with malignancy has been suspected.

S KEY SYNDROME

Lupus Erythematosus: This is a group of inflammatory disorders thought to share similar autoimmune pathophysiologies.

ACUTE CUTANEOUS LUPUS: Several lesions occur: an acute malar or generalized rash appears, precipitated by sunlight exposure; erythematous scaling papules and plaques on the extensor surface of the fingers (sparing the interphalangeal joints); urticaria with purpura; hypersensitivity vasculitis.

SUBACUTE CUTANEOUS LUPUS: The skin lesions are psoriasiform plaques or annular erythematous lesions on the trunk, shoulders, extensor surfaces of the arms, or other sun-exposed areas. Systemic involvement is uncommon.

CHRONIC CUTANEOUS LUPUS: DISCOID LUPUS: Sharply marginated plaques with adherent scales gradually expand in circles or ovals with central atrophy. The lesions may occur on the face, scalp, forearms, and phalanges. The trunk is less commonly involved. Follicular plugging is seen. DDX: Psoriasis, lichen planus, confluent actinic keratoses, and polymorphic light eruptions may be confused.

SYSTEMIC LUPUS: This is a systemic disease with prominent, life-threatening involvement of other organs, including the brain and kidneys. The skin findings are those of acute cutaneous lupus and subacute cutaneous lupus.

S KEY SYNDROME

Pyoderma Gangrenosum: Painful nodules develop in the skin that progress to necrotic ulcers with undermined edges. The base of the wound does not granulate. It is most common on the lower extremities, buttocks and abdomen, but may involve the face. Ulcers heal with thin scars. DDX: Ecthyma gangrenosum, necrotic soft-tissue infections, Wegener granulomatosis, stasis ulcers.

✓ *PYODERMA GANGRENOSUM—CLINICAL OCCURRENCE:* Most often idiopathic; when an association is identified, inflammatory bowel disease (ulcerative colitis > Crohn disease) is most common. Other associations are with paraproteinemia (myeloma and monoclonal gammopathy of unknown significance [MGUS]), leukemia, and chronic active hepatitis.

D KEY DISEASE

Porphyrias: *Pathophysiology:* Inherited or acquired enzyme defects in the metabolism of aminolevulinic acid to heme results in the tissue accumulation of specific porphyrins. Photosensitivity is the hallmark of the porphyrias with cutaneous manifestations. Severe mutilating photosensitivity and hypertrichosis occurs in *hereditary erythropoietic protoporphyria*. *Porphyria cutanea tarda* (PCT) is an acquired or inherited disorder. The acquired form is associated with liver disease (cirrhosis, hepatitis C, hemochromatosis) and chemical exposures; it presents as burning erythematous vesicles or blisters on sun-exposed areas, often the backs of the hands or wrists; the lesions heal with atrophic hypopigmented scars. *Variegate porphyria* is inherited; the skin signs are like PCT, but systemic disease similar to acute intermittent porphyria (AIP) does occur. AIP does not have skin lesions.

KEY SIGN

Sweet Syndrome: Painful papules and nodules appear rapidly and coalesce to form large plaques infiltrated with neutrophils, most commonly on the arms and face. The lesions heal with minimal scarring. It may be chronic and recurrent.

✓ *CLINICAL OCCURRENCE:* Hematologic malignancies, myelodysplasia, monoclonal gammopathy of unknown significance, *Yersinia* infections, idiopathic.

S KEY SYNDROME

Sarcoidosis: Granulomatous skin lesions are particularly common in sarcoidosis. They present as purple or brown papules or plaques on the torso and extremities; nodules may be more common on the face and eyelids. They do not completely blanch with pressure. They are asymptomatic.

D KEY DISEASE

Diabetes: Diabetes is associated with a wide variety of skin lesions. *Necrobiosis lipoidica diabeticorum* is most often seen in diabetics. It begins as a brownish-red papule on the shin that enlarges to a plaque, which spreads with a raised rolled border surrounding a depressed atrophic center, which commonly has a yellowish coloration. Lesions may be single or multiple and merge by expansion. Diabetic hand syndrome (*diabetic cheiropathy*) is a thickening of the subcutaneous tissues in the palmar aspect of the hand, leading to inability to completely extend the fingers as demonstrated by the prayer sign. *Diabetic dermopathy* is a chronic condition with crops of erythematous papules appearing on the shins and forearms that heal with atrophic scars. *Mucocutaneous candidiasis* is much more common in diabetics with poor blood sugar control.

S KEY SYNDROME

Calciphylaxis: *Pathophysiology:* It is believed to be an ischemic injury resulting from calcium deposition in the small arterioles in patients with advanced renal insufficiency and secondary hyperparathyroidism with abnormal calcium-phosphate metabolism. This uncommon disorder presents with painful indurated plaques with vascular mottling or livedo which progress to infarction and ulceration. The lesions gradually enlarge circumferentially.

D KEY DISEASE

Pseudoxanthoma Elasticum: *Pathophysiology:* This is an inherited disorder of elastic connective tissue. The skin lesions are yellowish papules which may form plaques on the skin folds of the neck, axillae, groin, and abdomen. The skin bruises easily.

D KEY DISEASE

Tuberous Sclerosis: *Pathophysiology:* This is an autosomal dominant disorder of ectodermal and mesodermal tissues with hamartoma formation in the skin, brain, and kidneys. The skin signs are hypopigmented skin spots that may be multiple and small or larger elongated macules, *ash-leaf spots.* Pink, fleshy nodules up to 5 mm in size appear on the central face. Similar lesions are common around the nails. *Shagreen patches* are plaques on the back or buttock that represent connective tissue nevi.

D KEY DISEASE

Neurofibromatosis (NF): *Pathophysiology:* Two forms, NF-1 and NF-2, are inherited as autosomal dominant disorders affecting the skin, bones, nervous system, and endocrine organs. Café au lait (coffee with milk) *spots* occur in childhood as uniform pigmented macules from a few millimeters to several centimeters in size. The lesions are often innumerable and particularly common in the axilla. *Neurofibromas,* brown, rounded, raised, often pedunculated, lesions that can be reduced below the skin surface with finger pressure (button-hole sign), are present. *Plexiform neuromas* are larger, soft, sagging, subcutaneous lesions that protrude from the skin surface; they may become huge.

Vascular Disorders

S KEY SYNDROME

Vasomotor Disorders: Raynaud Disease and Phenomenon: Peripheral vasospasm involves one or several fingers or toes and can involve an entire hand. It starts with pallor and progresses to suffusion with cyanosis. It is recurrent and precipitated by cold exposure. If it occurs alone, it is termed **Raynaud disease;** if it occurs as part of a systemic illness, it is **Raynaud phenomenon.** Abnormalities of the fingernail capillaries in patients with Raynaud phenomenon is associated with systemic sclerosis [Klippel JH. Raynaud's phenomenon. *Arch Intern Med* 1991;151:2389–2393]. Raynaud disease is associated with an increased incidence of migraine and Prinzmetal angina. See page 488 for a complete discussion.

S KEY SYNDROME

▼ **Warfarin Skin Necrosis: Protein C Deficiency:** *Pathophysiology:* Protein C deficiency leads to intravascular coagulation and skin necrosis on exposure to warfarin. Painful, indurated lesions appear within 1–2 days after starting warfarin and progress to necrosis and sloughing. Areas with large amounts of adipose tissue (and hence poor circulation) are primarily involved, for example, the breast, abdomen, buttocks, and thighs.

Skin Neoplasms

A high index of suspicion is required to diagnose skin cancers at an early stage. They are often picked up incidentally at the time of a visit for another problem. Always survey the visible skin in all patients and perform a complete skin exam on all patients periodically [Whited JD, Hall RP, Simel DL, Horner RD. Primary care clinicians' performance for detecting actinic keratoses and skin cancer. *Arch Intern Med* 1997;157:985–990].

S KEY SYNDROME

▼ **Cutaneous Nevi: Moles:** *Pathophysiology:* Nevi are benign proliferations of melanocytes within the epidermis or at the dermal–epidermal junction; there is a hereditary influence on the number and type of moles. Moles may be congenital; more commonly they begin to appear during puberty and adolescence. Congenital nevi occur commonly over the lower back and upper buttocks, the *Mongolian spot.* Congenital *hairy nevi* are large pigmented plaques with prominent hairs. Several different types of acquired nevi are described. *Junctional nevi* are brown to black macules a few millimeters in diameter. *Dermal nevi* are skin colored to reddish domed papules or nodules less than 1 cm in size. Compound nevi have features of both junctional and dermal nevi. Halo nevi are nevi surrounded by a halo of depigmented skin; they may undergo complete regression. *Blue nevi* are deep purple to almost black, firm, discrete nodules; the blue color is the result of their deeper location in the dermis. *Atypical moles* have unusual features (asymmetry, irregular border, mixed colors, >6 mm in diameter), which raise the suspicion of melanoma; if they have abnormal histologic features on biopsy, they are *dysplastic nevi* [Naeyaert JM, Brocke ZL. Dysplastic Nevi. *NEJM* 2003, 349:2233–2240]. Serial photography is the best way to follow multiple atypical moles; dermatology referral is advised.

D KEY DISEASE

Malignant Melanoma: *Pathophysiology:* Malignant proliferation of melanocytes is initially within the epidermis then progressively invades the reticular and papillary dermis; prognosis is related to the depth of invasion. Melanomas are usually pigmented, but amelanotic melanoma is not rare. The lesions are macules *(lentigo maligna)* or papules that become nodules which may ulcerate in advanced disease. Melanoma may arise from preexisting nevi or appear on otherwise normal skin. Risk factors include a family history of malignant melanoma, blond or red hair, marked freckling on the upper back, three or more blistering sunburns before the age of 20 years, a history of 3 years or more of an outdoor summer job, and the presence of actinic keratosis. The American Cancer Society uses the mnemonic ABCD to help distinguish between melanoma and benign moles. Melanomas have *a*symmetry, *b*order irregularity, *c*olor variegation, and a *d*iameter greater than 6 mm. Inquire about and observe for changes in color, shape, elevation, texture, surrounding skin, sensation, and consistency that are ominous characteristics of melanoma. Any suspicious lesion should be referred to a dermatologist [Whited JD, Grichnik JM. The rational clinical examination. Does this patient have a mole or a melanoma? *JAMA* 1998;279:696–701].

D KEY DISEASE

▶ **Basal Cell Carcinoma:** This is the most common type of skin cancer. Basal cell cancer arises on sun-exposed skin, most commonly the face and upper back, without a precursor lesion. The lesions are pearly papules, often with surface telangiectasias. They slowly enlarge and may ulcerate. They may have considerable local extension and tissue destruction, but do not metastasize. *Superficial basal cell cancers* are flat, indurated, pink plaques with a rolled border. Uncommonly, basal cell cancer presents as areas of sclerosing skin atrophy.

D KEY DISEASE

▶ **Squamous Cell Carcinoma:** *Pathophysiology:* These cancers arise on areas of sun damage from preexisting actinic keratoses or as a result of human papillomavirus infection, usually in the genital region. When limited to the epidermis *(squamous cell carcinoma in situ, Bowen disease)* they present as sharply demarcated, slightly scaling plaques that may be several centimeters in diameter. Invasive squamous cell carcinoma may present as an ulcerated area of indurated skin (common on the lip) or as an eroded exophytic growth. These cancers invade the dermis and metastasize to regional lymph nodes.

D KEY DISEASE

▶ **Kaposi Sarcoma:** *Pathophysiology:* Infection with human herpes virus type 8 is the cause. Endemic disease is described in Italy and Africa; this is limited to the feet and extremities, with thickened scaling skin, enlargement of the extremity, and ulceration. HIV infection greatly increases the risk for development of Kaposi sarcoma;

the pattern is distinct from endemic disease. HIV-associated Kaposi frequently involves the mucous membranes and viscera (lungs and gut). The initial lesions are nonblanching, red-blue or bluish-brown papules, plaques, and nodules anywhere on the skin surface; some of the lesions become spongy or compressible tumors moving centripetally from the extremities. Lymphadenopathy and lymphedema are late findings.

D KEY DISEASE

Keratoacanthoma: This lesion is difficult to distinguish from squamous cell cancer. It appears as a solitary lesion, which grows rapidly to become an exophytic nodule with a central keratin plug. Spontaneous regression occurs over months.

S KEY SYNDROME

Cutaneous T-Cell Lymphoma: Mycosis Fungoides, Sézary Syndrome: *Pathophysiology:* This is a multifocal proliferation of malignant T cells within the dermis and epidermis. In *mycosis fungoides,* the lesions are indurated, often scaling, plaques, reaching several centimeters in size. They may be brown or pink and may appear eczematous. The papules and plaques progress to nodules or large masses, the tumor stage of disease. The disease is limited to the skin and may be confused with eczema and psoriasis. In *Sézary syndrome* there is systemic disease with leukocytosis and lymphadenopathy; the skin infiltration produces erythematous indurated thickening of the dermis prominently in the face and brows (*leonine facies*).

S KEY SYNDROME

Metastatic Cancer: The skin may be involved with a metastatic lesion from carcinomas or lymphomas. Breast cancer, B-cell lymphomas, and metastatic melanomas are particularly common in the skin. Any suspicious cutaneous nodule or plaque should be biopsied.

ADDITIONAL READING

Fitzpatrick TB, Johnson RA, Wolff K. *Color Atlas & Synopsis of Clinical Dermatology: Common & Serious Diseases.* 4th ed. New York, McGraw-Hill, 2001.

7 The Head and Neck

At least eight clinical specialties have a major focus on the head and neck: neurology, neurosurgery, ophthalmology, otolaryngology, plastic surgery, radiology, radiation oncology, and dentistry. Each specialty has developed detailed examinations to meet their needs, often with the use of specialized instruments. We describe examinations that can be made with the resources available to the general clinician. Presentation of the entire range of potential diagnoses is beyond the scope of this book. *Traumatic disorders are not considered.*

Examination of the head, neck, and cranial nerves is an essential part of the neurologic examination. Interpretation of physical examination findings is done with an eye to both the local findings and the pattern of neurologic abnormalities. This chapter discusses the physical examination, symptoms, and signs of the head and neck; for signs of primarily neurologic significance, we refer the reader to the appropriate section of the neurologic examination in Chapter 14 to discuss the finding and its interpretation. The major syndromes specific to the head and neck organs, exclusive of the central nervous system, are discussed in this chapter, while the neurologic syndromes are discussed in Chapter 14. By necessity, these distinctions are somewhat arbitrary.

In the general head and neck examination, the examiner should: (a) identify signs of generalized disease; (b) recognize local lesions within the purview of the generalist; and (c) recognize local lesions requiring specialist care.

Major Systems of the Head and Neck and Their Function

The head and neck contain a complicated grouping of major structures that are all within close proximity to one another. The examiner must always be aware of the anatomy and functional physiology of the superficial and deep structures being examined.

The skull, facial bones, and scalp provide *protection and insulation* to the deeper structures. The scalp and face are rich in blood vessels that vasodilate in response to cold to maintain normal body temperatures within these vital structures. The head contains the *organs of special sense:* the eyes, ears, olfactory nerve, and taste buds of the tongue. Impairment of the special senses suggests either problems with the sensory organs, their cranial nerves, or the brain. The tongue, pharynx, and larynx are the *organs of speech.* Changes in articulation suggest anatomic or functional problems with these structures. The nose, mouth, pharynx, larynx, and trachea form *the upper airways;* any compromise of these structures may impair effective respiration and effect changes in the tone or volume of voice. The mouth, teeth, mandible and maxilla, tongue, salivary glands, pharynx, and upper esophagus are the *upper alimentary tract* necessary for mastication and swallowing of food. Impairment of these structures may result in nutritional deficiency. The head and neck are *highly vascular.* The superficial structures have rich anastomoses from branches of the external carotid, so ischemia is unusual in these structures. The internal carotid and vertebral arteries supply blood to the brain. The head and neck have a rich *lymphatic network* draining to several discrete regional lymph node beds. In addition, the tonsils and adenoids are lymphatic organs surrounding the upper aerodigestive tract. The neck contains the thyroid and parathyroid glands, major structures of the *endocrine system.*

Functional Anatomy of the Head and Neck

The Scalp and Skull

The scalp has five layers: the skin, the subcutaneous connective tissue, the epicranius, a subfascial cleft with loose connective tissue, and the pericranium (Fig. 7-1). Surgically, the outer three strata are a single layer, which is thick, tough, and vascular, whose strength is supplied by the

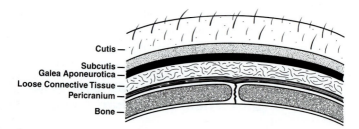

Cutis —
Subcutis —
Galea Aponeurotica —
Loose Connective Tissue —
Pericranium —
Bone —

Fig. 7-1 Layers of the Scalp. *For practical purposes, the cutis, subcutis, and galea aponeurotica constitute a single, thick, tough layer with fibrous bands compartmentalizing the more superficial tissue and binding it to the galea. Between the galea and the pericranium is a potential space with a little areolar tissue. Fluid and infection spread slowly through the compartments above the galea, but spread easily through the space beneath the galea and its attached muscles (the epicranius). The pericranium is the periosteal layer that covers the bones of the skull and dips inward at the suture lines. Subperiosteal fluid is limited to the area over a single bone.*

epicranius. The *epicranius* is a sheet of tissue covering the vertex of the skull; it consists of the *frontalis muscle* attached to the occiput by an intervening central aponeurosis, the *galea aponeurotica.* The skin and subcutaneous tissue are tightly bound to the galea by many fibrous bands that sharply limit the spread of blood and pus. The *pericranium* is the periosteal layer of the bones of the skull; it dips into the suture lines, limiting subperiosteal blood or pus to the surface of a single bone. Between the pericranium and the galea is a fascial cleft containing loose connective tissue. It is at this layer that the scalp can be lifted from the skull with minimal effort, either by accidental trauma or, formerly, by ritual scalping. In this space, blood or pus spreads under the entire epicranius. A useful pneumonic is *SCALP:* *s*kin, *c*onnective tissue, *a*poneurosis, *l*oose connective tissue, *p*eriosteum.

The scalp has three areas of *lymphatic drainage.* The forehead and the anterior portion of the parietal bone drain to the *preauricular lymph node.* The mid-parietal region drains first to the *postauricular node* and then into the nodes of the *posterior cervical triangle.* The occipital area drains first into the nodes at the origin of the trapezius, and then into the *posterior cervical triangle.*

The Face and Neck

The facial contour is determined by the frontal bone, which forms the forehead and the brows, by the maxilla and zygomatic arch, which form the cheeks and inferior orbital rim, and by the bony and cartilaginous nose, the external ears, and the mandible. The mandible articulates with the temporal bone anterior to the acoustic canal. The ramus drops inferiorly to the angle of the jaw from which the mandible turns anteriorly and medially with the two halves meeting in the midline to form the chin. The upper and lower teeth are important in determining vertical facial proportions. This bony superstructure is overlaid with muscles and soft tissues, including the lips, which give the face its rounded contours. Mild facial asymmetry is common. The anterior neck is dominated by the thyroid cartilage, which is more prominent in men (the Adam's apple), the cervical trachea, and the two bands of the sternocleidomastoid muscle arising on the mastoid process and inserting on the clavicle and manubrium. The posterior neck is enveloped in thick longitudinal muscles covering the cervical spine from the occiput to the upper back and the fan-shaped trapezius that forms the posterior lateral contour of the neck.

The Ears

The pinna, or auricle, and the external acoustic canal compose the *external ear;* the *middle ear* consists of the tympanic membrane and the tympanic cavity with its three ossicles. The *internal ear,* or labyrinth, is composed of the cochlea, the organ of hearing, and the semicircular canals, the sensory organ for maintaining balance; it is not accessible to direct examination.

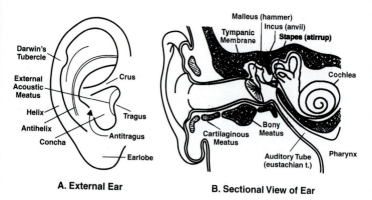

A. External Ear   **B. Sectional View of Ear**

Fig. 7-2 Pinna and Middle Ear Anatomy. *A. Surface of Pinna. The main features are depicted, but there are many individual variations. Darwin tubercle is only occasionally present.* **B. Middle Ear**: *A vertical section through the ear. Note the flexible cartilaginous and fixed bony segment of the external acoustic meatus. The plane of the tympanic membrane slants outward about 35 degrees from vertical; the conical apex points inward and upward.*

The External Ear

The *pinna or auricle* is a flattened funnel with crinkled walls of yellow fibroelastic cartilage. It has a wide external brim that narrows internally to the external *acoustic meatus.* Several prominent folds are readily identified, although there is considerable individual variation (Fig. 7-2A). The *helix* originates as the *crus,* which courses anteriorly and then winds upward, backward, and downward posteriorly to form the funnel's brim. Above the midpoint of its posterior vertical portion, a fusiform swelling occasionally develops, the *Darwinian tubercle.* An inner concentric fold, the *antihelix,* partially surrounding an ovoid cavity, the *concha,* is divided into an upper and lower portion by the transverse *helical crus.* From the anterior brim of the funnel, below the crus, the *tragus* points backward toward the lower concha as a small eminence. From the lower portion of the antihelix, another eminence, the *antitragus,* points forward across the *intertragal notch* to the tragus. The deep lower concha forms the *external acoustic meatus.* At the junction of the inferior limbs of the helix and antihelix is a pendant lobule of adipose and areolar tissue without cartilage, the *earlobe.*

The external acoustic meatus or canal is about 2.5 cm long, extending from the bottom of the concha to the tympanic membrane (see Fig. 7-2B). About one-third of the superficial canal is walled with cartilage, the deeper two-thirds runs through the temporal bone. From the concha, the canal forms a gentle S, tending inward, forward, and upward. About 20 mm in from the concha is a bony constriction in the canal, the *isthmus.*

The Middle Ear

Within the petrous portion of the temporal bone, the acoustic canal widens to form the *tympanic cavity,* surmounted by an attic providing room for movements of the ossicles. Separating the tympanic cavity and the external acoustic meatus is the *tympanic membrane,* an ovoid biconcave disk slanting across the canal in a plane 35 degrees from the vertical, its posterior superior portion more superficial than the anterior inferior attachment (see Fig. 7-2B). The *manubrium of the malleus* is firmly attached to the inner tympanic membrane; viewed from outside, the attached portion appears as a smooth ridge forming a radius of the membrane, slanting upward and slightly anterior. The tympanic membrane is a shallow cone whose apex points upward and inward into the tympanic cavity.

The Inner Ear

The inner ear, or *labyrinth,* consists of the spiral *cochlea* (the organ of hearing), the semicircular canals, ampullae, utricle and saccule (the organs of balance), and the acoustic nerve endings (cranial nerve VIII). These structures are contained in the bony labyrinth within the temporal bone adjacent to the middle ear. Two windows connect the middle and inner ear: the oval window contains the footplate of the stapes and communicates mechanical vibrations to the inner ear via the scala vestibuli; the round window covers the origin of the scala tympani.

The Eyes

The bony *orbits* are quadrilateral pyramids with bases facing anteriorly and apices pointing backward and medially. Their medial sides are parallel, while the lateral walls form a 90 degree angle (Fig. 7-3). The orbital roof is formed by the frontal and sphenoid bones. The medial wall

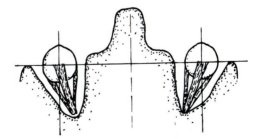

Fig. 7-3 Relationship of the Orbits and Globes. *A horizontal section through the orbits. The medial orbital walls are parallel. When the globes are in the primary position, the parallel optic axes are parallel with the medial orbital walls. Because the orbital apices and origins of the ocular muscles are medial to the optic axes in the primary position, the lateral rectus muscles are longer than the medial and the superior and inferior recti pull medially.*

is formed from portions of the maxilla, lacrimal, and sphenoid bones; the front of this wall contains the lacrimal groove for the lacrimal sac. The lateral wall is composed of the zygomatic and palatine bones. At the apex is the *optic foramen,* through which pass the optic nerve (CN II) and the ophthalmic artery. The *superior orbital fissure* is posterior between the roof and the lateral wall; it carries the middle meningeal artery, the ophthalmic vein, and four cranial nerves, the oculomotor (CN III), trochlear (CN IV), first (ophthalmic) division of the trigeminal (CN V1), and the abducens (CN VI) nerves.

Extraocular Movements

The eyeball is a globe with the optic axis passing between its two poles, the midpoint of the cornea and the back of the eye. Imagine a series of meridians between the poles, all transected by an equator. The globe is suspended at the front of the orbit by a fascia that prevents translation, that is, movements of all parts of the globe simultaneously in the same direction. Instead, rotation occurs about three axes intersecting perpendicularly at the center of rotation. Rotation about the vertical axis through the equatorial plane permits *abduction* and *adduction;* rotation about the horizontal axis through the equator produces *elevation* and *depression;* rotation of the uppermost meridian about the optic axis toward the nose is *inward deviation* (adduction); its movement away from the nose is *outward deviation* (abduction).

Six muscles effect these motions. The *four recti* originate in a fibrous ring around the optic foramen in the orbital apex (Fig. 7-4); these muscles insert slightly anterior to the global equator, spaced 90 degrees apart; the *superior* and *inferior recti* attach to the superior and inferior meridian, while the *lateral* (external) and *medial* (internal) *recti* are opposed on the horizontal meridians. The *superior oblique* muscle originates above the four recti at the optic foramen and runs anteriorly and medially to the trochlea, a fibrous pulley in the medial side of the anterior orbit, from which it runs laterally and posteriorly under the superior rectus

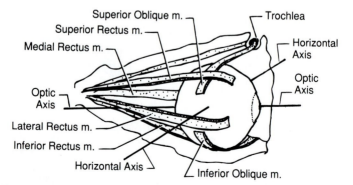

Fig. 7-4 The Extraocular Ocular Muscles.   *The right orbit viewed through the lateral wall.*

to insert behind the equator in the upper lateral quadrant of the posterior globe. Its physiologic point of action is at the pulley. The *inferior oblique* muscle originates anteriorly near the medial lacrimal groove, passes posteriorly and laterally between the inferior rectus and the orbital floor to its insertion in the posterior lower lateral quadrant near the superior oblique. The superior oblique is innervated by the trochlear nerve (CN IV), the lateral rectus by the abducens nerve (CN VI) and the other three recti and inferior oblique by the oculomotor nerve (CN III).

In the primary position, the globes are suspended with their optic axes horizontal in the sagittal plane. Because the rectus muscles pull toward the orbital apex, the lateral recti are longer than the medial recti. The superior and inferior recti do not pull exactly in the direction of the optic axes (Fig. 7-5A). Study Figure 7-5 to visualize the movements of the globe imparted by the six muscles starting from the primary position. Contraction of the medial rectus, with relaxation of the opposed lateral rectus, produces adduction; contraction of the lateral rectus and relaxation of the medial rectus results in abduction. Contraction of the superior rectus elevates and *intorts* the globe because the angular pull produces some rotation about the optic axis. Similarly, the inferior rectus causes depression and *extorsion*. The superior oblique depresses and intorts, assisting the depression while countering the extorsion of the inferior rectus. The inferior oblique assists the superior rectus in elevation, while its extorsion counters the intorting action of the superior rectus. Deviation from the primary position changes the relative effects of various muscles. When the eye is abducted (Fig. 7-5B) to a position where the direction of pull of the superior and inferior recti coincides with the optic axis, the recti produce pure elevation and depression, respectively.

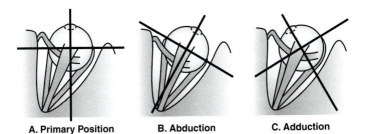

A. Primary Position   **B. Abduction**   **C. Adduction**

Fig. 7-5 Positions of the Right Globe in Relation to the Ocular Muscles. In all positions the lateral rectus produces abduction and the medial rectus causes adduction. With the optic axis in the primary position (A), the superior rectus elevates and intorts, the inferior oblique elevates and extorts, the inferior rectus depresses and extorts, and the superior oblique depresses and intorts. With the globe abducted so the optic axis coincides with the pull of the superior and inferior recti (B), these muscles produce elevation or depression without extorsion or intorsion. When adduction causes the optic axis to coincide with the pull of the oblique muscles along the equator (C), these muscles produce elevation and depression without intorsion or extorsion.

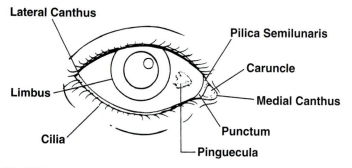

Fig. 7-6 External Landmarks of the Normal Right Eye.

Similarly, adduction can attain a position where the oblique muscles pull along the equator to produce pure intorsion or extorsion (Fig. 7-5C). Convergence is accomplished by contraction of the two medial recti.

The Eyelids

The area between the opened upper and lower eyelids is the *palpebral fissure* (Fig. 7-6); the two angles of the fissure are the *lateral* (temporal) and the *medial* (nasal) *canthi.* In the medial canthus is a small protuberance of modified skin, the *caruncle;* posteriorly is a tissue fold, the *plica semilunaris.* On an elevation of the lid margin, near the inner canthus, is the *punctum,* the entrance to the canaliculus draining into the *lacrimal duct;* each lid possesses a punctum. The *upper lid* extends upward from the fissure to the superior edge of the bony orbit, merging with dense tissue bound to the periosteum. The skin overlying the eyelids is the thinnest in the body; it is readily moved and picked up. During elevation, the upper eyelid invaginates between the eyeball and the upper border of the orbit. From the fissure the *lower lid* extends downward to the dense tissue and periosteum of the lower outer orbital margin; the lower lid is shorter and does not infold. Edema fluid in the lids is sharply limited by their orbital attachments. Within the lids are the circular fibers of the *orbicularis oculi* muscle, supplied by the facial nerve (CN VII). The upper lid also contains the vertical tendons of the *levator palpebrae superioris* muscle, which originates in the optic foramen and inserts in the tarsal plate. It is innervated by the oculomotor nerve (CN III). The lids are stiffened by *tarsal plates,* transverse dense plaques of elastic and connective tissue; the upper tarsus is much larger than the lower. Both tarsi are adherent posteriorly to the palpebral conjunctiva and contain many *meibomian glands* that run perpendicularly to the palpebral margins and empty through pinpoint openings in the lid margins. At the skin border of the lid margins is a double row of cilia or *eyelashes* with their hair follicles. The hairs are deeply pigmented and curve outward. Deep to the temporal side of the upper lid, beneath the frontal bone, lies the *lacrimal gland* that produces tears that lubricate the conjunctival surfaces.

The *epicanthus* is a semicircular fold of skin that lies vertically over the upper and lower lid of one or both eyes partially covering the medial canthus. It is present in about 20% of newborn white children, but it disappears by the age of 10 years in all but 3%. The epicanthus must be distinguished from the *mongolian fold* that originates in the upper lid and partially or completely overhangs the superior tarsus; this is horizontal, while the epicanthus is vertical. The mongolian fold is a normal characteristic of Far Eastern races and some individuals of other races. Epicanthus should not be confused with esotropia, in which there is excessive deviation of the visual axis toward the other eye.

The Conjunctiva and Sclera

The *palpebral conjunctiva* joins the skin at the anterior edge of the lid margins. It follows the inner surface of the lids into the *superior* and *inferior fornices*. Although firmly attached to the tarsal plates, it is quite loose in the fornices permitting movement of the globe. At the fornices the membrane is reflected anteriorly to cover the sclera as the *bulbar conjunctiva*. The larger *episcleral vessels* are normally visible peripherally through the transparent bulbar conjunctiva; they may be moved by sliding the conjunctiva over the sclera. At the limbus, the conjunctiva is firmly attached to the sclera and continues as the epithelium of the cornea. The superficial vessels of the bulbar conjunctiva run radially in tortuous courses (Fig. 7-44). The deeper vessels are not individually visible; they radiate near the limbus. A raised yellow plaque, the *pinguecula,* occurs normally on each side of the limbus in the horizontal plane. The nasal pinguecula is larger than the temporal; both increase in size with age.

The Cornea

The cornea is a convex tissue of five transparent avascular layers that joins the sclera at the *limbus.* Because its surface is highly reflective, inspection with oblique lighting (slit-lamp exam) is necessary to reveal small imperfections. Its diameter is about 12 mm, and its radius of curvature is slightly smaller than that of the globe, so it protrudes somewhat from the surface of the globe. Through it may be seen the iris and pupil.

The Sclera

Beneath the bulbar conjunctiva, the ocular globe is covered by a tough dense fibrous coat, the *sclera.* It is china white except for spots of brown melanin, varying in number with the individual's complexion and race. The sclera is pierced by the *scleral foramen,* for the optic nerve, the *long ciliary arteries* and *nerves,* the *short ciliary nerves,* and the *venae vorticosae.* The tendons of the ocular muscles attach to the sclera.

The Iris and the Pupil

The *pupil* is a circular hole surrounded by an optical diaphragm of loose pigmented stroma with a variable opening, the *iris.* The iris contains irregular holes, called *iris crypts.* Embedded in the central part of the iris is the *sphincter pupillae;* more peripheral is a radial muscle, the *dilator pupillae.*

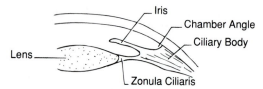

Fig. 7-7 Cross-Section of the Lens and Ciliary Body.

The Lens

The anterior and posterior surfaces of the lens are convex; the junction of the two curved surfaces is the *equator*. It is suspended behind the iris by a tough membrane, the *zonula ciliaris* (zonule of Zinn), that extends from the lenticular equator to the *ciliary body* on the choroid (see Fig. 7-7). When the eye is at rest, and thus suited for distant vision, the *ciliary muscle* is relaxed, so the pull of the zonula ciliaris diminishes the anteroposterior dimension. During accommodation, the ciliary muscle contracts, permitting the lens to thicken in response to its normal elasticity. Normally, the lens is highly transparent.

The Nose

The external nose is a triangular pyramid with one side adjoining the face (Fig. 7-8). The upper angle of the facial side is the *root*, connected with the forehead. The two lateral sides join in the midline to form the *dorsum nasi*; its superior portion is the *bridge* of the nose. The free angle or apex forms the *tip* of the nose. The triangular base is pierced on either side by an elliptic orifice, the *naris* (plural *nares*), separated in the midline by the *columella*, which is continuous internally with the *nasal septum*. Lining the margins of the nares, still hairs, the *vibrissae*, inhibit

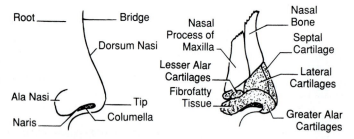

Fig. 7-8 The External Nose. *These diagrams show the topographic features and the skeleton. Note that the proximal half of the nose is bone and the distal half (stippled) is cartilage.*

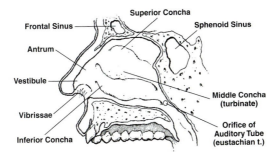

Fig. 7-9 Lateral Nasal Wall. *This parasagittal section shows the superior, middle, and inferior conchae; under each is its corresponding meatus. Posterior to the inferior meatus is the orifice of the auditory (eustachian) tube.*

inhalation of foreign bodies. The lateral nasal surface ends below in a rounded eminence, the *ala nasi* (plural, *alae nasi*).

The upper third of the lateral nasal wall is supported medially by the nasal bone and laterally by the nasal process of the maxilla. The lower two-thirds is supported by a framework of lateral cartilage, the *greater alar cartilage,* and several lesser alar cartilages. The *nasal septum,* also part bone and part cartilage, is formed deeply by the lamina perpendicularis of the ethmoid bone and superficially by the *quadrilateral septal cartilage.*

The nasal septum divides the *nasal cavity* into symmetrical air passages. Each passage begins anteriorly at the naris (Fig. 7-9) and widens into a *vestibule;* then it passes into a high, narrow chamber that communicates posteriorly with the *nasopharynx* by an oval orifice, the *choana.* Normally, the septal surface of the chamber is planar, while the lateral surface is thrown into convolutions by three horizontal, parallel, downward curving bony plates, the *superior, middle,* and *inferior turbinates* or *conchae.* The mucous membranes of the inferior turbinate are highly vascular and semierectile; it is most affected by vasoconstrictor drugs. Under each turbinate is a groove, the *superior, middle,* and *inferior meatus.* Above and posterior to the superior turbinate is the opening of the *sphenoid sinus.* The superior meatus contains the orifices of the *posterior ethmoid cells.* The middle meatus receives drainage from the *maxillary sinus,* the *frontal sinus,* and the *anterior ethmoid cells.* The inferior meatus contains the orifice of the *nasolacrimal duct.* The *auditory (eustachian) tube* opens into the nasopharynx just behind and lateral to the choana at the level of the middle meatus. Superior to the eustachian tube orifice in the nasopharynx is an aggregation of lymphoid tissue, the *pharyngeal tonsil,* or *adenoids.*

The endings of the *olfactory nerve* (CN I) are located high in the nasal chamber, above the superior turbinate. A vascular network on the portion of the nasal septum called *Kiesselbach plexus* is noteworthy because it is the site of most nosebleeds.

The Mouth and Oral Cavity

The mouth is surrounded by two fleshy *lips;* the *vermillion border* marks the transition from cornified epithelium of the skin to the noncornified squamous epithelium of the mouth. The *philtrum* is a vertical groove from nasal septum downward to vermilion border of the upper lip. Surrounding the mouth is the *orbicularis oris,* a circular band of muscle innervated by the facial nerve (CN VII); contraction closes and protrudes the lips. Each *lip* is anchored to its adjacent gum by a fold of mucosa, the *labial frenulum.* The *oral cavity* is a short tunnel with an arched roof formed by the *hard and soft palate,* walls of the cheeks and lateral teeth, and with a floor formed by the tongue. The double portals of the tunnel, the lips and teeth, are separated by a shallow *vestibule.* The tunnel's exit is the *isthmus faucium* between the *faucial pillars;* it opens into a vertical passage, the *oropharynx,* continuous above with the *nasopharynx.*

The anterior two-thirds of the roof is formed by the *hard palate,* comprised of maxilla and palatine bone covered by mucosa with a *median raphe.* A fold of mucosa and muscle, the *soft palate,* continues the roof posteriorly. It hangs free forming a curtain in the *isthmus faucium.* From the midline of its free border is suspended the conical or bulbous *uvula.* The lateral border of the soft palate splits into two vertical folds, the *pillars of the fauces.* Between the anterior and posterior pillars lies the *palatine tonsil,* a mass of lymphoid tissue containing deep crypts or clefts. Similar lymphoid tissue lies in the base of the tongue, the *lingual tonsil.*

The Teeth

Upper and lower semicircles of *teeth* are set in the maxilla and mandible, approximating at their contact surfaces. The bony *dental ridges* and necks of the teeth are covered by tough fibrous tissue and mucosa, the *gums.* The gum borders are called the *gingival margins.*

A child develops 20 *deciduous teeth:* from the midline on either side, uppers and lowers, they are two *incisors,* one *canine,* and a first and second *molar.* Gradually, these teeth are lost, to be replaced by *permanent teeth* with the addition of a first and second *premolar,* or bicuspid, and a third molar, making a total of 32 (Table 7–1). Dentists use a universal numbering system starting with the right upper third molar as 1 and

TABLE 7–1 Age at Tooth Eruption

	Deciduous (Months)	Permanent (Years)
First molars	15–21	6
Central incisors	6–9	7
Lateral incisors	15–21	8
First premolars		9
Second premolars		10
Canines	16–20	12
Second molars	20–24	12–13
Third molars		17–25

counting left to the opposite upper third molar as 16, then continuing down to the left lower third molar as 17 and counting right to 32 at the mandibular third molar. The eruption times of various teeth are shown in Table 7–1.

The Tongue

The *tongue* lies within the horseshoe curve of the mandible; its dorsal surface forms the floor of the oral cavity. The *tip* or apex is thin and narrow, resting against the lingual surface of the lower incisors. Posteriorly and inferiorly is the *root,* composed of muscle masses and their bony attachments. The common expression "tongue shaped" applies only to the visible tip and dorsal surface of the human tongue; like an iceberg, the greater bulk is submerged and is neither thin nor sinuous. The *extrinsic muscles* extend between the *symphysis mentis* of the mandible, the *hyoid bone,* and the *styloid process* of the temporal bone; they cause protrusion and retraction of the tip, convex and concave curving of the dorsum, and move the root upward and downward. The *intrinsic muscles* alter the length, width, and curvature of the dorsal surface. The lingual muscles are innervated by the hypoglossal nerve (CN XII).

The tongue is free at its tip, dorsum, sides, and anteroinferior surface (Fig. 7-10). A midline fold of mucosa, the *lingual frenulum,* attaches the tongue to the floor of the mouth and the lingual surface of the lower gum. Near its base, the frenulum swells to form twin eminences, the *carunculae sublingualis,* each surmounted by the orifice of a *submaxillary duct* (Wharton duct). Running from the carunculae laterally and posteriorly around the base of the tongue is a ridge of mucosa, the *plica sublingualis,* punctured at intervals by the duct orifices from the sublingual gland, lying deep to the ridges.

The *dorsum* of the tongue extends from its tip to the epiglottis. The *median sulcus* bisects the dorsum from tip to the posterior third, where it ends in a depression, the *foramen cecum,* at the closure site of the em-

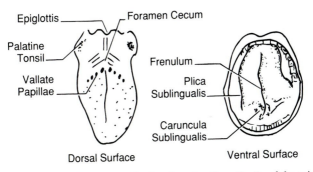

Fig. 7-10 Tongue Surfaces. *The dorsal surface from the tip of the epiglottis is depicted, showing the position of the palatine tonsils. The ventral surface is viewed from the outside of the mouth. The caruncula sublingualis is at the base of the frenulum; it contains the orifices of the submaxillary salivary ducts. In the plica sublingualis are some sublingual salivary gland orifices.*

bryonal *thyroglossal duct.* A *sulcus terminalis* extends forward and laterally from either side of the foramen cecum to form a V whose apex is
posterior. Slightly anterior and parallel is another V formed by a row of
8 to 12 *vallate papillae.* The vallate papillae are round, discrete eminences
with concentric fossae. The anterior two-thirds of the dorsum linguae is
textured like velvet by the protrusion of microscopic *filiform papillae.*
These papillae catch desquamated cells, bacteria, and particles of food
to form the coating of the normal tongue. Scattered among the filiform
papillae, at the tip and sides of the tongue, are the less numerous *fungiform papillae.* They are readily identified with the unaided eye as large,
raised, rounded, and deeper red. Microscopic taste buds are numerous
in the vallate and fungiform papillae, on the sides and back of the tongue,
in the soft palate, and on the posterior surface of the epiglottis. The sensory root of the facial nerve (CN VII), through the *chorda tympani,* supplies the taste buds in the anterior two-thirds of the tongue; the posterior third is innervated by the glossopharyngeal nerve (CN IX).

The Larynx

The larynx is immediately behind and below the oral cavity; in many
persons the epiglottic tip is directly visible through the mouth. Because
the larynx is on the anterior wall of the pharynx with the sloping plane
of its rim facing posteriorly, it is easily viewed in the laryngeal mirror
held behind it (see Fig. 7-28). The laryngeal apparatus may be visualized as three parallel stacked incomplete rings, one atop the other, held
together by ligaments. Topmost is the arched *hyoid bone,* which opens
posteriorly; suspended below are the arched *thyroid cartilage,* which also
opens posteriorly, and the *cricoid cartilage,* which is a complete ring affixed to the tracheal rings below. Although these structures are practically subcutaneous and palpable in the neck, their openings are posterior and well protected.

   The ability to phonate depends on the shape, position, and action of
the two *arytenoid cartilages* (Fig. 7-11). Each is a three-sided pyramid with
a triangular base. The base is slightly concave to glide on a convex joint
surface on the posterior rim of the cricoid cartilage, the *cricoarytenoid
joint,* which is surrounded by a capsule. The two pyramids stand erect
on either side of the midline of the cricoid. Muscles pull on the various
faces of the pyramids, causing their bases to rotate in the joints. The apex
of each pyramid is surmounted by a horizontal crescent of small cartilages and ligaments pointing medially toward its opposite and curving
anteriorly. From the curve of each crescent, a tough fibroelastic band,
the *true vocal cord* (vocal fold), extends forward to the midline of the thyroid cartilage. The two vocal cords thus form an opening into the trachea, the *rima glottidis.* When open, the rima is an isosceles triangle, with
apex anterior beneath the epiglottis and base posterior, formed by the
tissue bridge between the two arytenoid crescents. Rotation of the arytenoids brings the legs of the triangle together posteriorly to approximate the cords over their entire length.

   Lateral, parallel to, and above the true cords is a pair of tissue folds,
the *false vocal cords* (ventricular folds). A membrane covers the epiglot-

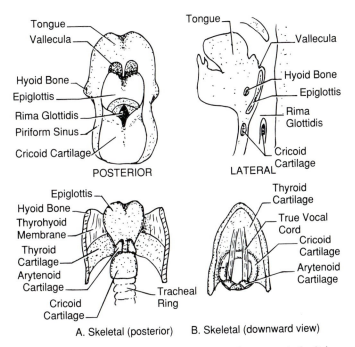

Fig. 7-11 Anatomy of the Larynx. *The larynx faces posteriorly; it is seen with the mirror behind the plane of the vocal cords. The arytenoid cartilages are small pyramids perched on the cricoid cartilage, to which they are connected by true joints. The arytenoid cartilages twist on their bases to vary vocal cord tension.*

tis and continues around posteriorly to envelop the crescents of the arytenoids, forming the *aryepiglottic folds.* Because the larynx protrudes slightly from the anterior pharyngeal wall, several pockets are formed: two *valleculae* between the epiglottis and the base of the tongue, and two *piriform sinuses,* one on either side of the cricoid. Most of the intrinsic muscles of the larynx are supplied by fibers of the *recurrent laryngeal nerve,* a branch of the vagus nerve (CN X).

The Salivary Glands

Parotid Gland

This is the largest of the salivary glands. Normally, it is not palpable as a distinct structure, but its location and extent must be known to recognize parotid enlargement (Fig. 7-12). A *superficial portion* lies subcutaneously extending from the zygomatic arch superiorly to the angle of the mandible inferiorly and from the external auditory canal posteriorly to the midportion of the masseter muscle anteriorly. A *tail portion* wraps around the angle and horizontal ramus of the mandible in the upper

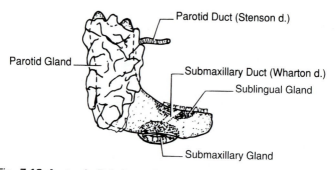

Fig. 7-12 Anatomic Relations of the Salivary Glands to the Mandible.
Note that the parotid gland lies on the lateral surface of the mandibular ramus,
curling behind its posterior margin. The submaxillary gland is on the medial
surface of the mandible with its lower margin protruding below the bone. The
sublingual gland is behind the medial mandibular surface near its superior mar-
gin. Using the jaw for a landmark, the glands can be located accurately by pal-
pation.

neck, and a *deep lobe* extends from the tail medial to the stylomandibu-
lar ligament and styloid muscles. The *parotid (Stensen) duct* is about 5
cm long and runs forward, horizontally on the superficial surface of the
masseter muscle, about one fingerbreadth below the zygomatic arch, in
a line drawn from the inferior border of the concha of the ear to the commissure of the lips. At the muscle's anterior border, it pierces the buccinator muscle to reach its orifice in a papilla on the buccal mucosa opposite the upper second molar.

Submaxillary Glands

About the size of a walnut, the gland lies medial to the inner surface of
the mandible; its lower portion can be palpated from beneath the inferior mandibular border somewhat anterior to the angle of the jaw. Bimanual palpation, with a gloved finger in the floor of the mouth and
the opposite hand on the corresponding skin, reveals the finely lobulated glandular architecture. The *submaxillary (Wharton) duct* is about 5
cm long; it courses upward and forward to the floor of the mouth, where
its orifice is crowned by the *caruncula sublingualis,* beside the lingual
frenulum.

Sublingual Glands

The smallest of the glands, it lies beneath the floor of the mouth, near
the symphysis mentis. It empties through several short ducts, some with
orifices in the plica sublingualis, some entering the submaxillary duct.

The Thyroid Gland

Knowledge of thyroid embryology is necessary to understand thyroid
disorders. A median diverticulum, evaginating from the ventral pha-

ryngeal wall (the future *foramen cecum* in the tongue), goes downward and backward in front of the trachea as a tubular duct (the *thyroglossal duct*), bifurcating and further dividing into cords that later fuse to form the thyroid isthmus and lateral lobes. Normally, the thyroglossal duct is obliterated, but remnants may persist in the adult to form thyroglossal sinuses or cysts. At the duct's superior end, a normally functioning lingual thyroid gland may form. Inferiorly, ductal tissue frequently forms a *pyramidal lobe* arising from the isthmus or a lateral lobe, usually the left. The pyramidal lobe may ascend in front of the thyroid cartilage as high as the hyoid bone. Occasionally, a normal glandular component, such as the isthmus or lateral lobe, may fail to develop. Rarely, the lingual growth may be the only active thyroid tissue in the body.

The thyroid is the largest endocrine gland. It consists of two lateral lobes whose upper halves lie on either side of the projecting prow of the thyroid cartilage; the lower halves are at the sides of the trachea (Fig. 7-13). A flat band of isthmus passes in front of the upper tracheal rings, joining the lateral lobes at their lower thirds. The major outline of the gland is trapezoidal, with a parallel top and bottom, and with the sides converging downward (the Greek thyroid means shield-shaped). The normal adult gland weighs approximately 25–30 g; it is slightly larger in the female. Each lateral lobe is an irregular cone about 5 cm long; the greatest diameter is about 3 cm, the thickness about 2 cm. The right lobe is normally one-fourth larger than the left. The lateral posterior borders touch the common carotid arteries. Usually, on the posterior lateral surfaces are the *parathyroid glands*. The *recurrent laryngeal nerves* lie close to the medial deep surface. Each lobe is covered anteriorly by the respective sternocleidomastoideus, while the isthmus lies on the tracheal rings and is practically subcutaneous. Pairs of *superior and inferior thyroid arteries* supply an exceedingly vascular parenchyma. The gland is firmly fixed to the trachea and larynx, so that it ascends with them during swallowing; this movement distinguishes thyroid structures from other masses in the neck. The thyroid actually lies in the upper anterior me-

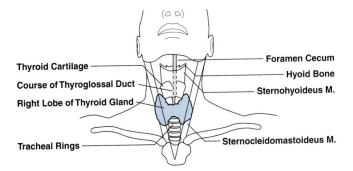

Fig. 7-13 Anatomic Relations of the Thyroid Gland, Anterior View. The blue structures are the thyroid gland and the course of the obliterated thyroglossal duct.

diastinum. Enlargement by downward growth extends behind the sternum, a retrosternal goiter. The *thymus gland* also occupies the anterior mediastinum. Thus, a tumor of the anterior mediastinum may arise from either gland.

Physical Examination of the Head and Neck

Examination of the Scalp, Face, and Skull

Examination is by inspection and palpation. *Inspect* for asymmetry of the skull, ears, eyes, nose, mouth, jaw, and cheeks. Use a tongue blade in the sagittal plane from the midline of the brows to the midline of the lips to detect nasal deformity. Observe the position of the ears, viewing from the front. Note any masses or deformities. Inspect the skin of the scalp by displacing the hair sequentially to reveal the roots. Inspect for actinic changes and lesions on the sun-exposed skin, especially the helix of the ear, the temples above the zygoma, the forehead, cheeks, and lips. Gently *palpate* the skull for irregularities. Run a fingertip around the orbital rim and along the zygoma on each side. Palpate the ramus, angle, and arch of the mandible.

Examination of the Ears, Hearing and Labyrinthine Function

Pinna

Inspect the pinna for size, shape, and color. Note serous, purulent, or sanguinous discharges from the meatus. Palpate the consistency of the cartilages and any swellings. Assess for pain with movement of the pinna and tragus.

External Acoustic Meatus

Prepare the canal for inspection by taking time to clean it properly. Remove liquid material with a cotton applicator. Remove solids through an ear speculum with either a cotton applicator or a cerumen spoon under direct vision. Use a speculum attached to a lighted otoscope or a speculum and a head lamp. Select the largest speculum that will fit the cartilaginous canal. Before inspection is attempted, tip the patient's head toward the patient's opposite shoulder to bring the canal horizontal. Insert the speculum while retracting the pinna upward and backward for adults so that the flexible cartilaginous portion is raised to coincide with the axis of the bony canal; use downward traction for infants and young children (Fig. 7-14). The lining epithelium of the bony canal is very sensitive, so use gentle manipulation.

Tympanic Membrane and Middle Ear

When a beam of light shines into the external acoustic meatus, the tympanic membrane reflects a brilliant wedge of light, the *light reflex*; its apex is the center or *umbo* and its legs extend peripherally in the ante-

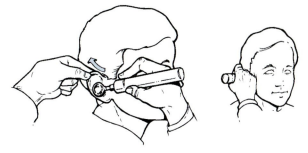

Fig. 7-14 Use of the Otoscope. *Insert the ear speculum by pulling the upper edge of the pinna upward and backward to straighten the cartilaginous meatus so that it coincides with the axis of the bony canal.*

rior inferior quadrant of the membrane, approximately at a right angle to the manubrium. Examine the normal landmarks of the drumhead: the *manubrium of the malleus* that forms a smooth ridge from the umbo or center and runs radially upward and forward toward the circumference and ends in the knob of the *short process;* the two *malleolar folds,* diverging from the knob to the periphery; the *shadow of the incus,* often showing through the membrane in the upper posterior quadrant; and, finally, look carefully around the entire circumference of the *annulus* for perforations just inside its border. Note the *color* and *sheen* of the membrane, which is normally shiny and pearly gray. Serum in the middle ear colors it *amber or yellow;* pus shows as a *chalky white* membrane; blood appears *blue.* Note changes in the *definition of the manubrium;* bulging makes the landmarks indistinct or completely obscures them. Inadequate function of the auditory (eustachian) tube produces *retraction* of the membrane that sharpens the outline of the manubrium and mallear folds; when fluid accumulates, the membrane looks *amber* and *air bubbles* may show through. The wedge of the light reflex may be distorted. When the incus is visible through the membrane, a normal middle ear is fairly certain.

Rough Quantitative Test for Hearing Loss

Difficulty understanding spoken questions during history taking may alert you to hearing loss.

WHISPER TEST. Test with the whispered voice by placing your mouth at the side of the patient's head, approximately 60 cm (2 ft) from her ear with the far ear covered. Whisper test numbers and have the patient repeat them, or whisper questions that cannot be answered yes or no. Test consistently with loud, medium, and soft tones. Alternatively, use the same intensity for all tests and find the maximal distance from the ear at which the whisper may be heard.

TUNING FORK. Hearing acuity may also be tested with the vibrations of a tuning fork. A fork with a frequency from 256 to 1024 cycles per second is preferred; the 128-cycle fork for testing vibratory sense is too low-pitched.

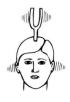
A. Weber Test

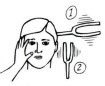
B. Rinne Test

Fig. 7-15 Tests of Hearing Perception and Conduction. A. Weber Test: The vibrating tuning fork is on the midline of the skull. Lateralization of the sound to one ear indicates a conductive loss on the same side, or a perceptive loss on the other side. B. Rinne Test: The handle of the tuning fork is first placed against the mastoid process then near the external ear. Each time the patient indicates when the sound ceases. Normally, air conduction persists twice as long as bone conduction.

Distinguishing Between Neurosensory and Conductive Hearing Loss

Use a tuning fork with frequencies of 256 to 1024 cycles per second. Set the fork in motion by gently tapping the base of the other hand.

THE WEBER TEST (FIG. 7-15A). Place the handle of the vibrating fork against the midline of the skull and ask the patient whether the sound is louder in one ear than in the other. With normal neurosensory hearing and no conductive loss, the sounds are equal in both ears.

THE RINNE TEST (FIG. 7-15B). Test one ear by pressing the handle of a vibrating fork first against the mastoid process (*bone conduction*), then direct the tines of the fork near the ear canal (*air conduction*). Ask the patient if it was louder behind the ear or at the ear canal. When air conduction is louder than bone conduction, the test is arbitrarily said to be *Rinne-positive*. The test is *Rinne-negative* when bone conduction is louder than air conduction. Have the patient indicate when they can no longer detect the sound by air conduction; see if you can hear the vibrating fork to compare their hearing to yours.

A conductive hearing loss is indicated when bone conduction is greater than air conduction. A conductive loss on a particular side is confirmed when the Weber lateralizes to that ear. If air conduction is greater than bone conduction bilaterally and the Weber lateralizes to one side, neurosensory hearing loss is suspected on that side.

Labyrinthine Test for Positional Nystagmus: Nylen, Barany, Hallpike Maneuver

Have the patient sit on the examination table and inspect the eyes carefully for spontaneous nystagmus. Then, keeping the eyes open, have the patient lie supine with the head extending beyond the head of the table, the chin elevated about 30 degrees and the head turned 45 degrees to the right. Observe the eyes for 30 seconds looking for nystagmus. Return the patient to the sitting position. After a short rest, redo the same

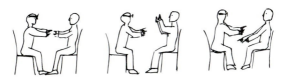

Fig. 7-16 Past Pointing Test for Labyrinthine Disorders.

test but with the patient turning the head to the left. Have the patient sit up and inspect the eyes for 30 seconds. A positive test induces nystagmus, often accompanied by intense nausea. The slow component of the nystagmus is in the direction of the endolymph flow; *the nystagmus is named for its fast component.*

Labyrinthine Test for Past Pointing

Have the patient sit facing you, keeping his eyes closed (Fig. 7-16). Have the patient point his forefingers toward you; place your forefingers lightly under the patient's forefingers. Hold your fingers in constant position; ask the patient to raise his arms and hands, then have him return his fingers to yours. Normally, this maneuver can be performed accurately. Past pointing indicates either loss of positional sense or labyrinthine stimulation.

Labyrinthine Test for Falling: Romberg Test

Have the patient stand with the inner aspects of the patient's feet close together (heel and toe) (Fig. 7-17). Encircle the patient's body with your arms but without touching the patient. Assure the patient that you will not let him fall, and then have the patient close his eyes. Normally patients will be steady, even with gentle, forewarned, pushes on the trunk. Falling during the test is the *Romberg sign.*

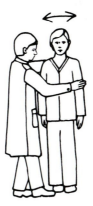

Fig. 7-17 Falling Test for Labyrinthine Disorders (Romberg Sign). *Normally the patient will waver somewhat, but not fall. With labyrinthine stimulation, the patient tends to fall in the direction of the flow of endolymph. Falling may also indicate loss of positional sense as in cerebellar deficits.*

Exam of the Eyes, Visual Fields and Visual Acuity

Remote Eye Examination

EXAMINE THE PALPEBRAL FISSURES AND POSITION OF THE GLOBE.   From a distance, note the width of the palpebral fissures (normal, increased, or diminished). Look for protrusion or recession of one or both globes by inspecting the eyes from the front, from the profile, and from above (looking downward over the forehead). Accurate measurement of the distance between the anterior surface of the cornea and the outer edge of the bony orbit can be made with a Hertel exophthalmometer; accurate use requires some practice. Individual variation is great, and there are familial and racial trends toward proptosis. The best evidence of pathologic exophthalmos lies in a series of accurate measurements showing progressive anterior displacement.

INSPECT FOR INFLAMMATION.   Inspect for redness and or swelling: Is it in one or both eyes? Does it involve the eyelid and/or the ocular surface?

TEST FOR LID LAG.   Use your finger or a penlight as a target. Start in the midline above eye level, about 50 cm (20 in) away, moving the target rapidly downward in the midline (Fig. 7-18). A lag is indicated by white sclera appearing between lid and limbus.

TEST EXTRAOCULAR MOVEMENTS.   Test the six cardinal positions of gaze for each eye by having the patient look to the right, right and up, left and up, to the left, left and down, right and down and then return to the primary position (see Fig. 14-16 page 832). Ask the patient to indicate if they see double as you test the six cardinal positions of gaze. When testing horizontally acting muscles hold the stimulus with the long dimension vertically; for testing vertically acting muscles, hold it horizontally. This allows the patient to easily see a doubled image. Finally, test convergence by holding the target in the midline and at eye level, about 50 cm (20 in) from the face, gradually moving the target toward the bridge of the nose; note the near point at which convergence fails, normally 50 to 75 mm (2 to 3 in).

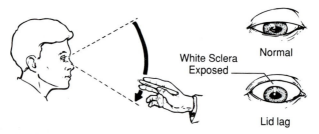

Fig. 7-18 Test for Lid Lag.

Tests for Gross Visual Fields Defects: Confrontation Methods

Use one or a combination of the following tests to detect visual field defects. Finger, face, and hand confrontation readily detect temporal field cuts. To detect nasal field cuts, test each eye independently.

FINGER CONFRONTATION. Fingers are presented in each quadrant on both sides of the vertical midline in each quadrant while the gaze is kept straight ahead. The patient is asked to sum the number of fingers seen. Because it is difficult to differentiate three fingers from four, it is best to use 1, 2, or 5 fingers. This testing tells whether there is an absolute defect in one quadrant. You can increase the sensitivity by decreasing the presentation time and increasing the distance from the patient.

FACE AND HAND CONFRONTATION. The patient is asked to look at the examiner's nose and then asked if the whole face appears clear. The patient may report various defects, such as the examiner's eye appearing blurry (which would represent a paracentral scotoma). With *hand confrontation* the patient fixes on the examiner's nose and the examiners hands are held on either side of the vertical midline first above then below the plane of gaze. The patient is asked if the hands appear the same. A cloudy or a faded-color appearing hand represents a relative and subtle defect along the vertical plane.

COLOR CONFRONTATION. This test is traditionally done with red caps of mydriatic bottles. (a) *Color comparison* about the vertical midline is performed as hand comparison above. This is a sensitive test for relative hemianopic defects. (b) For *central scotoma testing* of each eye, the subject is asked to look at one red cap and the other red cap is held in the patient's nasal field. The patient is then asked which cap is redder or brighter. A response that the peripheral cap is brighter, or that the caps are the same color, represents a central scotoma. Care should be taken not to hold the peripheral red cap in the temporal field as a cecocentral defect may confound interpretation, or you might place the cap in the patient's blind spot.

TEST FOR TUNNEL VISION (FIG. 7-19). Have the patient cover her left eye with her hand. Place your face in front of the patient's and at the same eye level, with your nose about 1 m (40 in) from the unmasked eye. Ask the patient to fix constantly on your eye. Cover your own right eye; fix your left eye on the patient's unmasked eye. Hold your left hand off to the side in the midplane between your faces. With a flicking finger or penlight for a target, bring it slowly toward the midline between you. Ask the patient to indicate when the target first appears and compare that with your own experience. Also test vertical and oblique runs. Test the nasal field with your right hand. Test the second eye similarly. This technique is less sensitive and specific than the first three because it will not detect scotomas within the visual field.

TECHNIQUES FOR LESS-COOPERATIVE PATIENTS. (a) For young children and obtunded adults, use the response to visually elicited eye move-

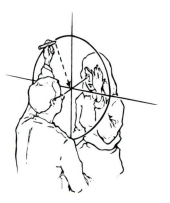

Fig. 7-19 Test for Tunnel Vision. *The patient fixes on the examiner's left eye. The examiner imagines a line of sight extending between the patient's open eye and the examiner's own eye; the two can be termed the opposing eyes. The examiner imagines radii that are perpendicular to the line of sight and center at a point equidistant between the two opposing eyes. A target on any point of such a radius will be equidistant between the opposing eyes at all locations. The examiner slowly moves a flicking finger or a penlight target along a radius from the periphery toward the center until the patient indicates that she can see it. Simultaneously, the examiner checks his view of the target.*

ments to novel targets. (b) For more obtunded adults, observe a blink in response to threat; try not to move air toward the cornea because this could stimulate the fifth cranial nerve and cause a corneal reflex. (c) Toddlers can be tested by finger mimicking.

Tests for Strabismus (Heterotropia)

Be sure the patient has useful vision in each eye.

ALTERNATE COVER TEST. Ask the patient to fixate on an object at the end of the room, or on your penlight, held about 33 cm (13 in) away. First cover the patient's left eye with your right hand (Fig. 7-20). Watch the uncovered right eye to see if it moves to take up fixation. Uncover the left eye and allow the patient to look with both eyes. Then cover the right eye and watch the uncovered left eye to see if it moves to fixation. If there is fixation movement, the patient has *heterotropia* (strabismus, squint). To *determine if the heterotropia is paralytic or nonparalytic,* ask the patient to follow your penlight in the six cardinal directions of gaze (both eyes look to right, right and up, left and up, left, left and down, right and down). If the eyes move equally without restriction, the deviation is nonparalytic. If one eye overshoots and the other fails to look the entire distance in one or more directions, the deviation is paralytic.

COVER–UNCOVER TEST. Have the patient fix on the object with both eyes; cover one eye for a few seconds, then uncover it while observing to see if it moves to reestablish fixation. If there is fixation movement, the eye has heterophoria.

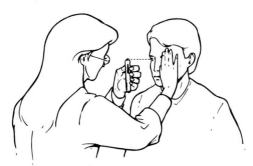

Fig. 7-20 Testing for Strabismus.

Close External Examination of the Eyes

EYELIDS. Look for swelling about the lids, above, below, and near the canthi. Note inversion or eversion of the lid margins. Examine the lid margins for scaling, excess or sparsity of secretions, purulent exudate, papules, or pustules. Look for lashes turned inward (*trichiasis*). Press on the lacrimal sac; if fluid can be expressed through the punctum, the tear duct is obstructed.

BULBAR CONJUNCTIVA AND SCLERA. Gently retract the lids with the thumb and forefinger; note the color of the sclera, whether white, blue, yellow, or hemorrhagic. Look for pigment deposits noting normal variations of complexion and race. Look for vascular engorgement. Distinguish the normal pinguecula from pterygium.

PALPEBRAL CONJUNCTIVA. *To evert the lower lid* (Fig. 7-21A) place the thumb tip on the loose skin beneath the margin and slide the skin down, pressing it gently into the orbit) and ask the patient to look up. Look for congestion, discharge, and other lesions. If indicated, *evert the upper lid* (Fig. 7-21B). Either face the patient or stand behind her while she is sitting, so her head rests against your body. Ask her to keep both eyes open and look downward to prevent elevation that reflexly accompanies closure of the lids. Grasp some eyelashes of the upper lid between your thumb and forefinger, pull the lid gently downward and away from the globe. With the tip of an applicator press against the upper lid just above the superior edge of the tarsal plate. Using this pressure point as a fulcrum, pull the eyelid quickly upward so that the tarsal plate turns on the fulcrum, its lower edge becomes uppermost, and the lid is everted. After the lid has been everted (to the astonishment of the patient), hold the lid with the left fingers, freeing the right hand. The normal position is regained merely by having the patient glance upward.

CORNEA. Shine light from a penlight obliquely on the cornea to search for scars, abrasions, or ulcers. The corneal light reflex should look smooth and regular as you play the light over the surface. Abrasions are readily demonstrated by fluorescein staining. Place the tip of a moistened fluorescein strip in the inferior fornix. After removing it, ask the

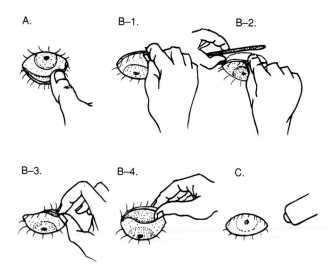

Fig. 7-21 Examination of the Eyelids. A. Eversion of the Lower Lid. B. Eversion of the Upper Lid: Tell the patient to look downward and proceed with four steps: (a) with the right thumb and forefinger, grasp a few cilia of the upper lid and pull the lid away from the globe; (b) lay an applicator along the crease made by the superior edge of the tarsal plate and the soft adjacent tissue; (c) quickly fold the lid over the applicator so the tarsal plate turns over and its upper edge faces downward; and (d) replace the right thumb and finger by the corresponding left ones to hold the lid. C. Testing Pupillary Reaction to Light.

patient to blink. Observe with a blue light; corneal abrasions appear green. The cornea may also be examined with a lens.

IRIS AND LENS.   Note the clarity of the iris, whether it appears distinct or muddy. Look for new vessels and deposits. Note the size, shape, and equality of the pupils. Test **pupillary reaction to light** by having the patient fix on a distant object (>3 m [10 ft] away) so that the patient does not fixate on the light and use accommodation. Shine a penlight into the pupil from the side (see Fig. 7-21C) while observing the *direct pupillary reaction;* remove the light and repeat the process, this time looking at the opposite (unlighted) pupil for *consensual reaction.* Repeat this sequence exposing the opposite eye to the light. Test **pupillary reaction to accommodation** by having the patient fix on her own finger as it is gradually brought closer to her nose. Shine the penlight obliquely through the lens to discover deposits on the surface and opacities in the matrix such as cataracts. **Testing for a relative afferent pupillary defect (RAPD).** Use the alternating light exam. As you shine light in the right eye, observe its iris for the force and amplitude of constriction; the left pupil should constrict as well, the normal *consensual response.* Swing the

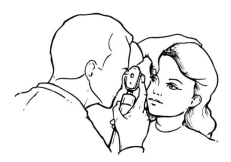

Fig. 7-22 Ophthalmoscopic Examination.

light slowly towards the left eye; observe the left pupil for dilatation as you swing the light across to it. In a normal eye, as the flashlight is swung to it from the other, there is a minimal dilatation, termed hippus, followed by constriction; again note the force and amplitude of constriction. If the left pupil dilates as the light moves toward it and remains dilated, it is termed a *Marcus-Gunn pupil,* indicating a defect in the detection or transmission of light by the left retina or optic nerve.

SCHIRMER TEST FOR LACK OF TEARS (FIG. 7-46D). A thin strip of filter paper is folded over the lower eyelid without anesthetic. Wetting of less than 10 mm of the paper after 5 minutes indicates keratoconjunctivitis sicca.

OPHTHALMOSCOPIC EXAMINATION (FIG. 7-22). The use of the ophthalmoscope requires supervised practice; do not hope to obtain meaningful information on your first attempt. Face the patient so that your right eye looks into her right eye; later, your left eye should examine her left eye. Examination of the right eye without dilating the pupils is described. Grasp the instrument with your right hand, your forefinger on the disk of lenses. Rest your left hand on the patient's forehead so that your thumb can pull up the upper lid slightly to uncover the pupil and prevent excessive blinking. Ask the patient to fix her eyes straight ahead on a distant object.

THE MEDIA (FIG. 7-22). Place the +8 or +10 diopter lens in the sight hole, bring it close to your eye or glasses, and move forward to about 30 cm (12 in) in front of the patient's eye. Shine the light into her pupil to see the red retinal reflex. A dull red or black reflex is produced by diffuse dense opacities. Look for black spots showing against the red; these are the shadows of opacities in the lens or vitreous made by the light reflected from the retina. Move forward or backward until the spots are clearly focused. While watching the opacities, ask the patient to elevate the eyes slightly; if the spots move upward, they are on the cornea or anterior part of the lens; little movement occurs when the location is near the lenticular center; downward movement indicates a location in the posterior lens or vitreous. Vitreous opacities appear more distinct when viewed obliquely with the white optic disk as a background.

THE FUNDUS (SEE FIG. 7-22).   When the media appears sufficiently clear, hold the instrument about 5 cm (2 in) from the patient's eye with your forehead near or touching your hand on the patient's forehead. The physician's right eye examines the patient's right; the physician's left eye is employed for the patient's left eye, so the physician's nose parallels the patient's cheek. The physician's right forefinger changes the lenses; the physician's left hand rests upon the head of the patient with the thumb gently retracting and holding the upper lid to prevent excessive blinking. Run the gamut of lenses in the sight hole from +10 to −5 to find the optimal focus for a distinct view of the retina. The selection is governed by the refractive error and the degree of accommodation in both patient and examiner. In the absence of both factors, the best view should be obtained when the sight hole is turned to zero. Minus lenses are required to correct for involuntary accommodation. When a cataract has been extracted without intraocular lens replacement, about +10 is needed for correction. High astigmatism cannot be corrected with the spherical lenses of the instrument; the fundi should then be examined through the patient's glasses. When the correct setting is found, examine the following regions (see Fig. 7-49A).

Optic Disk: The optic disc lies 10 degrees into the nasal retina. Therefore, angle the ophthalmoscope 10 degrees nasally from the line of sight to be in the vicinity of the optic disc. Note the shape and color of the optic disk. The shape is round or oval vertically. Most of the disk is red-orange, the color imparted by the capillaries around the nerve fibers. The *physiologic cup* is a pale area in the temporal side of the disk devoid of nerve fibers; it forms a depression whose base is the nonvascular *lamina cribrosa*. The size and shape of the cup vary greatly in normal eyes. It is measured by the *cup-to-disk ratio*, for example, 0.2/1.0. If the cup is not circular, the vertical ratio is used. The site of ingress and egress of vessels, called the *vessel funnel*, also lacks nerve fibers, so it is pale and white. The borders of the disk may merge gradually into the surrounding retina, or they may be sharply demarcated by a white scleral ring. Outside the ring, on the temporal side, a crescent of pigment may occur.

Retinal Vessels: The arteries are bright red with a central stripe, the *light reflex*. Note the width of the reflex stripe. Normally the veins are wider than the arteries in a ratio of about 4:3; they are darker red and lack a stripe. The vessel branching pattern shows great individual variation. As they emerge from the disk, the afferent vessels are true arteries; branches beyond the second bifurcation, about 1 disk diameter from the disk margin, are arterioles. Look for sheathing of the arteries. Observe the veins carefully at the arteriovenous crossings for nicking, deviation, humping, tapering, sausaging, or banking. Retinal veins normally pulsate; arteries in the retina do not.

Retina: The amount of pigmentation corresponds to the patient's complexion and race. The retina is thinner in the nasal periphery and therefore paler. Note areas of white or pigment from scarring. Look for hemorrhages and exudates. Express the size of abnormalities in disk diameters. Measure depression or elevation by the diopters of correction required to focus on an arterial reflex in the area.

Macula: The macula is slightly below the horizontal plane of the disk and from 2–3 disk diameters to the temporal side of its margin. Examination of the macula is usually fleeting because illumination of this region produces discomfort; examine it last. In the center of the macula, the *fovea* appears as a small darker-red area, set apart from visible vessels. In its center appears a small darker spot, the *foveola,* whose center gives off a speck of reflected light.

BEDSIDE TESTS FOR VISUAL ACUITY. Gross tests for visual acuity can be made without special equipment. Test a single eye at a time. Show the patient a newspaper or magazine, testing first with the fine print. If this is not perceived, show the larger letters. If the patient fails on large letters, hold up several fingers 1 m (3 ft) away and ask the patient to count them. If the patient cannot count them, determine if the patient can see movements of the hand. Failing this, flash a light beam into the eye, asking the patient to indicate when it appears. Test whether the patient can perceive the direction of the light source.

When gross visual acuity is fair, more accurate tests can be made with the standard *Snellen charts.* Be sure there are adequate illumination and the standard distance to the chart. Determine the smallest line of letters the patient can read without error with each eye, and then with both eyes together. Express the reading as a ratio of the distance at which the test is conducted and the distance at which the line of letters should be read by a normal eye. The distance is expressed in feet or meters; 20/20 feet and 6/6 meters are normal. If the patient could only read the line for 40 feet, her acuity is expressed as 20/40.

It should always be noted whether the patient's optical correction (glasses or contact lens) were used. If the visual acuity is abnormal, the potential acuity from an improved optical correction using lenses can be estimated by using the *pinhole test.* To perform this, a 1-mm hole (or series of holes) is made in a note card. The patient is then asked to read a Snellen chart through the pinhole. The patient then selects only those rays of light that are in focus. A close approximation to the patients best corrected visual acuity can then be recorded.

TESTS FOR COLOR VISION. Ask the patient to identify the colors of objects immediately available. For more precise testing, use a book of *Ishihara plates.* Remember that color vision is a mixture of red, blue, and green.

SLIT-LAMP MICROSCOPY. Slit-lamp examination requires special equipment and is reserved for an experienced ophthalmologist. A powerful light is focused in a narrow slit upon the various layers of the cornea, the anterior chamber, the lens, and the anterior third of the vitreous chamber, while the objects are examined through a corneal microscope. Accurate inspection of opacities and minute foci of inflammation can be made.

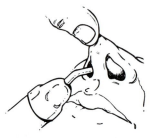
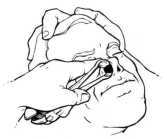

A. Transillumination of   B. Speculum Examination
   the Nasal Septum   of the Nose

Fig. 7-23 Examination of the Nasal Septum and Nares. A. Transillumination of the Nasal Septum. B. Speculum Examination of the Nose.

Examination of the Nose and Sinuses

Routine Nasal Examination

Inspect the contour of the nose for asymmetry and abnormalities of profile. Test the patency of each naris by closing the other with digital compression while the patient inhales with the mouth closed. *Transilluminate* the nasal septum: with the thumb, push the soft nasal tip upward, while a lighted penlight in the other hand closes one naris (Fig. 7-23A); through the open naris, view the transilluminated septum for deviations, perforations, and masses. Palpate the cheeks and supraorbital ridges for tenderness over the maxillary and frontal sinuses. If no significant abnormalities have been encountered thus far, no further examination of the nose is required.

Detailed Nasal Examination

The history or the findings from the routine examination may prompt a more thorough search with special methods and instruments.

EXAMINATION OF THE NASAL SEPTUM AND NARES USING THE NASAL SPECULUM. Examine the nasal chambers anteriorly by retracting the nares with the speculum and illuminating with a head mirror or head lamp. For either naris, hold the handles of the speculum in the left hand (see Fig. 7-23B); insert the closed blades about 1 cm into the vestibule; open the blades vertically, in the plane of the septum, with the left forefinger pressing the ala nasi against the superior blade to anchor it. This avoids painful pressure on the septum. The right hand is free to position the patient's head or to hold instruments. Only a small area can be viewed with a single position of the speculum, so explore the region by changing the direction of the speculum and the position of the patient's head. Examine the *vestibule* for folliculitis and fissures. Note the color of the *mucosa* and any swelling. Inspect the nasal septum for deviations, ulcers, or hemorrhages. Direct your attention to the lateral chamber wall. Locate the *inferior turbinate* to note swelling, increased redness, pallor,

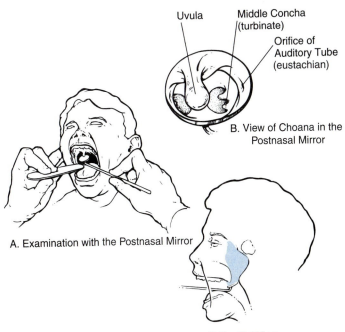

Uvula

Middle Concha
(turbinate)

Orifice of
Auditory Tube
(eustachian)

B. View of Choana in the
Postnasal Mirror

A. Examination with the Postnasal Mirror

C. Sagittal View

Fig. 7-24 Examination of the Nasopharynx. A. Examination with the Postnasal Mirror. In the drawing, all deep spaces are heavily stippled. B. View of the Choana in the Postnasal Mirror. C. Sagittal View.

or blueness. Identify the *middle turbinate* and its underlying *meatus.* Look particularly in the *middle meatus* for purulent discharge from frontal, maxillary, and anterior ethmoid sinuses.

EXAMINATION OF THE NASOPHARYNX USING THE POSTNASAL MIRROR (FIG. 7-24A). A head mirror or head lamp is required for illumination. Use a No. 0 (small) postnasal mirror, warming it by immersion in warm water; test its temperature by touching its back to your hand. Grasp the end of a tongue blade in the left hand so the thumb pushes upward from beneath, while the index finger and long finger press downward on the middle of the blade. Have the tongue tip placed behind the lower incisors. Depress the tongue by inserting the blade from the right corner of the mouth to rest upon the midpoint of the lingual dorsum; press the arched tongue downward and forward by depressing the middle of the blade with the two fingers and the upward push of the thumb serving as a fulcrum at the end. Steady the left hand by pressing the ring and little fingers against the patient's cheek. Have the patient breathe steadily through the nose with the mouth opened. Grasp the handle of the mirror in your right hand, like a pencil; steady your hand by bracing your

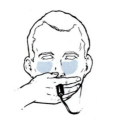

A. Maxillary Sinuses

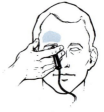

B. Frontal Sinuses

Fig. 7-25 Transillumination of the Nasal Sinuses. *A. Maxillary Sinuses. B. Frontal Sinuses.*

fingers against the patient's cheek. Insert the mirror from the left side of the mouth (opposite the tongue blade), with mirror upright, avoiding contact with tongue, palate, and uvula. Position it behind the uvula and near to the posterior pharyngeal wall. Turn the mirror upward, focus the light on it, and adjust it to view the various parts of the *choana* (Figs. 7-24B and 7-24C). Locate the posterior end of the *nasal septum,* the *vomer,* always found in the midline. Identify the *middle meatus;* pus draining posteriorly from this region comes only from the maxillary sinus. The *inferior meatus* is not well visualized posteriorly. The orifices of the *auditory (eustachian) tubes* are behind and lateral to the middle meatus. The orifice appears pale or yellow and is about 5 mm in diameter. The tubes are closed except during swallowing or yawning. Look for masses of *pharyngeal tonsil (adenoids)* hanging from the roof into the fossa of the tubal orifice, and for areas of inflammation, exudate, polyps, and neoplasms in the nasopharynx, uvula, and soft palate. If available, a fiberoptic instrument will simplify your examination.

TRANSILLUMINATION OF THE MAXILLARY SINUSES (FIG. 7-25A). Use a specially insulated electric lamp on a cord. In a darkened room, place the light in the patient's mouth and have the patient close his lips tightly about it. Put your hand over the patient's mouth to shield the light coming from the buccal cavity. Usually, the two maxillary sinuses and the orbits are illuminated. Alternatively, press a cool light against the each maxilla while observing the hard palate for transmitted light. Most significant is when one maxillary sinus lights up and the other is clouded.

TRANSILLUMINATION OF THE FRONTAL SINUSES (SEE FIG. 7-25B). Use the same arrangements, but place the light under the nasal half of the supraorbital ridge; with your hand, shield the orbit up to the eyebrow. Look for a bright area in the forehead.

Exam of the Lips, Mouth, Teeth, Tongue, and Pharynx

Examination is by inspection and palpation. Facing the patient, hold a tongue blade in the left hand and a penlight in the right. If a head lamp or mirror is used, your right hand is free to hold a nasal or laryngeal mirror. Completely inspect the oral cavity before beginning palpation.

Lips

Look for cleft lip and other congenital and acquired defects. Have the patient attempt to whistle, to reveal paralysis from facial nerve (CN VII) lesions. Note the color of the lips and look for evidence of angular stomatitis, rhagades, ulcers, granulomas, and neoplasms. Inspect the inner surface of the lips by retracting them with a tongue blade while the teeth are approximated.

Teeth

Note the absence of one or more teeth and the presence of caries, discoloration, fillings, and bridges. Notice abnormal dental shape, such as notching. Tap each tooth with a probe for tenderness.

Gums

Have the patient remove any dental appliances. Look for retraction of the gingival margins, pus in the margins, inflammation of the gums, spongy or bleeding gums, lead or bismuth lines, or localized gingival swelling.

Breath

Smell the breath for acetone, ammonia, or fetor.

Tongue

Have the patient protrude his tongue. Assess its size; look for deviation from the midline or restricted protrusion. Examine the coat of the tongue for color, thickness, and adhesiveness. Look for abnormalities on the dorsal surface. Describe local lesions and palpate them with gloved fingers. Have the patient raise the tip to the roof of the mouth; inspect the undersurface, including *frenulum* and *carunculae sublingualis.* Palpate the accessible portions of a tongue that is painful, or has restricted motion, for deep-seated masses. Have the tongue inside the teeth when palpating to relax the muscles. Palpate the region of the sublingual salivary glands and the submaxillary ducts for calculi.

Buccal Mucosa

Retract the cheek with the tongue blade. Look for melanin deposits, vesicles, petechiae, candida, Koplik spots, ulcers, neoplasms. Examine the orifices of the parotid duct, opposite the upper second molar.

Oropharynx

To depress the tongue, have the patient place the tip behind the lower incisors and breathe gently but steadily (Fig. 7-26A). Hold the tongue blade in your left hand with your middle finger over its midpoint and your thumb pushing upward on the nearer end of the blade; place the flat of the farther end about midway back on the tongue; pull down on the middle of the blade and push up with the thumb to depress the tongue and pull its root forward. Pressing the tongue farther back causes

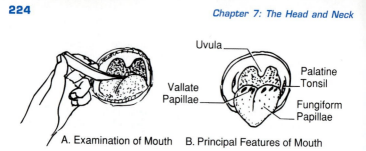

Uvula

Vallate Papillae

Palatine Tonsil

Fungiform Papillae

A. Examination of Mouth   B. Principal Features of Mouth

Fig. 7-26 Examination of the Oral Cavity. A. Use of the Tongue Blade. B. Principal Anatomic Features Seen in the Oral Cavity.

gagging; pressing anteriorly permits posterior bulging. An optimal view may require several placements of the blade transversely at the midpoint. Test for vagal nerve (CN X) paralysis by noting whether the uvula is drawn upward in the midline when the patient says "e-e-e."

Tonsils

Look for hyperplasia, ulcers, membrane, masses, and small, submerged tonsils.

Palpation of the Roof of the Tongue

If the patient gags readily, spray the throat with a topical anesthetic; otherwise, proceed without anesthesia. While wearing gloves, have the patient open his mouth wide. From the outside, with your left fingers, push a fold of the patient's right cheek between the patient's teeth to avoid having your fingers bitten. Insert your right forefinger to the back of the mouth and palpate the roof of the tongue, the valleculae, and the tonsillar fossae (Fig. 7-27).

EXAMINATION OF A LINGUAL ULCER.   Dry off the ulcer by pressing it gently with a cotton sponge and then inspect it carefully. Palpate the surrounding and underlying tissue with gloved fingers (you may be dealing with a chancre). Remember that the pain from lingual lesions may be referred to the ear.

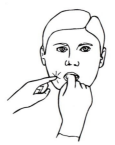

Fig. 7-27 Palpation of the Roof of the Tongue.

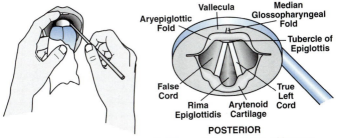

Vallecula

Median
Glossopharyngeal
Fold

Aryepiglottic
Fold

Tubercle of
Epiglottis

False
Cord

True
Left
Cord

Rima
Epiglottidis

Arytenoid
Cartilage

POSTERIOR

A. Mirror Laryngoscopy

B. Mirrored Appearance of Larynx

Fig. 7-28 Mirror Laryngoscopy. ***A. Hand and Instrument Positions for Laryngoscopy. B. Appearance of the Larynx in the Mirror.*** *This is the appearance with the cords abducted.*

Examination of the Larynx

Mirror Laryngoscopy

Use a head mirror or head lamp because both your hands must be free. To use the mirror, seat the patient in a chair with a clear 150W electric lamp immediately behind and to the right side of the patient's head. Reflect this light with your head mirror; practice is required. Have the patient sit quite erect with the chin somewhat forward, both feet on the floor, knees together. Seat yourself in front of the patient with your knees outside the patient's knees. Explain exactly what you are about to do and have the patient concentrate on breathing softly and regularly through the mouth (Fig. 7-28). Have the tongue protrude maximally over the lower teeth; with your left hand, wrap a piece of gauze over the tongue, grasp the wrapped portion between thumb and middle finger, bracing your hand against the patient's upper teeth with the forefinger; pull the tongue gently to the patient's right side. With thumb and forefinger of your right hand, grasp a No. 5 (large) laryngeal mirror at the midpoint of its handle. Heat the mirror over a lamp or in warm water to avoid subsequent steaming over; test the temperature by touching the mirror back to your left wrist. Holding the handle like a pencil and bracing your fourth and fifth fingers against the patient's cheek, insert the mirror in the patient's mouth from the patient's left side, with the face of the mirror downward and parallel to the tongue surface. Move it posteriorly until its back rests against the anterior surface of the uvula. Press the uvula and soft palate steadily upward; avoid touching the back of the tongue to prevent gagging. Have the patient breathe steadily while you inspect the larynx. While still viewing the vocal cords, ask the patient to say "e-e-e" or "he-e-e" in a high-pitched voice. Sing along with him in the desired pitch and for the proper duration. When looking in the mirror, remember that upward is anterior, downward is posterior. Examine the *vallate papillae, lingual tonsils, valleculae,* and *epiglottis* (Fig. 7-28B). Then look at the *false cords, true vocal cords, arytenoids,* and *piri-*

form sinuses. Finally, observe the true vocal cords during quiet respiration when the rima is tent-shaped. During phonation, watch the cords meet in the midline.

K, L, M Test for Dysarthria

To distinguish between cranial nerve deficits causing dysarthria, ask your patient to say: "Ka, Ka, Ka" (gutturals, CN IX and CN X); "La, La, La" (linguals, CN XII); and "Me, Me, Me" (labials, CN VII).

Examination of the Salivary Glands

Parotid Gland

If lateral facial swelling is present, see if it has the distribution of the parotid gland: swelling (a) in front of the tragus of the external ear, (b) in front of the auricular lobule, (c) behind the ear, pushing the pinna outward. Have the patient clench his teeth to tense the masseter muscle; palpate the swelling against the hardened muscle to determine extent, consistency, and tenderness of the mass. When fullness is present anterior to the tragus, ascertain whether it is continuous with the inferior mass, as in parotid swelling, or discontinuous, as in swelling of a preauricular lymph node. Feel for swelling behind the mandibular ramus, which is always present in parotid enlargement. Inspect the orifice of the parotid duct, opposite the upper second molar. While watching the orifice, press the cheek swelling, observing for pus from the duct. Palpate the parotid duct externally for calculus. With a gloved finger, feel the orifice and the region posterior to it, in a horizontal line, for calculus or other mass. The location of the parotid duct on the cheek is one fingerbreadth below the zygomatic arch, on a line between the inferior border of the concha of the ear and the commissure of the lips. The normal duct is thick enough to be felt when rolled against the tensed masseter.

Submaxillary Gland

Note a swelling under the mandible and slightly anterior to the angle of the jaw. When no mass is present but there is a history of a mass appearing after meals, have the patient sip some lemon juice and watch for the development of a swelling; the appearance of a mass or the enlarging of a preexisting swelling is diagnostic of ductal obstruction. Also compare the appearance of the ductal orifice with its homologue. Using bimanual palpation, with gloved finger in the floor of the mouth, feel for calculus or a mass; look for the drainage of pus when the mass is pressed in the submandibular triangle. Test both orifices for the secretion of saliva: place dry cotton under the tongue and let the patient sip lemon juice; then remove the swab and watch for salivary flow from each orifice.

Examination of the Temporomandibular Joint

Palpate over the temporomandibular joint, anterior to the tragus, while the patient opens and closes the mouth, feeling for clicking or crepitus (see Fig. 7-29). Corresponding noises may be heard by placing the bell

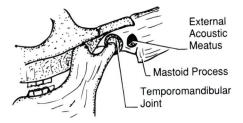

Fig. 7-29 Anatomy of the Temporomandibular Joint. *Note the nearness of the joint to the external acoustic meatus, so the joint may be palpated by a finger in the meatus (see Fig. 7-75).*

of the stethoscope over the joint during movement. To elicit joint tenderness, face the patient and place the tips of your forefingers behind the tragi in each external acoustic meatus. Pull forward while the patient opens her mouth.

Examination of the Neck

Examination of Cervical Muscles and Bones

If cervical fracture is suspected, and in trauma cases, immobilize the patient and obtain x-rays before trying to elicit physical signs. Have the patient's neck and shoulders uncovered. Face the patient looking for any swellings, especially in the sternocleidomastoideus and the cervical spine. Note any asymmetry of shoulder height and clavicles or fixed posture of the neck. Note the extent of movement and the pain elicited by cervical flexion, extension, lateral bending, and rotation of the head. Palpate the cervical vertebrae and the muscles for local tenderness, muscular tightness, and masses. See if massage of muscles brings relief. Special diagnostic maneuvers may be required.

Examination of the Thyroid Gland

The normal adult thyroid is often not palpable. In a thin neck, the normal isthmus may be felt as a band of tissue that just obliterates the surface outlines of the tracheal rings. A *goiter* is any enlarged thyroid gland.

INSPECTION. Have the patient seated in a good cross-light. Inspect the lower half of the neck in the anterior triangles. Have the patient swallow to note any ascending mass in the midline or behind the sternocleidomastoids. If the patient is obese or has a short neck, tilt the patient's neck back, supporting the occiput with the patient's clasped hands; ask the patient to swallow while in this posture.

PALPATION FROM BEHIND. Have the patient seated in a chair and stand behind her. Instruct the patient to lower her chin and relax her neck muscles. Place your thumbs in back of the patient's neck, curling your fingers anteriorly so their tips just touch while resting over the upper tracheal rings (Fig. 7-30A). It is a good practice to have the patient hold some water in her mouth and swallow on demand. Run the fingers up and down the tracheal rings, feeling for any tissue on their anterior sur-

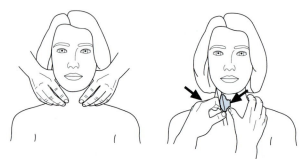

**A. Palpation of the Thyroid
from Behind**

**B. Palpation of the Thyroid
from in Front**

*Fig. 7-30 Palpation of the Thyroid Gland and Adjacent Structures. A.
Palpation from Behind. B. Frontal Palpation of the Thyroid Gland.*

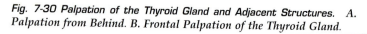

face; if found, it is likely to be a hyperplastic thyroid isthmus. Palpate
systematically the lower poles of both lateral lobes. During the examination, shift the inclination of the patient's head to relax the neck muscles, and have the patient swallow to test the adherence of palpated
masses to the trachea. Palpate the anterior surface of the lateral lobes
through the sternocleidomastoids with the patient's head slightly in-
clined toward the side being examined to relax the muscles. Occasionally, the thyroid is more easily felt when the neck is dorsiflexed.

FRONTAL PALPATION.   Face your patient placing the fingers of one hand
at the back of the neck with your extended thumb forward at the base
of the thyroid cartilage (see Fig. 7-30B). With the pulp of this thumb,
push the trachea gently away from the midline while the fingers of your
other hand are inserted behind the sternocleidomastoid of the opposite
side, where they can feel the posterior aspect of the displaced lateral
lobe; let the thumb feel medial to the muscle for the anterior surface of
the mass. Having the patient swallow or depress the chin may further
assist in the examination. Palpate the other lateral lobe in the same manner with the tasks of the two hands reversed. Ask the patient to swallow to test the adherence of the masses to the trachea.

AUSCULTATION OF A GOITER.   Always auscultate a goiter, using the bell
of the stethoscope to listen for a bruit or murmur.

Examination of the Lymph Nodes

See Chapter 5, page 104.

Examination of the Vascular System

See Chapter 8, page 365ff.

Symptoms

General Symptoms

▼ KEY SYMPTOM
◪ Headache: See Chapter 14, page 850ff, and page 316ff.

Skull, Scalp, and Face Symptoms

▼ KEY SYMPTOM
◪ Blushing and Flushing: *Pathophysiology:* Transient dilation of the superficial blood vessels of the head, face, and neck occurs with emotional, pharmacologic, or physical stimulation. *Flushing* is a normal response to exercise, hot environments, and ingestion of vasoactive substances such as capsaicin in hot peppers or alcohol. Flushing is common in patients with rosacea or carcinoid syndrome and in women at the menopause. *Blushing* is a term usually reserved for flushing associated with embarrassment or self-consciousness.

▼ KEY SYMPTOM
◪ Pain in the Face: Facial pain is usually well localized, indicating the structure involved. In some cases, it may present a difficult diagnostic problem. An anatomic approach to identifying the cause is useful.

✓ **CLINICAL OCCURRENCE:** *Nerves* trigeminal neuralgia, postherpetic neuralgia; *Blood Vessels* temporal arteritis, cavernous sinus thrombosis; *Teeth* periapical abscess, periodontitis, unerupted teeth; *Bones* sinusitis, osteomyelitis; *Joints* temporomandibular arthritis; *Salivary Glands* parotitis.

⬛ KEY SYNDROME
◪ Facial Pain: Trigeminal Neuralgia (Tic Douloureux): *Pathophysiology:* Usually an underlying cause is not found, but compression of the fifth nerve root by a vessel or neoplasm has been described. The patient experiences periodic pain, always unilateral, initially limited to one division of the trigeminal nerve (CN V). A normally nonpainful slight stimulus provokes a paroxysm of "hot" lancinating pain. The intense pain causes grimacing, hence the French term *tic*. Each patient has a special, adequate stimulus in the trigger area: a light touch, chewing, sneezing, a draft, or a tickling of the skin. The second, maxillary, division is most commonly involved, so the pain is in the maxilla, the upper teeth and lip and the lower eyelid. Uncommonly, the third, mandibular, division is involved with pain distributed in the lower teeth and lip, the oral portion of the tongue, and the external acoustic meatus. The ophthalmic branch is rarely affected. There are no motor or sensory changes. DDX: The initial stage of herpes zoster may suggest tic douloureux, but the diagnosis is made when herpetic vesicles appear.

D KEY DISEASE

Facial Pain: Herpes Zoster: Sharp burning pain may occur unilaterally in the distribution of a branch of the trigeminal nerve before vesicles indicate the diagnosis. Persistent pain after resolution of the skin lesions is post-herpetic neuralgia.

S KEY SYNDROME

▶ **Facial Pain: Acute Suppurative Sinusitis, Orbital Cellulitis:** See pages 325–326.

KEY SYMPTOM

Spasms of the Jaw Muscles: Trismus: See page 239.

KEY SYMPTOM

▶ **Pain With Chewing: Masseter Claudication:** *Pathophysiology:* Ischemia of the masseter and/or temporalis muscles is induced by chewing. The onset of jaw pain sometimes occurs after initiating chewing. Tough meats are especially problematic; the patient may have altered their diet. This should initiate a search for giant cell arteritis.

S KEY SYNDROME

Temporomandibular Joint (TMJ) Pain: *Pathophysiology:* The TMJ is a biconcave joint that is subject to considerable pressure with chewing. Symptoms include pain, which may be felt in the ear or temple, clicking, and occasionally locking. Trauma is associated with injury and crepitation. Physical examination is superior to MRI for diagnosis [Haley DP, Schiffman EL, Lindgren BR, et al. The relationship between clinical and MRI findings in patients with unilateral temporomandibular joint pain. *J Am Dent Assoc* 2001;132:476–481]. See also Syndromes page 317.

KEY SYMPTOM

Numb Chin Syndrome: *Pathophysiology:* Involvement of the mental or inferior alveolar nerve causes numbness in the chin. Patients present with a complaint of numbness of the chin; no other symptoms or signs may be present. If thorough oral exam doesn't identify a local cause of nerve injury, a search for neoplastic disease is indicated [Maillefert J-F, Gazet-Malillefert M-P, Tavernier C, Farge P. Numb chin syndrome. *J Bone Spine* 2000;67:86–93].

Ear Symptoms

KEY SYMPTOM

Tinnitus: Ringing in the ears or tinnitus is sufficiently distressing that it serves as a chief complaint in bringing the patient to the physician [Lockwood AH, Salvi RJ, Burkard RF. Tinnitus. *N Engl J Med* 2002;347:904–910]. Unilateral tinnitus may be the first symptom of an acoustic neuroma.

✔ *TINNITUS—CLINICAL OCCURRENCE:* *Outer Ear* cerumen, foreign body, polyp in the external acoustic meatus; *Middle Ear* inflammation, otosclerosis; *Inner Ear* Ménière disease, syphilis, fevers, suppuration of the labyrinth, fracture at the base of the skull, acoustic nerve tumor, acoustic trauma; *Drugs* quinine, salicylates, aminoglycoside antibiotics.

KEY SYMPTOM
Temporary Altered Hearing: Eustachian Tube Block: See page 244. The patient experiences mild intermittent pain, a feeling of fullness in the ear and altered hearing. The patient may hear a popping sound on swallowing or yawning. Inspection of the eardrum shows it to be retracted (Fig. 7-35B).

KEY SYMPTOM
Earache: *Pathophysiology:* The middle ear arises from the first and second pharyngeal pouches. Pain may arise from inflammation of structures in the ear or be referred from other pharyngeal sites, including the thyroid. Although the cause of acute pain in the ear is usually readily discovered, chronic earache may offer considerable challenge in diagnosis.

✓ *EARACHE—CLINICAL OCCURRENCE:* *Auricle* trauma, hematoma, frostbite, burn, epithelioma, perichondritis, gout, eczema, impetigo, insect bites, carcinoma, herpes zoster; *Meatus* external otitis, malignant external otitis, carbuncle, meatitis, eczema, hard cerumen, foreign body, injury, epithelioma, carcinoma, insect invasion, herpes zoster, trigeminal neuralgia (CN V3); *Middle Ear* acute otitis media, acute mastoiditis, malignant disease; *Referred Pain* (through CN V, IX, and X and the second and third cervical nerves) unerupted lower third molar, carious teeth, arthritis of temporomandibular joint, tonsillitis, carcinoma or sarcoma of pharynx, ulcer of epiglottis or larynx, cervical lymphadenitis, subacute thyroiditis, trigeminal neuralgia.

KEY SYMPTOM
Dizziness and Vertigo: See page 322.

Eye Symptoms

KEY SYMPTOM
Double Vision: Diplopia: *Pathophysiology:* Perception of two visual images results from abnormalities of refraction or, less commonly, nonconjugative gaze. A careful history should determine the pattern of the symptom (e.g., vertical or horizontal), precipitating activities, the field of vision where the diplopia is apparent, and the position of the head or gaze that relieves the diplopia. If the patient reports monocular diplopia or diplopia when one eye is covered, the cause is nearly always refractive. Diplopia also results from impairment of the CN III, CN IV, and/or CN VI, damage to or weakness of the extraocular muscles, or displacement of the globe. Careful physical examination should be able to differentiate between these causes. Important diagnostic considerations are myasthenia gravis, Graves ophthalmopathy, and ophthalmoplegias.

Dry Eyes: See page 264, Keratoconjunctivitis sicca.

Blurred Vision: *Pathophysiology:* Loss of sharp focus of light on the retina occurs with inability of the eye to accommodate the shape of the lens to near or far vision, or scattering of light as a result of opacities in the cornea, lens, or vitreous. The history is the key to identifying the problem. Pain in the eye suggests inflammation of one of the structures (keratitis, iritis, uveitis) or glaucoma. Abnormality of the oils in the tear film is a frequent cause of visual aberration. Use of topical and systemic drugs, especially anticholinergics, results in decreased accommodation and dilation of the pupil. Loss of vision in one eye may also be described as "blurred vision," meaning the vision is less distinct than normal because of loss of binocular sight. The pinhole test (see page 219) can be used to determine if the blurred vision is optical in origin, which can be improved by the a new spectacle correction [Shingleton GJ, O'Donoghue MW. Blurred vision. *N Engl J Med* 2000;343:556–562].

► **Pain in the Eye:** *Pathophysiology:* Pain in the eye results from inflammation, infection, trauma, and increased intraocular pressure. Inspect the lids, conjunctivae, and sclera for lesions. Careful examination of the cornea, anterior chamber, iris, and retina are mandatory in patients complaining of eye pain. Always assess visual acuity in each eye. Optimal exam requires an ophthalmologist.

✔ *CLINICAL OCCURRENCE:* *Endocrine* thyrotoxicosis, Graves ophthalmopathy; *Idiopathic* cluster headache; *Inflammatory/Immune* hordeolum (sty), chalazion, interstitial keratitis, iritis, iridocyclitis, episcleritis, scleritis, band keratopathy, optic neuritis (e.g., multiple sclerosis); *Infectious* infective keratitis (herpes simplex, zoster and others), sinusitis (ethmoid, frontal sphenoid); *Mechanical/Trauma* foreign body, corneal abrasion, entropion, glaucoma, eyestrain.

► **Visual Loss:** *Pathophysiology:* Injury or impairment to any portion of the visual pathways can lead to visual loss. Acute loss of vision is a medial emergency (see page 319). Chronic progressive loss of vision is common with diseases of the cornea, lens, or retina. Standard tests of visual acuity will quantitate the degree of impairment and formal visual field testing is required. Referral to an ophthalmologist is indicated.

Nose Symptoms

Loss of Smell: Anosmia: See page 281.

Abnormal Smell or Taste: Dysgeusia: This is a common complaint in patients who have loss of smell (*anosmia*). If it is paroxysmal and associated with behavioral symptoms, it suggests complex partial seizures.

Lip, Mouth, Tongue, Teeth, and Pharynx Symptoms

KEY SYMPTOM

Soreness of Tongue or Mouth: Pain or tenderness in the tongue or mouth is a presenting symptom for a number of disorders. Inspection and palpation will reveal clues to assist in the differential diagnosis [Drage LA, Rogers RS. Clinical assessment and outcome in 70 patients with complaints of burning or sore mouth symptoms. *Mayo Clin Proc* 1999;74:223–228].

✓ **CLINICAL OCCURRENCE:** *No Lesions* tobacco smoking, early glossitis from all causes, menopausal symptom, heavy metal poisoning; *Deep Lesions* calculus in duct of submaxillary or sublingual gland, foreign body, myositis of lingual muscles, trichinosis, periostitis of hyoid bone, neoplasm of lingual muscles; *Localized Superficial Lesions* biting the tongue, trauma to lingual frenulum, dental ulcer, injury while under anesthesia, foreign body (e.g., fish bone), epithelioma or carcinoma, ranula, tuberculous ulcer, herpes, Vincent stomatitis, leukoplakia, *Candida*; *Generalized Disease* pellagra, riboflavin deficiency, scurvy, pernicious anemia, atrophic glossitis, leukemia, erythematous disorders, collagen diseases, pemphigus, cicatricial pemphigoid, lichen planus, scarlet fever, heavy-metal poisoning, phenytoin, uremia, cancer chemotherapy, drug sensitivity; *Irradiation* Therapeutic irradiation for head and neck malignancy causes temporary or permanent loss of saliva production. Within 2–4 weeks of the beginning of treatment, and lasting 6 or more weeks, patients experience increasing dryness and generalized soreness of the mouth and throat.

KEY SYMPTOM

Difficult or Painful Swallowing: Dysphagia and Odynophagia: A disorder in swallowing is termed *dysphagia*. With *oropharyngeal dysphagia* the patient describes difficulty initiating a swallow or choking and coughing with swallowing. With *esophageal dysphagia,* the patient experiences a sense of obstruction at a definite level when fluid or a bolus of food is swallowed. *Neurogenic dysphagia* may be accompanied by regurgitation through the nose. Some varieties of dysphagia may cause localized pain (*odynophagia*); others are painless. Deglutition involves muscles in both the oropharynx and the esophagus. Pain from the oropharynx is accurately localized in the neck, but esophageal pain is dispersed in the thoracic six-dermatome band, so it presents as pain in the chest (see page 327 and Chapter 9 pages 533 and 563–564).

✓ **DYSPHAGIA AND ODYNOPHAGIA—CLINICAL OCCURRENCE:** **Oropharynx** *Painful dysphagia from intrinsic lesions:* glossitis, tonsillitis, stomatitis, pharyngitis, laryngitis, lingual ulcer, carcinoma, pemphigus, erythema multiforme, Ludwig angina, mumps, bee sting of the tongue, angioneurotic edema, candidiasis, sometimes Plummer-Vinson syndrome; *Painful dysphagia from local extrinsic lesions:* cervical adenitis, subacute thyroiditis, carotid arteritis, infected thyroglossal cysts or sinuses, pharyngeal cysts or sinuses, carotid body tumor, spur in cervical spine, pericarditis; *Painful dysphagia from systemic conditions:* rabies, tetanus, Plummer-Vinson syndrome; *Painless dysphagia from intrinsic lesions:* cleft palate, flexion of the neck from cervical osteoporosis, xerostomia in Sjögren syndrome, and magnesium deficiency; *Painless dysphagia from neurogenic lesions:* globus hystericus, postdiphtheritic paralysis, bulbar paralysis, myasthenia gravis, hepatolenticular degeneration (Wilson disease), paresis, parkinsonism, botulism, poisoning (lead, alcohol, fluoride); **Esophagus** *Painful dysphagia from intrinsic lesions (see Pain in the Chest, page 563):* foreign body, carcinoma, esophagitis, diverticulum, hiatal hernia; *Painless dysphagia from intrinsic lesions:* achalasia, congenital stricture, adult acquired stricture, scleroderma, dermatomyositis; xerostomia in Sjögren syndrome, amyloidosis, and thyrotoxicosis; *Painless dysphagia from extrinsic lesions:* aortic aneurysm, dysphagia lusoria (see page 329), vertebral spurs from osteoarthritis, enlarged left atrium.

TEST FOR ESOPHAGEAL OBSTRUCTION: Supply the patient with a glass of drinking water. Place the chest piece of your stethoscope over the patient's abdominal left upper quadrant. Measure the time elapsing between swallowing and the murmur produced by the bolus passing the cardia. Normally it should range from 7–10 seconds.

Larynx Symptoms

KEY SYMPTOM

Hoarseness: See page 304.

Salivary Gland Symptoms

KEY SYMPTOM

Dry Mouth: Xerostomia: See page 333.

Neck Symptoms

KEY SYMPTOM

Pain in the Neck: Pain in the neck is a common complaint whose cause is often readily diagnosed by a careful history, palpation of the neck, and examination of the oropharynx. Posttraumatic or postural cervical strain is the most common cause of pain in the neck. In palpation of the neck, each anatomic structure should be examined systematically. The enhancement of pain by certain bodily movements may be somewhat helpful in searching for the source of pain. Serious disorders may be overlooked without careful consideration.

✔ *NECK PAIN—CLINICAL OCCURRENCE:* **Neck Pain Increased by Swallowing** *Pharynx:* pharyngitis, Ludwig angina, inflamed thyroglossal duct or cyst; *Tonsils:* tonsillitis, neoplasm; *Tongue:* ulcers, neoplasm; *Larynx:* laryngitis, neoplasm, ulcer, foreign body; *Esophagus:* inflamed diverticulum, esophagitis (peptic, candida, HSV, pill, radiation); *Thyroid:* acute suppurative thyroiditis, subacute thyroiditis, hemorrhage into thyroid cystadenoma; *Carotid Artery:* carotodynia, carotid body tumor; *Salivary Glands:* mumps, suppurative parotitis; **Neck Pain Increased by Chewing** *Mandible:* fracture, osteomyelitis, periodontitis; *Salivary Glands:* mumps, suppurative parotitis; **Neck Pain Increased by Movements of the Head** *Sternocleidomastoideus:* torticollis, hematoma; *Nuchal Muscles:* viral myalgia, muscle tension, "crick" in neck; *Cervical Spine:* injury, herniated intervertebral disk, spinal arthritis, meningitis, meningismus, craniovertebral junction abnormalities; **Neck Pain Increased by Shoulder Movement** *Superior Thoracic Aperture:* cervical rib, scalenus anticus syndrome, costoclavicular syndrome; **Neck Pain Not Increased by Movement** *Skin and Subcutaneous Tissues:* furuncle, carbuncle, erysipelas; *Lymph Nodes:* acute adenitis. *Branchial Cleft Remnants:* inflamed pharyngeal cyst; *Salivary Glands:* calculus in duct; *Subclavian Artery:* aneurysm; *Nervous System:* poliomyelitis, herpes zoster, epidural abscess, spinal cord neoplasm. *Spinal Vertebrae:* herniated intervertebral disk, metastatic carcinoma; *Referred Pain:* Pancoast syndrome, angina pectoris, and other conditions in the six-dermatome band.

S KEY SYNDROME

Neck Pain: Carotodynia: The patient complains of constant or throbbing pain in the side of the neck that is intensified by swallowing. The pain may extend to the mandible or the ear. Onset frequently follows a viral pharyngitis with fever. Some patients have no generalized symptoms, others exhibit profound lassitude. Several relapses may occur within a few months. The carotid bulb is exquisitely tender, and the trunk of the common carotid may be tender. In some patients, the carotid bulb seems dilated and its pulsations exaggerated. Sudden digital compression of the carotid causes the pain to spread in the distal branches of the external carotid to the jaw, ear, and temple (*Fay sign*). One or both common carotid arteries may be involved. The pharynx and larynx may appear normal or slightly hyperemic and edematous. In a few cases, aphthous ulcers have been present. The diagnosis is made by demonstrating tenderness of the carotid artery.

KEY SYMPTOM

Neck Fullness: Tracheal Displacement from Goiter: Many patients with a small goiter complain of a sense of constriction or fullness in the neck. See page 335ff.

Head and Neck Signs

Scalp, Face, Skull, and Jaw Signs

KEY SIGN

Bleeding from Scalp Wounds: Wounds in the scalp bleed profusely because the tissue is extremely vascular. The wounded scalp does not gape unless the galea aponeurotica has been severed. If gaping is noted, one should suspect an open fracture of the skull; the wound should not be explored without strict asepsis.

KEY SIGN

Fluctuant Scalp Masses: Hematoma, Abscess, Or Depressed Fracture: When blood or pus accumulates in the skin or subcutaneous layer of the scalp, it is sharply localized and the mass readily slides over the skull. A boggy, fluctuant mass in the entire adult scalp results from blood or pus in the loose connective tissue under the aponeurosis; the same finding in a young child may also be evidence of parietal bone fracture. A fluctuant mass bounded by the skull suture lines indicates subperiosteal blood or pus or a depressed fracture. A hematoma under the periosteum usually has a soft center that is plastic, while the edges are firm and feel much like a depressed fracture.

S KEY SYNDROME

Cellulitis of the Scalp: The scalp is tender, soft, and boggy. The infection extends rapidly, causing edema of the eyelids and pinnae; the regional lymph nodes are tender and swollen.

KEY SIGN

Scalp Mass: Sebaceous Cyst (WEN): *Pathophysiology:* This is a sebaceous cyst arising from obstruction of the sebaceous gland's orifice. A common lesion, it is either single or multiple. Because it arises from the skin, it slides easily over the skull. The mass is firm, nontender, nonulcerative, often hemispheric (Fig. 7-31A). If suppuration occurs, the cyst bleeds easily and may be mistaken for a squamous cell carcinoma.

Scalp Mass: Lipoma: A fatty tumor in the subcutaneous layer feels smooth and soft; the finger slides around its edges. When it occurs beneath the pericranium, its movement is strictly limited, but the finger can detect a smooth, rounded border.

Scalp Masses: Rare Tumors: *Neurofibromas* may occur in the scalp in the generalized neurofibromatosis of von Recklinghausen. The lesions are discrete, sessile, or pedunculated tumors that look solid but seem to collapse with pressure. Rarely, a proliferating scalp tumor forms a festoon hanging from the head. Chronic cystic swellings of the scalp include *cirsoid aneurysm* (see Fig. 7-31B), a rare lesion that presents

    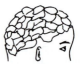

A. Sebaceous Cyst or Wen   B. Cirsoid Aneurysm   C. Turban Tumor

Fig. 7-31 Scalp Lesions.

as fluctuant sinuous vessels that may produce bruits, *cavernous hemangioma* from a meningocele, which slowly refills after being compressed and *pneumatocele,* which is tympanitic with percussion. The rare *turban tumor* (*cylindroma* of eccrine gland origin), grows slowly to produce a red, lobulated, fissured cap devoid of hair (see Fig. 7-31C).

KEY SIGN

Swelling of the Cheek: Parotitis: see page 308.

KEY SIGN

Swelling of the Cheek: Preauricular Abscess and Ulcer: *Pathophysiology:* An abscess forms in front of the tragus involving the preauricular lymph node; breakdown of the abscess produces an ulcer. The swelling is localized, tender, and sometimes warm. Search for the source of the infection in the region drained by the node: the side of the face, the pinna, the anterior wall of the external acoustic meatus, the anterior third of the scalp, the eyebrows, and the eyelids.

Swelling of the Cheek: Masseter Muscle Hypertrophy: Either one or both masseter muscles may undergo spontaneous hypertrophy producing swelling of the face that must be distinguished from parotid gland swelling. While palpating the mass, have the patient clench his teeth; if the entire mass hardens, the swelling is muscular.

Redness of the Cheek: Malar Lesions: Look for erythema, scaling, pustules, and tenderness. Consider sunburn, cellulitis, rosacea, seborrheic dermatitis, discoid or systemic lupus erythematosus, and acne vulgaris.

Wrinkling of the Forehead: Transverse wrinkles normally occur in the forehead with extreme upward gaze or in raising the eyebrows. Absence of such furrowing is a sign of hyperthyroidism. Deep wrinkling, with longitudinal furrowing and prominence of intervening tissue, constitutes the *bulldog skin* in pachydermatosis and some congenital disorders. Unilateral loss of wrinkling results from facial nerve (CN VII) paralysis.

Skull Malformation: Craniosynostosis: *Pathophysiology:* Premature union of specific cranial sutures leads to skull malformations. The shape of the skull indicates which sutures are fused. One example is oxycephaly caused by premature closure of the lambdoid and coronal sutures, producing a pointed vertex (Fig. 7-32A). Surgical treatment in infancy can prevent permanent deformity.

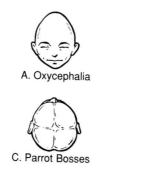
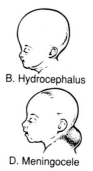

A. Oxycephalia

B. Hydrocephalus

C. Parrot Bosses

D. Meningocele

Fig. 7-32 Malformations of the Skull. **A. Oxycephalia, Oxycephaly, or Steeple Skull:** *The skull is pointed at the vertex as a result of premature fusion of the cranial sutures.* **B. Hydrocephalus:** *Enlargement of the calvarium as compared to the normal size of facial bones.* **C. Parrot Bosses or Hot-Cross-Bun Skull:** *This is notable for the bulging prominence of four parietal and frontal bones, leaving contrasting deep fissures at the suture lines.* **D. Meningocele:** *A fluctuating outpouching of the meninges in the vertex or occiput.*

KEY SIGN
Enlarged Infantile Skull: Hydrocephalus: *Pathophysiology:* The increased intracranial pressure from obstructed spinal fluid circulation occurring before the sutures are closed causes enlargement of the calvarium (see Fig. 7-32B). The bones of the face are normal in size. With early detection, appropriate surgical treatment can prevent progression.

Skull Malformation: Parrot Bosses (Hot-Cross-Bun Skull): *Pathophysiology:* An increased prominence of the frontal and parietal bosses produces intersecting grooves at the sagittal and transverse sutures (see Fig. 7-32C). This deformity is usually a stigma of congenital syphilis.

Skull Malformation: Meningocele: A fluctuating outpouching of the meninges occurs in the midline of the vertex or the occiput (see Fig. 7-32D).

KEY SIGN
Enlarged Adult Skull: Paget Disease (Osteitis Deformans): *Pathophysiology:* The bones of the skull thicken centrifugally as normal bone is replaced by disorganized bone with porous vascular osteoid. In addition to bone pain, the patient may complain that his hats have become too small. The calvarium is large compared with the facial bones. A bruit is sometimes heard in the skull. The porous bone may form arteriovenous shunts affecting the general

circulation. Other associated bone changes may be acquired: kyphosis, bowed legs, shortening of the stature from flattened vertebrae.

KEY SIGN
Mastoid Pain and Tenderness: Mastoiditis: See page 321.

Skull Masses: Frontal Osteomyelitis: Involvement of the frontal bone with osteomyelitis leads to a localized edematous swelling over the affected region. This condition is usually a sequelae of suppurative sinusitis.

Skull Masses: Neoplasms: An *osteoma* frequently occurs in the outer table of the skull, producing a hard, sessile eminence in the bone. A protuberance, soft or hard, in one of the bones of the vertex may be a *pericranial sarcoma,* diagnosed only by biopsy. Hard or soft masses in the cranial bones may be carcinomatous metastasis, lymphomas, leukemia, or multiple myeloma.

Skull Softening: Craniotabes: Firm digital pressure on the skull behind and above the pinna discloses yielding of the outer table of the skull. Softening of the outer table occurs in rickets, hydrocephalus, syphilis, and hypervitaminosis A.

KEY SIGN
▶ **Limited Jaw Opening: Trismus (Lockjaw) And Local Disorders:** *Pathophysiology: Trismus* is the forceful apposition of the jaws from spasm of the masticatory muscles. Failure of the mouth to open from causes other than true trismus is common. The sign is often associated with tetanus, but it has many other causes.

✓ *CLINICAL OCCURRENCE: Local Disorders* impacted third molar, arthritis of the temporomandibular joint, malignant external otitis, lymphadenitis, trigeminal neuralgia (tic douloureux), scleroderma or dermatomyositis of the face; *Disorders with Widespread Muscle Spasm* trichinosis, rabies, tetany, tetanus, strychnine poisoning, typhoid fever, cholera, septicemia; *Cerebral Disorders* encephalitis, epilepsy (transient), catalepsy, hysteria, malingering.

KEY SIGN
Inability to Close the Jaw: Temporomandibular (TMJ) Joint Dislocation: *Pathophysiology:* Because the TMJ joint is a shallow biconcave surface, it can easily partially sublux or completely dislocate. The jaw cannot be closed, usually after a wide yawn or an upward blow on the chin with the mouth opened widely. The mandible protrudes with the lower teeth overriding the upper. Palpation discloses an abnormal depression or pit anterior to the tragus. It is more obvious when bilateral; in unilateral dislocation, the pretragal depression occurs only on the affected side. Confirm the dis-

location by palpating through the external acoustic meatus: no movement of the mandibular head is felt on the affected side.

Ear Signs

External Ear Signs

KEY SIGN

Earlobe Crease: An earlobe crease, defined as a visible crease extending at least one-third of the distance from tragus to posterior pinna, has been associated with a higher rate of cardiac events in patients admitted to the hospital with suspected coronary heart disease [Elliott WJ, Powell LH. Diagonal earlobe creases and prognosis in patients with suspected coronary artery disease. *Am J Med* 1996;100: 205–211].

KEY SIGN

Malformations of the Pinna: The pinna may develop smaller than normal *(microtia),* or unusually large *(macrotia)* (Fig. 7-33). Rarely, the pinna is absent, usually in association with *atresia* of the external acoustic meatus. The pinna may protrude at a right angle to the head *(lop ear* or *bat ear).* Failure of development of the lobule produces *Aztec ear* or *Cagot ear.* When an eminence occurs near the upper third of the posterior helix, the effect is termed *Darwin ear.* A pointed pinna is a

A. Microtia and Atresia

B. Accessory Pinna

C. Aztec Ear

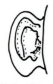
D. Bat or Lop Ear

E. Satyr Ear

F. Cauliflower Ear

Fig. 7-33 Malformations of the Pinna. **A. Microtia and Atresia:** *Associated congenital defects; only a ridge of skin and cartilage may represent the ear.* **B. Accessory Pinna:** *Usually small and rudimentary, it is commonly found anterior to the tragus of the well-formed ear.* **C. Aztec or Cagot Ear:** *Characterized by the absence of the lobe.* **D. The Bat or Lop Ear:** *Stands out from the head at a right angle.* **E. Satyr Ear:** *Has a point at the top of the helix.* **F. Cauliflower Ear:** *Fibrosis from trauma and hemorrhage results in a misshapen ear.*

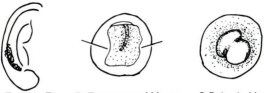

A. Gouty Tophi in Ear   B. Exostoses of Meatus   C. Polyp in Meatus

Fig. 7-34 Lesions of the External Ear. **A.** *Tophi*: Hard, irregular, painless nodules usually near the helix. Occasionally, the skin breaks down to exude chalky crystals of urates. **B.** *Bony Swellings*: Exostoses may protrude into the external acoustic meatus from the walls, so that the view of the eardrum is completely obscured. **C.** *Polyps*: These are occasionally seen in the external meatus.

satyr ear. Curling of the pinna is called *scroll ear*. A small rudimentary accessory pinna may develop. Untreated hematomas heal as nodular and bulbous irregularities of the helix and antihelix, the *cauliflower ear*.

Pinna Nodule: Darwin Tubercle:
A developmental eminence in the upper third of the posterior helix, this condition is harmless. It must be distinguished from acquired nodules, such as tophi.

KEY SIGN
Pinna Nodule: Gouty Tophus: *Pathophysiology:*
In long-standing gout, accumulations of sodium urate crystals may occur in the helix and antihelix; they also occur in the olecranon bursa, the tendon sheaths, and the aponeuroses of the extremities. The nodules are painless, hard, and irregular (Fig. 7-34A). They may open, discharging chalky contents.

Pinnal Nodule: Calcification of the Cartilage:
This is a rare complication of Addison disease. The nodule is not usually tender.

Other Painless Pinnal Nodules:
In addition to gouty tophi, these may be basal cell carcinomas, rheumatoid nodules, or leprosy.

KEY SIGN
Pinnal Mass: Hematoma: *Pathophysiology:*
Trauma or a hemostatic defect results in a hematoma arising as blood accumulates between the cartilage and the perichondrium. There is a tender, blue, doughy mass, usually without spontaneous pain. Early diagnosis is desirable because prompt incision and drainage avoids suppuration or cauliflower ear.

S KEY SYNDROME

Recurring Inflammation of Pinna: Relapsing Polychondritis: *Pathophysiology:* This is a rare disease, with inflammation leading to degeneration of cartilage, especially the pinna; the nasal septum, laryngeal cartilages, tracheal and bronchial rings, and joint cartilages may be affected. The etiology is unknown. The involved ear is painful, swollen, and reddened, except over the lobule, which remains normal because there is no underlying cartilage. Hoarseness indicates laryngeal involvement; blindness may result from involvement of the sclerae, and tinnitus and deafness from involvement of the middle ear. Rarely, degeneration of the aortic ring has led to aortic regurgitation or aneurysm; similar involvement of the mitral ring has caused mitral valve prolapse.

Post-Pinnal Mass: Dermoid Cyst: A favorite site is just behind the pinna. This lesion is soft and semifluctuant.

KEY SIGN

Pinna Neoplasms: Squamous cell carcinoma is common on the pinna; basal cell carcinoma is less frequent. Any small crusted, ulcerated, or indurated lesion that fails to heal promptly should be biopsied. In advanced stages, squamous cell carcinoma produces fungating lesions while the basal cell neoplasm tends to be flattened with elevated borders.

External Acoustic Meatus Signs

KEY SIGN

External Acoustic Meatus: Cerumen Impaction: *Pathophysiology:* Ear wax, which normally forms in the cartilaginous portion of the meatal canal, acidifies it and protects the epithelium by suppressing bacterial overgrowth and capturing foreign particles. The wax migrates to the concha because of epithelial migration of ear canal skin in that direction. The wax of Native Americans and East Asians is often drier and flakier, and more yellow than amber. Either excessive production of wax or a narrowed meatus leads to impacted cerumen, causing partial or complete obstruction of the canal. When obstruction is complete, partial deafness results. Tinnitus or dizziness may occur. A partial obstruction may suddenly become complete when water enters the meatus during bathing or swimming. The obstructing wax is easily seen in the external meatus.

KEY SIGN

Discharge from the Ear: Otorrhea: Discharge from the ear suggests different possibilities, depending on the nature of the discharge.

✓ *CLINICAL OCCURRENCE:* *Yellow Discharge* melting cerumen; *Serous Discharge* eczema in the meatal wall, early ruptured acute otitis media;   *Bloody Discharge*   trauma of the external canal from without or longitudinal temporal bone fracture causing tympanic membrane and external canal laceration;   *Purulent Discharge*   chronic external otitis, perforation of acute suppurative otitis media, chronic suppurative otitis media with or without cholesteatoma, tuberculous otitis media.

KEY SIGN

External Acoustic Meatus: External Otitis: See page 320.

KEY SIGN

External Acoustic Meatus: Dermatitis, Itching: *Pathophysiology:* The supply of wax becomes inadequate leading to dryness and pruritus. Seborrheic dermatitis commonly causes scaling and pruritus of the choana and meatus. Medicated ear drops can cause contact dermatitis.

External Acoustic Meatus: Exostoses and Chondromas: Exostoses form nodules in the osseous part of the meatus near the tympanic membrane (see Fig. 7-34B). They rarely produce obstruction, although the view of the drumhead may be partially obscured. A single bony osteoma may also occur. Rarely, chondromas arise from the cartilaginous portion of the canal, usually without obstructing it.

External Acoustic Meatus: Furuncle: These form in the outer half of the canal producing extreme pain. It appears as a red, tender eminence with or without a pustule.

External Acoustic Meatus: Foreign Body: Children often place objects in their ears. A purulent discharge from the canal or an earache may be the first indication.

External Acoustic Meatus: Insect Invaders: Occasionally, insects enter the canal, where their movements cause great distress. To remove one, place a drop of oil or a pledget soaked with ether in the canal and extract the immobilized creature. By contrast, we have seen maggots in the ear of a patient with chronic external otitis accompanied by the usual insensitiveness.

External Acoustic Meatus: Polyps: A polyp may form a bulbous, reddened, pedunculated mass arising either from the meatal wall or from the middle ear (see Fig. 7-34C). Gently moving the mass with the forceps frequently indicates its origin. In either site, the growth causes a foul purulent discharge.

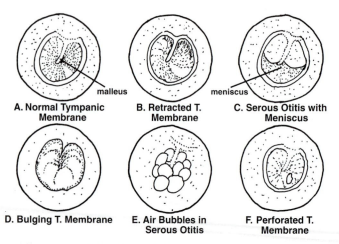

A. Normal Tympanic
Membrane

B. Retracted T.
Membrane

C. Serous Otitis with
Meniscus

D. Bulging T. Membrane

E. Air Bubbles in
Serous Otitis

F. Perforated T.
Membrane

Fig. 7-35 Lesions of the Tympanic Membrane. **A. Normal:** *The normal tympanic membrane is slanted downward and forward; its surface glistens and contains a brilliant triangle, the light reflex, with its apex at the center, or umbo, and its base at the annulus. The handle of the malleus makes an impression on the disk from the umbo upward and forward.* **B. The Retracted Eardrum:** *The light reflex is bent and the malleus stands out in sharper relief than normally.* **C. Serous Middle Ear Fluid:** *Hairline menisci curve from the handle of the malleus to the annulus.* **D. Bulging Drumhead:** *The curves in the membrane obscure the normal landmarks of the malleus and distort the light reflex.* **E. Serous Fluid Mixed with Air:** *Bubbles may be seen through the drumhead.* **F. Perforations** *of the membrane appear as oval holes with a dark shadow behind.*

KEY SIGN

External Acoustic Meatus: Carcinoma: *Pathophysiology:* Either squamous cell or basal cell carcinoma can involve the meatal epithelium. Pain and discharge are the presenting symptoms. In advanced stages, deafness and facial paralysis may occur. The appearance of the neoplasm here is similar to that in other regions.

Tympanic Membrane Signs

KEY SIGN

Retracted Tympanic Membrane: Serous Otitis Media: *Pathophysiology:* Swelling of the orifice of the auditory (eustachian) tube prevents access of air to the middle ear. Resorption of oxygen produces a negative pressure, leading to inward displacement of the membrane as a result of atmospheric pressure. With decreased pressure in the middle ear persisting for days, effusion develops. Initially, the membrane is retracted around the malleus, making it more distinct and curving the light reflex (Fig. 7-35B). Later, amber serous fluid may be seen through the membrane (Fig. 7-35C). When the middle ear is partially filled, a fluid meniscus appears as a fine black line. Sometimes air bubbles are visible (Fig. 7-35E). The condition usually accompanies upper respiratory infections, although it may occur alone. Reduction of barometric pressure, as in an airplane ride, may induce it [Hendley JW. Otitis media. *N Engl J Med* 2002;347:1169–1174].

KEY SIGN

Red or Bulging Tympahic Membrane: Acute Suppurative Otitis Media: *Pathophysiology:* Bacteria from the nasopharynx (*Streptococcus pneumonia, Haemophilus influenza, Moraxella catarrhalis*) enter the middle ear via the eustachian tube; fluid in the chamber favors purulent infection. Throbbing earache is a prominent symptom; frequently, there is fever. Hearing is impaired. Occasionally, slight dizziness and nausea occur. Before rupture, the tympanic membrane bulges obliterating the normal landmarks (see Fig. 7-35D); its surface is bright red and lusterless. Initial perforation is marked by rapid relief of pain. After rupture, pus appears in the canal; a pulsatile stream of discharge may be seen emerging from the perforation in the drum. Light pressure on the mastoid process may elicit pain if the infection has extended into the mastoid air cells. Movement of the pinna and tragus do not cause pain, unlike acute external otitis. The fever and signs of constitutional disease are more prominent in children than in adults.

KEY SIGN

Vesicles on the Tympanic Membrane: Bullous Myringitis: *Pathophysiology:* Infection with *Mycoplasma pneumoniae* is the cause. Severe ear pain is present. Examination shows an inflamed drum with vesicular change.

KEY SIGN

Perforated Tympanic Membrane: *Pathophysiology:* Previous suppurative middle ear infection has eroded through the membrane, producing holes. Other than some decrease in auditory acuity, chronic perforations are asymptomatic. The perforations appears as oval holes through which the darkened middle ear cavity is seen.

Hearing Signs

KEY SIGN

Weber Test Lateralizing to an Ear: Ipsilateral Conductive Hearing Loss or Contralateral Neurosensory Loss: *Pathophysiology:* When neurosensory hearing is intact bilaterally, the sound will lateralize to the side of conductive loss, which loses the masking effect of background noises. Neurosensory loss on one side results in a *louder* sound on the opposite side. Lateralization of sound to the right ear means conductive loss on the right or perceptive loss on the left.

Bone Conduction Greater Than Air Con-duction (Rinne-Negative Test): Conductive Hearing Loss: *Pathophysiology:* When amplification of sound vibrations by the ear drum and ossicles is impaired, direct transmission of vibrations through bone to the cochlea will be perceived as louder than sound transmitted through air. Conductive hearing loss results from obstruction of the auditory canal, damage to the tympanic membrane, and destruction or ankylosis of the ossicles.

Balance and Position Signs

Positive Past Pointing Test: Deviation to the right or left of the target fingers, past pointing, indicates either labyrinthine stimulation or loss of positional sense. The flow of endolymph is in the same direction as the past pointing.

Unsteady Romberg Test (Romberg Sign): Labyrinthine Disorder: *Pathophysiology:* Stable standing with the eyes closed requires normal labyrinthine function, position sense, and cerebellar function. Persistent labyrinthine stimulation or loss of positional sense leads to unsteadiness, elevation of the arms for balance or falling. With labyrinthine stimulation, the patient will fall in the same direction as the flow of endolymph. Inability to maintain balance with the eyes open suggests abnormalities of the labyrinth, position sense, or cerebellar function.

Eye Signs

Lid Signs

Lacrimation: Lacrimation usually refers to any condition resulting in tears, although strict usage indicates an overproduction. *Epiphora* means an overflow of tears from any cause.

✓ **CLINICAL OCCURRENCE:** *Increased Secretion of Tears* weeping from emotion, irritation from foreign body, corneal ulcer, conjunctivitis, coryza, measles, hay fever, poisoning (iodide, bromide, arsenic); *Obstruction of the Lacrimal Ducts* congenital, cicatrix, edema of the eyelids, lacrimal calculus, dacryocystitis; *Separation of the Puncta from the Globe* facial paralysis, aging, chronic marginal blepharitis, ectropion, proptosis from any cause.

Widened Palpebral Fissures: Lid Spasm (Dalrymple Sign): *Pathophysiology:* When the eyes are in the primary position, the upper lid covers the limbus, but a white scleral strip usually shows between the limbus and the lower lid. Widening of the palpebral fissure uncovers the upper border of the limbus to expose white sclera superiorly. The fissures may be widened by retraction of the lids (contraction of Mueller muscle) or by protrusion of the eyeballs. When there is no actual proptosis, widened fissures produce the optical illusion of global protrusion. A few normal persons seem to have widened palpebral fissures. The acquired type is usually noted when acquaintances have commented on "the change in the eyes."

KEY SIGN
Widened Palpebral Fissures: Lid Lag: See *Lid Lag (von Graefe Sign): Hyperthyroidism* page 248.

KEY SIGN
Widened Palpebral Fissures: Exophthalmos (Ocular Proptosis): Widened palpebral fissures present an optical illusion of global prominence, but actual proptosis must be proved by measurement (see page 214). Unilateral proptosis is recognized by comparing the two eyes. If both eyes seem equally prominent, the facial profile should be inspected (Fig. 7-36). Unilateral proptosis suggests orbital tumor or inflammation. When the globe is displaced medially, disease of the lacrimal gland should be suspected; upward displacement suggests disease in the maxillary sinus; lateral displacement can occur from a lesion in the ethmoid or sphenoid sinus. Graves disease is the most common cause of bilateral proptosis. Imaging studies of the orbit are usually required.

✓ *EXOPHTHALMOS—CLINICAL OCCURRENCE:* *Unilateral Exophthalmos* mucocele, orbital cellulitis and abscess, thrombosis of the cavernous sinus, orbital periostitis, Graves disease, myxedema, orbital fracture, hemangioma, meningocele, encephalocele, gumma, orbital neoplasm, tubercle of the orbit, arteriovenous aneurysm, aspergilloma, histiocytosis (Hand-Schüller-Christian disease); *Bilateral Exophthalmos* Graves disease, myxedema, acromegaly, thrombosis of the cavernous sinus, empyema of the nasal accessory sinuses, lymphoma, leukemia, oxycephaly, histiocytosis (Hand-Schüller-Christian disease and Letterer-Siwe disease), hyperpituitarism.

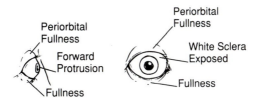

Fig. 7-36 Exophthalmos (Proptosis).

KEY SIGN

Lid Lag [Von Graefe Sign]: Hyperthyroidism:
Pathophysiology: The presence of lid lag indicates lid spasm, even
when the eyes do not show widened fissures in the primary position.
In the absence of wide palpebral fissures, the sign must be sought (see
page 212). Lid spasm occurs in hyperthyroidism and in Graves disease.
The mechanism is uncertain, but it is attributed to sympathetic stimulation. Usually the finding is bilateral; occasionally one fissure is much
wider than the other. *Other Lid Signs in Hyperthyroidism* *Stellwag
Sign:* infrequent blinking; *Rosenbach Sign:* tremor of the closed eyelids; *Mean Sign:* global lag during elevation; *Griffith Sign:* lag of
the lower lids during elevation of the globes; *Boston Sign:* jerking of
the lagging lid; *Joffroy Sign:* absence of forehead wrinkling with upward gaze, the head being tilted down.

KEY SIGN

**Narrowed Palpebral Fissures: Enophthal-
mos:** *Pathophysiology:* The globe is recessed in the orbit. When
bilateral, it is usually caused by decreased orbital fat (inanition, dehydration) or congenital microphthalmos. The causes of unilateral enophthalmos are trauma or inflammation. Enophthalmos is described as an
integral sign of *Horner syndrome;* actually, the accompanying droop of
the eyelid merely produces an optical illusion of globe recession.

KEY SIGN

**Failure of Lid Closure: Paralysis of Orbicu-
laris Muscle:** *Pathophysiology:* The facial nerve (CN VII) supplies the orbicularis oculi muscle. Disorder of this nerve, as in Bell palsy,
causes partial or complete paralysis of the orbicularis. When complete,
both upper and lower lids remain retracted so the eye is unprotected
and tears drain onto the face. *Bell phenomenon* occurs: the globes elevate
during attempted closure of the lids. Failure of lid closure is also present in severe grades of exophthalmos or lid spasm from sympathetic
stimulation.

KEY SIGN

Failure of Lid Opening: Ptosis of the Lid:
Pathophysiology: The congenital form is usually bilateral from paralysis of or failure to develop the levator palpebrae superioris. The acute
acquired condition usually results from disease of the oculomotor nerve
(CN III). In the congenital form, the eyelid will show lid lag as the child
looks down. With CN III lesion paralysis of other eye muscles may be
present.

✓*CLINICAL OCCURRENCE:* Supranuclear lesions (e.g., encephalitis),
Horner syndrome, paralysis of the levator muscle, levator dehiscence,
thinning of levator tendon (the lid drops, but it will show a full, normal
excursion of 15–18 mm).

KEY SIGN

Ptosis of the Lid: Horners Syndrome: *Pathophysiology:* Interruption of the cervical sympathetic chain interrupts sympathetic innervation of the eye and face. The complete syndrome has ptosis, miosis, and anhydrosis on the affected side. In this condition, the ptosis is incomplete, distinguishing it from paralysis of the levator muscle.

KEY SIGN

Epicanthal Fold: Down Syndrome: See page 318.

KEY SIGN

Shortened Palpebral Fissures: Fetal Alcohol Syndrome: The combination of shortened palpebral fissures, shortened nose with epicanthic folds and anteverted nostrils, and hypoplastic upper lip with thinned vermilion and flattened or absent philtrum, together with mental retardation, are stigmata of an individual born to a mother who has consumed excessive alcohol during pregnancy.

KEY SIGN

Lid Inversion: Entropion: *Pathophysiology:* Structural changes or muscular contraction turns the eyelashes inward to impinge upon the globe. **Spastic entropion** occurs only in the lower lid and is caused by increased tone of the orbicularis oculi, usually from inflammation of an eye with a scanty tarsal plate or disinsertion of lower eyelid retractors causing poor tissue tone. The lid turns in only when forcibly closed (Fig. 7-37A). **Cicatricial entropion** occurs in either lid by contracture of scar tissue, as in trachoma. Entropion from any cause may be accompanied by *blepharospasm* from irritation of the inverted eyelashes.

KEY SIGN

Lid Eversion: Ectropion: The lid turns outward (see Fig. 7-37B). Both lids may be affected by **spastic** or **cicatricial ectropion**, but **paralytic ectropion** involves only the lower lid. The spastic type is encountered in severe protrusion of the globe from staphyloma or palpebral edema. Senile atrophy of tissues sometimes results in ectropion rather than entropion.

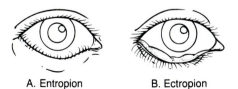

A. Entropion   B. Ectropion

Fig. 7-37 Pathologic Inversion and Eversion of the Eyelids.

Lid Redness: Local Active Hyperemia: Generalized reddening of the lids is nonspecific. Hyperemia of the nasal half of the upper lid suggests inflammation of the frontal sinus. Disease of the lacrimal sac sometimes causes reddening of the adjacent portion of the lower lid. Hyperemia of the temporal side of the upper lid should suggest dacryoadenitis. The lid is frequently red in the region of a sty.

Lid Cyanosis: Local Passive Hyperemia: Blueness of the eyelid occurs from thrombosis of the orbital veins, orbital tumors, and arteriovenous aneurysms of the orbit.

KEY SIGN

Violaceous Lids: Dermatomyositis: Heliotrope or violaceous discoloration of the periorbital skin occurs in dermatomyositis and after chronic quinacrine ingestion.

KEY SIGN

Lid   Hemorrhage: Palpebral   Hematoma: Trauma to the lids may result in extravasation of blood into the surrounding tissue, colloquially known as a "black eye." Palpebral hematoma can occur from nasal fracture. The appearance of hematoma many hours after head trauma suggests a skull fracture; the greater the time interval, the more remote the fracture site. Fractures of the basilar skull may produce hematoma of the lid several days later. Involvement of both eyes is called *raccoon sign.*

KEY SIGN

Lid Swelling: Palpebral Edema: Local infections cause *inflammatory edema* of the eyelids, which is readily identified by finding redness, warmth, and pain. *Noninflammatory edema* is frequent in acute nephritis, but uncommon in chronic nephritis and cardiac failure (Fig. 7-38A). It occurs early in the course of both myxedema and the exophthalmos of Graves disease. Palpebral edema is frequent in trichinosis. Angioedema frequently involves the lids. Contact dermatitis is often a baffling cause of palpebral edema. A patient may be able to tolerate contact with an allergen on the hands, but when transferred to the lids, swelling occurs.

KEY SIGN

Yellow Lid Plaques: Xanthelasma: Raised yellow plaques, painless and nonpruritic, occur on the upper and lower lids near the inner canthi (see Fig. 7-38B). They grow slowly and may disappear spontaneously. The lesion is a form of xanthoma frequently associated with hypercholesterolemia.

KEY SIGN

Lid Scaling and Redness: Marginal Blepharitis: Seborrheic blepharitis is an oily inflammation of the lid margins that produces greasy flakes of dried secretion on the eyelashes and red-

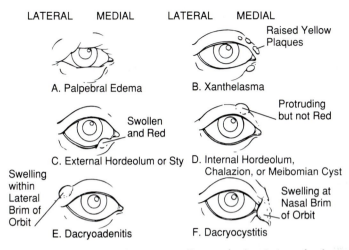

LATERAL MEDIAL   LATERAL MEDIAL

A. Palpebral Edema

B. Xanthelasma
Raised Yellow Plaques

C. External Hordeolum or Sty
Swollen and Red

D. Internal Hordeolum, Chalazion, or Meibomian Cyst
Protruding but not Red

E. Dacryoadenitis
Swelling within Lateral Brim of Orbit

F. Dacryocystitis
Swelling at Nasal Brim of Orbit

Fig. 7-38 Lesions of the External Eye. *(See text for descriptions of each condition.)*

dening of the lid margins. When ulceration of the lid margin occurs, it is termed *staphylococcal blepharitis*. *Angular blepharitis* is a specific disease caused by the diplococcus of Morax-Axenfeld, in which the margins near the temporal canthi are inflamed.

KEY SIGN
Lid Pustule: External Hordeolum (Sty): *Pathophysiology:* When a sebaceous gland near the hair follicle of an eyelash becomes inflamed, a pustule forms on the lid margin (see Fig. 7-38C). It may be surrounded by hyperemia and swelling. Many rupture and heal spontaneously.

KEY SIGN
Lid Protrusion: Internal Hordeolum, and Meibomian Cyst (Chalazion): *Pathophysiology:* Acute inflammation of a meibomian gland is termed an internal hordeolum or internal sty. A granuloma of the gland is known as a chalazion or meibomian cyst (see Fig. 7-38D). These lesions of internal sebaceous glands produce localized swelling that frequently causes a protrusion of the lid. Eversion of the lid shows hyperemia and perhaps a localized cyst or enlarged gland. Consider that Kaposi sarcoma may mimic chalazion in patients with HIV infection.

KEY SIGN
Lacrimal Gland Inflammation: Dacryoadenitis: *Pathophysiology:* Obstruction of the lacrimal duct produces acute inflammation of the lacrimal gland. This causes pain and tender-

ness within the temporal edge of the orbit; it must be distinguished from orbital cellulitis and hordeolum of the upper lid (see Fig. 7-38E).

KEY SIGN

Lacrimal Duct Inflammation: Dacryocystitis: *Pathophysiology:* Obstruction of the nasolacrimal duct leads to inflammation and infection. Patients present with pain and an overflow of tears onto the cheek (*epiphora*), which are increased by irritants such as wind, dust, or smoke. There are tenderness, swelling, and redness beside the nose, near the medial canthus (see Fig. 7-38F). The swelling sits anterior to the eyelid, distinguishing it from hordeolum of the lower lid. The swelling may extend to the eyelid. Fluid can be expressed with pressure on the puncta. Conjunctivitis and blepharitis may be present.

Eye Movement Signs

KEY SIGN

Repetitive Jerky Eye Movements: Nystagmus: *Pathophysiology:* Under many conditions of fixation, the eyes may drift slowly to one side, to be corrected by a quick movement back to the original position. This is termed nystagmus; it is named after the direction of the quick component. Nystagmus may be horizontal, vertical, rotatory, oblique, or mixed. When both eyes participate, the nystagmus is *associated;* movement of one eye only is *dissociated*. Fewer than 40 jerks per minute is considered slow; more than 100 jerks per minute is fast. Amplitudes of less than 1 mm are *fine;* amplitudes of more than 3 mm are *coarse.*

End-Position Nystagmus. The correctional jerks occur only with fixation far to the side; so nystagmus is always in the direction of fixation (Fig. 7-39A). There are several varieties. Damage to either the labyrinth, its connections to the cerebellum, or damage to the cerebellum will create instability when the patient stands with eyes open.

Fixation nystagmus occurs in many normal persons when they are required to fix to one side or the other; it is horizontal or horizontal-rotatory, moderate to coarse.

Labyrinthine end-position nystagmus usually occurs in disease of the semicircular canals; it is horizontal-rotatory and is initiated by fixation

A. End-position Nystagmus   B. Nystagmus in Primary Position

Fig. 7-39 Nystagmus. A slow drift of the eyes away from the position of fixation (indicated by the broken arrow) is corrected by a quick movement back (solid arrow). The direction of the nystagmus is named from the quick component. Nystagmus from the primary position is more likely to be of serious import than that from the end position.

in the end position, but it persists for some time after the primary position has been resumed.

Muscle-paretic nystagmus presents as a dissociated movement of an eye with a paretic muscle, when fixation is directed to the paralyzed side; the muscle attempts to renew its position with new impulses.

Gaze-paretic nystagmus appears in paralysis of conjugate movements. Both eyes show more nystagmus to one end position than to the other.

Primary Position Nystagmus occurs with fixation in the primary position or at a point away from the direction of the quick component (see Fig. 7-39B).

Peripheral labyrinthine nystagmus is horizontal-rotatory, with medium frequency and amplitude, commonly seen in Ménière syndrome, benign paroxysmal positional vertigo, viral or bacterial labyrinthitis, perilymphatic or labyrinthine fistula, and vestibular neuronitis.

Central nystagmus may be horizontal, rotatory, vertical, or mixed, usually in the direction of the diseased side. Commonly, it is found in multiple sclerosis, encephalitis, brain tumors, and transient or permanent vascular insufficiency states involving the vestibular nuclei or the medial longitudinal bundle.

Vertical nystagmus usually indicates a lesion in the midbrain.

Three types of nystagmus identify more localized lesions.

Convergence-retraction nystagmus occurs in the dorsal midbrain syndrome with lid retraction (*Collier sign*), limited up-gaze and light-near dissociation.

Seesaw nystagmus, found in parasellar lesions, is characterized by rising and intorting of one eye while the other falls and extorts.

Downbeat nystagmus typically signifies lesions at the foramen magnum such as the Arnold-Chiari malformation, but it may also be seen with other disorders, including magnesium depletion, Wernicke encephalopathy, and lithium intoxication.

Congenital nystagmus is characterized by unsystematic wandering movements, with various frequencies and amplitudes, in persons who have poor vision from birth. DDX: Other ocular instabilities that resemble nystagmus include ocular flutter, opsoclonus, and ocular bobbing. *Ocular flutter* is the arrhythmic and rapid movement of the eyes horizontally. When both horizontal and vertical components exist, it is termed *opsoclonus.* These conditions may be associated with vascular or neoplastic processes, underlying immune mechanism, or paraneoplastic syndrome, particularly neuroblastoma in children, or small cell lung cancer, breast cancer, or ovarian cancer in adults. *Ocular bobbing* is the intermittent, conjugate, rapid, downward movement of the eyes followed by a slow return to primary position and is often seen in comatose patients with pontine lesions.

Abnormalities of Gaze

KEY SIGN

Constant Squint Angle: Comitant Strabismus or Squint (Nonparalytic Heterophoria):
Pathophysiology: The muscles are normal; the disorder probably re-

sults from abnormal innervation in the nuclei of the cranial nerves, because the squint angle disappears during general anesthesia. The word *comitant,* when applied to strabismus, indicates that the angle between the two optic axes, the *squint angle,* remains constant in all positions assumed by the globes, no matter which eye fixates. Neither eye has limited motion (Fig. 7-40A). Because comitant strabismus occurs in the very young, children learn to suppress the image from one eye and do not have diplopia. In most cases the optic axes converge, which is termed *comitant convergent strabismus* or ***esotropia***. When hypermetropia causes excessive convergence, the condition is called *accommodative squint.* Occasionally the optic axes diverge, which is termed is comitant divergent strabismus or ***exotropia***.

KEY SIGN

Varying Squint Angle: Noncomitant Strabismus or Squint (Paralytic Heterotropia): *Pathophysiology:* This is caused by paralysis of one or more eye muscles. The squint angle changes with the direction of fixation. As opposed to comitant strabismus, the motions of the paralyzed eye are limited. The head is held toward the field of the paralyzed eye to avoid diplopia. The squint angle is greatest when the unaffected eye is fixed on the visual field requiring the action of the paralyzed muscle, *secondary deviation.* When paralysis is acquired during maturity, diplopia occurs at the onset, frequently accompanied by vertigo.

In the following discussions, only paralyses of the right eye are employed as examples to avoid confusion. In the figures, only the deficient movements of the eye are illustrated; all others are normal.

RIGHT LATERAL RECTUS PARALYSIS (SEE FIG. 7-40B): In the primary position, the optic axes may be parallel, or the right eye may converge slightly. The right eye cannot move laterally. The lateral rectus muscles are the most frequent site of isolated paralysis. The abducens nerve (CN VI) may be damaged in infectious diseases, periostitis of the orbit, fracture of the petrous portion of the temporal bone, aneurysm of the carotid artery within the cavernous sinus, and lesions of the posterior pons near the midline.

RIGHT MEDIAL RECTUS PARALYSIS (SEE FIG. 7-40C): In the primary position, the right eye deviates laterally; it cannot move medially. The head is turned to the left to avoid diplopia.

RIGHT SUPERIOR RECTUS PARALYSIS (SEE FIG. 7-40D): In the primary position, the right eye deviates downward; it cannot move upward to the right. The squint angle and the diplopia increase with fixation of the left eye upward to the right.

RIGHT INFERIOR RECTUS PARALYSIS (SEE FIG. 7-40E): In the primary position, the right eye deviates upward; it cannot move down to the right. With the left eye fixed downward and to the right, the squint angle and the degree of diplopia increase.

RIGHT SUPERIOR OBLIQUE PARALYSIS (SEE FIG. 7-41A): In the primary position, the right eye deviates upward; movement is limited down and

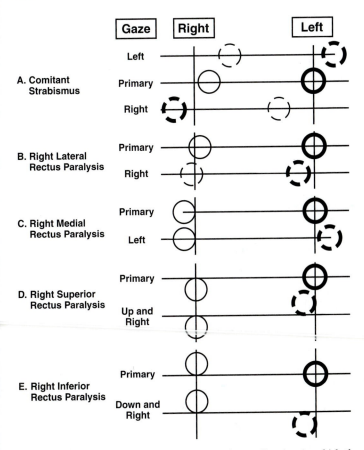

Fig. 7-40 Strabismus (Squint). This term refers to disorders in which the optic axes are not parallel. The diagrams illustrate positions of the patient's eyes as they appear to the observer. The unbroken circles connected by the unbroken lines show pairs in the primary position with the normal or fixing eye represented in heavier lines. Pairs with broken lines are in secondary positions with the heavier lines for the fixing eye. **A. Comitant Strabismus**: The squint angle between the two optic axes is constant in all positions regardless of which eye fixates. **B. Right Lateral Rectus Paralysis**: The right eye is unable to move laterally. **C. Right Medial Rectus Paralysis**: Right eye is lateral in the primary position; it fails to move medially. **D. Right Superior Rectus Paralysis**: The right eye is slightly depressed in primary position and fails to move farther upward. **E. Right Inferior Rectus Paralysis**: The right eye is elevated slightly in primary position; it cannot move downward.

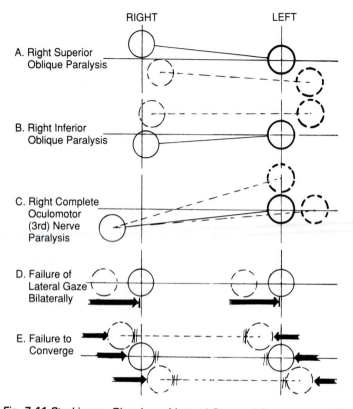

Fig. 7-41 Strabismus: Disorders of Lateral Gaze and Convergence. *Diagrams constructed as in Fig. 7-40.* **A. Right Superior Oblique Paralysis:** *In primary position, right eye slightly elevated and can only be slightly depressed.* **B. Right Inferior Oblique Paralysis:** *The right eye is slightly depressed in primary position; it can be elevated only slightly.* **C. Right Complete Oculomotor Nerve Paralysis:** *The right eye is fixed in depressed and lateral position.* **D. Failure of Lateral Gaze:** *Both eyes cannot be moved beyond the median to the left or right, as the case may be.* **E. Failure of Convergence:** *In no position can the two eyes converge.*

to the left. The squint angle is increased when the left eye is fixed downward and to the left. Most characteristic is the tilt of the head toward the left shoulder to compensate for the pronounced extorsion. This position results in the normal intorsion of the left eye correcting the torsional diplopia. If the head is tilted to the right side, the right eye rotates upward.

RIGHT INFERIOR OBLIQUE PARALYSIS (SEE FIG. 7-41B): In the primary position, the right eye deviates downward; its movement is limited upward and to the left. The squint angle increases when the left eye is fixed upward to the left.

KEY SIGN

Varying Squint Angle: The Ophthalmoplegias: *Pathophysiology:* Paralysis of two or more ocular muscles is termed ophthalmoplegia. Because only the oculomotor nerve (CN III) supplies more than a single muscle, partial ophthalmoplegia must be attributed to malfunctioning of that nerve. Unilateral total ophthalmoplegia can be caused only by involvement of all nerves in the superior orbital fissure or the cavernous sinus; a bilateral lesion could result only from a focus in the base of the brain. Recognition of *internuclear ophthalmoplegia,* with associated strabismus and diplopia, suggests multiple sclerosis or Wernicke encephalopathy.

VARYING SQUINT ANGLE: COMPLETE RIGHT OCULOMOTOR (CN III) NERVE PARALYSIS (SEE FIG. 7-41C): This produces paralysis of the levator, the superior, medial, and inferior recti, and the inferior oblique muscles (and the pupillary sphincter). Only the superior oblique and the lateral rectus muscles are functioning. In the primary position, the right eye is deviated downward and outward to the right. Motion to the left and upward is absent. The squint angle and the degree of diplopia are increased when the left eye is fixed to the left. Ptosis is present in the right eye from paralysis of the levator. The most frequent causes of third-nerve paralysis is an aneurysm in the circle of Willis and acute diabetic neuropathy (usually sparing the lid).

S KEY SYNDROME

Transient Weakness of Ocular Muscles: Myasthenia Gravis: *Pathophysiology:* Antibodies to the acetylcholine receptors on the motor endplate leads to muscle weakness, which worsens with repetitive firing. The most important question is, "Do you see single immediately after arising?" This is the time of day when the most acetylcholine is stored. The levator and, to a lesser extent, the other ocular muscles characteristically show normal strength after rest, but they fatigue as the day progresses, with ptosis and diplopia developing. Ptosis is quickly relieved by neostigmine, but the other paralyses do not respond as dramatically. DDX: *Absence* of diplopia is important in distinguishing myasthenia from other ocular motility disorders that also may worsen with muscle fatigue as the day progresses.

KEY SIGN

Restriction of Motion: Orbital Tumors and Exophthalmos: Movement of the globe may be restricted in all directions by orbital tumor or the increase in orbital contents in Graves disease.

KEY SIGN

Conjugate Failure of Lateral Gaze: *Pathophysiology:* A disturbance in the frontopontine pathway causes this disorder (see Fig. 7-41D). When the lesion is on the right, there is constant conjugate deviation to the right; the patient turns the head to the left to fixate in front. The optic axes are parallel in all positions, so there is no diplopia. Neither eye can move to the left of the midline. This is distinguished from combined paralysis of the left lateral rectus and the right medial rectus by retention of convergence. In partial failure of lateral gaze, the patient can *will* her gaze to the left, but cannot fix it, so there is bilateral nystagmus to the left.

KEY SIGN
Conjugate Failure of Vertical Gaze: *Pathophysiology:* The exact mechanism is unknown; it is thought to be a disorder of the rostral midbrain. The patient is unable to gaze upward. The eyes cannot move above the horizontal, so the patient tilts the head backward. There is no diplopia. When failure is incomplete, there is slight upward movement with upward nystagmus. Combined bilateral paralyses of the superior recti and the inferior obliques (innervated by CN III) produce similar findings, but vertical gaze palsy is distinguished by retention of the normal *Bell phenomenon:* reflex elevation of the globes when the lids close. This reflex is mediated by fibers between the nuclei of CN III and CN VII in the medial longitudinal bundle; CN III supplies the superior rectus and the inferior oblique, CN VII serves the orbicularis. Persistence of the reflex proves the intactness of both nuclei, so the lesion must be supranuclear. Rarely, upward failure is combined with downward failure, or failure of downward gaze may be present alone.

KEY SIGN
Disjunctive Movement: Failure of Convergence (see Fig: 7-41E): *Pathophysiology:* A lesion in the frontopontine pathway is responsible. All movements are normal except convergence. Normal abduction of both globes to the right and left proves the medial recti to be normal.

Visual Field Signs

KEY SIGN
Bilateral Visual Field Defects: Hemianopsia (Hemianopia): *Pathophysiology:* By definition, hemianopsia involves nerves projecting from both eyes. It is caused by a lesion in the optic chiasm, the optic tracts, or the brain. The optic nerves carry all the nerve fibers from the ipsilateral retina. At the optic chiasm the fibers from the nasal retinas cross the midline (decussate) to join the fibers of the lateral retina from the opposite side to form the optic tracts. The right optic tract carries all fibers to the right side of the brain, projecting the left visual field (Fig. 7-42). The left side of the brain serves both left retinae.

Homonymous Hemianopsia: The same side of each *field* contains a defect (Fig. 7-43A). A left homonymous hemianopsia can be caused by a lesion in the right optic tract or the right side of the brain. With a tract

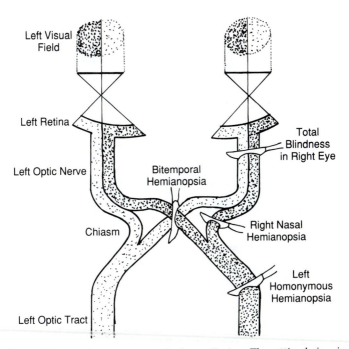

Left Visual Field

Left Retina

Left Optic Nerve

Bitemporal Hemianopsia

Total Blindness in Right Eye

Chiasm

Right Nasal Hemianopsia

Left Homonymous Hemianopsia

Left Optic Tract

Fig. 7-42 Neural Pathways from Retina to Brain. *The cutting knives indicate points of lesions and the resulting visual defects.*

lesion, the pupillary reflex is lost if the light is projected only into the blind hemifield; the pupil reacts when the lesion is in the brain.

Crossed Hemianopsia: Signals from symmetrical sides of both retinae are deficient, so the lesion is either *bitemporal or binasal.* A lesion of the decussating fibers in the chiasm causes *bitemporal hemianopsia* (see Fig. 7-43B) by injuring the fibers to both nasal retinae. The lesion at this site is commonly a tumor of the pituitary gland that enlarges from below, so the temporal sides of both fields are first affected, the temporal cut. *Binasal hemianopsia* is uncommon because it involves injury of both lateral halves of the optic nerves or optic tracts. When only a quadrant of each field is lost, it is termed *quadrantanopsia.* Transient homonymous hemianopsia may occur with migraine.

KEY SIGN
Bilateral Field Defects: Glaucoma: *Pathophysiology:* Early damage leads to nasal steps and arcuate defects. Later there is generalized constriction of the visual field from destruction of the optic nerve by increased intraocular pressure or vasculopathy of the nerve head (see Fig. 7-43C). Visual fields must be examined with automated perimetry to detect early changes in glaucoma and other conditions.

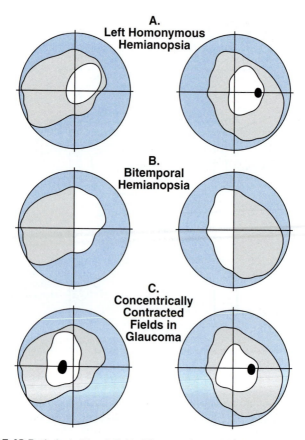

Fig. 7-43 Pathologic Visual Fields. *The normal visual field areas are gray and white in the blue background. Those areas obscured by pathologic conditions are gray, leaving white open areas that remain visible.*

KEY SIGN

Monocular Field Defects: Lesions of the Optic Nerve or Retina: *Pathophysiology:* Destruction of an optic nerve produces blindness in the eye. Optic neuritis may produce smaller field defects. Destructive lesions of the retina also result in monocular field defects. Retinal ischemia from emboli, arteritis, or stenosis of the ipsilateral internal carotid artery may produce transient monocular blindness *(amaurosis fugax)*. Retinal ischemia also results from ophthalmic artery or vein occlusion and optic nerve compression with idiopathic intracranial hypertension. Optic neuritis is a common initial presentation of multiple sclerosis.

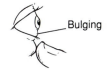

A. Scleral Vessels   B. Subconjunctival   C. Chemosis
                         Hemorrhage

Fig. 7-44 Vascular Disorders of the External Eye.   *A. Scleral Vessels:*
These are the most prominent vessels seen normally. **B. Subconjunctival Hem-**
orrhage: *Bright-red superficial blotches show through the sclera. They appear*
suddenly and painlessly. **C. Chemosis:** *The conjunctival edema may be dem-*
onstrated by pressing the lower lid against the globe, producing a bulge in the
boggy global conjunctiva above the point of compression.

Conjunctiva Signs

KEY SIGN
Subconjunctival Vessels: The scleral vessels may be
prominent in normal individuals. They run in from the sides (Fig.
7-44A).

KEY SIGN
Subconjunctival Hemorrhage: Bleeding under the
conjunctiva is obvious (see Fig. 7-44B). Bleeding may be induced by
coughing, sneezing, weight lifting, or defecation; frequently, the cause
is not apparent. The extravasation is harmless unless an excessive
amount of blood lifts the conjunctiva so that draining is required.

KEY SIGN
Conjunctival Edema: Chemosis: Usually associ-
ated with edema of the lids, the conjunctiva is swollen and transparent.
The edema may be demonstrated by looking at the globe in profile while
pressing the lower lid against the bulbar conjunctiva; the edge of the lid
pushes up a wave of edematous bulbar conjunctiva (see Fig. 7-44C). It
is frequent in Graves ophthalmopathy.

KEY SIGN
Global Hyperemia and Ciliary Flush: Hyperemia
of the global vessels reveals the circulation of the bulbar conjunctiva and
iris. The conjunctival vessels are readily visible as radii with tortuous
branches running from the fornices toward the center of the cornea (Fig.
7-45A). The vessels of the iris are deeper; they begin at the limbus and
run in straight radii toward the pupil. When congested, the vessels of
the iris and adjacent ciliary body dilate and produce a pink band sur-

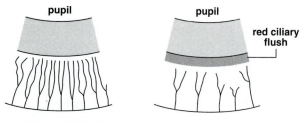

A. Conjunctival Vessels   **B. Iridic Vessels**

Fig. 7-45 Hyperemia and Congestion of the Globe.   A. Hyperemic Scleral Vessels are superficial, coursing radially from the periphery to the limbus in tortuous branches. B. Iritis: The vessels of the iris are deeper; when congested, individual vessels are not visible, but they produce a pink or red band around the limbus, the ciliary flush.

rounding the corneal limbus, the *ciliary flush* (Fig. 7-45B). Suffusion in the conjunctiva blanches with pressure; the ciliary flush does not blanch. Ciliary flush indicates inflammation of the uveal tract (see page 318).

KEY SIGN
Hyperemic   Conjunctiva: Conjunctivitis:
Pathophysiology: Inflammation with or without infection of the conjunctiva. The patient may complain of awakening with eyelids stuck shut and a gritty or burning sensation with excessive lacrimation. There is marked redness of the eye(s) from hyperemia of the palpebral and peripheral global conjunctival vessels. There are many causes; consider viral and bacterial infections, foreign-body reaction, allergies, and Reiter syndrome.

KEY SIGN
Hyperemic Conjunctiva: Conjunctival Calcification:
Pathophysiology: The lesions occur when the serum calcium-phosphorus product (calcium in milligrams × phosphorus in milligrams) exceeds 70 in patients with renal disease. The lesions have also been described in hypercalcemia with sarcoidosis.   *Conjunctival Lesions:* The segments from limbus to canthus at 7 to 10 o'clock and at 2 to 5 o'clock show hyperemic reddening, calcified plaques, and pingueculae. The eyes are painful or feel gritty. The affected areas contain calcium deposits, visible to the unaided eye or through the slit lamp.   *Corneal Lesions:*   These are called *band keratopathy*. White material is visible in the limbal arcs at 2 to 5 o'clock and 7 to 10 o'clock. The slit lamp reveals calcium deposits. Band keratopathy has been reported in disorders with hypercalcemia and in some patients with renal disease having conjunctival calcification.

KEY SIGN
Conjunctival New Growth: Pterygium: *Pathophysiology:*   Chronic irritation from wind and dust is thought to stim-

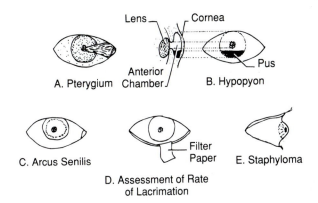

Fig. 7-46 Lesions of the Cornea and Iris. **A. Pterygium**: *This abnormal growth of the pinguecula appears as a raised, subconjunctival fatty structure, growing in a horizontal band toward a position over the pupil.* **B. Hypopyon**: *A collection of pus in the lowest part of the anterior chamber between the cornea and the iris.* **C. Arcus Senilis**: *A gray, opaque, circular band in the cornea, separated from the limbus by a narrow, clear zone.* **D. Assessment of Lacrimation: The Schirmer Test**: *See page 217.* **E. Staphyloma**: *Anterior protrusion of the cornea or sclera.*

ulate the growth of the pinguecula, resulting in the extension of a vascular membrane over the limbus toward the center of the cornea, called a pterygium. This appears as a raised, subconjunctival fatty structure, growing in a horizontal band toward a position over the pupil (Fig. 7-46A). Usually, it is bilateral; vision may be obstructed. This is identified by its firm attachment to the bulbar surface and being limited strictly to the horizontal meridian. A *pseudopterygium* is a band of scar tissue that may extend in any direction and adhere only partially to the bulbar conjunctiva, so a probe may be passed beneath it.

Pigmented Pingueculae: Gaucher Disease: Brownish pigmentation of the pingueculae occurs as one of the few physical signs of Gaucher disease; the other signs are hepatosplenomegaly, thrombocytopenic purpura, and patchy brown pigmentation of the skin of the face and legs.

Cornea Signs

KEY SIGN

Pus Behind the Cornea: Hypopyon: *Pathophysiology:* Inflammation in the iris or anterior chamber produces a purulent discharge. The purulent fluid is seen as an opaque fluid level within the anterior chamber, behind the cornea (see Fig. 7-46B). Iritis is a common cause.

KEY SIGN
Lusterless Cornea: Superficial Keratitis:
Pathophysiology: Inflammation of the cornea with loss of its epithelium occurs with trauma, exposure, toxic exposures, and infection. Most are characterized by early loss of the normal corneal luster with an underlying grayness of the anterior stroma. A ciliary flush is often present. Fluorescein staining demonstrates ulceration or denuded epithelium. *Disruption of the epithelium demands urgent expert therapy, because visual loss can occur rapidly.* A corneal ulcer is extremely painful and causes miosis and photophobia.

✔ *KERATITIS—CLINICAL OCCURRENCE:* Among the many causes of superficial keratitis are contact lens-related ulcers, infected epithelial scratches, spread of conjunctival infection, herpes simplex and zoster, corneal exposure from muscle paralysis or proptosis, injury to the trigeminal nerve (CN V), and tuberculosis.

Cloudy Cornea: Interstitial Keratitis, Congenital Syphilis:
The prototype is congenital syphilis, in which interstitial keratitis, deafness, and notched teeth constitute the *Hutchinson triad*. During the early stages of inflammation, between ages 5 and 15 years, a faint opacity begins in the central zone of the cornea together with a faint ciliary flush. Usually, pain and lacrimation occur as well. Later, the cornea becomes diffusely clouded, so the iris may be obscured. Blood vessels grow into the cornea. After the acute stage, there is more or less permanent corneal opacity. Acquired syphilis and tuberculosis occasionally cause this lesion.

KEY SIGN
Tearless Cornea: Keratoconjunctivitis Sicca (Sjögren Syndrome):
Pathophysiology: Inflammation of the conjunctivae occurs from lack of tears as a consequence of lymphocytic infiltration of exocrine glands (lacrimal and salivary). The diagnosis of Sjögren syndrome is probable if your patient has, without other cause, persistent dry eyes, dry mouth, and a positive Schirmer test (see page 217 and Fig. 7-46D). Autoantibodies in the sera to Ro/SS-A or La/SS-B support the diagnosis and are absent in patients with sicca syndrome and HIV infection or sarcoidosis.

KEY SIGN
Peripheral Corneal Opacity: Arcus Senilis:
The term arcus comes from the early stage, when only a segment of the circumference is involved; later the circle is completed. A gray band of opacity in the cornea, 1.0–1.5 mm wide, is separated from the limbus by a narrow clear zone (see Fig. 7-46C). The lesion is bilateral. It is present in some degree in most persons older than 60 years of age. An arcus before age 40 years is often a sign of hyperlipidemia. Regarded as a degenerative change, it has little clinical significance.

KEY SIGN
Peripheral Corneal Opacity: Kayser-Fleischer Ring, Wilson Disease: A circular band of golden-brown pigment, 2 mm wide, is seen on the posterior corneal surface near the limbus. It invariably accompanies the neurologic manifestations of hepatolenticular degeneration (Wilson disease). Although the rings may be seen with the naked eye, a slit lamp is often required for identification.

Central Corneal Opacity: This is usually the result of trauma or infection. Initially, blood in the anterior chamber following trauma may opacify the cornea. It also occurs in 75% of the cases of dysostosis multiplex (Hurler syndrome).

Dots in the Cornea: Fanconi Syndrome: Crystals of cystine are deposited throughout the stroma with no accompanying inflammatory reaction.

Sclera Signs

KEY SIGN
Yellow Sclera: Fat, Icterus: Commonly, deposits of fat beneath the sclera show through the membrane and impart a yellow color to the periphery, leaving the perilimbal area relatively white. The lipochrome is more obvious with advancing age and in patients with anemia. In obstructive jaundice, conjugated bilirubin infiltrates all body tissues and fluids; it colors the sclera evenly. The conjunctiva of the fornices is usually a deeper yellow because it is thicker.

Blue Sclera: Osteogenesis Imperfecta: *Pathophysiology:* The blue color results from thinning of the sclera so the choroid shows through. This finding is distinctive in osteogenesis imperfecta, but may be mimicked by long-term use of minocycline.

Brown Sclera: Melanin or Homogentisic Acid: Patches of melanin are commonly seen in the sclerae of many persons with dark complexions, especially in blacks. In alkaptonuria, homogentisic acid may color the sclera near the attachments of the ocular muscles upon the globe. Wedge-shaped areas of brown extend their apices toward the limbus.

Scleral Protrusion: Staphyloma: *Pathophysiology:* Scleral injury or increased intraocular pressure leads to a protrusion from the surface of the globe. In the region of the cornea or anterior sclera, an anterior staphyloma forms with a characteristic profile (see

Fig. 7-46E). A posterior staphyloma cannot be seen by external inspection.

KEY SIGN

Red Sclera: Scleritis and Episcleritis: *Pathophysiology:* Sterile inflammation of the sclera and/or Tenon capsule can produce loss of scleral integrity. *Scleritis* is typically diffuse or nodular and is frequently associated with autoimmune diseases. In natural daylight, the area of involvement will appear purple. The patient will often have severe, deep, boring pain. Suppurative scleritis is rare; it is usually metastatic from pyogenic inflammation elsewhere in the body. Tuberculosis, sarcoidosis, and syphilis cause a granulomatous scleritis in which localized elevation of the sclera with nodule formation occurs. Thinning of the sclera may be either nonnecrotizing, termed *scleromalacia perforans,* or necrotizing, with an acute inflammation around an ischemic area of sclera. The latter may develop frank ulceration. *Episcleritis* is a much milder form of inflammation involving Tenon capsule, and appears clinically as a salmon-colored nodule or a diffuse salmon pink color.

Pupil Signs

KEY SIGN

Normal Pupillary Reaction: *Physiology:* The sphincter pupillae is a circular muscle embedded in the iris near the pupillary margin. It is innervated by parasympathetic fibers from the Edinger-Westphal nucleus near the oculomotor nerve (CN III) nucleus (Fig. 7-47). The fibers enter the orbit in the third nerve and accompany its motor branch to the inferior oblique muscle, whence the parasympathetic fibers synapse in the ciliary ganglion; from there, other fibers enter the eye through the short ciliary nerves. The dilator pupillae is arranged radially in the peripheral two-thirds of the iris. It receives sympathetic fibers, arising in the cortex, descending to the hypothalamus to the ciliospinal center; new fibers go to the cervical sympathetic chain and ascend to the superior cervical ganglion to synapse with fibers that run to the carotid plexus, and then to the first division of the trigemi-

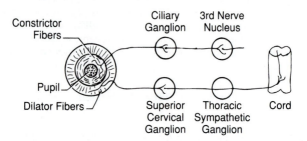

Fig. 7-47 Innervation of the Pupillary Muscles.

nal nerve (CN V) into the eye. Thus, the sphincter contracts the pupil through parasympathetic stimulation; the dilator widens the pupil by sympathetic stimuli. The size of the pupils frequently fluctuates from changes in tone; exaggerated wavering is termed *hippus,* or *physiologic pupillary unrest;* it is of little clinical significance. Patients with Cheyne-Stokes respiration may have pupils that dilate during the phase of hyperventilation and contract during the periods of apnea. *Mydriasis* is dilatation; *miosis* is pupillary constriction. Bright light causes constriction, accompanied by a consensual reaction in the unexposed eye. In older persons, the pupils may react sluggishly to light; the reaction is hastened after several stimulations. Miosis occurs when the eye is fixed on a near object, say 20 mm (0.8 in) away.

KEY SIGN
Unequal Pupils: Anisocoria: *Pathophysiology:* Inequality between the diameters of the two pupils occurs from either constriction and/or dilation of *one* pupil, or an asymmetric combination. Anisocoria can be without clinical significance. The best method to distinguish a pupil that is too small on one side from one that is too large on the other side, is to measure the pupils in both bright light and very dim light. If the one pupil is pathologically too large with a failure of the sphincter muscle, the difference between the pupils will be exaggerated in bright light. If the difference is greater in darkness, there is a failure of the dilator muscle, indicating that the small pupil is the pathologic one. Beware of the artificial eye.

✓ *ANISOCORIA—CLINICAL OCCURRENCE:* Miosis of one pupil with a large disparity in size suggests iritis, paralysis of the cervical sympathetics, or the use of a miotic drug (e.g., pilocarpine). Dilatation of a single pupil can be caused by a mydriatic drug (such as atropine), paralysis of CN III, or increased intraocular pressure in one eye. Inequality may occur congenitally or with syphilitic meningitis, tabes dorsalis, trigeminal neuralgia, carotid or aortic aneurysm, unilateral intracranial mass, glaucoma, or Adie pupils.

KEY SIGN
Sluggish Pupillary Reaction: Argyll Robertson Pupil: *Pathophysiology:* There is no agreement on the site of the lesion in the nervous system. The classic signs are (a) weak or absent contraction to light, (b) the contraction to light does not improve with dark adaptation, (c) normal or exaggerated contraction to accommodation, (d) miotic pupils, (e) failure to dilate with painful stimulation in other parts of the body, and (f) irregular and unequal pupils. The disorder cannot be demonstrated in a blind eye. The fully developed Argyll Robertson pupil is almost pathognomonic of tabes dorsalis or taboparesis. The pupil does not dilate with atropine.

KEY SIGN
Sluggish Pupillary Reaction: Tonic Pupil (Adie Pupil): Reaction to both light and near focus may initially

appear to be lost. Closer observation shows both to be present but extremely sluggish, with a prolonged latent period. Later, the response to light may be absent with a full but tonic response to a near stimulus. There may also be sectoral or vermiform movements of the pupillary border. It may be unilateral. It is most frequently encountered in young women with normal-sized pupils, in contrast to the requisite miosis in the Argyll Robertson pupil; whatever the degree of reaction in the Argyll Robertson pupil, its reaction is prompt. The tonic pupil dilates with atropine; the Argyll Robertson pupil usually does not.

KEY SIGN

Unreactive Pupil: Pupillary Paralysis (Ophthalmoplegia Internal):   The pupil lacks the ability to constrict from either light or accommodation. It is generally dilated, never miotic.

✓ *CLINICAL OCCURRENCE:*   Topical mydriatics are most common; less-common causes are luetic meningitis, vasculitis, virus encephalitis, diphtheria or tetanus toxin, lead poisoning, midbrain lesions, bilateral CN III involvement, Adie pupils, iris dysfunction from trauma, anticholinergic medications (e.g., scopolamine patches, benztropine mesylate).

KEY SIGN

Unilateral Miosis: Horner Syndrome: *Pathophysiology:*   This is caused by a lesion of the sympathetic pathway. It is accompanied by ptosis and anhydrosis on the affected side. See Chapter 14, page 878.

Lens Signs

KEY SIGN

Lenticular Opacity: Cataract: *Pathophysiology:* Deposits of opaque substances within the layers of the lens produce focal or diffuse lesions that can obstruct and/or scatter light before it reaches the retina. Because nearly all adults have some opacity of the lenses, a clinical definition of cataract implies a degree of clouding that interferes with vision. Some cataracts can be readily seen by shining a light beam obliquely through the lens (*focal illumination*), by ophthalmoscopic inspection against the red retinal reflex with 0 diopter magnification from approximately 40 cm (15.7 in), or by using +10 diopter magnification with close inspection (*direct illumination*). Many can only be identified with the slit lamp. Centrally placed cataracts can be seen without pupillary dilatation; those in the periphery can be visualized only after employment of a mydriatic. *This discussion is limited to the types detectable without mydriatics or the slit lamp.*

   Anterior Polar Cataract.   A small white plaque can be seen in the center of the pupil. It either is congenital or occurs after corneal ulceration.

   Nuclear Cataract.   Diffuse pigmentation occurs in the central portion of the lens. Ophthalmoscopic illumination shows a black reflection instead of the normal red retinal reflex.

Cortical Cataract. Wedge-shaped opacities, arranged radially in the periphery, appear gray with the penlight and black against the red retinal reflex through the ophthalmoscope.

Secondary Cataract. Occurring after incomplete removal of the lenticular capsule, this type shows as dense folds of tissue and clusters of clear vesicles.

Complicated Cataract. Associated with uveal disease or retinal detachment, opacities with rainbow colors extend toward the center as radii.

Diabetic Cataract. Older diabetic patients have an increased tendency to develop nuclear or cortical cataracts with no distinctive character. Juvenile diabetic patients acquire a distinctive snowflake cataract containing chalky white deposits; the entire lens subsequently becomes milky.

Posterior Subcapsular Cataract. This type of lesion is commonly seen after long-term use of corticosteroids.

KEY SIGN

Lenticular Displacement: Subluxation and Dislocation: *Pathophysiology:* Rupture of the zonula ciliaris (zonule of Zinn) permits the lens to move from its fixed position behind the pupil. Slight displacement, with the lens still backing the pupillary aperture, is termed *subluxation* (Fig. 7-48A); it is manifest by tremulousness of the iris (*iridodonesis*), when the eye moves horizontally. Viewed through the ophthalmoscope, the equator of the lens may show as a dark, curved line crossing the pupillary aperture; a double image of the retina with different magnifications may be seen, one through the lens, the other without the lens. When the lens is displaced completely from the aperture, the condition is called *dislocation.* The lens is readily seen when it emerges into the anterior chamber (Fig. 7-48B). Lenticular displacement is usually caused by trauma. Nontraumatic dislocation occurs in Marfan disease and homocystinuria.

KEY SIGN

Intraocular Pressure Changes: Increased tension occurs in glaucoma; decreased tension means extreme dehydration. Accurate assessment is made by measurement of pressure with the tonometer.

Retina Signs

The following article provides a good review of retinal diseases with pathophysiology and photographs of many retinal signs [D'Amico DJ. Diseases of the retina. *N Engl J Med* 1994;331:95–106].

A. Subluxation

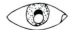
B. Dislocation

Fig. 7-48 Displacement of the Lens. *A. Subluxation. B. Anterior Chamber Dislocation.*

KEY SIGN

Increased Cup-to-Disk Ratio: Glaucoma:

Pathophysiology: Increased intraocular pressure leads to atrophy of the rim of nerve fibers in the disk producing enlargement of the cup. A progressive cup-to-disk ratio (e.g., 0.2/1.0 to 0.7/1.0), discovered by sequential observations, suggests increasing intraocular pressure.

KEY SIGN

Proliferation About the Disk: Myelinated Nerve Fibers: *Pathophysiology:* Myelination of the optic nerve fibers usually ends at the lamina cribrosa; infrequently myelin sheaths are retained by some nerve fibers until they reach well into the retina, causing this picture (Fig. 7-49B). Semiopaque white patches emerge from the borders of the optic disk and spread into one or two quadrants of the retina. The retinal borders appear frayed, and the underlying vessels are partially or completely obscured. Novices may think they are viewing a serious lesion, when actually it is a normal variation of no clinical significance.

KEY SIGN

Disk Pallor: Optic Atrophy: *Pathophysiology:* Damage to the optic nerve (ischemia, inflammation, or increased intracranial pressure) leads to atrophy of the nerve fibers and loss of normal vascularity (see Fig. 7-49C). The disk is pale pink or white from loss of nerve fibers and capillaries, the borders may be sharp or less distinct, and the physiologic cup and lamina cribrosa are variably seen. The emerging vessels may be surrounded by perivascular lymph sheathing, seen as white lines. Pigmented or gray patches in the retina attest to previous hemorrhages or exudates. These findings indicate increased intracranial pressure producing the optic atrophy. The common cause is brain tumor. In optic atrophy from chorioretinitis, the disk may have a yellow cast, and the surrounding retina may contain hemorrhages, areas of atrophy, and pigment. DDX: The distinction between optic atrophy as a result of intrinsic lesions of the optic nerve and that from increased intracranial pressure cannot be made reliably by the physical findings.

✔ *OPTIC ATROPHY—CLINICAL OCCURRENCE:* Intrinsic optic nerve lesions: tabes dorsalis, taboparesis, multiple sclerosis; increased intracranial pressure (e.g., idiopathic intracranial hypertension, brain tumors); conditions causing compression of the optic nerve without increased intracranial pressure; present in approximately 5% of patients with pernicious anemia.

KEY SIGN

Disk Edema: Papillitis, Optic Neuritis: *Pathophysiology:* When optic neuritis involves the portion of the optic nerve within the globe, papillitis, with loss of vision, is produced (see Fig. 7-49D). Papillitis causes edema of the disk that is indistinguishable from papilledema. However, visual loss occurs early in optic neuritis and usually later with papilledema. The disk is hyperemic and its margins may

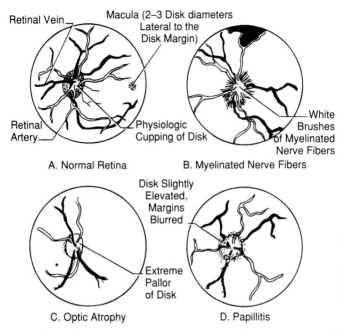

A. Normal Retina   B. Myelinated Nerve Fibers

C. Optic Atrophy   D. Papillitis

Fig. 7-49 Retinal Abnormalities I. *A. Normal Left Retina:* The background of the retina is red-orange; it contains a variable amount of black pigments, depending on race and complexion. Diverging blood vessels emerge from the optic disk to spread over the retina, usually in pairs of an artery and a vein. The veins are solid and dark red, and they may pulsate normally. The arteries are brighter red, contain central white stripes, and are pulseless. The width of an artery is usually about four-fifths that of the adjacent vein. The optic disk is lighter red, with sharp borders, often outlined by a strip of black pigment in the adjacent retina. The physiologic cup is white or pale yellow. The macula lies in the horizontal plane of the disk and from 2–3 disk diameters to the temporal side. The macular area is pale red with a central white or shining dot. *B. Myelinated Nerve Fibers:* White brushes of myelinated nerves emerge from the disk, obscuring segments of vessels and disk margins. *C. Optic Atrophy:* The disk is chalk-white with sharply defined borders. The blood vessels are normal. *D. Papillitis:* The disk is hyperemic and its borders are blurred.

be indistinct as a result of edema in the peripapillary nerve fiber layer. The disk surface is elevated above the surrounding retina, demonstrated by finding that a +1 or +2 lens correction is required to focus on the disk.

✔ *PAPILLITIS—CLINICAL OCCURRENCE:* Causes of optic neuritis include local inflammation (such as uveitis and retinitis), sympathetic ophthalmia, multiple sclerosis, meningitis, sinusitis, infectious diseases (e.g., syphilis, tuberculosis, influenza, measles, malaria, mumps, and pneumonia), metabolic conditions, pregnancy, and intoxications (e.g., methyl alcohol).

Disk Edema: Anterior Ischemic Optic Neuropathy (AION): *Pathophysiology:* This is an infarction of the optic nerve head caused by inadequate perfusion of the posterior ciliary arteries. AION occurs in two forms, the arteritic, related to giant cell arteritis, and the nonarteritic, which occurs in a slightly younger group of patients with vasculopathies such as hypertension or diabetes mellitus. The onset is usually sudden and painless, with profound visual loss, typically altitudinal, involving the upper and lower field. Vision may be lost progressively in some cases. The optic nerve appears edematous, with scant hemorrhage and more pallor than typical papilledema. If the patient is older than age 55 years, it is imperative to search for giant cell arteritis. The nonarteritic form is accompanied by a small to absent optic cup in the uninvolved eye and often a period of systemic hypotension.

Disk Edema: Papilledema (Choked Disk): *Pathophysiology:* Increased intracranial pressure causes the cerebrospinal fluid in the optic nerve sheath to compress the optic nerve, with resultant axoplasmic flow stasis and intraneuronal ischemia (Fig. 7-50A). In contrast to papillitis, central vision is unimpaired, but like glaucoma, there is usually peripheral loss. Early papilledema causes a C-shaped halo of nerve fiber layer edema that surrounds the disc with a gap temporally. With more advanced papilledema, the halo becomes circumferential; next there is obscuration of major vessels as they leave the disc; and later there is obscuration of vessels on the optic disc. The emerging vessels can be seen to bend sharply as they pass over the edge

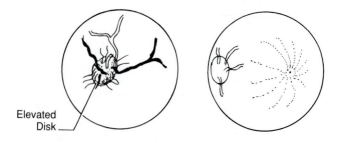

Elevated
Disk

A. Papilledema, Choked Disk   B. Star Figure of Macula

Fig. 7-50 Retinal Abnormalities II. A. Papilledema (Choked Disk): The disk surface is elevated, the nasal borders blurred. The vessels curve downward over the borders. The veins are distended and pulseless. Both arteries and veins in the disk may be obscured by the swollen structure. B. Star Figure of the Macula: Edema throws the retina into traction folds that radiate from the macula as white lines.

of the elevated disk. Edema of the retina in the macular region throws the retina into traction folds (*choroidal folds*), seen as white lines radiating from the macula (Fig. 7-50B).

✔ *PAPILLEDEMA—CLINICAL OCCURRENCE:*   The principal causes are brain tumor, hydrocephalus from any cause, and idiopathic intracranial hypertension. Less common causes are hydrocephalus, hypertensive, arteriosclerotic, or leukemic retinopathy, subarachnoid hemorrhage, meningitis, and salicylate poisoning. Rarely, papilledema occurs in polycythemia and macroglobulinemia.

KEY SIGN
Pseudopapilledema: Drusen   Bodies: *Pathophysiology:*   Drusen bodies (German for "geode") are granular deposits in the optic disk that cause pseudopapilledema. The distinctions between early papilledema and drusen bodies are reported as follows: drusen cause obvious irregular, lumpy, bumpy elevation of the disk; drusen are pink or yellow, the surface of papilledema is hyperemic; drusen cause the nerve fiber layer to glisten and often show a halo of feathery reflections, whereas the layer in papilledema is dull; drusen are in the disk center; in papilledema, the vessels show absence of venous pulsation and the light reflexes are dulled; drusen make the disk outline irregular and are more frequent in small, hypermetropic eyes.

KEY SIGN
Retinal Vessels: Venous Engorgement: Distention of the retinal veins suggests polycythemia vera, congenital heart disease, leukemia, diabetes, and macroglobulinemia.

KEY SIGN
Retinal Vessels: Hemorrhages: *Pathophysiology:* Hemorrhage may occur in any layer of the retina. The shape of the hemorrhage frequently reveals its source. A very large and deep hemorrhage in the choriocapillaris produces a dark, elevated area in the retina that looks like a melanotic tumor (Fig. 7-51A). These dark, greenish areas should make you suspect a *subretinal vascular membrane.* Subretinal vascular membranes are seen in association with macular degeneration. A smaller, more superficial hemorrhage appears as a round red spot, with blurred margins, called a *blot hemorrhage* (Fig. 7-51B). *Microaneurysms* are also round red spots, but their borders are distinct, they are not reabsorbed like hemorrhages, and they may occur in clusters about vascular sprigs (Fig. 7-51C). *Flame-shaped hemorrhages* occur in the nerve fiber layer of the retina; they are red and striated (Fig. 7-51D). In the *subhyaloid or preretinal hemorrhage,* a pool of blood accumulates between the retina and the hyaloid membrane to form a turned-up half-moon, with the straight upper side, a fluid level (Fig. 7-51E). These lesions sometimes organize slowly to form arcuate strands of white near blood vessels, a condition called *retinitis proliferans.* A small hemorrhagic spot with a central white area is called a *Roth spot* (Fig. 7-51F); it occurs in subacute bacterial endocarditis and leukemia.

A. Deep Retinal Hemorrhage B. Blot Hemorrhages C. Retinal Microaneurysms

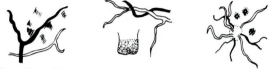

D. Flame Hemorrhages E. Subhyaloid Hemorrhages F. Roth Spots

Fig. 7-51 Hemorrhages and Similar Lesions in the Retina.

✓ *RETINAL HEMORRHAGES—CLINICAL OCCURRENCE:* Some of the many conditions producing retinal hemorrhages are hypertension, diabetes mellitus, choked disk, occlusion of retinal veins, subacute bacterial endocarditis, HIV, systemic lupus erythematosus, pulseless disease (Takayasu disease), macroglobulinemia, leukemia, polycythemia, sickle cell disease, and sarcoidosis.

Retinal Vessels: Cytomegalovirus (CMV) Retinitis: *Pathophysiology:* Immunosuppression from HIV infection is frequently accompanied by cytomegalovirus infection of the retina. Patients describe visual loss, blurring, floaters, and flashes of light. Look for whitening of the retina, cotton-wool spots, and intraretinal hemorrhages. Although less common, consider varicella zoster infection, toxoplasmosis, and syphilis [ET Cunningham, TP Margolis. Ocular manifestations of HIV infection. *N Engl J Med* 1998;339:236–244].

KEY SIGN
Retinal Vessels: Arterial Occlusion: *Pathophysiology:* Sudden loss of vision occurs when the central artery of the retina becomes completely occluded, usually from thrombosis, rarely from embolism. Early the retina is very pale from ischemic edema; the arteries are extremely narrowed, and the smaller ones are invisible (Fig. 7-52A). Although the veins are full, they are pulseless. Pressure on the eyeball induces no pulsation in either artery or vein, proving the lack of circulation. Retinal edema around the macula causes pallor; by contrast, after 36 hours, the macula appears as a *cherry-red spot,* which disappears within a few weeks with subsidence of the edema. Occlusion of a branch artery causes findings limited to its area of supply.

✓ *RETINAL ARTERY OCCLUSION—CLINICAL OCCURRENCE:* The common causes of arterial occlusion are vascular disease, syphilis, rheumatic fever, hepatitis, and temporal arteritis. Rarely, it is a complication of systemic lupus erythematosus, sickle cell disease, cryoglobulinemia, or thromboangiitis obliterans.

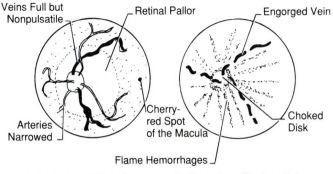

Fig. 7-52 Retinal Vascular Occlusions. *A. Retinal Artery Occlusion: The retinal background is white and the arteries are much narrowed. The veins are pulseless.* ***B. Retinal Vein Occlusion:*** *The affected veins are engorged and tortuous. Hemorrhages occur near the veins.*

KEY SIGN

Retinal Vessels: Venous Occlusion: *Pathophysiology:* Thrombosis of the central retinal vein is accompanied by engorgement and tortuosity of all visible veins (see Fig. 7-52B). This is not associated with sudden loss of vision. Variform hemorrhages appear throughout the retina. Edema of the disk is present. Occlusion of a branch of the central vein produces findings limited to the area of its drainage.

✔ *RETINAL VENOUS OCCLUSION—CLINICAL OCCURRENCE:* Venous occlusion is often the result of atherosclerosis, but other causes are diabetes, periphlebitis from tuberculosis, polycythemia, multiple myeloma, macroglobulinemia, and leukemia. In sickle cell disease, multiple venous thromboses may be accompanied by neovascularization.

KEY SIGN

Retinal Vessels: Arteriolar Sclerosis: The progress of the disease can be viewed through the ophthalmoscope, although the retinal changes do not necessarily parallel the changes elsewhere in the body, as the disease is spotty in its distribution.

Arterial Stripe. Normally, the retinal arteries contain a central white stripe from the light reflection off the curved blood column. Increases in mural thickness cause widening of the stripe and brightening of the reflex. In moderate disease, the walls look like burnished copper and the vessels are called *copper-wire arteries.* When the condition is far advanced, the entire width of the artery reflects as a white stripe, and the vessels are termed *silver-wire arteries.*

Vessel Sheaths. Normally the vessel walls are completely transparent, hence invisible. Mural thickening with lipoid infiltration produces

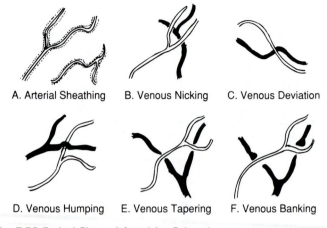

A. Arterial Sheathing   B. Venous Nicking   C. Venous Deviation

D. Venous Humping   E. Venous Tapering   F. Venous Banking

Fig. 7-53 Retinal Signs of Arteriolar Sclerosis.

a milky white streak on either side of the blood column, called *pipestem sheathing.*

Arteriovenous Crossings. As the arterial and arteriolar walls become more dense and less compliant, signs are produced where they cross the veins (Fig. 7-53). Concealment of the vein (*arteriovenous nicking,* Fig. 7-53B) occurs with thickening of the arterial sheath, so the vein is invisible for a short segment on either side of the overlying artery. *Deviation of the vein* is produced when the stiffened artery pushes the vein to assume a crossing at 90 degrees where the normal angle of the two vessels is acute (Fig. 7-53C). When the vein overlying the artery is elevated by the latter, it is called *humping* (Fig. 7-53D). *Tapering of the veins* results when the artery compresses the vein at the crossing (Fig. 7-53E). When venous flow is partially obstructed, dilatation occurs at the end of the vein segment, called *banking* (Fig. 7-53F).

The degree of involvement of the retinal vessels by the arteriolar sclerotic process has been variously scored. Table 7-2 represents the Kirkendall and Armstrong modification of the Scheie classification [Kirkendall WM, Armstrong ML: Vascular changes in the eye of the treated and untreated patient with hypertension. *Am J Cardiol* 1962;9:663].

TABLE 7–2   Grades of Retinal Arteriolar Sclerosis

Grade 1	Thickening of vessels with slight depression of veins at arteriolar-venular (AV) crossings.
Grade 2	Definitive AV crossing changes and moderate local sclerosis.
Grade 3	Venule beneath the arteriole is invisible; severe local sclerosis and segmentation.
Grade 4	To the preceding signs are added venous obstruction and arteriolar obliteration.

TABLE 7–3 Grades of Retinal Hypertension

Grade 1	Narrowing in terminal branches of vessels.
Grade 2	General narrowing of vessels with severe local constriction.
Grade 3	To the preceding signs are added striate hemorrhages and soft exudates
Grade 4	Papilledema is added to the preceding signs.

KEY SIGN
Retinal Vessels: Hypertensive Retinopathy:
Arterial hypertension produces distinctive retinal signs that often coexist with the signs of arteriolar sclerosis. For example, the appearance of a retina may be classified as "grade 3 arteriolosclerosis, grade 4 hypertension." The signs attributed to hypertension may also be graded by using the classification of Kirkendall and Armstrong (Table 7-3) [Kirkendall WM, Armstrong ML: Vascular changes in the eye of the treated and untreated patient with hypertension. *Am J Cardiol* 1962;9:663].

KEY SIGN
Retinal Spots: Cotton-Wool Patches: *Pathophysiology:* Thickening and swelling of the terminal retinal nerve fibers results from ischemic infarcts. Gray to white areas with ill-defined fluffy borders occur in disarray around the posterior pole of the retina. They are often accompanied by red dots, representing microaneurysms, that subsequently rupture to produce striate hemorrhages.

✓ *CLINICAL OCCURRENCE:* Hypertension, lupus erythematosus, dermatomyositis, HIV, occlusion of a central retinal vein, papilledema from any cause.

KEY SIGN
Retinal Spots: Hard Exudates: *Pathophysiology:* The cause is lipid deposition from leaking capillaries. Distinct from the superficial cotton-wool patches, these are small white spots with sharply defined edges. They are deeper than the superficial retinal vessels.

Retinal Spots: Pigmented Spots: The sites of old hemorrhages are marked by groups of pigmented spots over retinal vessels.

KEY SIGN
Refractile Spots in Retinal Arteries: Cholesterol Emboli: *Pathophysiology:* Ulcerated atherosclerotic plaque in the aorta or carotid artery shed cholesterol crystals that become lodged at the bifurcations of retinal vessels. Patients may be asymptomatic or present with transient monocular visual loss, *amaurosis fugax,* or transient ischemic neurologic attacks (TIA) in a carotid distribution. Finding cholesterol emboli proves plaque rupture with embolization.

White or Yellow Spots in Retinal Arteries: Deposits of Talc: These are seen in the retinae of intravenous drug users who have injected ground-up tablets containing talc. The granules seem to be harmless in the eye, but granules trapped in lung capillaries could be harmful.

Macular Region: Macular Degeneration: Although vision is much reduced, the only visible sign may be a few spots of pigment near the macula and blurring of the macular borders. In other cases, subretinal hemorrhages, patches of retinal atrophy, yellow drusen, and pigmented areas may be seen.

S KEY SYNDROME

Macular Region: Diabetic Retinopathy: In diabetes, the macular region is especially involved. *Microaneurysms* occur around the macula, seen as sharply defined small red spots, and need to be distinguished from blot hemorrhages with blurred borders. In advanced diabetic retinopathy, the picture is embellished by white or yellow waxy *exudates* with distinct, often serrated, borders. The exudates gradually coalesce to form a broken circle around the macular region. With advanced disease, *neovascularization* may be seen on the disk (NVD) or elsewhere in the retina (NVE). The signs of atherosclerosis and hypertension are sometimes superimposed. Patients with type 1 diabetes should have an indirect ophthalmoscopic screening examination 5 years after onset and at least annually thereafter. Patients with type 2 diabetes need an ophthalmoscopic screening examination when first diagnosed and annually thereafter. Women with gestational diabetes need a diagnosis or screening examination every 3 months until after delivery. Although microaneurysms around the macula are characteristic of diabetes, be aware that retinal microvasculopathy with cotton-wool spots, intraretinal hemorrhages, and microaneurysms occurs in many patients with HIV.

White Macular Region: Tay-Sachs Disease: Inherited in Jewish families, the disease is manifest in the retina by a white macular region containing a cherry-red spot in the fovea.

Pigmentary Retinal Degeneration: Retinitis Pigmentosa: *Pathophysiology:* Inherited singly or as a component of several syndromes, retinitis pigmentosa is manifest by diminution in the caliber of the retinal vessels and pigmentation of the retina. Night blindness is the earliest symptom; later, all types of vision are greatly impaired. Spidery strands of pigmented spots form a girdle about the global equator (Fig. 7-54A). Later, most of the retina is infiltrated with pigment. The condition may occur in the Laurence-Moon-Biedl syndrome, which includes obesity, polydactylism, hypogenitalism, and mental retardation.

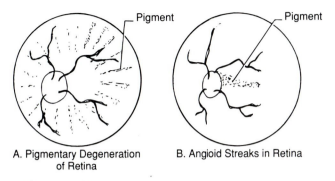

A. Pigmentary Degeneration of Retina

B. Angioid Streaks in Retina

Fig. 7-54 Retinal Pigmentation.

Angioid Streaks in the Retina: *Pathophysiology:* They probably represent degeneration of elastic tissue. Broad lines of pigment radiate from the optic disk, branching in the manner of blood vessels (see Fig. 7-54B). They occur in Paget disease and in pseudoxanthoma elasticum.

KEY SIGN

Retinal Detachment: Retinal detachments may be symptomatic or asymptomatic. Patients may complain of flashing lights followed by floaters and then a curtain crossing their vision. The earliest sign is elevation of a retinal area so that it is out of focus with the surrounding structures. The arteries and veins in the separated membrane appear almost black (Fig. 7-55). When widely separated, the retinal sheet is gray and frequently folded. Underlying inflammation may produce areas of choroiditis and vitreous opacities. A torn edge may be encountered, often shaped like a horseshoe. The cause of detachment is often undetermined (idiopathic), or a retinal hemorrhage or tumor may produce it.

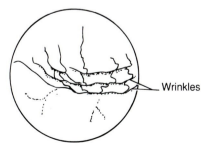

Wrinkles

Fig. 7-55 Retinal Detachment.

Nose and Sinus Signs

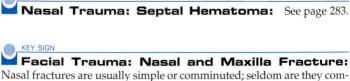

KEY SIGN

Epistaxis (Nosebleed): *Pathophysiology:* In the anterior nose, the most common site of bleeding is Kiesselbach plexus, a vascular network in the anterior nasal septum. Posteriorly, hemorrhage occurs frequently at the back third of the inferior meatus; vessels in the region are large and belong to the external carotid artery system. In some cases, there are multiple oozing points in the mucosa. Nosebleed can be a spontaneous and trivial occurrence or a sign of serious local or generalized disease. Hemorrhage from the external nares is obvious, but bleeding from the choana must be distinguished from hemoptysis and even hematemesis. The first problem is to ascertain the bleeding site and judge whether trauma or some predisposing disease is present. Inquire about trauma, predisposing local or systemic disease, and the amount of blood lost. Seat the patient in a chair and seat yourself in front of the patient. Observe universal precautions: use gloves, gown, and face protection to avoid blood contamination. Remove the clots by suction or have the patient clear the nose by blowing. Inspect the anterior nasal chambers, especially the septum. If hemorrhage is so profuse as to obscure the site, advance the sucker tip backward in small increments, clearing the blood at each step, until a point is reached where the passage immediately fills after clearing; this is the bleeding site. Blood-tinged fluid suggests a cerebrospinal fluid leak. Consult textbooks for methods of arresting hemorrhage.

✔ *EPISTAXIS—CLINICAL OCCURRENCE:* *Local Causes* coughing, sneezing, nose picking, fractures, lacerations, foreign bodies, adenoid growth, nasopharyngeal fibroma, angioma, rhinitis sicca. *Generalized Causes: Congenital* hereditary telangiectasia; *Inflammatory/Immune* Wegener granulomatosis, lethal midline granuloma; *Infectious* viral rhinitis, typhoid fever, scarlet fever, influenza, measles, infectious mononucleosis, diphtheria, pertussis, psittacosis, Rocky Mountain spotted fever, erysipelas; *Metabolic/Toxic* pernicious anemia, aspirin, scurvy; *Mechanical/Trauma* (see local causes) changes in atmospheric pressure (mountain climbing, caisson disease, flying) exertion; *Neoplastic* nasopharyngeal carcinoma and others, leukemia; *Vascular: Coagulopathies* cirrhosis, uremia, hemophilia, von Willebrand disease, thrombocytopenia; *Elevated Arterial Pressure* hypertension, coarctation of the aorta; *Elevated Venous Pressure* cor pulmonale, congestive heart failure, superior vena cava syndrome.

KEY SIGN

Nasal Trauma: Septal Hematoma: See page 283.

KEY SIGN

Facial Trauma: Nasal and Maxilla Fracture:
Nasal fractures are usually simple or comminuted; seldom are they com-

pound. A blow from the side displaces both nasal bones to the opposite side, producing an S-shaped curve in the dorsum nasi. The septum may be fractured with or without nasal bone fracture. Frontal blows depress the nasal bones. Palpation along the inferior border of the orbit may disclose an irregularity indicating fracture of the maxilla, with displacement of a fragment downward into the sinus. Backward displacement of the maxilla is indicated by malocclusion of the teeth. Fracture of the zygoma produces flattening of the cheek.

KEY SIGN

Loss of Smell: Anosmia: *Pathophysiology:* Lesions of CN I, often shearing of the nerve ending passing through the cribriform plate, or nasal obstruction produce loss of smell. Anosmia is invariably accompanied by a perceived change in the taste of food, which seems bland and unpalatable. The most common cause is closed head trauma [Cullen MM, Leopold DA. Disorders of smell and taste. *Med Clin North Am* 1999;83:57–74].

KEY SIGN

External Nasal Deformities: Congenital: Disturbances in development of the nose are myriad, but they are so obvious as to pose little problem in diagnosis. Perhaps the most common is cleft nose (Fig. 7-56B), a congenital defect from incomplete fusion at the tip and dorsum. The physician should recognize nasal deformities as sources of extreme psychological trauma that can be alleviated by rhinoplasty.

KEY SIGN

External Nasal Deformities: Acquired: Trauma, infection, and neoplasm produce classic types of acquired deformities. *Rhinophyma* is a bulbous enlargement of the distal two-thirds of the nose from multiple sebaceous adenomas of the skin, which may follow long-standing rosacea (see Fig. 7-56A). The nodular mass of tissue is covered by erythematous skin. These deformities are remediable

A. Rhinophyma   B. Cleft Nose   C. Saddle Nose

Fig. 7-56 External Nasal Deformities. A. Rhinophyma. B. Cleft Nose. C. Saddle Nose: Note the sinking of the dorsum with relative prominence of the lower third.

by plastic surgery. *Saddle nose* is distinguished by the sunken bridge (see Fig. 7-56C), which most commonly results from loss of cartilage secondary to septal hematoma or abscess. Rarely, it can follow relapsing polychondritis, Wegener granulomatosis, or either congenital or acquired syphilis. *Skewed nose* (the term is not in general use), with a curved or oblique dorsum nasi, results from fracture.

KEY SIGN

Nasal Vestibule: Folliculitis: Mild inflammation around the hair follicles is evident on inspection.

KEY SIGN

Nasal Vestibule: Furunculosis: *Pathophysiology: A small superficial abscess forms in the skin or mucous membrane.* Easily seen from the exterior, the lesion is typical of all furuncles. The area becomes extremely tender, swollen, and reddened. Swelling may involve the nasal tip, alae nasi, and upper lip (Fig. 7-57A). Avoid instrumentation or other trauma to pyogenic lesions within the triangle anterior to a line from the corners of the mouth to the glabella; this may cause spread of the infection directly to the cavernous sinus.

Nasal Vestibule: Fissure: Fissures often develop at the mucocutaneous junction. They become overlaid with crusts that cover tender surfaces.

KEY SIGN

Nasal Septum: Deviation: In the adult, the nasal septum is seldom precisely a midline structure. The cartilaginous and bony septum may deviate as a hump, spur, or shelf to encroach on one nasal chamber, occasionally causing obstruction. Columnar dislocation of the septum may occur.

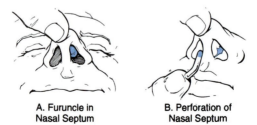

A. Furuncle in   B. Perforation of
Nasal Septum   Nasal Septum

Fig. 7-57 Lesions in the Nasal Vestibule. *A. Furuncle: Avoid trauma that might spread infection to the cavernous sinus. B. Perforation of Nasal Septum: Transillumination of the septum discloses a hole.*

KEY SIGN
Nasal Septum: Perforation: A hole in the nasal septum is commonly caused by chronic infection, with repeated trauma in picking off crusts or as a result of nasal surgery. Perforation was formerly attributed to tuberculosis or syphilis; however, these causes are now quite rare. Consider cocaine abuse as a cause. Perforation is readily demonstrated by looking in one naris while a light is shone in the other (see Fig. 7-57B). The cartilaginous portion is usually involved.

KEY SIGN
Nasal Septum: Hematoma: *Pathophysiology:* Even slight trauma to the nose may produce bleeding under the mucoperichondrium, usually causing bilateral hematomas. Nasal obstruction necessitates breathing through the mouth. The hematoma is seen as a violaceous, compressible, obstructive mass. The columella may be widened; the nasal tip pales from stretching of the skin. Pressure on the anterior ethmoidal nerve by the hematoma may cause anesthesia of the tip. Long-standing hematomas interfere with the blood supply of the septum, causing slow necrosis of the cartilage and a saddle nose deformity.

KEY SIGN
Nasal Septum: Abscess: The septum swells into both nasal chambers, and the overlying membranes become edematous. Infection of a septal hematoma invariably results in loss of cartilage; it must therefore be immediately incised, drained, and treated with appropriate antibiotics. There is risk of progression through the angular veins to produce cavernous sinus thrombosis.

S KEY SYNDROME
Bilateral Rhinorrhea: Acute Rhinitis: *Pathophysiology:* Rhinoviruses, and many others, infect the mucous membranes of the nose and sinuses causing inflammation and increased nasal secretions. Beginning with a watery discharge (*rhinorrhea*) and sneezing, the nasal secretion ultimately becomes purulent, possibly accompanied by fever and malaise. Nasal obstruction occurs from edema of the mucosa. A sore throat is not part of the picture. Severe local pain suggests a complication, such as bacterial sinusitis.

S KEY SYNDROME
Bilateral Rhinorrhea: Chronic Rhinitis: Chronic bilateral rhinorrhea suggests chronic environmental irritants (dust, smoke, perfume, dry or cold air), allergic rhinitis (seasonal or perennial), rhinitis medicamentosa or nasomotor rhinitis.

KEY SIGN
Dry Nasal Mucosa: Atrophic Rhinitis: The patient complains of nasal discomfort or "stuffiness." The membranes appear dry, smooth, and shiny; they are studded with crusts. A foul odor (*ozena*) may be present. The cause is unknown.

Unilateral Nasal Discharge: Choanal Atresia:
A congenitally closed orifice is occasionally encountered, usually in infants, demonstrated by obstruction when an attempt is made to pass a catheter from the external naris to the nasopharynx.

KEY SIGN
Unilateral Nasal Discharge: Foreign Body:
Children frequently put objects into the nose that remain for long periods and produce foul, purulent discharge.

KEY SIGN
Unilateral Nasal Discharge: Neoplasm: Often carcinoma produces a bloody discharge, in distinction to the brisk bleeding of epistaxis.

KEY SIGN
Unilateral Nasal Discharge: Cerebrospinal Rhinorrhea: *Pathophysiology:* A traumatic fistula occurs between the subarachnoid space and the nasal cavity. A unilateral discharge of clear spinal fluid may occur after head injury or surgery. The fluid may be blood-tinged but is readily distinguished from a brisk nosebleed. Compression of the jugular vein increases the flow. Spinal fluid also gives a positive test for sugar. There is substantial risk for meningitis; recurrent meningitis should stimulate a search for an occult cerebrospinal fluid leak.

KEY SIGN
Nasal Discharge: Acute Suppurative Sinusitis: See page 325.

KEY SIGN
Nasal Discharge: Chronic Suppurative Sinusitis: See page 326.

KEY SIGN
Sinusitis and Periorbital Edema: Periorbital Abscess: See page 326.

KEY SIGN
Sinusitis and Periorbital Edema: Orbital Cellulitis: See page 326.

KEY SIGN
Sinusitis and Ocular Palsies: Cavernous Sinus Thrombosis: See page 326.

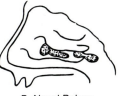

A. Cavernous Sinus Thrombosis   B. Nasal Polyps

Fig. 7-58 Lesions about the Nose. A. Cavernous Sinus Thrombosis: Early there is paralysis of a single ocular muscle, with the development of edema and proptosis (shown). B. Nasal Polyps: The parasagittal section shows the lateral wall with three polyps emerging from the middle meatus.

KEY SIGN

Intranasal Masses: Polyps: *Pathophysiology:* Nasal polyps are overgrowths of mucosa that may be either sessile or pedunculated, developing from recurrent episodes of mucosal edema. They are frequently seen in long-standing allergic rhinitis, aspirin-sensitive asthma, and cystic fibrosis. Polyps are commonly multiple, most frequently protruding from the middle meatus to present as smooth, pale, spheric masses of mucosa (Fig. 7-58B); they are mobile and insensitive to the probe, distinguishing them from swollen turbinates. Polyps may enlarge to obstruct the air passages; they frequently recur after removal.

Intranasal Masses: Mucocele and Pyocele: *Pathophysiology:* Permanent obstruction of the orifices of the frontal or ethmoid sinuses causes accumulation of mucus normally secreted by their lining membranes. A resulting sac or mucocele slowly enlarges; the pent-up mucus exerts pressure on the surrounding structures and erodes bone, thus behaving like a neoplasm. A sac from either site eventually erodes through the floor of the frontal sinus or the lateral ethmoid wall to produce a painless swelling beneath the supraorbital ridge, medial to the ocular globe (Fig. 7-59). The painless mass feels rubbery and slightly compressible. The globe is pushed downward and laterally, causing diplopia; proptosis may also occur. Upward and medial motions of the eye are restricted. Intranasal examination may be negative. Occasionally, a previous skull fracture is the cause. An infected mucocele is termed a pyocele. DDX: Swelling from the mucocele occurs above the inner canthus; dacryocystitis forms a swelling below the canthus.

KEY SIGN

Intranasal Masses: Neoplasm: Benign *papillomas* are often found in the vestibule. Slow-growing, benign neoplasms of the sinuses are usually *osteomas* or *chondromas*. They grow slowly and cause

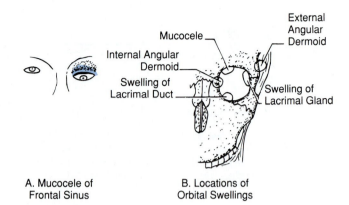

Fig. 7-59 Some Masses About the Orbit. *A. Mucocele of Frontal Sinus. An example of a mucocele, this occurring in the floor of the supraorbital ridge and presenting medially.* **B. Locations of Masses About the Eye.**

no symptoms until air passages or a sinus orifice is obstructed. X-ray films or CT scans of the skull frequently lead to the diagnosis. Sinus *carcinomas* cause obstruction, blood-stained discharge, and constant, boring pain. They invade bone: in the orbit, they may cause ocular disturbances; in the maxillary antral floor, upper teeth may become loose, a denture may no longer fit properly, or bulging and softness of the hard palate is seen.

D KEY DISEASE

► **Nasal Necrosis Without Systemic Disease: Midline Granuloma:** *Pathophysiology:* The cause is unknown, but some classify it as one of the angiocentric immunoproliferative lesions. The inflammation is attended by granuloma formation. It is most common in fifth and sixth decades, with a slight preference for women. Symptoms include sneezing, nasal stiffness, obstruction, and pain. Signs are rhinorrhea, nasal congestion, and paranasal sinusitis progressing to inflammation and ulcerations of the nasal septum, palate, and nasal ali. Advanced disease is indicated by destruction of midfacial structures including pharynx, mouth, sinuses, and eyes with death from cachexia, pneumonia, meningitis, or hemorrhage. Indolent ulceration and mutilation suggest the diagnosis. DDX: Unlike Wegener granulomatosis, here there is no systemic involvement or primary vasculitis.

D KEY DISEASE

► **Chronic Nasal Erosion with Systemic Disease: Wegener's Granulomatosis:** This is one of the segmental necrotizing vasculitides (see Chapter 8, page 422).

Breath Signs

KEY SIGN

Odor of the Breath: Detection of breath odors is a quick and important diagnostic procedure. There is great individual variation in olfactory acuteness. Description of odors is meaningless; the examiner must first smell the properly identified substance before it can be recognized. A foul breath odor, *fetor oris,* is common in dental or tonsillar infections, atrophic rhinitis, putrefaction of food in the stomach from pyloric obstruction, and infected sputum in bronchiectasis or lung abscess. *Acetone* can be detected on the breath, even when absent from the urine by chemical tests; it indicates ketonemia in diabetic or starvation acidosis. In some patients with uremia, *ammonia* is detected on the breath. A curious *musty odor* occasionally is smelled in patients with severe liver disease. *Hydrocyanic acid* is said to impart the odor of bitter almond to the breath following cyanide ingestion. When a person has inhaled or swallowed *volatile hydrocarbons,* the odor is detectable in the exhaled air (natural gas is odorless). *Alcohol* on the breath indicates that the person has been imbibing, but medical illness, trauma, or the ingestion of other drugs must be excluded in explaining the patient's symptoms and signs. A few patients in coma have no alcohol odor on the breath while the aspirated gastric contents smell strongly of alcohol. The breath of the chronic alcoholic may reek of *acetaldehyde* instead of alcohol. The odor of *paraldehyde* should be recognized. When *garlic* is eaten, the methyl mercaptan causing its odor is excreted in the lungs for more than 24 hours. The odor of *chloroform* on the breath can result from its use as an anesthetic or from poisoning with methylchloroform, used in industry as a substitute for carbon tetrachloride.

Lip Signs

Labial Deformity: Cleft Lip: *Pathophysiology:*   In the embryo, incomplete fusion of the frontonasal process with the two maxillary processes leaves a persistent cleft in one or both sides of the upper lip. This is incorrectly termed harelip, because the rabbit has a midline cleft. Cleft lip is sometimes accompanied by cleft palate.

Labial Enlargement: The lips may appear large in cretinism, myxedema, acromegaly, and collagen injections.

KEY SIGN

Labial Vesicles: Herpes Simplex (Cold Sores, Fever Blisters):   *Pathophysiology:*   Latent herpes simplex virus is reactivated producing local inflammation when the carrier develops another infectious disease, has local trauma, or is exposed to sunlight. Groups of vesicles containing clear fluid are surrounded by areas of erythema. Frequently, they occur on the lips. The lesions may burn or smart.

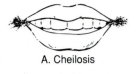
A. Cheilosis

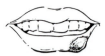
B. Epidermoid Carcinoma of Lip

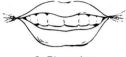
C. Rhagades

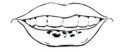
D. Labial Pigmentation of Intestinal Polyposis (Peutz-Jeghers Syndrome)

Fig. 7-60 Some Lip Lesions.   A. Cheilosis. B. Epidermoid Carcinoma of Lip: Notice the sharply demarcated elevated edges with the ulcerating base, typically located at the mucocutaneous junction. *C. Rhagades. D. Signs of Peutz-Jeghers Syndrome.*

KEY SIGN

Inflamed Labial Corners: Cheilosis (Angular Stomatitis):   Maculopapular and vesicular lesions are grouped at the corners of the mouth, on the skin, and at the mucocutaneous junction (Fig. 7-60A). Ulceration of the skin leads to crusting and fissuring. Often accompanying profuse salivation from any cause, it is specifically associated with riboflavin deficiency or ill-fitting dentures. Secondary candida infection is common. The entire labial surface may be inflamed from overexposure to sunlight, *actinic cheilosis.*

KEY SIGN

Local Labial Inflammation: Carbuncle: Painful localized swelling with erythema and increased skin warmth suggests early cellulitis or carbuncle. When it occurs on the upper lip, it may be exceedingly dangerous, because the veins drain into the cavernous sinus, where thrombosis may occur.

KEY SIGN

Labial Ulcer: Squamous Cell Carcinoma: Early, the lesion is indurated and discoid; later, it becomes warty and crusted, forming a shallow ulcer that slowly extends. The ulcerated border is elevated, sometimes pearly (see Fig. 7-60B). The regional lymph nodes are usually involved late; involvement of lymph nodes is less common when the lesion is warty and nonulcerating. It is more frequent in men, and in 95% of the cases, the lesion is on the lower lip. Any ulcer more than 2 weeks old should be biopsied.

Labial Ulcer: Chancre: *Pathophysiology:*   The initial lesion of syphilis occurs at the site of inoculation and is the first sign of the disease. The lip is the most common extragenital site of the primary syphilitic lesion; usually the upper lip is involved. The lesion is discoid, without sharply defined borders. Palpation with gloved fingers reveals a plaque that can be moved over the underlying tissues. The lesion soon ulcerates to exude a clear fluid, teeming with *Treponema pallidum* when examined with darkfield microscopy. The regional lymph nodes are involved early; they feel larger and softer than those with carcinoma. Serologic tests for syphilis are frequently negative while the chancre is present.

Labial Ulcer: Molluscum Contagiosum: A nodular growth in the lip may ulcerate to discharge caseous material. The ulcer border may be elevated. The lesion is caused by *Molluscipoxvirus*. The resemblance to carcinoma may be striking, so biopsy may be required.

Labial Scarring: Rhagades: These white radial scars about the angles of the mouth are stigmata of previous syphilitic lesions (see Fig. 7-60C).

KEY SIGN
Labial Scaling Lesion: Actinic Keratosis: A dry, flat, light-colored lesion occurs on the lip and produces scaling. It bleeds easily when traumatized. It is a precancerous growth.

KEY SIGN
Labial Pigmentation: Intestinal Polyposis (Peutz-Jeghers Syndrome): Multiple pigmented brown to black spots on the lips may resemble freckles, but they are suspect on the mucosa, where freckles are uncommon (see Fig. 7-60D). The lesions strongly suggest an autosomal dominant syndrome associated with intestinal polyposis. Their presence may furnish the clue for the cause of gastrointestinal hemorrhage.

Oral Mucosa and Palate Signs

KEY SIGN
Lack of Saliva: Xerostomia, Sjögren Syndrome: See page 318.

KEY SIGN
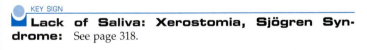
Buccal Pigmentation: Addison Disease (Chronic Adrenal Cortical Insufficiency): *Pathophysiology:* Cortisol deficiency leads to stimulation of proopiomelanocortin synthesis and adrenocorticotropic hormone (ACTH) release from the pituitary with secondary increase in melanocyte-stimulating hormone (MSH). Small patches of pigment in the buccal mucosa are common in blacks and other darkly pigmented races. In whites, however, dappled brown pigment in the lining of the cheek strongly suggests Addison disease or the intestinal polyposis of Peutz-Jeghers.

Buccal Mass: Retention Cyst: A mucous gland anywhere in the buccal surface may be obstructed to produce a blue-domed translucent cyst.

Buccal White Spots: Mucosal Sebaceous Cysts (Fordyce Spots): These appear in the mucosa of the lips, cheeks, and tongue as isolated white or yellow spots less than 1 mm in diameter and sometimes slightly raised. They are painless and harmless. Often a bit of white sebum may be expressed from the lesion.

KEY SIGN

Buccal White Spots: Koplik Spots in Measles: They are the earliest diagnostic sign of the measles. One or 2 days before the appearance of the exanthem (rubeola, morbilli), small white spots appear opposite the molars and sometimes elsewhere on the buccal mucosa (Fig. 7-61B). Each is surrounded by a narrow red areola. They are pathognomonic of measles.

KEY SIGN

Oral White Patches: Lichen Planus: The lesions are thin, bluish-white, spiderweb lines that can resemble leukoplakia. Circumscribed areas of flattened papules on the flexor surfaces of the wrists and the middle of the shins strengthen the diagnosis of lichen planus.

KEY SIGN

Oral White Patches: Leukoplakia: *Pathophysiology:* This often occurs at the site of chronic irritation from ill-fitting dentures or smokeless tobacco; it is precancerous. Tobacco and alcohol use are cocarcinogens. The first lesion is a whitened hyperkeratotic plaque. On the tongue, one or more areas on the dorsal surface are af-

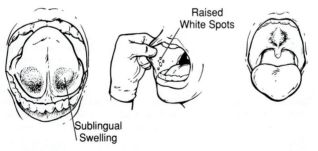

Raised
White Spots

Sublingual
Swelling

A. Sublingual   B. Koplik Spots   C. Torus Palatinus
Dermoid Cyst

Fig. 7-61 Some Lesions of the Oral Cavity.   *A. Sublingual Dermoid Cyst.*
B. Koplik Spots. C. Torus Palatinus.

fected by obliteration of the papillae with thin white lesions that are wrinkled and sometimes pearly. Early lesions coalesce; as they persist and enlarge, they become chalk-white and thick and are palpable as a more firm nodule than the compliant adjacent mucosa. Biopsy is indicated to ascertain if invasion has occurred.

KEY SIGN

Oral White Patches: Thrush, Candidiasis:
Pathophysiology: Infection of the oral mucosa with *Candida* spp. occurs in patients who are immunosuppressed or have received broad spectrum antibiotics. The lesions may be painless or the patient complains of mouth soreness. Exam reveals white plaques that are easily removed with a tongue blade. Less commonly, the oral mucosa appears erythematous and thinned, without the white plaques. Pain with swallowing suggests concomitant *Candida* esophagitis.

KEY SIGN

Buccal Red Spots: Osler-Weber-Rendu Disease:
The fine blood vessels of hereditary hemorrhagic telangiectasia blanch on pressure and are seen in the buccal mucosa, palate, uvula, tongue, lips, and skin of the trunk.

KEY SIGN

Oral Vesicles and Blisters: Herpes Simplex:
Primary infection with herpes simplex often causes severe stomatitis with painful vesicles that rupture to form shallow ulcers which heal slowly.

KEY SIGN

Oral Vesicles and Blisters: Cicatricial Pemphigoid:
Pathophysiology: Autoantibodies directed against the hemidesmosomes in the basal layer of the mucosa and skin lead to separation of the mucosal layers with blister formation. Pain is mild to moderate. The incidence increases with age; oral lesions may be accompanied by skin lesions. The course is chronic and recurrent.

KEY SIGN

Oral Vesicles and Blisters: Stevens-Johnson Syndrome:
Pathophysiology: This is a severe allergic reaction with generalized involvement of the skin and mucous membranes. The most common cause is medication exposure. Early recognition, withdrawal of the offending agent, and supportive therapy may be life saving.

KEY SIGN

Oral Ulcer: Aphthous Ulcer (Canker Sore):
A few small vesicles appear in crops on the tip and sides of the tongue and on the labial and buccal mucosa. When seen, the original vesicle has ruptured, so the lesion appears as a painful, small, round ulcer with white floor and yellow margins surrounded by a narrow erythematous

areola. The cause is unknown. Recurrent or persistent aphthous ulcers are seen in Crohn disease and Behçet syndrome.

KEY SIGN
Oral Ulcer: Mucous Patches (Condyloma Latum): *Pathophysiology:* This is the common lesion of secondary syphilis, occurring on the tongue and the buccal and labial mucosa regardless of the site of the primary lesion. The patches are round or oval, 5–10 mm in diameter, slightly raised, and covered by gray membrane. They may ulcerate slightly. Palpated with gloved fingers, they feel indurated and are painless. Regional lymphadenopathy occurs.

KEY SIGN
Chronic Oral Ulcerations: Cancer Chemotherapy: *Pathophysiology:* The bone marrow, and oral and intestinal mucosa are the most rapidly proliferating tissues in the body. Cytotoxic chemotherapy transiently stops proliferation and leads to impaired mucosal repair. Mouth ulcers commonly occur with cytotoxic chemotherapy, usually 5–10 days after treatment with intermittent bolus therapy. They can occur anytime in the course of chronic daily oral therapy with alkylating agents or antimetabolites.

KEY SIGN
Chronic Oral Ulcerations: Behçet's Syndrome: See page 473.

Chronic Oral Ulceration: Disseminated Histoplasmosis: A persistent oral ulcer can be the presenting sign of disseminated histoplasmosis. Diagnosis is made by biopsy.

Reddened Parotid Duct Orifice: Mumps: The parotid (Stensen) duct orifice, opposite the upper second molar, may become reddened in mumps or other acute parotitis.

KEY SIGN
Bony Palatine Protuberance: Torus: *Pathophysiology:* It is a developmental abnormality. A common anatomic variation, a bony knob or ridge occurs in the midline of the hard palate (see Fig. 7-61C). It is harmless.

KEY SIGN
Palantine Mass Carcinoma: The epithelium of the hard and soft palates can be the site of carcinoma. Do not confuse it with torus.

Palatine Mass: Mixed Tumor of Ectopic Salivary Gland: This occurs in the soft or hard palate. Unless noticed accidentally, it is silent until ulceration causes pain. It may invade the base of the skull.

Arched Palate: There are many causes for high-arched palate. Because of its association with Marfan and Turner syndromes, look for the other manifestations of these disorders.

Cleft Palate: *Pathophysiology:*   A midline opening in the hard palate is a congenital failure of fusion of the maxillary processes. It is usually associated with cleft lip but also occurs in isolation. Its severity varies from a complete cleft of the entire soft and hard palate, including the alveolar ridge, to a partial cleft of the soft palate alone. A submucous cleft in which only the underlying muscle is deficient is suggested by a bifid uvula.

Palatine Perforation: Tertiary syphilis is a common cause of a hole in the hard palate, but the deformity can result from radiation therapy or from postoperative breakdown after surgical repair of cleft palate.

Teeth and Gum Signs

Absent Teeth: Loss or Developmental Failure:
The absence of teeth should be noted in the record. An insufficient number may seriously impair nutrition.

Absent Tooth with Swelling: Odontoma: Failure of eruption of a tooth may be caused by a tumor arising from an odontogenic origin, producing an unexplained swelling.

Beveled Teeth: Worn Teeth: The biting surfaces may be worn down in patients with bruxism or by continuous chewing on hard substances, such as a pipe stem.

KEY SIGN
Widened Interdental Spaces: These may occur congenitally or they may be acquired when the jaw enlarges in a person developing acromegaly.

KEY SIGN
Eroded Teeth: Caries: Unusual sensitivity to hot or cold liquids may bring the patient to the dentist or physician. Usually the presence of cavities in the teeth is obvious. Occasionally, a mirror is required to see them.

KEY SIGN

Eroded Teeth: Loss of Enamel: Demineralized teeth from erosion by acidic stomach contents are seen in patients who have chronic emesis with bulimia nervosa and in swimmers who are exposed to pools with excessive chlorination.

KEY SIGN

Darkened Tooth: Devitalized Tooth (Dead Tooth): When the pulp of the tooth is no longer viable, the enamel appears less white than its companions. The tooth becomes insensitive to cold, which is tested by the application of ice.

KEY SIGN

Pigmented Teeth: Fluoride Pits: Opaque chalk-white spots, 1–2 mm in diameter, are seen scattered on the surface of multiple teeth. This is a harmless condition found in persons who have ingested large amounts of fluoride in the water during childhood.

KEY SIGN

Notched Teeth: Hutchinson Teeth: *Pathophysiology:* Notched teeth result from congenital syphilis interfering with the development of the permanent teeth. The permanent upper central incisors are misshapen (Fig. 7-62A). They are peg-topped, resembling the frustum of a cone, and smaller than normal; their tips are notched. Notching is one component of the *Hutchinson triad,* together with interstitial keratitis and labyrinthine deafness.

KEY SIGN

Bleeding Gums: *Pathophysiology:* Bleeding results from local lesions in the gums or from generalized disorders of the blood vessels or hemostasis. The patient may complain of brushing accompanied by bleeding, or may notice blood in expectorated phlegm. Other signs a systemic vascular or hemostatic process should prompt direct questioning about bleeding from the gums because many patients do not consider this abnormal.

✔ *BLEEDING GUMS—CLINICAL OCCURRENCE:* *Local Causes: Infectious* pyorrhea alveolaris, actinomycosis, stomatitis (aphthous, ulcerative, Vincent stomatitis), tuberculous gingivitis; *Traumatic* tooth brushing, lacerations, dental caries, tartar on the teeth; *Neoplastic* papilloma of gums, epulis, myeloma, epithelioma. *Systemic Causes: Infectious* syphilis; *Inflammatory/Immune* erythema herpetiformis, pemphigus, immune deficiency states; *Metabolic/Toxic* scurvy, metal poisoning (phosphorus, lead, arsenic, mercury); *Neoplastic* leukemia, Hodgkin disease; *Vascular and Blood Dyscrasia* thrombocytopenia, aplastic anemia, hemophilia, Christmas disease.

KEY SIGN

Tender Teeth: Periapical Abscess (Gum Boil): *Pathophysiology:* An abscess forms at the tip of the root

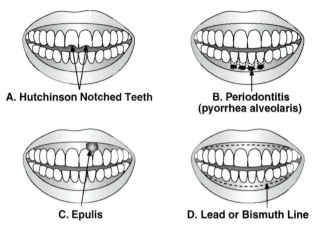

Fig. 7-62 Dental Abnormalities. A. Hutchinson Notched Teeth. B. Periodontitis: In the drawing, some of the lower teeth are involved: the gums are retracted and pus is exuding from behind the gingival margins. C. Epulis: It is sessile, lighter in color than the gums. D. Lead or Bismuth Line in the Gums.

within the bone. The inflammation produces a very painful increase in intraosseous pressure. An abscess in an alveolus is suspected when toothache pain is accentuated by tapping the tooth with a tongue blade or probe. Tender swelling occurs in the adjacent gum; a sinus tract may form to drain the pus.

KEY SIGN

Retracted Gums: Gum Recession: In older persons, the gingival margins may recede to expose the rough, lusterless cementum, proximal to the enamel border.

KEY SIGN

Purulent Gums: Periodontitis (Pyorrhea Alveolaris): *Pathophysiology:* Inflammatory pockets form between the teeth and gums destroying the dental ligament leading to recession; they may become infected and exude pus (see Fig. 7-62B). The gingival borders are reddened; pressing the gums against the teeth may express the pus. Anaerobic organisms predominate.

KEY SIGN

Inflamed Gums: Necrotizing Ulcerative Stomatitis (Trench Mouth, Vincent Stomatitis): *Pathophysiology:* Inflammation of the gums and adjoining mucosa is attributed to a symbiotic infection with *Borrelia vincentii* and *Fusobacterium plauti-vincenti*. The infection may remain localized in the gums or it may extend to involve all pharyngeal structures, including bone. On the gum mucosa, it produces punched-out ulcers covered with gray-yellow membrane that sometimes must be distinguished from diphtheria.

KEY SIGN
Swollen Gums: Scurvy (Scorbutus):   The gums are deep red or purple; they become swollen, tender, and spongy. They bleed easily as part of the general bleeding tendency, along with subperiosteal hemorrhages and purpura.

KEY SIGN
Swollen Gums: Gingival Hyperplasia: The volume of the gums increases. When severe they may cover the teeth. Several drugs occasionally induce the condition, notably phenytoin. A similar appearance is seen in monocytic leukemia, from infiltration with monocytes.

KEY SIGN
Mass in Gums: Epulis: *Pathophysiology:*   A fibrous tumor of the gum, it arises from the alveolar periosteum and emerges between the teeth as a nodular mass. It appears as a nontender sessile mass (see Fig. 7-63C), lighter in color than the gum; rarely, it is pedunculated. A similar tumor, but bright red, is a *fibroangiomatous epulis.*

Mass in Gums: Granuloma: A granuloma may occur in the gums spontaneously, or it may result from an ill-fitting denture. It is firm, pink, and nontender; it may break down to form an ulcer.

Blue Gums: Lead and Bismuth Lines: *Pathophysiology:*   With chronic exposure to lead (occupational) or bismuth (therapeutic), the heavy metals may be deposited in the gums, forming a blue line about 1 mm from the gingival margin. The metallic deposit appears as a solid line to the unaided eye (see Fig. 7-62D). Inserting a corner of white paper behind the gingival border aids in seeing the line. Viewing through a magnifying lens shows the line to be composed of small, discrete dots. Because the lead sulfide is formed only in the presence of bacterial infection, the deposit does not occur when the teeth are absent. Chronic quinacrine ingestion colors the gums diffusely blue or purple.

Tongue Signs

Dry Tongue Without Longitudinal Furrows: The lingual surface may be dry from mouth breathing or lack of saliva (*xerostomia*) in Sjögren syndrome and irradiation. The volume of the tongue remains normal, so no longitudinal furrows develop.

KEY SIGN
Dry Tongue with Longitudinal Furrows:
Pathophysiology: Longitudinal furrows develop in the lingual surface

from reduction of volume of the tongue. This is a reliable physical sign of volume depletion. In adults, this occurs regularly with a 3 L deficit of extracellular fluid. This degree of volume depletion is always accompanied by loss of skin turgor, but the latter also occurs in senile cutaneous atrophy or recent loss of body tissue.

KEY SIGN
Lingual Enlargement: The tongue is enlarged in Down syndrome, cretinism, and adult myxedema. It increases in size during the development of acromegaly and amyloidosis. Transient swelling occurs with glossitis, stomatitis, and cellulitis of the neck. Occlusions of the lymphatics by carcinoma and obstruction of the superior vena cava often produce enlargement. Transiently, it may be the site of angioedema or abscess. Hematoma results from trauma; look for bite marks on the lateral aspects of the tongue.

Lingual Tremor: *Pathophysiology:* Increased sympathetic activity is associated with fine tremor. A fine tremor of the tongue is often present in hyperthyroidism. A coarser tremor is frequently seen in anxious persons; it also occurs in alcoholism, paresis, and drug withdrawal, or it may accompany any debilitating disease.

KEY SIGN
Lingual Fasciculation: *Pathophysiology:* Denervation leads to spontaneous firing of motor units. It is a sign of denervation in bulbar poliomyelitis or amyotrophic lateral sclerosis.

KEY SIGN
Limited Lingual Protrusion: Shortened Frenulum (Tongue-Tied): *Pathophysiology:* The frenulum is congenitally short. This limits protrusion and prevents the patient from placing the tip of the tongue in the roof of the mouth, impairing articulation of lingual consonants.

KEY SIGN
Limited Lingual Protrusion: Carcinoma: *Pathophysiology:* Infiltration of the lingual muscles with neoplasm may limit protrusion of the tongue. Inspection usually reveals an ulcerated, whitish lesion that is hard on palpation compared with the surrounding muscle. A firm, nontender nodule in the base of the tongue may not be visually impressive, but it can represent squamous carcinoma. Palpation of the tongue discloses the buried neoplasm.

KEY SIGN
Lingual Deviation: Unilateral Carcinoma: A unilateral neoplasm may hinder muscles action on that side; the deviation is toward the side of the lesion. Palpation discloses the mass.

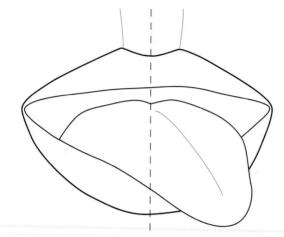

Fig. 7-63 Paralysis of the Left Side of the Tongue. *Deviation is toward the paralyzed side.*

Lingual Deviation: Paralysis of the Hypoglossal Nerve (CN XII): *Pathophysiology:* The tongue protrudes by tensing the two lateral muscle bundles; paralysis of one bundle causes the tongue to deviate to the paralyzed side (Fig. 7-63). With longstanding lesions, the two halves of the tongue are of unequal size because of muscle atrophy. Absence of a palpable mass excludes infiltration with carcinoma.

Lingual Fissures: Congenital Furrows (Scrotal Tongue): The median sulcus is deepened, the dorsal surface is interrupted by deep *transverse* furrows that are not inflamed (Fig. 7-64A). This is a harmless condition, frequently inherited. It must be distinguished from the longitudinal furrowing in syphilitic glossitis.

Lingual Fissures: Syphilitic and Herpetic Glossitis: The furrows of syphilitic glossitis are mainly *longitudinal* and deeper than the congenital type. The intervening epithelium is desquamated (see Fig. 7-64D). A similar lesion with painful inflamed tongue and longitudinal fissures has been described with herpes infection in HIV-infected patients [Grossman ME, Stevens AW, Cohen PR. Herpetic geometric glossitis. *N Engl J Med* 1993;329:1859–1860].

Lingual Coat: Geographic Tongue (Migratory Glossitis, Glossitis Areata Exfoliativa): *Patho-*

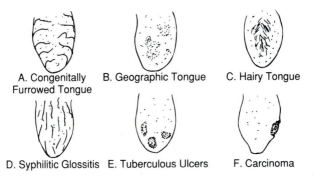

A. Congenitally Furrowed Tongue   B. Geographic Tongue   C. Hairy Tongue

D. Syphilitic Glossitis   E. Tuberculous Ulcers   F. Carcinoma

Fig. 7-64 Tongue Surface Patterns. **A. Congenitally Furrowed Tongue. B. Geographic Tongue. C. Black Hairy Tongue. D. Syphilitic Glossitis. E. Tuberculous Ulcers. F. Carcinoma:** *A typical location of carcinoma of the tongue is on the lateral edge.*

physiology: The normal lingual coating is interrupted by circular areas of smooth red epithelium without papillae, surrounded by rings of light-yellow piled-up cells (see Fig. 7-64B). The patches heal in a few days and are succeeded by new ones in other areas. This is a harmless condition of unknown cause [Assimakopoulos D, Patrikakos G, Foytika C, Elisaf M. Benign migratory glossitis or geographic tongue: An enigmatic oral lesion. *Am J Med* 2002;113:751–755].

KEY SIGN

Lingual Coat: Hairy Tongue (Furry Tongue, Black Tongue): *Pathophysiology:* The appearance is imparted by hyperplasia of the filiform papillae entangled with an overgrowth of mycelial threads of *Aspergillus niger* or *Candida albicans*. The distal two-thirds of the dorsum looks as if it were growing short hairs, usually black (see Fig. 7-64C). The condition is symptomless. Occasionally the color is green, either from the fungus or because the patient is chewing gum containing chlorophyll. Formerly, the finding was restricted to debilitated patients; now it often appears during treatment with antibiotics that inhibit the growth of normal bacteria and permit overgrowth of fungi.

KEY SIGN

Lingual Coat: Hairy Leukoplakia: *Pathophysiology:* Epithelial hyperplasia results from Epstein-Barr virus infection in patients with HIV infection. The sides of the tongue have elongated "hairy" filiform papillae.

KEY SIGN

Smooth Tongue: Atrophic Glossitis: *Pathophysiology:* Nutritional deficiency results in impaired mucosal proliferation. The patient may complain of dryness of the tongue, intermittent burning, and paresthesias of taste. The tongue becomes smaller, its surface slick and glistening, and the mucosa thinned. The color may be pink or red, depending on the hemoglobin concentration in the blood and the amount of local inflammation. In the advanced stages, there is considerable pain and swelling. The color is red or blue-red with atrophied hyperemic papillae that appear as small punctate red dots.

✔ ATROPHIC GLOSSITIS—CLINICAL OCCURRENCE: *Deficiency of Vitamin B_{12}* pernicious anemia, postgastrectomy syndrome, blind intestinal loop, extreme vegetarian diets, infestation with fish tapeworm (*Diphyllobothrium latum*); *Folic Acid Deficiency* megaloblastic anemia of pregnancy, chronic liver disease; *Other Causes* iron deficiency anemia, idiopathic gastritis, mixed B-complex deficiency, unknown causes.

KEY SIGN
Red Tongue: Pellagra: *Pathophysiology:* Deficiency of niacin (nicotinic acid and nicotinamide) results from nutritional deficiency. In the early stages, the patient complains of burning tongue when in contact with hot or spicy foods, but no signs are visible. Later, the burning is constant; diarrhea, delirium, and dermatitis may appear (the three Ds). The tongue becomes reddened at the tip and borders; later the erythema spreads and the tongue swells. The surface is denuded to present a fiery-red mucosa with ulcerations and indentations from the teeth. During remission, the lingual surface is pallid and atrophied.

KEY SIGN
Red Tongue: Nonspecific Glossitis: Localized infections of the pharynx may also involve the tongue, producing redness and swelling. The tongue may burn and feel tender.

KEY SIGN
Red Tongue: Strawberry Tongue (Raspberry Tongue): *Pathophysiology:* In streptococcal or staphylococcal infection with release of exotoxins (e.g., scarlet fever, toxic shock syndrome), the lingual papillae become swollen and reddened. According to Osler, the name strawberry tongue was given to the stage in which the inflamed and hyperplastic papillae show through the white coat. Later, the epithelium desquamates, carrying away the coat and leaving a fiery-red, denuded surface surmounted by hyperplastic papillae; this has also been termed a strawberry tongue, but others prefer the more accurately descriptive term raspberry tongue. During the desquamated period, the sense of taste is diminished.

Magenta Cobblestone Tongue: Riboflavin Deficiency: *Pathophysiology:* Riboflavin deficiency is a result of dietary insufficiency. Burning of the tongue is relatively mild; more discomfort is caused by the lesions of the lips and eyes. Swollen hyperemic fungiform and filiform papillae produce rows of reddened elevations that suggest the name cobblestone tongue. Edema at the bases of the papillae modifies the color to magenta, in contrast to the fiery red of the pellagrous tongue, in which the epithelium is denuded. Cheilosis and angular stomatitis are common, beginning as a painless gray papule at one or both corners of the mouth. The papule enlarges and ulcerates to produce indolent fissures with piled-up yellow crusts, leaving permanent scars. Similar lesions may occur at the ocular canthi and the nasolabial folds; the sebaceous glands in the nose become hyperplastic. Superficial keratitis and conjunctival injection are common.

Smooth, Burning Tongue: Menopausal Glossitis: *Pathophysiology:* This is ascribed to estrogen deficiency. Intense burning of the tongue and slight atrophy of the lingual mucosa often occur at menopause or in other states of estrogen deficiency. The symptoms and signs are improved when estrogens are administered.

KEY SIGN
White Lingual Patches: Leukoplakia: See *Buccal Leukoplakia*, page 290, and Fig. 7-65A. In the early stages, the areas are thin and white, often wrinkled or pearly; they obliterate the papillae. Later, the lesions coalesce, thicken, and become chalk white. In advanced stages, they look like dried, cracked white paint.

KEY SIGN
Lingual Ulcer: Chancre: A syphilitic primary lesion on the tongue is rare; it usually occurs on the tip. Starting as a small pustule, the top soon ruptures to form an ulcer. When examined with the gloved finger, its base is indurated, feeling like a small button embedded in tissue. In contrast to the aphthous ulcer, it is not very painful. Painless enlargement of the regional lymph nodes develops quickly; the submental or submaxillary nodes are usually involved.

KEY SIGN
Lingual Ulcer: Gumma: The lesion occurs in the anterior two-thirds of the tongue in the dorsal midline, whereas carcinoma is usually on the side, base, or ventral surface. Beginning as a painless nodule the mass goes on to ulcerate forming a punched-out area with

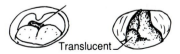

A. Lingual Leukoplakia   B. Lingual Thyroid   C. Ranula

Fig. 7-65 Tongue Lesions. *A. Lingual leukoplakia. B. Lingual thyroid. C. Ranula.*

little induration. Carcinoma forms an indurated ulcer with rolled-up margins.

Lingual Ulcer: Dental Ulcer: *Pathophysiology:* The ulcer results from irritation of a projecting tooth or an ill-fitting denture. These are always on the sides or undersurface of the tongue. Frequently, the ulcer is elongated, its base is sloughing, and its borders erythematous. The ulcer margin may be elevated and surrounded by induration, suggesting carcinoma. Removal of the irritating surface should result in a trend toward healing in a few weeks. Lacking improvement, biopsy is indicated.

Lingual Ulcer: Granuloma: One or more indolent nodules occur on the tip of the tongue or on its anterior sides (see Fig. 7-64E) without much surrounding inflammation. A rare lingual lesion, it is nearly always associated with pulmonary tuberculosis or histoplasmosis. Characteristically, tuberculous lesions are extremely painful. Later, the nodules ulcerate, forming bases with gray membranes; the margins may overhang slightly.

Lingual Ulcer: Carcinoma: The sites of predilection for carcinoma are the sides, base, and undersurface of the tongue (see Fig. 7-64F). Inquire about tobacco and alcohol abuse. The disease usually appears as an ulcer with rolled and everted margins. Palpation of the region discloses a discrete firm mass with some surrounding induration. It is not tender unless ulcerated. Inspection and palpation are the keys for establishing the diagnosis, although pain from the ulcer while drinking acidic or alcoholic beverages should arouse suspicion. If no lesions are visible, yet the patient complains of lingual discomfort or dysphagia, or if the tongue does not readily protrude, palpate the root of the tongue. Also feel the submental, submandibular, and deep cervical lymph nodes.

Posterior Lingual Mass: Lingual Thyroid: *Pathophysiology:* Aberrant thyroid tissue can occur anywhere in the course of the thyroglossal duct; a mass near the foramen cecum may be lingual thyroid. A round, smooth, red, nontender mass at the base of the tongue, near the foramen cecum, may be a lingual thyroid arising from the remnants of the thyroglossal duct (see Fig. 7-65B); it does not ulcerate. It may be the only site of functioning thyroid tissue, consider the possibility before attempting biopsy.

Sublingual Varices: Caviar Lesions: The superficial sublingual veins may develop varicosities with aging. Frequently, they resemble a mass of purple caviar under the tongue (see Fig. 6-14A). They are of no clinical significance.

Sublingual Mass: Dermoid Cyst: This is an opaque fluctuant cyst; when superficial, it may appear white. It may occur behind the frenulum or beside it (see Fig. 7-61A). Bimanual palpation allows assessment of size and demonstrates fluctuation.

KEY SIGN

▶ **Sublingual Mass: Carcinoma:** Because it is more sensitive to food and beverages, the patient often notices a carcinoma in the floor of the mouth. Ulceration produces pain and tongue motion may also cause discomfort. Secondary infection is common. It may begin as a leukoplakic area. Ulceration and a palpably discrete mass suggest carcinoma. Fixation to the mandible and metastases to submental or anterior jugular lymph nodes occur early.

Pharyngeal Signs

KEY SIGN

Tonsillar Enlargement: Hyperplasia: The normal adult tonsils seldom protrude beyond the faucial pillars; the tonsils are larger in children, shrinking at puberty. For adequate examination, take a tongue blade in each hand; depress the tongue with one and retract the anterior faucial pillar laterally with the other to disclose the anterior tonsillar surface. Normally, the color of the tonsil matches the surrounding mucosa; its surface is interrupted with deep clefts or crypts; these may contain white or yellow debris which is not a sign of infection. Hyperplasia is usually attributed to chronic infection, but it may be associated with obesity, hyperthyroidism, or lymphoma. Hyperplasia is usually bilateral.

KEY SIGN

▶ **Tonsillar Ulcer: Carcinoma:** The patient may complain of earache from referred pain. The breath is foul with a bleeding ulceration. Palpation of the tonsil discloses characteristic induration.

KEY SIGN

▶ **Tonsillar Swelling: Peritonsillar Abscess (Quinsy):** *Pathophysiology:* Pyogenic infection of the tonsil spreads into the peritonsillar and pharyngeal spaces. Usually the abscess occurs between the palatine tonsil and the anterior faucial pillar, so the swelling pushes the tonsil medially, displacing the uvula to the opposite side. Much edema surrounds the swelling. The affected side of the pharynx is very painful. Opening the mouth is always limited and may be difficult because of muscle spasm, or trismus. When the abscess is anterior, between the tonsil and the anterior faucial pillar, the anterior bulging is easily seen; the swelling also displaces the uvula to the opposite side (Fig. 7-66A). The adjacent soft palate is edematous and bulging. When the abscess is posterior to the tonsil, earache accompanies the sore throat and the tonsil is pushed forward; much of the swelling is hidden from direct vision. Surgical drainage is necessary.

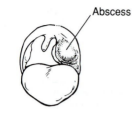
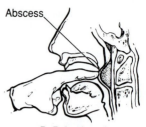

A. Peritonsillar Abscess
(quinsy)

B. Palpation of a
Retropharyngeal Abscess

Fig. 7-66 Lesions of the Oral Cavity. A. Peritonsillar Abscess (Quinsy). B. Palpation of a Retropharyngeal Abscess: The sagittal section shows the relation of the abscess to the palpating finger. The gloved finger feels a boggy indentable mass as it presses gently against the anterior surfaces of the vertebral bodies.

KEY SIGN

Posttonsillar Swelling: Retropharyngeal Abscess: *Pathophysiology:* An accumulation of pus occurs in the space between the pharynx and the prevertebral fascia. If the swelling is in the oropharynx, it may be seen directly through the mouth, with the tongue depressed, as an anterior swelling of the posterior pharyngeal wall. In the nasopharynx, or opposite the larynx, it is never directly visible. This should be suspected when nose breathing is impaired (often attributed to adenoids) or with laryngeal respiratory distress or swallowing difficulty. The abscess is demonstrated by gentle palpation (see Fig. 7-66B), which discloses a unilateral swelling that is soft and indentable. It usually occurs in children younger than 5 years old. Urgent surgical drainage is necessary to avoid airway obstruction by the expanding mass.

KEY SIGN

Edema of the Uvula: *Pathophysiology:* Inhalation of hot gases through the mouth causes a thermal burn to the soft palate and uvula. Localized edema of the uvula may result from allergic or nonallergic angioedema; it has occurred with thrombosis of an internal jugular vein containing a central venous line. Edema of the uvula together with bronchitis, asthma, and rhinopharyngitis, suggests inhalational injury, often from recreational drug use (e.g., recent heavy smoking of marijuana, crack cocaine, hashish).

Larynx and Trachea Signs

KEY SIGN

Hoarseness: *Pathophysiology:* Paralysis of a cord, or edema, infiltration, or masses on the vocal cords, change their vibrational response to airflow. More than any other sign, hoarseness focuses attention directly on the larynx. A multitude of disorders exhibit this sign.

✓*HOARSENESS—CLINICAL OCCURRENCE:* **Recent Onset** *Overuse* shouting, cheering; *Infections* upper respiratory infections, chlamydia, diphtheria, smallpox, measles; *Drugs* atropine-like drugs (dryness), strychnine (laryngeal spasm), aspiration of aspirin (chemical burn), potassium iodide (edema of cords), uremia (edema of cords); *Angioedema* insect bites, drug allergy, angiotensin-converting enzyme inhibitors, hereditary angioedema; *Foreign Body* food aspiration, after endotracheal intubation; *Laryngeal Spasm* croup, tetany, tetanus, tabetic crisis; *Burns* inhalation of irritant gases, swallowing of hot or caustic liquids; onset of all chronic conditions. **Chronic Course** *Occupational Overuse* in the clergy, orators, singers, teachers; *Foreign Body* food aspiration, after prolonged endotracheal intubation; *Lack of Mucus* Sjögren disease (keratoconjunctivitis sicca); *Chronic Vocal Cord Inflammation* nonspecific chronic laryngitis, alcoholism, gout, tobacco smoking; *Edema of Cords* myxedema, chronic nephritis; *Surface Lesions of Cords* keratosis, pachyderma, herpes, leukoplakia, pemphigus; *Ulcers of Cords* tuberculosis, syphilis, leprosy, lupus, typhoid fever, trauma, contact ulcer; *Neoplasm of Cords* vocal nodules, sessile or pedunculated polyp, vocal process granuloma, vallecula cyst, leukoplakia, carcinoma in situ, epidermoid carcinoma, papilloma, angioma; *Innervation of Cords* compression of recurrent laryngeal nerve by aortic aneurysm, large left atrium of the heart, mediastinal neoplasm, mediastinal lymphadenopathy, retrosternal goiter, severance of nerve in thyroidectomy; *Weakness of Cord Muscles* debilitating diseases, severe anemia, myasthenia gravis, myxedema, hyperthyroidism, normal aging process; *Laryngeal Bones and Cartilages* perichondritis of cricoid or arytenoids, ankylosis of cricoarytenoid joints (rheumatoid arthritis, syphilis); *Compression of Larynx* retropharyngeal abscess, caries of cervical vertebrae, neoplasm of pharynx, large goiters, actinomycosis of neck; *Irradiation of Neck Region.*

KEY SIGN

► **Stridor:** *Pathophysiology:* Narrowing of the extrathoracic airway is worsened when the transtracheal pressure increases during inspiration as a consequence of decreased intratracheal and constant atmospheric pressures. Inhalation is accompanied by a high-pitched sound that has the same pitch and intensity throughout the entire inspiratory effort. Its presence indicates a high degree of airway obstruction. It is almost always accompanied by significant dyspnea. It is caused by mass lesions, such as carcinoma, which restrict vocal cord mobility or reduce the size of the glottic aperture, by bilateral vocal cord paralysis, which limits the effective glottic opening, or by swelling of the epiglottis with acute epiglottitis or inhalation injury.

KEY SIGN

Laryngeal Edema: The usual signs of laryngeal obstruction are present, ranging through hoarseness, dyspnea, and stridor. Inspection through the mirror is diagnostic. Glistening, swollen mucosa may be seen on the vocal cords, the arytenoid prominences, and the epiglottis (Fig. 7-67A). The membranes may not be reddened, depending on the cause.

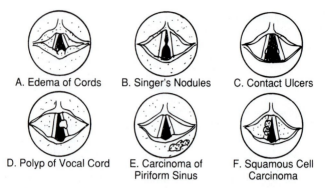

A. Edema of Cords   B. Singer's Nodules   C. Contact Ulcers

D. Polyp of Vocal Cord   E. Carcinoma of   F. Squamous Cell
                              Piriform Sinus   Carcinoma

*Fig. 7-67 Laryngeal Lesions in the Mirror. **A. Laryngeal Edema**: The mucosa on the vocal cords, arytenoid prominences, and epiglottis is swollen and glistening. **B. Singer's Nodules**: Apposing swellings on the free margins of the vocal cords at a distance one-third posteriorly in their extent. **C. Contact Ulcers** apposed on the free margins of the cords at their junctions with the arytenoid cartilages. **D. Laryngeal Polyp** on the free margin of the left cord. **E. Laryngeal Carcinoma** in the left piriform sinus. **F. Squamous Cell Carcinoma** along the anterior half of the right cord.*

✓ **LARYNGEAL EDEMA—CLINICAL OCCURRENCE:** Acute laryngitis, lymphatic obstruction by neoplasm or abscess, trauma to the larynx from instrumentation, radiation, anaphylaxis, angioedema, and myxedema.

KEY SIGN

Laryngeal Nodules: Vocal Nodules (Singer's Nodules): With voice overuse, apposing nodules may be seen on the free margins of the true cords at the junction of the anterior one-third and the posterior two-thirds (see Fig. 7-67B). Initially, the lesions may appear red; fibrosis later turns them white. Their size varies from 1 to 3 mm.

KEY SIGN

Laryngeal Contact Ulcer: *Pathophysiology:* Apposing ulcers occur on the free edges of both vocal cords at their junctions with the arytenoid cartilages. The irregular borders of the ulcers cause hoarseness (see Fig. 7-67C). They usually result from overuse trauma or instrumentation, for example, intubation. Granulation tissue may develop on one or both ulcers and become sizable enough to cause airway embarrassment.

KEY SIGN

Laryngeal Masses: Neoplasm: Tumors in the larynx may be benign or malignant, pedunculated or sessile, localized or infiltrative. Infiltrative lesions are malignant; localized masses must be biopsied for diagnosis (see Figs. 7-67E and F).

KEY SIGN

Laryngeal Leukoplakia: A superficial nonulcerative white membrane appears on one or both vocal cords. Hoarseness may occur, but pain is absent. This results from chronic irritation, such as smoking tobacco, and may proceed to carcinoma in situ and invasive epidermoid carcinoma.

KEY SIGN

Immobile Vocal Cord: Laryngeal Paralysis: *Pathophysiology:* The vocal cords are innervated by the recurrent laryngeal nerves, which are susceptible to injury in the neck and chest inferior to the larynx. In unilateral cord paralysis, the affected cord may be immobilized near the midline or slightly more laterally in the paramedian position. In the latter case, vocal cord approximation is poor and the voice is husky (Fig. 7-68A). During phonation, laryngoscopy shows the normal cord crossing the midline to meet the abducted immobile cord. In bilateral cord paralysis, the cords are usually fixed near the midline, so the voice is normal but dyspnea is extreme and inspiratory stridor with strenuous exertion is pronounced (Fig. 7-68B).

✓ *CLINICAL OCCURRENCE:* Following thyroidectomy (either or both sides), aneurysm of the aortic arch (left side), mitral stenosis with enlarged left atrium (left side), and mediastinal tumor (either or both sides).

KEY SIGN

Immobile Vocal Cord: Ankylosis of Cricoarytenoid Joint: *Pathophysiology:* Inflammatory or traumatic arthritis limits motion at the cricoarytenoid joint. Hoarseness and voice weakness are common, as in laryngeal paralysis. The mirror view shows limited or absent motion of the true cords, also resembling paralysis. Passive mobility, tested by an otolaryngologist, is absent in ankylosing, but present with paralysis. Arytenoid arthritis should be considered in any patient with rheumatoid arthritis and hoarseness. If the joints are not completely immobilized, crepitus over the larynx may

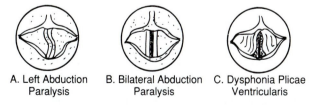

A. Left Abduction   B. Bilateral Abduction   C. Dysphonia Plicae
   Paralysis   Paralysis   Ventricularis

Fig. 7-68 Malfunctions of the Vocal Cords. **A. Left Abduction Paralysis**: *In attempting adduction, the right cord crosses the midline to meet its immobile mate.* **B. Bilateral Abduction Paralysis**: *The cords remain nearly in opposition but cannot be abducted.* **C. Dysphonia Plicae Ventricularis**: *The false cords move over the true cords, instead of remaining passive, causing the voice to break.*

be heard with the stethoscope. Traumatic arthritis may be induced by contact with an esophageal feeding tube. The condition may be so insidious that dyspnea is not recognized.

Polypoid Corditis: The entire free margins of the true cords are loose and sagging. Hoarseness results from imperfect approximation of the edematous cords. Causal factors include voice strain, irritation from alcohol and tobacco, and upper respiratory allergy or infection.

Salivary Gland Signs

KEY SIGN
Lack of Saliva: Xerostomia: Dry mouth is caused by mouth breathing, obstruction of the salivary gland ducts, irradiation, and Sjögren syndrome. An indication of Sjögren syndrome is called the *sour ball sign:* the patient sucks on sour candies to relieve oral dryness.

KEY SIGN
Salivation: Ptyalism: Ptyalism implies an excessive production of saliva, but the diagnosis is frequently extended to any condition in which saliva seems overabundant, from rapid secretion, inability to swallow, production of saliva that is more viscid (and more difficult to swallow), or failure of the lips to withhold it.

OVERPRODUCTION OF SALIVA: Drugs, intoxicants, and local inflammation stimulate salivary secretion.   *Drugs:*   mercury, copper, arsenic, antimony, iodide, bromide, potassium chlorate, pilocarpine, aconite, cantharides, carbidopa-levodopa. *Stomatitis:*   aphthous ulcers, septic ulcers, suppurative lesions, pyorrhea alveolaris, chemical burns. *Specific Oral Infections:*   variola, diphtheria, syphilis, tuberculosis. *Single Oral Lesions:*   alveolar abscess, epulis, salivary calculus. *Reflex Salivation:*   Gastric dilatation, gastric ulcer or carcinoma, acute gastritis, pancreatitis, hepatic disease.

KEY SIGN
Sublingual Mass: Ranula: *Pathophysiology:*   This is any cyst of the sublingual or submaxillary salivary gland, usually caused by obstruction of the duct. Hippocrates used the Greek word for "little frog" to describe this lesion, because it looks like a frog's belly. When the tongue is raised, a translucent mass is seen beside the frenulum linguae. The swelling may extend to the other side behind the frenulum (see Fig. 7-65C). Use bimanual palpation to identify extension of the mass to the submaxillary gland. Transillumination of the mass may show the submaxillary (Wharton) duct traversing the upper part of the cyst. It is readily distinguished by its location.

KEY SIGN
Painful Parotid Swelling: Acute Nonsuppurative Parotitis: There is brawny induration of the parotid region, with swelling in front of the tragus, back of the mandibular ra-

mus, and behind the ear, pushing it outward. The skin is warm, there is exquisite pain or tenderness and fever is common. The pain is accentuated by opening the mouth or chewing because of the proximity of the gland to the temporomandibular joint. The ductal orifice may be reddened, occasionally with a discharge of pus. One or both sides may be involved. Mumps is the usual cause; occasionally bacterial infection is responsible. Allergy to iodine can cause the same symptoms.

S KEY SYNDROME

Painful Parotid Swelling: Acute Suppurative Parotitis: *Pathophysiology:* Acute bacterial infection of the parotid gland, usually in a debilitated, immunosuppressed or postirradiated patient. The gland is swollen, tender, and painful; induration and pitting edema are often present. Local inflammation is accompanied by high fever. The ductal orifice discharges pus. Multiple abscesses may form, although fluctuation may be difficult to detect.

Painless Parotid Swelling: Chronic Suppurative Parotitis: Repeated episodes of ductal obstruction may produce chronic inflammation in the gland without fever or pain.

KEY SIGN

Painless Bilateral Parotid Swelling: The phenomenon is associated with a great diversity of conditions: its mechanism is unknown.

✔ *CLINICAL OCCURRENCE: Endocrine* diabetes mellitus, pregnancy and lactation, hyperthyroidism; *Idiopathic* bilateral fatty atrophy of the salivary glands; *Inflammatory/Immune* Sjögren syndrome, sarcoidosis, amyloidosis; *Metabolic/Toxic* malnutrition (cirrhosis, kwashiorkor, pellagra, vitamin A deficiency), poisoning (iodine, mercury, lead), drugs (e.g., thiouracil, isoproterenol, sulfisoxazole), obesity, starch ingestion; *Neoplastic* lymphocytic leukemia, lymphoma, salivary gland tumors; *Psychosocial* bulimia nervosa, stress

Neck Signs

KEY SIGN

Stiff Neck: Pain in the neck and limitation of its motion are direct attention to the muscles, bones, and joints of the neck. The disorders are too varied for a routine approach to diagnosis; the history will often give the best initial clues to the diagnosis. DDX: Be sure there are no mental status changes or signs of meningeal inflammation (see page 838) before evaluating for other causes.

✔ *STIFF NECK—CLINICAL OCCURRENCE: Congenital* torticollis; *Idiopathic* fibromyalgia, myofascial pain syndrome, stiff-man syndrome; *Inflammatory/Immune* osteomyelitis, epidural abscess, tuberculosis, prevertebral (retropharyngeal) abscess, rheumatoid arthritis, ankylosing spondylitis, polymyalgia rheumatica; *Infectious* pharyngitis, laryngitis, cervical lymphadenitis, meningitis; *Metabolic/Toxic* strychnine,

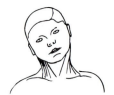

Fig. 7-69 Torticollis or Wryneck.

hypercalcemia,   tetanus;   *Mechanical/Trauma*   acquired   torticollis,
trauma to cervical vertebrae (fracture, dislocation, subluxation, disk herniation), muscles and soft tissues (e.g., whiplash), cervical spondylitis;
Neoplastic   thyroid cancer, lymphoma (Hodgkin and non-Hodgkin diseases), oropharyngeal carcinoma, metastatic carcinoma;   *Neurologic*
Parkinson disease;   *Psychosocial*   malingering, pending litigation secondary to injury.

S KEY SYNDROME

**Lateral Deviation of the Head: Torticollis
(Wryneck):** *Pathophysiology:* The congenital type is attributed
to hematoma or partial rupture of the muscle at birth resulting in unilateral muscle shortening. Dystonic reactions to phenothiazine drugs
may cause it. The head may be tipped to one side. The dystonic sternocleidomastoideus may be more prominent than the other. If tipping is
present but the muscles are not prominent, ask the patient to straighten
his head; this will cause the sternal head of one muscle to tense more
than the other (Fig. 7-69). If the torticollis is of long-standing, the face,
and even the skull, may be asymmetrical. DDX: The head tilt of torticollis must be distinguished from a head posture assumed to correct for
vertical squint or an ocular muscle palsy, *ocular torticollis.* To demonstrate the latter, slowly but firmly straighten the neck with your hands
while watching the eyes for the appearance of squint. Asymmetrical erosion of the occipital condyle from rheumatoid arthritis or neoplastic disease may result in cranial settling in a tilted position.

**Lateral Deviation of the Head: Hematoma of
the Sternocleidomastoideus:** A mass can be felt in the
belly of the muscle; it is usually a hematoma.

KEY SIGN

Stiff Neck with Dorsiflexion: Meningitis: The
neck is held stiffly in slight or extreme dorsiflexion from pain and reflex muscle spasm. Forcefully anteflexing the neck results in involuntary flexing of the hips, knees, and ankles, *Brudzinski sign,* an indication
of meningeal irritation. See Chapter 14, page 838.

KEY SIGN

**Neck Pain and Inflammation: Septic Throm-
bophlebitis of the Internal Jugular Vein
(Lemierre's Syndrome):** *Pathophysiology:* Local infec-
tion in the face or oropharynx leads to septic thrombophlebitis of the in-

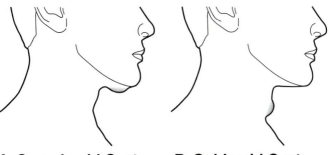

A. Suprahyoid Cyst   **B. Subhyoid Cyst**

Fig. 7-70 Thyroglossal Cysts and Sinuses.   A. Suprahyoid Cyst: This is above the hyoid bone. B. Subhyoid Cyst.

ternal jugular vein. This is a medical and surgical emergency, so early recognition is mandatory. The patient is systemically ill with fever, chills, and signs of septicemia. Septic emboli to the lungs may result in multiple pulmonary abscesses [Chirinos JA, Lichstein DM, Tamiriz LJ. The evolution of Lemierre syndrome. *Medicine (Baltimore)* 2002;81:458–465].

Nongoitrous Cervical Masses and Fistulas

After the thyroid gland has been excluded by inspection and palpation as the site of a cervical mass, consider the other neck structures.

KEY SIGN
Midline Cervical Mass: Thyroglossal Cysts and Fistulas: *Pathophysiology:* Cysts arise from midline remnants of the thyroglossal duct (see page 208–209). Normally, the thyroglossal duct becomes completely obliterated before birth; however, segments of the duct often persist and develop into cysts or even sinuses. Any of these derivatives will occur in the midline of the neck. A thyroglossal cyst may appear at any time in life. A few of the cysts are translucent. A fistula results from drainage of an inflamed cyst or the incomplete excision of a thyroglossal remnant; the sinus tract opening will be in or near the midline.

Cysts at various levels present specific challenges in diagnosis.

Suprahyoid Level (Fig. 7-70A). A thyroglossal cyst immediately above the hyoid bone must be distinguished from a sublingual dermoid cyst, which may be visible under the tongue as a white, opaque body shining through the mucosa.

Subhyoid Level (see Fig. 7-70B). The cyst is in the midline between the hyoid bone and the thyroid cartilage. Sometimes swallowing causes the mass to hide temporarily under the hyoid; ask your patient to dorsiflex her neck and open her mouth, at which point the cyst reappears.

Thyroid Cartilage Level. Only at this site does a thyroglossal cyst deviate from the midline, usually to the left; the forward pressure of the prow-like thyroid cartilage pushes it aside. To distinguish the mass from

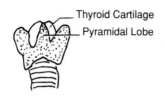

A. Pyramidal Lobe of Thyroid Gland   B. Delphian Nodes

Fig. 7-71 Thyroid-Associated Masses.   A. Pyramidal Lobe of Thyroid Gland. B. Delphian Nodes.

an enlarged lymph node, have the patient protrude her tongue maximally. If the mass is connected with the structures of the thyroglossal duct, this maneuver gives it an upward tug.

Cricoid Cartilage Level.   A thyroglossal cyst in this region must be distinguished from a mass of the thyroid pyramidal lobe. The cyst tugs upward with protrusion of the tongue.

Midline Cervical Mass: Pyramidal Lobe of Thyroid:
See the preceding discussion on thyroglossal cyst at the cricoid level. The pyramidal lobe may extend from the isthmus of the thyroid to the hyoid bone (Fig. 7-71A); true to its name, its base on the isthmus is usually wider and can be felt as an isthmic projection. It may be palpable in Hashimoto thyroiditis.

Mass in Suprasternal Notch: Dermoid Cyst:
Frequently, a nonpulsatile fluctuant mass in the suprasternal notch (*Burns space*) proves to be a dermoid cyst. The mass is not adherent to the trachea, nor does it move upward with protrusion of the tongue. The cyst may be confused with a tuberculous abscess.

Mass in the Suprasternal Notch: Tuberculous Abscess:
This has the same physical characteristics as a dermoid cyst, except that it is slightly less fluctuant. It may arise from an abscess in the lung apex or by drainage from the deep cervical chain of lymph nodes.

KEY SIGN
Fatty Mass in Suprasternal Notch: Dewlap:
In Cushing syndrome, excess adrenocorticosteroids may produce a soft, nontender, fatty mass in the suprasternal notch. The term dewlap has been suggested because of its resemblance to a fold of skin in the cow.

KEY SIGN
Pulsatile Mass in the Suprasternal Notch: Aorta or Innominate Artery:
Pathophysiology: Occasionally, elongation of the aortic arch or the innominate artery causes the vessel to bow upward into the suprasternal notch. This is not necessarily evidence of aneurysmal dilatation.

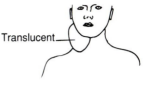

A. Branchial Cyst B. Cervical Hygroma

Fig. 7-72 Single Tumors of the Lateral Neck I. A. Branchial Cyst. B. Cervical Hygroma.

KEY SIGN

Lateral Cervical Cyst: Branchial Cyst: *Pathophysiology:* Remnants of the embryonic branchial clefts undergo cystic enlargement. A tumor usually appears in adult life, not in childhood. Commonly, there is a single cystic mass just anterior but deep to the upper third of the sternocleidomastoid (Fig. 7-72A). The mass feels slightly soft and resilient; intercurrent inflammation makes it tender and firm. Aspirated fluid appears to be pus, but if it is spread on a watch glass, oil droplets may be seen floating on the surface.

Lateral Cervical Cyst: Hygroma: *Pathophysiology:* The mass is formed by many cysts of occluded lymphatic channels. The soft, irregular, and partially compressible mass is usually present from childhood. It occupies the upper third of the anterior cervical triangle, but it may extend downward and under the jaw (see Fig. 7-72B). It is readily distinguished from all other cysts by its brilliant translucence. Its size may vary from time to time and it may become inflamed.

Lateral Cervical Cyst: Carotid Body Tumor: *Pathophysiology:* This arises from the chromaffin tissue of the carotid body; it can be familial or sporadic. The mass usually arises near the bifurcation of the common carotid artery. It appears in middle life and grows very slowly. The mass can be palpated near the bifurcation of the common carotid artery (Fig. 7-73A). Usually shaped like a potato (*potato tumor*), it is freely movable laterally, but it cannot be moved in the long axis of the artery. Although growing in the carotid sheath, it does not

A. Tumor of Carotid Body B. Intermittent Cervical Pouches

Fig. 7-73 Single Tumors of the Lateral Neck II. A. Carotid Body Tumor. B. Laryngocele.

always transmit arterial pulsations. Early it may feel cystic; later it becomes hard. Pressure on the tumor sometimes produces slowing of the heart rate and dizziness. Occasionally, the tumor produces vasoactive amines, and palpation can produce pupillary dilatation and hypertension, a useful diagnostic sign. In 20% of cases, regional extension eventually occurs upward along the carotid sheath.

Intermittent Lateral Cervical Cyst: Zenker's Diverticulum (Pharyngeal Pouch): *Pathophysiology: A diverticulum occurs proximal to the cricopharyngeus muscle.* The patient complains of gurgling in the neck, especially during swallowing. Regurgitation of food is common during eating or when lying on the side. An intermittent swelling in the side of the neck may be seen; usually the left side is involved. When not apparent, the swelling may be induced by swallowing water. Pressure on the filled pouch causes regurgitation of old food. The diagnosis is made from the esophagram.

Intermittent Lateral Cervical Cyst: Laryngocele: *Pathophysiology: Herniation of a laryngeal diverticulum through the lateral thyrohyoid membrane causes an intermittent swelling of the neck at that point (see Fig. 7-73B).* Blowing the nose will often induce an air-filled swelling that is resonant to percussion. Usually the condition occurs from chronic severe coughing or sustained blowing on a musical instrument.

Lateral Cervical Cyst: Cavernous Hemangioma: As in other parts of the body, the swelling is soft, compression partially empties the cavity of blood and refilling is slow. A faint blue color under the skin may be discerned.

Lateral Cervical Fistula: Branchial Fistula: In the same location as the branchial cyst, the fistula may be either congenital or have developed from an inflamed cyst. Probing of the tract usually discloses a blind end in the lateral pharyngeal wall. Fistulas become intermittently infected.

Thyroid Signs

KEY SIGN
Tracheal Displacement from Goiter: Although the caliber or the position of the trachea is not altered, a large or strategically located goiter may cause either tracheal compression or displacement or both (Fig. 7-74A). *Tracheal Compression:* Usually the trachea is narrowed in the transverse diameter. Small degrees of compression cannot be diagnosed by history or physical examination. With a greater degree of embarrassment, the *Kocher test* is helpful, where slight pressure on the lateral lobes of the thyroid produces stridor. *Tra-*

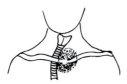

A. Tracheal Displacement
by Retrosternal Goiter

B. Venous Engorgement
by Retrosternal Goiter

Fig. 7-74 Two Physical Signs of Retrosternal Goiter. A. Tracheal Displacement: The retrosternal goiter on the patient's left compresses the trachea transversely pushing it to the right. The tracheal deviation can be demonstrated by palpation. B. Venous Engorgement: Compression of the external jugular vein by a retrosternal goiter produces engorgement of the superficial branches in the skin of the neck and clavicular regions.

cheal Displacement: Lateral deviation of the trachea can usually be shown by physical examination, except where the deviation begins at a level below the suprasternal notch.

KEY SIGN
Tender Thyroid: Acute Suppurative Thyroiditis: *Pathophysiology:* Infection of the thyroid gland by bacteria or fungi often extends from branchial cleft remnants. There is acute pain and fever. The gland is slightly enlarged, asymmetric, and fluctuance may be noted [Pearce EN, Farwell AP, Braverman LE. Thyroiditis. *N Engl J Med* 2003;348:2646–2655].

KEY SIGN
Tender Thyroid: Subacute Thyroiditis: See page 338.

KEY SIGN
Thyroid Bruit: Graves Disease: See page 335. *Pathophysiology:* When the thyroid undergoes hyperplasia, accelerated blood flow through the enlarged, tortuous thyroid arteries often produces vibrations, felt as a thrill, or heard with the bell of the stethoscope as a soft murmur, called a *thyroid bruit*. A bruit must be distinguished from a carotid murmur, which may be heard proximal to the gland, and an aortic murmur, which originates at the base of the heart. The bruit is often confused with a venous hum, but the hum has a different pitch and is abolished by light compression of the jugular vein. A bruit suggests Graves disease.

KEY SIGN
Thyroid Enlargement: Goiter: See page 335ff. *Pathophysiology:* Enlargement of the thyroid gland results from hy-

perplasia of thyroid tissue, infiltration with foreign substances (e.g., amyloid), infection, or neoplastic growth (primary thyroid cancers, lymphoma, or metastatic disease). The patient may complain of fullness or a mass in the neck, but, surprisingly, they are often unaware of thyroid enlargement. During examination, determine the size of each component of the gland, extension of the gland within the neck or into the retrosternal space, consistency (smooth, a single nodule, multinodular), fixation to surrounding structures, tenderness, and the presence or absence of regional lymph node enlargement. Also assess the state of thyroid function: hypothyroid, euthyroid, or hyperthyroid (see page 122ff). Clinical classification of goiters is based upon whether the goiter is diffuse or nodular and the level of the functional thyroid state, that is, is it a toxic goiter (hyperthyroid) or a nontoxic goiter (euthyroid or hypothyroid). See page 335ff for further discussion.

KEY SYMPTOM
Solitary Thyroid Nodule: See page 337ff.

KEY SIGN
Enlarged Delphian Lymph Nodes: *Pathophysiology:*   A few lymph nodes are regularly present in the *thyrohyoid membrane;* when enlarged, they are termed the *delphian nodes* because they may indicate metastases from thyroid carcinoma. Enlargement of the delphian nodes indicates either subacute thyroiditis or thyroid cancer (see Fig. 7-71B).

Head and Neck Syndromes

Scalp, Face, Skull, and Jaw Syndromes

KEY SYNDROME
Headache: For a full discussion of headache see Chapter 14, page 850ff. Discussed below are regional causes of headache related to extracranial disease.

HEADACHE FROM FEVER: Many febrile illnesses are associated with headache. The location varies; the pain may be slight or severe, throbbing or steady. Evidence suggests that distention of the cranial arteries is the cause of the pain.

HEADACHE: GIANT CELL ARTERITIS, TEMPORAL ARTERITIS: See Chapter 8, page 471.   *Pathophysiology:*   Temporal headache and scalp tenderness results from ischemia in the temporal artery distribution. The headaches are constant and relatively severe. Scalp tenderness is often present; exquisite scalp sensitivity is nearly diagnostic. Search for nodularity and/or decreased pulsations in the temporal artery.

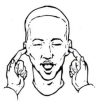

Fig. 7-75 Palpation of the Temporomandibular Joint (TMJ). *Place the tips of your index fingers in each external acoustic meatus and have the patient open and close his mouth. Clicking or crepitation is felt with TMJ arthritis; the joint will be tender if rheumatoid arthritis is the cause.*

HEADACHE: OCCIPITAL NEURITIS: *Pathophysiology:* Entrapment of the occipital nerve radiates pain in its distribution. Shooting sharp pain over the ear and posterior scalp suggests occipital neuritis.

LOCALIZED HEADACHE: PARANASAL SINUSITIS: See page 325.

ICE CREAM HEADACHE: Application of cold to the palate triggers intense pain felt in the medial orbital area. This common occurrence is precipitated by eating very cold foods, classically ice cream. It lasts 20–120 seconds, during which time the pain is intense. It may be more common in people with migraine.

S KEY SYNDROME

Temporomandibular Joint Pain: Rheumatoid Arthritis: This joint is often involved in rheumatoid arthritis. Ask your patient if stiffness restricts her from opening her mouth on arising. Tenderness in this location is distinguishes the disease from rheumatic fever (Fig. 7-75). Trismus may occur from muscle spasm.

S KEY SYNDROME

Temporomandibular Joint Pain: Osteoarthritis: Osteoarthritis produces joint crepitus with movement. The patient may hear grating while chewing or talking. Other diseases that occasionally affect the temporomandibular joint are systemic lupus erythematosus, gout, Sjögren syndrome, and Mediterranean fever.

Temporomandibular Joint Pain: Displaced Cartilage: The patient may hear a snap in the ear. Thereafter, an annoying click occurs with each opening of the mouth. The clicking may be palpated as a sudden movement in the joint. Occasionally, the joint locks, with sudden pain in the ear radiating to the pinna and the skin above, accompanied by salivation from stimulation of the auriculotemporal nerve. Pain persists until the cartilage is reduced.

Eye Syndromes

S KEY SYNDROME

▼ **Sjögren Syndrome: Keratoconjunctivitis Sicca:** *Pathophysiology:* There is lymphocytic infiltration of the salivary and lacrimal glands with loss of exocrine function. This is an autoimmune disorder first described as keratoconjunctivitis sicca, xerostomia in patients with rheumatoid arthritis. Primary Sjögren syndrome is a relatively common disorder with symptoms of fatigue, dry mouth, eyes, and other mucosal surfaces, arthralgias and arthritis, and nephritis. Both central and peripheral neurologic symptoms may be present. Other autoimmune diseases, in addition to rheumatoid arthritis, may accompany the syndrome. There is an increased risk of non-Hodgkin lymphomas.

D KEY DISEASE

▼ **Graves Ophthalmopathy:** *Pathophysiology:* Deposition of mucopolysaccharides within the extraocular muscles leads to forward displacement of the globe and impairs extraocular motion. Acquired bilateral exophthalmos is most commonly associated with Graves disease. In Graves disease, the proptosis occurs independently of the abnormalities of thyroid function; the patient may be hyperthyroid, euthyroid, or hypothyroid at the time of presentation. The proptosis is usually permanent, or at least it persists for many years. Other accompanying but transient signs may be palpebral edema and periorbital swelling. At onset, the proptosis may be unilateral, raising concern for other intraorbital pathology.

S KEY SYNDROME

▼ **Down Syndrome:** The four ocular signs of Down syndrome (trisomy 21) are an increased incidence of (a) epicanthic fold persisting after the age of 10 years; (b) unilateral or bilateral slanting eyes in which the lateral canthus is elevated more than 2 mm above a line through the medial canthi; (c) *Brushfield spots,* accumulations of lighter-colored tissues in the concentric band of the outer third of the iris; and (d) hypoplasia of the iris, showing as darker discolorations of the iris.

S KEY SYNDROME

► ▼ **Uveal Tract Inflammation: Uveitis (Iritis, Iridocyclitis, and Choroiditis):** *Pathophysiology:* Inflammation of the uvea may involve only the iris (iritis), extend to the ciliary body (iridocyclitis), or involve the choroid (choroiditis). *Iritis* is characterized by ciliary flush and miosis, accompanied by deep pain, photophobia, blurring, and lacrimation. The iris becomes adherent to the anterior lenticular surface, forming *posterior synechiae,* manifest by irregularities in the pupil. Cast-off cells sediment in the anterior chamber of the eye to form a sterile *hypopyon* (see Fig. 7-45B). If there is involvement of the ciliary body and choroid, deposits of yellow or white dots of aggregated cells occur on the posterior surface of the cornea, *keratic precipitates* (KP). *Uveitis* (inflammation of the uveal tract, the vascular layer of the eye) may be caused by trauma, infection, allergy, sarcoidosis, collagen vascular diseases, and ankylosing spondylitis. *Irido-cyclitis* in association with cytomegalovirus retinitis is relatively common in patients infected with HIV.

S KEY SYNDROME

▼ **Patients with Red Eye:** A red eye may result from benign self-limited conditions or be an indication of serious sight-threatening eye disease. DDX: Generalized redness of the bulbar and tarsal conjunctivae with minimal discharge and no visual loss is usually caused by viral conjunctivitis or blepharitis. Localized redness and swelling of a lid suggests hordeolum or chalazion. Severe photophobia or perilimbic injection suggest inflammation of the cornea or uveal tract requiring immediate ophthalmologic consultation. Pain, visual loss, elevated intraocular pressure, corneal haze, ciliary flush, acute proptosis, acute scleritis or severe photophobia require urgent evaluation by an ophthalmologist.

✔ *RED EYE—CLINICAL OCCURRENCE: Benign Disorders* viral conjunctivitis, external hordeolum (sty), internal hordeolum (chalazion), and blepharitis; *Serious Disorders* (urgent care of an ophthalmologist required): acute keratitis (herpes simplex, bacterial, trauma, foreign body), gonococcal and chlamydial conjunctivitis, acute glaucoma, acute iridocyclitis, uveitis, and acute scleritis.

S KEY SYNDROME

▼ **Glaucoma, Narrow Angle:** *Pathophysiology:* Obstruction to aqueous drainage from the anterior chamber is a result of the narrowing of the chamber angle and probably of increased production of aqueous. Acute symptoms are extreme ocular pain with loss of vision, nausea, and vomiting. Chronic symptoms include halos around lights, tunnel vision, ocular pain, and headache. Chemosis, corneal edema, ciliary flush, and a fixed dilated pupil are seen on exam [Coleman AL. Glaucoma. *Lancet* 1999;354:1803–1810].

S KEY SYNDROME

▼ **Glaucoma, Open Angle:** *Pathophysiology:* There is increased secretion of aqueous with obstruction to outflow with normal chamber angles. This is the most common type of glaucoma. It occurs in older persons who may see colored halos around lights and experience insidious, painless blindness. There are increased intraocular pressure, dilation of pupils, and cupping of the disks.

S KEY SYNDROME

▼ **Sudden Visual Loss:** This always requires the urgent care of an ophthalmologist. Visual loss is usually monocular resulting from retinal detachment, vitreous hemorrhage, retinal artery occlusion (embolus, thrombus, vasculitis), compression on optic nerve or anterior ischemic optic neuritis (arteritic and nonarteritic). Transient visual loss in one eye for 5–15 minutes (*amaurosis fugax*) usually results from embolic occlusion of the retinal artery. On funduscopic exam, refractile cholesterol emboli may be seen at the retinal artery bifurcations. Loss of vision in a single visual field (right or left hemianopsia) indicates a lesion between the optic chiasm and the visual cortex. Patients are often unaware of this visual field loss.

Ear Syndromes

S KEY SYNDROME
Acute External Otitis: *Pathophysiology:* A variety of organisms can cause the inflammation, but the usual offender is *Pseudomonas aeruginosa,* or, less commonly, streptococci, staphylococci, or *Proteus vulgaris.* This may result from an increased pH in the canal ("swimmer's ear"). Pain may be mild or severe; it is accentuated by movement of the tragus or pinna. The epithelium appears either pale or red; it may swell to close the canal and impair hearing; the tragus may also swell. An aural discharge often results. Fever is not uncommon. Tender, palpable lymph nodes may appear in front of the tragus, behind the pinna, or in the anterior cervical triangle.

S KEY SYNDROME
Chronic External Otitis: *Pathophysiology:* Bacteria and fungi are the chief causative agents, although the condition may accompany a chronic dermatitis, such as seborrhea or psoriasis. Instead of pain, pruritus is the chief symptom. Aural discharge may be present. The epithelium of the pinna and the meatus is thickened and red; it is abnormally insensitive to the pain of instrumentation.

S KEY SYNDROME
Malignant (Necrotizing) External Otitis: *Pathophysiology:* Pseudomonas aeruginosa invades the soft tissues, cartilage, and bone in patients with diabetes mellitus. Although some patients have minimal clinical findings, others may experience pain, discharge, and fever with swelling and tenderness of the tissues around the ear. Examination of the auditory canal may reveal edema, redness, granulation tissue, and pus obscuring the tympanic membrane. The process can advance to osteomyelitis of the mastoid, temporal bone and the base of the skull, involving the seventh and other cranial nerves and presenting with a facial palsy. CT or MRI permit an accurate diagnosis; an otolaryngology consult must be obtained.

Middle Ear Glomus Tumor: *Pathophysiology:* Fibrovascular tumors arise from the glomus bodies in the jugular bulb or the middle ear mucosa. They present with pulsatile tinnitus in the involved ear, or sometimes the glomus jugulare type is associated with paralysis of CN IX and CN XI, which pass through the jugular foramen. Glomus tumors appear as red masses behind the tympanic membrane. Identical tumors arise from the carotid artery bifurcation. Rarely, the tumors are multiple, malignant or secrete vasoactive amines. If biopsied, they bleed profusely. Familial forms occur.

S KEY SYNDROME

Acute Otitis Media with Effusion: Serous Otitis Media: See *Signs*, page 244.

S KEY SYNDROME

Acute Suppurative Otitis Media: See *Signs*, page 245.

S KEY SYNDROME

Acute Mastoiditis: *Pathophysiology:* The mastoid air cells communicate with the middle ear. Usually, infection of the mastoid cells results from inadequate treatment of acute suppurative otitis media. The symptoms of otitis gradually increase. There is low-grade fever with a thick, purulent discharge from the meatus. The eardrum is lusterless and edematous. Deep bone pain can be elicited by percussion on the mastoid process. Imaging confirms the diagnosis by showing clouding of the mastoid air cells and bony destruction, which is evident radiographically only after 2–3 weeks of suppuration. Extension can cause a subperiosteal abscess of the mastoid process. Less commonly, erosion of bone damages the facial (CN VII) nerve, with facial paralysis. Extension through the inner table can cause meningitis, epidural abscess, or abscess of the temporal lobe or cerebellum. Infection of the internal ear can produce labyrinthitis.

S KEY SYNDROME

Chronic Suppurative Otitis Media: *Pathophysiology:* By definition, the condition is associated with a permanent perforation of the eardrum. A marginal perforation of the annulus is more grave than a central defect. The chief symptom is painless aural discharge. Hearing is always impaired. The amount of discharge may wax and wane, but recurrence is invariable. Painless discharge accompanying an upper respiratory infection suggests previously existing perforation. Occurrence of pain or vertigo indicates development of a complication, such as subdural irritation, brain abscess, or labyrinthine involvement.

S KEY SYNDROME

Cholesteatoma: *Pathophysiology:* In chronic suppurative otitis media with a deep retraction pocket in the attic or posterior superior quadrant of the eardrum, the squamous epithelium of the meatus may grow into the attic of the tympanic cavity. Desquamation produces a caseous mass of cells, keratin, and debris, which becomes infected, and slowly enlarges, extending into the mastoid antrum. The mass may ultimately erode bone. Patients may have fullness in ear, pain, headache and hearing loss. Signs include chronic foul-smelling suppurative discharge from middle ear, hearing loss, and a pearly gray mass visible with otoscope.

S KEY SYNDROME

▼ **Hearing Loss:** *Pathophysiology:* Sensorineural loss (nerve deafness) results from disorders of the cochlea or the acoustic (CN VIII) nerve. Conductive loss occurs from failure in transmission of sound vibrations to the sensory apparatus. Some causes of **sensorineural loss** are hereditary deafness, congenital deafness, trauma, infections, drug toxicity, and aging (*presbycusis*). Unilateral hearing loss with unilateral tinnitus may be the first symptoms of an acoustic neuroma. **Conductive loss** occurs with obstruction of the external acoustic meatus, disorders of the eardrum and middle ear, and overgrowth of bone with fixation of the stapes (*otosclerosis*) [Nadol JB Jr. Hearing Loss. *N Engl J Med* 1993;329:1092–1102; Jackler RK. A 73-year-old man with hearing loss. *JAMA* 2003;289:1557–1565].

S KEY SYNDROME

▼ **Dizziness:** The patient has a sense of disturbed relation to space. Frequently it is described as being unsteady, weak, light-headed, or having a feeling of turning. There is no impression that the surroundings are whirling about as in true vertigo [Colledge NR, Barr-Hamilton RM, Lewis SJ, et al. Evaluation of investigations to diagnose the cause of dizziness in elderly people: A community based controlled study. *BMJ* 1996;313:782–792].

✔ *DIZZINESS—CLINICAL OCCURRENCE: Endocrine* hypothyroidism, pregnancy, hypoparathyroidism, aldosteronoma; *Idiopathic* multisystem atrophy; *Inflammatory/Immune* vestibular neuronitis; *Infectious* tabes dorsalis, meningitis, encephalitis, brain abscess, syphilis; *Metabolic/Toxic* nutritional: pellagra, alcoholism, vitamin B_{12} deficiency (e.g., pernicious anemia); cerebral hypoxia; fluid and electrolyte disturbances; *Mechanical/Trauma* ears: utricular trauma from skull fracture, otosclerosis, leaks from tears in the oval or round windows, perilymph fistula; eyes: muscle imbalance, refractive errors, glaucoma; *Neoplastic* brain tumors (primary and metastatic); *Neurologic* migraine, absence seizures, peripheral neuropathy; *Psychosocial* panic attack, generalized anxiety disorder; *Vascular* hypotension, orthostatic hypotension.

S KEY SYNDROME

▼ **Vertigo:** *Pathophysiology:* Persistent stimulation of the semicircular canals or vestibular nucleus when the head is at rest gives a hallucination of motion. When the eyes open, the patient's surroundings seem to be whirling or spinning about. With the eyes closed, the patient continues to feel in motion. Severe vertigo is accompanied by nausea and vomiting [Froehling DA, Silverman MD, Mohr DN, Beatty CW. The rational clinical examination. Does this dizzy patient have a serious form of vertigo? *JAMA* 1994;271:385–388].

✔ *VERTIGO—CLINICAL OCCURRENCE: Peripheral Labyrinthine System* serous labyrinthitis, perilymph fistula, labyrinthine (otic capsule) fistula, viral labyrinthitis, otosclerosis, otitis media with effusion, benign paroxysmal positional vertigo, idiopathic endolymphatic hydrops (*Ménière disease*), motion sickness, cholesteatoma, temporal bone fracture, postural vertigo; *Central Labyrinthine System* migraine, vertebrobasilar insufficiency, brainstem or cerebellar hemorrhage or infarction, cerebellopontine angle tumors, intraaxial tumors (pons, cerebellum, medulla), craniovertebral abnormalities causing cervicomedullary junctional compression, multiple sclerosis, intracranial abscess (temporal lobe, cerebellum, epidural, subdural); *CN VIII* infections (acute meningitis, tuberculous meningitis, basilar syphilitic meningitis), trauma, tumors; *Brainstem Nuclei* infections (encephalitis, meningitis, brain abscess), trauma, hemorrhage, thrombosis of the posteroinferior cerebellar artery, infarction of the lateral medulla (*Wallenberg syndrome*), tumors, multiple sclerosis.

D KEY DISEASE

Vertiginous Disorder: Acute Labyrinthitis: This is the most frequent cause of vertigo. The patient gradually develops a sense of whirling that reaches a climax in 24–48 hours. During the height of the symptoms, nausea and vomiting may occur. The patient seeks comfort in the horizontal position; raising the head may induce vertigo. The patient is incapacitated for several days. The symptoms gradually subside, and they disappear in 3 to 6 weeks. There is no accompanying tinnitus or hearing loss.

S KEY SYNDROME

Vertiginous Disorder: Benign Paroxysmal Positional Vertigo (BPPV): *Pathophysiology:* Calcium deposits in the labyrinth (otoliths) are dislodged and move in response to gravity eliciting a feeling of motion. This is most common in older individuals. The onset is sudden, often when rolling over in bed or arising in the morning. There is no headache or fever. There is often intense nausea and inability to stand. Symptoms are minimized by avoiding any head motion. Barany Hallpike maneuver causes profound symptoms.

Vertiginous Disorder: Vascular Disease: Transient vertigo may be caused by vascular spasm. More severe and prolonged symptoms occur from thrombosis or dissection of a brainstem artery. There is sudden vertigo with nystagmus, loud tinnitus, and sudden deafness. Partial recovery is usual in 3–4 weeks.

Vertiginous Disorder: Trauma: Skull fracture through the inner ear, concussion, or a loud noise may induce symptoms similar to a stroke. Tinnitus and hearing loss are present. Labyrinthine tests show delay and hypoactivity on the affected side.

D KEY DISEASE

Vertiginous Disorder: Labyrinthine Hydrops (Méniere Syndrome): *Pathophysiology:* Swelling of endolymphatic labyrinthine spaces with degeneration of the organ of Corti occurs with unknown cause. Symptoms are characterized by sudden attacks of whirling vertigo, tinnitus, and neurosensory hearing loss; there are intervals of complete freedom from vertigo, but the hearing loss and the tinnitus persist. An attack lasts hours but not days. Hearing loss predominates on one side and is fluctuating, but slowly progressive. Tinnitus also fluctuates, accentuating before an attack. The disease is self-limited. The cause of the hydrops is unknown. Labyrinthine tests are normal or hypoactive on the involved side.

Vertiginous Disorder: Damage to CN VIII or Brainstem Nuclei: Lesions at either level produce vertigo and nystagmus. Disorders of the eighth nerve (e.g., acoustic neuroma) are accompanied by hearing loss; this is absent with lesions of the brainstem except when other cranial nerves are also damaged.

Nose and Sinus Syndromes

S KEY SYNDROME

Infectious Rhinosinusitis: The Common Cold: *Pathophysiology:* Rhinoviruses, and many others, infect the mucous membranes of the nose and sinuses causing inflammation and increased nasal secretions. The onset is abrupt with a watery discharge (*rhinorrhea*) and sneezing, often with malaise and mild myalgia, but without fever. Nasal obstruction occurs from edema of the mucosa. A sore throat is not part of the picture. The sinuses are involved in 75% of patients [Fwaltney JM, Phillips CD, Miller RD, Riker DK. Computed tomographic study of the common cold. *N Engl J Med* 1994;330:25–30]. Symptoms last 3–10 days and most people have 4–6 such infections per year. Severe local pain suggests a complication, such as bacterial sinusitis.

S KEY SYNDROME

Allergic Rhinosinusitis: *Pathophysiology:* Immunoglobulin (Ig) E-mediated mast cell degranulation occurs with specific allergen exposure to which the patient has been sensitized by previous exposure. Itching of the nose and eyes, rhinorrhea, and lacrimation are accompanied by sneezing. Headache is common. The membranes are typically pale, swollen, and edematous; occasionally they are dull red or purplish. Allergic rhinitis may be seasonal or perennial. Common allergens are pollens, molds, animal danders, and house dust mite and cockroach antigens. Symptoms are associated with seasonal exposure to pollens (trees in the spring; grasses in the summer; ragweed in the fall) or to antigens associated with a specific environment. Perennial allergic rhinitis suggests exposure to environmental antigens such as house dust mite and animal danders (usually cats) in the home.

S KEY SYNDROME

Vasomotor Rhinitis: *Pathophysiology:* Nonallergic mucosal edema and rhinorrhea are associated with vasodilation of the nasal vessels, mucosal edema, and increased mucous production. This is associated with environmental, hormonal, and pharmacologic exposures. Environmental irritants such as smoke, perfumes, strong odors, and cold air trigger increased mucous production and mucosal edema.

Pregnancy and therapeutic estrogens and progestins have been associated. *Chronic vasomotor rhinitis* seems to result from an over reaction of the nasal and pharyngeal mucosa to environmental exposures.

S KEY SYNDROME

▼ **Bilateral Rhinorrhea: Rhinitis Medicamentosa:** *Pathophysiology:* Use of topical vasoconstrictors for more than a few days produces rebound hyperemia when they are stopped, triggering more medication use. The appearance is similar to allergic rhinitis. A history of using nasal vasoconstrictors and the absence of eosinophils in nasal secretions suggest the diagnosis.

S KEY SYNDROME

▼ **Suppurative Paranasal Sinusitis:** *Pathophysiology:* Most viral upper respiratory infections are accompanied by inflammation of the sinuses. Obstruction of the narrow sinus orifices leads to accumulation of mucous which becomes secondarily infected by bacteria (*Streptococcus pneumoniae, Haemophilus influenzae, Moraxella* spp.) leading to suppurative sinusitis. Severe pain in the face occurring 7–14 days after signs and symptoms of an acute upper respiratory infection suggests complicating acute suppurative bacterial sinusitis. Pain and pressure without fever earlier in the course of illness suggests sinus obstruction requiring decongestants [Williams JW, Simel DL. The rational clinical examination. Does this patient have sinusitis? Diagnosing acute sinusitis by history and physical exam. *JAMA* 1993;270:1242–1246; Engels EA, Terrin N, Barza M, Lau J. Meta-analysis of diagnostic tests for acute sinusitis. *J Clin Epidemiol* 2000;53:852–862].

Maxillary Sinusitis causes dull throbbing pain in the cheek and in several of the upper teeth on that side [Williams JW, Simel DL, Roberts L, Samsa GP. Clinical evaluation for sinusitis—Making the diagnosis by history and physical examination. *Ann Intern Med* 1992;117:705–710]. Thumb pressure discloses localized tenderness on the maxilla. Pain in the teeth with maxillary sinusitis must be distinguished from inflammation about a tooth; in the latter case, only one tooth is painful and may be tender when tapped with a probe. In sinusitis, examination of the affected side with a nasal speculum discloses a reddened, edematous mucosa and swollen turbinates. When the mucosa is shrunk by the application of a cotton pledget soaked with 3% ephedrine in saline solution, a purulent discharge may be seen; the drug may also be applied as a spray. During the first 2 days, the discharge may be tinged with blood. With shrinkage, pus in the posterior middle meatus may be seen in the nasopharyngeal mirror.

Frontal Sinusitis produces pain in the forehead above the supraorbital ridge; pressure in this region elicits tenderness. Edema of the eyelids on the affected side is infrequent.

Ethmoid Sinusitis pain is medial to the eye and seems deep in the head or orbit; there is no localizing tenderness, although palpebral edema is common.

Sphenoid Sinusitis generates pain either behind the eye, in the occiput, or in the vertex of the skull; no tenderness is produced.

Transillumination may reveal an opaque maxillary or frontal sinus; x-ray films may show clouding of the sinus or a fluid level. CT imaging is definitive. *There is no pain associated with chronic inflammation or infection of the paranasal sinuses.* DDX: Many patients with a history of recurrent "sinus headaches" actually have migraine. Persistent and progressive symptoms should raise consideration of more serious diseases such as Wegener granulomatosis, nasopharyngeal carcinoma, and lethal midline granuloma.

S KEY SYNDROME

Protracted Purulent Discharge: Chronic Suppurative Sinusitis: When a purulent nasal discharge persists for more than 3 weeks, subacute or chronic sinusitis should be suspected. Pain over the sinuses is not a prominent symptom, and tenderness is frequently absent. Examination of the shrunken membranes may disclose the source of the pus. Transillumination of the sinuses may assist in localization. The diagnosis of sinusitis is confirmed by CT imaging. DDX: Chronic sinusitis resistant to medical therapy should suggest the possibility of common variable immunodeficiency. The finding of chronic suppurative sinusitis, especially with unusual organisms (e.g., fungi like *Aspergillus* spp. or *Mucor* spp.), warrants a search for other immunodeficiency.

S KEY SYNDROME

▶ **Sinusitis and Periorbital Edema: Periorbital Abscess:** *Pathophysiology:* In suppurative ethmoid sinusitis, pus may extend through the lateral wall of the sinus to form an abscess between the ethmoid plate and the periosteum lining the orbit. This is accompanied by fever, pain on eye movement, and edema between the inner canthus and the bridge of the nose. The edematous region is tender and may extend to involve most of both lids. The pus may push the ocular globe slightly downward and laterally. No chemosis is present. Surgical drainage is essential.

S KEY SYNDROME

▶ **Sinusitis and Periorbital Edema: Orbital Cellulitis:** *Pathophysiology:* A periorbital abscess may extend to produce a diffuse cellulitis of the orbital tissue. Invasion may be heralded by a chill, high fever, and dull pain in the eye. The eyelids become edematous, particularly near the inner canthus. Chemosis develops. Ultimately, the eye becomes fixed. The patient appears very ill and requires the immediate surgical care.

S KEY SYNDROME

▶ **Sinusitis and Ocular Palsies: Cavernous Sinus Thrombosis:** *Pathophysiology:* Usually infection spreads from the nose through the angular vein to the cavernous sinus, where septic thrombosis occurs. This is the most feared complication of nasal infections because it can cause blindness or death. There are sudden chills and high fever; the patient becomes prostrate and may rapidly become comatose. The patient complains of pain deep in the eyes. Early, there is selective ocular palsy involving one of the nerves in the cavernous sinus, either the oculomotor nerve (CN III), the trochlear nerve (CN IV), or the abducens nerve (CN VI). Both eyes are involved fairly early, with immobilization of the globes, periorbital edema, and chemosis. Death may occur within 2 or 3 days. DDX: Selective ocular palsy occurs early in cavernous sinus thrombosis, whereas orbital abscess produces complete immobilization of the globe gradually, without preliminary disorder of a single nerve. Bilaterality strongly suggests cavernous sinus thrombosis.

Oral Syndromes (Lips, Mouth, Tongue, Teeth, and Pharynx)

S KEY SYNDROME

Difficulty Swallowing: *Pathophysiology:* Swallowing is a complex voluntary and reflex event requiring normal sensory and neuromuscular function of the tongue, mouth, and pharynx. Impairment of any of these structures can produce difficulty swallowing. Careful observation of the patients attempts to swallow thin and thickened liquids, soft foods and solid boluses will help to identify the site of the problem. Assistance of speech therapists and videofluoroscopy is often necessary. See also page 233, and Chapter 9 pages 533 and 563–564.

✔ *CLINICAL OCCURRENCE: Congenital* cerebral palsy, mental retardation; *Endocrine* hypothyroidism; *Inflammatory/Immune* amyloidosis, Sjögren syndrome, scleroderma; *Infectious* tonsillitis, quinsy, mononucleosis, epiglottitis, mumps, retropharyngeal abscess, chancre, gumma, actinomycosis, oral and esophageal herpes simplex and candida; *Mechanical/Trauma* fractures, dislocation of the jaw, ankylosis of the temporomandibular joint, irradiation; *Neoplastic* sarcoma of the jaw, carcinoma; *Neurologic* stroke, bulbar paralysis, pseudobulbar paralysis, bilateral facial nerve palsy, myasthenia gravis, palsy of the hypoglossal nerve, diphtheritic palsy, Parkinson disease, rabies, botulism; *Psychosocial* hysteria.

S KEY SYNDROME

Aberrant Right Subclavian Artery (Dysphagia Lusoria): *Pathophysiology:* Anomalous development of the aortic arch results in the right subclavian artery arising from the descending aorta, distal to the origin of the left subclavian artery (Fig. 7-76). To reach the right axilla, the anomalous artery crosses the midline obliquely upward, either posterior to the esophagus, between the esophagus and the trachea, or rarely anterior to the trachea. If the artery is in contact with the esophagus the aberrant vessel may produce intermittent pressure on the esophagus, resulting in difficulty swallowing solid food, the only symptom or sign leading to the diagnosis. Symptom onset is in adolescence or early adulthood. The condition is termed dysphagia lusoria from the Latin lusus naturae, "a natural anomaly." The diagnosis is made when dysphagia prompts an esophagram showing a pressure notch in the esophagus.

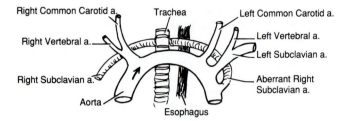

Fig. 7-76 Aberrant Right Subclavian Artery. *The right subclavian artery arises in the descending aorta, distal to the origin of the left subclavian artery. It crosses the midline either behind the esophagus, between the esophagus and the trachea, or anterior to the trachea. In either of the first two patterns, the artery may compress the esophagus producing difficulty in swallowing, "dysphagia lusoria." A transverse compression band in the esophagram suggests the diagnosis.*

S KEY SYNDROME

Acute Pharyngitis: Between 1892, when diphtheria antitoxin was discovered, and 1935, when sulfonamide drugs were introduced to therapeutics, the chief diagnostic problem was to distinguish between diphtheria and nondiphtheritic pharyngitis, for which there was no specific treatment. With the advent of antibiotics, the practical implications of diagnosis changed considerably; the chief problem was to distinguish between treatable bacterial pharyngitis and viral infections. More recently, the physician cares for immunosuppressed patients from HIV infection or immunosuppressive drug therapy so recognition of viral and fungal infections is essential. The physician relies on antigen detection and cultures from the throat to confirm the diagnosis and guide therapy [Bisno AL. Acute pharyngitis. *N Engl J Med* 2001;344: 205–211].

S KEY SYNDROME

Acute Pharyngitis: Viral Pharyngitis: *Pathophysiology:* Pharyngeal inflammation accompanies infection with a wide variety viruses but the most common are Ebstein-Barr virus (EBV), respiratory syncytial virus (RSV), parainfluenza, influenza, adenovirus, and coxsackievirus. The patient complains of sore throat, often with mild rhinorrhea and hoarseness. In influenza, the patient is febrile and usually complains of malaise, myalgia, and often a moderately sore throat and rhinorrhea. Inspection of the oral cavity discloses only swelling of lymphoid tissue in the mucosa of the posterior oropharyngeal wall, seen as elevated oval islands (Fig. 7-77). The mucosa may be dull red and the faucial pillars slightly edematous. Herpes simplex may produce painful ulcers of the posterior pharynx, soft palate, buccal mucosa, or tongue, whose punched out edges are surrounded by a rim of erythema. A pale, boggy mucosa of the posterior pharynx caused by adenovirus may accompany the scratchy sore throat preceding the coryza of a cold.

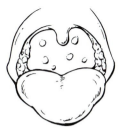

Fig. 7-77 Granular Pharyngitis in Viral Infections. *Elevated islands of lymphoid tissue are seen in the oropharyngeal mucosa. The mucosa is only slightly reddened; seldom is there any edema or exudate.*

S KEY SYNDROME

Acute Pharyngitis: Streptococcal or Staphylococcal Follicular Pharyngitis: The onset is often sudden; pain in the throat is severe; the temperature may rise to 39.5°C (103°F) or higher. The pharyngeal mucosa is bright red, swollen, and edematous, especially in the fauces and uvula; it is studded with white or yellow follicles. When the tonsils are present, they are swollen and stippled with prominent follicles. Tender, swollen cervical lymph nodes are common. This picture may be caused by either *Streptococcus* or *Staphylococcus*. *Scarlet fever* presents as an extremely painful throat with few follicles but brilliant red mucosa in the oropharynx, which extends forward to end abruptly near the back of the soft palate and fauces as if red paint had been applied. This is streptococcal until proved otherwise [Ebell MH, Simth MA, Barry HC, et al. The rational clinical examination. Does this patient have strep throat. *JAMA* 2000;284:2912–2918].

S KEY SYNDROME

Acute Epiglottitis: *Pathophysiology:* Bacterial infection of the epiglottis produces severe edema which can compromise the airway leading to asphyxiation. The condition is both more common and more dangerous in children. Patients present with sore throat and painful swallowing, decreased voice and signs of pharyngitis. Stridor and the need to sit erect to breathe indicate impending airway compromise [Frantz TD, Rasgon BM, Quesenberry CP Jr. Acute epiglottitis in adults: Analysis of 129 cases. *JAMA* 1994;272:1358–1360].

D KEY DISEASE

Acute Pharyngitis: Pharyngeal Diphtheria: The fauces first become dull red and a patch of white membrane appears on the tonsil; in the absence of tonsils, the membrane forms elsewhere. The pharyngeal mucosa becomes reddened, swollen, and edematous. Lifted with tongue blade, the membrane tenaciously holds to the mucosa; when separated, it discloses a bleeding surface. The membrane extends rapidly to involve other structures while turning gray or yellow. The cervical lymph nodes are enlarged and tender, and the patient appears quite ill, with severe constitutional symptoms. DDX: The throat is not nearly as sore as in follicular pharyngitis. A membrane limited to a tonsil must be distinguished from *Vincent angina* (acute necrotizing ulcerative stomatitis) in which the membrane does not extend beyond the tonsil and is not so tenacious. It is not accompanied by severe constitutional symptoms, but it is more locally destructive. A membrane in the pharynx requires culturing on media appropriate for the diphtheria bacillus.

D KEY DISEASE

Acute Pharyngitis: "Candida" (Moniliasis, Thrush): Shiny, raised white patches, surrounded by an erythematous rim, appear on the posterior pharynx, buccal mucosa, and tongue. They may be painful. An atrophic erythematous mucosal lesion without white exudate may occur also. Ask if there is pain on swallowing, because *Candida* esophagitis may accompany pharyngitis in the immunosuppressed patient.

S KEY SYNDROME

Acute Pharyngitis: Infectious Mononucleosis: *Pathophysiology:* An acute acquired infection of lymphocytes with Epstein-Barr virus (EBV) leads to lymphadenopathy and atypical circulating lymphocytes. An identical clinical picture can be caused by acute HIV, CMV, and toxoplasma infections. Sore throat is the most common symptom, accompanied by slight fever, malaise, cough, and headache. The pharynx is red and edematous, often with enlarged tonsils coated with exudate, making distinction from streptococcal infection difficult. The tonsils may reach the midline and impair speech and, rarely, respirations. There may be petechiae on the palate and uvula. The cervical lymph nodes are usually enlarged and tender. Disproportionate cervical lymph node enlargement suggests a generalized disease, so the physician should search for axillary and inguinal lymphadenopathy and splenomegaly. A morbilliform rash, conjunctivitis, splenomegaly and occasionally jaundice with a tender, enlarged liver may be seen.

D KEY DISEASE

Acute Pharyngitis: Herpangina: Infection with coxsackievirus 16 results in fever and sore throat. On examination, there are small vesicles or whitish papules on the soft palate.

Larynx Syndromes

S KEY SYNDROME

▶ **Acute Laryngeal Obstruction: Aphonia, Choking ("The Cafe Coronary"):** This diagnosis calls for instant treatment. Even physicians may fail to recognize and treat the condition in time to save life. *Immediate Diagnosis:* Usually during a meal, the victim rises suddenly with a look of panic or anguish, often with hand to throat, unable to speak or breathe. Ask the patient if she can speak. She may rush from the room, with face rapidly changing from pale to blue. This behavior is presumptive evidence of choking (in contrast, myocardial infarction permits speech and breathing), and there are fewer than 5 minutes in which to intervene before death.

The Heimlich Maneuver: *With the Victim Standing (Fig. 7-78):* Stand behind the victim and wrap your arms around the victim's waist. With your other hand grasp your fist and place its thumb side against the victim's abdomen, between the navel and the rib cage. Press your fist deep into the abdomen with a quick upward thrust. Repeat several times, if necessary. After an adult has aspirated a bolus during inspiration, Heimlich calculated that his maneuver could forcefully expel about 940 mL of residual and tidal air at an average pressure of 31 mmHg, enough to cause the bolus to pop out [Heimlich HJ. A life-saving maneuver to prevent food-choking. *JAMA* 1975;234:398–401].

S KEY SYNDROME

Acute Laryngitis: The most common cause of hoarseness, acute viral laryngitis, is often accompanied by an unproductive cough, producing pain or a burning dryness in the throat. Through the mirror, the true cords are reddened, their edges rounded by swelling. Erythema of the other laryngeal membranes is present; edema of the larynx is common. DDX: A white membrane in the larynx suggests infection with either streptococcus or the diphtheria bacillus.

S KEY SYNDROME

Croup: *Pathophysiology:* An acute obstruction of the upper airway occurs with infection, allergy, foreign body, or neoplasm and is accompanied by a hoarse, brassy cough and dyspnea. Children are usually affected. Parainfluenza virus infection causing acute laryngotracheobronchitis is the most frequent cause in children. *Inflammatory croup* is actually acute laryngitis. The cords may appear normal and edema may be greatest in the subepiglottic region. An attack produces a danger of asphyxia. In *spasmodic croup* (*laryngismus stridulus*), the child is awakened with a barking cough, dyspnea, and stridor. Cyanosis from air hunger is frequent. Recovery is sudden and complete. Viewed in the mirror, the larynx looks normal. The cause of the condition is unknown.

S KEY SYNDROME

Chronic Laryngitis: Hoarseness and unproductive cough are usually present. Pain is negligible. The true cords may appear dull and thickened or edematous and polypoid. Frequently, the false cords are similarly affected.

✓ *CLINICAL OCCURRENCE:* Chronic overuse of the cords; tobacco smoking; syphilis; tuberculosis of the cords complicating cavitary pulmonary tuberculosis.

Hysterical Aphonia: The organic causes of aphonia are readily diagnosed by inspection of the larynx. Even before laryngeal examination, hysterical aphonia may be distinguished by demonstrating that

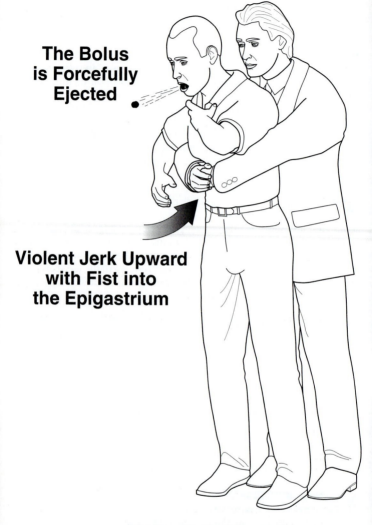

**The Bolus
is Forcefully
Ejected**

**Violent Jerk Upward
with Fist into
the Epigastrium**

Heimlich Maneuver

Fig. 7-78 Heimlich Maneuver.   *This is used to dislodge foreign bodies from
the larynx. Standing at the subject's back, encircle the subject's waist with your
arms. Grasp your fist with the other hand and give it a sudden forceful jerk
that thrusts the fist upward into the subject's epigastrium. Repeat until the obstructing bolus is forcefully expelled from the throat.*

the patient can make a sharp normal cough. When viewed through the mirror, the cords are morphologically normal. On attempted phonation, the cords promptly approximate but quickly diverge, or the arytenoids approximate while the free edges of the cords bow outward.

S KEY SYNDROME

Laryngeal Malfunction: Laryngeal Dyspnea: Shortness of breath has many causes other than laryngeal dysfunction (Chapter 8, page 375). In laryngeal disease, the occurrence of dyspnea is a mark of an advanced degree of obstruction, lesser degrees having been heralded by hoarseness. In laryngeal dyspnea, the harder the attempt to inhale, the greater becomes the obstruction, because the in rushing air forces the cords to approximate. Exhalation is unopposed, so quiet breathing is more efficient.

S KEY SYNDROME

Laryngeal Malfunction: Paradoxical Vocal Cord Motion: *Pathophysiology:* During attempted inspiration the vocal cords paradoxically close narrowing the airway to produce wheezing. Patients often present with episodic wheezing and shortness of breath unresponsive to treatment appropriate for asthma. Diagnosis requires direct visualization of the cords during an episode.

Dysphonia Plicae Ventricularis: *Pathophysiology:* Intermittent or chronic hoarseness results when the false vocal cords close over the true cords instead of remaining passive during phonation. A single examination of the cords may disclose no abnormality; subsequent examinations eventually coincide with an occasion when the false cords are seen to close partially or completely over the true cords (see Fig. 7-68C). When this occurs, the voice breaks, as in a boy whose "voice is changing." The false cords may also be active when the true cords are separated by tumor, cricoarytenoid arthritis, voice abuse, or emotional instability.

KEY SIGN

Disorders of Speech: See Chapter 14, page 875.

Salivary Gland Syndromes

KEY SIGN

Dry Mouth: Xerostomia: *Pathophysiology:* Generalized abnormalities of salivary gland function result in inadequate wetting of the mucosa. The patient complains of a dry mouth and difficulty swallowing dry foods such as crackers. The patient often consumes large amounts of liquids in an attempt to keep the mouth wet. In addition to the dry mucosa, extensive caries are frequently seen, often leading to loss of all the teeth. The common causes are anticholinergic drugs, head and neck irradiation, and immune destruction of the salivary glands in

Sjögren syndrome. Ask about dry eyes, *xerophthalmia,* which accompanies the latter.

Parotid Tumors: Parotid neoplasia may be either benign or malignant. *Pleomorphic Adenoma (Mixed Parotid Tumor)* presents as a firm, painless, nontender nodule, slightly above and in front of the mandibular angle. Less commonly, the site is just anterior to the tragus. It may remain benign for years, growing very slowly. Rarely, it suddenly becomes malignant, with rapid growth and metastases. The second most common benign neoplasm is the *Warthin Tumor (Papillary Cystadenoma Lymphomatosum),* which most commonly occurs in the tail of the parotid in older men and is bilateral more often than any other salivary gland tumor. Malignancy is suggested by pain and tenderness, rapid tumor growth, paralysis of a branch of the facial nerve, and fixation to the skin or underlying tissues. Biopsy is necessary because the biological behavior of the several tumor types requires different techniques for management.

Salivary Calculus: Sialolithiasis: *Pathophysiology:* Calcium phosphate stones frequently form in the salivary ducts. The cause is unknown. In about 85% of patients with salivary calculi, the stone is in the submaxillary gland or duct. The symptoms are pathognomonic: submandibular swelling, with or without pain, occurs suddenly while the patient is eating and subsides within 2 hours. The sequence may be invariable for several years. Occasionally, the gland becomes infected or the duct obstructed. In parotid duct stone, glandular swelling may persist for several days after onset. In all three glands, calculi are commonly identified by palpation. Approximately 80% of the calculi are calcified, so they can be seen by radiography without contrast. Intraoral dental radiographs are excellent for demonstrating the calculi because they can minimize the density of the mandible by positioning the film properly. An impalpable stone, without calcium, must be detected by sialography.

Diseases of the Submaxillary and Sublingual Glands: These glands are subject to the same diseases as the parotid, with slight variations. Rarely, mumps involves the submaxillary gland without affecting the parotid, although it is more common to have the submaxillary involved secondary to the parotid in mumps. Ranula involving the sublingual or submaxillary gland is described on page 308.

Thyroid Syndromes

Hypothyroidism: See Chapter 5, page 123.

● KEY SIGN
Hyperthyroidism: See Chapter 5, page 124.

S KEY SYNDROME
▼ **Thyroid Enlargement: Goiter:**   Enlargement of the thyroid has many different causes. It is essential to characterize the enlargement as focal or diffuse, nodular or smooth, and to make an assessment of the state of thyroid hormone production: euthyroid, hypothyroid, or hyperthyroid (toxic) [Siminoski K. The rational clinical examination. Does this patient have a goiter? *JAMA* 1995;273:813–817].

● KEY SIGN
▼ **Diffuse Nontoxic Goiter:** *Pathophysiology:* Thyroid-stimulating hormone (TSH) stimulation of thyroid tissue leads to diffuse hyperplasia, while defects in thyroid hormone synthesis limit effective hormone production. All parts of the gland are smooth, enlarged, and firm. The surface may be slightly irregular (*bosselated*); but circumscribed nodules are absent. This is frequently termed *colloid goiter,* or *endemic goiter,* although the terms are not always applicable, because sporadic cases occur in nongoitrous regions. The gland is often more than twice normal size. This size goiter may result from any cause of smaller diffuse glands, except that physiologic hyperplasia rarely becomes so large.

✔ *GOITER—CLINICAL OCCURRENCE:* *Physiologic Euthyroid Hyperplasia* (a) before menstrual periods, (b) from puberty in the female until 20 years of age, (c) during pregnancy; *Hypothyroid* iodine deficiency or with excessive doses of thiouracil drugs, thiocyanates, paraaminosalicylic acid, phenylbutazone, lithium, amiodarone; rarely, in certain patients taking iodides; inherited defects of thyroid enzymes; chronic thyroiditis.

S KEY SYNDROME
▼ **Nontoxic Multinodular Goiter:** *Pathophysiology:* The nodules are polyclonal proliferations, with less-efficient production of thyroid hormone than normal thyroid tissue. This is usually found in persons older than 30 years of age, most often women. The gland may be small or large. The significant feature is the presence of two or more distinct nodules in the parenchyma. The nodules may vary in consistency in the same goiter. Thyroid hormone secretion may be low or normal.

D KEY DISEASE
▼ **Diffuse Toxic Goiter: Graves Disease:** *Pathophysiology:* Thyroid-stimulating antibodies react with the thyroid-stimulating hormone (TSH) receptor to produce TSH-independent hyperplasia and increased release of thyroid hormone. Myxomatous infiltration of the extraocular muscles produces exophthalmos and abnormalities of gaze. Graves disease is an autoimmune disease characterized by goiter, exophthalmos, pretibial myxedema, and hyperthy-

roidism. The thyroid is diffusely enlarged, usually less than twice normal size. Usually the right lobe is larger than the left. Asymmetry may occur from congenital absence of a lobe or the isthmus. A bruit may be heard over the thyroid as a result of the increased blood flow through the tortuous thyroid arteries. The eye signs may be absent or occur any time in the course of the disease; they also can occur without abnormalities of thyroid hormone secretion. The entire spectrum of eye lesions may not occur in a single individual. Often the signs are initially unilateral, the other eye being involved some months later. The signs are lid lag, lid spasm, lacrimation, chemosis, periorbital edema, periorbital infiltration with mucopolysaccharides, and exophthalmos (proptosis) (see Fig. 7-36). Often there is paresis of extraocular muscles, usually involving one or two symmetrical pairs; isolated weakness of the two superior recti is common. The skin over the shins may be the site of circumscribed elevated areas that are firm, nontender, and pink. Paradoxically, this is called *pretibial myxedema;* it usually occurs in association with the ophthalmopathy. A similar finding is thickening of the skin on the dorsa of the fingers or toes (thyroid acropathy) [Weetman AP. Grave's disease. *N Engl J Med* 2000;343:1236–1248].

S KEY SYNDROME

Toxic Multinodular Goiter: *Pathophysiology:* Autonomous function of one or more nodules produces elevated hormone production. This often arises from a long-standing nontoxic multinodular gland. The onset is usually gradual with signs of hyperthyroidism (e.g., atrial fibrillation, weight loss, diarrhea) bringing the patient to the physician. The gland is bilaterally enlarged with multiple nodules apparent by palpation or ultrasound.

S KEY SYNDROME

Retrosternal Goiter (Substernal, Intrathoracic, or Submerged Goiter): When the lower border of a goiter cannot be definitely palpated in the neck, consider the possibility of retrosternal extension, most frequently encountered when the neck is short. Usually, careful palpation of the gland during swallowing will convince the examiner of the extension. Rarely, the goiter may be entirely retrosternal and rise only with increased intrathoracic pressure, as with coughing; this is termed a *plunging goiter.* An increase in retromanubrial dullness seldom occurs. Compression of the trachea may be inferred from the history of dyspnea, or from the *Kocher sign,* in which pressure on the lateral lobe produces stridor. The trachea may be displaced laterally by the goiter (Fig. 7-74A).

A goiter in the superior thoracic aperture may compress other structures, causing (a) cough; (b) dilated veins over the upper thorax from pressure on the internal jugular vein (Fig. 7-79B); also, rarely, edema of the face; (c) nocturnal dyspnea from a posture of the neck assumed during sleep in which the goiter impinges on the trachea; (d) dyspnea while awake, when the head is tilted to the side; and (e) hoarseness, from pressure on the recurrent laryngeal nerve. *Pemberton Sign.* Test the circulation by having the sitting patient hold her arms vertically, touching her face, for a few minutes. In this position, an obstructed thoracic inlet will cause venous suffusion and cyanosis of the face and dyspnea [Wallace C, Siminoski K. The Pemberton sign. *Ann Intern Med* 1996;125:568–569; Auwaerter PG. The Pemberton and Maroni signs. *Ann Intern Med* 1997;126:916 (picture)]. DDX: The internal jugular vein is rarely impaired, so the cyanosis of the face and edema of the neck associated with superior vena caval obstruction are not present. For unknown reasons, retrosternal goiter is associated with a high incidence of hyperthyroidism.

S KEY SYNDROME

Solitary Thyroid Nodule: *Pathophysiology:* A solitary nodule may be a benign or malignant neoplasm, a cyst, or a dominant nodule in a multinodular gland. Many nodules thought to be solitary by palpation are found to be part of a multinodular process by ultrasound. Fine-needle aspiration of solitary nodules is the diagnostic procedure of choice. Irradiation of the thyroid in childhood increases the risk for carcinoma. Finding an isolated nodule in an atrophic thyroid gland suggests a *Plummer nodule* or toxic adenoma [Singer PA, Cooper DS, Daniels GH, et al. Treatment guidelines for patients with thyroid nodules and well-differentiated tyroid cancer. American Thyroid Association. *Arch Intern Med* 1996;156:2165–2172; Mazzaferri EL. Management of a solitary thyroid nodule. *N Engl J Med* 1993;328:553–559].

S KEY SYNDROME

Solitary Thyroid Nodule: Toxic Adenoma: *Pathophysiology:* This benign tumor results when thyroid-stimulating hormone receptors are constitutively activated, with the resultant overproduction of thyroid hormone. The patient has symptoms and signs of hyperthyroidism, and examination shows a single nodule in an otherwise atrophic gland.

D KEY DISEASE

▶ **Solitary Thyroid Nodule: Epithelial Carcinoma:** *Pathophysiology:* Malignant thyroid cancers are classified as papillary, follicular, and anaplastic. Thyroid cancer is more common in women and in those exposed to radiation. It presents as a painless nodule in most cases. Anaplastic cancer spreads widely and rapidly, whereas papillary and follicular cancers spread regionally before widely metastasizing.

D KEY DISEASE

▶ **Solitary Thyroid Nodule: Medullary Carcinoma:** *Pathophysiology:* Neoplasia of the thyroid C cells, which produce calcitonin, is either sporadic or inherited alone, or associated with multiple endocrine neoplasia syndromes (MEN) 2A or 2B. This should be sought in all patients with a family history of MEN-2A or MEN-2B or those with a family history of medullary carcinoma.

S KEY SYNDROME

▼ **Subacute Thyroiditis: DE Quervain Thyroiditis, Viral Thyroiditis:** *Pathophysiology:* Acute inflammation of the thyroid from viral infection or postinfectious inflammation results in release of thyroid hormone from the damaged follicles producing hyperthyroidism with depressed thyroid-stimulating hormone and iodine uptake. The patient may complain of pain with swallowing. The pain is frequently referred to the ear, so the physician may be consulted for earache. The gland is unusually firm and rather small (20–30 g), but it frequently contains one or more, often tender, nodules. The patient may be euthyroid or hyperthyroid in the acute phase [Pearce EN, Farwell AP, Braverman LE. Thyroiditis. *N Engl J Med* 2003;348:2646–2655].

● KEY SIGN

■ **Subacute Thyroiditis: Hashimoto and Postpartum Thyroiditis:** These syndromes most often present with symptoms and signs of abnormal thyroid function. Although a goiter may be present, the thyroid is nontender and may not appear a likely source of the problems.

● KEY SIGN

■ **Chronic Thyroiditis: Reidel Thyroiditis:** *Pathophysiology:* The thyroid gland is densely fibrotic with fibrosis extending into the surrounding tissues; the cause is unknown. Patients may present with compressive symptoms of the esophagus, trachea, neck veins, or recurrent laryngeal nerves. Women in midlife are most often affected; thyroid function is usually preserved. The gland is hard and fixed.

ADDITIONAL READING

Jonathan D. Trobe. The Physician's Guide to Eye Care. San Francisco, *The American Academy of Ophthalmology*, 1993.

8 The Chest: Chest Wall, Pulmonary, and Cardiovascular Systems; The Breasts

Section 1 CHEST WALL, PULMONARY AND CARDIOVASCULAR SYSTEMS

Major Systems: Physiology and Respiratory Mechanics

The thorax encloses the visceral organs of the chest and is the mechanical platform for arm and neck motion and powers breathing. It is bounded anteriorly by the sternum and ribs, laterally and posteriorly by the ribs, and supported posteriorly by the spine. The inferior boundary is the diaphragm and rib margins. Superiorly it is bounded by the clavicles and soft tissues of the neck. The bony thorax is covered with skeletal muscles involved in spinal posture and motion and arm stability and motion. The intercostal muscles, diaphragm and, to a lesser extent, the major anterior neck muscles, power the thoracic bellows.

The Thoracic Wall

The thoracic wall includes the bodies of the 12 thoracic vertebrae, the 12 pairs of ribs, and the sternum. The bones are arranged as a cage covered by skin, subcutaneous tissue, fascia, and muscles, with accompanying blood vessels, nerves, and lymphatic channels. Certain anatomic facts are pertinent to the physical examination.

Bones of the Thorax

The **shape of the thorax** resembles a truncated cone whose varied circumferences are pairs of ribs, each pair having a greater diameter than that immediately above it, so the sternovertebral dimension is much smaller at the top than at the base. Each rib is separated from adjacent ones by intercostal spaces; the space takes its numbers from the rib above. The first rib slopes slightly downward from vertebra to sternum; each succeeding rib has a greater slope than the one above; thus, the width of the intercostal spaces increases progressively from top to bottom.

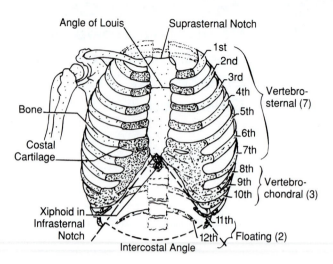

Fig. 8-1 The Bony Thorax. *The left clavicle is removed exposing the underlying first rib. The cartilages of the xiphoid and ribs are stippled. Note the surface landmarks: the suprasternal notch, the angle of Louis, and the infrasternal notch. The two lower rib margins form the intercostal angle.*

The **sternum** is a flat bone in the anterior midline of the thorax (Fig. 8-1). Shaped like an ancient Greek sword pointing downward, it consists of the manubrium (handle), the gladiolus (blade), and the xiphoid cartilage (tip). The manubrium is joined to the gladiolus by a fibrocartilage that sometimes develops a synovial cavity, but mobility is slight. The xiphoid cartilage is fixed to the lower end of the gladiolus and usually develops calcification during later life. Commonly, it is either lance-shaped or bifid and may be mistaken for an abdominal mass when it angulates forward.

Each **rib** is a flattened, arched bone. Its vertebral end has a head, neck, and double tubercle. The sternal end continues as a costal cartilage. In *typical ribs,* a bipartite arthrodial (gliding) joint binds the head to the bodies of the two adjacent vertebrae and their intervertebral disk. A second arthrodial joint connects the articular tubercle of the neck with the transverse process of the upper vertebra, so each rib has two connections with the vertebral column. The first, tenth, eleventh, and twelfth ribs are *atypical.* Each articulates with a single vertebra. The costal cartilages of the first to seventh ribs, inclusive, join the sternum. They are *vertebrosternal* or *true ribs.* The eighth to twelfth ribs are *false ribs.* The eight, ninth, and tenth ribs are *vertebrochondral,* each costal cartilage usually joining the cartilage of the rib above, although many variations are found. The eleventh and twelfth ribs, free at their anterior ends, are termed *vertebral or floating ribs.* The costal cartilage of the first rib articulates with the manubrium by a synarthrodial (fixed) joint. The other six true ribs attach to the sternum by arthrodial joints with synovial cavities. The second rib is exceptional in having two synovial cavities by which it makes contact with interfaces on both the manubrium and gladiolus at their fibrocartilage.

Muscles of the Thoracic Wall

The intercostal spaces contain the intercostales externi and interni. Each is a muscle sheet between adjacent edges of two ribs that draws the bones together. When the first rib is fixed by contraction of the scaleni, the externi and interni pull the ribs upward; the action is aided by the levatores costarum and the serratus posterior superior. When the last rib is fixed by contraction of the quadratus lumborum, the subcostales and the transversus thoracis draw the ribs downward.

The Respiratory System

The respiratory system in the chest is composed of the trachea entering superiorly, the lungs with their branching airways, arterial, venous, and lymphatic vascular channels, and the pleura, which lines both the lung (visceral pleura) and the chest wall and mediastinum (parietal pleura). The space between the two pleural layers is a potential space, normally with a negative pressure relative to atmospheric pressure. This negative pressure maintains lung distention and transfers the inspiratory forces of diaphragm flattening and chest expansion to the lung. Introduction of air into this space (pneumothorax) destroys mechanical coupling of chest motion to lung expansion. Expiration is largely passive relying on the elastic recoil of the lung and chest wall, although forced expiration through contraction of the abdominal and chest wall muscles can greatly accelerate airflow through normal airways.

Respiratory Excursions of the Thorax

At the end of expiration, the volume of the thorax is at its smallest. Inspiration expands the thoracic volume by increasing the dimensions of the cavity anteroposteriorly, transversely, and vertically. Each integrated component of this movement will be considered separately.

ANTERIOR BULGING OF THE THORAX. In Figure 8-2A, consider the geometry of a cylindrical pail with its wire handle bowed in a semicircle of slightly greater diameter than the cylinder. When the handle hangs down obliquely, the distance from its center to the cylindric axis coincides with the radius of the pail. As the handle is raised toward the horizontal, its periphery travels away from the sides of the pail. Now consider the model in Figure 8-2B, where a straight piece of wood represents the thoracic spine, and a vertical stick is the sternum in the position of expiration (*dotted*). The dotted hoop represents a pair of ribs, acting together as a circle, whose plane slants downward from the transverse axis of rotation through the spine. When the sternum and first rib are pulled upward, the costal ring rotates to push the sternum forward and upward. Anatomically, this movement is executed when the sternum and first rib are fixed by the scaleni, while contraction of the external and internal intercostal muscles narrows the interspaces. The ribs are pulled upward and the sternum thrust forward, increasing the anteroposterior dimension of the thoracic cavity.

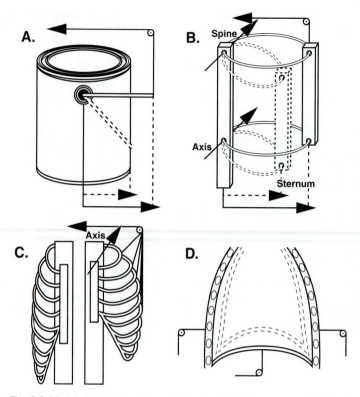

Fig. 8-2 Models Illustrating Thoracic Respiratory Movements.   A. At rest, the handle of a cylindric paint can hangs obliquely, so its center and the side of the pail are equidistant from the central axis of the cylinder. When the handle is raised to the horizontal, the center of the handle diverges from the side increasing the distance from the central axis. B. In this model, two parallel rigid hoops pierce two vertical sticks. Elevation of the front stick (representing the sternum) will increase the distance between it and the other stick (representing the spine). The differences in the points of the arrows show this change in the anteroposterior diameter. C. The semicircular ribs hang from the sternum and the spine, like the hoops in B and the bucket handle in A. The ribs move in such a way that elevation of the sternum and the lateral bows of the ribs during inspiration increases both the transverse (as in A) and the anteroposterior (as in B) diameters of the thorax. D. Inspiratory volume further augmented by depression of the diaphragm.

LATERAL EXTENSION OF THE THORAX.   Consider a similar model in Figure 8-2C, where the sternum and the first rib are fixed. Each rib of a pair is a separate semicircle rotating on an anteroposterior axis. During expiration, the planes of the hoops slant downward on either side of the axis. When the hoops are pulled upward toward the horizontal, each hoop acts as a pail handle by moving further from the center, increasing the transverse dimension. Anatomically, the narrowing of the interspaces by the intercostal muscles causes elevation of the rib curves to increase the transverse diameter of the thorax.

Thus, fixation of the first rib and manubrium by the scaleni and the narrowing of the interspaces by the intercostal muscles cause rotation of each rib, except the first, on both an anteroposterior and a transverse axis, which expands the corresponding dimensions of the thoracic cavity. Because the lower ribs are longer and more oblique, and the interspaces are wider, the amplitude of movement is greater in the lower thorax.

VERTICAL ELONGATION OF THE THORACIC CAVITY. The diaphragm is an elliptic sheet of muscle whose center is a fibrous aponeurosis. The edges of the sheet are fixed to the lower ribs while the center forms a dome into the thoracic cavity. After expiration, the dome is high and the thoracic walls are closest together (see Fig. 8-2D). During inspiration, the walls diverge, lowering the diaphragmatic dome. The dome is further flattened by contraction of the muscular diaphragm during inspiration. Lowering the diaphragm elongates the vertical dimension of the thoracic cavity to increase its volume.

It is important to remember that volume varies as the third power of changes in linear dimension. Therefore, relatively small changes in the height, width, and depth of the thoracic cavity lead to large changes in its volume.

The Lungs and Pleura

The airways of the respiratory system include the nasal passages and nasopharynx, the mouth and oropharynx, the larynx, the trachea, and the branches of the bronchial tree supplying the pulmonary alveoli. Surmounting the trachea, the larynx is a frequent site of obstruction, either from intrinsic swelling or by paralysis of its vocal cords.

The Bronchial Tree

The trachea bifurcates asymmetrically into the right and left bronchus at a dividing septum, the carina. The left bronchus diverges at a greater angle from the trachea than the right bronchus, explaining why foreign bodies are more likely to lodge in the right main stem bronchus. The right bronchus sends a lobar bronchus to each of three pulmonary lobes; the left bronchus forms two lobar bronchi. Each first branch of a lobar bronchus supplies a bronchopulmonary segment of lung. The heart lies in front of the tracheal bifurcation and the aorta arches over the left bronchus from front to back. Interposed between the aorta and bronchus is the left recurrent laryngeal nerve, which descends in front of the aortic arch, loops under it, and ascends beside the trachea to the neck. The dilated aorta may produce a tracheal tug by pulsating against the left bronchus, or it may compress the left recurrent laryngeal nerve against the left bronchus, with resulting paralysis of the left vocal cord.

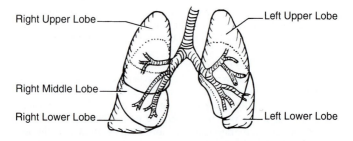

Fig. 8-3 The Lobes of the Lungs. *The transparent diagram shows the anterior aspects of the pulmonary lobes and their main bronchi. Note the three divisions of the right main bronchus and the more direct line with the trachea on the right side. The dotted line shows the posterior extent of the lower lobes.*

The Lungs

The lungs may be regarded as clusters of pulmonary alveoli around the subdivisions of the bronchial tree. The right lung has three major masses: the right upper lobe, the right middle lobe, and the right lower lobe. The left lung has two lobes: the left upper lobe and the left lower lobe. Each lobe is separated from the others in the same lung by a lobar fissure, an infolding of visceral pleura. Molded by the contour of the thoracic cavity, the shape of both lungs is similar, but the medial edge of the left lung has an inferior indentation, the cardiac notch. Each lobe is further divided into bronchopulmonary segments, consisting of the cluster of alveoli supplied by a single first branch of the lobar bronchus (Figs. 8-3 and 8-4). These divisions are not demarcated by fissures; their limits are demonstrable only by special dissections with injected preparations. When present, extra fissures do follow these boundaries. In the practice of thoracic surgery, the lingula tends to be regarded as a separate lobe, homologous to the right middle lobe.

The Pleura

The relations of a single lung to its pleura can be visualized by imagining a sphere of thin plastic material from which the air is being evacuated (Fig. 8-5). As the sphere collapses, one part invaginates to form a hollow hemisphere with convex and concave layers in apposition. The convex layer is cemented to the inside of the thoracic cavity representing the parietal pleura. Place the lung in the concavity of the hemisphere and cement its surface to the concave layer, representing the visceral pleura. Arrange the invagination of the sphere so the parietal pleura has a greater area than the visceral pleura, permitting the lung some mobility in the thoracic cavity. Anatomically, the parietal pleura is adherent to the thoracic wall; the visceral pleura is fixed to the lung surface and also lines the interlobar fissures. The two apposing layers form the pleural cavity, devoid of air and containing only enough fluid for lubrication. The parietal pleura has the greater area, extending inferiorly on the ribs and diaphragm some distance below the lower tip of the lung

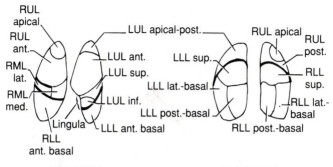

ANTERIOR   **POSTERIOR**

Fig. 8-4 Lung Segments. *Each lobe is divided into segments. The thick lines are the anatomical fissures, readily identified on inspection of the lung and often in radiographs. The thinner lines are established only by careful dissections of injected preparations. In the abbreviations the first capital letter designates "right" or "left"; the second, "upper," "middle," or "lower"; the third L is for "lobe." Note that the lingula, composed of the superior and inferior segments of the left upper lobe, is near the heart and corresponds in many respects to the right middle lobe.*

to form the costophrenic sinus. The lung descends part way into this sinus during deep inspiration.

Mechanics of the Lung and Pleura

When the otherwise normal lung is removed from the thoracic cavity, it partially collapses from the elastic recoil of its tissue. Even so, the lung

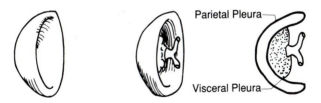

Fig. 8-5 Modelling the Relationship of the Pleura and Lung. *Deflate a rubber or plastic sphere so that it assumes a hemisphere with a concave and convex surface. Place a model lung in the concavity and cement the lung surface to the inner surface of the hemisphere. On the right, in cross section, the parietal pleura is represented by the convex surface of the hemisphere; the cemented layers represent the visceral pleura. To complete the model, exhaust the hemisphere of air, replacing it with a little fluid to lubricate the inner surface. This geometry should be visualized in the examination of the chest and when looking at x-ray films, remembering that the pleural surfaces are anterior, lateral, medial, and inferior.*

contains enough trapped air to make it float on water. The organ feels tough, elastic, spongy, light in weight, and crepitant, that is, it crackles from the movement of air bubbles under the pressing fingers. The volume of the collapsed lung is much smaller than the hemithorax from whence it came. When the lung is in the closed thorax, its volume is much greater because its surface is held against the thoracic wall by the apposition of the parietal and visceral pleurae. Contact between the two pleural layers is maintained because the pleural sac is devoid of air, so the layers are pressed together by the weight of the atmosphere on the thoracic wall and parietal pleura on one side, and the column of air under atmospheric pressure in the airway pressing through the alveoli on the other side. The atmospheric pressure resists any force tending to separate the pleural layers. The elastic recoil of the lungs exerts such a separating pull. If a needle attached to a water manometer is inserted into the empty pleural space, the pressure during expiration registers about 25 cm of water, roughly a measure of the elastic recoil of the lung and thorax. During inspiration, the negative pressure increases to about 215 cm of water because additional elastic recoil is produced by stretching the lung as the thorax expands.

The parietal pleura contains sensory nerve endings, but the visceral pleura is anesthetic. This is significant in performing thoracentesis.

The Cardiovascular System

The Circulation

The circulatory system includes the heart, the blood and its conducting vessels, the lymph and its ducts, and the vessel walls. Vascular phenomena are divided into those dependent on cardiac action and those caused by local disorders of blood vessels. The cardiovascular system extends to every part of the body, but the source of mechanical power to maintain circulation, the heart, is intrathoracic, as are the origins of the major arteries. Blood returning from the extremities enters the chest from the abdomen and lower extremities via the inferior vena cava (IVC), and from the arms and head via the axillary and jugular veins, which merge into the brachiocephalic veins and superior vena cava (SVC) in the mediastinum. The heart is suspended from the great vessels (aorta, pulmonary artery, pulmonary veins, IVC, and SVC) within the pericardium, which allows free motion of the heart during ventricular contraction.

The Cardiac Conduction System

The normal pacemaker of the heart is the sinoatrial (SA) node located in the right atrial wall near the entrance of the superior vena cava (see Fig. 4-1). It originates rhythmic waves of excitation that spread quickly through both atria until they reach the atrioventricular (AV) node near the posterior margin of the interatrial septum. The AV node delays conduction during atrial systole. The impulse then passes down the bundle of His, which divides into right and left bundle branches to the muscle of the right and left ventricles. Conduction is normally very rapid, arriving nearly simultaneously in both atria, and, after AV delay, in both ventricles. Deviations in the timing or pathways taken by these electrical waves cause changes in rate, rhythm and electrical pattern of the P, QRS, and T waves that can be analyzed with considerable accuracy by the electrocardiogram (ECG). Normal cardiac function results when these electrical signals trigger mechanical muscular contraction via the cellular process of electrical–mechanical coupling.

Heart Movement and Function

The myocardial muscle fibers form a complete spiral, so contraction produces a decrease in all diameters during systole. The apex rotates forward and to the right, approaching the chest wall and frequently causing a visible and palpable thrust, the *apical impulse.* Occurring early in systole, this thrust serves the examiner as a marker for the onset of cardiac contraction.

The heart has extremely high oxygen and energy requirements and the highest oxygen extraction of any organ in the body. As a result, it is particularly sensitive to decreases in blood supply. Blood flow within the heart and lungs is dependent upon complete functional separation of the cardiac chambers by intact interatrial and interventricular septa and functional valves. Valve closure, turbulent blood flow, and the mechanical contraction of the heart can be felt and auscultated through the chest wall.

Peripheral Arteries

Blood is distributed to the body through the major branches of the aorta, which are easily examined where they leave the chest (carotid and axillary arteries) or abdomen (femoral arteries). Measurement of blood pressure and estimates of the blood flow within the arterial tree are easily performed on physical examination.

Superficial Thoracic Anatomy

The Chest Wall

The anterior surface of the sternum is subcutaneous, so it presents landmarks for inspection and palpation. The separated heads of the clavicles form the sides of the *suprasternal notch* (jugular notch); its base is the superior edge of the manubrium (see Figs. 8-1 and 8-6). The junction of the manubrium and gladiolus produces a slight angle protruding anteriorly, the *angle of Louis* (angle of Ludwig, sternal angle). This marks the second rib articulating with the manubrium-gladiolus. At the inferior end of the gladiolus is a slight depression, the infrasternal notch, formed by the junction of the costal cartilages of the two seventh ribs. Immediately beneath this, the xiphoid cartilage may be felt and, sometimes seen.

Portions of most ribs can be seen or palpated, except the first rib, which is effectually overlaid by the clavicle. The pectoralis major and

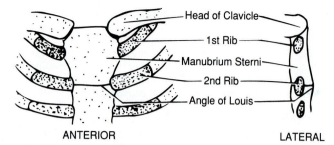

ANTERIOR   LATERAL

Fig. 8-6 The Angle of Louis. *The adjacent edges of the manubrium and gla-diolus form the angle of Louis. This is a landmark for counting ribs anteriorly because the second rib abuts the junction that forms the angle. The costicartilage of the second rib articulates with the fibrocartilage between the manubrium and the gladiolus and with the edges of both bones.*

the female breasts obscure palpation of parts of the ribs anteriorly; the latissimus dorsi covers some ribs in the axillary line. Posteriorly, the scapulae cover parts of the second to seventh ribs, inclusive. With the arms at the sides, the inferior border of the scapula is usually at the seventh or eighth intercostal space, serving as the usual landmark for counting ribs in the back (Fig. 8-7). The inferior margins of the seventh, eighth, and ninth costicartilages on the two sides meet in the midline to form the *infrasternal angle* (intercostal angle); the angle may be considerably more or less than 90 degrees. The diagram (see Fig. 8-1) shows that an oblique line drawn from the head of the clavicle to the anterior axillary line on the ninth rib locates approximately the costochondral junctions of the second to tenth ribs.

The bony thorax is a truncated cone narrowing superiorly. This narrowing is partially obscured by the overlying clavicles, the shoulders,

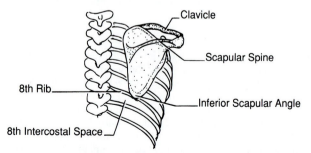

Fig. 8-7 Surface Landmarks of the Posterior Thorax. *Note the relation of the scapulae to the ribs. The inferior angle of the scapula is usually at the eighth interspace; this allows one to identify the eighth rib posteriorly to count ribs in the back.*

and muscles of the upper chest and arms, which give the body its broad shouldered, squared-off contour. The smaller radius of curvature and overlying muscles makes the upper ribs much less susceptible to mechanical injury than the lower ribs whose larger radii, superficial location, and extensive anterior cartilage make them vulnerable to injury. The clavicles, sternum, and lower ribs are palpable throughout their extent. The sternal angle of Louis is at the second intercostal space, a useful landmark for identifying ribs and interspaces. The scapula overlies the posterior chest wall lateral to the spine. It is overlaid with skeletal muscle and glides on the chest wall. Its medial border, inferior angle, lateral border, spine, acromion and coracoid process are easily palpable. The lungs extend to the thoracic apex and may extend superiorly into the base of the neck where they are vulnerable to penetrating injury. The pleural spaces coapt in the anterior superior mediastinum, but are separated posteriorly by the spine and mediastinum and anteriorly and inferiorly by the pericardial sack and heart. The heart lies retrosternally and to the left with the right ventricle in the retrosternal position and the left ventricle left lateral and posterior. The liver and spleen are positioned inferior to the diaphragm deep to the inferior ribs. Deep inspiration with flattening of the diaphragm pushes them toward the costal margins where the normal liver and enlarged spleen can be palpated. The axillary folds are formed by the pectoralis major anteriorly and the subscapularis and latissimus dorsi posteriorly.

The Lungs and Pleura

The topography of the five lung lobes has some clinical applications. In Figure 8-8, note that the anterior aspect of the right lung is formed almost entirely of the right upper and middle lobes; the posterior aspect contains only the upper and lower lobes. In the left lung, the upper and lower lobes present both back and front.

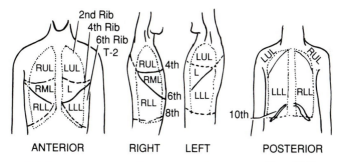

Fig. 8-8 Topography of the Five Lobes of the Lungs. *The solid lines are the pulmonary fissures; the broken lines are projections. The boundary of the lingula (L) is hypothetical.*

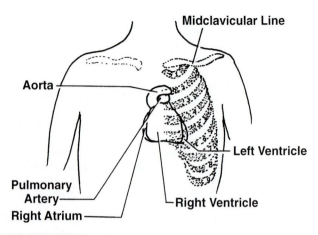

Fig. 8-9 Precordial Projections of the Anterior Surface of the Heart. *The entire central area of the precordium is a projection of the right ventricle. The left border and apex are formed by the left ventricle; the right atrium is the right border.*

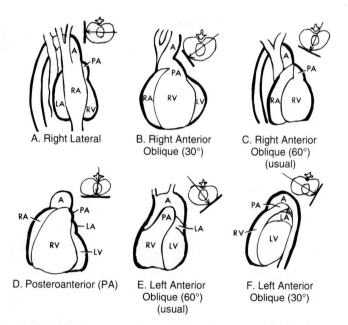

Fig. 8-10 X-Ray Silhouettes of the Heart. *The positions are named for the aspect of the patient's thorax that faces the cassette (except for the posteroanterior [PA] view). Angles are measured between the direction of the x-ray beam and the plane of the patient's back. The heavy lines on the silhouettes indicate distinctive segments used in diagnosis.*

The Heart and Precordium

The anterior surface of the chest closest to the heart and aorta is termed the precordium. Normally, this area extends vertically from the second to the fifth intercostal space, transversely from the right border of the sternum to the left midclavicular line in the fifth and sixth interspaces. The upper epigastrium is occasionally included. When the heart is enlarged or displaced, the boundaries of the precordium shift accordingly. In dextrocardia, all signs described herein are located in the opposite hemithorax.

The projections of the normal heart upon the precordium are depicted in Figure 8-9 and their projection on a chest radiograph are depicted in Figure 8-10. Behind the manubrium sterni are the arch of the aorta and other mediastinal structures. The right border of the heart corresponds roughly to the right edge of the sternum from the third to fifth interspaces. The right atrium forms the right border with the right ventricle anterior under the sternum and left lower ribs. The left ventricle forms the cardiac apex and a slender area of the left border, and sits posteriorly to the right ventricle. Thus, the right ventricle forms most of the anterior surface of the heart even though it forms neither lateral border.

Physical Examination of the Chest and Major Vessels

Examination of the Rib Cage and Thoracic Musculature

Inspection

INSPECTION OF THE THORACIC WALL.   Examine the skin over the thorax for lesions that restrict respiratory excursion. Note structural deformities of the thorax. Observe several respiratory cycles noting the respiratory rate, amplitude, rhythm, and movements of the chest. Look for labored inspiration, intercostal retraction, and forced expiration, while noting cough or noisy breathing. Palpate with the palms of the hands to confirm areas of dyskinetic chest wall motion. Note the amplitude of diaphragmatic movements. Be sure to inspect the chest wall of the supine patient from the foot of the bed. The findings from inspection are supplemented by signs obtained with palpation, percussion, and auscultation.

INSPECTION OF THE THORACIC SPINE.   Have the patient stand or sit; inspect the profile of the spine from the side for kyphosis, lordosis, and gibbus. From the back, look for lateral deviation of the spinous processes indicating scoliosis. When the curvature is slight, or the patient is very fat, palpate each spinous process and mark its location with a skin pencil to detect a deviation. Consider the possibility of kyphoscoliosis, a combination of lateral and anteroposterior deviation. This is sufficient examination of the spine to evaluate the thorax; a more detailed spinal examination is described in Chapter 13 on page 690–693.

Palpation

PALPATION OF THE TRACHEA.   Assess the position of the trachea by palpating its connections to the tissues in the suprasternal notch. Place your forefinger in the suprasternal notch and feel the space between the heads of the clavicles and the lateral border of the trachea. Alternatively, direct the finger posteriorly through the middle of the suprasternal notch until the fingertip touches the tracheal rings. If the apex of the rings touches the finger on the center of its tip, the trachea is in the midline.

PALPATION OF THE THORACIC WALL.   Palpation is indicated in the presence of (a) any pain in the chest, (b) masses seen in the chest wall, (c) masses apparently in the breast, and (d) draining sinuses in the thorax. Examine the soft tissues by pressing or pinching the large muscles of the thorax to elicit tenderness; if tender, try to determine the movements that elicit pain. Feel for soft-tissue crepitus. Palpate the interspaces for tenderness and masses. Examine the costal cartilages and palpate the costochondral junctions testing them for tenderness, swelling, and mobility. Palpate the ribs for point tenderness, swelling, bone crepitus, and remote pain on compression. Palpate the xiphisternal joint for tenderness.

TESTING EXCURSION OF THE UPPER THORAX.   Place a hand on each side of the patient's neck with palms against the upper anterior thoracic wall. Curl the fingers firmly over the superior edges of the trapezii. Move the palms downward against the skin, to provide slack, until the palms lie in the infraclavicular fossae. Then extend your thumbs so their tips meet in the midline (Fig. 8-11A). Have the patient inspire deeply, which permits your palms to move freely with the chest while your fingers are anchored firmly above on the trapezii. The upper four ribs move forward with inspiration, so your thumbs diverge from the midline. Normally, the thumbs move laterally for equal distances. Asymmetric excursions suggest a lesion on the lagging side in the chest wall, the pleura, or the upper lobe of the lung.

TESTING EXCURSION OF THE ANTERIOR MIDDLE THORAX.   With your fingers high in each axilla and your thumbs abducted, place the palms on the anterior chest. Move the hands medially, dragging skin to provide slack, until the thumb tips meet in the midline at the level of the sixth ribs (see Fig. 8-11B). Have the patient inspire deeply letting your hands follow the chest movements. The thumbs should move apart. A unilateral lag indicates a nearby lesion in the wall, pleura, middle lobe of the right lung, or lingula of the left lung.

TESTING EXCURSION OF THE POSTERIOR LOWER CHEST.   Have the patient sit or stand with his back toward you. Place your fingers in each axilla, with the palms applied firmly to the patient's chest, so your forefingers are one or two ribs below the inferior angles of the scapulae. To provide slack, press the soft tissues and pull your hands medially until your thumbs meet over the vertebral spines (see Fig. 8-11C). Have the patient inspire deeply, following the lateral movements of the chest with your

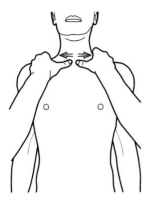

A. Testing of Upper Thorax

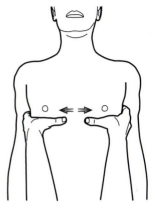

B. Testing of Expansion of Midthorax

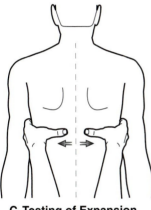

C. Testing of Expansion of Posterior Thorax

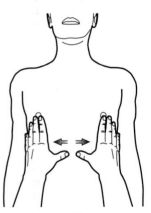

D. Testing Movements of Costal Margins

Fig. 8-11 Testing Thoracic Movement. A. The Upper Anterior Thorax. B. Expansion of the Anterior Mid-Thorax. C. Expansion of the Posterior Thorax. D. Movement of Costal Margins.

hands; your thumbs should move apart. A unilateral lag indicates a lesion in the nearby wall, pleura, or lower lobes of the lung.

TESTING EXCURSION OF THE COSTAL MARGINS. With the patient supine, place your hands so the extended thumbs lie along the inferior edges of the costal margins, with their tips nearly touching (see Fig. 8-11D). Have the patient inspire deeply, letting your thumbs follow the costal margins. Normally, the thumbs diverge. Diminished divergence indicates depression of the dome of the diaphragm; convergence results when the dome is considerably flattened.

Examination of the Lungs and Pleura

Some argue that physical examination of the lungs and pleura is no longer necessary, because x-ray examination is readily available and discloses many lesions without physical signs. While the usefulness of x-ray examination is acknowledged, it does not replace the physical examination of the lungs. Physical examination is rapid, can be performed in all clinical situations, and does not require additional equipment or remove caregivers from the patient. In addition, some clinical conditions are diagnosed only by physical examination, or may be apparent on examination before radiographic signs appear: for example, early pneumonia can be diagnosed by the clinician before x-ray signs appear; a fractured rib may be obvious to palpation weeks before callus is evident in the x-ray film; the radiologist cannot diagnose asthma; the friction rub of pleurisy can appear and subside without x-ray signs; and pulmonary emphysema may be evident clinically before the radiologist can recognize it.

The physical examination of the pleura seeks to detect evidence of pleural inflammation, pleural adhesions, increases in pleural thickness, and the presence of air or excessive fluid in the pleural cavity. The lungs are examined to judge their volume, distensibility, density, changes in airway caliber, and abnormal secretions in the airways. As already indicated, inspection and tactile palpation give some information. Examination is extended by observing the vibratory qualities of the thorax and its contents. Some vibrations may be perceived by vibratory palpation, by using the deep sensibility in the joints and muscles of the examiner's hands. Other vibrations are perceived as sound by the examiner's unaided ears in sonorous and definitive percussion or through the stethoscope in auscultation. Vibrations are produced by the patient's spoken voice and by the examiner tapping the patient's chest. The caliber of the airways and their contained secretions modify the breath sounds or produce extraneous noises heard through the stethoscope.

Examination of the Lungs and Pleura by Palpation

Vibratory Palpation of the Lungs and Pleura.　　Palpation reveals many different types of sensation to the examiner's hands. We have chosen to introduce a more selective term, *vibratory palpation,* to designate specifically the use of the examiner's vibratory sense. This seems justified because a different technique is required. Set a tuning fork in vibration and apply the handle first to the fingertip and then to the palmar base of the finger over the metacarpophalangeal joint; this readily demonstrates the superior sensitivity of the basal part of the finger to vibrations (Fig. 8-12).

During speech, the patient's vocal cords set up vibrations in the bronchial air column that are conducted to the chest wall through the lung septae, where they may be perceived by vibratory palpation, as *vocal (or tactile) fremitus*. Diminished vocal fremitus can be caused by blockage of the airways, or by sound screens of fluid or air in the pleural cavity, or by fibrosis of the pleura itself. Increased transmission of vo-

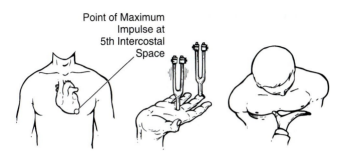

Point of Maximum
Impulse at
5th Intercostal
Space

Fig. 8-12 Vibratory Acuity in Various Parts of the Hand. *Place the handle of a vibrating tuning fork sequentially on the fingertip and the palmar aspect of the metacarpophalangeal joint: the palmar base is more sensitive. This part of the hand should be applied to the precordium to detect thrills.*

cal fremitus occurs with consolidation of the lungs; the density of the tissues is determined by percussion (see pages 356–358). Because the intensity of vocal fremitus is compared in various regions of the chest, equal pitch and loudness must be employed when each test word is spoken. Vocal fremitus is normally more intense in the parasternal region in the right second interspace where it is closest to the bronchial bifurcation. The interscapular region is also near the bronchi and registers increased fremitus. High-pitched voices produce unsatisfactory vibrations for vocal fremitus, so some women must be instructed to lower the pitch of the spoken test words.

PROCEDURE FOR VIBRATORY PALPATION. Ask the patient to sit or stand if the patient is able. Test for vocal fremitus by applying the palmar bases of the fingers of one hand to the interspaces (Fig. 8-13). Alternatively, the ulnar side of the hand and fifth finger may be used. Ask the patient to repeat the test words "ninety-nine" or "one-two-three," using the same pitch and intensity of voice each time. If vibrations are not well

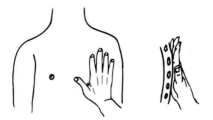

Fig. 8-13 Detection of Vocal Fremitus by Vibratory Palpation. *Symmetrical points on the chest are palpated sequentially with the same hand and the strength of vocal fremitus is compared in different regions. The palpating hand is applied firmly to the chest wall with palm in contact with the wall, and vibrations are sensed with the bases of the fingers.*

felt, have the patient lower the pitch of the voice. With the same hand, compare symmetrical parts of the chest sequentially, such as the left infraclavicular fossa, then the right; left fourth interspace, then right. It is easier to compare two sensations sequentially with the same hand than to compare simultaneous sensations from two hands. When the lower thorax is reached, use the ulnar surface of the hand in the interspaces to ascertain the point at which fremitus is lost. In the absence of a pleural lesion, this maneuver should indicate the position of the lung bases. This site should be compared with that obtained by percussion and the transmission of breath sounds by auscultation. With the same method, feel for pleural friction rubs (*friction fremitus*) over the thorax.

Percussion of the Lungs and Pleura

THORACIC PERCUSSION.   See Chapter 3, page 43 for a discussion of the techniques of percussion. Percuss the back with the patient sitting and the anterior chest with the patient sitting and supine. The borders of the heart are outlined, and both sonorous and definitive percussion are applied to the back. The entire examination can be conducted from the patient's right side. With the patient ill in bed and unable to sit, the patient must be examined in the right and left lateral decubitus positions. This position introduces problems in the interpretation of percussion sounds. Changing position may be painful for an ill patient and laborious for the attendant, so you may choose to inspect, palpate, percuss, and auscultate the front, then repeat the sequence on the next aspect that is presented on moving. A routine sequence for thoracic percussion is described; many other plans are equally good. A physician interrupts her routine whenever a finding is disclosed that needs further search or introduces new problems (Fig. 8-14).

For best results, press the pleximeter finger into the intercostal spaces between and parallel to the ribs, then strike a series of blows with the plexor.

PERCUSSION OF CARDIAC DULLNESS.   See page 361. Usually, we prefer to do this after inspection and palpation of the precordium; many clinicians use different sequences.

PERCUSSION OF THE ANTERIOR LUNGS.   This procedure calls for sonorous percussion with heavy indirect bimanual percussion. To make the lateral aspects of the thorax accessible in the supine position, the patient's arms should be slightly abducted; when standing or sitting, the patient's hands should rest on his hips. Starting under the clavicles, compare the percussion sound from each interspace sequentially with that from the contralateral region. Work downward to the region of hepatic dullness on the right and the Traube semilunar space on the left (see Fig. 8-14). Also percuss the lateral aspects of the thorax. The entire anterior region should be resonant, except for the area of cardiac dullness.

PERCUSSION OF HEPATIC DULLNESS.   The domed superior aspect of the liver normally produces a transverse zone of dullness from the fourth to the sixth interspaces in the right midclavicular line. Because a wedge of lung, edge downward, intervenes between the upper border of the

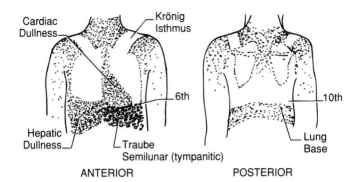

Cardiac Dullness — Krönig Isthmus

6th

Hepatic Dullness — Traube Semilunar (tympanitic)

ANTERIOR

10th — Lung Base

POSTERIOR

Fig. 8-14 Percussion Map of the Thorax.   The entire lung surface is normally resonant. At the apices, a band of resonance, known as the Krönig isthmus, runs over the shoulders like shoulder straps. Hepatic dullness ranges downward from the right sixth rib to merge into hepatic flatness. The Traube semilunar space of tympany extends downward from the left sixth rib; it is variable in extent, depending upon the amount of gas in the stomach. Posteriorly, the dullness below the lung bases begins at about the tenth rib.

liver and the chest wall, the transition in the sixth interspace from lung resonance to hepatic dullness is subtle and gradual. The lower border of the dull zone merges into hepatic flatness when percussion is carried below the edge of the lung.

PERCUSSION OF GASTRIC TYMPANY.   Normally, the stomach contains an air bubble of variable size that yields tympany in an area known as the *Traube semilunar space.* The upper tympanitic border is somewhat lower than the upper border of the liver on the opposite site, because the left diaphragm is lower. The anterior horn of the half-moon ends in the lower border of cardiac dullness. The variable volume of air in the stomach vitiates the diagnostic value of this area.

PERCUSSION OF SPLENIC DULLNESS.   The splenic dullness is an oval between the ninth and eleventh ribs in the left midaxillary line. Gastric or colonic tympany often obscures it completely. Also, the area of dullness in the region may be greatly enlarged by fluid or solids in the stomach or colon or by pleural effusion. The splenic area is worthy of percussion, however, because an enlarged spleen is seldom obscured by gas, and an increased area of splenic dullness prompts more searching palpation for the organ.

PERCUSSION OF THE LUNG APICES.   The patient must be sitting or standing. The apices of the lungs normally extend slightly above the clavicles, producing a band of resonance over each shoulder, widening at its scapular and clavicular ends. The narrowest part, termed the *Krönig isthmus,* lies on the shoulder top. Reproducibility of this finding is low. We merely sound each supraclavicular fossa by modified indirect percussion. For the pleximeter on the right, the examiner's left thumb is ap-

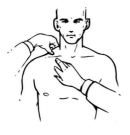
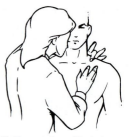

A. Percussion of Right Apex   B. Percussion of Left Apex

Fig. 8-15 Percussion of the Lung Apices. *Bimanual indirect percussion is applied in the usual fashion, except for the use of the pleximeter. See the text for descriptions.*

plied to the right supraclavicular fossa by sliding it down from the edge of the trapezius muscle (Fig. 8-15A). For the pleximeter in the left fossa, the examiner's left arm is put around the patient's back, and the left long finger is curled anteriorly over the trapezius muscle into the fossa, where it is struck by the plexor finger of the right hand (Fig. 8-15B). Fibrosis or infiltration of the lung narrows or obliterates the resonance.

PERCUSSION OF THE POSTERIOR LUNG. This is sonorous percussion with the patient sitting or standing. The patient's arms are folded in front and she is requested to pull her shoulders forward ("hump the shoulders"), with the spine slightly anteflexed. Percussion of each hemithorax is begun at the top, working downward to compare symmetrical regions sequentially. The scapular muscles and bones impair resonance in proportion to their mass, so interpretation of percussion notes is difficult, but symmetry should be preserved. The zone of resonance ends inferiorly at about the ninth rib, the left being lower than the right (see Fig. 8-14).

PERCUSSION OF THE POSTERIOR LUNG BASES. During quiet respiration, the inferior lung edges are relatively high in the costophrenic sulci, usually at about the ninth rib on the left and the eighth interspace on the right. The transition between lung resonance and muscle dullness or flatness is gradual over the wedge-shaped lung bases. Light percussion is required. After the lung bases have been located during quiet respiration, mark the level, and have the patient inspire deeply and hold her breath while you percuss the level after descent. Normally, the bases should move downward 5 or 6 cm.

DEFINITIVE PERCUSSION OF THE CHEST. In the examination of the thorax, definitive percussion is employed to outline the borders between lung resonance and dullness of the heart, the spleen, the upper border of the liver, and the lumbar muscles below the lung bases. The boundary between resonant lung and tympanitic gastric bubble outlines the Traube semilunar space. The Krönig isthmus over the lung apices is defined by percussing the area of resonance in the supraclavicular fossae.

Auscultation of the Lungs and Pleura

Movements of the tracheobronchial air column produces vibrations that are perceived as sounds. Sounds from the lungs and heart have a frequency range between 60 and 3000 cycles per second. Vibrations may occur from air eddies in quiet breathing through normal airways, from air moving in dilated or constricted tubes, from the behavior of fluid moved by the air, or from the vocal cords. The absence of the sounds normally produced by the tracheobronchial air column indicates blockage in the airways or an abnormal screening of sound in the pleural cavity.

PROCEDURE IN AUSCULTATION OF THE LUNGS AND PLEURA. Seek a quiet room, which should be warm to eliminate shivering as a cause of muscle sounds. Preferably, have the patient sit. When recumbent, the back should be examined by turning the patient from side to side. Demonstrate how you wish the patient to breathe through the mouth, deeper and slightly more forcefully than usual. Some normal persons cannot cooperate; when their attention is called to their respiration, they heave and puff irregularly, making noises with their mouths. Make certain that the patient is actually breathing deeply rather than making prodigious movements of the chest without exchanging much air. Start listening with the stethoscope diaphragm anteriorly at the apices and work downward, comparing symmetrical points sequentially. Then listen to the back, starting at the apices and working downward. Inferiorly, note where breath sounds disappear comparing these sites with those determined by vocal fremitus and percussion.

At all points on the chest, identify the breath sounds, whether vesicular, bronchovesicular, bronchial, asthmatic, cavernous, or absent, by their duration of inspiration and expiration, and by their quality and pitch (Fig. 8-16). If crackles are heard, note whether they persist or disappear after a few deep breaths. If crackles are not heard, test for posttussive crackles by listening to inspiration after the patient coughs at the end of expiration. If any abnormality is noted, go over the front and back again while the patient whispers test words, such as "one-two-

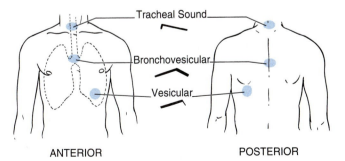

ANTERIOR   POSTERIOR

Fig. 8-16 Breath Sounds Map in the Normal Chest. *The areas of the lungs that are unlabeled have normal vesicular breathing.*

three" or "ninety-nine," to determine the absence or the presence of *whispered pectoriloquy* (page 394–395). Test similarly with the spoken voice for *bronchophony* (page 395). Listen for friction rubs, bone crepitus, and other special sounds.

Bedside Inspection of the Sputum

Inspection of the sputum discloses many valuable diagnostic clues to pulmonary disease. Have a clear plastic sputum cup on the bedside stand and order 24-hour collections of sputum, free from foreign materials. Estimate the daily volume. Note the color, turbidity, and viscosity. Ascertain if it is bloody, frothy, or odoriferous. Place a sample in a petri dish to look for caseous masses, mucous plugs, Curschmann spirals, bronchial casts, and concretions. Whenever indicated, send specimens to the laboratory for culture, cytology, and other examinations.

Examination of the Cardiovascular System

The examination of the cardiovascular system is presented here in a sequence you will find convenient. Assess the body by anatomic regions, so the heart and blood vessels are tested sequentially. Although you should direct special emphasis to the precordium in the physical examination, carefully examine the entire body for the remote signs of cardiovascular dysfunction. A complete cardiovascular examination includes history taking, physical examination and, when indicated, supplementary procedures such as electrocardiography, fluoroscopy, echocardiography, CT and cine-CT, MRI, cardiac catheterization, and angiography.

Physical Examination of the Heart and Precordium

Despite the vast improvements in diagnostic technology, the physical examination of the cardiovascular system remains an essential skill for the expert physician. It seems that practice under the mentorship of an expert is still the best way to learn heart examination, although technology improvements are augmenting the training [Richardson TR, Moody JM. Bedside cardiac examination: Constancy in a sea of change. *Curr Probl Cardiol* 2000;25:783–825]. The physical examination is both sensitive and relatively specific for the diagnosis of valvular heart disease [Roldan CA, Shively BK, Crawford MH. Value of the cardiovascular physical examination for detecting valvular heart disease in asymptomatic subjects. *Am J Cardiol* 1996;77:1327–1331].

PRECORDIAL INSPECTION. The examiner should stand or sit at the patient's right side. Illuminate the precordium from a single source, shining transversely toward the examiner across the anterior chest surface. Alternatively, have the single light source shining from the head or foot, with the observer on the right side. When possible, the patient should be examined both supine and erect. First, look for an *apical impulse,* it is visible in 20% of normal people; then shift your head so your line of sight is across the sternum to detect heaving of the precordium. Finally, inspect the manubrial area.

PRECORDIAL PALPATION. Pulsations, lifts, heaves and thrills can be felt in the precordium by the examiner's senses of touch and vibration. The palmar bases of the fingers are most sensitive to vibrations (see Fig. 8-12), so palpate the precordium with the palm of the hand. First, examine the areas where pulsations are visible; the palpable area should be no larger than 2 cm in diameter. If not visible, try to identify the *apical impulse* by palpation. The impulse is synchronous with the beginning of ventricular systole, in the left fifth interspace 7–9 cm from the midsternal line, or about 1–2 cm medial from the midclavicular line. Frequently, the impulse may be felt when it is not visible, although it often also is not palpable. The strength of the normal impulse must be learned by examining many hearts. Next, feel each part of the precordium systematically. Determine the presence and strength of right and left ventricular thrusts. Palpate over a visible thrust, if present. Pulsations over the base of the heart should be carefully felt. Thrills should be identified and timed as systolic or diastolic by their relation to the apical impulse. Recognize and time pleural and pericardial friction rubs.

PRECORDIAL PERCUSSION. The precordium is percussed to define the cardiac borders (*definitive percussion*). This may be helpful in the absence of a palpable apical impulse or the immediate availability of a chest x-ray. The left arm of the supine patient is abducted; the erect patient is asked to put her left hand on the hip. The sitting woman is requested to hold her left breast up with the left hand. Delineate the *left border of cardiac dullness (LBCD)* by percussing in the fifth, fourth, and third left interspaces sequentially, starting over resonant lung near the axilla and moving medially along an interspace until relative cardiac dullness is encountered (Fig. 8-17). Measure the distance from the midsternal line to the LBCD in the fifth interspace. Measure along a straight line parallel to the transverse diameter of the thorax, not following the curvature of the chest wall so the measurement can be directly compared with posteroanterior film of the chest.

The *right border of cardiac dullness (RBCD)* is sought near the right edge of the sternum. The change from resonant lung to cardiac dullness

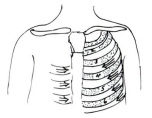

Fig. 8-17 Pattern of Precordial Percussion. *The fifth, fourth, and third intercostal spaces on the left are percussed sequentially, as indicated by the arrows, starting near the axilla and moving medially until cardiac dullness is encountered.*

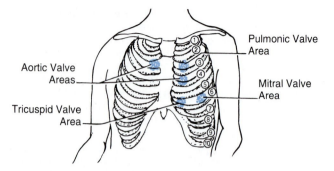

Fig. 8-18 Cardiac Valve Areas for Precordial Auscultation. These are the areas where the sounds originating from each valve is best heard; the areas are not necessarily closest to the anatomic location of the valves.

cannot be clearly discerned with a normally placed right border. When the RBCD is behind the sternum, the examiner cannot be certain of its position; it may be displaced leftward. When the right border is displaced rightward, the change in percussion note in the right hemithorax is definite. No conclusion about the size of the heart should be made by percussing only the left border. In the presence of hydrothorax or thickened pleura, percussion of the heart border may be impossible. In the examination of the precordium, the width of the *retromanubrial dullness* is conveniently measured. Normally, its width should not exceed 6 cm in the adult; an excessive width suggests a mass in the mediastinum.

AUSCULTATION OF THE PRECORDIUM. The stethoscope and its proper use are described in Chapter 3 on pages 45–47. The same principles apply to auscultation of the heart as to auscultation of the lungs. Listen in each of the primary valve areas (Fig. 8-18). If abnormal sounds are identified, map their strength and radiation across the precordium. Timing of cardiac sounds is especially important; use the apical impulse, or, if absent, the carotid upstroke to mark the onset of ventricular systole.

AUSCULTATION FOR CARDIAC RATE AND RHYTHM. The ventricular rate is measured by counting the number of heart beats per minute. Guessing at the heart rate is fallacious and fraught with error. In the same fashion, the arterial pulse rate may be counted, palpating the waves in a peripheral artery. If the rate is regular and not very slow, counting for 15 seconds and multiplying by 4 is sufficiently accurate. If comparison of the auscultated apical and palpated arterial rates reveals a discrepancy, it is termed a *pulse deficit*. Pulse deficit has been overemphasized as a sign of atrial fibrillation when, in fact, it occurs whenever ventricular contraction occurs before enough blood has accumulated to produce a pulse wave in the arteries; it is frequent in premature beats and bigeminal rhythm. We recommend that you auscultate the precordium to count the ventricular rate. Even this is less accurate than the ECG, as not all electrical events produce an audible mechanical event at high heart rates.

After counting the heart rate, listen carefully for several minutes for the presence of an *irregularity of rhythm*. The slower the rate, the longer and more intently one should listen; dysrhythmias are harder to detect when the diastolic intervals are either very long or very short. When irregularities are found, a *pattern* should be sought to determine if there is a relation to respiratory movements or if there is recurrence after a constant number of beats.

Auscultation of the Heart Sounds.   Auscultation of the precordium reveals paired sounds in seemingly endless repetition. Each member of a pair usually differs from its mate in intensity and pitch; each represents a heart sound and the pair correlates with a single cardiac cycle (see Fig. 8-36, page 411). Direct your attention toward the individual sounds. Positive identification of the first and second sounds must first be made because they serve as audible markers of the beginning and ending of cardiac systole. When an apical impulse is visible or palpable, the sound synchronous with it is the first sound; this is the best association to make. In the absence of an apical impulse, the carotid pulse wave may be palpated, realizing that there is a perceptible interval between cardiac systole and the arrival of the resulting wave in the neck. Never use the radial pulse in timing, because it is too far removed from the heart in distance and time, so it is misleading. If the ventricular rate is less than 100, diastole is longer than systole, so the first sound can be accepted as the first of the pair. When identification of the heart sounds or timing of murmurs is difficult because the tones are muffled or the rate is fast, slow the heart for a few beats by having the patient take a deep breath or by massaging either carotid sinus. The initial sound after a long pause must be the first sound followed by a systolic interval. Finally, at the base of the heart the second sound is almost invariably louder than the first.

When the two heart sounds have been identified at the base, move the stethoscope short distances toward the apex, called *inching,* tracing each sound across the precordium. Use separate passes to concentrate sequentially on the intensity (accentuated or diminished), the quality, the duration and the presence of splitting of the sounds. In examining for duration and splitting, think of the normal heart sound as being the shortest sound that can be perceived; any sound that exceeds this must be either prolonged, split, or a murmur. Prolonged sounds can be differentiated from murmurs by their abrupt beginning and ending, whereas murmurs have gradual onset and end. A sound that begins abruptly but ends gradually is probably a heart sound followed by a murmur. It takes considerable experience with listening to many normal and abnormal hearts to master cardiac auscultation and to learn to recognize ranges of normal and be able to identify the presence or absence of abnormal sounds.

Auscultation of Cardiac Murmurs.   Search for cardiac murmurs only after the heart sounds have been positively identified, so they may be employed as audible markers for the onset and ending of systole. Decide whether a sound of abnormal length is a split heart sound or a heart sound and murmur. Now turn your attention to the systolic interval between S1 and S2. Decide if there is any audible sound in this interval, by assuming that a heart sound is the shortest perceptible sound and that anything appreciably longer may be heart sound *and* murmur. In such a combination, remember that a heart sound begins and ends abruptly. A prolonged sound starting abruptly and dwindling is probably a heart sound followed by murmur; one developing gradually and ending abruptly is likely murmur and heart sound. Carefully examine each valve area on the precordium with both chest pieces (bell and diaphragm) of the stethoscope. Cover the intervening space on the precordium by inching. Once the presence of a murmur is established, ascertain the following characteristics: *Timing:*   Determine in what part of the cardiac cycle the murmur occurs, and whether it is early, middle, or late in the interval, by reference to the first and second heart sounds. *Location:*   Ascertain where on the precordium the murmur exhibits maximum intensity.   *Intensity:*   Grade intensity by the following scale:

Grade I: Barely audible with greatest difficulty
Grade II: Faint but heard immediately upon listening
Grades III, IV, V and VI: Progressively louder
Grade IV: Characterized by the presence of a thrill
Grade V: Loud enough to be heard with the stethoscope placed on its edge
Grade VI: So loud it can be heard with the stethoscope off the chest

The recording of grade III, for example, should be grade III/VI to show that the scale of VI is being used.   *Pattern or Configuration:*   Decide if the murmur is uniform in intensity throughout or whether the pitch increases (*crescendo*), or diminishes (*decrescendo*), or both (*crescendo-decrescendo*). The term *diamond-shaped murmur* is taken from the graphic representation on the screen of the phonocardiograph; the maximum intensity is midsystolic, with crescendo preceding and decrescendo following the peak (see Fig. 8-40).   *Pitch:*   Determine whether the murmur is high or low pitched. To the inexperienced and nonmusical examiner, the simplest method is to determine whether the murmur is heard better with the bell (low pitched) or the diaphragm (high pitched). Remember, the bell should be applied lightly and the diaphragm should be pressed firmly against the skin. Last, but important, ask whether the pitch seems more like a murmur or a pericardial friction rub. The latter, being rare, is frequently misdiagnosed as a murmur; the only distinction is by the quality of the sound.   *Posture and Exercise:*   When possible, auscultate the heart in both the supine and erect positions. In addition, employ the left lateral decubitus position, especially when listening at the cardiac apex to demonstrate the murmur of mitral stenosis and the gallop rhythms. Exercise sometimes brings out otherwise inaudible murmurs. After the systolic interval has been thoroughly explored, turn your attention to the diastolic interval; carry out the same procedures and ask the same questions.

Listening for Abnormal Systolic Sounds.   After identifying systole and diastole by using S1 and S2 as markers and noting any murmurs, the examiner listens for extra sounds in the systolic interval. Any abnormal sound must be either a murmur or a systolic click (see Fig. 8-37B).

LISTENING FOR DIASTOLIC SOUNDS.   After the systolic interval has been examined, examine the diastolic interval between S2 and S1. Sounds in diastole can be murmurs, opening snaps, third heart sounds, fourth heart sounds, or pericardial knocks (see Fig. 8-37B).

Physical Examination of the Blood Vessels

In performing the physical examination, the physician must have precise knowledge of the location of the accessible arteries and veins, their relations to other parts of the vascular system, and their responses to cardiac contraction. The arteries, usually palpable, are the temporal, common and external carotid, brachial, radial, ulnar, abdominal aorta, common iliac, femoral, popliteal, dorsalis pedis, and posterior tibial (Fig. 4-2). The veins that are frequently visible in the normal person are the external jugular, cephalic, basilic, median basilic, great saphenous, and the veins on the dorsa of the hands and feet. Other veins become visible during increases in general venous pressure or in the formation of collateral circulations.

MEASUREMENT OF ARTERIAL BLOOD PRESSURE.   See Chapter 4, page 82ff.

VENOUS PRESSURE.   Central venous pressure is measured at the level of the right atrium. In the erect position, the level of the right atrium is at the fourth intercostal space. Vertically from this point, a direct venous channel extends through the superior vena cava, the two subclavian veins, and then to the two external jugulars that emerge from the thorax at the superior borders of the clavicles to become subcutaneous and visible in the neck. With normal venous pressure in the erect position, a column of blood distends the superior vena cava to a height of about 10 cm above the right atrium (Fig. 8-19A). Any peripheral veins anatomically below this level are normally filled with blood; those above are collapsed. In most adults, the upper border of the clavicles is from 13 to 18 cm above the right atrium, so the visible segment of the external jugular veins in the neck is collapsed when the patient is erect (Fig. 8-19C). The visible veins in the dependent arms and forearms are distended with blood up to the same level as in the vena cava. When the thorax reclines at 45 degrees the column of blood rises higher in the venous channel, so the head of the column may be visible in the jugulars (Fig. 8-19B). In the horizontal position, all peripheral veins are filled (Fig. 8-19A). If the arm is raised slowly, the distal portions of the veins collapse as they attain the height of 10 cm above the level of the right atrium.

ESTIMATING CENTRAL VENOUS PRESSURE.   Because the superior border of the clavicle in the adult is usually from 13 to 18 cm above the fourth interspace, distention of the external jugular vein in the neck when the body is vertical is valid evidence of increased venous pressure, provided that there is no compression of the venous channel proximal to the atrium. Factors that increase intrathoracic pressure must be excluded, for example, coughing, laughing, crying, and other movements involving the Valsalva phenomenon. A large cervical or retrosternal goiter may cause venous obstruction. The presence of venous waves in the jugular excludes obstruction centrally; but tense distention of the jugulars may

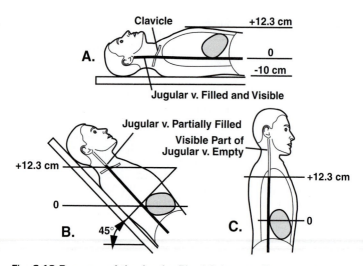

Fig. 8-19 Response of the Jugular Blood Column to Changes in Posture.
The anteroposterior diameter of the thorax at the fourth interspace is 20 cm;
from this point, the vertical distance to the superior border of the clavicle is 15
cm in the erect position. The right atrium is located at the midpoint of an an-
teroposterior line from the fourth interspace to the back. In any posture, a hor-
izontal plane through this point is the "phlebostatic" or "zero level." In this
*figure, a slightly elevated venous pressure of 12.3 cm is assumed. **A.** With the*
patient supine, the horizontal plane 12.3 cm above the zero level is above the
*neck; at normal venous pressure the jugular vein is filled. **B.** With the thorax*
at 45 degrees, the blood column extends midway up the jugular, so the head of
*the column is visible. **C.** In the erect position, the head of the column is con-*
cealed within the thorax, 2.7 cm below the upper border of the clavicle.

prevent venous waves from being apparent. A few persons do not develop peripheral veins that are large enough to inspect.

INDIRECT MEASUREMENT OF VENOUS PRESSURE.   When the head of the
blood column is visible in the vertical position, and obstruction or temporary increases in pressure are excluded, the vertical distance in centimeters from the head of the column to the right atrium is an approximate measure of venous pressure. When the jugulars are collapsed in
the vertical position, put the patient on an examining table or hospital
bed with a movable backrest. Starting from the sitting position, slowly
lower the thorax until the head of the blood column appears in the jugular vein. Establish the location of the right atrium in this position by
running an imaginary anteroposterior line from the anterior fourth interspace halfway to the back; a horizontal plane through this point is
the zero level for measurement of venous pressure (see Fig. 8-19B). The
vertical distance in centimeters from this plane to the head of the blood
column gives an approximation of the venous pressure. Another standard reference point in estimating the height of the jugular venous col-

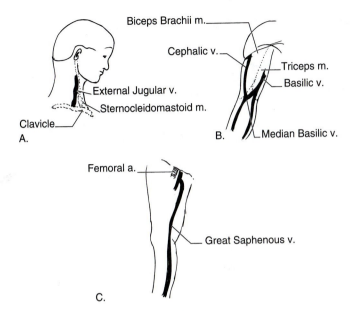

Fig. 8-20 Visible Veins and Venous Pressure Measurements. A. Veins of the Neck. B. Veins of the Arm. C. Veins of the Thigh and Leg.

umn is the angle of Louis (sternal angle); this is assumed to be about 6 cm above the atrium in most positions, although this is not always the case [Seth R, Magner P, Matzinger F, van Walraven C. How far is the sternal angle from the mid-right atrium? *J Gen Intern Med* 2002;17:852–856]. Jugular venous pulsations >3 cm vertically above this landmark indicate elevated venous pressure [McGee SR. Physical examination of venous pressure: A critical review. *Am Heart J* 1998;136:10–18].

ALTERNATE INDIRECT MEASUREMENT. The thorax can be at any angle. Establish the zero level, as previously described, and then raise the patient's arm slowly until a position is found where the distended veins in the arm or hand collapse. The vertical distance from the zero level to the point of collapse should give the venous pressure. Unfortunately, there is great individual variation in the caliber and superficiality of the veins of the arms. For observation, veins should be selected as close to the heart as possible so as to exclude blockage by valves; this is less likely in the cephalic, basilic, or median basilic veins (Fig. 8-20B).

VENOUS PULSATIONS. *Physiology:* Under ideal conditions, one can see three components of the wave (Fig. 8-21) and two prominent descents. *The a wave* results from rebound of atrial systole; *the c wave* is caused by the bulging backward of the tricuspid valve cusps at the beginning of ventricular systole and, in the jugular veins, transmission of the underlying carotid pulses; *the v wave* is produced by filling of the atria while the atrioventricular (AV) valves are still closed, together with the upward (hence backward) movement of the AV valve ring at the end of

Jugular Pulse (sphygmogram)

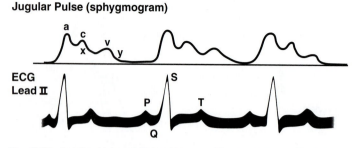

Fig. 8-21 Jugular Veinous Pulse Waves. *Heart action is reflected in the jugular vein. The waves should be timed with the apical impulse or heart sounds, remembering that a perceptible time elapses between cardiac events and their signs in the neck. The **a wave** is the rebound from atrial systole. The bulging of the tricuspid valve cusps early in ventricular systole produces the **c deflection**. The **v wave** results from atrial filling while the valves is closed, together with an upward movement of the atrioventricular (AV) valve ring at the end of ventricular systole. The **x descent** comes with atrial relaxation and the **y descent** with opening of the tricuspid valve.*

ventricular systole. The a wave is the only direct physical sign of atrial contraction. The c wave is followed by an *x descent* related to atrial relaxation and downward movement of the tricuspid valve with right ventricular systole. The v wave is followed by the *y descent* associated with opening of the tricuspid valve with onset of right ventricular diastole. The venous pulse wave is a normal phenomenon that can be demonstrated in the external jugular veins. Venous pulsations can also be seen by the expansion of the neck which occurs with filling and collapse of the internal jugular veins and their tributaries. This is best seen from the foot of the bed. In a few persons, pulsations occur in the superficial veins of the arms, forearms, and hands. Venous pulsation is readily distinguished from an arterial pulse by being impalpable. Venous pulses are best seen at the head of a blood column, but visibility depends on the amount of overlying tissue. Occasionally, a disproportion in the number of a waves and ventricular systoles gives direct indication of a dysrhythmia, but the waves are difficult to see consistently. When the geometry of posture has been so arranged as to expect a normal pulse wave, the absence of venous pulse is a sign of obstruction of the channel to the right atrium.

CAPILLARY PULSATION.   This has been widely advertised as a sign of aortic regurgitation, despite the repeated demonstrations of Thomas Lewis and others that it is a normal phenomenon, seen in most normal persons. To elicit it, press down on the tip of the fingernail until the distal third of the pink nail bed has paled: with each heartbeat the border of pink extends and recedes. When seen in aortic regurgitation, it is known as *Quincke pulse.*

Physical Exam of Arterial Circulation in the Extremities

We shall consider large arteries as those with anatomic names and normally visible or palpable pulses, whose occlusion can be recognized by the region of ischemia produced. Because smaller arteries and the arterioles are observable only in the superficial layers of the skin or in the retina, methods of their examination are quite different. In the routine physical examination, most physicians test the circulation of the extremities by (a) palpation of the walls of the brachial or radial arteries; (b) palpation of the pulse volume in the pairs of brachial, radial, femoral, dorsalis pedis, and posterior tibial arteries; (c) palpation for temperature changes; (d) inspection for varicose veins, edema, pallor, cyanosis, and ulceration of the arms and legs; and (e) inspection of the retinal vessels. Complaints of pain, coolness, or numbness in an extremity, or signs of enlarged veins, masses, swellings, localized pallor, redness, or cyanosis, lead to special examinations of the peripheral circulation. When you find a circulatory deficit, seek the cause from the history, the distribution of the deficit, and the state of the vessel walls.

When the affected part is below heart level, the pooled venous blood masks the effect of arterial flow to the part. Venous pressure rarely sustains a pressure higher than 30 cm above that of the right atrium, whereas the systolic arterial pressure produces a pressure more than 150 cm above the same reference point. Thus, when the hand or foot is lifted above the right atrium to a height exceeding the venous pressure, the masking venous blood pool is drained, permitting evaluation of the tissue color produced by the arterial blood. The most reliable sign of regional perfusion abnormality is a temperature or perfusion discrepancy between symmetrical parts when they have been sufficiently exposed to the same external temperature. If the pair are affected equally, judge the change in color from experience with other patients.

Skin Color is imparted by the blood in the venules of the subpapillary layer and the melanin content of the skin. Examination for circulatory changes in dark-skinned individuals is difficult; focus attention on the mucous membranes, nail beds, and the palms of the hands. When the arterial flow is nil and the veins empty, the skin is chalky white. Partial but inadequate arterial supply may produce red or cyanotic skin, depending on the effect of external temperature and amount of pooled blood in the venules. Because the degree of deoxygenation varies directly with the temperature, the same pooled blood may be red in the cold and blue at higher temperatures.

Skin Temperature is a reliable indicator of dermal perfusion. Normally, flow is governed principally by the constriction or dilatation of the arterioles. The internal body temperature is maintained within narrow limits, partly by the regulated dissipation of heat from the dermal vessels. In clothed persons, the skin of the head, neck, and trunk is warmer than that of the extremities and the digits are colder than their respective hands and feet. Peculiarly, the normal digits adjust their temperature to only one of two levels. The fingers are somewhat cooler (32°C [90°F]) than blood temperature (37°C [98°F]) when the air temperature exceeds 20°C (68°F). If the room temperature is below 16°C (60°F), the fingers adjust to a level of about 22°C (72°F); there are no intermediate levels of adjustment. Thus, distinguish between physiologic responses to external temperatures and the results of disease.

DERMAL EXAMINATION FOR ARTERIAL DEFICIT.   In a draft-less room at about 22°C (72°F) place the patient on an examining table or bed and expose the extremities for 10 minutes. If the room temperature much exceeds 26°C (78°F), coldness in the skin should not be demonstrable. Have the patient sit, hanging the legs from the table or bed; compare the *skin color* of both feet looking for pallor, deep redness, pale blueness, deep blueness, or a violaceous color (Fig. 8-43). With the back of your hand or fingers, feel the *skin temperature* from the feet up the legs. Compare similar sites on each leg in sequence; in moving proximally, note whether the increase in temperature is gradual or sharply demarcated. Have the patient lie supine. Grasp both of the patient's ankles and elevate the feet more than 30 cm (12 in) above the right atrium. Note any change in the color of the feet. If the color does not change, have the patient dorsiflex the feet five or six times, wait several minutes, then observe the feet for latent color changes induced by exercise. Allow the feet to hang down again and note the time for the return of color to the skin. Note rapidity of return of color to an area blanched by finger pressure. Inspect the feet carefully for *evidence of malnutrition*, for example, atrophy of the skin, loss of lanugo hair on the dorsa of the toes, thickening or transverse ridging of the nails, ulceration, patches of gangrene. Apply the same methods in examining the upper extremities. Expose the hands for 10 minutes and then observe the color in dependency and when elevated well above heart level. Have the hands opened and closed to disclose latent color changes. Note the time of return of color in dependency. Seek evidence of dermal malnutrition.

EXAMINATION OF LARGE ARM AND LEG ARTERIES.   Palpate the walls of accessible arteries for increased thickness, tortuosity, and beading. A spastic artery feels like a small cord. Systematically compare the pulse volumes at symmetric levels of the arteries.

UPPER EXTREMITIES.   Palpate the *subclavian artery* in the supraclavicular fossa, feeling for a thrill, and listen for a bruit. The arteries of the arm and forearm are palpable only in a segment of the brachial artery in the upper arm and segments of the radial and ulnar arteries in the wrist. With the forearm in about 90 degrees of flexion, palpate the *brachial artery* on the medial aspect of the arm, in the groove between the biceps and triceps muscles (Fig. 8-22A). Feel the *radial artery* on the flexor surface of the wrist, just medial to the distal end of the radius. Palpate the *ulnar artery* on the flexor surface of the wrist, just lateral to the lower end of the ulna; it lies deeper than the radial artery and frequently it is impalpable in the normal subject. Examine the patency of the radial and ulnar arteries with the *Allen test* (Fig. 8-22B): Have the patient sit with her hands supinated on her knees; stand at the patient's side with your fingers around each of her wrists and your thumbs on the flexor surfaces of her wrists. Have the patient make a tight fist, and then compress the tissue over both the radial and ulnar arteries with your thumbs.

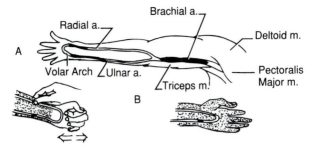

Fig. 8-22 Testing Patency Arm Arteries. A. Palpable Segments of the Arm Arteries (segments in solid black). Frequently the ulnar pulse is not palpable in normal persons. B. Allen Test. See the text for details.

Have the patient open the hand; the skin should be pale and remain so if both arteries are compressed. Take your thumb off the radial artery; the palm and fingers should quickly turn pink as flow returns. Delayed flush or no flush indicates partial or complete obstruction of the radial artery. Repeat the process, this time removing pressure from the ulnar artery. Return of flow is normally somewhat slower from the ulnar artery, but absence of flush is pathologic. Repeat this sequence on the other hand.

LOWER EXTREMITIES.   Palpate the *abdominal aorta* deeply between the xiphoid and the umbilicus, where the aorta bifurcates. Feel the *common iliac arteries* from the bifurcation to the midpoint of the inguinal ligaments. Palpate the *common femoral arteries* just below the inguinal ligaments, equidistant between the anterior superior iliac spines and the pubic tubercles (Fig. 8-23). Feel for the pulse of the *popliteal arteries* with the patient supine and the legs extended. Place one of your hands on each side of the patient's knee with your thumbs anteriorly near the patella and the fingers curling around each side of the knee so that the tips rest in the popliteal fossa. Firmly press the fingers of both hands forward to compress the tissues and the artery against the lower end of the femur or the upper part of the tibia; feel for pulsation of the artery. Frequently, the pulse of a normal popliteal artery is impalpable. For the pulse of the *posterior tibial artery,* feel in the groove between the medial malleolus and the Achilles tendon. It may be more accessible with passive dorsiflexion of the foot. Locate the *dorsalis pedis artery* on the dorsum of the foot, just lateral to and parallel with the tendon of the extensor hallucis longus. In apparently normal persons older than age 45 years, either the dorsalis pedis or the posterior tibial pulses frequently will be impalpable, but not both on the same foot. In feeling for the patient's pulse, carefully guard against mistaking the pulse in your own fingertips for that of the patient. Test the patency of the dorsalis pedis and posterior tibial arteries with the Allen maneuver by using the same principles as described for the pulses of the wrist, except compress the

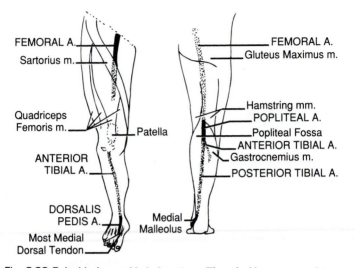

FEMORAL A.
Sartorius m.

Quadriceps
Femoris m.

ANTERIOR
TIBIAL A.

DORSALIS
PEDIS A.
Most Medial
Dorsal Tendon

Patella

FEMORAL A.
Gluteus Maximus m.

Hamstring mm.
POPLITEAL A.
Popliteal Fossa
ANTERIOR TIBIAL A.
Gastrocnemius m.
POSTERIOR TIBIAL A.

Medial
Malleolus

Fig. 8-23 Palpable Lower Limb Arteries. *The palpable segments of the arteries are in solid black. The **femoral artery** is palpable only a short distance below the inguinal ligament at the midpoint between the anterior superior iliac spine and the pubic tubercle. The **popliteal artery** lies vertically in the popliteal fossa; it can be felt only by compressing the contents of the fossa from behind against the bone. The **posterior tibial artery** can be felt as it curls forward and under the medial malleolus. The palpable segment of the **dorsalis pedis artery** lies just lateral to the most medial of the dorsal tendons of the foot (the flexor of the great toe) over the arch of the foot.*

pedal arteries while the foot is elevated, and then let the foot hang down when you release pressure to observe the color change. Check the **ankle-brachial index (ABI)** by measuring the systolic blood pressure in the brachial artery and the posterior tibial and/or the dorsalis pedis artery. The ABI is the ratio of the ankle systolic pressure to the brachial systolic pressure. Normal is >0.9, 0.75–0.9 is mild, 0.6–0.75 is moderate, and <0.6 is severe ischemia. ABI <0.5 is limb threatening. Use of Doppler (see *Doppler Ultrasound Examination* below) may be necessary. With the dorsal aspects of your fingers, palpate the skin of the thighs and legs for abnormal distribution of *skin temperature,* comparing symmetric areas. When the feet are abnormally cold, look for a sharp line of demarcation with a proximal region of normal temperature. Feel for a warm area over the knees or the anteromedial aspect of the thighs indicating collateral circulation via the geniculate artery. If peripheral arterial deficits are detected, be sure to inspect the *retinal arteries.*

DOPPLER ULTRASOUND EXAMINATION. Small portable instruments for use at the bedside make it possible to evaluate the arterial circulation more precisely, especially when the pulses are not readily palpable.

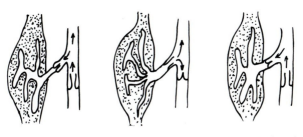

Muscle Relaxed　　　Muscle Contracted　　　Muscle Relaxed

Fig. 8-24 Muscle Contraction and Venous Flow. When the muscle is relaxed, it is filled with blood, but no blood emerges into the collecting veins. Muscle contraction expels blood into the collecting veins and closes the valves so the blood is propelled toward the heart. Thus venous return from muscles depends upon patent vessels, competent valves, and muscular contractions.

Exam of the Large Limb Veins

Adequate drainage of blood from the extremities requires (a) patency of the venous lumina, (b) voluntary muscle contractions to furnish the pumping action by compressing the adjacent veins (Fig. 8-24), and (c) competent valves in the veins so venous compression moves the blood proximally. A defect in any of these three may result in venous stasis with increased filtration pressure in the distal capillaries and post-capillary venules producing edema of the extremities, stasis pigmentation of the skin, and/or ulceration of the skin.

EXAMINATION OF LARGE ARM AND LEG VEINS.   With the patient supine, look for signs of venous stasis. Have the patient stand, and look for dilated veins in the arms and legs. Demonstrate venous occlusion by elevating the extremity to determine whether the veins collapse promptly. If occlusion is present, palpate the venous walls for hard plugs of thrombus or hard cords of fibrosis. If patent varicose veins are present, use the special tests for incompetency of valves.

LABORATORY EXAMINATION OF THE LARGE LIMB VEINS.   Techniques such as ultrasonic Doppler, impedance plethysmography, venography, and MRI permit experienced laboratory personnel to determine the patency and competence of the large limb veins.

Chest, Cardiovascular and Respiratory Symptoms

General Symptoms

KEY SYMPTOM

Pain in the Chest: Thoracic pain has many different causes and, unless obviously the result of trauma, is likely to be accompanied by fear of heart disease. Chest pain may be associated with no physical signs, so diagnosis requires careful attention to history, especially the attributes of pain (*PQRST = provocative-palliative factors, quality, region, severity, and timing*). Always ask your patient to point to the site of the pain. The diagnostic approach is twofold: first to assess the risk for major vascular disease and acute coronary events, and second, to develop the differential diagnosis of noncardiovascular explanations [Lee TH, Goldman L. Evaluation of the patient with acute chest pain. *N Engl J Med* 2000;342:1187–1195]. Acute coronary events may be missed in younger patients, women, and people with normal ECGs, so careful risk factor assessment and a high index of suspicion are necessary. Reassurance based upon the exclusion of cardiovascular disease is often the most effective therapy for the patient. See *Six-Dermatome Pain Syndromes*, page 456–464.

KEY SYMPTOM

Deep Retrosternal or Precordial Pain: A Symptom of the Six-Dermatome Band: Deep visceral pain behind the sternum or in the precordial region is not specific for cardiac disorders. Rather, it is the primary symptom for the entire region supplied by dermatomes T1 to T6. The neuroanatomy of the region furnishes the structural basis for this concept, which clinical experience confirms. *Pathophysiology:* Dermatomes T1 to T6 cover the thoracic surface from the neck to beneath the xiphoid process and extend down the anteromedial aspects of the arms and forearms (Fig. 8-25). The upper four dermatomes are supplied by sensory afferent fibers to the posterior roots of T1 to T4, the lower cervical and upper thoracic sympathetic ganglia. In the ganglia and spinal cord the fibers communicate with one another superiorly and inferiorly. Practically all the tho-

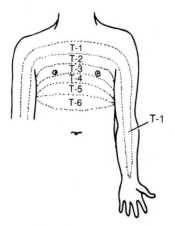

Fig. 8-25 The Six-Dermatome Band. *Dermatomes T1 to T6 form a band that covers most of the thorax and extends down the anteromedial aspect of the arms and forearms. Sensory pathways from the viscera of this entire region are so interconnected axially that stimulation of any part can produce the same patterns of chest pain.*

racic viscera are served by sensory fibers in these pathways: myocardium, pericardium, aorta, pulmonary artery, esophagus, and mediastinum. Lesions in any of these structures produce pain of the same quality: deep, visceral, poorly localized. Usually such pain is maximal in the retrosternal region or the precordium; it often extends with lesser intensity upward into the neck and downward on the anteromedial aspects of one or both arms and forearms. The band made by dermatomes T5 and T6 comprises fibers from the lower thoracic wall, the diaphragmatic muscles and their peritoneal surfaces, the gallbladder, the pancreas, the duodenum, and the stomach. Inflammation in these structures causes deep, visceral, poorly localized pain precisely similar in quality to that from the upper band. Usually, the maximal intensity is in the xiphoid region and in the back, inferior to the right scapula. But the pain may extend to the upper band of T1 to T4 through posterior connections in the sympathetics, so that the pattern may be indistinguishable from that arising above the diaphragm. (For a comprehensive review see the following reference [Castell DO (ed). Chest pain of undetermined origin; proceedings of a symposium. *Am J Med* 1992;92(suppl 5A):1–129].) To determine the cause of deep chest pain, (a) ask the location of the pain, accepting the location of the pain as indicating only that the source is somewhere in the six-dermatome band (the myocardium, pericardium, aorta, pulmonary artery, mediastinum, esophagus, gallbladder, pancreas, duodenum, stomach, or subphrenic region); (b) ask the patient to state the intensity of the pain on a scale of 1 to 10; (c) shorten the list of possibilities by carefully searching for provocative-palliative factors and timing; and (d) make appropriate tests to distinguish between the disorders on the shortened list [Pryor DB, Shaw L, McCants CB, et al. Value of the history and physical in identifying patients at increased risk for coronary artery disease. *Ann Intern Med* 1993;118:81–90].

✓ *PRECORDIAL PAIN—CLINICAL OCCURRENCE: Congenital* hypertrophic cardiomyopathy; *Endocrine* retrosternal thyroid; *Idiopathic* esophageal spasm, gastroesophageal reflux; *Inflammatory/Immune* esophagitis, pericarditis, pleuritis, myocarditis, postcardiotomy syndrome, pancreatitis, cholecystitis, gastritis; *Infectious* infectious pericarditis and pleuritis, myocarditis, subphrenic abscess; *Metabolic/Toxic* acid or alkali ingestion; *Mechanical/Trauma* pneumothorax, esophageal rupture, esophageal obstruction (extrinsic, foreign body, neoplasm, web, or ring), esophageal diverticulum, gastric perforation; *Neoplastic* carcinoma (primary or metastatic) of the esophagus, pericardium, lung, mediastinum, pleura; lymphoma; thymoma; teratoma; testicular cancer; *Neurologic* postherpetic neuralgia, diabetic radiculopathy, intercostal neuritis; *Psychosocial* somatization disorder, panic attack, hypochondriasis, malingering, Munchausen syndrome; *Vascular* myocardial ischemia (coronary atherosclerosis, spasm, embolism, thrombosis, vasculitis), pulmonary embolism and infarction, aortic dissection.

KEY SIGN

▶ **Shortness of Breath: Dyspnea:** *Pathophysiology:* Dyspnea results from abnormalities of gas exchange (decreased oxygenation, hypoventilation, hyperventilation), and increased work of breathing because of changes in respiratory mechanics and/or anxiety [Manning HL, Schwartzstein RM. Pathophysiology of dyspnea. N Engl J Med 1995;333:1547–1553]. Dyspnea means difficult breathing; it is both a symptom and a sign. The patient's complaint is likely to be "shortness of breath," "quickly out of breath," "can't take a deep breath," "smothering," or "tightness in the chest." Dyspnea is often accompanied by tachypnea, increased respiratory excursions, tensing of the scaleni and sternocleidomastoidei, flaring of the alae nasi, and facial expressions of distress. Sometimes the patient is not conscious of being dyspneic, and the first clue encountered by the examiner is that the patient pauses for breath in the middle of a sentence. It is useful to distinguish several degrees, ranging from exertional dyspnea to dyspnea at rest and orthopnea. A diagnostic classification of the causes of dyspnea may be based on anatomic and physiologic criteria. Often more than one mechanism is involved, for example, pneumonia causes hypoxia and increases the work of breathing. Patients may complain of dyspnea disproportionate to any identifiable physiologic or anatomic abnormality: anxiety with hyperventilation or unsuspected decreases in respiratory compliance should be suspected.

✓ *DYSPNEA—CLINICAL OCCURRENCE:* **Decreased Fraction of Inspired Oxygen (FIO2)** high altitudes; **Airway Obstruction** *Larynx and Trachea* infections (laryngeal diphtheria, acute laryngitis, epiglottitis, Ludwig angina), angioedema, trauma (hematoma or laryngeal edema), neuropathic (abductor paralysis of vocal cords), foreign body, tumors of the neck (goiter, carcinoma, lymphoma, aortic aneurysm), ankylosis of the cricoarytenoid joints; *Bronchi and Bronchioles* acute and chronic bronchitis, asthma, retrosternal goiter, aspirated foreign bodies, extensive bronchiectasis, bronchial stenosis. **Abnormal Alveoli** *Alveolar Filling* pulmonary edema from left ventricular failure or acute lung injury, pulmonary infiltrations (infectious and aspiration pneumonia, carcinoma, sarcoidosis, pneumoconioses), pulmonary hemorrhage, pulmonary alveolar proteinosis; *Alveolar Destruction* pulmonary emphysema, pulmonary fibrosis, cystic disease of the lungs; *Compression of the Alveoli* atelectasis, pneumothorax, hydrothorax, abdominal distention; **Restrictive Chest and Lung Disease** paralysis of the respiratory muscles (especially the intercostals and the diaphragm), thoracic deformities (kyphoscoliosis, thoracoplasty), scleroderma of the thoracic wall, pulmonary fibrosis; **Abnormal Pulmonary Circulation** pericardial tamponade, pulmonary artery stenosis, arteriovenous shunts in heart and lungs, pulmonary thromboemboli and infarction, other emboli (fat, air, amniotic fluid), arteriolar stenosis (primary pulmonary hypertension-Ayerza disease, irradiation); **Oxyhemoglobin Deficiency** anemia, carbon monoxide poisoning (carboxyhemoglobinemia), methemoglobinemia and sulfhemoglobinemia, cyanide and cobalt poisoning; **Abnormal Respiratory Stimuli** pain from respiratory movements, exaggerated consciousness of respiration (effort syndrome), hyperventilation syndrome, secondary respiratory alkalosis (increased intracranial pressure, metabolic acidosis).

KEY SYMPTOM

Paroxysmal Dyspnea: *Pathophysiology:* There is a transient increase in pulmonary capillary pressure associated with redistribution of fluid from edematous extremities to the lungs with recumbency, or ischemia-induced transient decreases in left ventricular performance. This is characterized by sudden paroxysms of breathlessness. When sleep is interrupted, it is termed *paroxysmal nocturnal dyspnea*. These attacks are attended by orthopnea and coughing. The patient often finds that walking a few minutes relieves the dyspnea, permitting the patient to resume sleep. This can be distinguished from true asthma by finding that the lungs do not clear when the patient inhales a bronchodilator.

KEY SYMPTOM

Shortness of Breath When Lying Down: Orthopnea: *Pathophysiology:* Redistribution of extracellular fluid from the periphery to the lungs, elevation of the diaphragm from obesity or ascites, and muscular weakness all contribute to dyspnea when lying flat. Orthopnea is dyspnea associated with recumbency leading the patient to assume a resting position that elevates the head and chest. Many patients experience awakening severely short of breath in the supine position (*paroxysmal nocturnal dyspnea*). Severity may be judged by the number of pillows the patient requires to achieve a comfortable position. Orthopnea is often overlooked if the patient does not mention it and is only examined in the seated position; the physician must specifically ask about it or observe the patient supine.

Chest Wall Symptoms

KEY SYMPTOM

Chest Pain with Tenderness: See *Chest Wall Signs*, pages 381 and 444.

Lung and Pleural Symptoms

KEY SYMPTOM

Shortness of Breath: Dyspnea: See page 375.

KEY SYMPTOM

Respiratory Pain: Intercostal Neuralgia: Irritation of an intercostal nerve produces sharp, lancinating, stabbing pain along the nerve's course. The pain is frequently intensified by respiratory motion or movements of the trunk; exposure to cold may accentuate it. Tenderness along the nerve is diagnostic. Usually the tenderness is maximal near the vertebral foramen, in the axilla, or at the parasternal line; these points correspond to the major cutaneous branches of the nerve.

✔*INTERCOSTAL NEURALGIA—CLINICAL OCCURRENCE:* Associated conditions are onset of herpes zoster, diabetes mellitus, tabes dorsalis, mediastinal neoplasm, neurofibroma (where an intercostal mass may be felt), vertebral tuberculosis or obesity with nerve stretching.

KEY SYMPTOM
Respiratory Pain: Herpes Zoster (Shingles):
See Chapter 6, page 179. This produces a specific type of intercostal neuralgia. There is sudden onset of the neuralgic pain followed by the development of vesicular skin lesions on an erythematous base.

KEY SYMPTOM
Cough: *Pathophysiology:* A cough is a sudden, forceful, noisy expulsion of air from the lungs. The three stages of coughing are preliminary inspiration, glottal closure and contraction of respiratory muscles, followed by sudden glottal opening to produce the outward blast of air. The sensory nerve endings for the cough reflex are branches of the vagus in the larynx, trachea, and bronchi; but cough may also be induced by stimulation in the external acoustic meatus that is supplied by the auricular nerve (Arnold nerve), a branch of the vagus. Stimuli to coughing include exudates in the pharynx or bronchial tree, irritation of foreign bodies, and inflammation. Coughing may be voluntary or involuntary, single or paroxysmal. A cough in which sputum is raised is *productive*. A *brassy cough* is unproductive and has a strident quality. It occurs in any condition that narrows the trachea or glottal space, most commonly laryngitis or epiglottitis, but also laryngeal paralysis, neoplasm of the vocal cord, or aortic aneurysm. In pertussis, the cough is characterized by a long strident inspiratory noise, a *whoop*, preceding the cough. Chronic unexplained coughs are most commonly related to one or a combination of chronic post-nasal drip, gastroesophageal reflux or cough-variant asthma [McGarvey LP, Heaney LG, Lawson JT, et al. Evaluation and outcome of patients with chronic non-productive cough using a comprehensive diagnostic protocol. *Thorax* 1998;53:738–743].

✔*COUGH—CLINICAL OCCURRENCE: Congenital* tracheoesophageal fistula, mediastinal teratoma; *Endocrine* substernal thyroid; *Idiopathic* emphysema; *Inflammatory/Immune* inhaled allergens, asthma, chronic bronchitis, vasculitis, Goodpasture syndrome, relapsing polychondritis, endobronchial amyloidoma; *Infectious* sinusitis, pharyngitis, laryngitis, epiglottitis, tracheobronchitis (measles, pertussis), pneumonia (viral, bacterial, fungal, tuberculosis, nontypical mycobacteria, pneumocystis), typhoid, bronchiectasis, lung abscess, subphrenic abscess; *Metabolic/Toxic* tobacco smoking, inhaled irritants, angiotensin-converting enzyme inhibitors; *Mechanical/Trauma* cervical osteophytes, inhaled foreign bodies, acute and chronic aspiration, mediastinal mass and lymphadenopathy; *Neoplastic* cancer of the larynx and lung, endobronchial adenoma, thymoma, mediastinal lymphoma, metastases to the lung; *Neurologic* gastroesophageal reflux, tympanic membrane irritation; *Psychosocial* cough tics and habits; *Vascular* congestive heart failure, vasculitis (Wegener, Churg-Straus), aortic aneurysm, pulmonary embolism and infarction, pulmonary hemorrhage.

KEY SYMPTOM
Chest Pain Intensified by Respiratory Motion: See *Chest Syndromes*, page 444ff.

Cardiovascular Symptoms

KEY SYMPTOM
Chest Pain: See pages 373–375.

KEY SYMPTOM
Palpitation: When the patient is conscious of heart action, whether it be fast or slow, regular or irregular, the term palpitation is applied. The sensation is usually described as "pounding," "fluttering," "flip-flopping," "skipping a beat," "missing a beat," "stopping," "jumping," or "turning over." The frequency, regularity, rate, and intensity depend on the underlying cause. Begin evaluating palpitations by taking a history. Be sure to ask your patient to describe whether the sensation is a single "extra beat or pause" or a series of beats. If the latter, ask them to describe whether they recall if it starts and ends abruptly or gradually, whether it is fast or slow, and whether it is regular or irregular. Ask them to tap out the rhythm with their finger. Be sure to have them describe the circumstances when the palpitations occur and any associated symptoms that precede or accompany the palpitations (such as lightheadedness, paresthesias, dyspnea). Then perform a physical examination and obtain a 12-lead ECG. If you find no evidence of heart disease and the palpitations are well tolerated and not sustained, reassure your patient. Ambulatory monitoring is recommended in patients who tolerate the palpitations poorly, have heart disease or sustained palpitations. Although often caused by trivial disorders, palpitations nevertheless frighten the patient, as does any symptom referable to the heart. Identification of the cause and careful explanation are often the only treatment necessary. When questions remain, obtain cardiology consultation.

KEY SYMPTOM
Exertional Limb Pain: Claudication: *Pathophysiology:* Exercising muscle has high oxygen and energy requirements; energy is stored, but oxygen must be continuously delivered to meet the increased demand. Inability to increase muscular blood flow with exertion produces ischemic pain relieved by rest. The patient complains usually of calf pain, which requires him to stop or sit for relief, at a fixed distance of walking. It is consistently reproducible. Claudication can occur in any exercising muscle, so the examiner must be alert to reproducible exertional extremity or gluteal pain.

✓ *CLINICAL OCCURRENCE:* Atherosclerotic obstruction of major arteries to the lower extremity is most common. Exertional pain in the buttocks and/or thighs may represent true claudication or pseudoclaudication because of spinal stenosis.

Cold Hands and/or Feet: *Pathophysiology:* This common problem is probably caused by regional vasoconstriction to conserve heat. Examine carefully for any diminution in the peripheral pulses or skin changes suggesting decreased nutrition. Absent of these findings, the patient can be reassured. The head is the greatest site of heat loss; have the patient wear a warm hat.

Chest, Cardiovascular and Respiratory Signs

Chest Wall Signs

KEY SIGN

Thoracic Spine Deformity: Abnormalities of the Thoracic Spine: See *Musculoskeletal Signs*, Chapter 13, for a complete discussion. It is important to remember that deformities of the thoracic spine and chest wall may decrease chest compliance, severely limit respiratory excursions, and increase the work of breathing. In either curved or angular kyphosis (Fig. 8-26A), the spinal flexion may force the thorax to assume permanently the inspiratory position, with increased anteroposterior diameter and horizontal ribs. The thoracic distortion is identical with the barrel chest of pulmonary emphysema. In

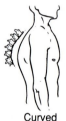
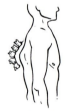
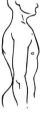

Curved   Angular
A. Kyphosis   B. Lordosis

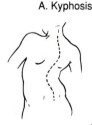
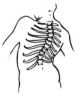

C. Scoliosis

Fig. 8-26 Curvatures of the Spine Affecting the Thorax. A. Kyphotic Thorax. B. Lordotic Thorax. C. Scoliotic Thorax. Note the narrowing of the rib interspaces on the right and the accentuation of the interspaces, posterior humping of the chest, and elevation of the shoulder on the left.

this case, the auscultatory signs of emphysema are absent. Accentuation of the lumbar curve throws the thoracic spine backward and the thoracic cage becomes flattened from the pull of the abdomen, causing an expiratory position to be assumed (Fig. 8-26B). Lateral curvature of the thoracic spine is usually accompanied by some rotation of the vertebral bodies, but only the lateral deviations of the spinous processes are visible (Fig. 8-26C). Minor functional scoliosis forms a single lateral curve, usually with convexity to the right. With structural changes, the lateral curve in the thorax produces an opposite compensatory curve inferiorly, so the line of spinous processes forms an S-shaped curve. The spinous processes always rotate toward the concave side. On the convex side, rotation of the vertebral bodies causes flattening of the ribs anteriorly and bulging of the chest posteriorly, raising of the shoulder, and lowering of the hip. Viewed from the patient's back, the posterior bulge is augmented with anteflexion of the spine.

KEY SIGN

Respiratory Pain with Tenderness: *The distinction between respiratory pain and chest pain with tenderness is somewhat artificial; the conditions may present in either manner, or with both pain at rest and with respirations.* The patient complains of pain associated with breathing. Careful examination of the chest discloses tenderness of specific structures.

RESPIRATORY PAIN WITH TENDERNESS: PERIOSTEAL HEMATOMA OF RIB: This is very painful and tender. It usually follows direct trauma, and fracture is expected, but not found on x-ray.

RESPIRATORY PAIN WITH TENDERNESS: PERIOSTITIS OF RIBS: Inflammation of the periosteum is extremely painful. Trauma or acute osteomyelitis produces periostitis with exquisite tenderness and severe sharp pain, often affected by motion. It persists for hours and is often worse at night. Acute osteomyelitis is usually accompanied by fever and leukocytosis.

RESPIRATORY PAIN WITH TENDERNESS: SLIPPING CARTILAGE: *Pathophysiology:* The interchondral ligament between the ninth and tenth costicartilages becomes weakened and elongated, or has been fractured, permitting the tenth rib to override the ninth. The costal cartilage slips over the adjacent rib causing pain with respiratory motion or movement of the shoulder girdle. The slipping may be accompanied by an audible or palpable click (Fig. 8-27). The tenth rib is usually affected. The slipping rib may cause pain, falsely attributed to intraabdominal disease.

RESPIRATORY PAIN WITH TENDERNESS: STITCH OF THE INTERCOSTAL MUSCLES: A sharp pain in the chest wall following severe exercise may be relieved by rest. The mechanism is unknown; it has been attributed to spasm of the diaphragm.

RESPIRATORY PAIN WITH TENDERNESS: INTERCOSTAL MYOSITIS: Severe aching pain, intensified by thoracic motion, results from inflammation of the intercostal muscles. The muscles are tender; induration and palpable nodules may ultimately appear.

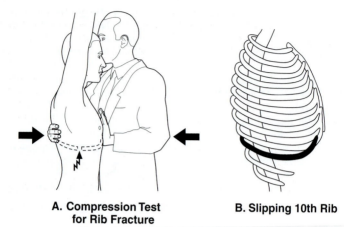

A. Compression Test
for Rib Fracture   **B. Slipping 10th Rib**

*Fig. 8-27 Examining for Rib Pain. **A. Compression Test for Rib Fracture**. When the site of suspected rib fracture is located by point tenderness, the sternum is pushed toward the spine with one hand while the other hand supports the patient's back. The maneuver will elicit pain at the untouched fracture site. **B. Slipping Tenth Rib**. When the tenth rib lacks an anterior attachment, it can slip forward upon the ninth rib during respiratory movements and cause pain.*

RESPIRATORY PAIN WITH TENDERNESS: STRAIN OF THE PECTORALIS MINOR: Irritation of this muscle from overuse, such as elevation of the arm, carrying a backpack, or lifting a baby, causes pain in the upper anterior lateral chest. The involved muscle is tender.

RESPIRATORY PAIN WITH TENDERNESS: DISORDERS OF THE SHOULDER GIRDLE: Shoulder disease may cause pain in the upper chest, augmented by arm and chest motion.

● KEY SIGN
Chest Pain with Tenderness: *The distinction between respiratory pain with tenderness and chest pain with tenderness is somewhat artificial; the conditions may present in either manner, or with both pain at rest and with respirations.* The patient may recognize the pain as superficial, sharp, and well localized. Almost always, this type of pain is accompanied by localized tenderness. The structures involved are the skin and subcutaneous tissues, the fat, skeleton, or the breasts.

CHEST PAIN WITH TENDERNESS: SKIN AND SUBCUTANEOUS STRUCTURES: Inflammation, trauma, and neoplasm in these tissues offer no special diagnostic problems, provided that they are considered and searched for. The presence of bruises, lacerations, ulcers, hematomas, masses, or tenderness is usually diagnostic.

CHEST PAIN WITH TENDERNESS: CHEST WALL SYNDROME: Ask your patient to point to the region of pain. Next, perform four maneuvers: (a)

Palpate the chest wall for tenderness by applying firm, steady pressure to the sternum, the costosternal junctions, the intercostal spaces, the ribs, and the pectoralis major muscles and their insertions; (b) flex the arms horizontally by lifting one arm after the other by the elbow and pulling it across the chest toward the contralateral side, with the head rotated toward the ipsilateral side; (c) extend the neck by having the patient look toward the ceiling as the arms are pulled backward and slightly upward; and (d) exert vertical pressure on the head. If any of these tests reproduces the patient's pain, review the history to ascertain whether your patient forgot recent minor trauma or strain of the chest muscles.

CHEST PAIN WITH TENDERNESS: COSTOCHONDRITIS OF RIB AND TIETZE SYNDROME: This is a common cause of chest pain. The onset may be sudden or gradual. The pain is usually dull; it may be intensified by respiratory motion and movements of the shoulder girdle. The sole physical sign is tenderness at the costochondral junction of bone and cartilage. There is no swelling and there are no x-ray findings. In **Tietze syndrome** the pain is accompanied by tender, fusiform swelling of one or more costicartilages, often that attached to the second rib. The overlying skin is reddened. Pain may radiate to the shoulder, neck, or arm. There is no lymphadenopathy. It may subside in a few weeks or persist for months. The swelling may persist for months after the pain and tenderness subside. The cause is unknown and the condition must be distinguished from osteitis, periostitis, rheumatic chondritis, and neoplasm of the ribs.

CHEST PAIN WITH TENDERNESS: FRACTURED RIB: The history may suggest pleurisy. The patient complains of pain in the chest with breathing. Movement of rib fragments causes well-localized, sharp, lancinating pain. Inspiration is limited and palpation discloses point tenderness on a rib. There may be a history of direct chest trauma; if not, ask about recent severe coughing which the patient may not recognize as a cause of fracture. The edges of the fracture may be felt, but bone crepitus is absent when the fragments are well opposed. With one hand supporting the back, compression of the sternum with the other elicits pain at the untouched fracture site (see Fig. 8-27A). The diagnosis is made readily when the patient gives a history of trauma to the thorax. Fractures of several contiguous ribs are usually caused by external violence; the chest wall may be so weakened as to produce the flail chest.

CHEST PAIN WITH TENDERNESS: FRACTURED RIB, COUGH FRACTURE: *Pathophysiology:*   Any rib from the fifth to the tenth is likely to break. The fracture is usually anterior to the attachments of the serratus anterior that pulls the rib upward, and posterior to the fixations of the abdominal external oblique muscle that pulls the rib downward creating a shearing force on the rib. A single cough is not enough to produce fracture; breaking is attributed to the fatigue (stress fracture) from repeated coughing. Cough fracture was described by Robert Graves sometime before 1833. The patient has been coughing for some time and pain begins to occur with respiratory movements and coughing. The typical signs of fracture of a rib are present. When palpation of the ribs is not performed, the condition is usually diagnosed as pleurisy.

CHEST PAIN WITH TENDERNESS: TENDER STERNUM: Many normal persons have slight tenderness in the lower third of the sternum, elicited when the finger is drawn over it.

CHEST PAIN WITH TENDERNESS: FRACTURED STERNUM: The profile of the sternum usually has abnormal angulation, the site of which is tender. Pain prompts the patient to bend the head and thorax forward with the shoulders rotated inward.

CHEST PAIN WITH TENDERNESS: THROMBOPHLEBITIS OF THE THORACOEPIGASTRIC VEIN (MONDOR DISEASE): The pain is felt along the anterolateral chest wall with radiation to the axilla or inguinal region. A tender cord, 3–4 mm in diameter, is usually palpable and often visible when the skin is stretched. The disease is self-limited and lasts 2–4 weeks.

CHEST PAIN WITH TENDERNESS: TENDER MUSCLE IN THE THORAX: Frequently, a tender muscle is mistaken by the patient and the physician for intrathoracic disease.

CHEST PAIN WITH TENDERNESS: FAT: In a rare form of obesity, symmetrical fat lobules on the trunk and limbs are painful and tender. The condition is known as *adiposis dolorosa* (Dercum disease). If inflammation is present, consider one of the forms of panniculitis.

CHEST PAIN WITH TENDERNESS: BREASTS: Painful lesions are fissures of the nipples, cystic mastitis, fibroadenosis, acute breast abscess, and, occasionally, breast carcinoma.

CHRONIC CHEST PAIN WITH TENDERNESS: XIPHISTERNAL ARTHRITIS: The pain may be ascribed to myocardial ischemia unless the xiphoid cartilage is palpated and the pain reproduced.

KEY SIGN
Chest Pain with Dysesthesia: Herpes Zoster (Shingles): See page 179. The pain of herpes always precedes the rash by 2–3 days. Other causes of intercostal neuritis need to be considered until the diagnostic rash appears.

KEY SIGN
Pain in the Chest: Palpable Pleural Friction Rub: *Pathophysiology:* The inflamed pleural surfaces lose their lubricating fluid ("dry pleurisy") and rub together during movements of the lungs. Sometimes the vibrations from the two rubbing surfaces can be felt, similar to that of two pieces of dry leather rubbing together. The rub is also heard with the stethoscope or the unaided ear as a creaking sound.

Restrictive Soft Tissue: Atrophy or Myopathy:
Muscle weakness and atrophy producing decreased respiratory excursions may be sequelae of poliomyelitis and various myopathies involving the respiratory muscles.

Restrictive Soft Tissue: Cicatrix: Extensive scarring of the skin and soft tissue of the thorax from burns, operations, or lacerations may seriously restrict inspiratory capacity.

Restrictive Soft Tissue: Scleroderma: Diffuse cutaneous scleroderma may, rarely, affect the chest wall sufficiently to cause respiratory impairment. More commonly, scleroderma syndromes produce restrictive pulmonary parenchymal disease.

KEY SIGN
Thoracic Deformity: Rachitic Rosary: A prominent structural feature of rickets is failure of hardening of the bones. The sternal ends of rachitic ribs bulge at their costochondral junctions. The bulging is mostly inward, but in severe cases, there is enough outward bulging to be perceived as knobs at the costochondral junctions (Fig. 8-28A). The condition exists only during the activity of the rickets in the first 2 years of life; healing obliterates the knobs without a trace.

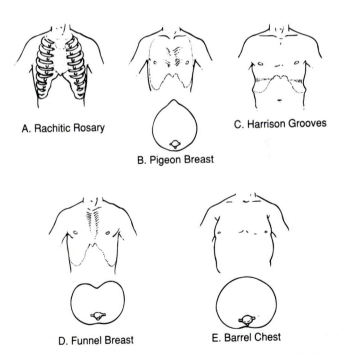

A. Rachitic Rosary

B. Pigeon Breast

C. Harrison Grooves

D. Funnel Breast

E. Barrel Chest

Fig. 8-28 Deformities of the Thorax. A. Rachitic Rosary. B. Pigeon Breast. C. Harrison Grooves. D. Funnel Breast. E. Barrel Chest.

Thoracic Deformity: Pigeon Breast (Pectus Carinatum):

During active rickets, the softened upper ribs bend inward, forcing the sternum forward increasing the anteroposterior dimension at the expense of the width. The sternum protrudes from the narrowed thorax like the keel of a ship (see Fig. 8-28B). Vertical grooves are formed in the line of the costochondral junctions, as depicted in the cross section. The deformity persists after healing of the rickets. Pigeon breast also occurs in Marfan syndrome. Similar distortion occurs in severe primary kyphoscoliosis, but the sides of the thorax are not symmetric. Fusion abnormalities in the midline resembling pectus carinatum also occur in some forms of congenital heart disease.

Thoracic Deformity: Harrison Groove (Harrison Sulcus):

During active rickets, the protuberant rachitic abdomen pushes the plastic lower ribs outward on a fulcrum formed by the costal attachments of the diaphragm. The line of bending forms a groove or sulcus in the rib cage, extending laterally from the xiphoid process, with flaring of the cage below the groove (see Fig. 8-28C). The deformity remains when the rickets heals, but its significance is only cosmetic.

Thoracic Deformity: Funnel Breast (Pectus Excavatum):

The reverse of the pigeon breast, the lower costal cartilages, inferior sternum and xiphoid process are retracted toward the spine. In its rudimentary form, an oval pit occurs near the infrasternal notch. A more extensive distortion (see Fig. 8-28D) is formed when the entire lower sternum sinks, significantly diminishing the anteroposterior dimension of the thoracic cavity. Rickets and Marfan syndrome are known causes, but many cases are unexplained.

Thoracic Deformity: Barrel Chest:

Both the anteroposterior and transverse dimensions of the thorax are enlarged, without bulges or depressions, so the arched ribs tend to form perfect circles in cross section (see Fig. 8-28E). Emphysema causes increased residual volume which is suspected on finding increased anteroposterior diameter of the chest, horizontal ribs, depressed diaphragm, prolonged expiration, and decreased breath sounds. Senile kyphosis of the thoracic spine produces a similar posture in the ribs, but is distinguished from emphysema by an absence of lung signs.

Movement of the Chest in One Piece:

During respiratory movements, the entire thorax appears to move as a unit. This may result from increased lung volume in pulmonary emphysema or ankylosis of the joints of the thoracic cage.

KEY SIGN

Inspiratory Retraction of Interspaces: *Pathophysiology:* Airway obstruction or decreased lung compliance leads to inspiratory collapse of the intercostal spaces because of the excessively negative inspiratory intrapleural pressure. The inward intercostal movement is usually more evident in the lower thorax. Sudden, violent retractions occur in tracheal obstruction and severe paroxysms of asthma.

KEY SIGN

Diminished Local Excursion of the Thorax: This points to a lesion in the underlying wall, pleura, or lung; causes include pain, fibrosis, or consolidation. The restricted movement may be best observed from the foot of the bed.

KEY SIGN

Diminished Local Excursion of the Thorax: Tension Pneumothorax: See page 402.

KEY SIGN

Localized Bulging of the Thorax During Expiration: Flail Chest: *Pathophysiology:* Fracture of several contiguous ribs or the separation of several contiguous costal cartilages results in loss of chest wall integrity. The negative intrathoracic pressure during inspiration pulls the injured segment inward while the rise in intrathoracic pressure during expiration causes it to bulge outwards. The paradoxical chest movements decreases minute ventilation and, if extensive, produces respiratory failure.

KEY SIGN

Inspiratory Convergence, or Less Divergence of Costal Margins: *Pathophysiology:* When the dome of the diaphragm is flattened, the direction of its pull on the costal margins is changed from upward to inward. The degree of outward flare of the margins is lessened or, in extreme cases, the margins are pulled inward. Lowering of the diaphragm may be caused by pulmonary emphysema or by accumulations of fluid or air in the pleural space.

Exaggerated Costal Margin Flare During Inspiration: *Pathophysiology:* Elevation of the dome of the diaphragm increases the upward pull of the diaphragm during inspiration. The most common causes are hepatomegaly and subphrenic abscess.

KEY SIGN

Lateral Deviations of the Trachea: Lateral tracheal deviation at the level of the clavicle may be caused by a mass higher in the neck, such as cervical goiter or enlarged lymph nodes (see Fig. 7–78). Below the suprasternal notch, a retrosternal goiter, eccentrically located, may push the trachea to one side. The trachea and mediastinum deviate to the opposite side with pleural effusion and pneumothorax. Displacement of the trachea to the ipsilateral side occurs in pulmonary atelectasis or fibrosis of the lung or pleura. Carcinoma of the lung rarely causes displacement except by producing atelectasis.

KEY SIGN

Fixation of the Trachea: While the patient's head is held in the customary position, the examiner palpates the cricoid cartilage or tracheal rings with the thumb and index finger and asks the patient to swallow. Normally, this lifts the larynx and trachea cephalad and there is considerable axial mobility. Grasp the trachea gently and move it side to side; usually, it is easily mobile. Fixation of the trachea occurs normally when the neck is dorsiflexed, and abnormally in pulmonary emphysema, adhesive mediastinitis, aortic aneurysm, and mediastinal neoplasm.

KEY SIGN

Soft-Tissue Crepitus: Subcutaneous and Mediastinal Emphysema: *Pathophysiology:* Trauma to the chest may produce subcutaneous emphysema of the thoracic wall. Air may invade the chest wall from the neck or directly from the lung. Rupture of pulmonary alveoli permits air to travel beneath the visceral pleura to the hilum of the lung, then along the trachea to the neck. The thoracic wall is involved secondarily by migration from the neck. When a fractured rib or penetrating foreign body punctures the pleura, air travels across the pleura to the thoracic wall causing emphysema in the deep muscle layers and later the subcutaneous tissues. Soft-tissue crepitus may be the first clue to rupture of the alveoli, pleura or esophagus. Crepitus is a sensation imparted to the pressing finger by small globules of air moving in the tissues. The air may invade the mediastinum, where it produces a distinctive systolic crunching in the precordium known as *Hamman sign.* Vomiting with esophageal rupture produces this sign. Compression of the soft tissues of the neck can occur, producing massive swelling of the neck and face accompanied by cyanosis.

Mass in the Interspace: Fluctuant Masses: These are usually abscesses. A cold abscess, so named because it lacks surrounding inflammation, is usually tuberculosis arising from a nearby rib. Actinomycosis frequently produces abscesses in the lung that burrow through the chest wall. An abscess may result when an untreated pleural empyema points through the interspaces, termed empyema necessitatis.

Mass in a Rib: Some causes of masses on ribs are callus around an old fracture or fibrous dysplasia, neoplasm of ribs (e.g., chondrosarcoma), myeloma, desmoid tumor, metastasis of carcinoma, angioma, eosinophilic granuloma, and bone cysts, including osteitis fibrosa cystica. A neurofibroma arising from an intercostal nerve causes a swelling near the neck of the rib. Imaging usually distinguishes the various lesions.

Sinuses in the Thoracic Wall: Chronic sinuses discharging through the intercostal spaces may result from a variety of conditions, including empyema, tuberculosis, actinomycosis, and necrosis of ribs. The sinus tract should be probed from the exterior to ascertain the extent and direction. Actinomycosis produces a sinus with a peculiar dusky color around its mouth. Imaging is necessary for more detailed information about all sinuses.

Lung, Pleura, and Respiratory Signs

Inspection

KEY SIGN
Shortness of Breath: Dyspnea: See page 375.

KEY SIGN
Hiccup, Hiccough (Singultus): *Pathophysiology:* Hiccup is a sudden, involuntary diaphragmatic contraction producing an inspiration interrupted by glottal closure to emit a characteristic sharp sound. It is thought to be mediated centrally through the phrenic nerve, by direct stimulation of the phrenic nerve, or by direct irritation of the diaphragm. The contractions occur two or three times each minute. A variety of clinical conditions are associated with hiccup prompting the inference that it may be initiated centrally or peripherally.

✔ *HICCOUGH—CLINICAL OCCURRENCE:* *Hiccough Without Organic Disease* excessive laughter, tickling, aerophagia, excessive tobacco smoking, excessive intake of alcohol, hysteria (persisting for weeks, but ceasing during sleep); *Diseases of the Central Nervous System* encephalitis, meningitis, vertebrobasilar ischemia, intracranial hemorrhage, intracranial tumor, uremia, degenerative changes in brain and medulla, tabes dorsalis; *Mediastinal Disorders* trauma to phrenic nerve, enlargement of mediastinal lymph nodes (tuberculosis, malignant neoplasm, fibrosis), bronchial obstruction, adherent pericardium, cardiac enlargement, myocardial infarction, esophageal obstruction; *Pleural Irritation* pneumonia with pleurisy; *Diaphragmatic and Abdominal Disorders* diaphragmatic hernia of stomach, subphrenic abscess, subphrenic peritonitis, involvement of liver (neoplasm, gumma, abscess), carcinoma of stomach, splenic infarction, acute intestinal obstruction, acute hemorrhagic pancreatitis, after operations in the upper abdomen, diaphragmatic stimulation by an implanted cardiac pacemaker.

KEY SIGN
► **Hemoptysis: Coughing or Spitting Blood:** Spitting or coughing of blood is hemoptysis. The bleeding lesions may be anywhere from the nose to the lungs. Expectorated blood usually

comes from the upper respiratory tract while blood in the bronchial tree induces coughing. However, the patient may not be able to distinguish which of the two is occurring, so both upper and lower respiratory tract disorders must be considered.

✔ *HEMOPTYSIS—CLINICAL OCCURRENCE:* *Upper Respiratory Tract* epistaxis from the nasopharynx, bleeding from the oropharynx, bleeding from the gums, laryngitis, laryngeal carcinoma, hereditary hemorrhagic telangiectasia; *Bronchial Tree* acute and chronic bronchitis, trauma from coughing, bronchiectasis, bronchial carcinoma, broncholiths, foreign body aspiration, erosion by aortic aneurysms; *Lungs* infections (pneumonia, especially caused by *Klebsiella*, lung abscess, tuberculosis, fungal infections, amebiasis, hydatid cyst), pulmonary embolism with infarction, trauma, pulmonary hemorrhage (vasculitis especially Wegener, Goodpasture syndrome), idiopathic pulmonary hemosiderosis, lipoid pneumonia; *Cardiovascular* mitral stenosis, congestive heart failure, arteriovenous fistula, anomalous pulmonary artery, hypertension; *Hematologic* thrombocytopenia, leukemia, hemophilia.

KEY SIGN
Noisy Breathing: Snoring: Snoring is the common and harmless noise produced by vibrations of the lax soft palate during sleep. It also occurs in association with obstructive sleep apnea (see page 449). A similar sound results from vibrations of secretions in the upper respiratory tract. When this occurs during severe illness, it is frequently a grave prognostic sign, the "death rattle."

KEY SIGN
▶ **Noisy Breathing: Stridor:** A high-pitched whistling or crowing sound is caused by passage of air through the partly closed glottis. It occurs in edema of the vocal cords, neoplasm, diphtheritic membrane, abscess of the pharynx, and foreign body in the larynx or trachea. It may signal impending airway closure and asphyxiation.

Palpation

KEY SIGN
Vocal Fremitus Diminished or Absent: *Pathophysiology:* Palpable vibrations are transmitted from the bronchotracheal air column through the pulmonary septa and pleura. Damping of vibratory transmission occurs when lung tissue is destroyed, the pleura is thickened or the pleural surfaces are separated by air or fluid. Failure of the vocal cords or blockage of the airways results in absent vocal fremitus. The interposition of filters of variable quality such as thickened pleura, pleural effusion, pneumothorax or loss of lung parenchyma (e.g., emphysema) obstructs transmission of vibration through the chest wall, with diminished or absent vocal fremitus.

KEY SIGN
Vocal Fremitus Increased: *Pathophysiology:* Increased tension in the lung septa increases transmission of vibrations. Consolidated tissue in pneumonia or inflammation around a lung ab-

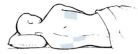

Fig. 8-29 Areas of Percussion Dullness Created by the Lateral Decubitus Position. *The lowest blue-shaded area is dull from compression of the thorax against the mattress. Immediately above, dullness is produced by compression of the lung from the body weight. In the opposite lung, dullness results by lateral deviation of the spine as it follows the sag in the mattress and compresses the lung.*

scess, when in contact with a bronchus or cavity in the lung, transmits bronchotracheal air vibrations with greater efficiency than do the air-filled pulmonary alveoli; hence, vocal fremitus is increased.

Percussion

KEY SIGN

Abnormal Percussion Notes: Normal Dullness in the Lateral Decubitus Position: When the patient cannot sit up in bed, the best compromise is frequently to percuss the back while the patient lies on one side or the other. The position is not optimal because it is difficult to interpret the percussion sounds. The damping effect of the mattress causes a band of dullness in the part of the thorax nearest the bed (Fig. 8-29). Directly above this band is an irregular area of dullness caused by compression of the downward lung by the body weight. The lengthwise sag of the mattress from the body weight flexes the spine laterally to compress the thoracic wall and underlying lung on the upward hemithorax, yielding another area of dullness.

KEY SIGN

Abnormal Percussion Notes: Modified Tympanitic Notes: Modified tympanitic notes have limited value in special situations. In suspected pneumothorax, the coin test may be used. An assistant percusses the front of the affected hemithorax by holding a coin flat to the chest wall and striking it with the edge of a second coin (Fig. 8-30). The examiner listens with the stethoscope over the back on the same side for a clear ringing note, termed *bell tympany*. Although not always present, bell tympany is diagnostic of pneumothorax. Percussion over a pneumothorax, or a large pulmonary cavity, sometimes yields a hollow, low-pitched sound, termed *amphoric*. Occasionally, a superficial pulmonary cavity has a small bronchial exit through which percussed air is forcefully expelled to produce *cracked-pot resonance*. The name is descriptive, as the sound is dull, clinking, and closely approximates the effect obtained by percussing the cheek when the mouth is slightly opened. The zone of lung above a level of pleural fluid may be tympanitic: the sound is termed *skodaic tympany*. It arises from dilated air sacs in the lung just above the part compressed by the pleural fluid.

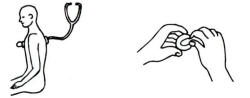

Fig. 8-30 Coin Test for Pneumothorax. *An assistant places a coin flat on the anterior chest wall and strikes it with the edge of a second coin. The examiner applies the chest piece of his stethoscope to the back of the same hemithorax. In pneumothorax, the note is transmitted as a clear ringing sound, called bell tympany.*

 KEY SIGN

Abnormal Percussion Notes: Abnormal Distribution: An abnormal distribution of sounds of normal quality can be pathologic. The lung is normally resonant. As consolidation occurs its density increases to yield, successively, impaired resonance, dullness, and flatness. Ordinarily, the pleura contributes little to the percussion note, but fluid in the pleural cavity produces a dense layer that gives dullness to flatness in a characteristic distribution.

ABNORMAL PERCUSSION NOTES: DULLNESS REPLACING RESONANCE IN THE UPPER LUNG: This finding suggests neoplasm, atelectasis or consolidation of the lung.

ABNORMAL PERCUSSION NOTES: DULLNESS REPLACING RESONANCE IN THE LOWER LUNG: To the causes in the upper lung must be added pleural effusion, pleural thickening, and elevation of the diaphragm.

ABNORMAL PERCUSSION NOTES: FLATNESS REPLACING RESONANCE OR DULLNESS: Almost invariably, flatness in the thorax results from massive pleural effusion.

ABNORMAL PERCUSSION NOTES: HYPERRESONANCE REPLACING RESONANCE OR DULLNESS. When lung resonance is replaced by hyperresonance and the area of hepatic and cardiac dullness is encroached upon, either pulmonary emphysema or pneumothorax are suggested.

ABNORMAL PERCUSSION NOTES: TYMPANY REPLACING RESONANCE: This occurs almost exclusively with a large pneumothorax.

Auscultation of Breath Sounds

Several types of breath sounds with distinctive qualities are recognized. All are characterized by rising pitch during inspiration and falling pitch during expiration (Doppler effect). Duration of inspiration and expiration affects the breath sounds: the longer the phase, the louder the sound in that phase.

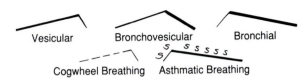

Fig. 8-31 Distinguishing Features of Breath Sounds. In the diagrams, the vertical component indicates rising and falling pitch, the thickness of the lines indicates loudness, and the horizontal distance represents duration. Inspiration is longer in vesicular breathing, expiration in bronchial breathing. Bronchovesicular breathing is a mixture of the two. Normally vesicular breathing is heard over most of the lungs, except that bronchovesicular breathing occurs over the thoracic portion of the trachea, anteriorly and posteriorly. Bronchial breathing does not occur in the normal lung. In cogwheel breathing, the inspiratory sound is interrupted with multiple breaks. Asthmatic breathing is characterized by a much prolonged and higher-pitched expiratory sound than is found in bronchial breathing. Asthmatic breathing is usually, but not always, accompanied by wheezes.

KEY SIGN
Normal Breath Sounds: Vesicular Breathing: Shallow breathing during quiet respiration produces a whishing noise over the surface of the lungs. Vesicular breath sounds are characterized by having a long inspiratory phase and a short expiratory phase (Fig. 8-31). They are heard normally over the entire lung surface, except beneath the manubrium and in the upper interscapular region, where they are replaced by bronchovesicular breathing. The breath sounds are faintest over the thinner portions of the lungs.

Breath Sounds: Cogwheel Breathing: This is identical with vesicular breathing except that the inspiratory phase is broken by short pauses, giving the impression of jerkiness (see Fig. 8-31). The pauses are attributed to irregular inflation of the alveoli; it has no pathologic significance.

KEY SIGN
Abnormal Breath Sounds: Bronchial Breathing (Tubular Breathing): *Pathophysiology:* This results from consolidation or compression of pulmonary tissue that facilitates transmission of sound from the bronchial tree. In contrast to vesicular breathing, bronchial breath sounds have a short inspiratory phase and a long expiratory phase (see Fig. 8-31). They are usually louder, but not always; intensity should not be relied on to distinguish them. Bronchial breathing does not occur in the normal lung. The closest normal counterpart is tracheal breathing, heard in the suprasternal notch and over the sixth and seventh cervical spines. It is harsher and more hollow than true bronchial breathing and has no pathologic significance.

KEY SIGN

Abnormal Breath Sounds: Bronchovesicular Breathing: *Pathophysiology:* Bronchovesicular breathing is pathologic and indicates a small degree of pulmonary consolidation or compression that transmits sounds from the bronchial tree with increased facility. As the name indicates, this is intermediate between vesicular and bronchial breathing. The two respiratory phases are about equal in duration (see Fig. 8-31), although expiration is frequently a bit longer. Normally, it is heard at the manubrium and in the upper interscapular region. As the degree of compression or consolidation increases, bronchovesicular breathing is converted to bronchial breathing.

KEY SIGN

Abnormal Breath Sounds: Asthmatic or Obstructive Breathing: *Pathophysiology:* See *Wheezing,* page 395. Like bronchial breathing, inspiration is short and expiration prolonged, but there is no confusing the two (see Fig. 8-31). In asthma, the expiratory phase is several times longer than in bronchial breathing, and the pitch is much higher. The listener is aware that expiration is active, not passive, and may require significant effort. Frequently, but not always, asthmatic breathing is accompanied by wheezes audible without the stethoscope. Emphysema produces a similar pattern of breath sounds, but wheezing is absent and the intensity of sound is diminished.

KEY SIGN

Abnormal Breath Sounds: Amphoric Breathing: *Pathophysiology:* This sound is produced by a large empty superficial cavity that communicates with a bronchus or an open pneumothorax. The Latin word for jug is amphora. Amphoric breath sounds have the quality generated by blowing air over the mouth of a bottle. When the pitch is relatively low and the sound hollow, it is called *cavernous breathing,* with the same pathologic significance.

Abnormal Breath Sounds: Metamorphosing Breathing: The breath sounds suddenly change in intensity in different parts of the cycle. This is usually caused by movement of a loose bronchial plug.

Auscultation of Voice Sounds

KEY SIGN

Voice Sounds: *Pathophysiology:* In the normal lungs, whispered words are faint and their syllables are not distinct, except over the main bronchi. Increases in loudness and distinctness have clinical significance, indicating consolidation, atelectasis, or fibrosis, which improve transmission of vibrations. Because of their pitch and loudness, whispered and spoken voice sounds are somewhat more valuable than breath sounds in detecting pulmonary consolidation, infarction, and atelectasis. Spoken voice sounds are not as useful as whispered sounds because they are too loud for careful distinction.

KEY SIGN
Abnormal Voice Sounds: Whispered Pectoriloquy: Pulmonary consolidation transmits whispered syllables distinctly, even when the pathologic process is too small to produce bronchial breathing. This sign is particularly valuable in detecting early pneumonia, infarction, and pulmonary atelectasis.

KEY SIGN
Abnormal Voice Sounds: Bronchophony: Normally, the spoken syllables are indistinctly heard in the lungs. In the presence of pulmonary consolidation, syllables are heard distinctly and sound very close to the ear.

KEY SIGN
Abnormal Voice Sounds: Egophony: This is a form of bronchophony in which the spoken "Eee" is changed to "Ay," which has a peculiar nasal or bleating quality. Often the tone quality is imparted by compressed lung below a pleural effusion, although it occasionally is heard in pulmonary consolidation.

Auscultation of Adventitious Sounds

Abnormal (adventitious) sounds, including crackles (rales), wheezes, rhonchi, rubs, and bruits, are heard in the lungs of patients with various illnesses.

KEY SIGN
Adventitious Sounds: Crackles (Rales): *Pathophysiology:* Crackles result from the opening and closing of alveoli and small airways during respiration. In pulmonary edema, fine rales may be produced by air bubbling through fluid in the distal small airways. Inspiratory crackles (fine rales) resemble the sound of several hairs being rubbed together between thumb and forefinger. They are heard in the bases of patients with interstitial lung disease, fibrosing alveolitis, atelectasis, pneumonia, bronchiectasis, and pulmonary edema, and in the apices with tuberculosis.

KEY SIGN
Adventitious Sounds: Wheezes (Musical Rales): *Pathophysiology:* Wheezes arise from turbulent airflow and the vibrations of the walls of small airways in which there is partial obstruction to airflow. Wheezes are heard predominantly during expiration. They occur when airways are narrowed by bronchospasm, edema, collapse, or by intraluminal secretions, neoplasm, or foreign body. They are diffuse in asthma and bronchitis, usually accompanying a prolonged expiratory phase of respiration. An isolated wheeze heard in just one area may be a sign of bronchial obstruction by a tumor or foreign body. Use of wheezing to either detect or exclude obstructive airways disease is not advised [King DK, Thompson BT, Johnson DC. Wheezing on maximal forced exhalation in the diagnosis of atypical asthma: Lack of sensitivity and specificity. *Ann Intern Med* 1989;110:451–455].

KEY SIGN
Adventitious Sounds: Rhonchus: Rhonchi occur as low-pitched gurgling sounds when there is liquid within the larger airways from inflammatory secretions or drowning and in agonal states (death rattle). They clear or change significantly after an effective cough.

KEY SIGN
Adventitious Sounds: Rubs (Pleural Friction Rub): Pleural friction rubs occur when inflamed, unlubricated surfaces of pleurae rub together during respiration. They are characterized as the "creaking of new leather." Listen at the spot where the patient feels pleuritic pain. Rubs may be ephemeral and disappear after several respiratory cycles.

KEY SIGN
Adventitious Sounds: Continuous Murmur: The continuous murmur of a pulmonary arteriovenous fistula increases in intensity with inspiration. In patients with coarctation of the aorta, continuous murmurs may be heard below the left scapula and over the intercostal and internal mammary arteries from the collateral circulation. These are rare findings.

Adventitious Sounds: Special Sounds in Hydropneumothorax: *Pathophysiology:* Movement of fluid is noiseless in a cavity devoid of air. When the cavity contains both air and fluid, body movements cause a succussion splash, audible to the patient and the examiner. Hippocrates described the sign. To elicit it, the physician grasps the patient's shoulders and shakes the thorax while listening with or without a stethoscope. The *succussion splash* is normally present in the stomach or bowel. It occurs in hydropneumothorax, where its presence is diagnostic. A fluid-filled stomach protruding into the thorax through a diaphragmatic hernia may also produce the splash. The physician should hesitate to shake a very ill patient. Occasionally, one hears a *falling-drop sound*, resembling a drop of water hitting the surface of fluid; it is occasionally encountered in the collapsed lung. A *metallic tinkle* may be heard when air bubbles emerge through a small bronchopleural fistula below the fluid level; when the fistula is larger, the air may gurgle, a *lung-fistula sound*.

Adventitious Sounds: Bone Crepitus: The movements of fractured ends of a rib may produce a grating sound, leading to a correct diagnosis.

Adventitious Sounds: Systolic Popping, Clicking, or Crunching Sounds: Hamman sign; see page 463.

Interpretation of Pulmonary and Pleural Signs

The findings disclosed by inspection, palpation, percussion, and auscultation of the lungs and pleura may now be synthesized to suggest a pathophysiologic process or diagnosis. Frequently, the signs of altered density serve as a starting point for the differential diagnosis, so the subject will be presented in terms of altered density and the transmission of vibrations to the chest wall.

KEY SIGN

Dullness and Diminished Vibrations: Pleural Fluid: *Pathophysiology:* Fluid accumulates in the pleural space due to transudation of fluid from the pleural and pulmonary vessels (increased venous hydrostatic pressure, decreased oncotic pressure, capillary leak), increased production of pleural fluid (inflamed pleura or pleural neoplasm), decreased pleural absorption of fluid (lymphatic obstruction, systemic venous hypertension), or by bleeding into the pleural space. All produce certain physical exam findings (Fig. 8-32). During the physical examination any liquid in the pleural cavity is called "fluid." Subsequent thoracentesis reveals the liquid to be clear (transudate or exudate), purulent (pyothorax or empyema thoracis), bloody (hemothorax), or chylous (chylothorax) [Light RW. Pleural effusion. *N Engl J Med* 2002;346:1971–1977]. See procedural texts for instructions on thoracentesis and *Harrison's Principles of Internal Medicine*, 16th edition for discussion of the differential diagnosis of transudates and exudates. Pleural effusion can be detected with chest CT or MRI in the absence of physical findings. The pleural fluid produces a dull or flat note to percussion. The lung immediately over the fluid may be hyperresonant (*skodaic resonance*) from distention of the alveoli above a compressed region. The distribution of dullness is dependent. With large amounts of fluid, the trachea may be pushed to the unaffected side (Fig. 8-32). Vocal fremitus is absent. Occasionally, loud bronchial breathing is heard through

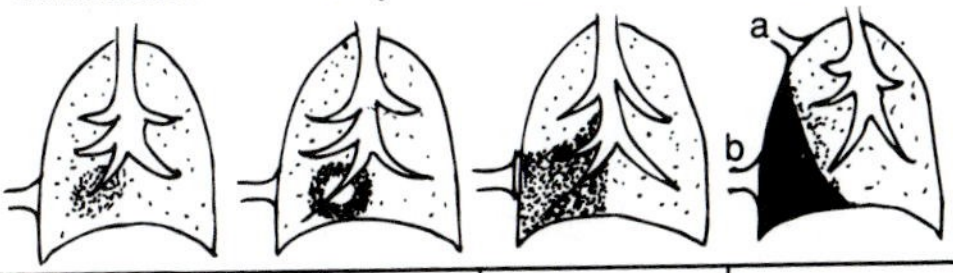

	Small Consolidation	Thick-walled Cavity	Massive Consolidation	Large Pleural Effusion
Tracheal Deviation	O	O	O	→
Fremitus	N or Λ	N or Λ	Λ	O
Percussion	Slight Dullness	Slight Dullness	Dull or Flat	(a) Hyperresonant (b) Flat
Breath Sounds	Bronchovesicular or Bronchial	Bronchovesicular or Amorphic	Bronchial	O or Loud Bronchial
Whisper Sounds	N, O, or Λ	Pectoriloquy	Λ	O or Λ
Voice Sounds	N, O, or Λ	Λ	Λ	O or Λ
Rales	+ or O	+	+	O

Legend: O = Absent   N = Normal   + = Present   Λ = Increased   ← = Direction of Deviation

Fig. 8-32 Thoracic Disorders with Dullness and Accentuated Vibration.

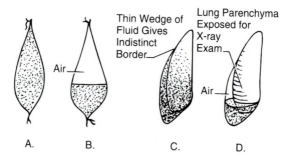

Fig. 8-33 Models Illustrating Pleural Effusion and Pneumothorax. **A**. *Suspend a plastic bag filled with water, noting its contour.* **B**. *When air is introduced, a fluid level forms, the contour changes, and a succussion splash occurs with shaking.* **C**. **An Uncomplicated Pleural Effusion**: *Note the tapering upper wedge, or meniscus, of fluid.* **D**. **Hydropneumothorax**: *When air is introduced, a fluid level forms and the meniscus largely disappears.*

the fluid from the compressed lung; the unwary mistake it for consolidation. Fluid is distinguished from consolidation by noting diminished breath sounds and absence of fremitus with fluid, and bronchial breath sounds with "E" to "A" changes in consolidation. Massive pleural effusion obscures the lung fields on radiographs, so that no appraisal of the parenchyma is possible. If air has entered the pleural cavity, producing a hydropneumothorax, when the patient stands, the fluid level falls below much of the lung, permitting its visualization (Fig. 8-33) Case with differential diagnosis: Case records of the Massachusetts General Hospital. Case 8–2002. *N Engl J Med* 2002;346:843–850].

✓ *PLEURAL EFFUSION—CLINICAL OCCURRENCE*: *Increased Transudation* congestive heart failure, hypoalbuminemia (cirrhosis, nephrotic syndrome), pulmonary embolism, superior vena cava syndrome; *Increased Production* mesothelioma, metastatic cancer, infections (bacteria, mycobacteria, viral, parasites, fungi), pulmonary infarction, pancreatitis, mediastinitis, collagen-vascular diseases (e.g., rheumatoid arthritis, systemic lupus erythematosus, drug-induced lupus, vasculitis), after heart or lung surgery, uremia, Meigs syndrome, pleuropericarditis peritoneal dialysis; *Decreased Absorption* lymphatic obstruction (lymphoma, lymphatic carcinomatosis, irradiation, surgical injury), heart failure, superior vena cava syndrome; *Bleeding* ruptured aortic aneurysm or dissection, trauma, postoperative.

KEY SIGN

Dullness and Diminished Vibrations: Small Pleural Effusion or Pleural Thickening (Fig. 8-34): Unless the fluid is loculated, dullness always occurs in the lowermost part of the thorax. The dull region is a transverse band that

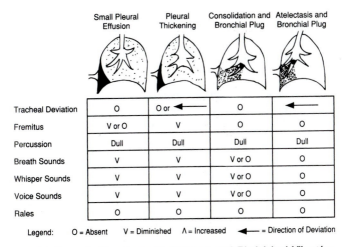

	Small Pleural Effusion	Pleural Thickening	Consolidation and Bronchial Plug	Atelectasis and Bronchial Plug
Tracheal Deviation	O	O or ⟵	O	⟵
Fremitus	V or O	V	O	O
Percussion	Dull	Dull	Dull	Dull
Breath Sounds	V	V	V or O	O
Whisper Sounds	V	V	V or O	O
Voice Sounds	V	V	V or O	O
Rales	O	O	O	O

Legend: O = Absent   V = Diminished   Λ = Increased   ⟵ = Direction of Deviation

Fig. 8-34 Thoracic Disorders with Dullness and Diminished Vibration.

is broadest posteriorly and laterally because the costophrenic sulcus is higher in front. The superior border of the dullness may be difficult to percuss accurately because the fluid layer is an upward-pointing wedge. Shifting dullness is not usually demonstrable. Because air is absent, there is no succession splash. With a small amount of fluid, the respiratory excursions of the thorax are normal. In pleurisy, an antecedent friction rub disappears when fluid forms. Pleural fluid baffles vibrations from the bronchotracheal column of air, so vocal fremitus, breath sounds, whispered and spoken voice are transmitted poorly to the stethoscope. The mediastinum is not shifted with small pleural effusions. Unless the fluid has recently appeared, the signs cannot be distinguished from thickened pleura. Because pleural fibrosis results from the organization of pleural effusion, the distribution of dullness is the same. The pleura may attain a thickness of 5 or 6 cm. The thicker it is, the more it obstructs air transmission and the more the percussion note indicates denseness. Extensive fibrosis may pull the trachea to the affected side. Ultrasound and decubitus radiography distinguish the two. Any longstanding pleural effusion may organize. Neoplastic involvement may simulate thickening. Asbestosis and/or mesothelioma may cause thickening.

KEY SIGN
Dullness and Diminished Vibration: Pulmonary Consolidation with Bronchial Plug:
Pathophysiology: The consolidated lung produces dullness. A bronchial plug prevents vibrations of the air column, so there is absence of vocal fremitus, breath sounds, whispered and spoken voice (Fig. 8-34). The trachea is not displaced. Plugging of a bronchus is usually a

transitory occurrence in lobar pneumonia, so it is recognized by the sudden loss of air transmission. X-ray films can usually distinguish between pleural effusion and pulmonary consolidation. If the dullness is in the upper lobe, effusion is excluded on physical examination.

KEY SIGN

Dullness with Diminished Vibration: Atelectasis with Bronchial Plug: *Pathophysiology:* The volume of the atelectatic lung is diminished; the dense mass is pulled toward the chest wall by the negative intrapleural pressure, so the trachea shifts to the affected side. The collapsed lung is dull because its density is increased. The bronchial plug prevents air vibration, so vocal fremitus and breath and voice sounds are absent (Fig. 8-34). The tracheal deviation distinguishes atelectasis from consolidation with bronchial plug and from pleural effusion. Usually, atelectasis is accompanied by fever that distinguishes it from thickened pleura with fibrotic traction on the mediastinum.

KEY SIGN

Dullness with Accentuated Vibration: Pneumonia with Small Consolidation: *Pathophysiology:* A small, deeply placed region of consolidation may produce impaired resonance or dullness, depending on its size and depth from the chest wall. The dense lung transmits the air column with increased facility, so vocal fremitus is increased and bronchovesicular or bronchial breathing and crackles may be heard (Fig. 8-32). Symptoms of fever, chills, and productive cough are accompanied by tachypnea and tachycardia. Whispered pectoriloquy and bronchophony are produced by the consolidation. Small regions of consolidation must be distinguished from a small cavity lying near a bronchus. X-ray films are required for definitive diagnosis. Pneumonia, granulomatous infiltrates of the lung, neoplasm about a bronchus, rheumatoid arthritis, and sarcoidosis may all produce these findings [Metlay JP, Kapoor WN, Fine MJ. The rational clinical examination. Does this patient have community-acquired pneumonia? Diagnosing pneumonia by history and physical examination. *JAMA* 1997;278:1440–1445].

KEY SIGN

Dullness with Accentuated Vibration: Pneumonia with Lobar Consolidation: *Pathophysiology:* The dense lung yields dullness or flatness on percussion. The consolidated lung in contact with a bronchus transmits vibrations with increased facility, so vocal fremitus is pronounced, there is bronchial breathing, and whispered and spoken voice produce pectoriloquy and bronchophony (Fig. 8-32). Crackles (rales) are frequently present. The lung volume is unchanged, so the trachea remains in the midline. Occasionally consolidation may be confused with a thick-walled cavity, and the distinction must be made by imaging. These finding are seen classically in lobar pneumonia but occasionally in neoplasms of the lung and pulmonary infarction. Massive pleural effusion gives dullness and may transmit loud bronchial breath sounds above the effusion, but the trachea is usually displaced to the unaffected side.

KEY SIGN

Dullness with Accentuated Vibration: Thick-walled Cavity: The signs of pulmonary consolidation are present: dullness, increased vocal fremitus, bronchovesicular breathing, and pectoriloquy (Fig. 8-32). Usually distinctive, but most infrequent, is amphoric breathing or cracked-pot resonance. Even these signs may be present in consolidation without cavity.

KEY SIGN

Resonance and Hyperresonance: Pulmonary Emphysema: *Pathophysiology:* Loss of interstitial elasticity and interalveolar septa leads to air trapping, so the volume of the lungs is increased. The augmented volume holds the thoracic walls continuously in the inspiratory position, producing the increased anteroposterior diameter of the barrel chest. The diaphragm is pushed downward so the costal margins move out sluggishly or actually converge during inspiration (Fig. 8-35). The lungs are hyperresonant throughout because of their low density. Air pockets are poor transmitters of vibrations; thus vocal fremitus, breath sounds, heart sounds, and whispered and spoken voice are impaired or absent. When the breath sounds are audible, they are faint and harsh, lacking the rustling quality of vesicular breathing. This absence of the vesicular quality is distinctive; it may antedate recognizable x-ray evidence of emphysema. The expiratory phase of respiration usually exceeds the inspiratory phase. Rales are not necessarily present and wheezes are not heard.

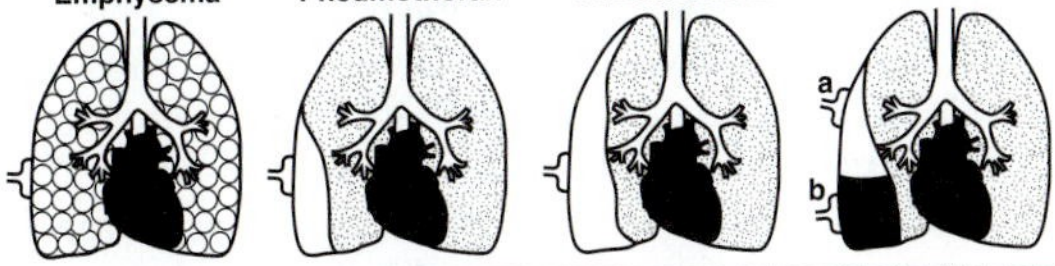

	Pulmonary Emphysema	Closed Pneumothorax	Tension Pneumothorax	Hydropneumothorax
Tracheal Deviation	O	O	→	→
Fremitus	V	O	O	O
Percussion	Hyperresonant	Resonant or Hyper	Hyperresonant	(a) Hyperresonant (b) Flat
Breath Sounds	V or O	V or O	V or O	O
Whisper Sounds	V or O	V or O	V or O	O
Voice Sounds	V or O	V or O	V or O	O
Rales	+ or O	O	O	O
		Coin Sound	Coin Sound	Coin Sound
				Succussion Splash
				Shifting Dullness

Legend: O = Absent V = Diminished + = Present → = Direction of Deviation

Fig. 8-35 Thoracic Disorders with Resonance Impaired Vibration.

KEY SIGN

► **Resonance or Hyperresonance: Closed Pneumothorax:** *Pathophysiology:* When the air leak between lung and pleura becomes sealed or when air is instilled into the pleural cavity for diagnosis or therapy, a *closed pneumothorax* is formed. If the volume of enclosed air is small, the lung remains partially inflated and the mediastinum is not displaced. In an open pneumothorax, a similar situation may be created by pleural adhesions, which prevent collapse of the lung and displacement of the trachea (Fig. 8-35). Vocal fremitus, breath sounds, and whispered and spoken voice are usually inaudible or impaired. The chest wall is resonant or hyperresonant. Frequently, pneumothorax cannot be distinguished from a normal or emphysematous chest by percussion. The disparity between the breath sounds on the two sides is the clue that leads to making the diagnosis. There may be a pendular deviation of the trachea toward the affected side during inspiration. The tear in the pleura may be spontaneous or the result of trauma to the thorax [Sahn SA, Heffner JE. Spontaneous pneumothorax. *N Engl J Med* 2000;342:868–874].

KEY SIGN

► **Resonance or Hyperresonance: Open Pneumothorax:** *Pathophysiology:* With continual communication between lung and pleural cavity, the air in the *open pneumothorax* is under atmospheric pressure (Fig. 8-35). The collapse of the affected lung is complete, and the mediastinum may be drawn toward the unaffected side by the contraction of the normal lung. Overlying the pneumothorax, the chest wall is hyperresonant or tympanitic. Fremitus and breath and voice sounds are absent. Usually, the patient is severely dyspneic and may be cyanotic.

KEY SIGN

► **Resonance or Hyperresonance: Tension Pneumothorax:** *Pathophysiology:* A one-way tissue valve permits air to be forced into the pleural space during inspiration and prevents its expulsion during expiration. Thus, the pressure in the cavity builds up in excess of the atmosphere. The affected lung is collapsed and the increasing intrapleural pressure causes extreme tracheal deviation, compression of the unaffected lung, and decreased venous return to the heart (Fig. 8-35). The physical signs of tension pneumothorax resemble those of the open pneumothorax, although the condition is actually a modified closed type. The signs of decreased respiratory excursion of a distended tympanitic hemithorax combined with tracheal deviation away from the immobile side are diagnostic of pneumothorax with tension. This situation is accompanied by deep cyanosis, severe dyspnea, and shock that demands aspiration of air from the cavity as a lifesaving measure.

KEY SIGN

Resonance and Hyperresonance: Hydropneumothorax: Hyperresonance or tympany in the upper part of the thorax, with dullness inferiorly, suggests either hydropneumothorax or a massive pleural effusion (Fig. 8-35). In either case, the trachea may be displaced to the unaffected side. In hydropneumothorax, the hyperresonant region does not transmit fremitus, breath sounds, or voice sounds, whereas the lung over a simple hydrothorax transmits well. When hydropneumothorax is present, the fluid level can be sharply demarcated by percussion; the level is vague in simple effusion. Shifting dullness is readily demonstrated by percussion in the presence of hydropneumothorax; this is not the case in hydrothorax. The air-filled cavity carries bell tympany, and a succession splash may be demonstrated.

Sputum Signs

KEY SIGN

Bloody Sputum: Blood in the sputum usually impresses patients enough to bring them to the physician. The first problem is to identify the anatomic site of hemorrhage. *Blood-Streaked Sputum* is usually caused by inflammation in the nose, nasopharynx, gums, larynx, or bronchi. Sometimes it occurs only after severe paroxysms of coughing and may be attributed to trauma. *Pink Sputum* usually results from blood mixing with secretions in the alveoli or smaller bronchioles; it most frequently occurs in pneumonia or pulmonary edema. *Massive Bleeding* occurs with erosion of a bronchial artery by cavitary pulmonary tuberculosis, aspergilloma, lung abscess, bronchiectasis, pulmonary infarction, pulmonary embolism, bronchogenic carcinoma or a broncholith. *Alveolar Hemorrhage,* as in Goodpasture syndrome, does not produce bloody sputum in all cases. Not infrequently, frank bleeding from the lungs occurs in mitral stenosis.

Bloody Gelatinous Sputum: Currant-Jelly Sputum: Copious quantities of tenacious, bloody sputum are almost pathognomonic for pneumonia caused by *Klebsiella pneumoniae* or *Streptococcus pneumoniae.*

Rusty Sputum: Prune-Juice Sputum: Purulent sputum containing changed blood pigment is typical of pneumococcal pneumonia but it is frequently preceded by small amounts of frank blood.

Stringy Mucoid Sputum: Increased mucous production and formation of mucous plugs occur in asthma; during resolution of an acute attack, retained mucous is mobilized.

KEY SIGN

Frothy Sputum: Pulmonary Edema: *Pathophysiology:* Fluid from the pulmonary capillaries enters the alveoli and is expectorated. A thin secretion containing air bubbles, frequently colored with hemoglobin, is typical of pulmonary edema. Both acute lung injury and left ventricular failure produce this sign.

KEY SIGN

Purulent Sputum: *Pathophysiology:* Inflammatory cells, predominately polymorphonuclear leukocytes, enter the airways and alveoli in response to lower airway infection. The exudate may be yellow, green, or dirty gray. Small amounts are typical of acute bronchitis, pneumonia during resolution, small tuberculous cavities or lung abscess. Copious purulent sputum suggests lung abscess, bronchiectasis, or bronchopleural fistula communicating with an empyema. Fetid sputum suggests anaerobic infection and/or lung abscess. Many lung abscesses do not yield much sputum because their bronchial communications are inadequate for complete drainage. In bronchiectasis, the daily volume is often from 200 to 500 mL. On standing, bronchiectatic sputum typically separates into three layers, with mucus on top separated by clear fluid from pus on the bottom. Copious sputum from a patient with signs of pleural effusion suggests a bronchopleural fistula.

Broncholiths: Occasionally, calcified particles are found in the sputum either by the patient or the physician. These are usually broncholiths, derived from calcified lymph nodes eroding the bronchi or from calcareous granulomas in silicosis, tuberculosis, or histoplasmosis. Their discovery may explain the source of pulmonary hemorrhage.

Cardiovascular Signs

Inspection

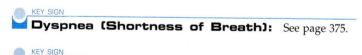
KEY SIGN

Dyspnea (Shortness of Breath): See page 375.

KEY SIGN

Pallor: See Chapter 6, page 158.

KEY SIGN

Cyanosis: See Chapter 6, page 159.

Palpation

KEY SIGN

Edema: *Pathophysiology:* The distribution of water between blood and interstitial tissues is maintained by a net equilibrium between hydrostatic and oncotic pressures. Normally, fluid flows into the extravascular interstitial space in response to hydrostatic pressure in the precapillary arterioles and capillaries (intravascular > interstitial), which is only partially offset by the opposing oncotic pressure (intravascular > interstitial). In the postcapillary venules, the lowered intravascular hydrostatic pressure is more than compensated by the intravascular oncotic pressure, resulting in return of interstitial water to the intravascular space. Interstitial fluid, proteins, and cells are also removed from the interstitial space and, ultimately, returned to the blood through the lymphatics. Alteration of any of these forces upsets the equilibrium. An increase in the systemic venous pressure in congestive heart failure produces generalized edema; occlusion of a vein may result in localized edema. Obstruction of lymphatic channels produces lymphedema. Reduction in the plasma albumin (the plasma protein with the highest contribution to oncotic pressure) results in lowering the oncotic pressure of the plasma, permitting edema to form; this type of edema may first appear in areas of decreased tissue pressure such as the periorbital tissues. Increased capillary permeability may cause edema that is not dependent. Tissue inflammation by bacterial, chemical, thermal, or mechanical means increases capillary permeability to make localized edema. Excessive accumulation of interstitial fluid, either localized or generalized, is termed edema. When the amount of generalized edema is great, the condition is termed *anasarca* or *dropsy*. In the adult, about 4.5 kg (10 lb) of fluid accumulates before it is detectable as pitting edema. To demonstrate the presence of edema, gently press your thumb into the skin against a bony surface, such as the anterior tibia, fibula, dorsum of the foot, or sacrum. When the thumb is withdrawn, an indentation persists for a short time.

The *distribution of edema* should be noted; the amount of fluid is roughly proportional to its extent and thickness. Because *dependent edema* responds to gravity, it first appears in the feet and ankles of the walking patient or over the posterior calves or sacrum of the supine patient. As the amount of dependent fluid increases, a fluid level may be detected under the skin; seldom does dependent edema rise higher than the heart. Anasarca can be recognized at a glance by the obliteration of superficial landmarks under the skin. Chronic edema of the legs leads to fibrosis of the subcutaneous tissues and skin, so they no longer pit on pressure; this is sometimes called *brawny edema* (i.e., muscle-like). Symmetric edema affecting both legs suggests that the problem is in the pelvis or more proximally, while edema limited to the arms and head suggests superior vena cava obstruction. Edema limited to one extremity suggests a local problem with vascular channels or local inflammation.

The processes involved in edema formation are the same whether the edema is generalized or local. To evaluate local edema, the examiner must consider the local anatomy of the arteries, veins, lymphatics and soft tissues, the presence of any local inflammatory or structural disease and then form hypotheses as to the likely mechanism and anatomic site of the local problem.

Because exclusive dependence upon clinical information may miss cardiovascular causes of bilateral leg edema, consider measurement of B-type natruretic peptide and/or echocardiographic evaluation with estimation of pulmonary artery pressure, right and left ventricular size and function and tricuspid valve function [Blankfield RP, Finkelhor RS, Alexander JJ, et al. Etiology and diagnosis of bilateral leg edema in primary care. *Am J Med* 1998;105:192–197]. The following approach, based upon the anatomic distribution of edema, is diagnostically useful.

✓ *EDEMA—CLINICAL OCCURRENCE:* **Localized Edema** *Inflammation* infection, angioedema, contact allergy; *Metabolic Causes* gout; *Insufficiency of the Venous Valves* (with or without varicosities); *Venous Thrombosis* postoperative, prolonged air or automobile travel; *Venous or Lymphatic Compression* malignancies, constricting garments; *Chemical or Physical Injuries* burns, irritants and corrosives, frostbite, chilblain, envenomation (insects, snakes, spiders); *Congenital* amniotic bands, arteriovenous fistulas, Milroy disease; **Bilateral Edema Above the Diaphragm** superior vena cava obstruction; **Bilateral Edema Below the Diaphragm** *Congestive Cardiac Failure* with elevated jugular venous pressure including elevated pulmonary artery pressures caused by left heart abnormalities, intrinsic pulmonary disorders, right heart abnormalities, and constrictive pericarditis; *Portal Vein Hypertension or Obstruction* cirrhosis, portal vein thrombosis, schistosomiasis; *Inferior Vena Cava Obstruction* thrombosis, extrinsic compression, pregnancy; *Loss of Venous Tone* drugs (calcium channel blockers, angiotensin-converting enzyme inhibitors, other vasodilators), convalescence, lack of exercise; **Generalized Edema** *Hypoalbuminemia* nephrotic syndrome, cirrhosis, chronic liver disease, protein losing conditions (e.g., enteropathy, burns, fistulas); *Renal Retention of Salt and Water* corticosteroids, nonsteroidal antiinflammatory drugs (NSAIDs); *Increased Capillary Permeability* sepsis, systemic inflammatory response syndrome (SIRS), interleukin (IL)-2.

IDIOPATHIC EDEMA: Recurrent and chronic edema may be observed in women in the 3rd to 5th decades in the absence of cardiac, hepatic, or renal abnormalities or of venous or lymphatic obstruction. Affective disorders and obesity may coexist. Possible mechanisms include exaggerated capillary leakage on assuming the upright posture and inappropriate chronic diuretic administration started initially for minor degrees of peripheral edema (*diuretic-induced edema*). Both mechanisms probably lead to inappropriate activation of hormones involved in salt and water retention.

TROPICAL EDEMA: Pitting edema of the ankles often occurs abruptly in normal adults within 48 h after they have traveled from a temperate climate to the heat of the tropics or in temperate zones when weather changes from cool and dry to warm and humid. It spontaneously resolves in a few days of acclimatization.

▶ **ANGIOEDEMA:** Subcutaneous soft-tissue edema begins abruptly and spreads to involve several centimeters of tissue with diffuse borders. Erythema is not prominent. Angioedema often involves the face, lips, or tongue, and is life-threatening when the larynx is involved. Causes include hereditary absence of C1 esterase, exposure to allergen, and angiotensin-converting enzyme inhibitors.

The physical signs from inspection, palpation, and percussion of the precordium depend for their interpretation on relatively normal anatomic relations between the heart and the chest wall. In gross distortions of the thoracic cage, such as kyphoscoliosis, funnel breast, or thoracoplasty, conclusions must be formed cautiously.

KEY SIGN

Apical Impulse: Increased Amplitude: *Pathophysiology:* Increased force of left ventricular myocardial contraction increases the amplitude of the apical impulse. This may be caused by left ventricular hypertrophy (arterial hypertension, aortic stenosis, aortic regurgitation, mitral regurgitation). An increased impulse is also associated with heightened myocardial tone (exertion, emotion, hyperthyroidism).

KEY SIGN

Enlarged and Sustained Apical Impulse: *Pathophysiology:* A left ventricle ejecting against increased afterload ejects more slowly than normal. Aortic valvular stenosis and arterial hypertension produces an enlarged sustained impulse rather than the normal brief tapping impulse.

KEY SIGN

Apical Impulse: Displaced to the Left: *Pathophysiology:* Volume overload of the left ventricle leads to left ventricular dilation, but does not interfere with ejection. Volume overload from aortic or mitral regurgitation or from cardiac shunts produces ventricular impulses that are enlarged, brisk, and displaced laterally but are not sustained. A weak myocardium produces an apical impulse of lesser intensity, although dilatation of the heart may cause it to be perceived over a wider area than normal. Other causes of leftward displacement are right pneumothorax, left pleural adhesions, or volume loss in the left lung.

Apical Impulse: Displaced to the Right: The location may be shifted to the right with left pneumothorax, right pleural adhesions, volume loss of the right lung, and dextrocardia.

Apical Impulse: Shifted to Downward: Severe pulmonary emphysema may force the heart downward to give an epigastric impulse just inferior to the xiphoid cartilage.

KEY SIGN

Right Ventricular Impulse: *Pathophysiology:* The contraction of the normal right ventricle does not produce a palpable impulse on the chest wall, but a dilated or hypertrophied or forward displaced right ventricle frequently does. Any palpable impulse in the precordium medial to the apex near the left edge of the sternum and in the third, fourth, or fifth interspace, originates in the right ventricle, and is nearly always abnormal. Slight impulses only pulsate the interspaces; with advanced disease, the lower sternum may heave with the heartbeat.

✓*RIGHT VENTRICULAR IMPULSE—CLINICAL OCCURRENCE:* *Right Ventricular Hypertrophy (Pressure Overload)* pulmonic stenosis, pulmonary hypertension, mitral stenosis; *Right Ventricular Dilation (Volume Overload)* tricuspid or pulmonary valve insufficiency, left-to-right intracardiac shunts; *Forward Displacement of the Heart* tumors behind the heart, enlarged left atrium; *Protuberance of the Right Ventricle* aneurysm of the right ventricular wall; *Hyperdynamic Circulation* exertion, emotion, hyperthyroidism.

Precordial Bulge: In both children and adults, a protrusion of the bony thorax over the right ventricle may result from marked cardiac enlargement in some forms of congenital heart disease. In the adult, a bulge near the upper sternum may be produced by erosion from a syphilitic aneurysm of the aorta.

Retraction of the Fifth Interspace: In some normal persons, a systolic retraction of the fifth interspace near the apex can be noted. This is not a reliable sign of disease. It is often present with considerable right ventricular hypertrophy.

Epigastric Pulsation: This occurs in many normal persons, especially after exertion. Occasionally, displacement of the heart in pulmonary emphysema causes it. Most frequently it is produced by pulsation of a normal abdominal aorta; aneurysmal dilation should be excluded.

Pulsations at the Base: In pulmonary hypertension an impulse may be felt over the pulmonary conus in the second or third interspace just to the left of the sternum. Pulsations in the right second interspace may occur from an aneurysm at the base of the aorta.

KEY SIGN
Thrills: *Pathophysiology:* Turbulent blood flow through an abnormal heart or arteries produces vibrations that are transmitted to peripheral structures, which are audible as murmurs and palpable as thrills. These vibrations are felt over the precordium, similar to the sensation felt by holding a purring cat. In the human body, the closest normal analogy is the sensation when the thorax is palpated while the person is speaking (tactile fremitus). Thrills have the same significance as murmurs and are usually associated with them since the ear is more sensitive to vibrations of this frequency. They should be located accurately and timed with respect to their sequence in the cardiac cycle, employing the apical impulse or carotid pulse for reference. DDX: In mitral stenosis, diastolic and presystolic thrills may be felt at the apex. Severe aortic stenosis causes a systolic thrill in the second right interspace and in the carotid arteries. Thrills may accompany other organic murmurs, such as a ventricular septal defect felt at the fourth and fifth interspaces near the left edge of the sternum. Thrills may be produced by a ruptured chorda tendinea or valve leaflet.

Palpable Friction Rubs (Friction Fremitus): A friction rub occasionally may be felt, although auscultation is more sensitive. The tactile sensation is like two pieces of leather being rubbed together. See *Pleural Rub* (page 396) and *Pericardial Rub* (page 418).

Percussion

KEY SIGN
Cardiac Dullness: Shifted Borders: Although precordial percussion can estimate the distance of the cardiac apex from the midsternal line in the fifth interspace with fair accuracy, only gross changes in cardiac silhouette can be detected [Heckerling PS, Wiener SL, Moses PK, et al. Accuracy of precordial percussion in detecting cardiomegaly. *Am J Med* 1991;91:328–334; Heckerling PS, Weiner SL, Wolfkiel CJ, et al. Accuracy and reproducibility of precordial percussion and palpation for detecting increased left ventricular end-diastolic volume and mass. *JAMA* 1993;270:1943–1948].

KEY SIGN
Cardiac Dullness: Widened Area: The area of cardiac dullness is judged to be expanded when you find (a) lateral displacement of the right or left border with the opposite border normally situated or (b) lateral displacement of both borders in opposite directions. An expansion of the area is caused by either cardiac dilatation or pericardial effusion. Indirect definitive percussion is accurate when compared to CT [Heckerling PS, Weiner SL, Wolfkiel CJ, et al. Accuracy and reproducibility of precordial percussion and palpation for detecting increased left ventricular end-diastolic volume and mass. *JAMA* 1993;270:1943–1948].

LEFT BORDER SHIFTED TO LEFT: The left border of cardiac dullness (LBCD) is normally 7–9 cm to the left of the midsternal line (MSL). Causes of a leftward shift include dilatation of the left ventricle (right border of cardiac dullness [RBCD] normally placed or shifted to right), pericardial effusion (RBCD shifted to right, muffled heart sounds, paradoxical pulse), and displacement of a normal-sized heart to left by right pneumothorax, right hydrothorax, left pleural adhesions, or atelectasis of left lung with mediastinal shift to left.

LEFT BORDER SHIFTED TO RIGHT: This finding should lead you to consider pulmonary emphysema with a normal heart in the midline, a prominent lingula of lung preventing accurate percussion of LBCD, displacement by atelectasis of right lung, left pneumothorax, or left hydrothorax.

RIGHT BORDER SHIFTED TO RIGHT: Causes include cardiac dilatation and pericardial effusion, left pneumothorax, left hydrothorax, right lung atelectasis, right pleural adhesions, and dextrocardia.

RIGHT BORDER SHIFTED TO LEFT: Distinguish between left atelectasis, left pleural adhesions, right pneumothorax, and right hydrothorax.

Retromanubrial Dullness: Widened: Width in excess of 6 cm suggests aortic aneurysm, retrosternal goiter, thymic tumor, lymphoma, or metastatic carcinoma.

Auscultation of Intracardiac Sounds

In writing this section, the authors have depended heavily on several publications to which you are referred for more details [Shaver JL, Leonard JJ, Leon DF. *Examination of the Heart, Part IV: Auscultation of the Heart.* Dallas, TX, American Heart Association, 1990; Perloff JK. The physiologic mechanisms of cardiac and vascular physical signs. *J Am Coll Cardiol* 1983;1:184–198].

KEY SIGN

Normal Heart Sounds: *Physiology:* At the onset of systole, ventricular contraction rapidly increases intraventricular pressure, closing the atrioventricular valves (mitral and tricuspid) and, shortly thereafter, opening the aortic and pulmonic valves (Fig. 8-36). Tensing of the atrioventricular valves is associated with the first heart sound (S1); tensing of the aortic and pulmonic valves is associated with the second heart sound (S2). The normal heart sounds are not caused by slapping together of the leaflets. Rather, the high-frequency components of these sounds are probably caused by tensing of the closed valves producing abrupt deceleration of blood with vibrations of the entire cardiohemic system. Ventricular ejection forces blood silently into the aorta and the pulmonary artery until the ventricles relax and the intraventricular pressure falls. Initial apposition of the aortic and pulmonic valve leaflets occurs prior to the high-frequency components of the second heart sound. The gradient of pressure between the artery and the more rapidly declining ventricular pressure leads to an abrupt stretching of the elastic leaflet tissue which is responsible for the second heart sound. The sound occurs when flow in the artery has fallen to near zero but just before brief retrograde flow occurs [Sabbah HN, Stein PD. Investigation of the theory and mechanism of the origin of the second heart sound. Circ Res 1976;39:874–882]. The heart sounds are usually loudest in the precordium nearest their point of origin: the first sound from the atrioventricular valves at the apex and lower left sternal border; the second sound from the semilunar valves at the base. Invariably, the second sound is louder than the first at the base. Occasionally, S2 at the apex may be as loud as or louder than S1. The intensity of the heart sounds changes when more or less stress is put on the valve leaflets.

KEY SIGN

First Heart Sound (S1): Onset of Systole: Normally heard over the entire precordium, S1 is usually louder than S2 at the cardiac apex (left fifth interspace near the midclavicular line). At the base it is fainter than S2. S1 marks the beginning of ventricular systole and is approximately synchronous with the visible apical impulse and the palpable precordial thrust. *Splitting of S1:* The two high-frequency components of the first sound are probably related to the mitral and tricuspid valves; the asynchrony of their closure probably accounts for the split.

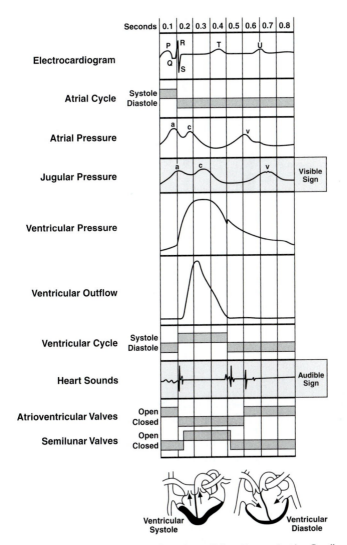

Fig. 8-36 Relation of the Heart Sounds to Other Events in the Cardiac Cycle. Of all these phenomena, only one visible and one audible sign are produced.

KEY SIGN

Second Heart Sound (S2): Onset of Diastole: *Physiology:* Tensing of the closed semilunar aortic (A2) and pulmonic (P2) valves produces the second heart sound; normally, A2 slightly precedes P2. The relative difference in the compliance or distensibility of the pulmonary artery versus that of the aorta and the effect of respiration upon this compliance explains both the fact that A2

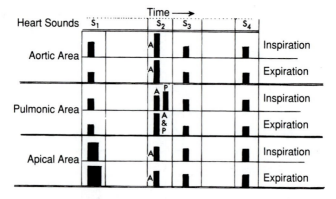

Fig. 8-37 Normal Physiologic Variations in the Heart Sounds. *Duration is represented on the horizontal axis, and intensity of the heart sounds on the vertical axis. The first sound (S1) is prolonged during inspiration. The aortic component of the second sound (A2) is audible over the entire precordium, but (P2) the weaker pulmonic component is heard only in the left second intercostal space. During expiration, the aortic and pulmonic components of are fused. With inspiration the splitting of S2 widens. Splitting of S2 is normal only in this pulmonic area; it is pathologic elsewhere.*

precedes P2 and that normally the splitting between the two widens during inspiration. The more compliant or distensible an artery is, the less faithfully the pressure in the artery will follow temporally the rise and fall of the pressure in the ventricle ejecting into that artery, a phenomenon known as *hangout* [Curtiss EI, Matthews RF, Shaver JA. Mechanism of normal splitting of the second heart sound. Circulation 1975;51:157–164]. Thus, the lesser compliance of the aorta as compared with the usually greater compliance of the pulmonary artery causes the interval between the completion of left ventricular systole and A2 to be much shorter than that between the completion of right ventricular systole and P2; therefore, A2 precedes P2 (Fig. 8-37). The intensity of A2 normally should be greater than that of P2. This follows logically from the normally much higher pressures in the aorta distending the aortic leaflets compared with the pressure in the pulmonary artery. The only truly reliable way to judge the relative intensities is by comparing the relative intensities of the two components when heard in the second left intercostal space. In adults, only A2 is present at the cardiac apex; if both components are heard at the apex, this should suggest that P2 is abnormally loud.   *Respiratory Effect*   The pulmonary valve closes later during inspiration than expiration because of the increased venous return to the right heart and change in pulmonary compliance created by the negative intrathoracic pressure. This produces inspiratory splitting of S2. In children and adolescents, the normal respiratory splitting of S2 is wider than that in older adults, probably as a result of changes in aortic compliance as we age. In young persons in recumbency, the splitting of S2 may not fuse into a single sound with expiration. However, in the sitting position, fusion should occur during expiration. Failure to fuse should suggest that the splitting is unusually wide. With advancing age, the splitting of S2 with inspiration may not be detectable even in recumbency due to the narrowness of the normal split.

KEY SIGN

Prosthetic Heart Valves: Prosthetic heart valves are very common. It is advisable for the clinician to be familiar with the various types of valves and their auscultatory features [Vongpatanasin W, Hillis LD, Lange RA. Prosthetic heart valves. *N Engl J Med* 1996;335:407–416].

KEY SIGN

Accentuated First Heart Sound (S1): *Pathophysiology:* Thickening with preserved mobility of the bellies of the mitral valve leaflets or increased force of left ventricular contraction accentuate S1. This occurs in mitral stenosis, tachycardia from fever, hyperthyroidism, exercise, emotion, and hypertension.

KEY SIGN

Diminished First Heart Sound (S1): *Pathophysiology:* When the mitral and tricuspid valves are more closely approximated at the onset of systole, their tensing is less forceful. Soft tissue attenuation of sound from the heart to the chest wall also diminishes the sound. This occurs with the thick chest wall of an obese person, pulmonary emphysema, pericardial effusion and pleural effusion. Other causes include weak ventricular contraction, aortic insufficiency, prolonged PR intervals, and heavily calcified mitral valve leaflets.

KEY SIGN

Varied Intensity of the First Heart Sound (S1) (Bruit de Canon): *Pathophysiology:* Variable diastolic ventricular filling and asynchrony of atrial and ventricular contraction change the intensity of valve tensing from beat to beat. Atrial fibrillation, atrial flutter with varying degrees of block, complete AV block, frequent premature beats, and ventricular tachycardia can each be a cause.

Widening or Splitting of the First Heart Sound (S1): *Pathophysiology:* S1 splits when tensing of the tricuspid and mitral valves are asynchronous. Slight splitting of S1 is a common normal finding. Wide splitting classically occurs with right bundle-branch block, which delays right ventricular contraction.

KEY SIGN

Accentuated Aortic Component of the Second Heart Sound (A2): *Pathophysiology:* Increased pressure against the closed aortic valve increases A2. Arterial hypertension is most common, but aneurysm of the ascending aorta can be associated.

A.

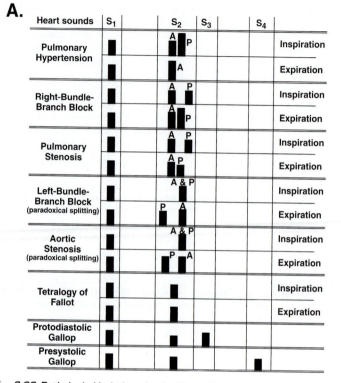

Fig. 8-38 Pathologic Variations in the Heart Sounds. A. *Pulmonary hypertension causes an increased P2. Right bundle-branch block delays right ventricular emptying, increasing the normal split and accentuating P2. Pulmonic stenosis also delays P2, but decreases its intensity. In left bundle-branch block and aortic stenosis, left ventricular ejection is delayed so A2 coincides with P2 and the normal expiratory movement of P2 causes paradoxic splitting during expiration.* B. *Timing of Heart Sounds, Clicks, Opening Snap, and Murmurs Within the Cardiac Cycle.* ICS = intercostal space; SB = sternal border; S2-A = S2-in aortic area; S2-P = S2 in pulmonic area.

Diminished Aortic Component of the Second Heart Sound (A2): *Pathophysiology:* A2 is decreased when the valve is rigid and immobile. It is found with heavily calcified aortic valves, as occur in adults with aortic stenosis.

KEY SIGN

Accentuated Pulmonic Component of the Second Heart Sound (P2): *Pathophysiology:* See accentuated A2 page 413. An accentuated P2 is seen in primary or secondary pulmonary hypertension, atrial septal defect, truncus arteriosus and in adolescence (Fig. 8-38A).

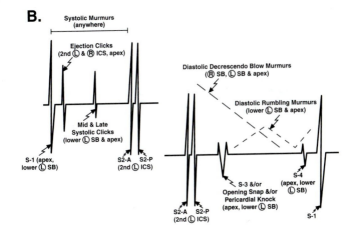

B.

Fig. 8-38 (continued).

KEY SIGN

Diminished Pulmonic Component of the Second Heart Sound (P2): *Pathophysiology:* Diminished pulmonary artery pressure reduces tension on the pulmonic valve. Pulmonic stenosis is the most common cause (Fig. 8-38A).

KEY SIGN

Widened Inspiratory Splitting of the Second Heart Sound (S2): *Pathophysiology:* Either delayed tensing of the pulmonic valve or early tensing of the aortic valve. P2 delay occurs with right bundle-branch block, atrial septal defect and pulmonic stenosis. Early closure of the aortic valve occurs with severe mitral regurgitation (Fig. 8-38A).

KEY SIGN

Reversed or Paradoxic Splitting of the Second Heart Sound (S2): *Pathophysiology:* A delay of left ventricular ejection causes A2 to coincide with or occur after P2. There is a single sound, or more closely approximated sounds, during inspiration; expiration is associated with increased splitting of the second heart sound. It is seen in hypertrophic cardiomyopathy with left ventricular outflow obstruction (idiopathic hypertrophic subaortic stenosis), valvular aortic stenosis or left bundle-branch block (Fig. 8-38A).

KEY SIGN

Gallops or Triple Rhythms: These low-pitched sounds are easily missed unless specifically listened for in a quiet room. Listen for triple heart sounds, couplets alternating with single sounds resembling a horse's gallop. The couplet may be either a normal S2 followed closely by an audible S3 or an audible S4 preceding a normal S1. Differentiating S3 from S4 requires accurate identification of S1 and S2.

If the ventricular rate is less than 90, listening at the base helps to identify the louder S2. At the apex, the louder sound is likely to be S1. If the heart rate exceeds 90, consider using brief carotid pressure to slow the rate for a better exam.

KEY SIGN

Early Diastolic Sound: Audible Third Heart Sound (S3) (Ventricular or Protodiastolic Gallop): *Pathophysiology:*

S3 occurs at the transition from the rapid phase of ventricular filling to the slow-filling phase, as the walls reach the limits of diastolic excursion. The resulting reverberations of ventricular muscle and blood mass cause the sound (Fig. 8-38B). An audible S3 closely follows S2 in early diastole. It has the cadence of "Tennessee." If from the left ventricle, it is best heard at the apex with the patient lying on the left side. Third heart sounds are best heard in expiration and are accentuated by exercise, abdominal pressure, or flexing the knees on the abdomen, all of which increase venous return. An S3 is normal in children and young adults. After the third decade, it indicates myocardial systolic dysfunction, with increased left ventricular end-diastolic pressure and elevated left atrial pressure. It is also seen, although of less concern, when caused by a hyperkinetic circulatory state as with fever, anemia, hyperthyroidism, or by excessively rapid ventricular filling from mitral regurgitation.

KEY SIGN

Late Diastolic Sound: Audible Fourth Heart Sound (S4) (Atrial Sound; Presystolic or Atrial Gallop): *Pathophysiology:*

An audible S4 is caused by vibrations of the left ventricular muscle, the mitral valve apparatus, and the left ventricular outflow tract as a result of atrial contraction (Fig. 8-38B). Fourth heart sounds occur after atrial contraction but before S1. They have the cadence of "Kentucky." These are the most difficult to hear of all heart sounds; listening at apex with patient in left lateral decubitus position is mandatory. They are low-pitched sounds, essentially identical to S3. The S4 often reflects a decrease in ventricular compliance. S4 is heard with thickened, "stiff" left ventricles, as occur with aortic stenosis, subaortic stenosis, hypertension, and acute ischemia or infarction from coronary artery disease.

KEY SIGN

Diastolic Sound: Summation Gallop, Mesodiastolic Gallop:

The sounds of S3 and S4 are so close together that they give the impression of a single sound or a rumbling murmur. Vagus stimulation by carotid pressure may slow the rate enough to distinguish four sounds per cycle.

Auscultation of Extracardiac Sounds

Because they are relatively uncommon and are heard in the precordial region, the extracardiac sounds are very often mistaken for murmurs.

Once the possibility is considered, the distinctions can usually be found. The conclusive difference is that extracardiac sounds may vary within a specific part of the cardiac cycle.

Systolic Click: Aortic Ejection Click: *Pathophysiology:* This is attributed to sudden tensing of the root of the aorta at the onset of ejection. In other cases, sudden doming of a stenotic yet flexible aortic valve may cause it (Fig. 8-38B). A click is heard in early systole, at the onset of left ventricular ejection. It is heard at the base and apex, although usually louder at the base, and is unaffected by respirations. Ejection clicks occur with aneurysm of the ascending aorta dilating the aortic root, coarctation of the aorta, hypertension with aortic dilatation, valvular aortic stenosis, and aortic regurgitation.

Systolic Click: Pulmonic Ejection Click: *Pathophysiology:* See *Aortic Ejection Click* above (Fig. 8-38B). This is a click at the onset of pulmonary ejection, occurring when there is pulmonary valve stenosis or when the pulmonary artery is dilated. It is heard best at the base of the heart in the left second interspace, early in systole. In some cases with a loud click, the latter is fused with S1 and S1 is interpreted as loud. Pulmonic clicks may decrease or disappear with inspiration.

KEY SIGN
Midsystolic Click with or Without Apical Late Systolic Murmur: Mitral Valve Prolapse: It is heard at the apex in mid or late systole and may be intermittent (Fig. 8-38B). It is unchanged by respiration, but may be delayed or disappear with increased left ventricular filling following a squat from standing or raising the legs of a supine patient. It is sometimes associated with a late systolic murmur of mitral insufficiency. It occurs with increased frequency in Marfan syndrome with myxomatous changes of the mitral valve (see also page 428).

KEY SIGN
Diastolic Snap: Mitral Opening Snap: *Pathophysiology:* When stenotic mitral valve leaflets are tethered at the orifice but still flexible (noncalcified), they buckle or bow outward into the left ventricle when ventricular pressure drops below left atrial pressure, producing a snap. The diastolic rumble begins a few hundredths of a second later (Fig. 8-38B). The snap is best heard at the apex, but may radiate to base and left sternal border, where it may simulate a widely split S2. This sign is characteristic of rheumatic mitral stenosis.

Diastolic Snap: Tricuspid Opening Snap: *Pathophysiology:* See *Mitral Opening Snap* above (Fig. 8-38B). Usually this is difficult to identify, because it is associated with other valve abnormalities of rheumatic heart disease.

KEY SIGN

Diastolic Sound: Pericardial Knock: *Pathophysiology:* In constrictive pericarditis, ventricular filling stops abruptly early in diastole, producing audible vibrations. Pericardial knocks are heard widely over the precordium. They are more high-pitched than the S3 and similar in character to an opening snap. They may occur slightly earlier in diastole than an S3 and may increase with inspiration (Fig. 8-38B).

KEY SIGN

Systolic and Diastolic Rubs: Pericardial Friction Rub: *Pathophysiology:* The sound arises from rubbing together two inflamed pericardial surfaces. This does not preclude the existence of rubs with a pericardial effusion; the effusion often does not cover the entire pericardial sac. Have the patient prone or sitting and leaning forward; listen at the precordium during deep expiration. Rubs are often scratchy, grating, rasping, or squeaky. In about half the cases, the sound is triphasic, heard in systole and early and late diastole. In about one-third of patients it is systolic and late diastolic. In the remainder, it is heard only in systole; often it is intermittent. Through the stethoscope, the sounds seem closer to the ear than murmurs. Causes are infectious pericarditis, myocardial infarction or cardiac surgery, uremia, carcinoma metastatic to pericardium, and, rarely, pulmonary infarction.

KEY SIGN

Systolic and Diastolic: Mediastinal Crunch (Hamman Sign): See page 463.

KEY SIGN

Systolic and Diastolic: Venous Hum (Humming Top Murmur) (Bruit de Diable): *Pathophysiology:* High-velocity flow in the internal jugular veins, especially the right, produces vibrations in the tissues that are heard as sound. Hums are usually heard in both supraclavicular fossae, often in the second and third interspaces near the sternum. They are low pitched throughout the cardiac cycle, frequently with augmentation during diastole. Hums are intensified by the patient sit or stand; they do not vary with respirations. The hum is readily abolished by light pressure on the jugular veins beside the trachea. The hum is frequently mistaken for an intracardiac murmur. Venous hums occur in some normal children and adults. They are more common with hyperthyroidism and anemia. The combination of a venous hum and an intracranial bruit suggests the presence of intracranial arteriovenous malformation.

Auscultation of Heart Murmurs

KEY SIGN

Heart Murmurs: *Pathophysiology:* In normal vessels and heart chambers, blood flow at rest is laminar and silent. Audible murmurs result from vibrations set up by turbulence (vortices) developing near the mural interfaces of the bloodstream after it passes an obstruction or dilatation (vortex-shedding theory). For a model, attach 60 cm (24 in) of pliable rubber tubing to a laboratory water faucet. Palpate the tubing with the thumb and finger of one hand and turn on the water with the other. A velocity can be attained that will not vibrate the walls of the tubing, because the flow is laminar and smooth. At this velocity, constricting the tubing slightly with the fingers will cause vibrations distally. Also, with no constriction, increasing the velocity of flow will induce turbulence. One can also demonstrate that a less-viscous fluid, such as alcohol, will set up vibrations at less velocity than water. In a normal heart, murmurs may be induced when the velocity of normal blood is increased by exercise or hyperthyroidism, i.e. a flow murmur. In anemia, blood with lessened viscosity may produce murmurs at normal velocity. Normal blood flowing over obstructions or through unusual openings in the circulation sets up turbulence and collision currents that result in murmurs. Careful observation of these murmurs for their location, pitch, and relations to the cardiac cycle can lead to remarkably accurate diagnoses of the anatomic derangements within the heart and vessels. The quality of murmurs is of some diagnostic value. Ventricular filling murmurs (for instance those involving diastolic flow across the atrioventricular valves) are relatively low pitched because they are produced by blood flowing under relatively little pressure; blood flowing through narrow orifices under higher pressure causes high-pitched murmurs (Fig. 8-38B).

Systolic Murmurs (Fig. 8-39)

These are described according to the part of the systolic interval in which they occur: early systolic (or protosystolic), midsystolic, and late systolic. When the murmur occupies the entire systole, it is termed pansystolic (or holosystolic). Leatham has taught us a more interpretive classification of systolic murmurs by associating the configuration of the murmurs with the pressure relations that produce them. When vibrations are set up by forcing blood from regions of high pressure to those with initially low but rising pressure, ejection murmurs are produced. An example is aortic stenosis, where the murmur starts soon after S1, intensifies to a maximum at mid-systole, and tapers off to disappear before S2 when the intraventricular pressure equals that in the aorta. In contrast, regurgitant murmurs occur when blood flows continuously from a high-pressure region to one of low pressure during systole, producing a pansystolic murmur of almost uniform intensity. This is typified in mitral regurgitation. With these criteria it is possible to distinguish many of the systolic murmurs of organic disease from those occurring only in early systole or perhaps mid-systole that are of little significance and are benign [Etchells E, Bell C, Robb K. The rational clinical examination. Does this patient have an abnormal systolic murmur? *JAMA* 1997;277:564–571].

KEY SIGN

Basal Systolic Murmur: Benign Murmurs (Innocent, Physiologic, Functional, Nonpathologic): *Pathophysiology:* Some authors believe that most of these

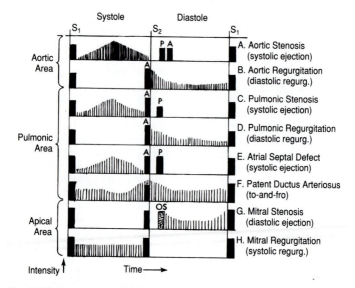

Fig. 8-39 Common Pathologic Heart Murmurs. *The diagrams are drawn to represent intensity of the heart sounds and murmurs on the vertical axis and duration on the horizontal axis. Pitch is depicted by the spacing of the shading: wider spacing lower pitch. "A" and "P" refer to the aortic and pulmonic components of the second sound (S2). "OS" indicates the opening snap of the mitral valve in mitral stenosis. Note that the systolic ejection murmurs are inaudible at either end of systole and attain maximum intensity at mid-systole (in this diagram they form the upper halves of "diamond-shaped" figures of the phonocardiogram). Systolic regurgitant murmurs are pansystolic. The configuration of the diastolic ejection murmur of mitral stenosis terminates in a crescendo caused by superimposition of atrial contraction. Although the diastolic regurgitant murmurs are pandiastolic, in aortic and pulmonic regurgitation, the late diastolic part is seldom heard.*

murmurs are produced by increases in velocity or decreases in viscosity of the blood. Most common in the second left interspace, they are characterized as medium-pitched and generally grade I or II, although occasionally louder. Usually they are short, occurring early in systole. When maximum in the second interspace, they are infrequently transmitted to the neck. They are best heard in the supine position and tend to disappear with sitting or standing. Have the patient sit upright with the shoulders back. The murmur may persist if the patient sits in a "slouched" position. Functional murmurs occur in normal adults with anemia, fever, emotional disturbances, exercise, hyperthyroidism, or pregnancy. About 50% of normal children have functional systolic murmurs. DDX: Their short duration without accompanying abnormalities of history and cardiovascular exam assists to distinguish these murmurs from those of organic disease.

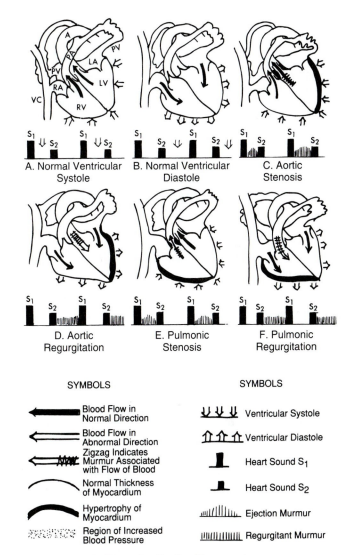

A. Normal Ventricular Systole

B. Normal Ventricular Diastole

C. Aortic Stenosis

D. Aortic Regurgitation

E. Pulmonic Stenosis

F. Pulmonic Regurgitation

SYMBOLS

⬅ Blood Flow in Normal Direction

⬅ Blood Flow in Abnormal Direction

⬅〰 Zigzag Indicates Murmur Associated with Flow of Blood

⌒ Normal Thickness of Myocardium

⬛ Hypertrophy of Myocardium

▨ Region of Increased Blood Pressure

SYMBOLS

⬇⬇⬇ Ventricular Systole

⬆⬆⬆ Ventricular Diastole

▮ Heart Sound S_1

▃ Heart Sound S_2

⏚ Ejection Murmur

⏚ Regurgitant Murmur

Fig. 8-40 Anatomic Bases for Cardiac Murmurs I.

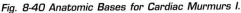

KEY SIGN

Basal Systolic Murmur: Valvular Aortic Stenosis: *Pathophysiology:* Progressive fusion of the valve commissures and fibrosis of the valve leaflets results in narrowing of the valve orifice and impedance to left ventricular ejection (Fig. 8-40C). *The Murmur* Classically the murmur is heard in the second right interspace, but almost as often it is audible along the left sternal border in the third and fourth interspaces and at the apex. In approximately 15% of cases, it is loudest at the apex. Regardless of the area of maximal intensity, it is transmitted to the carotid arteries. Loud murmurs are often accompanied by systolic thrills over the base and in the carotids. It is a typical ejection murmur with onset a short interval after the first sound, during the rise of the intraventricular pressure; it ceases before the second sound, when the intraventricular pressure falls below aortic pressure. Its configuration in the phonocardiogram furnishes the murmur with its description of diamond-shaped; the first half rises in pitch *(crescendo),* and the latter half falls in pitch *(decrescendo)* (see Fig. 8-39A). The murmur is usually medium-pitched, so it is audible with either the bell or the diaphragm. Although usually harsh, occasionally it has a peculiar quality that prompts the term *seagull murmur,* like the call of a gull or the cooing of a dove. If severe stenosis causes a decrease in left ventricular contractility, the murmur may decrease in intensity.   *Heart Sounds*   In moderate or severe stenosis accompanied by significant valvular calcification, A2 is diminished or absent. This is best appreciated by noting the second heart sounds at the apex to be faint or absent. If the valve is stenotic but not calcified (as in congenital aortic stenosis), S2 may be split during expiration (paradoxically) from delayed closure of the aortic valve (Fig. 8-38A). When the valve remains flexible although stenotic, the murmur is preceded by an ejection or early systolic sound caused by doming of the valve in early systole; this disappears when the valve becomes calcified. An S4 is frequently audible at the apex, producing a presystolic gallop.   *Precordial Thrust*   Hypertrophy of the left ventricle produces an accentuated precordial apical thrust. In the left lateral decubitus position, a double (bifid) apical thrust is sometimes felt; the first impact comes from atrial contraction, the second from left ventricular systole.   *Arterial Pulse*   Severe aortic stenosis produces a slowly rising carotid pulse contour *(tardus or anacrotic pulse,* Fig. 8-42D) and diminished pulse pressure. A decrease in the rate of rise is appreciated as a "sustained caress" to the finger rather than the normal brief "tap." A decrease in amplitude is often perceptible but is best judged by the pulse pressure noted when taking the arterial blood pressure. Physical findings may not always allow precise estimation of the severity of aortic stenosis [Munt B, O'Legget ME, Draft CD, et al. Physical examination in valvular aortic stenosis: Correlation with stenosis severity and prediction of outcome. *Am Heart J* 1999;137:298–306].   *Symptoms* Aortic stenosis may be asymptomatic until constriction of the orifice is severe, when exercise induces dyspnea, angina, or syncope. The most common etiologies for aortic stenosis are rheumatic valvulitis, calcific disease of the aortic valve, and congenital bicuspid valve.   *X-Ray Findings*   Calcification of the aortic valve may be seen on the films. DDX: The systolic murmur of aortic sclerosis (atherosclerosis of the aortic valve) is accompanied by normal heart sounds at the base and is briefer. The apical systolic murmur of aortic stenosis is diamond-shaped; but the murmur of mitral regurgitation is of a "blowing" quality and is often pansystolic or holosystolic. A systolic diamond-shaped murmur may occur in valvular aortic stenosis or hypertrophic subaortic stenosis [Carabello BA. Aortic stenosis. *N Engl J Med* 2002;346:677–682].

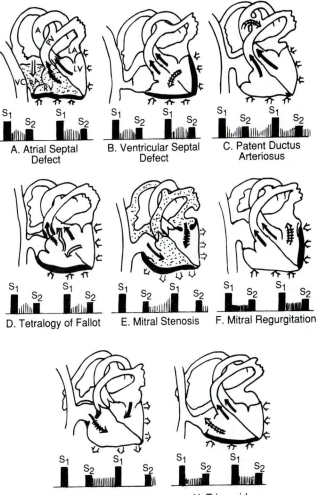

Fig. 8-41 Anatomic Basis for Cardiac Murmurs II. *(Same symbols as in Fig. 8-40.)*

KEY SIGN

Basal Systolic Murmur: Hypertrophic Obstructive Cardiomyopathy (Idiopathic Hypertrophic Subaortic Stenosis, IHSS): *Pathophysiology:* This results from asymmetric hypertrophy of the left ventricle with prominent hypertrophy of the basal interventricular septum. Dynamic obstruction occurs shortly after the onset of systole from apposition of the anterior leaflet of the mitral valve to the hypertrophied septum. A family history with autosomal dominant inheritance is often present; unexplained sudden deaths in the family should suggest the diagnosis of hypertrophic cardiomyopathy, with or without obstruction. The condition should be suspected when the signs of aortic stenosis are atypical. *The Murmur* A systolic ejection murmur is heard along the left sternal border and the apex, rather than in the right second interspace and the carotids. The murmur may be holosystolic at the apex. The murmur varies with changes in peripheral resistance and the influence of inotropic agents. The dynamic outflow obstruction and murmur are intensified by standing and/or the Valsalva maneuver, whereas the murmur of fixed valvular aortic stenosis diminishes under such circumstances. *Arterial Pulse* In contrast to the pulse of valvular stenosis with its diminished amplitude and delayed upstroke, the arterial pulse wave has a sharp upstroke. Pulsus bisferiens may be present. *Heart Sounds* As in valvular stenosis, a presystolic gallop is frequent. Absence of a systolic ejection click is distinctive in subaortic stenosis. *Symptoms* The symptoms are identical to those of severe aortic valvular stenosis. The diagnosis is confirmed by echocardiography.

Basal Systolic Murmur: Supravalvular Aortic Stenosis: *Pathophysiology:* A rare congenital anomaly, this is the result of narrowing of the ascending aorta, or a small-holed diaphragm distal to the valve. It produces most of the signs of valvular stenosis, but A2 is accentuated and the carotid murmurs are unusually loud. The finding of a systolic blood pressure that is more than 10 mmHg greater in the right arm than the left is typical of supravalvular aortic stenosis. The diagnosis is confirmed by cardiac catheterization.

KEY SIGN
Basal Systolic Murmur: Hypertension or Atherosclerosis: *Pathophysiology:* Aortic sclerosis is caused by the thickening of the aortic leaflet (sclerosis) without significant obstruction (stenosis). A murmur of medium pitch and moderate intensity is frequently heard in the aortic region of persons with hypertension or arteriosclerosis. It may be transmitted to the apex. It is usually not so loud as murmurs of aortic stenosis. It is often brief and confined to early systole. The murmur may be faintly heard in the carotids. A2 is usually present at the apex. DDX: Aortic stenosis is easily excluded, because the murmur is seldom loud or long, or accompanied by abnormality of the carotid pulse. Preservation of A2 at the apex speaks against severe calcific aortic valvular stenosis.

KEY SIGN
Basal Systolic Murmur: Valvular Pulmonic Stenosis: *The Murmur* This is a systolic ejection murmur, with diamond-shaped contour, maximal in the second left interspace (Figs. 8-40E and 8-39C). It is otherwise similar to that of aortic stenosis in intensity, configuration, and pitch. Transmission may be into the carotids, the left side more than the right. *Heart Sounds* Slowed ejection

through the pulmonic orifice delays P2 and the decreased pulmonary arterial pressure decreases its intensity; the S2 is widely split, but the pulmonic component is difficult to hear (Figs. 8-38A and 8-39C). Commonly, there is an ejection click; its presence marks the lesion as valvular rather than infundibular pulmonic stenosis. *Palpation* Right ventricular hypertrophy may be detectable as an accentuated precordial thrust. DDX: The murmur is similar to the pulmonary flow murmur with atrial septal defect. In the latter, the wide splitting of second heart sound is fixed, and the pulmonary component is not diminished in intensity. Pulmonary stenosis is usually congenital, either singly or in the tetralogy of Fallot. It can be acquired with carcinoid tumors.

Basal Systolic Murmur: Infundibular Pulmonic Stenosis: *Pathophysiology:* The funnel-shaped portion of the right ventricular chamber that leads to the pulmonary artery is the infundibulum. Congenital narrowing of the funnel produces a form of pulmonic stenosis. *The Murmur* In contrast to valvular stenosis, the ejection murmur and the systolic thrill are usually in the third left interspace and there is no ejection sound (click). Although this lesion may be isolated, it is usually accompanied by a ventricular septal defect, as in the tetralogy of Fallot.

Basal Systolic Murmur: Atrial Septal Defect (ASD) at the Ostium Secundum: *Pathophysiology:* The systolic murmur is produced when the blood flows with high velocity through the pulmonic valve from a right ventricle overfilled because of a congenital left-to-right interatrial shunt (Fig. 8-41A). *The Murmur* A medium-pitched murmur is nearly always heard in the second or third left interspace. The configuration frequently resembles that of pulmonic stenosis, with maximum intensity a little before mid-systole (see Fig. 8-39E). The pulmonary outflow tract murmur is sometimes accompanied by a low-pitched diastolic flow murmur heard along the lower left sternal border, resulting from increased flow through the tricuspid valve. *Heart Sounds* S2 is widely split. The split is fixed and the pulmonic component is not diminished. DDX: Sometimes the murmur is indistinguishable from that of pulmonic stenosis, but it usually peaks earlier in systole and is lower-pitched, leaving a longer pause before the second sound. The murmur rarely becomes very loud, in contrast to that in pulmonic stenosis. The wide splitting of S2 is the same during inspiration and expiration (the split is fixed) with a normal or accentuated intensity of the pulmonic component of S2.

Basal Systolic Murmur: Atrial Septal Defect from Persistent Ostium Primum: *Pathophysiology:* A congenital opening in septum near atrioventricular (AV) valves is often associated with a cleft mitral valve leaflet. *The Murmur* There is a harsh systolic murmur at left sternal border and an apical systolic murmur transmitted to axilla if mitral regurgitation is present. Sometimes an apical mid-diastolic murmur is heard. *Heart Sounds* S2 is accentuated with fixed splitting during inspiration and expiration. The chest may be rounded, rarely with a precordial bulge, and the precordial apical thrust is accentuated.

KEY SIGN

Basal Systolic Murmur: Coarctation of the Aorta:
Pathophysiology: The most common site of coarctation is just distal to the origin of the left subclavian artery, so the circulation to the head and arms is unaffected. Perfusion of tissues distal to the coarctation is maintained via high resistance collaterals in the chest wall perfused at the cost of sustained central arterial hypertension. See also page 478ff. *The Murmur* The site of constriction is remote from the precordium, so the murmur is faintly heard, if at all, on the anterior chest. When a murmur is audible anteriorly, it is usually a brief early systolic ejection murmur caused by an associated bicuspid aortic valve. This murmur is faint and maximal in either the left or right second interspace. The murmur of the coarctation itself is heard best in the interscapular area posteriorly. A continuous bruit can sometimes be heard over the sternum from the dilated internal mammary arteries. *Arterial Pulses* When the back is not routinely auscultated for murmurs, the condition is first suggested by finding diminished or absent femoral pulses. The pulse waves in the distal aorta and its branches are impaired; this is most easily discovered by routinely palpating the femoral arteries. The collateral circulation develops through the internal mammary and the intercostal arteries. The latter become dilated enough to be palpated in the intercostal spaces in the back of the thorax (which is diagnostic) and to produce notching in the inferior rib margins posteriorly visible in x-ray films.

Basal Systolic Murmur: Benign Thoracic Outlet Bruit:
Most common in well-developed, muscular young men, this systolic bruit is maximal in the supraclavicular fossa. It is usually heard in the first right intercostal space as well, but attenuates as the aortic area is approached. It may also radiate to the right carotid. Having the patient sit with elbows placed to the scapular tips usually decreases the bruit. It has no clinical significance, but has been confused with aortic stenosis.

KEY SIGN

Mid-Precordial Systolic Murmur: Ventricular Septal Defect (VSD):
Pathophysiology: Blood flows at high pressure through an opening in the interventricular septum from the left ventricle into a region of much lower pressure in the right ventricle or pulmonary outflow tract. Those with a very small defect have been called Maladie-de-Roger. Paramembranous defects are more common than defects in the muscular septum (see Fig. 8-41B). *The Murmur* Typically, the murmur is pansystolic with peak intensity in mid-systole in the third or fourth left interspace. The pitch is high and loud murmurs are accompanied by thrills. The murmur may be transmitted over the entire precordium and to the interscapular region. With the devel-

opment of pulmonary hypertension, the intensity and harshness of the murmur diminish and the midsystolic accentuation is lost. *Heart Sounds* When the defect is large, S2 may be accentuated. DDX: In the presence of pulmonary hypertension, ventricular septal defect may require cardiac catheterization or imaging techniques to distinguish it from patent ductus arteriosus in which the diastolic murmur has been lost because of high pulmonic pressure. Faint murmurs must be distinguished from benign systolic murmurs [Ammash NM, Warnes CA. Ventricular septal defects in adults. *Ann Intern Med* 2001;135:812–824].

✓ *VSD—CLINICAL OCCURRENCE:* Congenital septal defects occur alone and in the syndromes of Eisenmenger and Fallot. VSD may complicate myocardial infarction, typically at the cardiac apex; large defects are rapidly fatal.

KEY SIGN
Mid-Precordial Systolic Murmur: Tricuspid Regurgitation: *Pathophysiology:* This is a systolic regurgitant murmur in which the regurgitation occurs throughout the entire systolic interval (see Fig. 8-41H). *The Murmur* Faint murmurs are early systolic; loud ones are heard throughout systole. The pitch is high, the quality blowing, and the murmur is heard best with the diaphragm firmly pressed. Inspiration may make the murmur audible or accentuate it. *Palpation* The point of maximum intensity is nearly always along the inferior left sternal border. It may be sharply localized or transmitted to the apex. Right ventricular hypertrophy may be present with a palpable right ventricular precordial thrust. In severe tricuspid insufficiency, striking engorgement of the neck veins with prominent v-waves and a pulsating liver may occur. *Heart Sounds* There are no characteristic changes in the heart sounds. DDX: The location of maximum intensity and the effect of inspiration are characteristic and diagnostic.

✓ *CLINICAL OCCURRENCE:* Congenital tricuspid regurgitation occurs with Ebstein anomaly. The acquired form may be seen with rheumatic heart disease, right-sided cardiac failure from any cause, endocarditis, carcinoid tumor, and pulmonary embolism.

KEY SIGN
Apical Systolic Murmur: Mitral Regurgitation: *Pathophysiology:* This is the prototype systolic regurgitant murmur. Blood is forced backward through the mitral orifice with almost constant velocity during the entire systolic interval. In extreme degrees, the left ventricle empties prematurely, so the aortic component of the second sound is early, causing a widened splitting of the second sound (Fig. 8-41F). *The Murmur* A loud, high-pitched, pansystolic murmur with maximum intensity at the apex is typical (Fig. 8-39H). The murmur begins with the first sound, which it may mask, and continues at approximately the same intensity throughout systole until it meets the second heart sound. Occasionally, the murmur begins with S1 and ends in early to mid-systole or begins in mid to late systole and ends with the second heart sound. Fainter murmurs are well localized; louder murmurs of central mitral insufficiency are transmitted to the axilla.

Murmurs from eccentric jets may produce unusual radiation to the base and carotids or to the lung bases and spine. There is little variation with the phases of respiration or irregularities of rhythm. An early diastolic murmur from increased flow across the mitral valve may be heard. *Heart Sounds* S1 is often diminished; there may be increased splitting of S2 with severe regurgitation. A third heart sound is sometimes found in moderate or severe cases. *Palpation* Left ventricular hypertrophy and dilatation may be present, as indicated by accentuation and lateral displacement of the apical thrust. An increased thrust or lift at the left parasternal line may sometimes result from systolic expansion of the left atrium rather than from right ventricular dilatation and hypertrophy. DDX: The murmur must be distinguished from that of aortic stenosis, which is often loud at the apex, as well as at the base. The duration and quality of the murmur and comparison of murmurs at the apex and base will make differentiation possible. Benign murmurs at the apex are usually short and limited to a segment of the systolic interval; they are usually medium-pitched [Otto CM. Evaluation and management of chronic mitral regurgitation. *N Engl J Med* 2001;345:740–746].

✔ *MITRAL REGURGITATION—CLINICAL OCCURRENCE:* This results from myxomatous change in the valve, endocarditis, rheumatic valvulitis, chordal rupture, papillary muscles ischemia, myocardial infarction, and dilatation of the mitral valve ring by any condition producing left ventricular dilatation.

KEY SIGN

Apical Late Systolic Murmur after Midsystolic Click: Mitral Valve Prolapse: *Pathophysiology:* The valve undergoes myxomatous degeneration, producing redundant valve tissue (especially the posterior leaflet), enlargement of the valve annulus and elongation of the chordae tendineae. Systole causes one or more scallops of the valve leaflets to billow and prolapse backward into the atrium to produce mitral regurgitation. This is believed to be a very common condition (perhaps 2–5% of the population) and more frequent in women. It can be inherited, probably as an autosomal dominant with reduced male expressivity. *The Murmur* The systolic murmur classically occurs late in systole, heard best at the apex. It is usually short and relatively high-pitched, giving the impression of a crescendo sound. It may be transmitted to the back, left of the spine. Its quality is described as "cooing," "honking," or "whooping." It may be inaudible or so loud it can be heard away from the chest without a stethoscope. It typically moves closer to S1 with the patient standing, and becomes shorter and later in systole with the patient squatting. Auscultation in the erect position during a Valsalva maneuver may elicit a murmur that could not be heard at rest with the patient supine. *Heart Sounds* A snapping or clicking sound is heard and sometimes palpated during mid-systole; at the same time, a retraction of the apical region may be observed. *Associated Dysrhythmias* Ventricular premature beats, paroxysmal atrial tachycardia, atrial fibrillation, sinus bradycardia, periods of sinus arrest and positional atrial flutter can all occur in association. *Noncardiac Signs* Although usually normal, some patients show stigmata of Marfan syndrome with arachnodactyly, hyperextensible joints, and ecto-morph build. *Symptoms* Most persons are without symptoms. The minority develop easy fatigue, shortness of breath, nonanginal chest pain, palpitation, or syncope. Cerebral transient ischemic attacks, rup-ture of chordae tendineae, congestive cardiac failure, endocarditis, and sudden death occur with increased frequency, but are uncommon.

KEY SIGN

Abrupt Loud Systolic Murmur: Rupture of Interventricular Septum, Papillary Muscle or Chordae Tendineae: A sudden loud systolic murmur sug-gests rupture of the interventricular septum rupture of a chordae or se-vere dysfunction or rupture of a papillary muscle. With severe dys-function or rupture of a papillary muscle or rupture of major chordae there is sudden onset of a grade II–IV/VI pansystolic murmur often ac-companied by a precordial thrill; sudden massive pulmonary edema fol-lows. Severe mitral insufficiency may be associated with a surprisingly soft murmur. With a ruptured septum, signs of right-sided failure, as well as low cardiac output with poor peripheral perfusion, occur. These situations are grave emergencies, and prompt diagnosis is needed.

Diastolic Murmurs

(See Fig. 8-39.) These are practically always pathologic. They are classi-fied as early diastolic (protodiastolic), mid-diastolic, and late diastolic (presystolic). Nearly all diastolic regurgitant murmurs (for instance aor-tic insufficiency) begin with the second heart sound and many are pro-longed because the pressure in the great vessels remains higher than that in the ventricles throughout diastole. The diastolic murmur of mi-tral stenosis does not start with the onset of diastole (S2) because pres-sure in the ventricle must continue to fall before becoming less than that in the atrium.

KEY SIGN

Basal Diastolic Murmur: Aortic Regurgita-tion: *Pathophysiology:* The decrescendo murmur contour results from the decreasing transvalvular pressure gradient as the initial high aortic pressure decreases as blood regurgitates into the left ventricle, de-creasing the rate of flow with diminution of the murmur. A2 is accen-tuated by the initial high aortic systolic pressure. The high pitch is caused by blood being forced through a relatively small orifice at high pressure (Fig. 8-40D). *The Murmur* The murmur is decrescendo starting with A2. It is a high-pitched blowing murmur, heard best with the diaphragm of the stethoscope held firmly against the chest wall. The point of max-imum intensity is in either the second right or the third left interspace. The murmur immediately follows the second sound and exhibits a rapid decrescendo during the first third or so of diastole; it disappears or is pandiastolic with very low intensity (Fig. 8-39B). When faint, the mur-mur is best heard during full exhalation with the patient leaning for-ward. Usually, there is an accompanying aortic systolic murmur. Trans-mission down the right rather than the left sternal border should suggest aneurysmal dilatation of the aortic root.   *Heart Sounds*   The first heart sound is usually normal; A2 is often accentuated.   *Palpation*   Accentuation of the precordial apical thrust and its displacement laterally indicate the accompanying left ventricular hypertrophy and dilatation.   *Arterial Pulses*   Usually there are signs of vasodilatation, high pulse pressure, and pistol-shot sounds. DDX: The quality and location of the murmur along the left sternal border cannot distinguish it from the murmur of pulmonic regurgitation, but the maximal intensity in the aortic area, an accentuated and displaced precordial apical thrust, increased pulse pressure with a brisk carotid pulse, pulsus bisferiens, and Duroziez sign all favor the diagnosis of aortic regurgitation [Choudhry NK, Etchells EE. The rational clinical examination. Does this patient have aortic regurgitation? *JAMA* 1999;281:2231–2238].

✓ *AORTIC REGURGITATION—CLINICAL OCCURRENCE:*   Common causes are rheumatic valvulitis, congenitally bicuspid aortic valve, and endocarditis. Syphilitic aortitis is increasingly uncommon. Marfan syndrome, aortic dissection, aneurysm of the sinus of Valsalva, and annular ectasia of the aorta are less common.

KEY SIGN
Basal Diastolic Murmur: Pulmonic Regurgitation in the Presence of Pulmonary Arterial Hypertension: *Pathophysiology:*   This is practically always caused by dilation of the pulmonic valve ring by hypertension in the pulmonary circuit (Fig. 8-40F).   *The Murmur*   This is frequently termed the *Graham Steell murmur.* It is indistinguishable in quality and timing from the high-pitched murmur of aortic regurgitation (see Fig. 8-39D). It is usually less loud and is transmitted less widely than the aortic murmur. The point of maximum intensity is usually in the second or third left interspace. In the absence of pulmonary hypertension, as occurs after pulmonary valvotomy, the murmur of pulmonary regurgitation is medium- to low-pitched.   *Heart Sounds*   The P2 may be accentuated.   *Palpation*   A precordial thrust of the right ventricle may be palpated. DDX: Usually the diagnosis is made by the signs of right ventricular hypertrophy and the absence of peripheral signs of aortic regurgitation.

✓ *PULMONIC REGURGITATION—CLINICAL OCCURRENCE:*   This occurs with pulmonary hypertension from any cause (mitral stenosis, left-sided heart failure, pulmonary emphysema, idiopathic pulmonary hypertension, congenital heart lesions, obstructive sleep apnea, chronic pulmonary emboli) or postpulmonary valvotomy.

KEY SIGN
Mid-Precordial Diastolic Murmur: Tricuspid Stenosis: *Pathophysiology:*   Atrial   contraction   against   a stenotic valve orifice causes the presystolic accentuation and giant a-waves. Impedance to right ventricular filling leads to elevated central venous pressure (CVP). Because right ventricular filling is augmented during inspiration, the murmur becomes louder (Fig. 8-41G).   *The Mur-*

mur   The diastolic murmur is low-pitched and rumbling with a presystolic crescendo when atrial fibrillation is absent. It is best heard with the bell lightly placed. In lesser degrees, the murmur is late diastolic; with greater degrees, it also occupies mid-diastole and even early diastole. *Venous Pulse*   Giant a-waves will be seen at the appropriate timing; the CVP will be progressively elevated as stenosis worsens.   *Heart Sounds* The first heart sound is accentuated at the apex. Sometimes an opening snap of the tricuspid valve can be identified.   *Palpation*   The point of maximum intensity is quite sharply localized at the lower-left sternal border in the fourth or fifth interspace. In severe stenosis signs of central venous congestion (elevated CVP, hepatomegaly, ascites, edema) will be found, which can be mistakenly diagnosed as right ventricular failure. DDX: The murmur can usually be distinguished from that of mitral stenosis by its location and accentuation during inspiration. A murmur identical to the mid-diastolic rumble of tricuspid stenosis is the diastolic flow rumble that accompanies severe tricuspid regurgitation or a large atrial septal defect.

✓ *TRICUSPID STENOSIS—CLINICAL OCCURRENCE:*   Rheumatic valvulitis, congenital heart disease, and carcinoid tumor produce this lesion.

KEY SIGN

Apical Diastolic Murmur: Mitral Stenosis: *Pathophysiology:*   In mild *mitral stenosis,* ventricular filling is only slightly delayed and the period of rapid filling is shortened, so a mid-diastolic murmur is produced; because there is adequate ventricular filling, the pressure gradient is little increased by atrial contraction, and no presystolic murmur is produced. With *moderate or severe stenosis,* ventricular filling is prolonged, so atrial systole increases the pressure difference across the valve, producing a presystolic crescendo murmur; this presystolic accentuation may be absent in atrial fibrillation. The accentuated S1 is caused by the prolonged filling time, which places the valves low in the ventricle so they are snapped shut by systole. Pulmonary hypertension produces the accentuated P2. The audible opening snap of the mitral valve is attributed to the elevated atrial pressure (Fig. 8-41E). *The Murmur*   This murmur is heard best in the left lateral position. It is usually sharply localized near the apex; the audible area may be small, so the bell must be placed directly on the apex. Sometimes, only by carefully inching the bell over the entire apex will a loud murmur be discovered. The murmur is low-pitched and rumbling, sometimes only heard with the bell held lightly. The sound may resemble the roll of a drum. In mild stenosis, the murmur occurs in mid-diastole. As the orifice narrows, the murmur starts earlier and ends later, until it almost covers the diastolic interval; however, there is always a pause after the second sound before the onset of the murmur. The long murmur often has a presystolic crescendo (see Fig. 8-39G). The murmur is often accompanied by a thrill at the apex when the patient is in the left decubitus position.   *Heart Sounds*   S1 at the apex is accentuated. If there is pulmonary hypertension, P2 is accentuated, appears earlier and is normally delayed with inspiration. When the murmur is loud, there is usually a mitral opening snap shortly after A2, heard best at the left sternal border between the second and fourth interspaces. This is commonly mistaken for a split second sound. The opening snap disappears when the mitral cusps become rigid due to calcification. *Palpation* Often there is a palpable right ventricular thrust indicating right ventricular hypertrophy. DDX: Tricuspid stenosis produces a similar murmur, but it is localized nearer the sternum. A similar diastolic apical rumble may be heard with increased mitral diastolic flow due to severe mitral regurgitation. The murmurs of aortic and pulmonic regurgitation also occur at the apex. Echocardiogram examination resolves diagnostic questions [Thibault GE. Studying the classics. *N Engl J Med* 1995;333:648–653].

✓ *MITRAL STENOSIS—CLINICAL OCCURRENCE:* This nearly always results from rheumatic heart disease, but is rarely congenital.

Apical Diastolic Murmur: Shuddering of the Anterior Leaflet of the Mitral Valve (Austin Flint Murmur):

Pathophysiology: On echocardiograms, aortic regurgitation is often associated with fluttering of the anterior leaflet of the mitral valve. However, neither this phenomenon nor others accompanying chronic aortic regurgitation (such as premature closure of the mitral valve causing "functional" mitral stenosis, diastolic mitral regurgitation, and turbulence associated with the mixing of mitral inflow and the aortic regurgitant jet) seem consistently to correlate with the murmur. One study presented evidence that the murmur is caused by the abutment of the aortic regurgitant jet against the trabeculated left ventricular endocardium [Landzberg JS, Pflugfelder PW, Cassidy MM, et al. Etiology of the Austin Flint murmur. J Am Coll Cardiol 1992;20:408]. *The Murmur* Some patients with severe grades of aortic regurgitation and normal mitral valves have murmurs at the cardiac apex, which are similar in pitch and timing to those produced by organic disease of the mitral valve. The examiner confronted with a combination of aortic and mitral murmurs must decide if the mitral valve is normal. Authors vary on the criteria for diagnosis; the methods of Levine and Harvey are cited here. When the aortic lesion is undoubtedly syphilitic, the murmur is the Flint type (Fig. 8-40D). The presence of atrial fibrillation favors an organic lesion of the mitral valve, as the dysrhythmia is rarely associated with an aortic lesion. *Heart Sounds* S1 is not accentuated with the Flint murmur. Accentuation of S1 or P2 favors organic mitral stenosis. The opening snap of the mitral valve is absent in the Flint murmur. *ECG* Notching of the P waves in the ECG favors an organic lesion of the mitral valve. *Amyl Nitrite Test* When tachycardia and diminished systolic blood pressure have been produced by the inhalation of amyl nitrite, the apical diastolic rumbling of the Flint murmur becomes fainter, but the murmur of organic mitral stenosis becomes louder.

✓ *AUSTIN FLINT MURMUR—CLINICAL OCCURRENCE:* Aortic regurgitation from rheumatic valvulitis, syphilis, or acute endocarditis.

Continuous Murmurs

Murmurs heard throughout the cardiac cycle indicate that turbulent flow is occurring without interruption. Therefore, the flow must be from a continuous high pressure source to a low pressure sump, that is, from the aorta to the pulmonary artery or a vein, or across a fixed obstruction in the aorta.

KEY SIGN
Basal Continuous Murmur: Patent Ductus Arteriosus: *Pathophysiology:* A patent ductus is an arteriovenous fistula, between an arterial circuit of high pressure (aorta) and an arterial system of lesser pressure (pulmonary artery). The continuous murmur results from blood flowing continuously into the pulmonary artery during the entire heart cycle. The greater pressure during ventricular systole produces a higher pitch to the murmur. The pressures may be modified by the presence of other congenital anomalies (Fig. 8-41C). *The Murmur* A murmur heard continuously throughout systole and diastole in the second or third left interspace is typically caused by a patent ductus. Usually there is a crescendo late in systole and a decrescendo after the second sound, producing a machinery murmur (see Fig. 8-39F). Occasionally the murmur is transmitted down the left sternal border; sometimes it can be heard at the apex. Most frequently, transmission is to the interscapular region. The murmur is medium-pitched and rumbling, heard with either bell or diaphragm. Louder murmurs are harsh. Tricuspid regurgitation may develop from the pulmonary hypertension. The increased volume of left-sided flow through the mitral orifice may produce a diastolic rumble simulating mitral stenosis. *Heart Sounds* Sometimes the noise runs from first sound to first sound, with a second sound buried in the crescendo. Frequently there is a short pause between the first sound and the onset of the murmur. *Palpation* The precordial thrust of both the right and left ventricles may be accentuated. *Arterial Pulses* If the leak is large, the peripheral pulse wave may be collapsing as encountered in aortic regurgitation. DDX: When the diastolic component of the murmur is absent because of pulmonary hypertension, the condition can be distinguished from pulmonic stenosis only by cardiac catheterization. The continuous murmur should be distinguished from a venous hum in the internal jugular vein.

KEY SIGN
Basal Continuous Murmur: Coarctation of Aorta: See page 478ff and 426.

Mid-Precordial Continuous Murmur: Coronary Arteriovenous Fistula or Ruptured Sinus of Valsalva Aneurysm:

Similar physical signs in these two conditions require diagnostic imaging for differentiation. *The Murmur* A continuous murmur with late systolic accentuation (machinery or to-and-fro) is audible at the lower portion of the sternum, on either or both sides. It is often accompanied by a systolic or continuous thrill. DDX: Although the to-and-fro murmur has the same quality as that in ductus arteriosus, the location is sufficiently different to be distinctive. A mid-precordial to-and-fro murmur can occur with the combination of inter-ventricular septal defect and aortic regurgitation, but this murmur lacks the late systolic accentuation. Although a venous hum may be audible behind the upper sternum, its accentuation is diastolic and it is abolished by pressure on the internal jugular vein.

Vascular Signs of Cardiac Activity

Cardiac contraction maintains blood pressure in both veins and arteries. Left ventricular contraction produces pulses in all accessible arteries. Movements of the right heart originate venous pulses only in the upper part of the body. Because arterial pressure is normally about 16 times as high as pressure in the large veins, visible arterial pulsations are palpable; venous pulsations are usually not palpable. This observation is useful in determining the origin of visible pulsations in the upper part of the body.

ARTERIAL SIGNS OF CARDIAC ACTION. The pump function of the ventricles is reflected in the contour of the arterial blood pressure, modified by the vessels in the arterial tree. The contour of the arterial pulse wave is affected by the contractility of the left ventricle, the distensibility of the aorta, and the condition of the aortic valve orifice. Abnormalities of the other heart valves do not have this effect.

KEY SIGN

Pulse Contour: Normal Arterial Pulse: The primary wave starts with a swift upstroke to the peak systolic pressure, followed by a more gradual decline. A second, and normally smaller, upstroke, *the dicrotic wave,* occurs at approximately the end of ventricular systole, caused by a rebound against the closed aortic valve (see Fig. 8-42A). Normally, the dicrotic wave is not palpable; one feels only a sharp upstroke and a more gradual downstroke. The systolic blood pressure measures the peaks of the waves, and the diastolic pressure the troughs.

KEY SIGN

Pulse Contour: Twice Peaking Pulses: There are two types of arterial pulses with two palpable pulse waves per cycle (see Fig. 8-42B). Most common is *pulsus bisferiens* with two palpable waves that occur during systole. Less common is the *dicrotic pulse,* which has one wave palpable in systole and a second wave palpable in diastole.

✓ *CLINICAL OCCURRENCE:*   *Pulsus Bisferiens*   severe aortic regurgitation especially when associated with moderate aortic stenosis, hypertrophic subaortic stenosis, and hyperkinetic circulatory states such as hyperthyroidism;   *Dicrotic Pulse*   any very low cardiac output, such as might accompany a dilated cardiomyopathy or cardiac tamponade, especially in patients with an aorta of normal pliability.

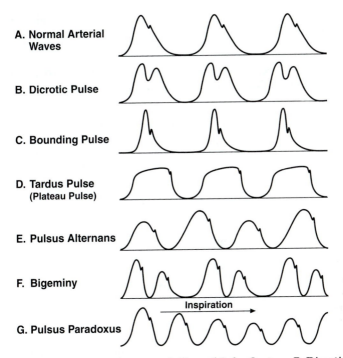

A. Normal Arterial Waves

B. Dicrotic Pulse

C. Bounding Pulse

D. Tardus Pulse (Plateau Pulse)

E. Pulsus Alternans

F. Bigeminy

Inspiration

G. Pulsus Paradoxus

Fig. 8-42 Arterial Pulse Contour. A. Normal Pulse Contour. B. Dicrotic Pulse. C. Bounding or Collapsing Pulse. D. Plateau Pulse. E. Pulsus Alternans. F. Pulsus Bigeminus. G. Pulsus Paradoxus.

KEY SIGN

Pulse Contour: Bounding or Collapsing Pulse (Corrigan Pulse, Water-Hammer Pulse): *Pathophysiology:* This is caused by a vigorous upstroke of the pulse wave because of a large stroke volume and/or vigorous contraction associated with a rapid runoff of blood from the aorta. With high pulse pressure, the upstroke of the waves may be very sharp, while the downstroke falls precipitously (see Fig. 8-42C). It may be accompanied by the pistol-shot sound.

✔ *CLINICAL OCCURRENCE:* This type of pulse wave is encountered in hyperthyroidism, emotional states, aortic regurgitation, patent ductus arteriosus, and arteriovenous fistula.

KEY SIGN

► **Pulse Contour: Plateau Pulse (Pulsus Tardus):** *Pathophysiology:* This is encountered in severe degrees of aortic stenosis, where ejection through the narrowed orifice is seriously impaired. The upstroke of the wave is gradual and the peak is delayed toward the latter portion of systole (see Fig. 8-42D). This pulse, best appreciated in the carotid arteries, is a gentle, sustained caress, lifting the palpating finger, in contrast to the normal brief tap of the pulse.

KEY SIGN

▶ **Pulse Volume Changes: Absent Pulses, Pulseless Disease:** See Takayasu aortitis, page 472.

KEY SIGN

▶ **Pulse Volume Changes: Pulsus Alternans:** *Pathophysiology:* This is a sign of decreased myocardial contractility. With normal rhythm and a normal interval between beats, the pulse waves alternate between those of greater and lesser volume (see Fig. 8-42E). In lesser degrees, the difference may not be palpable, but it is readily detected while measuring the blood pressure by auscultation. As the cuff is slowly deflated, the sounds from alternate beats are audible first. With further deflation, the number of sounds is suddenly doubled. DDX: This phenomenon must be distinguished from bigeminal rhythm, in which a normal beat is followed by a premature beat.

KEY SIGN

Pulse Volume Changes: Pulsus Bigeminus (Coupled Rhythm): *Pathophysiology:* The second or premature beat of the pair will have less volume than the preceding normal beat if contraction occurs before complete ventricular filling. A normal beat is followed by a premature beat and a pause (see Fig. 8-42F). Occasionally, the premature beats follow regular beats so closely that they do not produce waves in the peripheral arteries, so the radial pulse rate is half the ventricular rate. Errors in diagnosis may be avoided if the rhythm is first evaluated over the precordium by auscultation.

KEY SIGN

▶ **Pulse Volume Changes: Pulsus Paradoxus:** *Pathophysiology:* Normally, inspiration diminishes the intrathoracic pressure, so more blood flows into the thorax and right ventricle. While the right ventricular output is augmented, the inspiratory expansion of the pulmonary bed diminishes left ventricular filling resulting in decreases in left ventricular stroke volume and systolic blood pressure. With pericardial tamponade, the pericardial fluid creates a tense parietal pericardium; when inspiration increases right heart inflow and volume, left heart filling is further reduced leading to an exaggerated fall in left ventricular stroke volume and systolic blood pressure. Hyperinflated lungs in obstructive airway disease also produces a paradoxical pulse. Under normal resting conditions, there is an inspiratory fall of less than 10 mmHg in the arterial systolic pressure and an accompanying inspiratory fall in venous pressure. These changes are scarcely perceptible on the physical examination. A paradoxical pulse is said to exist when inspiration creates more than a 10 mmHg drop in systolic arterial pressure. The exaggerated waxing and waning in the pulse volume may sometimes be detected by palpation (see Fig. 8-42G); more often, it can only be detected by use of the sphygmomanometer. A paradoxical pulse can only be said to be present when there are no other reasons for variation in the left ventricular stroke volume; specifically, the rhythm must be regular with consistent atrial and ventricular synchrony [Bilchick KD, Wise RA. Paradoxical physical findings described by Kussmaul: Pulsus paradoxus and Kussmaul's sign. *Lancet* 2002;359:1940–1942].

✓ *PULSUS PARADOXICUS—CLINICAL OCCURRENCE:* Pericardial tamponade, pulmonary emphysema, severe asthma.

KEY SIGN

Pulse Volume Changes: Inequality of Contralateral Pulses: Disparity between the volumes of right and left arterial pulses may be detected by simultaneous palpation. If possible, confirm a suspicion of inequality by taking the blood pressure in both arteries. A diminution in one pulse suggests atherosclerotic obstruction, dissecting aneurysm or other arterial obstruction.

Disordered Changes in Pulse Volume or Rhythm: See Chapter 4, page 67ff. Many dysrhythmias produce arterial beats of greater or lesser volume and disordered timing. It is preferable to evaluate the disturbance from the precordial findings rather than attempting a judgment from the peripheral pulse alone. You should realize that any ventricular contraction occurring before the ventricle has had time to fill will produce a peripheral pulse wave of diminished volume, or none at all. *The ECG is the only way to accurately diagnose rhythm disturbances.*

KEY SIGN

Arterial Sound: Arterial Murmur or Bruit: Normally, arteries are silent when auscultated with the bell chest piece placed lightly over them. Interference with the normal laminar blood flow through the vessel may cause eddies that set the arterial wall in vibration, heard as a systolic murmur and palpated as a thrill. Although murmur and bruit are literally synonymous, there is a tendency among Americans to reserve bruit for arterial sounds. The presence of a bruit does not necessarily indicate limitation of flow [Sauvé, S-S, Laupacis A, Østbye T, et al. The rational clinical examination. Does this patient have a clinically important carotid bruit? *JAMA* 1993;270:2843–2845].

✓ *ARTERIAL BRUIT—CLINICAL OCCURRENCE:* Arteries become tortuous from arteriosclerosis or other circumstances or dilate with aneurysm. They may be constricted congenitally, by intimal proliferation, or by an atherosclerotic plaque. Dilatation of the thyroid arteries with increased blood flow occurs in Graves disease (here, the word bruit is often used). Blood flow through an arteriovenous fistula or large arterial collaterals, as in aortic coarctation, is often accompanied by bruits. A continuous murmur is produced by an arteriovenous fistula or a partially obstructed artery when the collateral circulation is poor and the diastolic pressure is quite low distal to the obstruction.

Arterial Sound: Pistol-Shot Sound: *Pathophysiology:* This is produced by the front of an arterial pulse wave of higher than normal pulse pressure striking the arterial wall in the region of auscultation. When the stethoscope bell is placed lightly over an artery, particularly the femoral, a sharp sound like a gunshot may be heard.

✓ *PISTOL-SHOT SOUND—CLINICAL OCCURRENCE:* Although commonly associated with aortic regurgitation, it also occurs in other conditions with high pulse pressure, such as hyperthyroidism, and anemia.

KEY SIGN
Arterial Sound: Duroziez Sign: *Pathophysiology:* Formerly attributed to retrograde flow of blood in the vessel, the second murmur only occurs when a dicrotic pulse wave is present, suggesting that the second phase is caused by onward acceleration of blood flow. When the femoral artery is compressed by pressure on the overlying stethoscope bell, eddies are created producing a systolic murmur in normal persons. Whenever such compression produces a second murmur in diastole closely following the first and giving the impression of a to-and-fro murmur, it is Duroziez sign. Listen through the stethoscope while pressure on the bell is gradually increased. First the normal systolic murmur appears; with further pressure a critical point is reached when the second murmur becomes audible. Most commonly encountered in aortic regurgitation of severe grades, it may also occur in other conditions with high pulse pressure (see Chapter 4, page 88).

Venous Signs of Cardiac Action

Cardiac action produces physical signs in the venous system by (a) alteration of the venous pressure in the periphery, (b) production of venous congestion in the viscera, or (c) alteration of the venous pulse waves.

KEY SIGN
Elevated Central Venous Pressure (CVP): *Pathophysiology:* Elevated central venous pressure indicates either overfilling of the intravascular space, exceeding venous capacitance, or impedance to filling of the right atrium or right ventricle. Impedance to right ventricular filling often occurs as a result of impaired outflow from the right ventricle causing elevated right ventricular end-diastolic pressure. When the venous pressure exceeds 10 or 12 cm of water under resting conditions, it should be considered elevated. DDX: A generalized increase in venous pressure must be distinguished from superior and/or inferior vena cava obstruction. Always assess whether the venous pressure appears uniformly elevated above and below the diaphragm, because it must be if the *central* venous pressure is elevated; absence of signs below the diaphragm suggests superior vena cava obstruction [Cook DJ, Simel DL. The rational clinical examination. Does this patient have abnormal central venous pressure? *JAMA* 1996;275: 630–634].

✓ *ELEVATED CVP—CLINICAL OCCURRENCE:* *Overfilling of the Vascular Space* kidney failure, rapid infusion of fluids and blood products, chronic congestive heart failure with edema; *Impedance to Right Heart Filling* tricuspid stenosis, tricuspid regurgitation, pericardial tamponade, constrictive pericarditis; *Impaired Outflow from the Right Ventricle* pulmonary hypertension, pulmonary embolus, pulmonic stenosis, right ventricular infarction.

KEY SIGN
Diminished Venous Pressure: *Pathophysiology:* This occurs in peripheral circulatory failure that is part of the shock syndrome, usually associated with hypovolemia, diminished venous tone and/or peripheral pooling. The peripheral veins are collapsed when the patient is supine. See the discussion of *Hypotension*, Chapter 4, page 86.

KEY SIGN
Venous Pulse Giant A Waves: Tricuspid Stenosis: See page 430.

KEY SIGN
Venous Pulse Cannon A-Waves: Atrioventricular Dyssynchrony: *Pathophysiology:* Atrial contraction against a closed tricuspid valve produces retrograde ejection of atrial blood into the central venous channels. Prominent venous pulsations are visible in the neck veins, *cannon a-waves*. They are identified as a-waves by being asynchronous with the apical impulse and carotid upstroke. They are easily obliterated by gentle pressure at the base of the neck insufficient to diminish the carotid pulse. DDX: Irregular cannon a-waves suggests that at least some atrial contractions are occurring simultaneously with ventricular contractions. A regular pattern of cannon a-waves suggests a fixed pattern of atrioventricular (AV) block, for example, atrial flutter with 2:1 block. An irregular pattern with variable a-waves volume suggests AV dissociation, for example, complete heart block. *An ECG is required to diagnose the rhythm.* Regular giant a-waves occurring consistently in synchrony with the heart sounds and arterial pulse suggests impedance to right atrial outflow, for example, a noncompliant right ventricle or tricuspid stenosis.

KEY SIGN
Large V-Waves in the Venous Pulse: Tricuspid Regurgitation: *Pathophysiology:* Tricuspid insufficiency allows the right ventricle to eject blood retrograde into the central venous channels. Large v-waves are visible in the jugular veins and there may be palpable pulsation of the liver. The waves are identified as v-waves by being synchronous with the apical impulse and carotid upstroke with collapse at S2. There may be a right ventricular thrust reflecting the volume overload on the right ventricle. See page 427.

Facial Suffusion with Arms Elevated: Pemberton Sign: *Pathophysiology:* Retrosternal goiters obstruct the thoracic inlet compressing the brachiocephalic veins when the arms are raised over the head. Have the patient raise and hold his arms over his head. Purple venous suffusion of the skin on the head and neck with distention of the jugular veins suggests a high anterior retrosternal mass.

KEY SIGN

► **Hepatojugular Reflux and Kussmaul Sign:** *Pathophysiology:* These phenomena are caused by inability of the right heart to accommodate increased venous return. Place the patient on a bed with movable backrest; lower the thorax until the head of the blood column is just visible in the jugular veins above the clavicle. Have the patient breathe at the normal rate and depth. Place the right hand on the right upper quadrant of the abdomen, and press firmly upward under the costal margin for at least 10–15 seconds. The *hepatojugular reflux* sign is "positive" if displacement of this small amount of blood from the abdomen causes a rise in the head of the blood column in the neck for as long as the abdominal pressure is continued. *Kussmaul sign* is present when distention, rather than collapse, of jugular veins occurs during inspiration. A positive hepatojugular reflux sign is most commonly seen with early right heart failure. Both signs may be seen with severe right heart failure, constrictive pericarditis, and right ventricular infarction [Bilchick KD, Wise RA. Paradoxical physical findings described by Kussmaul: Pulsus paradoxus and Kussmaul's sign. *Lancet* 2002;359: 1940–1942; Wiese J. The abdominojugular reflux sign. *Am J Med* 2000; 109:59–61].

Arterial Circulation Signs

The tissue effects of arterial blood flow must be distinguished from those of venous drainage. Arterial deficits cause dermal pallor, coldness, and tissue atrophy. Small-vessel disturbances are recognizable as patterns in the skin and are detected by the methods of dermatologic description. Diseases of the larger vessels cause regional hypoperfusion syndromes; diseases, such as the vasculitides, which affect smaller vessels tend to be more diffuse [McGee SR, Boyko EJ. Physical examination and chronic lower-extremity ischemia: A critical review. *Arch Intern Med* 1998;158: 1357–1364].

Feet Dependent: Warm Skin: Normal skin temperature indicates adequate arterial flow. The normal color of the nail beds is red or pink. If warm feet have blue nail beds, the warmth has been externally applied to feet with inadequate arterial flow.

KEY SIGN

Purpura: Atheroembolic Disease: *Pathophysiology:* Disruption of an arterial atherosclerotic plaque leads to embolization of cholesterol-rich atheroma to the small arteries of the organs, muscles, and skin, producing hemorrhagic infarcts. The lesions may be painless or accompanied by pain. Hemorrhagic cutaneous infarcts, which may be palpable, range from 1 mm to 2 cm in size; toes and finger tips may become necrotic. Livedo reticularis may be seen.

✓ *CLINICAL OCCURRENCE:* This most commonly follows passage of intravascular catheters during diagnostic or therapeutic procedures, or follows the initiation of warfarin therapy.

KEY SIGN
Palpable Purpura: Vasculitis: *Pathophysiology:* Inflammation of the small arterioles or venules in the skin associated with immune complex deposition produces inflammation with punctate edema and hemorrhage, *palpable purpura.* The patient may be well or have symptoms and signs of a systemic disease, including visceral involvement. The pattern and size of involved arteries and/or veins is characteristic of each vasculitis syndrome (see page 470).

KEY SIGN
Skin Pallor and Coldness: Chronic Arterial Obstruction: *Pathophysiology:* Chronic progressive arterial obstruction allows development of collateral circulation and tissue accommodation to ischemia. Pallid cool skin strongly suggests regional hypoperfusion. It is normal in a cold environment, but should rapidly resolve on exposure to warm air or water. Failure to do so suggests that the abnormality is not limited to the skin vessels but involves a major trunk artery. Pain may be present with exertion of the part (*claudication*). The distribution of the arterial deficit will depend upon the site of the obstruction and the presence and extent of collateral circulation. Other useful signs are prolonged venous filling time, abnormal pedal pulses and a femoral bruit [McGee SR, Boyko EJ. Physical examination and chronic lower-extremity ischemia: A critical review. *Arch Intern Med* 1998;158:1357–1364].

✓ *CLINICAL OCCURRENCE:* Atherosclerosis is most common; less common causes are vasculitis of large vessels (e.g., Takayasu aortitis, giant cell arteritis), Buerger disease, vasospastic disorders, and ergotism.

KEY SIGN
Dependent Rubor and Coldness: Chronic Arterial Obstruction: *Pathophysiology:* When the skin and nail beds are blue or purple, the inadequate arterial flow has been unable to displace the venous blood that contains reduced hemoglobin. Raise the part above heart level to drain the blue venous blood away to unmask tissues made pallid by insufficient arterial flow (Fig. 8-43). When the elevated foot is lowered, the pink color normally returns in 20 seconds. Return of color in 45 to 60 seconds confirms an arterial deficit. See page 487.

KEY SIGN
Acute Pain with Skin Pallor and Coolness: Arterial Embolus or Thrombosis: *Pathophysiology:* Acute occlusion of a major peripheral artery causes cutaneous and muscular ischemia producing skin and nail bed pallor, decreased temperature, and ischemic pain. The pain is severe and unremitting with changes

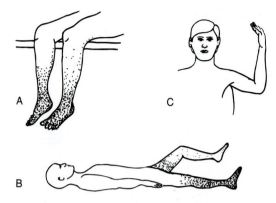

Fig. 8-43 Circulation of the Skin in the Extremities. *A.* *The legs are dependent to observe the color of the skin and nail beds. Arterial deficit produces a violaceous color from pooling of the blood in the venules because of loss of venomotor tone as a result of hypoxia.* *B.* *While the patient is supine, the foot is elevated above the level of venous pressure (15 cm [6 in] above the right heart or 25 cm [10 in] above the table when the patient is supine). Elevation drains the foot of venous blood so the skin color reflects only the presence of arterial blood. The elevated leg is compared with the opposite extremity.* *C.* *The hand is raised above the heart level so the skin color is produced exclusively by arterial blood.*

in position. Embolic arterial occlusion is most common in native vessels, whereas thrombus in prosthetic vascular channels is more common. Urgent relief of the obstruction is necessary to preserve the part. See page 486.

✓ *CLINICAL OCCURRENCE:* The embolic source is usually in the heart (endocarditis, prosthetic valve, atrial fibrillation); less commonly, it may arise from thrombus within an aortic aneurysm or paradoxical embolism from a vein via a patent foramen ovale.

KEY SIGN
Skin Atrophy: The skin is thinner than normal, as demonstrated by its shiny appearance and the fine texture of the wrinkles produced when it is pinched. The normal fine furrows in the epidermis are absent. The lanugo hair on the backs of the hands and feet and the dorsa of the fingers and toes fails to grow.

Malnourished Nails: The nails grow slowly or not at all. They are dry, brittle, and contain transverse ridges. Later, they become thickened (Fig. 8-44B).

Skin Scars: On an extremity with arterial deficiency, the skin may contain round scars, covered with atrophied skin that may be pig-

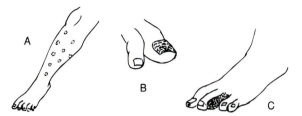

Fig. 8-44 Dermal Lesions from Arterial Deficit. **A. Atrophy.** *The skin over the legs contains round areas of dermal atrophy, with or without pigmentation. These result from small superficial infarctions.* **B. Dystrophic Nails.** *The toenails grow more slowly than normal and the nail plates become thickened and laminated; the layers form transverse ridges.* **C. Necrosis.** *Gangrene of the distal parts may develop from arterial deficit. The sketch shows a round spot of gangrene on the tip of the great toe, and the middle toe blackened from dry gangrene.*

mented (Fig. 8-44A). These develop without trauma as the result of obstruction of small arteries.

KEY SIGN

Skin Ulcers: Ischemic ulcers occur over the tips of the toes, the malleoli, the heels, the metatarsal heads, and the dorsal arches. They are termed cold ulcers because they lack the warm erythematous areola characteristic of warm ulcers caused by infection. Frequently, the borders of cold ulcers appear punched out. They are seen in diabetes mellitus with severe neuropathy and sickle cell disease.

KEY SIGN

Retiform Necrosis: Necrotic skin in a scalloped (retiform) pattern suggests obstruction of the dermal arteriole feeding the area. Vasculitis should be suspected.

KEY SIGN

Skin Gangrene: In the earliest stage, the lesions are round, less than 1 mm in diameter, with pitted centers of black skin (Fig. 8-44C). The areas may spread to involve the entire foot. When the skin is black, wrinkled, and dry, the condition is termed dry gangrene. If secondary infection occurs, the dead area becomes swollen with fluid oozing onto the surface; this is wet gangrene.

KEY SIGN

Nodular Vessels: Polyarteritis Nodosa: See page 472.

Syndromes

Chest Wall Syndromes

Chest Pain Intensified by Respiratory Motion

Thoracic movements displace ribs, muscles, nerves, and pleural surfaces. Pain is accentuated by breathing, coughing, laughing, or sneezing when these structures are inflamed or injured. As with superficial pain, the region may also be tender. The structures to be considered are ribs, cartilages, muscles, nerves, and pleurae. A systematic inventory of causes of pain in each of these tissues should be considered in the examination.

S KEY SYNDROME

Pleuritis and Pleurisy: *Pathophysiology:* The visceral pleura is anesthetic, but the parietal pleura contains many sensory fibers that join the trunks of adjacent intercostal nerves, giving off twigs to the overlying skin. Pleural pain is caused either by stretching of the inflamed parietal pleura or by separation of fibrous adhesions between two pleural surfaces. It is difficult to credit the concept that pain is produced by the rubbing together of two pleural surfaces; pain often occurs without a friction rub, and a rub is often present without pain. Inflammation of the pleura (*pleuritis*) produces knife-like or shooting pains in the skin of the adjacent thoracic wall. The pain is intensified by breathing, coughing, and laughing. Feel and listen for a friction rub; this is not constantly present, so perform several examinations. Signs of pleural effusion may develop. The diagnosis of *pleurisy* is made from the typical pain history or the presence of a friction rub after excluding other causes of pleuritis, rib fractures, myositis, and neuritis. A friction rub may precede x-ray findings diagnostic of pneumonia.

✔ *PLEURISY—CLINICAL OCCURRENCE:* Bacterial and viral pneumonia, tuberculosis, empyema, viral pleuritis, pulmonary infarction from embolus, mesothelioma, primary and metastatic lung neoplasm, and connective-tissue diseases.

Diaphragmatic Pleuritis and Pleurisy: *Pathophysiology:* The peripheral portion of the diaphragmatic pleura is supplied by the fifth and sixth intercostal nerves, so involvement of their regions produces pain near the costal margins. The central area of the diaphragm (thoracic and peritoneal) is innervated by the phrenic nerve (C3–4); these cervical roots also innervate the neck and supraclavicular fossae. Thus, pain in the neck may result from irritation of the diaphragmatic pleura by a subphrenic abscess, splenic infarction, splenic rupture or pericarditis (Fig. 8-45). There is sharp shooting pain in the epigastrium, lower retrosternal region, or shoulder, intensified by thoracic motions, especially deep breathing, coughing, or laughing. It may be localized along the costal margins, epigastrium, lumbar region, or neck at the superior border of the trapezius or the supraclavicular fossa. The painful areas are all on the same side. A pleural or pericardial friction rub may be present.

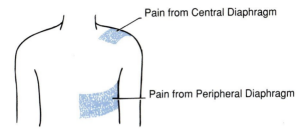

Fig. 8-45 Referral of Left Diaphragmatic Pain.

✔ *DIAPHRAGMATIC PLEURITIS AND PLEURISY—CLINICAL OCCUR-RENCE:* The diagnosis of *pleurisy* is suggested when pain is accompanied by fever and friction rub; later, pleural effusion may appear. Other causes of diaphragmatic pleuritis (e.g., subphrenic abscess perforating the diaphragm) must be excluded. A previous history of dysphagia or intraabdominal disease should suggest disorders of the esophagus, subphrenic abscess, peptic ulcer, or pancreatitis. Occasionally, gastric herniation through the esophageal hiatus of the diaphragm may produce similar pain. Pericarditis with pleuritic pain (pleuropericarditis) should be considered.

D KEY DISEASE

Epidemic Pleurodynia: Bornholm Disease, Devil's Grip: *Pathophysiology:* The usual cause is an infection with group B coxsackievirus, although group A or an echovirus is occasionally implicated. After a nondescript prodrome of 1–10 days, the patient is suddenly seized with apparently catastrophic sharp, knife-like pains in the walls of the thorax or abdomen, intensified by breathing and other bodily motions; the thorax may be splinted and the thighs flexed on the belly. Paroxysms of intense pain are separated by intervals of complete comfort. Headache and fever are frequent. Cases may appear sporadically or in an epidemic. Mild pharyngitis is often noted. The muscles of the neck, trunk, and limbs may be tender. In 25% of cases, a friction rub is detected. Orchitis or pericarditis may complicate the condition. The sudden retrosternal pain reminds the physician of myocardial infarction or dissecting aneurysm. The fever suggests pneumonia or acute appendicitis. Lacking an epidemic, the correct diagnosis may be suspected from the normal leukocyte counts. A period of several days of worried observation, until symptoms subside, is the usual method of diagnosis.

Chest Wall Twinge Syndrome (Precordial Catch): The patient experiences brief episodes of sharp pain or "catches" in the anterior chest, usually on the left side. No association with exertion is noted, although some patients report the onset while assuming a bent-over posture. The pains last from 30 seconds to 3 minutes; they are aggravated by deep breathing and relieved by shallow respirations. The cause is unknown, but speculation has considered intercostal muscle spasm and fleeting costochondral pains. The condition is common and harmless, but the patient must be reassured that it is not heart disease.

D KEY DISEASE

Rib Fracture, Periosteal Hematoma, Periostitis, Intercostal Myositis: See page 381–384.

Respiratory Syndromes

S KEY SYNDROME

Pneumothorax: *Pathophysiology:* Rupture of a subpleural bleb or penetrating chest trauma allows alveolar air to enter the pleural space separating the lung from the chest wall leading to failure of respiratory mechanics and collapse of the lung. *Symptoms* Frequently, there is sudden severe pain in the chest, often unilateral, rarely localized. Sometimes it is painless. Onset is immediately followed by progressive dyspnea; cyanosis and shock may ensue. *Signs* See page 402. When a large amount of air enters the pleural cavity, the physical signs are distinctive. Percussion is hyperresonant on the affected side. The trachea is deviated away from the affected side, while fremitus and transmission of voice and breath sounds are reduced or absent. There are decreased respiratory movements of the ribs with persistent distention of the hemithorax in expiration. The coin sign may be present. When *tension pneumothorax* develops, urgent diagnosis and treatment are necessary to prevent suffocation. When the air leak is small, the only physical sign may be decreased breath sounds. Then pneumothorax must be distinguished from pulmonary embolism, myocardial infarction, and acute pericarditis. *Chest X-Ray* Lung markings are absent where there is enough air to separate the layers of pleura; often, the line of the visceral pleura can be identified. DDX: Pneumothorax results from rupture of a pleural bleb in pulmonary emphysema, and, occasionally, from nonsuppurative disease of the lungs, such as sarcoidosis, fibrosis, or silicosis. Puncture of the lung by a fractured rib is the most common traumatic cause. It is not rare in slender, healthy young persons with no discernible pulmonary lesion.

Spontaneous Pyopneumothorax: There is usually a known history of bronchiectasis, lung abscess, or tuberculosis with cavitation. The sudden spillage of pus into the pleural cavity produces severe prostration, chills, fever, or shock. The physical signs and x-ray examination show evidence of hydropneumothorax, and pus can be aspirated from the pleural sac.

S KEY SYNDROME

Pneumonia: *Pathophysiology:* Infection or inflammation of the lung is called pneumonitis or pneumonia. The process may be limited to the airways and alveolar airspaces, or involve the pulmonary interstitium and vascular channels. The diagnostic challenges are to separate infectious from noninfectious forms of pneumonia, and then to identify the specific etiology of each. Onset may be sudden or gradual, depending upon the etiology. Patients present with cough, dyspnea, fatigue, and, especially with infection, high fever, often with rigors. Physical findings range from minimal signs of airspace disease (bronchophony, whispered pectoriloquy) to respiratory failure with multilobar consolidation (see page 400). Infectious pneumonia is separated into community- or hospital-healthcare-associated categories. An approach to the diagnosis of specific etiologies of pneumonia is beyond the scope of this text. *For a complete discussion see Harrison's Principles of Internal Medicine, 16th edition (HPIM-16), Chapters 119 and 239.*

✓ *PNEUMONIA—CLINICAL OCCURRENCE:* *Congenital* pulmonary sequestration (may be confused with pneumonia on chest x-ray); *Idiopathic* idiopathic interstitial pneumonia, eosinophilic pneumonia (acute and chronic); *Inflammatory/Immune* hypersensitivity pneumonitis, vasculitis, lymphomatoid granulomatosis, Goodpasture syndrome, lipoid pneumonia, collagen vascular diseases; *Infectious* bacterial, viral, tuberculosis, nontuberculous mycobacteria, rickettsia, fungi, nocardia, pneumocystis, parasites, primary alveolar proteinosis; *Metabolic/Toxic* inhalational injury, drug reactions, pneumoconioses; *Mechanical/Trauma* aspiration; *Neoplastic* endobronchial neoplasm with post obstructive infection; *Vascular* vasculitis (Churg-Strauss, Wegener).

S KEY SYNDROME

▼ **Severe Acute Respiratory Syndrome (SARS):** *Pathophysiology:* Infection with a novel coronavirus causes severe lung inflammation leading to hypoxia and respiratory failure. First recognized in early 2003, this virus appears to have originated in China and spread rapidly to other countries. The initial symptoms are those of a flu-like illness, followed by rapidly progressive pneumonia. The case fatality rate is approximately 15%, higher in patients over age 50. Spread is by droplets and contact with infected persons and contaminated surfaces. To make the diagnosis, a high index of suspicion is necessary with careful questioning about contact with infected or potentially infected people and travel to known areas of ongoing transmission. Current information is available at the Centers for Disease Control web site, www.cdc.gov.

S KEY SYNDROME

▼ **Aspiration Pneumonia:** *Pathophysiology:* Aspiration of oral secretions, food, or regurgitated stomach contents causes mechanical obstruction of the airways with secondary inflammation (especially with gastric contents at low pH) and secondary infection often with anaerobic flora from the oral cavity. The right middle and apical segment of the right lower lobe are commonly affected. Aspiration is common in association with impaired consciousness of any cause and with impairment of oropharyngeal function. Coughing in association with meals and nocturnal regurgitation with cough and dyspnea are suggestive of chronic aspiration. Necrotizing anaerobic infections may lead to lung abscess with fetid sputum. Aspiration should be suspected in any patient with a history of impaired consciousness or oropharyngeal neurologic dysfunction who presents with pneumonia [Marik PE. Aspiration pneumonitis and aspiration pneumonia. *N Engl J Med* 2001; 344:665–671].

S KEY SYNDROME

Bronchiectasis: *Pathophysiology:* Severe acute or chronic pulmonary infections results in multiple dilatations of the smaller bronchi, which are chronically infected. Cough with purulent sputum and occasionally hemoptysis or recurrent pneumonia are the presenting symptoms. Sputum is copious and purulent. In a resonant chest, with coarse crackles at the lung bases, bronchiectasis should be considered. Clubbing of the fingers may be present. Chronic infection with non-tuberculous mycobacteria is common. High-resolution CT imaging is diagnostic [Barker AF. Bronchiectasis. *N Engl J Med* 2002;346:1383–1393].

S KEY SYNDROME

Lung Abscess: *Pathophysiology:* Infection with necrotizing organisms destroys lung tissue, creating cavities with low oxygen tension, which is ideal for growth of microaerophilic or anaerobic organisms. A history compatible with aspiration is often present. The sputum is scant to intermittently copious, purulent, and foul smelling. Signs of consolidation may be present; amphoric breath sounds may be heard if the cavity communicates with a bronchus and is only partially filled (see page 394). Old abscess cavities my become colonized with *Aspergillus* to produce a fungus ball.

S KEY SYNDROME

Pulmonary Embolism: *Pathophysiology:* Thrombus dislodged from a site of deep venous thrombosis occludes the main pulmonary artery bifurcation or one of its branches. Deep venous thrombosis develops after surgery (particularly total hip and knee replacement), prolonged bed rest and air travel, immobilization by a cast, and venous stasis from venous insufficiency or congestive heart failure. Thrombophilia (factor V Leiden, prothrombin gene mutations, antiphospholipid syndrome, protein C or S deficiency, mucinous adenocarcinomas, estrogens, pregnancy, etc.) increases the risks of deep venous thrombosis. Large emboli obstruct the pulmonary circulation producing acute pulmonary hypertension, right ventricular pressure overload, and failure with circulatory collapse. Infarction of lung tissue results in local inflammation. Hypoxia occurs from ventilation-perfusion mismatching and intrapulmonary shunts. Less-common emboli are fat emboli (from the marrow of fractured bones), air, amniotic fluid (when the fluid contains meconium, it is especially dangerous), and tumor tissue. Patients may be minimally symptomatic or present with sudden dyspnea, chest pain in the six-dermatome distribution and circulatory failure.   *Symptoms*   The pain is either pleuritic or a deep, crushing sensation in the six-dermatome band. Sudden dyspnea is the key symptom. There may be dyspnea or tachypnea without pain. Sometimes painless dyspnea resembles asthma; this has been attributed to the release of serotonin from platelets in the blood clot. Massive pulmonary embolus may present with syncope and no other symptoms. *Signs* Systemic effects may predominate, with weakness, prostration, sweating, nausea, and vomiting. Tachycardia is constant and fever occurs with infarction. Dyspnea, tachypnea, and cyanosis may be extreme. When present, hemoptysis, a pleural friction rub, and bloody pleural effusion strongly support the diagnosis. Massive infarction is indicated by the onset of shock, jaundice, or right-sided heart failure. Pulmonary hypertension is marked by the increasing loudness of P2 and the appearance of a palpable precordial thrust of the right ventricle. Sudden death is not uncommon. Occasionally, pulmonary embolism may be accompanied by board-like rigidity of the abdomen, usually in the upper quadrant beneath the lung involved with the embolism. This is involuntary muscle spasm, so the region is not tender. Its occurrence is confusing because it tends to focus attention upon the abdomen. The evaluation for pulmonary emboli is controversial, but the clinician must have a high index of suspicion and pursue the diagnosis aggressively since recurrent emboli may be fatal. Chronic recurrent pulmonary emboli leads to chronic pulmonary hypertension [Fedullo PF, Auger WR, Kerr KM, Rubin LJ. Chronic thromboembolic pulmonary hypertension. *N Engl J Med* 2001;345:1465–1472]. DDX: Sudden onset of pain in the chest or dyspnea, tachypnea, or unexplained sinus tachycardia in a patient with a predisposing condition should raise the question of pulmonary embolism with or without infarction. The symptoms and signs may suggest asthma, bronchopneumonia, pleurisy, pericarditis, spontaneous pneumothorax, myocardial infarction, acute pancreatitis, or perforated peptic ulcer [Lchunilal SD, Eikelboom JW, Attia J, et al. Does this patient have pulmonary embolism? *JAMA* 2003;290:2849–2858].

S KEY SYNDROME

Sleep-Disordered Breathing: Obstructive and Central Sleep Apnea: *Pathophysiology:* Sleep-disordered breathing results from either mechanical obstruction caused by redundant, lax oropharyngeal soft tissues (*obstructive sleep apnea*) or by decreased medullary respiratory drive (*central sleep apnea*). Hypoventilation and hypoxia at night produce frequent arousals, disrupting effective sleep. Patients are often, but not always, obese. They have daytime hypersomnolence and irritability, and frequently have morning headaches and hypertension; snoring is prominent, but may not have been noted by the patient. History from the bed partner is critical. In severe disease, pulmonary hypertension develops as a consequence of severe hypoxia, leading to signs of right heart failure.

S KEY SYNDROME

Chronic Cough: *Pathophysiology:* Chronic nonproductive cough results from chronic upper or lower airway, or esophageal, irritation. Patients present with complaints of chronic irritating cough, but the physical findings in the chest are normal. The most common causes, accounting for 90% of cases, are chronic postnasal drip, unsuspected asthma, and gastroesophageal reflux. Specific evaluation for each entity is required. Angiotensin-converting enzyme inhibitors also cause chronic cough, which may begin months after starting the medication.

S KEY SYNDROME

Pleural Effusion: See page 397.

D KEY DISEASE

Lung Cancer: *Pathophysiology:*   Most primary lung cancers result from cigarette smoking or exposure to ionizing radiation. Patients present with symptoms and signs related to the chest (cough, hemoptysis, dyspnea, pneumonia, pleural effusion), regional symptoms (lymphadenopathy, superior vena cava syndrome, brain mass) or systemic symptoms (weight loss, weakness, hypercalcemia, hyponatremia). Endobronchial lesions may present as recurrent or slowly resolving pneumonia or atelectasis. Bronchioloalveolar cell carcinoma presents with cough, hypoxia and diffuse infiltrates, often mistaken for an infection. Early detection strategies are controversial [Patz EF, Goodman PC, Bepler G. Screening for lung cancer. *N Engl J Med* 2000;343:1627–1633]. *See HPIM-16, Chapter 75.*

D KEY DISEASE

Asthma: *Pathophysiology:*   Asthma is an acquired syndrome of increased airway responsiveness to both allergic and nonallergic stimuli, airway inflammation, bronchospasm, hyperplasia of mucous-producing cells, and bronchial smooth muscle hypertrophy. Airway obstruction leads to incomplete expiration with hyperinflation of the lungs. Even when patients are asymptomatic, there is active airway inflammation. Between attacks, the patient is well and the chest findings are normal. A paroxysm of asthma frequently begins with an unproductive cough and rapidly progressing dyspnea. Awaking at night with episodic attacks of coughing and chest tightness is commonly experienced. The patient rises to a sitting position, frequently leaning over a table or chair back. The respiratory rate does not increase, but the inspiratory phase is short while expiration is prolonged and labored; the patient is often anxious. The previously resonant chest becomes hyperresonant and the diaphragm descends. The thorax maintains the inspiratory position. The costal margins only diverge slightly, or they may actually converge during inspiration. In severe asthma attacks, the sternocleidomastoid and platysma muscles tense and the alae nasi flare with each expiratory effort. Wheezing may be readily heard at a distance, but becomes less prominent as the attack worsens. Auscultation discloses decreased air movement, wheezes, and coarse crackles. Localized disappearance of breath sounds can occur from bronchial plugging. As the attack subsides, clear tenacious sputum is raised, and the breathing gradually becomes less labored. Asthma can occur without the distinctive wheezing. The only sign that consistently identifies severe impairment of pulmonary function is tensing of the sternocleidomastoid muscle. DDX: Although most writers describe this clinical picture as distinctive, it can be confused with other conditions. Wheezing occurs in acute bronchitis, without the labored respiration. When wheezing is limited to a single region, bronchial obstruction from foreign body or neoplasm should be considered. The sudden occurrence of left-sided cardiac failure may closely simulate asthma: there are wheezes and crackles, and labored breathing may obscure auscultation of the heart. Vocal cord dysfunction (i.e., paradoxical closure of the cords during inspiration) may be identified by examination of the glottis during an attack. The symptoms and signs of asthma are often relieved in a few minutes by inhaled bronchodilators, and reversible airway obstruction can be demonstrated with pulmonary function testing. *See HPIM-16, Chapter 236*.

S KEY SYNDROME

▼ **Pulmonary Edema:** *Pathophysiology:* Edema of the lung interstitium leading to alveolar flooding may be caused by left-sided cardiac failure, pulmonary disease, or acute lung injury. An acute increase in left ventricular end-diastolic pressure is transmitted across the mitral valve to the left atrium and pulmonary veins. The increased hydrostatic pressure in the pulmonary capillaries causes transudation of fluid into the pulmonary interstitium and subsequently the alveoli. Increased fluid in the lung leads to stiffening of the lung with decreased pulmonary compliance, shortness of breath, and cough. As the alveoli are flooded, hypoxia and extreme respiratory distress ensue. Intense dyspnea is accompanied by crackles, rhonchi and gurgles throughout the lungs. Breathing is labored, with cyanosis and frothy sputum, often pink, occasionally bloody. The chest is resonant, but the bronchi are filled with bubbling crackles and sometimes wheezes. In chronic heart failure, the condition is often relapsing and the diagnosis fairly obvious. It may occur suddenly with acute myocardial infarction, especially with papillary muscle necrosis and flail mitral valve. DDX: Occasionally, paroxysmal nocturnal dyspnea in cardiac patients may closely resemble asthma with a prolonged expiratory phase and wheezing. The distinction may be made on the basis of findings from the history, cardiovascular examination, and chest x-ray.

✓ *PULMONARY EDEMA—CLINICAL OCCURRENCE:* *Idiopathic* high altitude; *Inflammatory/Immune* mismatched blood transfusion, hypertransfusion syndrome, systemic lupus erythematosus; *Metabolic/Toxic* acute lung injury (inhalation of noxious gases, aspiration, radiation, hemorrhagic pancreatitis, sepsis, drugs, fresh water drowning, etc.), intravenous heroin, snakebite; *Mechanical/Trauma* left ventricular failure-systolic and diastolic dysfunction (myocardial infarction, cardiomyopathies, tachy- and bradyarrhythmias), mitral stenosis, mitral and aortic insufficiency (especially acute), pulmonary embolism, hanging, suffocation; *Neoplastic* bronchioloalveolar cell carcinoma (not true pulmonary edema, but may appear similar radiographically), lymphangitic carcinoma or lymphoma; *Neurologic* postictal, head trauma, subarachnoid hemorrhage; *Vascular* severe hypertension, intravascular volume overload (crystalloid, colloid, transfusions, kidney failure, salt ingestion).

S KEY SYNDROME

▼ **Interstitial Lung Disease:** *Pathophysiology:* Inflammation with cellular infiltration, interstitial edema, and/or collagen deposition leads to thickening of the alveolar walls and septa, decrease in lung compliance, reduction in lung volume, and impairment of gas exchange. The inflammation may involve the entire alveolus; granuloma formation is characteristic of some of the diseases and is diagnostically important. Patients usually present with chronic cough and dyspnea, with little or no sputum production. A thorough occupational and avocational exposure history is critical to the identification of respiratory irritant, toxins, and allergens. Physical examination shows normal lung density to percussion, decreased breath sounds, and crackles of varying intensity, often at end inspiration and usually most prominent at the bases. X-ray films show increased interstitial markings, with or without alveolar signs [Gong MN, Mark EJ. Case records of the Massachusetts General Hospital. Case 40–2002. *N Engl J Med* 2002;347:2149–2157]. High-resolution CT may be diagnostic with characteristic patterns for specific entities [Gross TJ, Hunninghake GW. Idiopathic pulmonary fibrosis. *N Engl J Med* 2001;345:517–525].

✓ *INTERSTITIAL LUNG DISEASE—CLINICAL OCCURRENCE: After HPIM-15, chapter 259. Inhaled Toxic Substances* asbestosis, fumes and gases, aspiration pneumonia; *with granulomas*—hypersensitivity pneumonitis (organic dusts, e.g., farmer's lung), inorganic dusts (beryllium, silica); *Lung Injury* after acute respiratory distress syndrome, radiation; *Connective-Tissue Diseases* systemic lupus erythematosus, rheumatoid arthritis, ankylosing spondylitis, systemic sclerosis, CREST (calcinosis cutis, Raynaud phenomenon, esophageal motility disorder, sclerodactyly, and telangiectasia) syndrome, Sjögren syndrome, polymyositis-dermatomyositis; *Pulmonary Hemorrhage Syndromes* Goodpasture syndrome, idiopathic pulmonary hemosiderosis; *Congenital Diseases* tuberous sclerosis, neurofibromatosis, Niemann-Pick disease, Gaucher disease; *Miscellaneous* drugs (antibiotics, amiodarone, gold, bleomycin and other chemotherapy agents), eosinophilic pneumonia, lymphangioleiomyomatosis, amyloidosis, graft-versus-host disease, with gastrointestinal or liver disease (Crohn disease, ulcerative colitis, primary biliary cirrhosis, chronic active hepatitis); *Idiopathic Interstitial Pneumonia* idiopathic interstitial pneumonia (usual interstitial pneumonia), desquamative interstitial pneumonia, respiratory bronchiolitis-associated interstitial lung disease, acute interstitial pneumonia, cryptogenic organizing pneumonia, nonspecific interstitial pneumonia.

S KEY SYNDROME

Hypersensitivity Pneumonitis: *Pathophysiology:* Exposure to organic dusts in the work or home environment elicits a chronic inflammatory response in the lung which may progress to irreversible fibrosis. Patients present with cough, shortness of breath, and increasing dyspnea, often with airflow obstruction precipitated by exposure to the agent. Lung signs may show crackles and wheezes or be normal. A careful history is the key to diagnosis.

S KEY SYNDROME

Pulmonary-Renal Syndromes: *Pathophysiology:* Antibodies to basement membrane of the glomerulus and pulmonary capillaries (Goodpasture), or vasculitis involving the lung and glomeruli (Wegener), leads to glomerular injury and pulmonary inflammation and/or hemorrhage. Patients often present acutely with dyspnea, hemoptysis, and cough in Goodpasture syndrome. Wegener granulomatosis may be either acute or subacute. Each entity may present in only one of the two organs. Prompt diagnosis and treatment is required to preserve renal function.

S KEY SYNDROME

▼ **Sarcoidosis:** *Pathophysiology:* Noncaseating granulomatous inflammation involves many organs singly or in combination. The cause is unknown. The lungs and hilar and mediastinal lymph nodes are most commonly affected. Patients may be asymptomatic or present with nonproductive cough and dyspnea accompanied by fever, malaise, weight loss, and night sweats. Lung exam may be normal or show crackles; hepatosplenomegaly, lymphadenopathy, uveitis, cutaneous placques and salivary gland enlargement may be present.

S KEY SYNDROME

▶ ▼ **Tracheal or Bronchial Obstruction:** *Pathophysiology:* Complete obstruction of the trachea is incompatible with life. Partial tracheal obstruction by a foreign body, neoplasm, diphtheritic membrane, or other plug produces violent prolonged inspiratory movements with extreme retraction of the intercostal spaces, suprasternal notch, supraclavicular fossae, and epigastrium. A low-pitched rhonchus, or stridor, may be heard over the chest and at the opened mouth during inspiration and expiration. In a ball–valve obstruction, the rhonchus occurs only during inspiration. An isolated wheeze in the lung, without generalized wheezing, suggests the presence of a localized bronchial obstruction; look for a bronchial adenoma, carcinoma, or foreign body. Another indication of partial bronchial obstruction is the *bagpipe sign:* When the patient is required to cut short a forced expiration while the stethoscope is on the chest, the sound of expelling air is heard to continue after the patient's effort has ceased. If the inspiratory rhonchus is audible on both sides of the chest, the affected side is the one with the palpable rhonchus. In obstruction of a large bronchus, or with a large pneumothorax, there is a pendular movement of the trachea, moving toward the affected side during inspiration and away from it with expiration. Movements of a foreign body may cause an audible slap with coughing or breathing. Slow development of bronchial obstruction may be symptomless; sudden closure causes severe dyspnea. Higher-pitched rhonchi arise from smaller bronchi.

✔ *MAJOR AIRWAY OBSTRUCTION—CLINICAL OCCURRENCE:* Aspirated foreign bodies, intraluminal neoplasms (benign [bronchial adenoma, amyloidoma] or malignant [primary lung cancer]), relapsing polychondritis, extrinsic compression from mediastinal masses (retrosternal goiter, neoplasms, teratoma), laryngeal mass or paralysis, tracheomalacia following prolonged endotracheal intubation.

S KEY SYNDROME

▼ **Acute Bronchitis:** *Pathophysiology:* Acute infection is usually viral; less commonly, it is an atypical organism. Airway inflammation, often with shedding of bronchial epithelium, produces persistent cough and often retrosternal burning pain. Fever is absent. Secretions in the bronchi and trachea produce rhonchi and, occasionally, wheezing. Secretions high in the trachea produce rhonchi that are heard throughout the thorax. The cough may be unproductive; tenacious or mucoid sputum may be raised. Usually, there is no impairment of the airways, so breath sounds are normal. DDX: In epidemics, influenza and respiratory syncytial virus should be considered. Chest x-rays are normal.

S KEY SYNDROME
Chronic Obstructive Pulmonary Disease: Chronic Bronchitis: *Pathophysiology:* Chronic inflammation and secondary infection of the airways results from chronic exposure to tobacco smoke. Airways obstruction is prominent and hypoxia common. Patients present with chronic cough with >60 mL/d of sputum (chronic bronchitis with or without bronchiectasis) and progressive dyspnea. Lung exam shows diminished breath sounds and prolongation of expiration; wheezing and inspiratory crackles may be present. Physical finding are poorly correlated with the severity of airflow obstruction or abnormalities of gas exchange.

S KEY SYNDROME
Chronic Obstructive Pulmonary Disease: Emphysema: *Pathophysiology:* Smoking leads to the destruction of alveolar walls with loss of alveolar surface area and loss of elastic recoil produces airways obstruction. Patients present with progressive dyspnea, often accompanied by gradual weight loss. They often exhale with pursed-lips, especially with exertion. The chest is hyperresonant with decreased breath sounds and prolonged expiration (see page 401). Wheezes and crackles are uncommon unless infection supervenes. Physical findings are poorly correlated with the severity of airflow obstruction or abnormalities of gas exchange. Early detection of obstructive airways disease in patients with symptoms or risk factors is best accomplished by spirometry [Straus SE, McAlister FA, Sackett DL, et al. The accuracy of patient history, wheezing, and laryngeal measurements in diagnosing obstructive airway disease. *JAMA* 2000;283: 1853–1857; Holleman DR Jr, Simel DL. The rational clinical examination. Does the clinical examination predict airflow limitation? *JAMA* 1995; 273:313–319].

Churg-Strauss Disease: See page 473.

Lymphomatoid Granulomatosis: *Pathophysiology:* A variegated array of lymph cells, atypical lymphocytoid, plasmacytoid, and reticuloendothelial cells invade various tissues and vessels. Nodules of various sizes occur in the lungs, skin, kidneys, and central nervous system; usually spared are the spleen, lymph nodes, and bone marrow. In contrast with Wegener granulomatosis, the lung is always involved but the upper respiratory tract is seldom involved. Transition to malignant lymphoma is common.

Bronchopleural Fistula: *Pathophysiology:* A communication between bronchus and pleural cavity, which is usually caused by an empyema draining through a bronchus or a lung abscess invading the pleural cavity. Patients present with a chronic cough with a large volume of purulent sputum. Dullness and absent breath sounds in lower hemithorax with a resonant region above—the whole devoid of breath sounds—suggest the diagnosis. A succussion splash may be heard.

Cardiovascular Syndromes

Fourfold Diagnosis of Heart Disease

A proper assessment of the patient with heart disease necessitates a diagnosis that includes four categories: the etiology, the anatomic abnormalities, the physiologic disorders, and the functional capacity. A formal statement of the diagnosis should follow this example: "rheumatic heart disease, inactive; mitral stenosis, right ventricular hypertrophy and dilatation, pulmonary congestion; atrial fibrillation; functional class II."

ETIOLOGIC DIAGNOSIS. Common causes include congenital defects, infections, rheumatic fever, hypertension, and atherosclerosis.

ANATOMIC DIAGNOSIS. Abnormalities of the aorta and pulmonary arteries, coronary arteries, endocardium and valves, myocardium and pericardium are listed. Congenital anatomic abnormalities are listed as either cyanotic or noncyanotic (i.e., with or without significant right-to-left shunt).

PHYSIOLOGIC DIAGNOSIS. Disturbances in cardiac rhythm and conduction, myocardial function (e.g., systolic or diastolic dysfunction), and clinical syndrome (e.g., anginal syndrome, congestive heart failure, cardiac tamponade) are listed.

FUNCTIONAL CARDIAC DIAGNOSIS. Two commonly used functional classification systems are:

New York Heart Association
Class I (No Incapacity). Although the patient has heart disease, the functional capacity is not sufficiently impaired to produce symptoms.
Class II (Slight Limitation). The patient is comfortable at rest and with mild exertion. Symptoms occur only with more strenuous activity.
Class III (Incapacity with Slight Exertion). The patient is comfortable at rest but dyspnea, fatigue, palpitation, or angina appears with slight exertion.
Class IV (Incapacity with Rest). The slightest exertion invariably produces symptoms, and symptoms frequently occur at rest.

Canadian Cardiovascular Society (use restricted to patients with angina)
Class I. No angina with ordinary activity but angina occurs with strenuous or rapid or prolonged exertion.
Class II. Slight limitation of ordinary activity (e.g., walking more than two level blocks or climbing more than one flight of stairs at a normal pace).

Class III. Marked limitation of ordinary activity (walking one to two blocks on the level and climbing one flight of stairs).

Class IV. Inability to carry on any physical activity without angina; angina *may* also be present at rest.

Six-Dermatome Pain Syndromes [see Six-Dermatome Pain, page 374]

S KEY SYNDROME

► ▼ **Six-Dermatome Pain: Angina Pectoris (Heberden's Angina, Effort Angina):** *Pathophysiology:* Classic stable exertional angina results when a temporary increase in myocardial oxygen demand in some portion of the myocardium exceeds oxygen supply. Angina may result from inadequate oxygen supply, excessive demand, or a combination of both. Abnormalities of oxygen delivery can be best remembered by rearrangement of the Fick equation: $MVO_2 =$ coronary blood flow $\times$ myocardial arteriovenous oxygen difference. Because the arteriovenous oxygen difference is already nearly maximal at rest, decrements in oxygen delivery are most often related to relative decrements in coronary flow. Flow is directly proportional to the pressure difference driving blood through the coronary arteries. For the left ventricle, this driving pressure is principally the aortic diastolic pressure. Flow will be inversely proportional to the flow resistance in the coronaries. This resistance can be at the epicardial or arteriolar vessel level or be related to postcapillary pressures (coronary sinus and left ventricular end-diastolic pressure). An increased myocardial oxygen demand is always related to an increase in heart rate, myocardial contractility, ventricular systolic pressure, and/or ventricular cavity radius. The increase in oxygen demand occurs whether or not there is a change in cardiac output or stroke volume. Clinically important examples of these determinants include sinus tachycardia and pathologic atrial or ventricular tachycardias for rate; digitalis and other inotropic agents for contractility; systemic arterial hypertension, aortic stenosis, and regurgitation for systolic pressure; and aortic regurgitation and congestive heart failure for cavity radius. This is a deep, steady pain or discomfort for 1–10 minutes in the six-dermatome region.

PQRST: *Provocation* anginal pain has several classic provocations: (a) *Exertion,* for example, walking, climbing, lawn mowing. An important characteristic of exertional angina is the *lag period:* some activity must be sustained before the pain occurs, and the pain subsides only after a period of rest has elapsed. Exertional pain without a lag period suggests a source in the musculoskeletal system. (b) *Postprandial,* after eating a hearty meal, especially with exertion after a meal. (c) Intense emotion, which provokes increases in heart rate and blood pressure. (d) *Tachycardia* of any cause. (e) *Cold environment,* with or without exertion, such as walking while breathing cold air or sleeping in cold bedclothes. (f) *Sleep and rest pain.* In a minority of cases, angina occurs with rest or sleep. Angina at rest or during sleep indicates *unstable angina.* It may occur when blood pressure or heart rate increase during rapid eye movement

(REM) sleep. Also, *vasospastic (Prinzmetal) angina* is more likely to occur during rest than during activity. (g) *Hypoglycemia,* spontaneous or from insulin. (h) *Positive inotropic or chronotropic effects of drugs* (caffeine, catecholamines, etc.). (i) *Anemia* with reduced oxygen-carrying capacity when the hemoglobin is less than 10 g/dL.

Palliation (a) Rest, (b) warm environment, (c) the administration of nitroglycerin, and (d) the Valsalva maneuver. **Complete relief of pain or other discomfort in the six-dermatome band after the administration of nitroglycerin is strongly suggestive of angina pectoris but it is not diagnostic.** The tablets of the drug should be fresh; age and exposure to light cause deterioration in potency. Flushing and headache prove the dose is pharmacologically adequate for the individual. Instruct the patient to dissolve the tablet under the tongue at the onset of an attack of discomfort, using one 0.4 mg tablet every 5 minutes for three trials. If flushing, headache, or the cessation of chest pain occurs, stop further administration. Relief of pain with a dose that causes flushing or headache is strong evidence for angina pectoris. However, the pain of esophageal spasm may also respond to nitroglycerin. When headache or flushing occurs without relief of discomfort, stable exertional angina is unlikely.

Quality Angina is usually described as crushing, aching, or a sense of tightness or pressure. To illustrate the sense of constriction, the patient frequently clenches the fist, a sign emphasized by Samuel A. Levine.

Region The pain may occur anywhere in the six-dermatome band. Often it is most intense behind the sternum or in the precordium, radiating upward into the neck or throat, or down the medial aspect of either arm, forearm, or hand. Ischemic pain arising from muscle in the distribution of the right coronary artery may radiate to the interscapular or high dorsal region of the back. Less frequently, the pain occurs in the thoracic vertebrae and the right shoulder and arm. Occasionally, the patient denies having chest pain but complains of pain in the limbs or neck exclusively.

Severity The discomfort may be mild, moderate, or severe. It may be so slight as not to arouse concern of either patient or physician, or the patient may have a sense of impending death.

Timing The pain is continuous, not fleeting or lancinating. The duration of pain is usually more than 1 minute but less than 10 minutes.

PHYSICAL SIGNS. No physical findings may be present. Fourth heart sounds frequently occur during angina because of decreased compliance of the ischemic ventricle. Less commonly, a third heart sound may appear. If transient ischemia of a papillary muscle occurs, an apical systolic murmur of mitral insufficiency may be heard. The presence of an ectopic rhythm suggests a cause for the pain. In some cases, a precordial bulge or thrust at the cardiac apex may be palpated. The phenomenon is attributed to temporary dyskinesia of the left ventricle from myocardial ischemia. Signs of aortic stenosis, syphilitic aortitis, or free aortic regurgitation suggest other causes for the angina. **See HPIM-16, Chapter 226.**

DDX: The brevity of anginal attacks (less than 10 minutes) usually excludes myocardial infarction, dissecting aneurysm, pulmonary embolism, and neoplasm. The most common cause of angina is impaired oxygen delivery as a result of abnormalities of the coronary arteries. Usually this is caused by atherosclerotic narrowing that restricts the normal increase in coronary flow induced by increments in myocardial oxygen demand. Cold or exertionally induced vasospasm may be superimposed upon such atherosclerotic narrowing. Less-common causes of reduced coronary flow include tachy- and bradyarrhythmias, vasculitis (e.g., polyarteritis nodosa or syphilis at the coronary ostia), aortic regurgitation (reduces flow because of the very low diastolic arterial pressures), left ventricular hypertrophy (hypertrophic cardiomyopathy, aortic stenosis, or regurgitation) when a relative decrease in capillary density occurs, and anemia or arterial oxygen desaturation. Pain with swallowing and a sensation of food sticking suggest an esophageal source. The supine position often initiates the pain of gastroesophageal reflux ("heartburn"). Pain from cholecystitis often occurs after meals but without concurrent exertion; finding epigastric and/or right upper quadrant tenderness often indicates gallbladder disease. Walking induces pains in the shoulder girdle or spine, as well as angina; lack of a lag period favors muscle pains.

S KEY SYNDROME

▶ ▼ **Six-Dermatome Pain: Variant Angina Pectoris (Prinzmetal Angina):** *Pathophysiology:* Coronary artery spasm with ST-segment elevations may occur in the absence of angiographically detectable coronary narrowing, or may be superimposed upon obvious atherosclerotic narrowing. The quality and location of the chest pain resemble classic angina, but the onset occurs at rest with no initiating factors. The pain recurs in cycles, waxing and waning, often at the same time each day. During a paroxysm the ST segments of the electrocardiogram (ECG) are transiently elevated, suggesting myocardial injury. The pain is promptly relieved by nitroglycerin. Definitive diagnosis can be made by demonstrating the coronary spasm during angiography. There is an increased prevalence of migraine and Raynaud phenomenon in patients with variant angina.

S KEY SYNDROME

▼ **Six-Dermatome Pain: Acute Coronary Syndromes (Unstable Angina and Myocardial Infarction):** *Pathophysiology:* There is almost always disruption of the endothelium overlying an atherosclerotic coronary plaque, which exposes the plaque contents to platelets and procoagulants. This initiates formation of a platelet plug, a fibrin clot, and release of vasoconstrictor substances leading to intermittent or prolonged obstruction of the artery. Myocardial necrosis occurs with prolonged severe ischemia. Lesser degrees of ischemia result in unstable angina syndromes and myocardial hibernation (decreased contractile function without pain or necrosis). Less-common causes of acute coronary syndromes are coronary artery embolism and vasculitis. The transition from severe ischemia to infarction is gradual and depends upon the collateral coronary

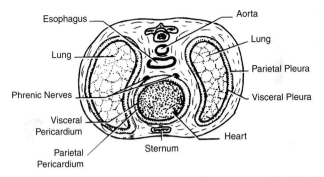

Esophagus — Aorta
Lung — Lung
— Parietal Pleura
Phrenic Nerves — Visceral Pleura
Visceral Pericardium —
Parietal Pericardium / Sternum — Heart

Fig. 8-46 Pleuropericardial Relationships. *A transverse section of the lower thorax with anesthetic serosal surfaces represented by heavy beaded lines and pain-sensitive surfaces by lighter beaded lines. Note the proximity of the phrenic nerves and esophagus to the parietal pericardium, so pericarditis can produce pain in the phrenic nerve distribution or pain on swallowing.*

flammation can cause dysphagia and phrenic pain. All these regions supply nerve fibers to the six-dermatome band. Because afferent sensory fibers from the central area of the diaphragm run in the phrenic nerve, irritation of the lower pericardium may cause pain in the neck at the superior border of the trapezius. *Symptoms* Deep constant or pleuritic pain occurs in the six-dermatome band or the phrenic distribution, often with pericardial friction rub or ECG signs. The location and quality of pain often resembles that of myocardial infarction. It is usually accentuated by breathing or coughing, worse in recumbency, and lessened while sitting and leaning forward. It may be intensified by swallowing. Pleuritic pain referred to the shoulder, particularly the left trapezius ridge, is quite suggestive of pericarditis (see Fig. 8-45). The chest discomfort may be prolonged for many hours; it is not relieved by nitroglycerin. Rarely, the pain is throbbing and synchronous with the heartbeat. *Signs* The onset of pain may be followed by fever. A transient pericardial friction rub is often heard. *Electrocardiogram* Widespread elevation of the ST segments followed by inversion of T waves, when present, is fairly diagnostic. The ECG signs of pericarditis must be differentiated from the injury currents of infarction and from early repolarization changes that represent a normal variant. DDX: Pericarditis may result from almost any infectious agent, malignancy, rheumatic fever, collagen vascular diseases, trauma, uremia, or following myocardial infarction or radiation to the chest. Until a pericardial friction rub appears or ECG signs develop, the steady pain suggests myocardial infarction, dissecting aneurysm, pulmonary infarction, cholecystitis, or peptic ulcer. Pain on swallowing may suggest an esophageal lesion. The pleural pain must be distinguished from that of pleurisy, subphrenic abscess, and splenic infarction [Spodick DH. Acute pericarditis: Current concepts and practice. *JAMA* 2003;289:1150–1153].

S KEY SYNDROME

▶ ▼ **Six-Dermatome Pain: Pulmonary Artery Embolism and Pulmonary Infarction:** See page 448.

S KEY SYNDROME

▶ ▼ **Six-Dermatome Pain: Aortic Dissection:** *Pathophysiology:* Cystic medial necrosis and intramural hemorrhage lead to secondary intimal rupture, or intimal tears may be the primary event. The intimal tear occurs most commonly in the lateral wall of the proximal ascending aorta, or, less commonly, just distal to the ligamentum arteriosum in the descending aorta. Blood from the lumen penetrates the weakened media to produce a hematoma that splits the vessel wall into two layers. During progression, the mouths of the aortic branches may be occluded sequentially, with ischemia in the parts supplied. A second intimal tear may occur distally to provide egress from the false lumen in the media; thus the aorta may consist of two concentric tubes, a double-barreled aorta. Pain is sudden, sharp, and crushing in the six-dermatome band. There is progressive diminution of pulses in the aortic branches and loss of specific nerve functions. *Symptoms* In 80% of cases, the onset is sudden, with excruciating pain that is felt in the precordium and/or the *inter*scapular region, and that may shift successively to the lower back, abdomen, hips, and thighs. The pain often suggests myocardial infarction. In the remainder, the onset is gradual, often without chest pain. *Signs* Arterial blood pressure is usually sustained, in contrast to the hypotension in myocardial infarction. Shock may result, with hypotension and collapse, especially with rupture into the pericardium or left pleural space. *Proximal Progression:* When the hematoma extends proximally from a tear in the aortic arch, it may (a) distort the aortic valve ring to separate the commissures and cause a murmur of aortic regurgitation, often transmitting down the right sternal border; (b) occlude the coronary ostia and cause myocardial infarction; (c) produce hemopericardium with a pericardial friction rub and cardiac tamponade with dyspnea, cyanosis, low-volume pulses, and hypotension; or (d) swell the base of the aorta, causing a pulsating sternoclavicular joint. This sign distinguishes dissection from myocardial infarction; it also occurs with ruptured saccular aneurysm of the aorta, persistent right aortic arch or fusiform aneurysms of the innominate, carotid, or subclavian artery. *Distal Progression:* When the hematoma extends away from the heart, progression may be indicated by sequential asymmetrical diminution or loss of arterial pulses in aortic branches and signs of deficient function in the nerves of these regions. Occlusion of the carotid artery causes cerebral ischemia with localizing neurologic signs. Obstruction of the spinal arteries is indicated by paraplegia and anesthesia. Occlusion of the renal artery may be marked by pain simulating renal colic, anuria, or hematuria. Aortic dissection may be rapidly fatal. In some, healing occurs. One of us had a patient who died of another disease, having lived for years with an aorta composed of two concentric blood-filled tubes with communication at the proximal and distal ends [Klompas M. The rational clinical examination. Does this patient have an acute thoracic aortic dissection? *JAMA* 2002;287:

2262–2272]. *Chest X-Ray* Widening of the aorta, an enlarged aortic knob or separation of calcified intimal plaques from the outer border of the aortic wall all suggest dissection. Imaging studies should be performed urgently if dissection is suspected; they are necessary for diagnosis and to show the extent of the dissection. DDX: Most commonly, dissection occurs in association with cystic medial necrosis of the aorta, especially in patients with Marfan and Ehlers-Danlos syndromes. It occurs with less frequency in patients with hypertension, with advancing age, during labor, and in those who have experienced direct or blunt trauma. Rarely, dissection occurs in a thoracic aortic aneurysm afflicted with aortitis from bacteria, syphilis, or giant cell arteritis.

S KEY SYNDROME

▶ ▼ **Six-Dermatome Chest Pain: Spontaneous Esophageal Rupture (Boerhaave Syndrome):** During a period of vomiting, a sudden pain occurs in the chest or upper abdomen, accompanied by extreme dyspnea. Subcutaneous emphysema in the supraclavicular fossae and mediastinal emphysema may appear, including a crunching sound in the precordium (*Hamman sign*). Chest x-ray shows air in the mediastinum. DDX: The symptoms are common to myocardial infarction, perforated peptic ulcer, cholecystitis, pancreatitis, esophagitis, hepatitis, nonperforating ulcer, and pneumonia. The demonstration of mediastinal emphysema should exclude all the foregoing in favor of ruptured esophagus.

S KEY SYNDROME

▼ **Six-Dermatome Pain with Dysphagia:** See Chapter 9, page 564.

S KEY SYNDROME

▼ **Six-Dermatome Pain: Mediastinal Tumors:** Although mediastinal lesions rarely cause pain in the chest, they are considered here because of their location in the six-dermatome band. Most mediastinal masses attract attention by compression of normal structures or are found incidentally on chest x-ray. Physical signs suggesting mediastinal tumors are dyspnea from retrosternal goiter, hoarseness and brassy cough from compression of the recurrent laryngeal nerve, *Horner syndrome* (unilateral ptosis of the eyelid, miosis of the pupil, and lack of facial sweating) from involvement of the superior cervical ganglion, edema of the arms and neck with cyanosis from obstruction of the superior vena cava and chylous pleural effusion. Lymph nodes are enlarged in Hodgkin disease, non-Hodgkin lymphoma, carcinoma, or tuberculosis. Other locations of neoplastic tissue are retrosternal goiter, thymoma, and teratoma (dermoid cyst). When a dermoid forms a tracheal fistula, it may produce the elegant sign of coughing hair, or *trichoptysis*. Superior sulcus tumors (neoplasms in the pulmonary apex, the upper mediastinum, or the superior thoracic aperture) produce **Pancoast syndrome** in which there is severe pain in the neck or shoulder or down the arm.

S KEY SYNDROME

Six-Dermatome Pain: Spontaneous Pneumothorax: See page 402 and 446.

S KEY SYNDROME

Six-Dermatome Pain: Mediastinal Emphysema: See page 388 and 463.

S KEY SYNDROME

Six-Dermatome Pain: Spontaneous Pyopneumothorax: See page 446.

S KEY SYNDROME

Six-Dermatome Pain: Subphrenic Diseases:
Although lesions below the diaphragm usually produce abdominal pain, frequent exceptions make it imperative to consider subphrenic disorders in the context of pain in the six-dermatome band. It is dangerous to the patient and embarrassing to the physician to overlook this possibility. Subphrenic abscess, acute cholecystitis, peptic ulcer, acute pancreatitis, and splenic infarction need to be considered.

Other Cardiovascular Syndromes

S KEY SYNDROME

▶ ## Generalized Pulmonary Edema: See page 451.

S KEY SYNDROME

Cardiac   Dilatation: *Pathophysiology:* Dilatation is caused by enlargement of the cavity radius in response to either poor systolic function or chronic volume overload. The heart of trained athletes dilates to accommodate a larger stroke volume to maintain a high cardiac output at relatively low heart rates, minimizing myocardial oxygen demand. Enlargement of the heart detectable by physical examination (apical impulse and borders of cardiac dullness) or chest x-rays usually implies dilatation of a cardiac chamber. The elongated fibers of the dilated heart with depressed contractility produce a weak apical impulse, which may be more diffuse than normal. Displacement of the apical impulse to the left with a normal right heart border suggests left ventricular dilation. DDX: Pericardial effusions will enlarge the heart silhouette and borders of dullness, but the apical impulse is usually undetectable and the heart sounds are diminished.

✓ *CARDIAC DILATATION—CLINICAL OCCURRENCE:*   *Left Ventricular Dilation*   aortic insufficiency, mitral insufficiency, ischemic cardiomyopathy, after myocardial infarction, dilated cardiomyopathy, viral myocarditis; *Right Ventricular Dilation*   pulmonic insufficiency, tricuspid insufficiency, atrial septal defect with left-to-right shunt, right ventricular infarction, pulmonary hypertension with right ventricular failure.

S KEY SYNDROME

Cardiac   Hypertrophy: *Pathophysiology:* Hypertrophy occurs with or without an increase in cavity radius because of pres-

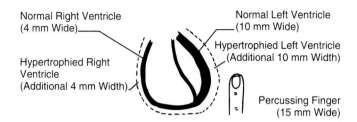

Fig. 8-47 Contribution of Myocardial Hypertrophy to the Area of Cardiac Dullness. *Without dilatation of the chambers, concentric hypertrophy of the cardiac muscle to twice its normal thickness and weight cannot cause enough increase in an area of cardiac dullness to exceed the width of the percussing finger. Therefore, increase in the area of dullness must be attributed to dilatation when pericardial effusion is excluded.*

sure and/or volume overload or hypertrophic cardiomyopathy. Hypertrophied left ventricular myocardium, with or without cavity dilatation, produces a more powerful apical impulse than normal. Enlargement of the chamber on physical exam is not present without concomitant dilation (Fig. 8-47). A palpable thrust along the left sternal edge, over the right ventricle, may be produced by right ventricular hypertrophy.

✓ **CARDIAC HYPERTROPHY—CLINICAL OCCURRENCE:** *Left Ventricular Hypertrophy* valvular aortic stenosis, mitral or aortic insufficiency, hypertension, hypertrophic cardiomyopathy; *Right Ventricular Hypertrophy* pulmonic stenosis, pulmonary hypertension, hypertrophic cardiomyopathy.

▶ **S** KEY SYNDROME

Congestive Heart Failure (CHF): *Pathophysiology:* Chronically decreased left ventricular contractility leads to dilation of the left ventricle to maintain stroke volume, increased left ventricular end-diastolic pressure (LVEDP), left atrial hypertension and dilation, and dilation of the pulmonary veins. Decreased cardiac output with renal hypoperfusion leads to retention of salt and water, weight gain, and edema. The ventricular ejection fraction is low when systolic function is impaired but not when congestion is principally caused by diastolic dysfunction, that is, increased muscle wall stiffness. Symptoms and signs are attributable to decreased cardiac output and volume expansion with pulmonary and peripheral vascular congestion. Early symptoms of left ventricular failure are pulmonary congestion with dyspnea, orthopnea, nocturia, and cough. Crackles are heard in the lung bases. Retrograde congestion causes right-ventricular failure with elevated central venous pressure, indicated by engorged jugular veins [Butman SM, Ewy GA, Standen JR, et al. Bedside cardiovascular examination in patients with severe chronic heart failure: Importance of rest or inducible jugular venous distension. *J Am Coll Cardiol* 1993;22:968–974]. Even before the increase in venous pressure, a hepatojugular reflux sign can be demonstrated. Frequently an S3 develops [Drazner MH, Rame

JE, Stevenson LW, Dries DL. Prognostic importance of elevated jugular venous pressure and a third heart sound in patients with heart failure. *N Engl J Med* 2001;345:574–581; Badgett RG, Lucey CR, Mulrow CD. The rational clinical examination. Can the clinical examination diagnose left-sided heart failure in adults? *JAMA* 1997;277:1712–1719]. Later, the liver becomes large, tender, and painful. After hepatomegaly from congestion has been present for some time, the liver capsule becomes thickened, tenderness disappears, and parenchymal fibrosis may occur. Edema fluid accumulates as right-sided or bilateral hydrothorax, ascites, and pitting edema of the ankles, legs, genitals, and abdomen. The lips, ears, and nail beds may be cyanotic. Impaired cerebral circulation may result in mental aberrations and periodic breathing. Findings on physical examination have independent prognostic value [Marantz PR, Tobin JN, Wassertheil-Smoller S, et al. Prognosis in ischemic heart disease. Can you tell as much at the bedside as in the nuclear laboratory? *Arch Intern Med* 1992;152:2433–2437]. DDX: A patient with portal hypertension may present a similar syndrome, except that they may lie flat comfortably and jugular venous distention is absent. Occasionally, a patient with cardiac failure is unaccountably comfortable in the reclining position, and one with cirrhosis may be dyspneic from hydrothorax or massive ascites. Metastasis from carcinoma may produce fluid in the abdominal and thoracic cavities with a distribution similar to that in cardiac failure [Jessup M, Brozena S. Heart failure. *N Engl J Med* 2003; 348:2007–2018].

✔ *CHF—CLINICAL OCCURRENCE:* The most common cause is chronic ischemic coronary artery disease. Dilated cardiomyopathy (pregnancy and postpartum, alcohol, hemochromatosis, idiopathic, secondary to viral infections) is also common, especially in younger patients. Diastolic heart failure is common in longstanding hypertension with LVH and hypertrophic cardiomyopathies.

S KEY SYNDROME

▼ **Right Ventricular Failure and Cor Pulmonale:** *Pathophysiology:* Right ventricular failure occurs because of damage to the myocardium, volume overload, and/or pressure overload. The right and left ventricles function together, so left ventricular failure also may be accompanied by some impairment of right ventricular function. In congestive failure when venous pressure exceeds 22 cm, the liver is always enlarged; above 25 cm, there are always ascites, edema, and orthopnea. The venous pressure is always high with increasing failure, but it falls before other signs of failure diminish. The most frequent cause of right ventricular failure is advanced ischemic heart disease. Right ventricular failure caused by primary disease in the lungs is called *cor pulmonale.* It occurs as a consequence of pulmonary vasoconstriction from chronic hypoxemia or obliteration of the pulmonary vascular bed.

✔ *CLINICAL OCCURRENCE: Impaired Myocardial Function* ischemic heart disease (especially right ventricular infarction), hypertrophic and dilated cardiomyopathies, endomyocardial fibrosis (e.g., drugs, carcinoid syndrome), restrictive myocardial disease (e.g., amyloidosis); *Vol-*

ume Overload tricuspid regurgitation, atrial septal defect with left-to-right shunt, pulmonic insufficiency; *Pressure Overload* primary pulmonary hypertension, secondary pulmonary hypertension—cor pulmonale (hypoxia caused by emphysema, cystic fibrosis, interstitial pulmonary diseases, pneumoconioses, hypersensitivity pneumonitis, pulmonary fibrosis, etc.), pulmonary embolus, pulmonic stenosis, Eisenmenger complex, mitral stenosis, pulmonary venoocclusive disease.

S KEY SYNDROME

Restrictive Cardiomyopathy: *Pathophysiology:* Cardiac output is limited by impedance to left ventricular filling as a result of decreased myocardial compliance leading to elevated left ventricular end-diastolic pressure. Systolic function is preserved. Patients present with dyspnea exacerbated by exertion, signs of intermittent pulmonary congestion. Signs of right ventricular failure with edema, elevated venous pressure, and ascites may predominate. The heart is not enlarged on exam or x-ray. S4 gallops are common. Causes are ventricular diastolic dysfunction, infiltrative disease of the heart (amyloid, sarcoid, hemochromatosis), and endomyocardial fibroelastosis. DDX: This must be distinguished from hypertrophic cardiomyopathy and constrictive pericarditis.

S KEY SYNDROME

Hypertrophic Cardiomyopathy: *Pathophysiology:* Inherited defects in the myocardial contractile proteins lead to progressive hypertrophy, disorganization of myocardial architecture, impaired diastolic function, ventricular conduction abnormalities and dysrhythmias. Asymmetric septal hypertrophy and hyperdynamic systolic function may produce dynamic obstruction to left ventricular outflow during early systole. A family history of sudden death is common. Patients present with dyspnea, angina, and presyncopal symptoms. The carotid upstrokes may show a bisferiens pattern. S4 gallop is common and a characteristic murmur, augmented with Valsalva, is heard when outflow obstruction is present (see page 423). Idiopathic forms of the disease exist, or may represent spontaneous mutations. Echocardiography is diagnostic.

S KEY SYNDROME

Hypertrophic Obstructive Cardiomyopathy: Idiopathic Hypertrophic Subaortic Stenosis (IHSS): See page 423.

S KEY SYNDROME

Infective Endocarditis: *Pathophysiology:* Infection of the heart valves leads to the formation of vegetations of fibrin and platelets harboring the infective agent. Low virulence organisms (e.g., viridans streptococci, HACEK [*Haemophilus aphrophilus*, *Actinobacillus actinomycetemcomitans*, *Cardiobacterium hominis*, *Eikenella corrodens*, and *Kingella*] organisms) present with subacute disease; high virulence organisms (e.g., *Staphylococcus aureus*, fungi) present with acute symptoms and rapid valvular destruction and/or systemic emboli. *Subacute Bac-*

terial Endocarditis Patients present with a subacute or chronic illness with fever, weight loss, arthralgia, myalgias, and signs of immune complex disease. *Acute Endocarditis* Patients have fever and rigors and often a history of injection drug use. Peripheral emboli with organ infarction and metastatic infection are common. Systemic illness with diffuse manifestations, especially with a new insufficiency murmur, should always trigger an evaluation for endocarditis. The Duke criteria are sensitive and specific for the diagnosis [Durack DT, Lukas AS, Bright DK. New criteria for diagnosis of infective endocarditis. *Am J Med* 1994; 96:200–209].

S KEY SYNDROME

▶ ▼ **Non-infective   Endocarditis: Nonbacterial Thrombotic Endocarditis (NBTE):** *Pathophysiology:* This results from inflammation of the endocardium with sterile vegetations. Multiple large emboli suggest *marantic endocarditis* associated with occult neoplasms, most often a mucin-secreting adenocarcinoma. Libman-Sacks lesions on the valves and endocardium occur with systemic lupus erythematosus and antiphospholipid syndrome. Patients may be asymptomatic, have peripheral emboli to the brain and elsewhere, or present with progressive valvular stenosis or regurgitation.

S KEY SYNDROME

▼ **Valvular Heart Disease:** These clinical conditions are discussed with their physical findings under *Cardiovascular Signs, Auscultation of Heart Murmurs*, page 418ff.

VALVULAR AORTIC STENOSIS: See page 421.

AORTIC REGURGITATION: See page 429.

VALVULAR PULMONIC STENOSIS: See page 424.

TRICUSPID STENOSIS: See page 430.

TRICUSPID REGURGITATION: See page 427.

MITRAL VALVE STENOSIS: See page 431.

MITRAL REGURGITATION: See page 427.

MITRAL VALVE PROLAPSE: See page 428.

ATRIAL SEPTAL DEFECT: See page 425.

VENTRICULAR SEPTAL DEFECT: See page 426.

PATENT DUCTUS ARTERIOSUS: See page 433.

COARCTATION OF AORTA: See page 426 and 478.

Congenital Complex: Eisenmenger Syndrome: This consists of pulmonary hypertension in the presence of a septal or aortic to pulmonary artery defect with reversal of the shunt to a right-to-left direction. It may be suspected when valvular signs are coupled with cyanosis, right-to-left shunt, and clubbing of the fingers. Diagnostic imaging is required to make an exact diagnosis.

Congenital Complex: Tetralogy of Fallot: The components of the tetralogy are a ventricular septal defect, obstruction to right ventricular outflow (usually infundibular pulmonic stenosis), an overriding aorta, and right ventricular hypertrophy (see Fig. 8-42D). The condition should be considered when multiple lesions are associated with cyanosis, polycythemia, and clubbing of the fingers. Imaging studies must make the diagnosis.

Congenital Complex: Lutembacher Complex: This is a combination of acquired mitral stenosis and congenital interatrial septal defect. It should be suspected when the pertinent physical signs are encountered in a patient with a childhood history of heart disease.

Congenital Complex: Ebstein Anomaly of the Tricuspid Valve: A congenital deformity of the tricuspid valve occurs in which the cusp is extremely thin and inadequate. There is downward displacement of a portion of the valve below the level of the AV ring, producing "ventricularization" of the right atrium. Tricuspid regurgitation is not a prominent feature; dysrhythmias are common.

S KEY SYNDROME

Constrictive Pericarditis: *Pathophysiology:* Progressive fibrosis of the pericardium following acute or chronic injury leads to thickening and restriction of cardiac diastolic filling. Symptoms are shortness of breath and fatigue. Signs are those of right heart failure: jugular venous distention, dependent edema, ascites, and hepatic congestion. Pericardial injury results from pericarditis (viral, tuberculous, neoplasm), cardiac surgery, mediastinal irradiation, and uremia. DDX: It must be distinguished from restrictive cardiomyopathies and right ventricular failure.

S KEY SYNDROME

Pericardial Tamponade: *Pathophysiology:* Rapid accumulation of fluid within the relatively noncompliant pericardium leads to compression of the heart chambers, preventing diastolic filling of the atria and ventricles. Cardiac output falls and central venous pressure is elevated. Patients complain of shortness of breath and fatigue that may rapidly progress to hypotension and circulatory failure due to decreased cardiac output. The key physical signs are an elevated central venous pressure with clear lung fields, no stigmata of chronic right ventricular failure, and a drop in systolic blood pressure during inspiration of >10 mmHg (paradoxical pulse) (see page 436). The heart size is usually normal by exam and chest x-ray. Tamponade must be urgently evaluated by echocardiography anytime it is suspected. DDX: Conditions that may be confused with tamponade are acute pulmonary embolism, right ventricular infarction, and constrictive pericarditis.

S KEY SYNDROME

▶ ▼ **Sudden Cardiac Death: Cardiac Arrest:** This condition demands immediate treatment for any chance of survival. Most patients have severe coronary artery disease, although in 25% of patients sudden cardiac death is the first symptom of the disease. Less-common causes are hypertrophic cardiomyopathy (especially in young male athletes), coronary artery emboli, right ventricular dysplasia, Brugada syndrome, long QT syndrome, and anomalous coronary artery anatomy. Public education seeks to teach all adults in basic cardiopulmonary resuscitation (CPR). Increasingly, automated defibrillators are present in public places for use by trained individuals to reverse these dysrhythmias. All health care personnel should be trained in basic CPR, and nurses and physicians should be trained in Advanced Cardiac Life Support (ACLS).

Disorders of the Arterial and Venous Circulations

S KEY SYNDROME

▼ **Vasculitis:** In 1866, Kussmaul and Maier described the first case of periarteritis nodosa (now called classic polyarteritis nodosa), which became the prototype for a large group of vasculitides. The present working classification has proven helpful in selecting appropriate treatment for many patients [Jennette JC, Falk RJ, Andrassay K, et al. Nomenclature of systemic vasculitides: Proposal of an international consensus conference. *Arthritis Rheum* 1994;37:187–192]. Vasculitides are classified by the size of the involved vessel. *Pathophysiology:* Large vessel vasculitides are of unknown etiology. Vasculitis of medium-sized arteries may be associated with infection (polyarteritis nodosa with hepatitis B and C) or specific immunologic markers (Wegener and c-ANCA [cytoplasmic antineutrophil cytoplasmic antibody]). Small-vessel vasculitides are associated with immune complex deposition in the walls of the vessels. In some cases the association with a specific infection is strong, for example, mixed cryoglobulinemia and chronic hepatitis C infection, while in others there is a strong association with serologic markers, for example, microscopic polyangiitis and p-ANCA (perinuclear antineutrophil cytoplasmic antibody). Each involves inflammation of the vessel wall leading to vascular obstruction and end-organ damage.

The clinical manifestations depend upon the size and distribution of the vessels involved. Symptoms and signs are related to local ischemia and signs of systemic inflammation. Cutaneous involvement is usually seen as palpable purpura, with or without skin infarction, whose extent correlates with the size of the vessel involved. Involvement of arteries to other organs is manifest as signs of specific organ dysfunction, for example, renal failure, transient ischemic attacks, stroke, and pneumonitis. The pattern of involvement suggests the size of the vessel and the specific vasculitis syndrome [Weyand CM, Goronzy JJ. Medium- and large-vessel vasculitis. *N Engl J Med* 2003;349:160–169].

TABLE 8–1 Systemic Vasculitis Syndromes*

Size of the Vessel	Specific Diseases
Large arteries	Giant cell arteritis
	Takayasu arteritis
	Primary central nervous system vasculitis
Medium arteries†	Polyarteritis nodosa
	Kawasaki disease
	Churg-Straus syndrome
	Wegener granulomatosis
Small vessels	Leukocytoclastic vasculitis
	(e.g., Henoch-Schonlein purpura,
	cryoglobulinemia, infections, drugs)
	Microscopic polyangiitis
	Urticarial vasculitis
	Systemic rheumatic syndromes
Pseudovasculitis‡	Antiphospholipid syndrome
	Embolic phenomena (atrial myxomas,
	cholesterol, nonbacterial thrombotic
	endocarditis/Libman-Sacks endocarditis)
	Bacterial endocarditis
	Endovascular lymphoma

*After Coblyn JS, McCluskey RT. Case 3-2003: Case records of the Massachusetts General Hospital. A 36-year-old man with renal failure, hypertension, and neurologic abnormalities. *N Engl J Med* 2003;348:333–342.
†May involve small vessels as well.
‡May involve vessels of any size.

S **KEY SYNDROME**

▶ ▼**Vasculitis, Large Vessel: Giant Cell Arteritis (GCA), Temporal Arteritis:** *Pathophysiology:* The cause is unknown. Histologic examination shows patchy medial necrosis of temporal artery segments, with diffuse mononuclear infiltration and giant cells throughout the vessel walls (giant cell arteritis). Thromboses are frequent. GCA affects major arterial branches of the proximal aorta, especially the external carotid. Patients older than age 50 years present with fever and weight loss and may have headache, jaw claudication, or scalp tenderness. Visual symptoms forebode irreversible visual loss as a consequence of inflammation of the retinal and ophthalmic arteries. The headache is severe, persistent, and throbbing. Polymyalgia rheumatica frequently antedates other manifestations or may occur simultaneously. Systemic symptoms (fever, profound weakness, malaise, and prostration) are common and may be the only clues to the disease. Prompt diagnosis and treatment may prevent loss of vision. Aortic aneurysms and dissection occur with increased frequency. Physical signs are few, but scalp tenderness and tortuous, tender, or nodular temporal arteries may be identified. The overlying skin is often red and swollen. Vision is often impaired and ophthalmoplegia may occur, temporarily or permanently. The retina may be normal or show evidence of retinal ischemia. The typical ophthalmic finding is anterior ischemic optic neuropathy (AION, see page 272). The disk appears pale and swollen because of closure of the posterior ciliary arteries that supply the nerve head [Salvarani C, Cantini F, Boiardi L, Hunder GG. Polymyalgia rheumatica and giant cell arteritis. *N Engl J Med* 2002;347: 261–271].

S KEY SYNDROME

Vasculitis, Large Vessel: Takayasu Aortitis: *Pathophysiology:* This is an inflammatory condition of the aorta and its major branches producing markedly reduced flow and thrombosis in the involved vessels. Patients are usually young women who present with arterial ischemic symptoms. A characteristic triad of signs is (a) absent pulse in vessels of the upper extremity or the neck (*pulseless disease*), (b) carotid sinus sensitivity wherein movements of the head induce syncope, and (c) ocular disorders, such as cataract and retinal defects.

S KEY SYNDROME

Vasculitis, Medium Vessels: Polyarteritis Nodosa: *Pathophysiology:* Small and intermediate muscular arteries are involved with transmural inflammation and necrosis, which sometimes extends to adjacent veins and arterioles. Involvement is segmental with a predilection for arterial bifurcations and branch points. Vascular occlusion leads to ischemia and necrosis. Aneurysms up to 1 cm in diameter are frequent. Symptoms include fever, weight loss, malaise, and pain in viscera and muscles. Cutaneous lesions, especially on the legs, are common, and subcutaneous nodules may be palpable along the course of vessels or nerves. Frequently involved organs are the kidneys (renal failure, hypertension), gastrointestinal tract (visceral infarction), heart (myocardial infarction, pericarditis), liver (acute to chronic hepatitis), peripheral nerves (mononeuritis multiplex), skin (subcutaneous nodules on superficial vessels, palpable purpura, livedo reticularis), joints and muscles (myalgias, arthralgias, arthritis). The lungs are rarely involved [Stone JH. Polyartertitis nodosa. *JAMA* 2002; 288:1632–1639; Coblyn JS, McCluskey RT. Case records of the Massachusetts General Hospital. Case 3–2003. A 36-year-old man with renal failure, hypertension, and neurologic abnormalities. *N Engl J Med* 2003; 348:333–342].

S KEY SYNDROME

Vasculitis, Medium Vessels: Wegener's Granulomatosis: *Pathophysiology:* The cause is unknown. Inflammation of small arteries and veins is associated with granuloma formation; neutrophil anticytoplasmic antibody (c-ANCA) to proteinase 3 is highly specific. Patients present with fever, malaise and signs of upper airway disease (sinusitis, obstructive and/or destructive symptoms and signs), pulmonary involvement and/or progressive renal failure. Other organ systems may be involved. Disease may be limited to the upper airway. It is most common in the fourth and fifth decades in either sex. Sinus pain and epistaxis arise from erosion of the nose (with a resulting saddle deformity), sinuses, palate, nasopharynx. The lungs may have infiltrates, nodules, and cavitations; the kidney lesion is a glomerulonephritis.

S KEY SYNDROME

Vasculitis, Medium Vessels: Churg-Strauss Syndrome, Allergic Angiitis and Granulomatosis: *Pathophysiology:* The cause is unknown. Eosinophilia is associated with nodular lung infiltrates and asthma; systemic symptoms and signs mimic polyarteritis nodosa. Patients present with signs and symptoms of asthma in association with eosinophilia and persistent slowly evolving abnormalities on the chest x-ray.

S KEY SYNDROME

Vasculitis, Small Vessels: Henoch-Schönlein Purpura: *Pathophysiology:* Thought to represent a postinfectious condition. There is inflammation of the small vessels of the skin, gastrointestinal tract, and kidneys. See page 160. Patients present with palpable purpura on the abdomen and lower extremities, abdominal pain, fever, and hemoccult-positive stools. Children are more often affected than adults.

S KEY SYNDROME

Vasculitis, Small Vessels: Microscopic Polyangiitis: *Pathophysiology:* The cause is unknown. There is a high prevalence of anticytoplasmic antibodies (p-ANCA) to myeloperoxidase. Patients present with systemic symptoms of fever and malaise and symptoms and signs of palpable purpura, pulmonary, and/or renal involvement.

Behçet Syndrome: This is a vasculitis of unknown cause, most prevalent in patients from the Mediterranean littoral and Japan. It is characterized by the triad of relapsing iridocyclitis, ulcerations in the mouth, and ulcers on the genitalia. The great majority of cases have come from Greece, Cyprus, Turkey, the Middle East, and Japan, but an increasing number of US natives are being found to have the disease. The disease is associated with a high incidence of erythema nodosum and arthritis. A characteristic sign is *pathergy*, the formation of sterile pustules at sites of needle punctures of the skin. Almost one-third of the patients have had thrombophlebitis, neurologic disorders, or intestinal involvement. The disease lasts for many years with relapses and remissions, but it can often be suppressed by corticosteroids.

S KEY SYNDROME

Arteriovenous Fistula, Acquired: *Pathophysiology:* A communication between an artery and an adjacent vein may be induced surgically to facilitate venous access or be caused by a stab or gunshot wound, diagnostic catheterization of the vessel, or erosion from neoplasm or infectious arteritis. Hemorrhage after the inciting

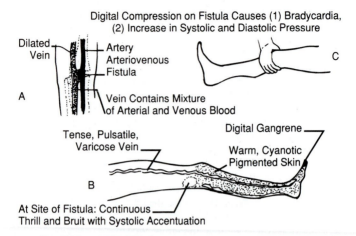

Fig. 8-48 Signs of Arteriovenous Fistula. *A fistula between the popliteal artery and vein is represented. A. Shows the communication between artery and vein behind the knee joint. B. The lesion is in the left leg. The superficial veins are greatly dilated from blood under arterial pressure; they are tense to the touch and sometimes pulsatile. Distal to the fistula, the skin is warm from the arterial blood in the veins, cyanotic, and pigmented from hemostasis. Distal gangrene may occur. At the site of the leak a thrill and bruit may be felt. These are continuous throughout the cardiac cycle, with systolic accentuation. The arterial pulse pressure is greater than normal if the orifice of the fistula is large enough. C. Closure of the fistula by digital compression produces slowing of the heart rate (Branham bradycardiac sign) and augmentation of both systolic and diastolic arterial pressures in the general circulation.*

trauma is profuse but easily controlled. A thrill and bruit may develop some hours later. After wound healing has occurred, the signs of chronic circulatory disturbance develop. Although fistulas may occur in many parts of the body, the greatest variety of signs are evident when an extremity is involved (Fig. 8-48). Venous congestion is manifest by varicose veins in the extremity, peripheral edema, stasis pigmentation of the skin, stasis ulceration, and indurative cellulitis. Ulcers are usually in the distal parts, in contradistinction to simple varicose ulcers, which are over pressure points. Arterial disorders produce gangrene of the distal parts and hypertrophy of the extremity when the injury occurs before the epiphyses have closed. A thrill and bruit are present locally throughout the cardiac cycle, with systolic accentuation. The skin temperature is increased distal to the fistula. Paradoxically, these signs assure that an arteriovenous shunt established surgically to facilitate venous access has remained patent. When the shunt is large, the dilated superficial veins may be less compressible than normal, the venous pressure may approach the arterial pressure, the velocity of venous blood is increased, and the right heart becomes dilated. Cardiac failure may result. The diastolic arterial pressure may be lowered by an extensive shunt. Compression closing the fistula, produces a sharp slowing of the pulse rate, called the *Branham bradycardiac sign*. Shunts deep in the abdomen or thorax yield only the bruit and the remote effects on venous and arterial pressure as diagnostic signs.

Arteriovenous Fistula, Congenital: Developmental shunts from arteries to veins may occur in many parts of the body, but they are most accessible to examination in the extremities. Cutaneous birthmarks are found in one-half of the cases, so the question of arteriovenous fistula should be raised when one sees port-wine spots, blue-red cavernous hemangiomas, or diffuse hemangiomas. The signs are evident at an early age, and there is no history of trauma to the part. Frequently, congenital fistulas are quite small, so the signs associated with the acquired type are not evident: thrills and bruits may be absent and the bradycardiac sign of Branham is less pronounced. The affected limb may be hypertrophied, and it may exhibit increased sweating and hypertrichosis.

Disorders of Circulation in the Head, Neck, and Trunk

The large arteries and veins in the head, neck, and trunk are less accessible to examination than are those in the extremities, so vascular disorders in these regions frequently must be inferred from evidence less direct than inspection and palpation of the vessels (Figs. 8-49 and 8-50A). In many instances, complexes of physical signs serve to indicate vascular lesions.

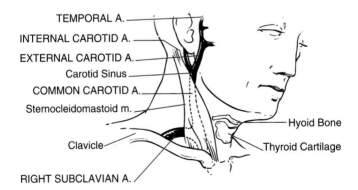

Fig. 8-49 Large Superficial Arteries of the Head and Neck. *The accessible arterial segments are diagrammed in solid black; inaccessible parts are stippled. The temporal artery courses anterior to the ear and upward to the temporal bone. The carotid arteries are deep to the anterior margin of the sternocleidomastoid muscle. The carotid sinus, at the bifurcation of the common carotid, is located by being level with the upper margin of the thyroid cartilage. A short segment of the subclavian artery is often palpable in the supraclavicular fossa.*

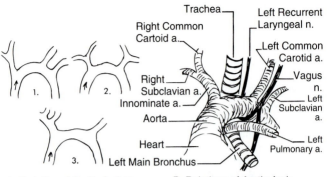

A. Varieties of Aortic Arches   B. Relations of Aortic Arch

Fig. 8-50 The Aortic Arch. A. Aortic Arch Variations. The "normal" pattern (1) is only slightly more common than the other two; it has a right innominate artery, branching into the subclavian and common carotid. There is no left innominate artery; the left subclavian and common carotid originate from the aorta itself. There may be both a right and left innominate (2) or the right innominate may give off the left common carotid (3), in addition to the right carotid and subclavian. B. Anatomic Relations of a Dilated Aortic Arch. Aneurysm of the aortic arch or dilatation of the left atrium may compress the left recurrent laryngeal nerve against the vertebrae or the left main bronchus to produce paralysis of the left vocal cord, resulting in hoarseness or a brassy cough. Expansion of the arch downward impinges upon the left main bronchus so the trachea is depressed with each pulse wave, giving a physical sign called the tracheal tug.

S KEY SYNDROME

▶ **Arterial Aneurysms:** *Pathophysiology:* Permanent abnormal dilatations of arteries occur as congenital anomalies or from weakening of the vessel walls from cystic medial necrosis, atherosclerosis, hypertension, vasculitis, and infection. The forms of aneurysms are fusiform, saccular, and dissecting. Aneurysms may consume platelets and clotting factors lowering their concentrations in the blood. Similar physical signs are produced by fusiform and saccular dilatations, but the dissection of an artery presents an entirely different clinical picture (see page 462).

S KEY SYNDROME

▶ **Arterial Aneurysms: Thoracic Aneurysms:** *Pathophysiology:* The cause of thoracic aneurysms is multifactorial. Breakdown of structural proteins (elastin, collagen, and fibrillin) in the aortic media and adventitia plays a central role. The process also leads to smooth muscle necrosis and development of cystic spaces filled with mucoid material (cystic medial necrosis). Predisposing factors include genetic abnormalities (e.g., Marfan syndrome, which is associated with a mutation in the fibrillin gene), hypertension, pregnancy, inflammation of the aorta (e.g., giant cell arteritis, syphilis, and other infections) and possibly atherosclerosis. Thoracic aneurysms are divided into those involving the ascending aorta, with or without involvement of the arch and distal aorta, and those only involving the aorta distal to the left subclavian artery, with or without involvement of the abdominal aorta. The signs and symptoms associated with thoracic aneurysm are related to compression or distortion of adjacent structures and pain related to dissection of the media and perhaps to sudden dilation of the aorta without dissection. Dissection may occur prior to aneurysmal dilatation. *Ascending Aortic Aneurysms* may produce aortic regurgitation from either dilation of the ascending aorta or dissection extending proximally to the valve ring and leaflets. The murmur characteristically transmits down the right sternal border rather than the left. A palpable thrust may develop in the right second or third intercostal spaces. The width of retromanubrial dullness is increased. Erosion of ribs and protrusion of a pulsatile mass may occur in the region. Compression signs include hoarseness (recurrent laryngeal nerve traction), and cough, wheezing, or hemoptysis (compression and/or erosion of bronchi). Acute "six-dermatome" chest pain may occur directly from dissection, or result from involvement of the coronary ostia (usually the right) by the dissection. Dissection can also extend proximally with rupture into the pericardium, producing acute, usually fatal, tamponade. *Aneurysms of the Aortic Arch* Retrosternal pain is frequent, radiating to the left scapula, the left shoulder, or the left neck. Dilatation of the arch may compress the left recurrent laryngeal nerve against the trachea or the left main bronchus to cause hoarseness and a brassy cough (see Fig. 8-50B). Partial obstruction or dissection of the left subclavian artery may cause delay of the pulse wave to the left arm, a reduction of blood pressure by more than 20 mm in the left arm, and a palpable diminution in pulse volume in the left radial artery. The dilated aortic arch may push down the left main bronchus with each pulsation to produce a tracheal tug, perceived by lightly grasping the cricoid cartilage with the thumb and forefinger and feeling the trachea dip with each pulse (see Fig. 8-50B). *Aneurysms of the Descending Aorta* Frequently, these are silent and are discovered incidentally on chest x-ray. They may erode the bodies of the vertebrae, causing pain in the back radiating around the chest via the intercostal nerves. When associated with dissection, the spinal arteries may be occluded leading to paraplegia. Pain with dissection of descending thoracic aneurysms is similar to that of acute myocardial infarction or dissection of the ascending aorta. However, the vast majority present with pain in the back with or without anterior chest pain.

S KEY SYNDROME

▶ **Abdominal Aortic Aneurysm (AAA):** *Pathophysiology:* AAA involves all three layers of the aorta; the risk of rupture is directly related to the diameter of the aneurysm. Atherosclerosis is uniformly present in the aorta and often widespread. These are the most common aortic aneurysms. AAA is uncommon in individuals younger than 60 years of age, but increases in prevalence with each decade thereafter. Major risk factors are atherosclerosis, cigarette smoking, and male sex. Family clustering has been noted. Estimate the width of the aneurysm on physical examination; this is only an estimate [Arnell TD, de Virgilio C, Donayre C, et al. Abdominal aortic aneurysm screening in elderly males with atherosclerosis: The value of physical exam. *Am Surg* 1996;62:861–864]. Imaging is required for reliable tracking of aneurysm size over time. Locate the pulsatile mass just cephalad to the umbilicus and place the fingers on the lateral walls. The expansile nature is demonstrated by showing lateral, as well as anteroposterior, movement, to distinguish it from a solid tumor in front of the aorta transmitting the pulsation [Rink HA, Lederle FA, Roth CS, et al. The accuracy of physical examination to detect abdominal aortic aneurysm. *Arch Intern Med* 2000;160:833–836]. The presence or absence of abdominal or femoral bruits has no predictive value for the presence or absence of AAA. Pain in the mid to lower abdomen and appearance of a pulsatile epigastric mass suggest recent expansion or possibly leaking of the aneurysm; rapid enlargement in size may, however, be asymptomatic. Rupture is associated with severe pain, which may be felt in the abdomen, back, and/or inguinal areas, accompanied by hypotension. The sensitivity of abdominal palpation for the detection of AAA depends upon the size of the aneurysm and the body habitus of the patient. Aneurysms >5 cm in diameter have a high risk of rupture and should be considered for elective surgical intervention; physical examination is only about 75% sensitive for detecting aneurysms of this size. Diagnostic imaging is the preferred method of detection, and high risk patients should be considered for screening [Lederle FA, Simel DL. The rational clinical examination. Does this patient have abdominal aortic aneurysm? *JAMA* 1997;1997;281:77–82; Lin PH, Lumsden AB. Small aortic aneurysms. *N Engl J Med* 2003;348:19; Ashton HA, Buxton MJ, Day NE, et al. The Multicentre Aneurysm Screening Study (MASS) into the effect of abdominal aortic aneurysm screening on mortality in men: A randomised controlled trial. *Lancet* 2002;360:1531–1539]. Aneurysms of the iliac arteries are not rare and may rupture. They are identified as pulsatile masses in the lower quadrants of the abdomen on deep palpation [van der Wliet JA, Boll APM. Abdominal aortic aneurysm. *Lancet* 1997;349:863–866].

S KEY SYNDROME
▶ **Dissecting Aneurysm of the Aorta:** See page 462.

Mycotic Aneurysms: *Pathophysiology:* These are saccular aneurysms caused by weakening of the arterial walls from infectious processes other than syphilis. Mural involvement may develop as an extension of localized suppuration, actinomycosis, or tuberculosis. More frequently, an embolic arteritis occurs in the course of subacute bacterial endocarditis or septicemia. Mycotic aneurysms usually involve vessels subject to much bending and lightly protected by overlying muscles, such as the axillary, brachial, femoral, and popliteal arteries.

S KEY SYNDROME
Coarctation of the Aorta: *Pathophysiology:* Congenital strictures of the aortic arch occur either proximal or distal to the

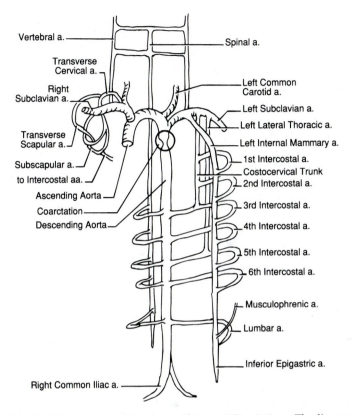

Fig. 8-51 Coarctation of the Aorta: Collateral Circulation. *The diagram shows the collateral channels causing dilatation of the intercostal arteries from the costocervical trunk and the internal mammary artery. The circulation around the scapula is augmented by blood through the transverse cervical artery. The pulse volume in the arms is normal; in the femoral arteries it is diminished. The dilated scapular and intercostal arteries may be palpated in the back.*

point where the ductus arteriosus joins the aorta (preductal or postductal). Usually, the constriction is distal to the origin of the left subclavian artery. When associated with an open ductus, there are usually additional congenital defects that cause early death; so almost invariably, the adult type has a closed ductus. Coarctations with closed ductus form extensive collateral arterial circulations via the left internal mammary artery and other branches of the left subclavian to the left intercostal arteries (excepting the first two), the musculophrenic and the superior epigastric arteries (Fig. 8-51). In most cases, the collateral circulation is adequate for symptomless living into adult life. Arterial hypertension develops in the upper limbs; there is slight hypotension in the lower extremities where the diminished pulse waves can be identified by palpation. Sometimes a blowing systolic murmur, reflecting turbulence at the coarctation, may be heard in the interscapular area. In many patients, nothing in the history or in the examination of the chest reveals the abnormality. A bicuspid aortic valve is a commonly associated anomaly so that an aortic systolic and/or diastolic murmur, often with an ejection click, may be heard. Bruits originating in the internal mammary arteries may be mistaken for intracardiac murmurs. The diagnosis of coarctation is first suspected when routine abdominal examination discloses diminution in pulse volume in both femoral arteries; for this reason, palpation of the femoral pulses should be an invariable routine in abdominal examination. The suspicion of coarctation increases when hypertension in the arms is coincident with weak femoral pulses and a marked disparity in blood pressures between the upper and lower extremities. A careful search should then be made for palpable arterial pulses in the left scapular region and under the lower edge of each of the left ribs posteriorly to detect the dilated arteries of the collateral circulation. When the femoral pulses have good volume, the coarctation may be suspected when the peak of the femoral pulse lags behind that of the radial artery. An x-ray film of the chest may reveal notching of the lower costal edges from erosion by the intercostal arteries. Hypertension in a young man or woman should suggest the possibility of aortic coarctation. Coarctation of the aorta is common in patients with the gonadal dysgenesis syndrome (*Turner syndrome*).

Aberrant Right Subclavian Artery (Dysphagia Lusoria): See Chapter 7, page 327.

Subclavian Stenosis: Subclavian Steal Syndrome: *Pathophysiology:* Patients have atherosclerotic stenosis of either subclavian artery, proximal to the origin of the vertebral artery. In addition to the expected low-volume flow in the affected arm, retrograde flow occurs in the ipsilateral vertebral artery inducing cerebral ischemia in the brainstem and consequent neurologic signs (Fig. 8-52B). On the occluded side, a bruit can be heard in the supraclavicular fossa; occasionally, a thrill is felt in the same place. The arterial pulse volume and blood pressure are diminished in the affected arm. Manifestations of cerebral ischemia are intermittent or continuous; they range from vertigo and vague dizziness to slurring of speech and hemiparesis. The cerebral signs and symptoms can be induced by exercising the affected arm.

S KEY SYNDROME

Subclavian: Compression Syndromes: Although compression of the subclavian artery is primarily a circulatory disturbance, the concomitant pressure on the brachial plexus produces symptoms (paresthesias) and signs that bring the patient to the physician. Hence, the true nature of the disorder is usually diagnosed by considering the causes of peripheral neuritis in the upper extremities and making appropriate maneuvers that demonstrate brachial compression.

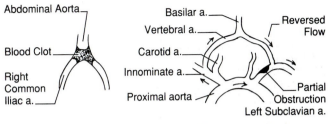

A. Closure of Aortic Bifurcation   B. Subclavian Steal

Fig. 8-52 Two Syndromes of Large Artery Obstruction. *A. Obstruction at the Aortic Bifurcation (Leriche Syndrome):* *A short thrombus closes the lower part of the abdominal aorta and extends a variable distance down the common iliac arteries. The accessible segments of the femoral, popliteal, dorsalis pedis, and posterior tibial arteries are pulseless. Pain in the legs and intermittent claudication are the common symptoms.* *B. Subclavian Steal Syndrome:* *The most common site of narrowing is the left subclavian artery, although other sites have also been reported.*

SUBCLAVIAN COMPRESSION: SCALENUS ANTICUS SYNDROME: *Pathophysiology:* The anterior side of a cervical triangle is formed by the belly of the scalenus anticus muscle stretching from the third, fourth, fifth, and sixth cervical vertebrae anteriorly and downward to the first rib (Fig. 8-53A). The posterior side is formed by the scalenus medius muscle and the base is the first rib. Between the two scaleni emerge the subclavian artery and the brachial plexus, where they are susceptible to compression. This condition is suggested by intermittent or constant pain in the ulnar aspect of the arm and hand, numbness or tingling in the same distribution and wasting or weakness of the arm or hand muscles. *Adson Test* Have the patient sit with pronated forearms on the knees, chin raised high and pointed toward the side being examined, holding the breath during inspiration; determine whether the radial pulse is abolished or diminished by this posture. Check with the breath held in similar fashion but the head held pointed straight forward. The latter posture should not cause compression.

✓*SUBCLAVIAN: COMPRESSION SYNDROMES—CLINICAL OCCURRENCE:* Hypertrophy or edema of the muscle may occur after unusually vigorous use in normally sedentary persons or in those with unusual occupations, such as weight lifters. Spasm of the muscle may result from poor posture, anomalous first rib, or cervical rib.

Subclavian Compression: Cervical Rib: In addition to producing spasm of the scalenus anticus muscle (see *Subclavian Compression: Scalenus Anticus Syndrome* above), a cervical rib may directly compress the subclavian artery producing diminution in the radial pulse in any position (see Fig. 8-53B). Occasionally, the extra rib may be palpated directly in the supraclavicular fossa, but usually the examiner is

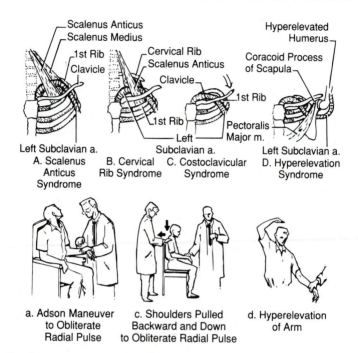

Left Subclavian a.
A. Scalenus Anticus Syndrome

Subclavian a.
B. Cervical Rib Syndrome   C. Costoclavicular Syndrome

Left Subclavian a.
D. Hyperelevation Syndrome

a. Adson Maneuver to Obliterate Radial Pulse

c. Shoulders Pulled Backward and Down to Obliterate Radial Pulse

d. Hyperelevation of Arm

Fig. 8-53 Compression Syndromes of the Superior Thoracic Aperture.
*A. Scalenus Anticus Syndrome: The scalenus anticus muscle has attachments to the transverse processes of the cervical vertebrae above and below to the first rib. Posteriorly and behind the subclavian artery, the scalenus medius attaches to the same bones. Hypertrophy of the bellies of the two muscles causes compression of the artery between them, with motions such as turning the head to the ipsilateral side. This is tested by the **Adson maneuver (a)**, where the patient sits with chin raised, head rotated to the left, and chest held in the inspiratory position. A positive test is marked by diminution or disappearance of the left radial pulse. The other side is tested similarly. B. Cervical Rib Syndrome: The diagram shows a cervical rib compressing the left scalenus anticus muscle and indirectly the subclavian artery. This may produce diminution in the radial pulse or a peripheral neuritis of parts of the brachial plexus. C. Costoclavicular Syndrome: The geometry of the aperture may be such that rotation of the clavicles downward and backward compresses the subclavian arteries against the first rib. This is tested (c) by having the patient seated in a chair and the examiner standing behind him. The physician pushes the shoulders downward and backward while an assistant feels for diminution of the radial pulses. D. Hyperelevation of the Arm: The geometry of the thorax in some persons is such that hyperelevation of the arm causes the coracoid process of the scapula to impinge and compress the subclavian artery. This is tested by (d) demonstrating that the radial pulse is lost with hyperelevation.*

uncertain; therefore, one must rely on the radiography for the diagnosis. The rib may also compress the brachial plexus to produce pain or paresthesias in the hand.

Subclavian Compression: Costoclavicular Syndrome: The symptoms are similar to those produced by compression of the scalenus anticus muscle. *Costoclavicular Maneuver* This tests for compression of the subclavian artery by the first rib. Have the patient sit with his radial pulses palpated by an assistant; stand behind the patient and force his shoulders downward and backward, so that the thoracic outlet is narrowed (see Fig. 8-53C). If there is sufficient compression to cause symptoms, the pulse volumes will be diminished. Later studies show that the maneuver just described does not disclose the costoclavicular syndrome in many patients. An additional test is recommended in which the patient stands with elbows flexed at 90 degrees. In the coronal plane of the body (arms in abduction), the arms are placed successively in three positions, at 45 degrees, 90 degrees, and 135 degrees of elevation (the last position by placing the hands on the head). At each position, the radial pulse is palpated and a point beneath the midportion of the clavicle is auscultated. In a series of normal subjects, 5% had obliteration of the radial pulse at 90 degrees elevation and 15% at 135 degrees. Patients with costoclavicular syndrome had pulse obliteration in at least one of the three positions; but in positions where the pulse was palpable, partial obstruction was shown by the presence of a subclavicular systolic murmur [Winsor T, Brow R. Costoclavicular syndrome. *JAMA* 1966;196:967].

✓ *COSTOCLAVICULAR SYNDROME—CLINICAL OCCURRENCE:* Situations in which the shoulders are forced downward and backward, such as a long walk with a heavy backpack on the shoulders.

SUBCLAVIAN COMPRESSION: ISCHEMIA FROM HYPERELEVATION OF THE ARM: *Pathophysiology:*   In some persons, elevation of the arm causes compression of the subclavian artery by the coracoid process of the scapula (see Fig. 8-53D). The patient usually complains of numbness and tingling in one or both hands or arms, either intermittent or constant. The patient often sleeps supine with arms elevated, so that the hands are behind or over the head, or the patient has engaged in some occupation requiring elevation of the arms, such as painting ceilings. *Hyperabduction Test* Lift the patient's hand over his head in approximately the position assumed in sleeping; have him open and close his hand several times; note whether the radial pulse volume is diminished or abolished.

S   KEY SYNDROME

► **Superior Vena Cava (SVC) Obstruction: SVC Syndrome:**   The principal signs are intense cyanosis of the head, neck, and both arms, edema of the face, both arms, and the upper third of the thoracic wall, and engorgement of the veins in the cyanotic region without venous pulsations normally transmitted from

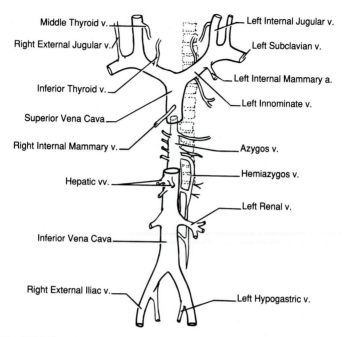

Middle Thyroid v.
Right External Jugular v.
Inferior Thyroid v.
Superior Vena Cava
Right Internal Mammary v.
Hepatic vv.
Inferior Vena Cava
Right External Iliac v.

Left Internal Jugular v.
Left Subclavian v.
Left Internal Mammary a.
Left Innominate v.
Azygos v.
Hemiazygos v.
Left Renal v.
Left Hypogastric v.

Fig. 8-54 Superior and Inferior Venae Cavae.

the right atrium (Fig. 8-54). The circumference of the neck is enlarged by nonpitting edema (*Stokes collar*).

✓ *SVC SYNDROME—CLINICAL OCCURRENCE:* Mediastinal neoplasms; cervical or retrosternal goiter; aortic aneurysms in the thorax; chronic mediastinitis from tuberculosis, histoplasmosis, syphilis, or pyogenic organisms; thrombophlebitis, thrombosis from an indwelling intravenous catheter.

S KEY SYNDROME

► **Inferior Vena Caval (IVC) Obstruction:** *Pathophysiology:* Occlusion of the IVC retards venous drainage from the lower extremities and pelvis and leads to development of collateral veins in the hemorrhoidal complex and abdominal wall. Renal vein thrombosis causes acute renal failure (see Fig. 8-54). *Acute IVC Obstruction* may be asymptomatic until lower extremity edema develops. Rapidly progressive edema of both legs symmetrically without evidence of heart or kidney disease should suggest mechanical obstruction to the inferior vena cava. *Chronic IVC Obstruction* is suggested by the presence of dilated superficial collateral veins with cephalad flow on the abdomen. The superficial veins may be more easily seen by viewing them through red goggles. Visible evidence of collaterals may appear within a week after complete obstruction, and the veins may attain maximal size in 3 months. To localize the site of obstruction, the vena cava is considered in three segments. *Lower Segment (below the renal veins):* Venous collaterals are distributed over thighs, groins, lower abdomen, and flanks. Edema of lower limbs is originally pitting, progressing to brawny induration of the skin with dermatitis, varicosities, and ulcers. Pelvic congestion may produce low back pain and edematous genitalia. *Middle Segment (above the renal veins and below the hepatic veins):* The venous collaterals are large central abdominal veins without lateral abdominal collaterals. Occlusion of the renal veins produces nephrotic syndrome with generalized edema. Gastrointestinal manifestations include nausea, vomiting, diarrhea and abdominal pain. The malabsorption syndrome may develop. *Upper Segment (above the hepatic veins):* Venous Collaterals form a prominent periumbilical plexus and large veins appear over the xiphoid region. **Budd-Chiari syndrome** develops with hepatosplenomegaly, ascites, jaundice, and elevated transaminases.

✓ **IVC OBSTRUCTION—CLINICAL OCCURRENCE:** *Intraluminal* thrombosis, embolism, neoplastic invasion or extension from renal cell carcinoma; *Intramural* rare benign or malignant neoplasms of the venous wall; *External Pressure* enlargement of the liver, paravertebral lymphadenopathy, aortic aneurysm, surgical ligation, pregnancy.

Disorders of Large Limb Arteries

Arterial disorders are either occlusive or nonocclusive. The occlusion may be partial or complete. When an arterial circulatory deficit has been demonstrated, one of four mechanisms is involved: (a) extrinsic compression; (b) vasospasm; (c) luminal obstruction by intimal thickening, or plugging of the lumen by thrombus or embolus; or (d) intrinsic disease of the artery (vasculitis, atherosclerosis) that promotes occlusion. Frequently, compression of an artery is related to the position of the extremity and is temporary. The compression may be demonstrated by maneuvers based on knowledge of the skeletal and muscular anatomy. Vasospasm is also transient; it is frequently recognized by the sharp border produced between ischemic and normal tissue. Usually, proliferation of the arterial intima is inferred when the blood flow is diminished but still present. When the occlusion is complete, the cause is usually embolism or thrombosis. The onset of thrombosis is usually gradual and painless, whereas embolism occurs suddenly, with severe localized pain. Underlying intrinsic arterial disease is usually inferred from the total clinical picture, the demonstration of characteristic findings in accessible arterial walls, the distribution of lesions in the arterial tree, and the extent of organ and tissue involvement.

In examining a major artery occlusion, the proximal extent of the occlusion is first determined by noting the presence or absence of pulses along the course of the vessel. When the entire vessel is not accessible, inferences are made from its branches and the proximal vessels. Afterward, the vessel walls are palpated for signs of intrinsic disease. Imaging with Doppler ultrasound, MR angiography, or contrast angiography is definitive.

▼ **Atherosclerosis:** The term arteriosclerosis includes three entities: (a) atherosclerosis, (b) medial calcification of Mönckeberg, and (c) arteriolar sclerosis. Of the three, atherosclerosis is the only process that causes plugging of medium-sized arteries. *Pathophysiology:* It is characterized by medial degeneration and fibrosis, together with occlusive proliferation of the intima. Occlusion may also be caused by the formation of intimal plaques composed of lipoid material and calcium salts. The walls become less compressible; the unyielding tactile sensation is interpreted as thickening. The arterial segments lengthen. When the ends of a segment are anchored by surrounding tissue, the elongated vessel buckles in the middle, producing visible and palpable tortuosity. The disease may be spotty throughout the body; frequently it is much more advanced in the vessels of the lower extremities. Atherosclerosis is the most likely cause of major arterial obstruction when the patient is older than age 45 years. In diabetes mellitus, atherosclerosis frequently occurs at a much earlier age. Hyperhomocysteinemia, congenital or acquired (as in folate deficiency), is also a risk factor for atherosclerosis and thromboembolic events. Atheromatous plaques may be felt in the walls of accessible arteries, and the calcium can be seen in x-ray films, but plaques are not common in the vessels of the upper extremities. Noninvasive vascular examination with Doppler ultrasonography and plethysmography are required for accurate diagnosis; angiography with contrast or MRA is anatomically definitive. DDX: Atherosclerosis must be distinguished from Mönckeberg medial calcification, which is characterized by annular calcified plaques in the media of larger vessels. The plaques are readily palpated in the brachial and radial arteries as beads or rings. However, this disease does not cause occlusion and seldom involves smaller vessels. It frequently coexists with atherosclerosis, but not invariably. Its plaques are readily seen in x-ray films. Arteriolar sclerosis is a disorder of small vessels, associated with arterial hypertension, but it does not cause occlusive vascular disease of large arteries.

ACUTE ARTERIAL OBSTRUCTION: Occlusion of arteries to the organs of the head, thorax, and abdomen present with symptoms referable to those organs, for example, stroke, acute myocardial infarction, pulmonary embolism, mesenteric, renal, or splenic infarction.

▼ **Acute Arterial Obstruction of an Extremity: Embolism and Arterial Thrombosis:** Usually, the patient experiences sudden excruciating pain in the extremity, followed by numbness and weakness in the part. This is most common in the legs, but can occur in the arms as well. Occasionally, anesthesia and muscle weakness precede the pain which appears more gradually. The distal portion of the extremity becomes pallid and pulseless. One or 2 hours later, the distal skin becomes blue, while mottling occurs proximally. Cyanosis lessens when the limb is elevated. The skin of the affected part soon becomes colder. The pulseless artery may be felt as a tender cord that must be distinguished from a similar finding caused by reflex vasospasm in arteries adjacent to inflamed veins. Tenderness in the calf muscles or the anterior leg indicates involvement, respectively, of the posterior tibial or the anterior tibial artery. Occasionally, the pain may be quite mild. Early, the muscles are flaccid; later the foot assumes plantar flexion.   *Distinction Between Thrombosis and Embolism*   Thrombosis is inferred when there are signs elsewhere of diffuse vascular disease or the history discloses symptoms of arterial insufficiency, such as claudication. Embolism from the left atrium is suspected when atrial fibrillation is present.

✔ *ACUTE ARTERIAL OCCLUSION—CLINICAL OCCURRENCE:*   *Thrombosis* atherosclerosis; thromboangiitis obliterans; vasculitis; blood sludging from polycythemia, hemoconcentration, cryoglobulinemia, and hyperglobulinemia; infection; trauma;   antiphospholipid syndrome   *Embolism*   atrial fibrillation, mitral stenosis, endocarditis (infectious and nonbacterial thrombotic endocarditis) myxomas of the left atrium, a mural thrombus in the ventricle following myocardial infarction, dislodgment of a thrombus or atherosclerotic plaque from a traumatized artery or aneurysm.

S KEY SYNDROME

▼ **Chronic   Arterial   Obstruction: Occlusive Vascular Disease:**   This is most common in the lower extremities, but may involve the arms. The patient complains of claudication and coldness of the part, progressing to continuous pain and night pain.   *Skin*   Arterial insufficiency may cause skin pigmentation, pallor, purplish discoloration that fades with elevation, coldness, warm areas of collateral circulation, local hair loss, malnutrition of toenails, ulceration, or gangrene (see Figs. 8-43 and 8-44).   *Arterial Pulses*   Absence of pulsations in the affected and distal arteries.   *Muscles*   Atrophy may be present. With occlusion of the popliteal artery, collateral circulation may develop in the branches of the geniculate artery, producing the combination of cold feet and warm knees. The unusually warm skin from these collaterals may be on the knee or in an area on the anteromedial aspect of the lower thigh, while there are pulseless popliteal, posterior tibial, and dorsalis pedis arteries. Assess the ankle-brachial index (ABI); see page 372.

S KEY SYNDROME

▼ **Pulseless   Femoral   Artery   (Leriche   Syndrome):**   (see Fig. 8-52). Always palpate the femoral arteries after examination of the abdomen. A decrease in, or absence of, the femoral pulse may point to the diagnosis of coarctation of the aorta, thrombosis of the distal aorta (Leriche syndrome), thrombosis of the common iliac artery, or dissecting aortic aneurysm. When the femoral pulse is diminished or absent, palpate the iliac pulses up to and including the aortic bifurcation. The aorta divides about 2 cm below and slightly to the left of the umbilicus. Lines drawn from the bifurcation to the midpoints of the lines between anterior superior iliac spines and symphysis pubis delineate the course of the iliac arteries; the upper third represents the common iliac, the lower two-thirds marks the external iliacs. These vessels may not be palpable in normal persons, but discrepancies in pulsations between the two sides are particularly significant. The significance of an absent or diminished femoral pulse must also be judged by the presence or absence of the pulses distal to the femorals. The syndrome is also caused by the chronic use of methysergide or ergot.

S KEY SYNDROME

▼ **Thromboangiitis Obliterans (Buerger Disease):** *Pathophysiology:* The process begins as an acute panarteritis involving all three layers of some medium-sized arteries. Granulation tissue in the intima ultimately causes gradual arterial plugging, producing arterial deficiency in the tissues. The onset of thromboangiitis is usually between 20 and 40 years of age, younger than in atherosclerosis. The disease occurs predominantly in males. Cigarette smoking is the major risk factor. Thromboangiitis is often associated with venous involvement manifest as superficial migrating thrombophlebitis. Commonly, only segments of an artery or arteries are affected. DDX: There are no physical signs, as such, that distinguish Buerger disease from atherosclerosis. The distribution of affected vessels may differ from that in atherosclerosis: in addition to the vessels of the lower extremities, thromboangiitis has a predilection for the radial, ulnar, or the digital arteries of one or more fingers, as demonstrated by the Allen test [Olin JW. Thromboangiitis obliterans (Buerger's disease). *N Engl J Med* 2000;343:864–869].

S KEY SYNDROME

▼ **Raynaud Disease and Phenomenon:** *Pathophysiology:* The pallor is produced by tight constriction of the digital and smaller arteries. Soon the capillaries dilate and fill with stagnant deoxygenated blood, producing the blue skin. Release of vascular spasm is associated with flushing and return of warmth. Paroxysmal constriction of the digital arteries and minute dermal vessels usually occurs bilaterally, commonly affecting the fingers and involving the toes in half the cases. Approximately 80% of the patients are young women. The attacks are induced by exposure to cold or emotional stress. Eventually, the digits of the hands and feet are symmetrically affected. Early attacks may involve only the tips of the digits; later, the process may extend proximally. From one to four fingers of each hand may be included, rarely the thumbs. In the classic picture, lasting from 15 to 60 minutes, the terminal digits become chalk-white and numb (Fig. 8-55A). The pallid skin is covered with sweat. Soon the pallor is succeeded by intense cyanosis and pain. Sometimes either pallor or cyanosis is absent, rarely are both absent. During recovery, either spontaneously or after immersion in warm water, projections of hyperemia from the unaffected skin invade the cyanotic regions until all blueness has been replaced by brilliant red. Hyperemia is accompanied by tingling, throbbing, and some swelling of tissues. After many attacks, trophic changes may appear in the nails and adjacent skin. Small areas of gangrene may develop on the tips of the fingers and toes (Fig. 8-55B). The term *Raynaud disease* is re-

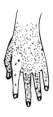
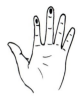

A. Blanching of Finger   B. Gangrene on Fingertips

Fig. 8-55 Signs of Raynaud Disease. **A.** *Blanching of the finger induced by exposure to cold may produce the classic sequence of color changes where a sharply demarcated area at the end of a finger becomes chalky white, then blue, and finally red, before it returns to normal. It may not be very painful.* **B.** *In long-standing cases, gangrenous spots at the fingertips occur; the area around the fingernail may ulcerate.*

served for cases in which the classic color changes are symmetric and there is no other associated disease. The same signs are called *Raynaud phenomenon* when they are associated with thromboangiitis obliterans, atherosclerosis, scleroderma, trauma to nerves of the arms from crutches or air hammers or cervical ribs, disseminated lupus erythematosus, polyarteritis, and various types of peripheral neuritis. Always inspect the nailbed capillaries (page 134); abnormal capillaries are highly suggestive of scleroderma. Raynaud phenomenon occurs more frequently in patients with migraine (26%) than in persons without migraine (6%) and may represent the expression of a generalized vasospastic disorder. Cold hands may precede the headache in patients with migraine. There is also an increased prevalence of chest pain and migraine in patients with Raynaud disease [O'Keeffe SJ, Taspatsaris NP, Beethan WP Jr. Increased prevalence of migraine and chest pain in patients with primary Raynaud disease. *Ann Intern Med* 1992;116:(12 pt 1):985–989]. DDX: The sequence of pallor, cyanosis, and redness is diagnostic when induced by exposure to cold [Wigley FM. Raynaud's phenomenon. *N Engl J Med* 2002;347:1001–1008].

S KEY SYNDROME

▼ **Blue Hands and Feet: Acrocyanosis:** *Pathophysiology:* The excessive arteriolar constriction is ascribed to increased tone of the sympathetic nervous system, although humoral agents may contribute. This is a benign condition in which the skin of the hands and feet is persistently cyanotic, cold, and sweating. It is most common in young women; it is seldom encountered in middle age except in patients with myeloproliferative diseases. The skin is uniformly blue; the color is intensified by exposure to cold. The cyanosis is abolished when the part is elevated or when the patient sleeps. There is no discomfort; the patient consults the physician because of the cosmetic effect.

S KEY SYNDROME

Gangrene of Digital Tips: Gangrene of the finger and toe tips can be caused by any disease or condition impairing peripheral perfusion.

✓ *CLINICAL OCCURRENCE:* Scleroderma, pneumatic hammer disease, obstruction of the superior thoracic aperture (scalenus anticus syndrome, cervical rib, mediastinal tumor or abscess), atherosclerosis, thromboangiitis obliterans, cold agglutination causing blood sludging, cryoglobulinemia, atheroemboli, sepsis, meningococcemia, vasopressor medications, antiphospholipid syndrome, warfarin skin necrosis (protein C deficiency), ergotism, methylsergide medication, chronic renal failure, and hemodialysis, possibly hyperphosphatemia, thrombocythemia.

Symmetrical Gangrene of the Digits: Ergotism:
Pathophysiology: An intense constriction of the peripheral blood vessels is caused by the ingestion of large amounts of ergot by normal persons or of small amounts by those who are sensitive. Ergot may be taken as a drug to treat migraine or eaten in grain that has been contaminated with the fungus. The first symptom is often burning pain in the extremities (*St. Anthony fire*) with loss of arterial pulses in the hands or feet. Mottled cyanosis of the extremities and coldness of the skin follow. Finally, symmetrical gangrene of the fingers and toes occurs, which may extend proximally. Symptoms of headache, weakness, nausea, vomiting, visual disturbances, and angina pectoris may accompany the signs.

Cavernous Hemangioma of the Leg: This congenital tumor may occur anywhere in the body. When a massive angioma involves the leg, it may be confused with varicose veins. The affected leg is usually enlarged circumferentially. The dilated, ill-defined blood sinuses raise the surface of the normal skin, under which are seen purplish masses that are readily compressible. They are distinguished from varicosities by their distribution, which does not correspond to that of the large leg veins. With the patient in the erect position, enough blood may be pooled to cause orthostatic hypotension. Massive cavernous hemangiomas (Kasabach-Merritt syndrome) trap platelets to produce thrombocytopenia, purpura, and bleeding.

Aneurysms of the Upper Limbs: The subclavian, axillary, and brachial arteries are most commonly affected; the carotids are rarely involved. Trauma to the vessel wall is the most common cause; rarely, the vessels are involved by mycotic, necrotizing, or atherosclerotic aneurysms. The dilatations may be readily palpated in this region.

Aneurysms of the Lower Limbs: The most common sites are the femoral artery in the Scarpa triangle and the popliteal artery in its fossa. Atherosclerosis is the most common cause. The lesions are readily palpable.

Disorders of the Major Extremity Veins

S KEY SYNDROME

Deep Vein Thrombosis (DVT): Phleboth-rombosis: *Pathophysiology:* See *Pulmonary Embolism*, page 448. Immobilization in bed or by casting following extremity trauma or surgery is a common precipitating event. Hip and knee surgery have particularly high incidence of associated DVT. This term is usually applied to thrombosis of the deep veins of the legs. Absence of inflammation facilitates dislodgment of clots; leg veins are the most common identified source of pulmonary embolism. Deep venous thrombosis requires timely diagnosis to initiate appropriate therapy, the goals of which are to prevent pulmonary embolus, diminish damage to the valves and endothelium of the veins, which predisposes to future thrombosis and stasis damage to the skin, and relieve pain. The history and physical examination will enable you to make an accurate diagnosis less than half the time; therefore reliance on the vascular laboratory equipped for definitive testing with Doppler ultrasound, impedance plethysmography, or venography is essential [Anand SS, Wells PS, Hunt S, et al. The rational clinical examination. Does this patient have deep vein thrombosis? *JAMA* 1998;279:1094–1099; Kearon C, Julian JA, Newman TE, et al. Noninvasive diagnosis of deep venous thrombosis. *Ann Intern Med* 1998; 128:663–677]. Early diagnosis can be lifesaving.

Symptoms   Pain or a sense of fullness in the leg, aggravated by standing or walking is often present.   *Signs*   Deep venous thrombosis is often accompanied by *cyanosis* of the skin on the lower third of the leg or on the foot, especially when the leg is dependent. Pitting *edema* of the foot, ankle, or leg persisting after a good diuresis or 2 weeks after the removal of a plaster cast suggests deep venous thrombophlebitis.   *Venous Engorgement*   of the feet that remains distended when the legs are elevated to 45 degrees suggests deep venous thrombosis. The *Pratt sign* is the presence of three dilated veins over the tibia, called sentinel veins. The venous distention should persist when the legs are elevated to 45 degrees. Small dilated veins just below the knee or above the ankle are usually communicating veins between the long and short saphenous systems, distended by blockage of intramuscular veins.

Pain   in the leg along the course of the thrombosed vein can be induced by sneezing or coughing (*Louvel sign*). The pain disappears with digital compression of the vein proximal to the obstruction. Palpate the leg to detect local tenderness of vein segments. The deep veins of the plantar surface drain mainly into the posterior tibial vein, deep to the Achilles tendon. The anterior tibial vein lies in a groove between tibia and fibula; it penetrates the interosseous membrane to join the popliteal vein. Because the majority of deep veins of the calf are in the soleus muscle, the following regions should be palpated for tenderness: the soles, the region deep to the Achilles tendon, in the groove between tibia and fibula (anterior tibial vein), bimanual palpation of the soleus muscle below the largest swelling of the calf made by the gastrocnemius, in the popliteal fossa, over the adductor muscles of the medial thigh, over the femoral veins above and below the inguinal ligaments, and digital examination of the rectum to test for tenderness of the iliac veins. *Calf Spasm (Homan Sign)* The patient's knee is put in flexion and the examiner forcefully and abruptly dorsiflexes the ankle. This produces pain in the calf or popliteal region in approximately 35% of the patients with deep venous thrombosis. The sign is also positive with herniated low intervertebral disk and other lumbosacral affections. The absence of bone tenderness excludes the skeletal causes of the Homan sign. Recurrent deep venous thrombosis may precede the diagnosis of cancer [Prandoni P, Lansing AWA, Buller HR, et al. Deep-vein thrombosis and the incidence of subsequent symptomatic cancer. *N Engl J Med* 1992;327:1128–1133].

✓ *DVT—CLINICAL OCCURRENCE: Congenital* Suspect congenital thrombophilia in patients who have DVT at a young age, at an unusual site (upper extremity, mesenteric vessels, etc.), with a history of previous thromboses or emboli, with a family history, or with minimal trauma or minor surgery. Look for resistance to activated protein C, factor V Leiden mutation, protein C deficiency, protein S deficiency, dysfibrinogenemia, homocystinuria, antithrombin III deficiency, and sickle cell disease. *Acquired* Antiphospholipid syndrome (lupus-like anticoagulant, anticardiolipin antibodies), heparin-induced thrombocytopenia and thrombosis (HITT syndrome), leg fractures, limb surgery, trauma, prolonged inactivity (bed rest, international air travel, automobile travel), infection, cancer (especially mucin producing adenocarcinomas), hyperhomocysteinemia, estrogen-containing medications, pregnancy, obesity, venous stasis and insufficiency, diabetes mellitus, polycythemia vera, idiopathic thrombocythemia, and paroxysmal nocturnal hemoglobinuria.

KEY SIGN

Deep Vein Thrombosis (DVT): Thrombophlebitis: *Pathophysiology:* See *Pulmonary Embolism*, page 448. As the name implies, thrombosis and inflammation of the venous walls are associated; inflammation may either precede or follow clot formation. The lesion may be spontaneous or result from mechanical or chemical trauma, immobilization, medications (estrogens, oral contraceptives), thrombophilia, suppurative disease, ischemia, anemia, polycythemia, or leukemia. When acute, the veins are painful and tender and the overlying skin is red and hot. Cramps are incited in adjacent muscles. Fever and leukocytosis are common. Involved superficial veins feel like firm cords. When thrombophlebitis involves an extremity, edema and dependent cyanosis result from venous occlusion. Expose the lower limbs to the room air for 10 minutes and then test the *skin temperature* of both legs with the back of your hand, comparing the two limbs. In half the cases of thrombophlebitis, there is elevated skin temperature around the ankle or calf. The history and physical findings are essential to the diagnostic evaluation [Miron MJ, Perrier A, Bounameaux H. Clinical assessment of suspected deep vein thrombosis: Comparison between a score and empirical assessment. *J Intern Med* 2000;247:249–254].

In a chronic process, pain and tenderness are slight and less reddening and heat occur in the overlying skin. Sudden thrombophlebitis of the femoral vein presents a clinical picture termed ***phlegmasia alba*** *dolens*, because of the excruciating pain, massive edema of the extremity, and pallor from arterial spasm. These signs suggest arterial embolism, but the pallor is less intense, there is more cyanosis, the femoral vein is tender, and no anesthesia is produced. When the arterial pulses are impalpable, they can usually be demonstrated by Doppler examination. A rare variant is ***phlegmasia cerulea dolens***, caused by the involvement of the entire venous return of an extremity. It is characterized by extreme pain, massive edema, and deep cyanosis of the entire limb. Circulatory collapse may abolish the arterial pulses, but the deep blue of the skin distinguishes the condition from arterial embolism. Obtain help from a vascular laboratory to make the diagnosis.

KEY SIGN

Superficial Thrombophlebitis: *Pathophysiology:* See *Deep Vein Thrombosis (DVT): Thrombophlebitis,* above. Thrombosis and inflammation occurs in the superficial veins, either alone, or extending from the deep veins. The patient complains of tender red nodules or cords under the skin. Often there is a history of recent trauma, though it may be incidental to the problem. Superficial thrombophlebitis may mask the coincidental occurrence of deep venous disease. Superficial thrombophlebitis is not usually associated with life-threatening pulmonary embolus. A Doppler study should be used to rule out deep venous thrombosis. DDX: Lymphangitis and other skin and soft-tissue infections can be confused with superficial thrombophlebitis.

SUPERFICIAL MIGRATING THROMBOPHLEBITIS: Successive episodes of thrombophlebitis involve different veins in widely separated parts of the body. In a single episode, a segment of vein becomes tender, reddened, and indurated. Involution begins in a few days and the adjacent tissues become successively blue and yellow, often resolving with some pigmentation of the skin. Veins of the extremities are most commonly involved, but the subcutaneous veins of the abdomen and thorax may be affected. Although the lesions do not cause serious discomfort, this complex should prompt a search for an underlying disease.

✓ *SUPERFICIAL THROMBOPHLEBITIS—CLINICAL OCCURRENCE:* Antiphospholipid syndrome, thromboangiitis obliterans, carcinoma of the pancreas or other abdominal organs, and thrombophilic hematologic disorders, especially paroxysmal nocturnal hemoglobinuria.

S KEY SYNDROME

Venous Stasis: *Pathophysiology:* Venous stasis results from vein occlusion or incompetence of the valves. Occlusion is caused by external compression of the walls or from plugging of the lumina by fibrosis, thrombi, or neoplasms growing in the vessel cavities. Dilation of vessels exacerbates stasis. Dilated superficial veins drain poorly into smaller communicating veins. Dilatation of deeper veins leads to incompetence of their valves. Decreased capillary flow produces poor skin nutrition, inflammation, and fibrosis. Signs of venous stasis are pitting edema, stasis pigmentation (hemosiderin), erythema, fibrosis and decreased elasticity of the skin and ulceration. The pumping action of voluntary muscles is inhibited by bed rest and by immobilizing an extremity.

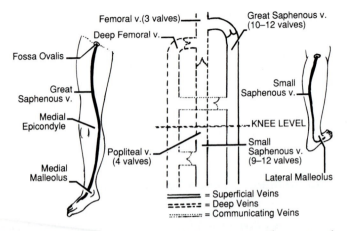

Fig. 8-56 Large Superficial Veins of the Lower Limb. The great saphenous vein begins on the medial aspect of the foot, courses backward under the medial malleolus, up the medial aspect of the calf, behind the medial epicondyle, and then obliquely across the anterior thigh to the femoral vein as it enters the femoral canal beneath the inguinal ligament. The small saphenous vein begins on the lateral side of the foot, curves backward beneath the lateral malleolus, and then upward on the posterior surface of the calf to enter the popliteal fossa and join with the popliteal vein. The middle figure diagrams the communications between the superficial veins (heavy solid lines) and the deep veins (broken lines) and the communicating vessels (dotted lines).

S KEY SYNDROME

Varicose Veins: *Anatomy:* Because varicosities are most common in leg veins, their anatomic relations are important to an examination (Fig. 8-56). The great saphenous vein begins at the mediodorsal side of the foot and courses upward along the medial edge of the subcutaneous aspect of the tibia, going medial to the patella and posterior to the median epicondyle of the femur. In the thigh, its course is slightly lateralward and upward to the femoral canal, where it empties into the femoral vein. The small saphenous vein begins at the lateral side of the foot, curving under and back of the lateral malleolus, going upward to assume a position in the midline of the belly of the gastrocnemius muscle; finally abandoning its superficial location, it dives deeply into the popliteal fossa to empty into the popliteal vein. Several communicating veins run between the great saphenous and the femoral vein. To summarize: the great saphenous vein emerges from the femoral canal and runs down the anteromedial aspect of the lower extremity to the medial side of the foot; the small saphenous vein emerges from the popliteal fossa and runs down the posterior aspect of the calf to curl under the lateral malleolus. The term varicose vein is usually applied to dilated veins from all causes except angiomas. Primary varicosities are venous dilatations that develop spontaneously; secondary varicosities are dilatations resulting from proximal obstruction in pregnancy, trauma, thrombophlebitis, compressing tumors, congestive heart failure, portal obstruction, or arteriovenous fistulas. Whenever varicose veins occur in only one extremity, the possibility of local compression or an arteriovenous fistula should be considered. In the latter condition, pulsations are frequently present in the dilated veins. When varicose veins are massive, standing may pool enough blood to cause orthostatic hypotension and faintness. Tests for patency and valvular competence of the large limb veins by physical examination are less accurate than ultrasonography and plethysmography. Baseline data helps direct treatment and enables you to evaluate whether subsequent symptoms represent new disease or progression of previous injury.

S KEY SYNDROME

Thrombosis of the Axillary Vein: This usually follows trauma or intensive use of the arm in hyperabduction, such as throwing. The entire arm swells and aches. The tissues are firm and there is no pitting edema. The superficial veins at the superior thoracic aperture may be dilated. Poor collateral circulation produces cyanosis of the skin. Axillary vein thromboses are less likely to lead to lethal pulmonary emboli than deep venous thromboses in the legs, but it does occur. DDX: In chronic cases, it must be distinguished from lymphedema. Both conditions produce solid, nonpitting swelling, but venous obstruction causes some cyanosis of the skin; the skin is pallid in lymphedema. Lymphedema of the arm is common after radical mastectomy.

Section 2   THE BREASTS

Breast Physiology

The Female Breast

Embryologically the breast is a skin structure, a highly complex and specialized sweat gland. The mammary glands are normally rudimentary in children and men. In the woman, maximal development occurs in the early childbearing years, when the breasts become conical or hemispheric, extending from the second to the sixth or seventh ribs. Ductal growth in the adolescent female follows the production of estrogenic hormones by the ovary. With onset of ovulation, the secretion of progesterone results in alveolar development. Other hormones including prolactin, adrenocorticotropic hormone (ACTH), corticosteroids, growth hormone, thyroxine, and androgens appear to play facultative roles in the completion of breast development and milk production. The breast contains from 15 to 20 subdivided lobes, arranged radially, each with its own excretory lactiferous tubule discharging through a separate orifice in the nipple. Considerable fat surrounds the glands, so discrete lobes are not ordinarily palpable. Fibrous bands vertically infiltrate the breast tissue, forming suspensory ligaments (Cooper ligaments), which pass from the fascia of the pectoralis muscle through the breast parenchyma to the skin of the breast. A fascial cleft separates the deep surface of the breast from the thoracic wall, permitting some mobility.

The glandular portion of the breast responds to the cyclic hormones of the pituitary and ovary. In the adult, it has four major components: stroma, ductal epithelium, glandular acini, and the myoepithelium, each influenced by a variety of hormonal signals. During the follicular phase of the menstrual cycle estrogens stimulate minimal mitotic activity. Progesterones provoke significantly greater cellular division during the luteal phase. Prior to the onset of menses, the breasts increase in size. If conception takes place, extensive alveolar and ductal proliferation occurs under the influence of estrogens, progesterones and prolactin. With parturition, the epithelium becomes actively secretory, and the release of progesterone inhibition of prolactin causes milk to be released.

The Male Breast

Because of its rudimentary structure, the male breast is more easily examined than the woman's. Unfortunately, examination is frequently neglected because the physician does not realize that the male breast may be the site of serious disease. The principles of examination are similar to those described for women. Residual anlage for breast development may remain in males and can be responsive to hormonal influences at any time during life from adolescence to old age. Breast development may occur secondary to abnormal endocrine influences, including hyperthyroidism, prolactin-secreting adenomas, acromegaly, tumors of the testes and adrenals, and a variety of drugs including, of course, estrogens. It is not infrequently observed in alcoholic males, as liver disease leads to increased circulating estrogenic hormones.

Superficial Anatomy of the Breasts

Lying against the pectoral fascia, the breast tissue forms a circular area of contact; from this circle, *the axillary tail* of gland tissue projects laterally and superiorly along the axillary and serratus anterior fascia (Fig. 8-57). This extension is important in evaluating axillary masses.

The conical or cylindrical *nipple* lies slightly below and lateral to the center of the breast. The overlying skin is wrinkled and pigmented; it is roughened with papillae containing the orifices of the lactiferous tubules. The skin of the nipple extends for a radius of 1–2 cm or more onto the surface of the breast to form the *areola*. Both nipple and areola vary from pink to brown, depending on the individual's complexion and parity. After the second month of pregnancy the color darkens progressively and the areola enlarges. Small elevations in the surface of the areola are produced by the sebaceous glands of Montgomery (areolar glands), which secrete a lipoid material to protect the nipples dur-

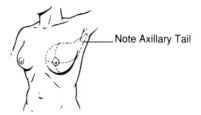

Note Axillary Tail

Fig. 8-57 Quadrants of the Breast. *The hemisphere of the breast is divided into quadrants by imaginary vertical and horizontal lines intersecting at the nipple. The quadrants are named upper medial, upper lateral, lower medial, and lower lateral. Popularly, these quadrants are also named, respectively, upper inner, upper outer, lower inner, and lower outer. Note the protrusion of the upper lateral quadrant, called the axillary tail, in which breast tissue extends to the axilla.*

ing nursing. Radial and circular muscle fibers are embedded in the subcutaneous tissue of the areola; light friction or massage stimulates them to contract, producing erection of the nipple.

Physical Examination of the Breasts

The importance of adequate breast examination in women is apparent from the prevalence of breast cancer, the high mortality rate in those women with advanced disease, and the improved survival of patients diagnosed with small tumors. The American Cancer Society and other groups provide guidelines for periodic physical examination and mammography for breast cancer screening.

The male breast must also be examined because breast cancer does occur in men and is easily identified if examination is performed.

In the routine physical examination, the breasts are usually inspected and palpated with the patient supine. Whenever the patient complains of a breast lump or a possible mass is detected, further evaluation is required. The breasts may engorge premenstrually, and usually do so during pregnancy, making examination both more painful and more difficult.

Breast Examination

The patient is examined sequentially both sitting and supine. Inspection of the breast includes observation of the surface and transillumination of masses. Be certain to examine the creases under and between the breasts.

PATIENT SITTING WITH ARMS DOWN (FIG. 8-58A). Have the patient strip to the waist and sit on the table or in a chair facing you. Compare

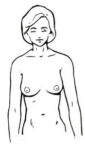
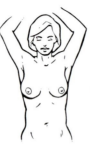
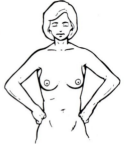

A. Patient Standing   B. Standing with   C. Pushing on Hips to
   with Arms Down   Arms Elevated   Tense Pectoral Muscles

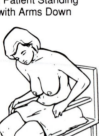
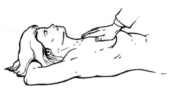

D. Bent Forward so   E. Breasts Palpated against
   Breasts Hang Free   Pectoral Muscles

Fig. 8-58 Patient Positions for Breast Examination. *The patient is stripped to the waist and sits facing the examiner. **A.** The patient stands with arms at sides; the examiner looks for elevation of the level of a nipple, dimpling, bulging, and peau d'orange. **B.** When the patient raises her arms, dimpling and elevation of the nipple are accentuated when there is a mass fixed to the pectoral fascia. **C.** The patient pushes her hands down against her hips to flex and tense the pectoralis major muscles; the examiner moves the mass to determine fixation to the underlying fascia. **D.** When the breasts are large and pendulous, the patient is asked to lean forward, so the breasts hang free from the chest wall; retraction and masses become more evident. **E.** In the supine position, the examiner presses the breasts against the chest wall with the flat of his hand; the normal nodosity from the lobules is less prominent and significant masses are more distinctly felt.*

the size and shape of the breasts, remembering that the left may normally be slightly larger. Look for abnormal bulging or flattening of the lateral contour. Inspect for retraction of the nipple, skin dimpling or unilateral dilated superficial veins as evidence of underlying disease. Observe if the two nipples are symmetrically placed; asymmetry suggests retraction. Examine for *peau d'orange,* evidence of cutaneous edema. If the patient has noted a lump, ask her to point it out, then palpate the

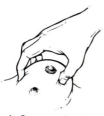

A. Compression to
Show Dimpling

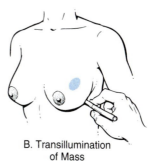

B. Transillumination
of Mass

Fig. 8-59 Further Breast Examination. A. Breast Compression to Accent Dimpling: *Dimpling is a sign of shortening of the suspensory ligaments of the breast from neoplasm or inflammation.* **B. Transillumination**: *The density of a mass may, on occasion, be ascertained by transillumination of the breast; transparency probably means a cyst full of fluid; other masses are opaque.*

opposite breast first. Palpation is performed by compressing breast tissue between the fingers and the chest wall with the hand flat, between the flats of both hands, and between thumb and forefinger. Palpate the tissue carefully in all four quadrants of both breasts searching for increased heat, tenderness, and masses. Squeeze the breast between thumb and finger to bring out dimpling (Fig. 8-59A). If a mass is found, ascertain its location, size, mobility, and consistency. Grasp the mass between thumb and forefinger moving it back and forth transversely, then up and down, to test for fixation to the underlying muscles. Repeat this test after tensing the pectoralis muscle (see below). Gently pinch the overlying skin to determine fixation of the mass to the skin. Transilluminate the mass to determine whether it is opaque or translucent (Fig. 8-59B). When carcinoma of the breast is suspected, metastases to the regional lymph nodes are sought (see page 105).

PATIENT SITTING WITH ARMS RAISED (SEE FIG. 8-58B).   Have the patient raise her arms over her head while you look for a shift in the relative position of the nipples, dimpling, or bulging.

PATIENT SITTING WITH HANDS PRESSING HIPS (SEE FIG. 8-58C).   Have the patient tense the pectoral muscles by pressing her hands downward on her hips. This maneuver may bring out dimpling by putting tension on the breast ligaments, which arise from the pectoralis major fascia. When the mass lies in the axillary tail, tense the serratus anterior muscle by having the patient press her hand downward on your shoulder.

PATIENT SITTING WITH TRUNK BENT FORWARD (SEE FIG. 8-58D).   When the breasts are large and pendulous, have the patient lean forward, supporting herself with her hands on chair arms or on her knees, so the mammae hang free from the chest wall. This posture sometimes facilitates inspection and palpation.

PATIENT SUPINE (SEE FIG. 8-58E).   When the breast is dependent, it may feel nodular because of the constituent fat lobules. The nodularity is less apparent when the patient lies supine and the breast is pressed against the chest wall with the flat of the examining hand. Thus, significant masses become more distinct.

Nipple Examination

Inspect the skin of the anterior trunk for supernumerary nipples. Look for retraction or deformity of the nipple; recent deformities suggest acquired disease. Look for fissures in the nipples. Search for discharge from the nipples by gently compressing the nipple and areola between the thumb and forefinger; note the color of the discharge. Look for dry scaling and red excoriation of the nipple. Palpate the periphery of the areola for tender nodules or cords.

Breast Symptoms

KEY SYMPTOM

Pain in the Breast: The patient with pain or a lump in the breast often fears cancer. It is estimated that more than half of all women will at some time experience breast discomfort significant enough to cause them to seek a physician's advice [Barton MB, Elmore JG, Fletcher SW. Breast symptoms among women enrolled in a health maintenance organization: Frequency, evolution, and outcome. *Ann Intern Med* 1999;130:651–657]. The physical examination helps make the diagnosis, but often confirmation by radiologic and/or pathologic means is required. Common causes of breast pain are engorgement during the luteal phase of the menstrual cycle, pregnancy, hematoma, cysts, mastitis, abscess, galactocele and nipple disorders including fissures, inflammation, and epithelioma. Chronic breast pain (mastodynia) without evident pathology is common.

Breast Signs

KEY SIGN

▶ **Breast Masses:**   *Pathophysiology:*   Masses in the breast may arise from cystic changes, benign proliferation of ductal or acinar tissue, infection, inflammation or fibrosis of the breast stroma, and neoplastic change in the ductal epithelium (ductal carcinoma) or the acinar tissues (lobular neoplasia). Masses in the breast, as elsewhere, must be accurately described noting their location (use the nipple as the center of a clock face: state the o'clock position and the radial distance from the nipple), size, shape, consistency (hard, firm, fluctuant, soft), texture (smooth, irregular), mobility (mobile, fixed to the breast tissue, fixed to the pectoral fascia) and the presence of tenderness. Always thoroughly examine the regional lymph nodes (axillary, infraclavicular and supraclavicular) for lymphadenopathy. Masses in the breast identified by the patient on self-examination or the clinician should never be ignored or assumed to be benign; the patient's age and other risk factors for breast cancer do not play a role in selecting when to evaluate a breast mass.

> *All masses that persist through one complete menstrual cycle, and all masses in postmenopausal women, require evaluation by a clinician experienced in the diagnosis and management of diseases of the breast and breast cancer. The finding of a normal mammogram, or nonvisualization of a palpable mass by ultrasonography, do not exclude the presence of a cancer.*

See page 504 for a discussion of common breast masses.

KEY SIGN
Tender Breasts: *Pathophysiology:* During the luteal phase of the menstrual cycle and with pregnancy and lactation, the breasts undergo glandular proliferation and become larger and more engorged. These changes are associated with increased tenderness. Many women of child-bearing years have persistent tenderness that may vary with the menstrual cycle, but never resolve completely. The breasts may be more firm and lobular on examination, but distinct masses are not felt. The finding is normal and not a cause of concern.

KEY SIGN
Tender Breast Mass: Cyst: *Pathophysiology:* Cystic change in the breast creates single or multiple tender fluid-filled cysts. The patient complains of tenderness that fluctuates with the menstrual cycle. Examination discloses one or more smooth, usually mobile tender tense masses that may be fluctuant or firm. Ultrasonography or needle aspiration confirms the cystic nature of the lesion.

Supernumerary Nipples (Polythelia) and Breasts (Polymastia): *Pathophysiology:* Extra nipples occur frequently in both sexes as minor errors in development; rarely are they associated with glandular tissue to form a complete breast. Commonly, supernumerary nipples are smaller than normal. Often they are mistaken for pigmented moles, but close examination usually discloses a miniature nipple and areola. Most occur in the mammary or milk line on the thorax and abdomen; rarely are they found in the axilla or on the shoulder, flank, groin, or thigh. Their only importance is to distinguish them from moles.

Retraction of Nipples: Inverted Nipples: A common developmental anomaly results in the nipple having a crater-like depression, a harmless variation. Appearance of retraction after maturity should arouse suspicion of underlying neoplastic or inflammatory disease.

▶ KEY SIGN

Retraction of Skin or Nipple: *Pathophysiology:* New onset of retraction of the nipple and skin dimpling are consequences of shortening of the suspensory ligaments of the breast because of underlying tumor or inflammation. Normally the breast is mobile on the chest wall. Inflammatory or malignant disease may cause retraction of breast tissue and/or fixation of the breast to the underlying pectoral fascia. Always examine for skin and nipple retraction. Determine which are present and carefully examine for an underlying mass and regional lymphadenopathy. This can result from previous mastitis; it should only be assumed so if the evolution from acute mastitis to fixation and retraction has been personally observed. Absent this history, this finding should be pursued as you would pursue a breast mass.

Nipple Fissures: Breaks in the skin are usually caused by local infection; their presence may indicate an unsuspected abscess.

Duct Fistula: A chronic draining wound close to the nipple and areola may herald a fistulous tract between an underlying duct and the skin.

KEY SIGN

Breast Secretions: Abnormal secretions from the breast result from a large number of causes. It is important to determine if the secretion is spontaneous or induced. The former is usually of greater consequence than the latter.

KEY SIGN

Serous, Bloody, or Opalescent Breast Fluid: Such secretions may occur with benign or malignant lesions. Benign causes are significantly more common than malignant ones. Bilateral secretion without pregnancy is usually a result of hormonal influences. When unilateral discharge is present, an underlying pathologic condition is more likely. If the cause is not evident from the history or physical examination, cytologic examination of the fluid or biopsy of the breast tissue may be necessary.

✓ *CLINICAL OCCURRENCE:*   Common causes of breast discharge are intraductal papilloma, fibrocystic disease, and sclerosing adenosis. Less-common causes are chronic cystic mastitis, duct ectasia, galactocele, papillary cystadenoma, breast abscess, keratosis of nipple, fat necrosis, acute mastitis, tuberculosis, toxoplasmosis, and eczema of the nipple. Invasive cancers of the breast do not ordinarily cause discharges. Malignant lesions include ductal carcinoma, lobular carcinoma, adenofibrosarcoma, fibrosarcoma, neurosarcoma, and Paget disease of the nipple.

KEY SIGN

Scaling and Excoriation of the Nipple: Paget Disease: *Pathophysiology:* A deep-seated invasive malignancy is present in half the cases, the cells of which have extended along the ductal system and the lactiferous tubules onto the surface of the nipple. As Paget described in his report of 1874, patients experience "tingling, itching, and burning." A scaling eczematoid lesion involves the nipple. Later, the nipple becomes reddened and excoriated; complete destruction of the structure may result. The process extends along the skin as well as in the ducts.

KEY SIGN

Tender Nodule in the Areola: Abscess of the Areolar Gland: The sebaceous glands of Montgomery may become inflamed, forming tender, palpable abscesses in the periphery of the areola. Usually single, these infections may become quite large and invade the breast tissue proper unless incised and drained early. After drainage, a biopsy ought to be performed to rule out an underlying cancer with secondary infection.

Breast Syndromes

The Female Breast

S KEY SYNDROME

Abnormal Lactation: Galactorrhea: *Pathophysiology:* Lactation depends on prolactin from the anterior pituitary and progesterone and estrogen from the ovaries and placenta. Milk ejection is initiated by mechanical stimulation sending afferent impulses to the hypothalamus, causing release of oxytocin from the posterior pituitary. Prolactin levels must be checked in patients with galactorrhea or amenorrhea. Pituitary prolactinomas cause elevated prolactin levels leading to galactorrhea and suppression of ovulation. Many physiologic states, clinical disorders, and drugs may be associated with the secretion of milk [Fiorica JV. Nipple discharge. *Obstet Gynecol Clin North Am* 1994;21:453–460].

✔ *GALACTORRHEA—CLINICAL OCCURRENCE:* *Endocrine* pregnancy, adolescence, hypothyroidism, hyperthyroidism; *Idiopathic* uterine atrophy with amenorrhea and lactation (Frommel disease); *Inflammatory/Immune* mastitis; *Infectious* herpes zoster, postencephalitis; *Metabolic/Toxic* drugs (phenothiazines, reserpine, methyldopa, oral contraceptive, tricyclic antidepressants, antihistamines, opiates); *Mechanical/Trauma* mechanical stimulation of the nipples, suckling, trauma to the chest wall, thoracoplasty, pneumonectomy, mammoplasty, irradiation; *Neoplastic* pituitary prolactinoma.

S KEY SYNDROME

► ▼ **Breast Masses:** *Pathophysiology:* Breast abnormalities may occur when a hormonal signal is abnormal, either too great or too small, or the hormone receptor is unable to respond normally. It may be overly responsive to a completely normal signal, in what has been called "hyperestrinism." *Benign Masses* **Fibrocystic disease** has, in both the professional and lay vernacular, been used to describe a broad spectrum of benign, nonmalignant, pathologic conditions of the female breast. A specific pathologic diagnosis depends on the preponderance of one component over others. If the pathology is confined to stromal proliferation, fibroadenoma, virginal hypertrophy of the breast, and intracanalicular fibroadenoma may be diagnosed. When an abnormal ductal system predominates, microcystic or macrocystic disease, cystic mastitis, sclerosing adenosis, intraductal papilloma, and ductal ectasia involving the lactiferous sinus are terms that are used to describe the changes. If the main source of changes is in the terminal ductules and glandular elements, lobular hyperplasia is identified. Finally, hyperplasia of the myoepithelium leads to a diagnosis of myoepithelial hyperplasia of Reclus. *Premalignant and Malignant Masses* Malignant neoplasms usually arise from the ductal epithelium and have a strong genetic contribution (*BRCA-1, BRCA-2*). The finding of **atypical ductal hyperplasia** is associated with an increased risk of subsequent **in situ or invasive ductal carcinoma**. Neoplasia of the acinar lobules is called **lobular neoplasia**. It is usually noninvasive, but is associated with an increased risk for invasive ductal carcinoma. **Malignant lymphoma** may involve the lymph nodes and other tissues of the breast. For the patient and clinician, it is essential to remember that the primary distinctions are between malignant and nonmalignant conditions and invasive and noninvasive malignancies. Biopsy of discrete, dominant lesions is necessary for correct diagnosis. Only the pathologist can make a histologic diagnosis. Neither the surgeon nor the radiologist can speak with the certainty of the microscopist. Normal or nondiagnostic mammography must not prevent biopsy of a clinically suspicious mass. The only virtue in diagnosing a benign breast condition lies in excluding malignancy. The evaluation of breast masses and their management is constantly evolving. Expert consultation is advised and many specialty breast clinics exist for just this purpose [Donegan WL. Evaluation of a palpable breast mass. *N Engl J Med* 1992;327:937–942].

► **SOLITARY NONTENDER BREAST MASS: CARCINOMA OF THE BREAST:** Usually there is a dominant nontender mass in the breast [Barton MB, Harris R, Fletcher SW. The rational clinical examination. Does this patient have breast cancer? The screening clinical breast exam: Should it be done? How? *JAMA* 1999;282:1270–1280]. Involvement of the suspensory ligaments results in retraction, revealed by dimpling, deviation of the nipples, and fixation to the pectoral muscles. Flattening of the nipple and a bloody or clear discharge indicates the presence of disease in the lactiferous tubules. Lymphatic obstruction produces edema of the skin, manifest by peau d'orange (Fig. 8-60). Lymphatic spread is marked by regional lymphadenopathy. A solitary breast mass mandates a diag-

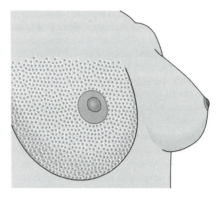

Fig. 8-60 Peau d'Orange. *Cutaneous edema of the breast is indicated by skin that is indented deeply with holes, the accentuated orifices of the sweat glands. This gives the appearance of an orange skin or a pig's skin.*

nostic biopsy. Occasionally, the presenting signs are bloody discharge without a mass, enlarged lymph nodes in the axilla without a mass, or dermal inflammation without a mass. The age of the patient with a palpable breast abnormality can assist in estimating the probable pathology. While the incidence of cancer in a woman younger than 30 years of age is 1%, there is a steady rise with increasing age, and it is now estimated that 1 in 9 or 10 women will eventually develop breast cancer. The median age at which the various pathologic breast abnormalities appear in women is known, and on that basis probabilities are estimated. The data in Table 8-2 is from patients operated on at New York Medical College-Flower Fifth Avenue Hospitals during the period 1960–1975 [Leis HP Jr. The diagnosis of breast cancer. *CA Cancer J Clin* 1977;27:209–232]. *For a complete discussion of breast cancer, see HPIM-16, Chapter 76.*

▶ **INFLAMMATORY MASS: INFLAMMATORY BREAST CARCINOMA:** Malignant neoplasm may present as an acute inflammatory disease, especially in the lactating breast. The signs are similar to those of acute mastitis except that the entire breast is swollen and there is early involvement of the axillary lymph nodes. This is in contrast to acute mastitis, in which the inflammation is usually limited to a single breast quadrant and lymphadenopathy is uncommon.

TABLE 8-2 *Relationship of Breast Abnormalities and Age*

Diagnosis	Age Range (Median)
Fibrocystic disease	20–49 (30)
Fibroadenoma	15–39 (20)
Intraductal papilloma and ductal ectasia	35–55 (40)
Carcinoma	40–71 (54)

FLUCTUANT BREAST MASS: CYST, LIPOMA, ABSCESS: Cysts are very common and must be distinguished from other fluctuant masses, for example, lipomas and abscesses. Fluctuation can be demonstrated by holding the periphery of the mass tight to the chest wall with one hand and pressing the center of the mass with the fingers of the other. Abscess is often quite tender and has other evidence of inflammation, while true lipomas are exceedingly rare, accounting for less than 1% of all breast lesions. Transillumination suggests a cyst while ultrasound or aspiration confirms the diagnosis.

SOLITARY NONTENDER BREAST MASS: FIBROADENOMA: This is usually found in a young woman with large breasts. The ovoid or lobulated nodule is firm, elastic, or rubbery in consistency. It may be the size of a pinhead or quite large. The mass is nontender and freely movable, causing it to slip easily in the breast tissue. The mass must be distinguished from dysplasia, carcinoma, and cystosarcoma phyllodes.

SOLITARY NONTENDER BREAST MASS: FAT NECROSIS: *Pathophysiology:* Breast trauma may produce a hematoma and fat necrosis resulting in a scar that adheres to the surrounding tissue and causes retraction. The finding may suggest carcinoma. A history of trauma should not weigh too heavily in the diagnosis because a common inclination of patients is to attribute neoplastic masses to some remote traumatic incident. Even though this lesion is inconsequential of and by itself, excisional biopsy may be necessary.

INFLAMMATORY MASS: ACUTE MASTITIS: The breast is flushed, tender, hot, swollen, and indurated, frequently accompanied by chills, fever, and sweating. Usually a single breast quadrant is involved. Often the inflammation proceeds to abscess formation. In about two-thirds of the cases, the disease occurs during lactation. Inflammatory carcinoma must be considered, especially in the presence of non-tender axillary lymphadenopathy.

INFLAMMATORY MASS: ACUTE ABSCESS: Usually this is the sequel of acute mastitis. There is a localized, hot, exquisitely tender and painful fluctuant mass frequently accompanied by chills and fever with leukocytosis.

SOLITARY NONTENDER BREAST MASS: CHRONIC BREAST ABSCESS: Pus may become enclosed by a thick wall of fibrous tissue, presenting a nontender, irregular, firm mass requiring biopsy to distinguish from carcinoma.

INFLAMMATORY MASS: JUVENILE MASTITIS: This disease occurs in young boys and in women between 20 and 30 years of age. Signs of inflammation are present in a firm mass beneath the nipple. Usually the involvement is unilateral. The course is a few weeks.

The Male Breast

D KEY DISEASE

Carcinoma of the Male Breast: Approximately 1–2% of carcinomas of the breast occur in men; there is an increased risk with the *BRCA2* mutation. The mass is apparent early because of the paucity of breast tissue. The lesion begins as a painless induration with retraction of the nipple and fixation to the skin and deep tissues. The mass does not transilluminate. It must be distinguished from gynecomastia. Fine-needle aspiration biopsy or excision should be used if doubt exists. Mammography in the male is usually not helpful.

S KEY SYNDROME

▼ **Gynecomastia:** *Pathophysiology:* Breast development is controlled by the circulating level of estrogens. Increased estrogen levels associated with puberty, diseases of the liver, drugs, and endocrine abnormalities can lead to proliferation of breast tissue in men. Gynecomastia is defined as a transient or permanent noninflammatory enlargement of the male breast [Braunstein GD. Gynecomastia. *N Engl J Med* 1993;328:490–495]. Physical examination reveals a finely lobulated subareolar mass that is mobile on the chest wall and is often tender. Increased sensitivity of the nipple is frequently noted by the patient. The mass may be small and unilateral, or can develop bilaterally to the same dimensions as the female breast. Hard masses or those with fixation to the skin or chest wall must be excised to exclude carcinoma.

✔ *GYNECOMASTIA—CLINICAL OCCURRENCE:* The idiopathic type frequently appears at puberty and is usually unilateral. Hormonal stimulation causes bilateral enlargement, for example, administration of estrogens, after castration, Cushing syndrome, and in choriocarcinoma of the testis. Enlargement of the breasts may also occur in cirrhosis of the liver, probably from incomplete hepatic destruction of estrogen. Refeeding gynecomastia occurs when patients with severe malnutrition are given food. Gynecomastia may occur in association with leukemia, lymphoma, pulmonary carcinoma, familial lumbosacral syringomyelia, and Graves disease. Among the drugs occasionally causing gynecomastia are digitalis, isoniazid, spironolactone, phenothiazine, and diazepam.

S KEY SYNDROME

▼ **Acute Mastitis in the Male Breast:** This usually occurs from trauma. The signs are similar to the condition in women. Irritation and chafing of the nipple and breast occur in active sports, like jogging and similar activities.

S KEY SYNDROME

▼ **Inflammatory Mass: Juvenile Mastitis:** This disease occurs in young boys and in women between 20 and 30 years of age. Signs of inflammation are present in a firm mass beneath the nipple. Usually the involvement is unilateral. The course is a few weeks.

9

Abdomen, Perineum, Anus, and Rectosigmoid

Symptoms implicating one or more abdominal organs as the site of disease are common in clinical practice. Because the likelihood of serious disease, its probable site, a possible pathophysiologic scenario for the patient's illness, and the selection of appropriate laboratory and imaging studies to confirm a diagnosis are all judgments based primarily on the history and physical examination, mastering the abdominal evaluation is essential. Diagnosis of abdominal disease relies heavily on an accurate and thorough history. It is essential to delineate the sequence of the patient's symptoms. In addition to the basic examination, the skillful examiner uses special maneuvers to further evaluate findings from the basic examination. Frequent repetition of the abdominal exam and correlation with the patient's symptoms are essential. Correct assessment of abdominal findings requires familiarity with anatomic pathology and pathophysiology. Surgeons must excel in abdominal examination because their findings influence the decision to operate.

In the supine position, the abdominal cavity is a shallow oval basin with a rigid W-shaped bottom of vertebral column and back muscles. Heavy flank muscles constitute the long sides and the diaphragm and pelvic floor muscles close either end. The brim is formed by the lower rib margins at one end, and the pubes and ilia at the other. The cover is formed by the flat muscles and fascia of the anterior abdominal wall, reinforced by two parallel bands of rectus muscles attached to the ends of the basin.

The abdominal viscera are solid or hollow. The solid viscera are the liver, spleen, kidneys, adrenals, pancreas, ovaries, and uterus. Most of these organs retain their characteristic shapes and positions as they enlarge. Many are clustered under the protecting eaves of the lower ribs. The hollow viscera are the stomach, small intestines, colon, gallbladder, bile ducts, fallopian tubes, ureters, and urinary bladder. They are normally not palpable, but when distended by gas or fluid they may be felt.

Two systems have been used to describe abdominal topography (Fig. 9-1). Most physicians prefer the simpler division into quadrants by an axial and a transverse line through the umbilicus; we use that plan in this book.

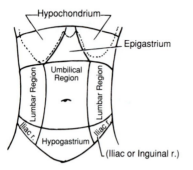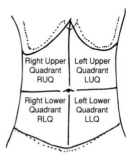

Fig. 9-1 Topographic Divisions of the Abdomen. *On the left are the regions of the abdomen as defined in the Basle Nomina Anatomica (BNA) terminology. Most of the nine regions are small, so that enlarged viscera and other structures occupy more than one. On the right is a simpler plan with four regions; it is preferred by most clinicians and is employed in this book. Many occasions arise when the quadrant scheme needs supplementing by reference to the epigastrium, the flanks, or the suprapubic region.*

Major Systems and Their Physiology

Alimentary System

The alimentary system is responsible for converting ingested foodstuffs into biologically available nutrients and fuels, and for eliminating solid wastes while maintaining a barrier to an enormous variety of microorganisms, parasites, and toxic molecules. This is a complex process involving ingestion, mastication, bulk transport, storage, mixing, digestion, and absorption of nutrients coordinated with production, storage, transport, and carefully timed release of digestive enzymes and bile acids. The alimentary system starts at the mouth and ends at the anus. The oral cavity and pharynx, were discussed previously. Most of the alimentary system is located in the abdomen, extending from the gastroesophageal junction at or near the diaphragmatic hiatus to the anus. Normal motility and digestion are dependent upon coordination of muscular and secretory functions via local and systemic neural and endocrine mechanisms. The bowel is a muscular tube suspended by a mobile mesentery (stomach, small intestine, cecum, transverse and sigmoid colon) or anchored to the posterior abdominal wall (duodenum, ascending and descending colon) or pelvic floor (rectum). It is susceptible to intraluminal obstruction at narrow points (gastroesophageal junction, pylorus, ileocecal valve), to extraluminal obstruction by compression anywhere in its course, and to twisting or kinking when suspended on a mesentery (especially the small bowel, cecum, and sigmoid). Disruption of this system by local or systemic disease results in symptoms and signs referred to the abdomen. Symptoms include changes in appetite and interest in food, changes in abdominal sensations, including pain, and alterations in stool character and frequency. Physical signs are reflective of changes in overall nutrition, abnormal abdominal contour, evidence of altered intestinal motility or obstruction, solid-organ enlargement, increased peritoneal fluid, and localized mass or tenderness.

Hepatobiliary and Pancreatic System

The hepatobiliary–pancreatic system arises from condensation of mesenchymal tissues around embryonic evaginations of the gut (biliary and pancreatic ducts). The pancreas produces bicarbonate and digestive enzymes (amylase, lipase, and proteinases), which are released in response to ingestion of specific foodstuffs and changes in duodenal contents. It also contains the endocrine islets of Langerhans, which release insulin, glucagon, and somatostatin in response to changes in the blood glucose level and a variety of other stimuli. The liver receives venous blood from the gut, pancreas, and spleen via the portal vein, and percolates it from the portal triads through a radial array of sinusoids to the central vein. From the central vein, blood passes to the heart via the hepatic vein and inferior vena cava. Hepatocytes perform three general functions: (a) They remove toxic molecules derived from the intestinal contents and systemic metabolism, process them, and release them back into the circulation or secrete them with the bile. (b) They synthesize many of the molecules necessary for maintenance of systemic homeostasis including albumin, coagulation factors, lipoproteins, and transport molecules. (c) They synthesize and secrete the bile salts that are necessary for digestion and absorption of fats. Kupffer cells are found within the sinusoids. They are phagocytic antigen-presenting cells that clear bacteria from the portal circulation and release cytokines, which enter the systemic circulation. Symptoms related to the hepatobiliary-pancreatic system are changes in general and specific food interest, pain or discomfort associated with the ingestion of food, and maldigestion with changes in bowel function, stool consistency, and frequency. Physical signs relate to (a) changes in the size, consistency, and shape of the liver; (b) to localized pain and masses; and (c) to local and systemic changes caused by alterations in hepatobiliary–pancreatic function, such as jaundice, weight loss, bleeding, and ascites.

Spleen and Lymphatics

See Chapter 5, page 104 for a discussion of the lymph nodes.

The spleen is the largest lymphatic organ. It has a complex sinusoidal structure that serves several functions. Arterial blood is distributed into sinusoids where senescent red blood cells, intracellular inclusions, and membrane abnormalities are removed. The spleen is important in the generation of specific humoral immune responses to encapsulated bacteria and their removal from the blood. The abdominal organs are rich in lymphatics. The lymphatic capillaries drain into regional lymph nodes located at the hila of solid organs and in the mesentery of the bowel. These drain into the periaortic nodes, which also receive lymph from

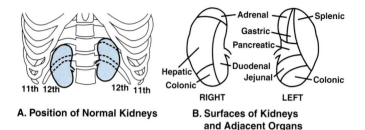

A. Position of Normal Kidneys

B. Surfaces of Kidneys and Adjacent Organs

Fig. 9-2 Anatomic Relations of the Normal Kidneys. A. The Position of the Normal Kidneys as viewed from the anterior surface of the abdomen. Note that the right kidney is lying in front of the twelfth rib, while the slightly higher left kidney is in front of the eleventh and twelfth ribs. B. The Anterior Surfaces of Both Kidneys, showing the regions touched by overlying viscera.

the lower extremities and pelvis. The periaortic nodes drain cephalad toward the thoracic duct. Few specific symptoms arise from alterations in these organs. Enlargement of the spleen will be felt as upper abdominal fullness, and retroperitoneal lymph node enlargement can present as flank and back pressure or pain. Fever, weight loss, and sweats may be the only symptoms of intraabdominal lymphoma. Moderate splenomegaly can be detected by physical exam, but intraabdominal lymph nodes are rarely palpable.

Kidneys, Ureters, and Bladder

See the discussion of urogenital function in Chapter 10. The kidneys are located in the retroperitoneum deep to the lower ribs (Fig. 9-2). The ureters course in the retroperitoneum along, then over, the psoas muscle, over the pelvic brim, and into the pelvis, where they enter the bladder. Symptoms referred to the abdomen arise mostly from obstruction of the renal pelvis or ureter, giving rise to deep, poorly localized visceral pain in the abdomen, flank, pelvis, or testicles. Symptoms referred to the back and flanks include fullness and pain because of kidney enlargement or invasion of adjacent structures by inflammatory, infectious, or neoplastic masses. Physical signs are palpable enlargement of the kidney or bladder, or pain on deep palpation over these structures.

Superficial Anatomy

The Abdomen

It is mandatory to have a thorough mental picture of the location and relative relationships of all abdominal organs, the bowel mesentery and its attachment to the posterior abdominal wall, and the arterial, venous,

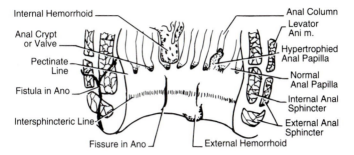

Fig. 9-3 Anatomy of the Anal Canal: Interior and Cross-Section. The anal columns (columns of Morgagni) descend vertically from the rectum and end in anal papillae that fuse to form the pectinate or dentate line; behind are the anal valves (crypts of Morgagni). The cut walls show the internal anal sphincter surrounded by the external sphincter that extends distally. The junction between the edges of the two sphincters forms the intersphincteric line. Internal hemorrhoids arise proximal to the pectinate line, external hemorrhoids distally. Two anal fissures are shown, one distal to a resulting hypertrophied papilla. A fistula (black and irregular) drains from an abscess in a rectal crypt (or valve) to the skin near the anus.

and lymphatic vascular supply of each organ. Next, it is necessary to anchor this picture to the superficial landmarks used during the physical examination: the spine, ribs and costal margins, umbilicus, rectus muscle, inguinal ligament, ilia, and pubes. Lastly, you must accurately associate this picture with the images presented by plain x-ray films, ultrasonography, CT, and MRI images. This is neither simple nor intuitive. The only way to become expert is to repeatedly study textbooks of gross anatomy, review the details of imaging studies with your radiologist, and validate your picture by attending autopsies, reviewing gross dissections, and observing surgical procedures.

The Anus

Figure 9-3 depicts the structure of the anal canal. It is 2.5 to 4 cm long in the adult and is surrounded by two concentric layers of striated muscle—the voluntary external sphincter and the involuntary internal sphincter. A small band of the external sphincter overrides the distal end of the internal sphincter and thus is felt first by the entering finger. The name of the external sphincter refers to its position surrounding the internal sphincter, rather than to its more distal position in the anal canal. The mucocutaneous junction may be inspected without a speculum by everting the anal mucosa.

The Rectum

The rectum is the terminal 12 cm of the colon. It begins at the rectosigmoid junction and ends at the entrance to the anal canal. Near its distal end, it dilates to form the rectal ampulla. In the rectum are found semilunar transverse folds, the valves of Houston, which are inconstant in number and position. Because the combined length of the anal canal and the rectum is approximately 16 cm, the examining finger cannot reach the entire length. The upper two-thirds of the rectum is covered by peritoneum. In men, the anterior peritoneal reflection extends downward as the rectovesical pouch to within 7.5 cm of the anal orifice, so it is potentially accessible to the examining finger. In women, the rectouterine pouch extends downward anteriorly to within 5.5 cm of the anal orifice.

The Sigmoid and Descending Colon

The descending colon starts at the splenic flexure and descends in the retroperitoneum to the left iliac fossa where it becomes the sigmoid colon at the iliac flexure. The sigmoid colon, suspended on its mesentery, extends from the iliac flexure to the rectum. In the pelvis, the sigmoid runs transversely from the left ileum toward the right side of the pelvis, then, doubling on itself, it passes leftward toward the midline, and then downward to meet the rectum at the level of the third sacral vertebra, frequently forming a crude S, from which the name is derived.

Physical Examination of the Abdomen, Perineum, Anus, and Rectosigmoid

The abdomen is usually examined in the following sequence: inspection, auscultation, percussion, palpation. Ensure a warm room and adequate covering so that the patient does not chill and tense the abdominal wall. Have the patient lie supine on the examination table or bed with a pillow under the head. A pillow under the knees, to support passive hip and knee flexion, may add additional comfort and relax the abdominal wall muscles. When orthopnea is present, raise the back rest to support the trunk. Patients with kyphosis require more elevation of the head and shoulders. Drape the abdomen with a sheet or blanket, covering the lower limbs up to the pubes (Fig. 9-4). Cover a woman's breasts with a folded towel or gown. For most purposes, stand at the patient's right side.

The Abdomen

Inspection

Don't slight this informative step in the physical exam because of an urge to start palpating. Effort and discipline are required to inspect properly, thoroughly, and unhurriedly (Fig. 9-5). Arrange a single source of light to shine across the abdomen toward you, or, alternatively, have the light shine lengthwise over the patient. Inspect the abdomen sequentially for distention, contour, scars, engorged veins, visible peri-

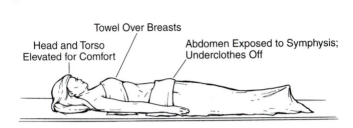

Fig. 9-4 Draping for Abdominal Examination. *The patient lies supine on the examining table with a sheet or blanket covering the lower extremities up to the pubes. For women, the breasts are covered with a folded towel or gown. A small pillow supports the head. To further relax the abdominal muscles, a pillow can be placed to support the knees in slight flexion.*

stalsis, and masses. Additional inspection from the foot of the table can reveal asymmetry of the abdomen and thorax.

THE DISTENDED ABDOMEN. Experience with hundreds of examinations is necessary to learn the normal range of abdominal contour and what constitutes abnormal abdominal distention. Abdominal distention may be caused by several simultaneous conditions, so be thorough and consider all potential contributing conditions.

Auscultation

Auscultation of the abdomen must not be omitted. Only by auscultating as part of *every* abdominal exam can you learn to distinguish normal from abnormal peristaltic sounds and correlate the variety of abnormal sounds with different types of abdominal pathology. Auscultate the abdomen before palpation alters the baseline bowel activity. The patient should be in a quiet room, supine, with the abdominal muscles re-

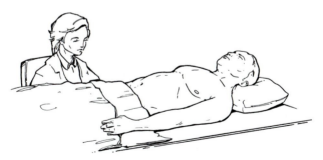

Fig. 9-5 Abdominal Inspection. *The patient is supine with a single source of light shining across from feet to head, or across the abdomen toward the examiner. The examiner should sit in a chair at the right of the patient with her head only slightly higher than the abdomen. In this manner, the physician can concentrate on the abdomen for several minutes, if needed.*

laxed. Listen with the bell of the stethoscope in all four quadrants and the midline.   *Peristaltic Sounds.*   Place the stethoscope bell just below and to the right of the umbilicus and listen. If bowel sounds are not audible, sit and listen for at least 5 minutes. Occasional weak tinkles are not evidence of good peristaltic activity. High-pitched tinkling sounds and rushes may be heard in partial obstruction.   *Abdominal Murmurs.* A murmur indicates turbulent blood flow in a dilated, constricted, or tortuous artery. A murmur is often, but not always, present in an aortic aneurysm.

Percussion

First, ask the patient to point to the area of maximum tenderness. Then ask her to suck in her abdomen while indicating any areas of discomfort. Next, position your hand about 15 cm over the abdomen and ask her to push her stomach out toward your hand, again while indicating any areas of discomfort. Finally, ask her to cough. Because these maneuvers cause movement of peritoneal surfaces without contact by the examiner, pain implies peritoneal inflammation. Percussion of the abdomen is performed as in percussion elsewhere (Chapter 3, page 43). Dullness over the liver in the right upper quadrant (RUQ) and a hollow tympanic note in the left upper quadrant (LUQ) over the stomach should be expected. The remainder of the abdomen usually gives a flat percussion note. Gas in the abdomen or bowel increases the area of tympany. Enlargement of the spleen and bladder is suggested by percussion dullness in the LUQ over the lower ribs (Traube space) and the suprapubic area, respectively. Pain elicited by percussion, especially pain remote to the immediate site of percussion suggests peritoneal inflammation (rebound). Gentle *fist percussion* performed with the heel of the hand on the ribs overlying the liver, spleen, and kidneys (Fig. 9-6) is useful to identify pain caused by stretching or inflammation of the capsules surrounding these organs.   *Percussion and Palpation for Costovertebral Angle Tenderness:*   This is elicited by palpation with one

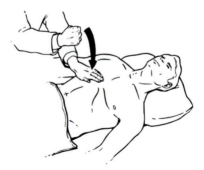

Fig. 9-6 Fist Percussion Over the Liver.   *The palm of the left hand is applied anteriorly to the lower ribs of the right hemithorax. The back of the applied hand is struck lightly with the fist of the right hand.*

finger or thumb. The finger is pressed in a radial direction into the soft tissues enclosed by the costovertebral angle between the spine and the twelfth rib (see Fig. 9-2). Alternatively, the heel of the palm may be used to strike the same point to cause jarring of the surrounding tissues in the area of the kidney.

Palpation

The anterior abdominal wall muscles resist palpation proportionally to their strength and tone. To minimize this resistance, be gentle and reassuring. Conversation with the patient sometimes relaxes her. Reassurance against pain can be imparted with soothing words and a deliberately careful manner. When the usual measures fail, the examiner may press hard on the lower sternum with the left hand while palpating the abdomen with the right. When the patient attempts inspiration against this pressure, she must relax her abdominal muscles.

POSTURE OF THE PATIENT.   Although the abdominal examination is usually performed with the patient supine with flexed hips and knees, be willing and able to employ other positions. Palpation with the patient on either side or in the knee–elbow posture can reveal masses not otherwise discernible. The standing position may be desirable and is mandatory in the proper examination for some hernias.

LIGHT ABDOMINAL PALPATION.   Always palpate the entire abdomen lightly before attempting deep palpation. This scouting expedition will reveal regions of tenderness and increased resistance to be examined later in detail, and sometimes discloses masses that cannot be felt when pushing harder. To palpate lightly, place the entire palm with fingers extended and approximated on the surface of the abdomen. Press the fingertips gently into the abdomen to a depth of about 1 cm (Fig. 9-7A). Begin at the pubes and work upward to the costal margins so that a huge liver or spleen is not missed because the lower edge is not felt. If symptoms or inspection has directed attention to a particular region, examine this area last. Watch the patient's face for evidence of discomfort as you palpate. Forewarned by this gentle preliminary, you can reduce pain and voluntary muscle rigidity that would otherwise limit deeper palpation.   *Ticklishness.*   Some persons, especially children, exhibit tenderness or ticklishness from the lightest abdominal palpation. They flinch, grimace, or tense the muscles so the examiner cannot evaluate underlying tenderness or masses. Such patients usually tolerate an equal amount of pressure from the stethoscope, which can be used to elicit tenderness. Alternatively, have the patient place her fingers on your palpating fingers and follow the motions (Fig. 9-7C); this has the effect of substituting the patient's fingers for yours, to which the patient is not ticklish.

DEEP ABDOMINAL PALPATION.   Pursue the findings from inspection, auscultation, percussion, and light palpation, and search for deep tenderness and masses not previously suspected. Continue to watch the patient's face as you palpate. *Single-handed palpation* is employed with the approximated fingers pressed more deeply than for light palpation. The

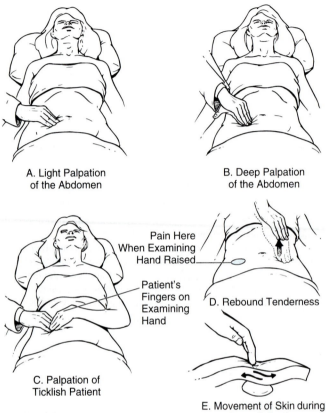

A. Light Palpation
of the Abdomen

B. Deep Palpation
of the Abdomen

Pain Here
When Examining
Hand Raised

Patient's
Fingers on
Examining
Hand

D. Rebound Tenderness

C. Palpation of
Ticklish Patient

E. Movement of Skin during
Deep Palpation

Fig. 9-7 Abdominal Palpation.　A. Light Palpation: Care should be taken
to avoid digging into the wall with the tips of the fingers. *B. Deep Palpation.*
C. Palpation of the Ticklish Abdomen. D. Rebound Tenderness: The hand
is slowly pushed deep into the abdomen remote from the suspected tenderness,
and then abruptly withdrawn. Pain in the affected region results from rebound
of the tissue, usually a sign of peritoneal irritation. *E. Exploration During*
Palpation: When palpating the abdomen, especially deeply, the hand is moved
in a special manner. The fingers remain relatively fixed to a place on the skin,
and the wall of the abdomen is carried with the fingers in a slow gentle to-and-
fro motion to distinguish underlying masses and surfaces. The fingers do not
glide over the skin but carry the skin with them.

hand should be placed so most tactile sensations are received on the
pads of the fingers. In addition to downward pressure, the fingers
should move slowly, laterally, and longitudinally, 4 or 5 cm, causing the
abdominal wall to glide over the underlying structures (Fig.
9-7E). When the muscular resistance is strong, *reinforced palpation* is em-

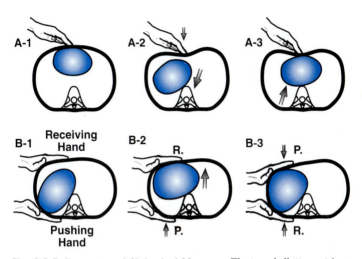

Fig. 9-8 Ballottement of Abdominal Masses. *The term ballottement is applied to two somewhat different maneuvers.* **A. One Hand Ballottement**: *The approximated fingers are abruptly plunged into the abdomen and held there; a freely movable mass will rebound upward and be felt with the fingers. This is most commonly employed to feel a large liver obscured by free fluid in the abdominal cavity.* **B. Bimanual Ballottement**. *B1–2: This is used to determine the size of a large mass in the abdomen. One hand (P) pushes the posterior abdominal wall, while the receiving hand (R) palpates the anterior abdomen. **B3**: The receiving hand is now in the flank, the pushing hand compresses the mass to get an estimate of its thickness.*

ployed. The fingers of the left hand press on the distal phalangeal joints of the right; thus, the left hand produces the pressure while the right hand receives the tactile sensations with its muscles and tendons relatively passive (Fig. 9-7B). When a mass is small, its thickness is determined by grasping it between the thumb, middle, and index fingers; when large, bimanual palpation is employed by placing a hand on each side of the mass. When ascites is present, *ballottement* is useful. The fingers are thrust rapidly and sequentially more deeply into the abdomen in the region of the suspected mass. The mass may tap the tips of the examining fingers (Fig. 9-8).

ATTRIBUTES OF MASSES. When you feel a mass in the abdomen, you must decide which anatomic structure is involved and the nature of the pathologic process. Nearly all masses arise from previously normal tissues. Many inferences may be drawn from the characteristics of a mass. During the examination a complete description of the mass must be obtained; omission of any attribute may lead to erroneous conclusions. *Location.* The location of an abdominal mass suggests the organs to be considered; for example, a mass in the left upper quadrant may be spleen, left kidney, stomach, or colon. *Size.* This gives insight into the pathologic process, its extent and change over time. *Shape.* Some organs have a characteristic shape; for example, kidney, spleen, and liver.   *Consistency.*   The pathologic process may be inferred from the resistance of the mass to pressure; for example, carcinoma may be stony hard, lymphoma rubbery, and abscess soft and fluctuant.   *Surface.*   A smooth surface implies a diffuse homogeneous process, while a nodular surface suggests metastases, granulomas, or irregular fibrosis.   *Tenderness.*   This may be caused by an inflammatory process (infectious or sterile), distention of the capsule of a viscus (e.g., an acutely distended liver), or ischemia.   *Mobility.*   Abdominal viscera suspended by long mesenteries permit them to move. Movement with diaphragmatic respiration suggests association with the liver or spleen or a mobile abdominal organ rather than a retroperitoneal location.   *Pulsatility.* This implies vascular, usually major arterial, association with the mass. Aneurysmal dilation of the aorta or one of its major branches must be assumed until excluded by imaging. Solid masses and tense cysts can transmit normal aortic pulsations, simulating aneurysms.

PALPATION OF THE LEFT UPPER QUADRANT.   Normally, no organs are palpable in this region. The normal spleen lies posterior laterally under the left diaphragm with its surface separated from the chest wall by the lung during deep inspiration. In this position it is not palpable (Fig. 9-9). Its long axis lies parallel to the tenth rib in the midaxillary line. Because of its oblique orientation, the width determines the vertical extent of the area of splenic dullness in the midaxilla. Percussion of this area (Traube space) is a desirable routine. Extension of the area of splenic dullness to obliterate the tympany over the gastric air bubble may be caused by fluid in the stomach or feces in the colon, but finding it should prompt the examiner to search more carefully for a large spleen [Barkun AN, Camus M, Green L, et al. The bedside assessment of splenic enlargement. *Am J Med* 1991;91:512–518]. To feel for a moderately enlarged spleen or left kidney, stand at the right side of the supine patient and use *bimanual palpation*, with the right hand palpating under the costal margin while the left hand lifts gently from the back and the patient inspires deeply (Fig. 9-10). To begin, lay the palm of the right hand on the abdominal wall in the left upper quadrant and place the tips of the approximated index and middle fingers 4–5 cm inferior to the rib margin in the anterior axillary line. Place the palm of the left hand on the left midaxillary region of the thorax, with the fingers curling posteriorly to support the thoracic wall at the eleventh and twelfth ribs. Ask the patient to take a slow deep breath. During inspiration, bring the two hands closer together by lifting the posterior wall with the left hand while gently, but firmly, pushing the approximated fingers of the right hand posteriorly and upward behind the costal margin. When the movement of both hands coincides with the rhythm of inspiration, the descending margin of an enlarged spleen will touch the palpating fingertips. Repeat the procedure with the patient lying partially on his right side. The spleen is more superficial than the left kidney, which is deeper and closer to the midline. Greatly enlarged spleens may be felt without bimanual palpation. The two-handed method is also employed with a type of ballottement (see Fig. 9-8). Place the hands in the position previously described; lift the posterior chest wall with the left hand, but let the right

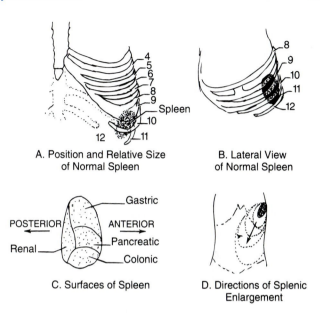

A. Position and Relative Size
of Normal Spleen

B. Lateral View
of Normal Spleen

C. Surfaces of Spleen

D. Directions of Splenic
Enlargement

Fig. 9-9 Anatomic Relations of the Normal and Enlarged Spleen. A. Position of the Normal Spleen, Anterior View: The area of splenic dullness is in the left posterior axilla and usually does not exceed a vertical distance of more than 8 or 9 cm. B. Normal Spleen, Left Lateral View: The spleen lies obliquely with its long axis along the tenth rib, its long borders coinciding with the ninth and eleventh ribs. C. Anterior Surface of the Spleen: The regions touching other viscera are indicated. D. Splenic Enlargement: The directions in which the spleen enlarges are indicated by the dotted lines; the long axis of enlargement points downward and obliquely toward the symphysis pubis.

hand passively receive the impulse from the mass that is pushed forward. In the *Middleton method* for palpating the spleen, the patient lies with his left fist beneath the left thorax (Fig. 9-11). Stand on the patient's left side, facing the patient's feet, and curl your fingers over the left costal margin so that your fingertips are pointing cephalad under the ribs. Feel for the splenic edge during a deep inspiration.

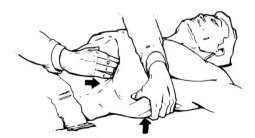

Fig. 9-10 Bimanual palpation of the Left Upper Quadrant.

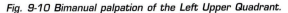

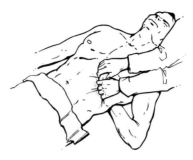

Fig. 9-11 Palpation of the Spleen, Middleton method.

PALPATION OF THE RIGHT UPPER QUADRANT.   The liver, gallbladder, hepatic flexure of the colon, and right kidney are the organs in this region. *Bimanual palpation* is used to detect a normal or mildly enlarged liver. The right hand with fingers adducted is inserted under the right rib margin with the volar surface of the hand touching the abdominal surface; the tactile sensations are received with the fingertips of this hand. The supinated left hand is placed under the right lower thorax. When the patient inspires deeply, the right hand is moved farther upward and inward as the height of inspiration is approached. Simultaneously the right thorax is lifted by the left hand in the direction of the arrow (Fig. 9-12). The maneuver is employed especially in feeling for the liver or right kidney. To avoid missing the edge of an enlarged liver, start palpation in the right lower quadrant (RLQ) and move cephalad.

PALPATION OF THE LOWER QUADRANTS.   Palpation of the right and left lower quadrants is straightforward. There are normally no palpable organs here, except for stool in the colon. Remember that the spine and posterior sacral prominence are easily palpable in thin individuals and should not be confused with masses. Psoas and obturator signs should be performed in patients with abdominal pain (Fig. 9-13). To elicit the *psoas sign*, lay the patient supine or on their side and put the hip through a full range of motion in flexion and extension. Pain suggests inflammation of the psoas muscle or the overlying peritoneum. Repeat on the opposite side. The *obturator sign* is elicited with the patient supine, and

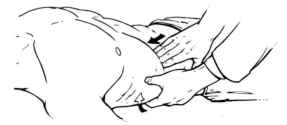

Fig. 9-12 Bimanual Palpation of the Right Upper Quadrant.

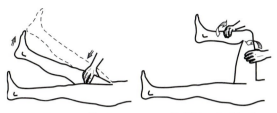

A. Iliopsoas Test   **B. Obturator Test**

Fig. 9-13 Tests for Irritation of the Iliopsoas and Obturator Muscles.
Abscesses in the pelvis may be localized by demonstrating irritation of the more lateral iliopsoas or the medial obturator internus muscles. **A. Iliopsoas Test***: The supine patient keeps his knee extended and is asked to flex the thigh against the resistance of the examiner's hand. Pain in the pelvis indicates irritation of the iliopsoas.* **B. Obturator Test***. The supine patient flexes the right thigh to 90 degrees. The examiner moves the hip in internal and external rotation. Pelvic pain indicates an inflamed muscle. Examine from the side of the limb being tested.*

the hip and knee flexed to 90 degrees. Put the hip through a full range of internal and external rotation; deep pelvic pain suggests inflammation of the obturator muscle or pelvic peritoneum.

EXAMINATION OF THE ABDOMEN AND PELVIS PER RECTUM AND VAGINA. (See Chapter 11, page 626, for the description of the female pelvic exam and Chapter 12, pages 527 and 657, for the description of the male rectal exam). Because the peritoneal cavity extends into the pelvis, masses in the lower abdomen must always be palpated from below the pelvic brim as well as from above (Figs. 9-14 and 9-15). Digital palpation via the rectum and vagina serves three purposes: (a) to detect intrinsic disease of the rectum and vagina; (b) to gain information about adjacent structures of the male and female genitourinary tract; and (c) to examine the lower part of the peritoneal cavity. Errors in the diagnosis of abdominal conditions are notoriously common because these examinations have not been performed. We urge routine vaginal examination as part of every abdominal examination of symptomatic women. When speculum exam cannot be performed, bimanual vaginal exam must still be done. The lithotomy position is preferred for both vaginal and rectal exams because masses will tend to fall upon the examining finger. Have the patient empty her bladder prior to the exam and insist on the presence of a chaperone. With the patient lying supine, have the thighs and knees flexed so the feet rest on the bed or in stirrups. Wear gloves and lubricate the exploring fingers, the index finger for a rectal examination, the index and long fingers for the vagina. In women, palpate the vagina first, then the rectum. Spread the labia minora with the index and long fingers; if the hymen allows, insert both fingers into the vagina. Palpate the cervix, body, and fundus of the uterus, the adnexa, and bladder. Palpate the lateral fornices and the rectouterine pouch of Douglas for masses and tenderness. For the abdominal–rectal examination of both sexes,

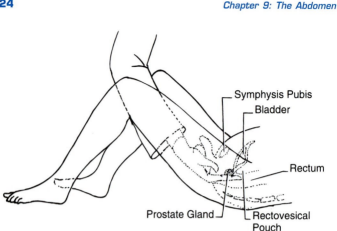

Fig. 9-14 Palpation of the Male Abdomen Per Rectum. *The examining hand is supinated. Anteriorly, the finger pad feels the prostate gland and seminal vesicles. Superiorly on the anterior rectal surface, the fingertip reaches the location of the rectovesical pouch of the peritoneum. Normally, this pouch is not palpable; in the presence of pus or a tender mass it may be perceived. Cancer cells may settle in this pouch from the abdominal cavity, producing a hard, nontender, transverse ridge, called a rectal shelf or Blumer shelf.*

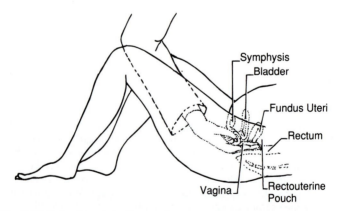

Fig. 9-15 Palpation of the Female Abdomen Per Rectum. *The finger pad feels the cervix uteri and the fundus uteri through the anterior rectal wall. Passing the finger inward, superior to the cervix, the fingertip reaches the location of the rectouterine pouch (Douglas pouch). Normally, this is not palpable; a tender mass is evidence of pus. See legend of Fig. 9-14 for Blumer shelf.*

place the palm of the examining hand toward the perineum and lay the pad of the index finger on the anus, gently pressing toward the perineal body so the anal sphincter relaxes to admit the tip of the finger. To avoid anal spasm be gentle while slowly advancing the finger into the anal canal as far as possible (see also *anal palpation*, page 526). To accomplish bimanual palpation, palpate between the fingers of the left hand pressing into the suprapubic region of the abdominal wall. Be ready to perform tests for occult fecal blood. When the exam is complete, either wipe the anus or provide papers or sponges for the patient to do so.

EXAMINATION FOR ABDOMINAL HERNIAS. (See pages 602ff.) Hernias are protrusions of abdominal contents through a weak point in the abdominal wall. In most cases, the hernia has a peritoneal sac, which may contain bowel, stomach, omentum, urinary bladder, colon, or even liver.

Inspection is the first procedure in examination for hernia. If the patient has suspected a problem, have the patient demonstrate his observation. Many hernias are encountered unexpectedly during routine examination of the supine patient. A bulge may be seen at rest, or it may appear during maneuvers that increase intraabdominal pressure. Palpate the defect in the abdominal wall and its contents; insert a finger in the defect and feel for an impulse when the patient coughs or performs a Valsalva maneuver. Omentum feels soft and nodular, whereas bowel is smooth and fluctuant. Gas in a herniated loop may cause crepitation and peristaltic sounds. If the hernia can be easily pushed back into the abdomen, it is said to be reducible; if it cannot be easily pushed back into the abdomen, the hernia is irreducible or incarcerated.

ZIEMAN INGUINAL EXAMINATION. This procedure reveals direct and indirect inguinal hernias, as well as hernias of the femoral triangle. With the patient standing, stand at the patient's right side and place the palm of your right hand against the right lower abdomen. Spread your fingers slightly so that your long finger lies along the inguinal ligament with its pulp in the external inguinal ring, your index finger is over the internal inguinal ring, and your ring finger palpates the region of the femoral canal and the opening of the saphenous vein (Fig. 12-5B). Have the patient take a deep breath, hold it, and bear down, as if to have a bowel movement. Then repeat the maneuver, standing at the patient's left side and palpating the patient's left groin with your left hand. A hernia in any of the three sites is perceived either as a gliding motion of the walls of the empty sac or as a protrusion of a viscus into the sac. When the internal ring is closed by the palpating finger, any herniating mass cannot be an indirect inguinal hernia.

Examination of the Perineum, Anus, Rectum, and Distal Colon

The patient may be examined in several positions, each with its advantages and disadvantages (Fig. 9-16). The standing position, with the patient leaning over and resting the trunk on a table, may be employed for speculum examination and palpation of the rectum. The left lateral

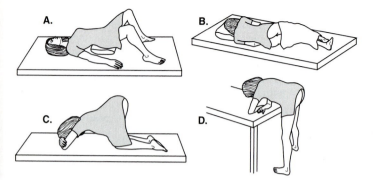

Fig. 9-16 Positions of the Patient for Rectal Examination. *A. Modified Lithotomy Position. B. Left Lateral Prone Position (Sims Position). C. The Knee–Chest Position. D. Bent Over the Table.*

prone (Sims) and bent-over-table positions permit adequate inspection of the perianal region and the anal mucosa with a speculum, and palpation of the anal canal and rectum is feasible. These positions are inadequate for bimanual palpation of the peritoneal contents through the rectum (see page 523). The lithotomy position can be used when inspection of the anal canal is not required. Examination in this position is facilitated by having the buttocks raised on an overturned bedpan or pillow. The knee–chest or knee–elbow position is uncomfortable for the patient and should be reserved for anoscopy and sigmoidoscopy.

INSPECTION OF THE PERINEUM. Whatever position is selected for the patient, the buttocks should be spread wide apart. Inspect the skin of the perineum and perianal region for signs of local inflammation, sinuses, fistulas, excoriations, hemorrhoids, masses, and cutaneous lesions.

Examination of the Anus

ANAL PALPATION. Reassure the patient and have the patient breathe normally through the patient's mouth. After gloving both hands, palpate the perineum gently around the orifices of sinuses and fistulas feeling for subcutaneous cords that indicate the direction of tracks. Palpate any bulges in the perineal tissue and the tissue around the anal orifice seeking firm fluctuant or tender abscesses. Palpate carefully between the anus and the ischial tuberosities searching for ischiorectal abscesses. Next, lubricate the gloved examining finger and place the pad of the finger on the anal sphincter (Fig. 9-17). Exert gentle pressure, directed inward and somewhat anteriorly, until the sphincter relaxes, admitting the pad followed by the tip of the finger. Gradually insert the finger as far as possible while palpating the walls and estimating the length of the canal and the sphincter tone. When inserting a finger or instrument it is important to remember that the anal canal slants anteriorly, so the

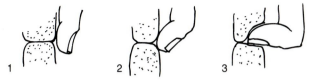

Fig. 9-17 Insertion of the Gloved Finger into the Anus. *(1) The pad of the gloved index finger is placed gently over the orifice, until the external sphincter is felt to relax. (2) and (3) Rotate the tip of the finger into the axis of the canal and insert gently. The entire procedure should be slow and gentle.*

axis of entry should point toward the umbilicus. Proper examination is not painful unless a fissure in ano or a thrombosed hemorrhoid is present. To feel the abscess causing a fistula, use bidigital palpation between the index finger in the canal and the thumb on the skin of the perineum. Be sure that there is a clear indication before performing a rectal examination on a patient with neutropenia.

ANOSCOPIC EXAMINATION. The anal canal is not inspected routinely and can only be viewed with a speculum. This is indicated when external signs, palpable masses in the canal, sphincter spasm, pain, or bleeding direct attention to the region. Although the proctoscope or the sigmoidoscope may be used, the anoscope is specifically designed for the procedure. It is a tube fitted with an obturator whose tip is conical; it is available in many styles and sizes. Plastic disposable anoscopes have the advantage of allowing visualization through the walls of the speculum. Anoscopic examination can only proceed after palpation has demonstrated no obstruction. The patient is placed in the left lateral, the knee–chest, or standing position (see Fig. 9-16). A good light must be available. With the obturator in place and the instrument well lubricated, the tip and tube are gently inserted through the sphincter, aiming toward the umbilicus. With the tube fully inserted, the obturator is removed and the walls of the canal are inspected as the tube is slowly withdrawn.

Examination of the Rectum

Three distinct and separate purposes are served in examination of the rectum: (a) palpation of the contents of the lower peritoneal cavity; (b) palpation of the adjacent internal genital organs in males and females; and (c) examination of the walls of the rectum itself. Although these three purposes are served in one examination, it is useful to consider each separately: as a part of the abdominal examination (see page 523), as a procedure in the examination of the genital organs, or as a search for intrinsic disease of the rectum.

RECTAL PALPATION. This is a continuation of palpation of the anal canal; the finger is merely pushed beyond the rectoanal junction, and the walls

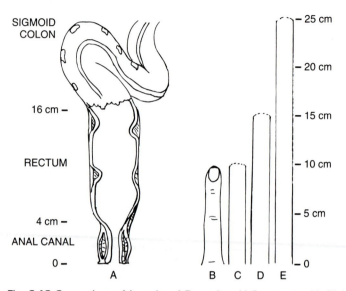

*Fig. 9-18 Comparison of Lengths of Rectosigmoid Segments with Rigid Examining Instruments. All lengths are drawn to scale. **A.** The rectosigmoid is shown with the anal canal of 4 cm, the rectum and valves of Houston of 12 cm, and the lower part of the sigmoid colon, whose total length is 40 cm. **B.** An average index finger, 10 cm long and 22 mm in diameter. **C.** A typical anoscope, 9 cm, with an added 1 cm of curved obturator. **D.** A proctoscope of 15 cm. **E.** Rigid sigmoidoscope of 25 cm. The fiberoptic flexible instruments are considerably longer.*

of the ampulla are felt. After entering the rectum in the male, the finger sequentially palpates on the anterior wall, the prostate gland, the seminal vesicles, and the rectovesical pouch. Posteriorly is the hollow of the sacrum and the coccyx. The lateral walls are also examined. On the anterior wall of the female, one encounters, in sequence, the uterine cervix, the uterine fundus (if retroverted), and the rectouterine pouch. The rectal wall is palpated for masses and narrowing of the lumen.

Examination of the Sigmoid Colon

The rectosigmoid and descending colon are accessible to inspection through the sigmoidoscope. The flexible sigmoidoscope has replaced rigid instruments, which restricted inspection to about 25 cm (Fig. 9-18). The flexible sigmoidoscope gives the examiner a wide field of view and can usually be advanced without anesthesia to the splenic flexure. Sigmoidoscopic examination is an exceedingly useful aid in diagnosing colonic disease. Because the sigmoidoscopy is employed without anesthesia, it should be considered part of the examination of the abdomen.

Specific indications for sigmoidoscopy are beyond the scope of this text. Please refer to appropriate texts for techniques of examination and interpretation of findings at sigmoidoscopy.

Abdominal, Perineal and Anorectal Symptoms

General Symptoms

KEY SYMPTOM

Six-Dermatome Pain: Esophageal Discomfort: See *Six Dermatome Pain*, Chapter 8, page 374, and page 563.

KEY SYMPTOM

▶ **Acute Abdominal Pain:** See also page 562ff. *Pathophysiology:* It is important to understand the physiology of pain specific to each organ and site in the abdomen. For instance, distention of the bowel produces pain, whereas mechanical laceration does not. In general, pain arising in the viscera and transmitted in the vagal visceral afferent nerves and sympathetic afferent nerves give sensations of deep, boring, poorly localized pain that is frequently accompanied by autonomic features such as nausea, vomiting, and diaphoresis. Pain transmitted via the spinal somatic afferent nerves innervating the body wall and peritoneum is generally described as sharp and well localized to the anatomic site of the inflammation or injury. This is a complex subject, the details of which are beyond the scope of this book, but knowledge of the innervation of each abdominal organ (somatic versus visceral, vagus, and/or sympathetic) will help the examiner understand the nature and pattern of the patient's pain history. Severe, acute abdominal pain can herald a variety of disorders from the benign to the immanently life-threatening; this situation is known in surgical slang as the acute abdomen. The specific diagnosis must be sought with a sense of urgency, because early surgical intervention may be lifesaving in some disorders (leaking abdominal aortic aneurysm, appendicitis) and contraindicated in others (acute intermittent porphyria, sickle cell crisis). Great reliance is necessarily placed on history and physical examination. Some assistance is obtained from imaging examinations, while laboratory tests are less important. A careful history and personally repeated examinations over a few hours, be it day or night, are mandatory. Of particular importance are the locations of the pain and tenderness (Fig. 9-19), any change in location, and their variations in quality during the period of observation. Relatively few findings may distinguish several conditions. For example, the patient with intraabdominal visceral pain may walk about, but when the viscus perforates, causing peritonitis, the patient lies very still in bed. Usually the severity of the symptoms brings the patient to the physician within a few hours of onset. Acute processes or acute complications of chronic diseases are most

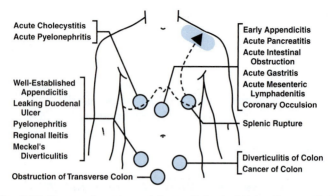

Fig. 9-19 Common Locations of Acute Abdominal Pain. *In general, the painful spot is also tender, but not always. Note especially that the pain of acute appendicitis is in the epigastrium early and later in the right lower quadrant. Pain in the spleen commonly radiates to the top of the left shoulder. These pains are ordinarily constant, in contrast to the intermittent pain of colic.*

likely. Pain increased with walking, jumping, sneezing, or coughing is equivalent to the jar test (page 551) and suggests the presence of peritoneal inflammation [Spiro HM. An internist's approach to acute abdominal pain. *Med Clin North Am* 1993;77:963–972]. A pregnancy test must be obtained in *all* women of childbearing age with acute abdominal pain.

✓ **CLINICAL OCCURRENCE:**   See *Acute Abdominal Pain Syndromes* pages 562.

◢ KEY SYMPTOM
◣ Chronic   and   Recurrent   Abdominal   Pain:
Pathophysiology: Chronic pain is physiologically different from acute pain. The role of conditioning in the spinal cord and thalamus in the setting of chronic pain are under study, as is the decreased threshold to the perception of pain with visceral stimulation in some individuals with chronic abdominal pain. The pattern of pain and associated symptoms will help to make inferences about the possible pathophysiology, while the location of the pain suggests the organs involved. Pain that is vague in onset but steadily worsens over time suggests a progressive anatomically advancing obstructive lesion or mass effect. Intermittent pain separated by periods free of pain suggests painful smooth-muscle contraction or dynamic obstruction, recurrent inflammation or ulceration, and relapsing infection. Careful history is required to identify precipitating factors (e.g., meals and type of food), timing (e.g., relation to menstrual cycle, starting new medications), and previous surgeries, symptoms, or illnesses that could help explain the current problem (e.g., adhesions from surgery or irradiation, trauma, infections, and travel). It is important to recognize that nonspecific abdominal and pelvic pain is a common symptom in persons with histories of current or previous abuse.

An empathetic, nonjudgmental history with specific questions relating to current safety, sexual practices, sexual abuse, and physical or emotional abuse is essential. Up to 30% of women presenting to a physician in the ambulatory setting have a history of abuse, and and one-third of these have been abused within the last 12 months. The link between abuse and abdominal pain is not clear; it is clear that many thousands of dollars are frequently wasted on fruitless undirected laboratory and imaging investigations when an explanation can be found with a few minutes of history and physical examination. If the history and physical exam do not suggest specific leads for further investigation, a barrage of laboratory and imaging tests are extremely unlikely to be helpful. There is a tendency to project pain inward to intraabdominal structures when it actually arises from the abdominal wall. Make the effort to think of disorders of the abdominal wall; this will avoid many unnecessary studies.

✓ **CLINICAL OCCURRENCE:** See *Chronic Abdominal Pain Syndromes* pages 576ff.

KEY SYMPTOM

Abdominal Wall Pain: *Pathophysiology:* Injury to the muscles, nerves, skin, and soft tissues of the abdominal wall, and referral of pain from the bones, nerve roots, and soft tissues of the spine, commonly present as complaints of abdominal pain. Well-localized (finger-tip precise) pain suggests somatic pain in the body wall. Band-like pain described as wrapping around the body suggests neuropathic pain or sclerotomal pain from bone lesions at that segmental level. Make the effort to think of disorders of the abdominal wall; this will avoid many unnecessary studies.

✓ **CLINICAL OCCURRENCE:** *Congenital* urachus abnormalities; *Idiopathic* xiphodynia; *Inflammatory/Immune* suture abscess, mononeuritis, polyneuritis, diabetic polyradiculopathy and amyotrophy, myositis; *Infectious* abscess, herpes zoster, pyomyositis; *Metabolic/Toxic* diabetic neuropathy; *Mechanical/Trauma* abdominal cutaneous nerve entrapment (rectus abdominis nerve entrapment syndrome), abdominal wall hernia, abdominal wall muscle tear, rib cartilage injury, rib tip syndrome, spinal disc herniation, burns, retention sutures, foreign bodies; *Neoplastic* desmoid tumors, lipoma, sarcoma, metastases; *Neurologic* complex regional pain syndrome, postherpetic neuralgia, mononeuritis multiplex, diabetic amyotrophy; *Psychosocial* abuse, somatization, malingering; *Vascular* vasculitis with mononeuropathy or polyneuropathy.

KEY SYMPTOM

Regurgitation: See *Heartburn*, page 533. *Pathophysiology:* Regurgitation is reflux of esophageal and stomach contents back into the mouth or upper airway without active vomiting. It is passive and occurs under the influence of normal body positions and activities, suggesting loss of function of the normal esophageal sphincters or increased intraabdominal pressure. Unlike vomiting, regurgitation may not be volunteered by the patient as a major complaint; you must seek it in the history. Particular attention should be paid to regurgitation at night, with recumbency and after meals. Regurgitation of stomach contents while fasting produces a sour bitter taste (water brash or pyrosis), whereas regurgitation after eating will return food. Regurgitation of food more than 2 hours after eating suggests delayed gastric emptying.

✔ *REGURGITATION—CLINICAL OCCURRENCE:* *Congenital* abnormal lower esophageal sphincter (LES) and upper esophageal sphincter tone; *Idiopathic* decreased LES tone with or without hiatal hernia; *Inflammatory/Immune* esophagitis; *Metabolic/Toxic* alcohol, tobacco, caffeine, uremia; *Mechanical/Trauma* achalasia, gastric outlet and upper intestinal obstruction, gastroparesis; *Neoplastic* esophageal or gastric cardia cancer.

KEY SYMPTOM
◤Nausea and Vomiting: *Pathophysiology:* Nausea is an unpleasant sensation referred to the stomach and suggesting that vomiting is imminent. Vomiting is an involuntary integrated movement of pharyngeal and thoracoabdominal smooth and voluntary muscles to expel stomach contents. Nausea and vomiting are triggered by cortical (emotional), gastrointestinal, vestibular, and chemical (via the CNS chemoreceptor trigger zone) stimuli, and vomiting is coordinated by the brainstem. The violence and discomfort of nausea and vomiting often make them a presenting complaint. Vomiting is usually preceded by nausea. The history should include inciting events and exposures, the nature of the vomitus and its relationship to meals. **Variants of Vomiting:** *Projectile Vomiting* is a particularly forceful type associated with increased intracranial pressure and lacking antecedent nausea. *Retching* involves all movements of vomiting except that gastric contents are not expelled.

✔ *CLINICAL OCCURRENCE:* *Congenital* pyloric stenosis; *Endocrine* adrenal insufficiency, pregnancy; *Idiopathic* peptic ulcer, pyloric stricture, gastroparesis, other GI motility disorders (e.g., scleroderma, pseudoobstruction), Ménière disease, glaucoma; *Inflammatory/Immune* numerous disorders of the alimentary canal, biliary system, and pancreas, for example, hepatitis, pancreatitis, peritonitis; *Infection* viral gastroenteritis, CNS infections; *Metabolic/Toxic* bacterial food poisoning; opiates, ipecac, chemotherapy agents, macrolide antibiotics, chemical toxins, many more; uremia, hepatic failure, ketoacidosis; *Mechanical/Trauma* upper gastrointestinal obstruction; *Neoplastic* brain tumors, primary or metastatic; *Neurologic* autonomic reflexes associated with visceral stimulation, for example, myocardial infarction, ureteral stone, biliary colic, postvagotomy, head injury with concussion, intracranial mass; *Psychosocial* offensive tastes, odors, and sights; severe pain; psychogenic; *Vascular* myocardial infarction, superior mesenteric ischemia (arterial or venous), migraine.

KEY SYMPTOM
◤Abdominal Bloating: See *Distended Abdomen*, page 541. *Pathophysiology:* The sensation of bloating can be caused by increased

gaseous distention of the bowel, increased sensitivity to normal bowel gas, enlargement of abdominal or pelvic organs, ascites, or masses. Patients often try to induce burping, during which they swallow more gas. Smoking and chewing gum are other causes of swallowed gas. Patients with the irritable bowel syndrome have pain and complaints of distention at volumes of intestinal gas not sensed by others.

Site-Attributable Symptoms

KEY SYMPTOM
Belching, Flatus and Sensible Peristalsis: See *Bloating Syndromes*, page 581, and *Tympanites*, page 549.

KEY SYMPTOM
Heartburn: *Pathophysiology:* Regurgitation of gastric acid or bile produces chemical imitation in the esophagus with or without esophagitis. Patients complain of burning retrosternal pain aggravated by alcohol, tobacco, caffeine and obesity, frequently occurring after meals. Symptoms increase with recumbancy and are decreased by antacids. Gastroesophageal reflux due to decreased lower esophageal sphincter tone is the most common cause.

KEY SYMPTOM
Difficulty Swallowing: Dysphagia: See also Chapter 7, page 233. *Pathophysiology:* Swallowing is a complex neuromuscular act involving both striated muscles under conscious control and smooth muscle innervated by the autonomic system and the intestinal myenteric plexus. Abnormalities in voluntary motor function of the pharynx, smooth-muscle function, salivary function, or mechanical obstructions in the pharynx or esophagus lead to complaints of dysphagia. Have the patient indicate the level where they feel the difficulty. Ask if the problem is more with liquids or solids. DDX: Ask whether they have coughing or choking with swallowing, which indicates a pharyngeal or laryngeal problem. If they regurgitate food after meals, it may indicate esophageal obstruction by mass or achalasia. If pain is present (odynophagia), then infection, neoplasm, or erosive disease is likely.

KEY SYMPTOM
Dysphagia with Six-Dermatome Pain Dysphagia: Dysphagia Lusoria (Aberrant Right Subclavian Artery): See Chapter 7, page 327. Pain is rarely present, and dysphagia is the only symptom. This prompts the making of an esophagram that shows a transverse band of indentation in the esophagus produced by the anomalous right subclavian artery.

KEY SYMPTOM
Pain with Swallowing: Odynophagia: See *Six-Dermatome Pain with Dysphagia in Syndromes*, page 563–564.

►
Hematemesis: *Pathophysiology:* Blood in the emesis indicates recent or active bleeding in the nose, oral cavity, pharynx, esophagus, stomach, duodenum, or, less frequently, the tracheobronchial tree. Bright red blood is arterial whereas dark blood is either venous or has been in the stomach for some time. Gastric acid and pepsin give blood a brown "coffee grounds" appearance after a longer period of time. Ask the patient to estimate the volume of blood lost. Patients frequently overestimate the amount, especially if mixed with water, as in a sink or toilet bowl. Occasionally, the patient has difficulty in distinguishing between hematemesis and hemoptysis (coughing up blood), especially when coughing induces vomiting. Hematemesis following prolonged and violent retching or vomiting is characteristic of a linear tear of the mucosa at the esophagogastric junction (Mallory-Weiss tear). If a bleeding site is not evident in the nose, mouth, or pharynx, upper endoscopy should be performed for diagnosis and possible therapy.

✓ *HEMATEMESIS—CLINICAL OCCURRENCE:* *Congenital* hereditary hemorrhagic telangiectasia (Osler-Weber-Rendu); *Endocrine* gastrinoma (Zollinger-Ellison syndrome), hyperparathyroidism; *Idiopathic* peptic ulcer, duodenal diverticulum, gastritis; *Inflammatory/Immune* gastritis, esophagitis; *Infectious* *Helicobacter pylori* ulcers; *Metabolic/Toxic* NSAID (nonsteroidal antiinflammatory drug) gastropathy; *Mechanical/Trauma* Mallory-Weiss tear, portal hypertension (esophageal and gastric varices), foreign bodies, gallstone erosion; *Neoplastic* cancer of the esophagus, stomach, and pancreas; *Psychosocial* factitious; *Vascular* arteriovenous malformations, gastric antral vascular ectasia (GAVE), esophageal and gastric varices, portal gastropathy, thrombocytosis, coagulation defects.

Small Intestine and Colon

▼
Diarrhea: Diarrhea is defined as >200 g of stool per day on a Western low-residue diet. It is also used to describe watery or loose stools, and some patients will use the term to describe increased stool frequency. *Pathophysiology:* Increased volume of fecal output accompanied by increased water loss in the stools has several general pathophysiologic causes. **Osmotic diarrhea** results from ingestion of nonabsorbable osmotically active solutes that draw water into the bowel and retain it there. **Secretory diarrhea** results when the normal secretions into the bowel are increased (e.g., Zollinger-Ellison syndrome) or the bowel abnormally secretes fluid into the lumen (e.g., cholera). **Inflammatory/immune diarrhea** results from inflammation of the bowel wall leading to exudation of fluid, proteins and cells into the lumen, usually combined with increased motility and decreased absorption because of the same injury. **Increased bowel motility** from any cause will decrease the time available for absorption of solutes (small intestine) or water (colon) leading to diarrhea (e.g., dumping syndrome, laxative abuse). **Malabsorption and maldigestion** result in diarrhea, the former from loss of effective absorptive surface (e.g.,

celiac disease), the latter from inadequate digestion of ingested food (e.g., pancreatic insufficiency). **Short bowel syndrome** results in loss of absorptive surface from surgical resection or surgical or pathologic fistulas and from bile acid malabsorption producing colonic irritation. First, determine exactly what the patient means by diarrhea, and decide if the diarrhea is acute, chronic, or recurrent. Second, obtain a detailed description of the stools, their frequency and pattern. Ask specifically about nocturnal diarrhea, which is always pathologic. Third, focus the history on exposures, such as travel and drugs, previous surgery, dietary habits, contact with others with a similar illness, and associated symptoms such as anorexia, nausea, vomiting, fever, weight loss, or abdominal pain. You should have a good working hypothesis as to the pathophysiologic mechanism of the diarrhea on completion of the history. On physical exam look for fever and signs of weight loss or volume depletion, increased bowel motility (borborygmi), and abdominal tenderness. For suspected viral diarrhea, laboratory evaluation is usually not required. If you suspect a bacterial or protozoal etiology, stool culture and tests for bacterial and protozoal antigens are necessary. You should always inspect a typical stool yourself. Diarrhea in persons infected with HIV is a complex clinical problem with multiple infectious and noninfectious causes. Consultation with a specialist in HIV-related diseases is recommended. *Patterns:* Recognition of several relatively distinct diarrheal syndromes can be helpful in forming a concise differential diagnosis: acute diarrhea; dysentery syndrome; diarrhea with maldigestion/malabsorption; steatorrhea; diarrhea with weight loss; diarrhea with bloody stools. See Diarrhea Syndromes, page 582ff, for discussion of these syndromes and specific diseases.

KEY SYMPTOM

Constipation: *Pathophysiology:* Bowel motility is under autonomic control and requires an intact myenteric plexus. Multiple factors, including luminal contents, drugs, emotional state, physical activity level, and acquired habits (bowel training), affect the frequency of stooling and the character of the stool. Each of these factors must be investigated in the evaluation of constipation, and several may be operative at one time. First, determine by history of the patient's baseline bowel movement pattern, the onset of the current difficulty, and any therapeutic interventions they have undertaken. Patients and physician use the term "constipation" to mean any combination of infrequent stools, hard desiccated stools, or stools that are difficult to pass for whatever reason. Many people do very well with two or three evacuations a week. Patients often describe the gradual development of a sensation of abdominal fullness. Acute or subacute constipation developing on a lifelong history of normal movements requires investigation; chronic constipation of years' duration may indicate an underlying disorder of the bowel wall or a gut motility problem.

✔ **CONSTIPATION—CLINICAL OCCURRENCE:** *Congenital* Hirschsprung disease; *Endocrine* hypothyroidism, hyperparathyroidism, pregnancy;

Idiopathic intestinal pseudoobstruction; diverticulosis, diverticulitis; *Inflammatory/Immune* scleroderma (progressive systemic sclerosis), amyloidosis; *Infectious* Chagas disease, toxic megacolon; *Metabolic/Toxic* drugs, including opiates, anticholinergics, tricyclic antidepressants, and many others; hypokalemia, hypomagnesemia, hypocalcemia; *Mechanical/Trauma* excessive fiber intake, mechanical obstruction by stricture or mass, irradiation, anal fissure; *Neoplastic* colon polyps and cancers; *Neurologic* spinal cord injury, sacral plexus lesions, multiple sclerosis, Parkinson disease, irritable bowel syndrome; *Psychosocial* eating disorders, substance abuse (opiates), depression; *Vascular* stroke.

KEY SYMPTOM
Fecal Incontinence: *Pathophysiology:* Loss of control of defecation can result from severe diarrhea of any cause, rectal inflammation, damage to the anal sphincters, or loss of normal sensory, autonomic, or voluntary muscle function. Vaginal delivery commonly injures the anal sphincter and pelvic nerves accounting for the large female predominance of this problem [Sultan AH, Kamm MA, Hudson CN, et al. Anal-sphincter disruption during vaginal delivery. N Engl J Med 1993;329:1905–1911]. Fecal and urinary incontinence are most common in women, especially those in institutions [Chassagne P, Landrin I, Neveu C, et al. Fecal incontinence in the institutionalized elderly: Incidence, risk factors, and prognosis. *Am J Med* 1999;106:185–190]. Evaluation of mental status, vaginal speculum and bimanual exam, and neurologic exam, including anal sensation and sphincter tone and strength during rectal exam, are necessary. Look for dementia, a flaccid anal sphincter, rectocele, rectal prolapse, impacted feces, mass, and neurologic deficit of the sacral nerves. Further evaluation requires specialty consultation [Rudolph W, Galandiuk S. A practical guide to the diagnosis and management of fecal incontinence. *Mayo Clin Proc* 2002;77: 271–275; Hirsh T, Lembo T. Diagnosis and management of fecal incontinence in elderly patients. *Am Fam Physician* 1996;54:1559–1564, 1569–1570].

✔ *FECAL INCONTINENCE—CLINICAL OCCURRENCE:* *Congenital* cerebral palsy, mental retardation, meningomyelocele; *Endocrine* hyperthyroidism; *Idiopathic* amyloidosis; *Inflammatory/Immune* ulcerative colitis, Crohn disease, ulcerative proctitis, microscopic colitis, amyloidosis; *Infectious* herpes simplex, gonorrhea or cytomegalovirus proctitis, dysentery syndrome caused by bacterial infection, infectious diarrhea, perirectal abscess; *Metabolic/Toxic* drugs, especially cathartics, laxative abuse; *Mechanical/Trauma* fissure, fistula, fecal impaction, pelvic floor relaxation, rectal prolapse, rectocele; *Neoplastic* anal or rectal carcinoma, metastatic invasion of the sacral plexus or spinal cord; *Neurologic* dementia, cauda equina syndrome, transverse myelitis, sacral plexopathy, weakness or immobility, peripheral neuropathy including diabetes, postherpetic neuralgia; *Psychosocial* psychosis; *Vascular* ischemic colon, stroke.

◢ **Pruritus Ani:** Although pruritus is a symptom, the signs of chronic itching are evident in the perianal skin containing excoriations and thickening (lichenification). Patients may have a maddening, uncontrollable desire to scratch, but relief is very short-lived. Pinworms are common in children and in adults with young children. When the involved skin is moist, the etiology may be infection with bacteria or fungi (*Candida*). Poor hygiene, contact allergies, irritation from bathroom tissue, and perianal dermatitis of unknown cause are also common.

◢ **Pain with Bowel Movements:** See *Anal Fissure*, page 556.

Pelvic Symptoms

◢ **Pain in the Perineum:** *Pathophysiology:* Perineal pain accompanies many disorders in the pelvis and can involve somatic or sacral sympathetic afferents. Take a history and perform a thorough physical exam looking for any pathology involving the rectum, anus, scrotum and its contents, vagina, pelvic floor muscles, pelvic bones, and perineal skin.

✓ **CLINICAL OCCURRENCE:** *Inflammatory/Immune* eczema, nonbacterial prostatitis, Bartholin gland inflammation; *Infectious* intertrigo, candidiasis, condyloma, vaginitis, cervicitis, urethritis, cystitis, prostatitis, epididymitis; *Mechanical/Trauma* thrombosed hemorrhoids, fissure in ano, fistula in ano, anal ulcer, cystocele, rectocele, testicular torsion or trauma, proctalgia fugax; *Neoplastic* anal, rectal, bladder, prostate, vaginal, cervical, or uterine cancer.

◢ **Pelvic Pain:** See *Abdominal Pain*, pages 529ff and 562ff, and *Pelvic Pain*, Chapter 11, page 630.

Stool Symptoms

◢ **Blood in the Feces:** *Pathophysiology:* Blood in the bowel eventually passes in the feces. Its appearance depends on the volume of blood, the site of bleeding and its transit time in the GI tract. Partially digested blood, depending upon quantity, rate, and site of bleeding can take on any character from bright blood through black loose stools to frank melena. Small amounts of blood loss insufficient to change the color or character of the stool is occult bleeding. The stool guaiac test is a screening test for the presence of blood in the stool. Readings are either positive or negative. The test is not designed to quantify the amount of blood detected. Therefore, terms such as "weak positive" and "strong positive" should not be used. Numerous foods, such as red meats and horseradish root, will give false-positive stool guaiac tests.

KEY SYMPTOM

▶ ✓**Black Tarry Stools: Melena:** *Pathophysiology:* 50–60 mL of blood in the stomach produces a black, sticky (tarry) stool because of the effect of gastric acid and digestive enzymes. Black, but not tarry, stools also occur with ingestion of iron and bismuth and some fruits (e.g., black cherries and blueberries) or leafy green vegetables (e.g., spinach and collard greens). Difficulty cleaning the anus after a stool because of the sticky quality of the stool is characteristic of melena and not present with other causes of black stools. Melena may have a slight reddish hue and an acrid-sweet odor that is similar to creosote.

KEY SYMPTOM

▶ ✓**Bloody Red Stools: Hematochezia:** *Pathophysiology:* Blood unchanged by passage through the gut usually has entered the bowel in the colon, or passed very quickly through the gut. Because blood in the bowel is cathartic, large bleeds stimulate rapid passage. History and physical exam should try to determine whether the blood is mixed in the stool or on the outside of an otherwise normal stool. Blood mixed in the stool suggests bleeding onto a semiformed stool in the colon, whereas blood on the outside suggests a source near the anus.

✓ **GASTROINTESTINAL BLEEDING—CLINICAL OCCURRENCE:** *Congenital* congenital polyps and hamartomas; hereditary hemorrhagic telangiectasia; pseudoxanthoma elasticum; von Willebrand disease; hemophilia; Meckel diverticulum, hematobiliar; *Idiopathic* arteriovenous malformations, colonic diverticulosis, duodenal diverticulum; *Inflammatory/Immune* immune thrombocytopenia, ulcerative colitis, Crohn disease, gastritis; *Infectious* see dysentery syndrome, page 584, *Clostridium difficile* colitis, typhoid enteritis, leptospirosis, *Herpes simplex* esophagitis and proctitis, parasites; *Metabolic/Toxic* vitamin K deficiency, scurvy, heavy metal poisoning, nonsteroidal antiinflammatory drugs; *Mechanical/Trauma* Mallory-Weiss tear, ulcers, intussusception, anal fissure, anal fistula, fecal impaction, epistaxis, swallowed blood; *Neoplastic* polyps or cancer anywhere in the GI tract, cancer invading the bowel wall, for example, pancreatic cancer, gastrinoma (Zollinger-Ellison syndrome); *Psychosocial* factitious; *Vascular* thrombocytopenia, arteriovenous malformations, ischemic bowel, erosion of abdominal aortic aneurysm into the gut, gastric antral vascular ectasia (GAVE), esophageal varices, gastric varices, portal gastropathy, hemorrhoids.

KEY SYMPTOM

✓**Red Stools with Negative Guaiac Test:** *Pathophysiology:* Passage of red pigments from ingested fruits and vegetables. The patient often presents with a complaint of blood in the stool. This should always be confirmed by a positive guaiac test. When negative, history will often identify ingestion of beets or certain fruits, usually in large quantity.

Abdominal, Perineal, and Anorectal Signs

Abdominal Signs

Inspection

KEY SIGN

Jaundice: Jaundice refers to the staining of tissues and fluids by bilirubin. Yellow skin is also caused by carotene and rare chemical toxins, conditions that must be distinguished from jaundice. Although jaundice merely means "yellow," medical use reserves the term for bilirubin staining. Bilirubin stains all tissues, but jaundice is most intense in the face, trunk, and sclerae. Jaundice is usually visible when the concentration of conjugated bilirubin exceeds 3 mg/dL in serum. Jaundice is less visible in artificial light than daylight. When the jaundice is of long standing, the deep yellow may acquire a green hue.

Physiology: *Normal Bile Pigment Cycle.* When senescent erythrocytes are destroyed in the spleen and other reticuloendothelial tissues, hemoglobin is metabolized to unconjugated bilirubin, iron, and globin. Unconjugated bilirubin is insoluble in water and circulates bound to albumin, hence it cannot be filtered by the kidneys. The liver takes up the unconjugated bilirubin, combines it with glucuronic acid to form water-soluble conjugated bilirubin, excretes it into the gut with the bile, where bacterial enzymes convert it to urobilinogen. Most urobilinogen is lost in the feces, but small amounts are reabsorbed by the intestine and reexcreted, some in the bile (enterohepatic circulation) and some in the urine. Excess water-soluble conjugated bilirubin in the blood is filtered by the kidneys and excreted in the urine. *Pathophysiology:* Jaundice occurs when there is a marked increase in production of unconjugated bilirubin, with impairment of hepatocellular uptake, conjugation or excretion of bilirubin, or obstruction of the intra- or extrahepatic bile ducts.

Scleral Color. Bilirubin is distributed uniformly throughout the sclera, in contrast to the yellow subscleral fat that collects in the periphery, farthest from the limbus. Carotene does not stain the sclerae, but it accumulates in the skin of the forehead, around the alae nasi, and in the palms and soles.

Pruritus. Itching leading to cutaneous excoriation often accompanies obstructive jaundice and biliary cirrhosis; it may become excruciating. The intensity of the itching is usually proportional to the bilirubin concentration and the duration of jaundice.

Urine color. Conjugated, but not unconjugated, bilirubin is excreted in the urine. High concentrations of conjugated bilirubin in the urine impart a dark-yellow to brown color. Shaking a specimen in a test tube produces yellow foam because of the ability of the bile salts to lower the surface tension of water. Jaundice without darkening of the urine suggests unconjugated bilirubinemia.

Acholic Feces. In complete biliary obstruction or severe hepatocellular degeneration, the stools are malodorous and appear white or gray, that is, clay colored.

UNCONJUGATED HYPERBILIRUBINEMIA. *Pathophysiology:* This is usually caused by hemolysis producing unconjugated bilirubin at a rate exceeding the maximal rate of liver conjugation and excretion. The stools are normal in color. The increase in bilirubin excretion into the gut leads to an increase in urinary urobilinogen. The urine contains no bilirubin because only water-soluble conjugated bilirubin is excreted in the urine. Tests for intrinsic liver disorders are negative. Less often, unconjugated bilirubinemia is caused by diminished hepatic uptake or a defect in hepatic conjugation.

✓ *CLINICAL OCCURRENCE:* *Increased Production:* *Hemolysis of normal red cells* autoimmune hemolytic anemia, transfusion hemolysis, hemolysis from chemicals, drugs, or infections; *Red cell defects* sickle cell disease, thalassemia, glucose-6-phosphate dehydrogenase (G-6-PD) deficiency, pyruvate kinase deficiency, paroxysmal nocturnal hemoglobinuria; *Ineffective erythropoiesis* thalassemia major, folate, and vitamin B_{12} deficiency; *Miscellaneous* absorption of hematoma, pulmonary infarction. *Deficient Hepatic Uptake:* sepsis, fasting, hypotension, and drugs. *Deficient Hepatic Conjugation:* *Congenital* Gilbert syndrome, Crigler-Najjar syndromes; *Acquired* advanced hepatocellular disease, sepsis, competitive inhibition by drugs metabolized to glucuronides.

CONJUGATED HYPERBILIRUBINEMIA. *Pathophysiology:* This results from impaired excretion of conjugated bilirubin from the hepatocyte into the bile canaliculi or obstruction of the biliary flow through the canaliculi, intrahepatic, and extrahepatic bile ducts to the duodenum. The feces may be acholic. The urine lacks urobilinogen but contains bilirubin. The serum alkaline phosphatase is elevated out of proportion to the transaminases. Clinically, it is important to distinguish mechanical extrahepatic obstruction from intrahepatic obstruction that results from either mechanical obstruction or altered hepatocyte and canalicular function. In most cases of extrahepatic obstructive jaundice, dilatation of the bile ducts can be detected by ultrasonography.

✓ *CLINICAL OCCURRENCE:* *Intrahepatic Cholestasis:* *Congenital* Dubin-Johnson syndrome, Rotor syndrome; *Acquired* hepatocellular disease, drugs (especially sex steroids), sepsis, hypotension, primary biliary cirrhosis. *Extrahepatic Obstruction:* *Intrinsic* gallstones, biliary sludge, biliary carcinoma, sclerosing cholangitis, stricture, parasites; *Extrinsic* pancreatic carcinoma, portahepatis lymphadenopathy, pancreatitis, pancreatic pseudocyst.

MIXED HYPERBILIRUBINEMIA. This results from a combination of hepatocellular and biliary tract injury. This is common in advanced hepatobiliary disease of almost any etiology, as these diseases are complex dynamic processes whose clinical and biochemical patterns evolve over time. The clinician should attempt to distinguish the primary etiology of hepatobiliary injury from the secondary consequences (e.g., cirrhosis or pigment stones). More than one process may be present, for example, alcohol, viral hepatitis, and drug effects. The diagnosis is made on

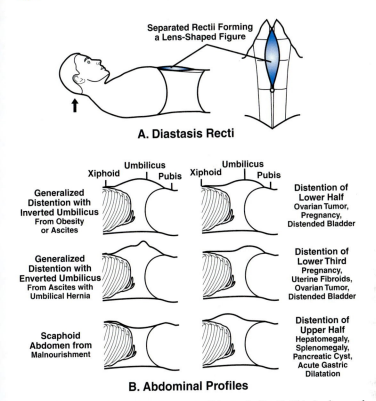

A. Diastasis Recti

B. Abdominal Profiles

Fig. 9-20 Visible Abdominal Signs. A. Diastasis Recti: This is abnormal separation of the abdominal rectus muscles. It is frequently not detected when the patient is supine unless the patient's head is raised from the pillow so that the abdominal muscles are tensed. B. Abdominal Profiles: Careful inspection from the side may give the first clue to abnormality, directing attention to a specific region and prompting search for more signs.

the basis of a careful history supported by serologic testing and liver biopsy. The plasma will contain both conjugated and unconjugated bilirubin; the serum transaminase level will depend upon the degree of active liver injury and the remaining hepatocyte mass; the alkaline phosphatase is variably elevated. The stools may be acholic.

KEY SIGN

Distended Abdomen: *Pathophysiology:* The abdomen becomes distended by the accumulation of normal or abnormal fluids or tissue (Fig. 9-20). These can be categorized as adipose tissue (obesity), gas (tympanites), peritoneal fluid (ascites), organomegaly of solid organs caused by tissue hypertrophy or cysts (e.g., hepatomegaly, splenomegaly, polycystic kidneys, ovarian cysts, fibroids), obstruction of hollow organs (stomach, small and large intestine, bladder, gallbladder), neoplasms (benign or malignant), and pregnancy.

KEY SIGN

Distended Abdomen: Obesity: *Pathophysiology:* Abdominal obesity results from excessive caloric intake and/or redistribution of adipose tissue caused by hormonal factors, especially glucocorticoids. Obesity causes a uniformly rounded abdomen with an increase in girth (Fig. 9-20). The umbilicus is buried deeply in the wall because it is adherent to the peritoneum. Excess fat is usually evident in other parts of the body, although men disproportionately deposit fat into the abdominal viscera and mesentery. Estimate the thickness of the panniculus by grasping a double layer between thumb and index finger; measure in centimeters half the thickness of the resulting fold at the base. The girth of the belly also reflects fat in the mesentery, omentum, and retroperitoneum. Because generalized obesity is obvious, the problem usually is to determine if any other causes of abdominal distention are present.

KEY SIGN

Distended Abdomen: Ascites: *Pathophysiology:* Ascites results from an increased accumulation of peritoneal fluid by any one or more of several mechanisms: transudation of fluid from the splanchnic circulation as a result of increased portal venous pressure (portal hypertension); obstruction of the normal lymphatic drainage of the peritoneum, or decreased plasma oncotic pressure; increased production of peritoneal fluid from peritoneal carcinomatosis or inflammation, usually infectious. Each of these mechanisms produces a recognizable clinical pattern discernible by history and physical examination. Unless distorted by surgical scars, diastasis recti, or hernia, the profile of the fluid-filled abdomen describes a single curve from xiphoid process to pubes (see Fig. 9-20). The umbilicus is sometimes everted.

Four signs are characteristic of free fluid: (a) *Bulging flanks* are produced in the supine position from weight of the fluid pressing on the side walls (Fig. 9-21B). (b) An area of *tympany* at the top of the abdominal curve is caused by gas-filled, mobile intestines floating to the uppermost surface of the fluid, regardless of the position of the patient (Fig. 9-21A). (c) Free fluid produces *shifting dullness*. With the patient supine, percuss the level of dullness in the flanks and mark it on the skin. Then turn the patient on one side for a minute and percuss the new level of dullness; considerable shift indicates the probability of fluid (Fig. 9-21C). (d) A *fluid wave* can be demonstrated by tapping a flank sharply with the right hand while the left hand receives an impulse when placed against the opposite flank. There is a perceptible time lag between the tap and reception of the impulse (Fig. 9-21D). Fat in the mesentery produces a similar wave, so the fat must be blocked by having the patient or an assistant press the ulnar surface of the hand into the midline of the abdomen. A wave passing this block is usually caused by free

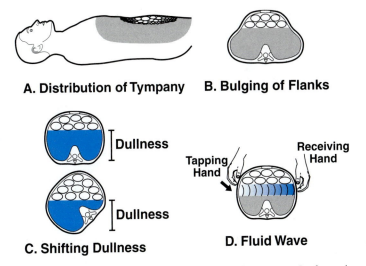

A. Distribution of Tympany

B. Bulging of Flanks

Dullness

Dullness

C. Shifting Dullness

Tapping Hand

Receiving Hand

D. Fluid Wave

*Fig. 9-21 Signs of Ascites. **A. Distribution of Tympany:** In the supine position, free fluid causes the gas-filled gut to float, so an area of tympany forms at the top of the bulging wall. **B. Bulging Flanks:** The weight of free fluid pushes the flanks outward so they bulge toward the table or the bed; fat in the mesentery also will cause this when the abdominal muscles are weak. **C. Shifting Dullness:** The dependent fluid causes an area of dullness in the lowest part; this shifts to remain lowest with changes in position of the body. **D. Fluid Wave:** A wave in the fluid, elicited by tapping one side of the abdomen, is transmitted to the receiving hand laid on the opposite side; the wave takes perceptible time to cross the abdomen.*

fluid. These signs will not detect less than 500 mL of peritoneal fluid [Williams JW, Simel DL. The rational clinical examination. Does this patient have ascites? How to divine fluid in the abdomen. *JAMA* 1992;267: 2645–2648].

ASCITES: AN APPROACH TO DIFFERENTIAL DIAGNOSIS: Listed below is a useful physiologic approach to the differential diagnosis of ascites based upon an assessment of the likely mechanism of ascitic fluid accumulation:

Increased Central Venous Pressure: Right ventricular failure from any cause, pulmonary hypertension (primary or secondary), constrictive pericarditis, tricuspid stenosis, or obstruction.   *Hepatic Vein Obstruction:*   Budd-Chiari syndrome, thrombosis, proximal inferior vena cava obstruction or thrombosis.   *Obstruction of the Hepatic Sinusoids and Intrahepatic Portal Veins:*   cirrhosis from any cause, primary biliary cirrhosis, amyloidosis, schistosomiasis, neoplastic infiltration.   *Obstruction of the Portal Vein:*   portal vein thrombosis, pylephlebitis, extrinsic compression by lymph nodes or masses in the portahepatis. *Peritoneal Irritation:*   acute or chronic peritonitis, neoplastic implants

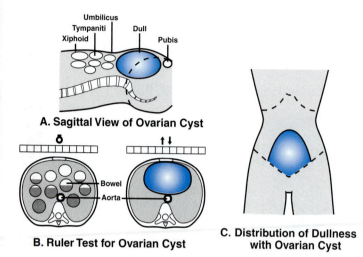

Fig. 9-22 Signs of Ovarian Cyst. *A. Abdominal Profile: The profile of the abdomen shows a curve more pronounced in the lower half. The gas-filled intestines, producing tympany, fill the superior half of the cavity, instead of floating to the top.* **B. The Ruler Test. C. Distribution of Dullness.**

(especially ovarian cancer), tuberculosis. *Decreased Oncotic Pressure:* nephrotic syndrome, hepatocellular dysfunction, repeated large volume paracentesis, protein-losing enteropathy, malnutrition. *Obstruction of the Thoracic Duct or Lymphatics (Chylous Ascites):* lymphoma, metastatic neoplasm, trauma, surgical injury, trauma to thorax or abdomen, tuberculosis, filariasis, intestinal lymphangiectasia. *Miscellaneous:* myxedema, benign ovarian adenoma with ascites and hydrothorax (Meigs syndrome), starvation edema, and wet beriberi (thiamine deficiency and hypoproteinemia are only contributing factors).

KEY SIGN

Distended Abdomen: See Abdominal Distention, page 581ff and Tympanites, page 549.

KEY SIGN

Distended Abdomen: Ovarian Cyst: *Pathophysiology:* Large ovarian cysts can fill much of the abdominal cavity and must be distinguished from ascites. Because they are thin-walled and filled with fluid, they can evert the umbilicus and produce a fluid wave and shifting dullness. The pelvic examination is not diagnostic. Three signs help identify these cysts (Fig. 9-22): (a) careful inspection of the abdominal profile reveals two curves instead of one; (b) when a ruler is pressed transversely across the abdomen, the pulsations of the abdominal aorta are not transmitted with free fluid. If the fluid is enclosed in a tight cyst, the aortic pulsation will move the ruler (*the ruler test*);

(c) in the supine position the tympanitic intestines are pushed superiorly, so the lower abdomen may be dull.

KEY SIGN
Distended Abdomen: Pregnancy: See Fig. 9-20. In pregnancy, the uterus can resemble a large ovarian cyst. The breasts are engorged, fetal movements and parts may be felt, the cervix is softened, and the fetal heart should be audible. With a molar pregnancy, there will be no signs of a fetus.

KEY SIGN
Abdominal Distention: Feces: *Pathophysiology:* An accumulation of large amounts of feces, as in megacolon, may cause distention. Chronic abuse of laxatives, disorders of the myenteric plexus, advanced age, and use of anticholinergic drugs are frequent causes. A history of chronic constipation or laxative use is common. A review of the patient's medication history is essential. The plastic nature of the masses can often be palpated through the abdominal wall and rectal exam may show stool in the vault. Tympanites is usually absent.

KEY SIGN
Depressed Abdomen: Scaphoid Abdomen: *Pathophysiology:*   In extreme malnutrition, the abdominal wall sinks inward toward the vertebral column, forming a depression, pointed superiorly by the costal angle and inferiorly by the wings of the ilia. This has the shape of an ancient Greek boat called a skaphe (see Fig. 9-20). The abdominal contents are more visible and more readily felt than normal. Be careful not to overestimate the size and significance of structures that are unfamiliar because they are normally not palpable.

KEY SIGN
Cutaneous Scars and Striae: See Chapter 6, *The Skin*, page 147.

KEY SIGN
Engorged Veins: *Pathophysiology:*   Ordinarily, the veins in the abdominal wall are scarcely seen unless the subcutaneous fat is thin. Distention of the abdominal wall veins occurs when collateral flow through the abdominal and thoracic wall veins increases as a result of obstruction to normal venous drainage. Because the venous system normally has a low pressure (<30 cm H_2O) it is easily obstructed by extrinsic compression; the low flow velocities in veins also increases the risk of thrombosis. Obstruction of venous drainage from the abdominal viscera is most common (see the discussion of portal hypertension, page 560). Obstruction of the inferior vena cava distal to the hepatic vein, iliac veins, the femoral veins, the superior vena cava, the brachiocephalic, and subclavian veins can each lead to collateralization on the chest and abdominal wall. Because the abdominal wall veins do not have valves, flow can be in either direction. The direction of flow is away from the site obstruction. Engorged veins are often visible through a normal ab-

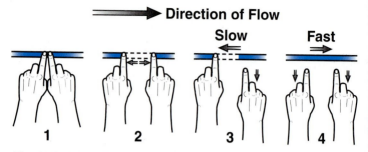

Fig. 9-23 Testing Direction of Blood Flow in Superficial Veins. *(1) The examiner presses the blood from the veins with his index fingers in apposition. (2) The index fingers are slid apart, milking the blood from the intervening segment of vein. (3) The pressure upon one end of the segment is then released to observe the time of refilling from that direction. (4) The procedure is repeated and the other end released first. The flow of blood is in the direction of the faster flow.*

dominal wall. Above the umbilicus, the venous flow is normally cephalad; below the navel, it is caudad. The direction of flow can be determined by identifying the direction of most rapid refilling of an empty venous segment (Fig. 9-23). Obstruction of the inferior vena cava causes a cephalad flow in the lower abdomen (flow reversal). Portal obstruction causes an increase in normal cephalad flow in the upper abdomen and caudad flow in the lower abdomen. Obstruction of the superior vena cava causes caudad flow in the upper abdomen (reversal). Very rarely, engorged veins form a knot around the umbilicus called *caput medusae.* The pattern of distended veins on the abdomen, chest and extremities together with the direction of flow can accurately predict the site of venous obstruction. The differential diagnosis will be developed on the basis of the patient's history, the site(s) of venous obstruction, and the other physical findings.

✓*ENGORGED ABDOMINAL VEINS—CLINICAL OCCURRENCE:*   *Mechanical/ Trauma*   extrinsic compression from mass lesions (superior vena cava, inferior vena cava, and their major tributaries), obliteration of hepatic sinusoids (portal hypertension), strictures caused by traumatic or iatrogenic injury (surgery, instrumentation, or irradiation); *Vascular* thrombosis caused by intravenous catheters or pacemakers (subclavian, jugular, brachiocephalic, femoral), spontaneous thrombosis from congenital or acquired thrombophilia (any vein, superficial or deep).

KEY SIGN

Visible Peristalsis: *Pathophysiology:* When the abdominal wall is thin, normal contractions of the stomach and intestines may be visible as slow undulations under the skin. Visible peristaltic waves through a wall of normal thickness usually reflect increased amplitude and strength of peristalsis. Peristaltic waves in the stomach or small bowel sometimes can be seen in the upper abdomen. They usually appear as oblique ridges in the wall that begin near the left upper quadrant and gradually move downward and rightward. Occasionally parallel ridges form a "ladder" pattern. The waves are slow; to see them, watch the abdomen for several minutes. Sit beside the bed with your eyes near the level of the abdominal profile. Visibility may be caused by normal waves showing through a thin abdominal wall or by abnormally powerful waves beneath a normal wall. The latter indicates obstruction of a tubular viscus. Borborygmus, intestinal rumblings heard without a stethoscope, in conjunction with visible peristalsis and evidence of pain are most suggestive of intestinal obstruction, either partial or complete. Common causes are pyloric obstruction and obstruction of small or large bowel. It can be normal in some thin persons.

KEY SIGN

Visible Pulsations: *Pathophysiology:* Normally, the abdominal aorta causes a slight pulsation in the epigastrium. The amplitude is increased with widened pulse pressure, tortuous aorta, or aneurysm. The pulse may be transmitted to the surface with increased facility by a solid mass overlying the aorta. Aortic tortuosity may be distinguished from dilatation by palpation. Feeling a pulsatile mass raises the question of aneurysm or a solid structure adjacent to the aorta. An aneurysm is expansile laterally as well as anteroposteriorly. A murmur near the mass suggests aneurysm. Ultrasonography or computed tomography are diagnostic.

Diastasis Recti: This occurs when the two abdominal rectus muscles lack their normal fibrous attachment in the midline. With the supine abdomen relaxed, no abnormality may be noted. When the patient raises his head from the pillow, the abdominal recti tense revealing the separation. This may be visible, but also may only be evident on palpation (see Fig. 9-20A).

Everted Umbilicus: Without a hernia, this is a sign of increased intraabdominal pressure from fluid or masses in the cavity.

Umbilical Fistula: This may discharge (a) urine through a patent urachus, (b) pus from a urachal cyst or tract or an abscess in the abdominal cavity, or (c) feces from a connection with the colon.

Umbilical Calculus: In persons with poor hygiene, a hard mass of dirt and desquamated epithelium may accumulate in the umbilical cavity and cause inflammation.

Bluish Umbilicus (Cullen Sign): A faintly blue coloration may occur as the result of retroperitoneal bleeding from any cause.

Chapter 9: The Abdomen

KEY SIGN

► **Ecchymoses on Abdomen and Flanks (Grey Turner Sign):** This results from dissection of blood along the extraperitoneal tissue planes to the skin surface. Nontraumatic ecchymoses may occur in the skin of the lower abdomen, groin, and flanks as a result of massive retroperitoneal hemorrhage. The color may be blue-red, blue-purple, or green-brown, depending on the degree of degradation of the hemoglobin. First associated with hemorrhagic pancreatitis, it also occurs with strangulated bowel, extravasation of hemorrhages from abscesses, or retroperitoneal hemorrhage from any cause.

Auscultation

KEY SIGN

Decreased or Absent Peristaltic Sounds: *Pathophysiology:* Absence of bowel sounds is a sign of ileus, which can have many causes. Listen for at least 5 minutes by the clock before accepting a total absence of bowel sounds. Occasional weak tinkles are not evidence of good peristaltic activity. High-pitched tinkling sounds and rushes may be heard in partial obstruction. Except in intestinal pseudoobstruction, ileus is never a primary problem, but the sign of a metabolic/toxic, inflammatory, or infectious process.

✓ *DECREASED BOWEL SOUNDS—CLINICAL OCCURRENCE:* *Endocrine* myxedema; *Idiopathic* intestinal pseudoobstruction; *Infectious* peritonitis; *Metabolic/Toxic* electrolyte abnormalities: hypokalemia, hypomagnesemia, hypocalcemia; uremia; drugs: opiates, anticholinergics; *Mechanical/Trauma* advanced intestinal obstruction; *Neurologic* spinal cord injury; *Vascular* mesenteric thrombosis.

KEY SIGN

Increased Peristaltic Sounds: *Pathophysiology:* Increased peristalsis indicates irritation of the bowel usually as a result of luminal toxins, irritants, or early obstruction. Correlation of the ausculatory findings with the patient's history and other findings on physical exam will readily differentiate between diarrheal illness or obstruction.

Succussion Splash: The combination of air and fluid in the normal stomach produces audible splashes with movement or palpation. A very loud splash and distention suggests obstruction in the stomach with gastric dilatation.

KEY SIGN

Peritoneal Friction Rub: *Pathophysiology:* Its presence indicates peritoneal inflammation (Fig. 9-24). Like its pleural counterpart, this sound resembles that of two pieces of leather rubbing together. It may be elicited with breathing, movement, peristalsis, or palpation.

✓ *PERITONEAL FRICTION RUB—CLINICAL OCCURRENCE:* *Infectious* liver or splenic abscess, perihepatitis (Fitz-Hugh-Curtis syndrome);

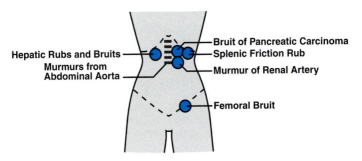

Fig. 9-24 Abdominal Bruits and Rubs. *Blue shading indicates the optimum areas for the auscultation of these abdominal sounds.*

Mechanical/Trauma after liver biopsy; *Neoplastic* hepatocellular carcinoma, liver metastases, peritoneal mesothelioma; *Vascular* splenic infarction.

KEY SIGN

Abdominal Bruits: *Pathophysiology:* Bruits imply arterial flow through a narrowed or tortuous artery (generally systolic only), or large volume flow from high to low pressure as in an arteriovenous malformation (both systolic and diastolic). Hepatocellular carcinoma frequently produces an arterial bruit that is harsh and either purely systolic or continuous with systolic accentuation. Rarely, a venous hum may be audible over a hemangioma in the liver or in the dilated periumbilical circulation in Cruveilhier-Baumgarten syndrome. A continuous systolic–diastolic bruit may occur from an arteriovenous fistula in renal vessels. Renal artery stenosis is found in about two-thirds of patients with systolic renal artery bruits. These murmurs are soft, medium- or low-pitched, and most commonly heard just above and slightly to the left of the umbilicus (see Fig. 9-24) [Turnbull JM. The rational clinical examination. Is listening for abdominal bruits useful in the evaluation of hypertension? *JAMA* 1995;274:1399–1401].

Percussion

KEY SIGN

Tympanitic Percussion: Tympanites: *Pathophysiology:* Tympanites is the presence of excessive gas within the bowel or free in the peritoneal cavity. Tympanites is synonymous with intestinal obstruction and ileus, conditions in which the flow of intestinal contents is diminished, reversed, or arrested. The physical signs are abdominal distention and a large area of tympany. The abdominal profile describes a single curve (Fig. 9-20B). Gastric distention from proximal obstruction results in distention of the left upper abdomen and localized LUQ tympany. The causes of obstruction are either mechanical (intraluminal mass, extraluminal compression, intussusception, volvulus), or nonmechanical (decreased bowel motility, which can be diffuse or segmental). Tympanites is not necessarily seen in intestinal obstruction proximal the ligament of Treitz, where the gut is too short to contain much air and is mechanically fixed in the retroperitoneum and left upper quadrant. Mechanical obstruction commonly produces vomiting and colicky pain. These symptoms are lacking in nonmechanical obstruction, although anorexia and nausea are common. Both types of obstruction may occur sequentially or together. Voluntary or involuntary muscle spasm of the abdominal wall may be present, especially with perforation. Learn to recognize the following clinical patterns: noisy tympanites with colic and vomiting; silent tympanites without colic or vomiting; tympanites with normal bowel sounds and no vomiting (see obstruction syndromes, page 591ff).

Tympanitic Percussion: Pneumoperitoneum: A small amount of gas in the peritoneal cavity cannot be identified by physical exam. With a larger quantity, the area of tympany is extended. Pain and peritonitis may be absent, depending on the presence of contaminants; gut motility is normal if peritonitis is absent.

✔ *PNEUMOPERITONEUM—CLINICAL OCCURRENCE: Idiopathic* ruptured diverticulum, perforated ulcer, pneumocystoides; *Inflammatory/Immune* perforated megacolon; *Infectious* typhoid fever with perforation; ruptured diverticular abscess; *Mechanical/Trauma* perforating abdominal wounds, perforating ingested foreign bodies, volvulus with perforation, postparacentesis, postlaparoscopy, perforated diverticulum, posthysterosalpingogram, peritoneal dialysis; *Neoplastic* perforated colon cancer; *Vascular* ischemic bowel with perforation.

Tympanitic Percussion: Intraluminal Gas: Increased gas in the intestinal lumen is common, but less so than symptomatic complaints of excessive gas. Aerophagia is common and has many causes, including chewing gum, ingestion of carbonated beverages, and inducing eructation.

✔ *INTRALUMINAL GAS—CLINICAL OCCURRENCE: Congenital* lactase deficiency, fructose malabsorption; *Idiopathic* intestinal pseudoobstruction, lactase deficiency; *Inflammatory/Immune* megacolon from ulcerative colitis or Crohn disease; *Infectious* bacterial overgrowth in the small bowel; *Metabolic/Toxic* toxic megacolon, lactase deficiency; *Mechanical/Trauma* volvulus, ileus, endoscopic procedures, air contrast barium enema, aerophagia, carbonated beverage ingestion, bowel obstruction; *Neurologic* ileus from spinal cord injury; *Psychosocial* factitious disorders; *Vascular* ileus from ischemia.

KEY SIGN
Abdominal Pain with Percussion: *Pathophysiology:* Percussion sends a wave of movement through the free wall of the abdomen and peritoneal surface. Pain induced by percussion, especially when referred to areas remote from the point of percussion suggests peritoneal inflammation. See rebound tenderness, below.

KEY SIGN

Costovertebral Tenderness: Tenderness in this region indicates inflammation of the kidney or the paranephric region, as in pyelonephritis.

Palpation

KEY SIGN

Rebound Tenderness (Blumberg Sign): *Pathophysiology:* The inflamed peritoneum is painful when disturbed by direct pressure or movement, especially when two inflamed peritoneal surfaces slide over one another. Because the peritoneum has somatic sensory afferents, the site of pain is well localized. Press the approximated finger tips gently into the abdomen, then suddenly withdraw them (see Fig. 9-7D). Pain worsened after withdrawal is rebound tenderness. The pain may occur at the site of pressure or remote from it. If a site of inflammation is suspected, do your first maneuver in the other quadrants. An alternate and less-painful method is the use of light percussion. Rebound tenderness is a reliable sign of peritoneal inflammation. Another test for peritoneal irritation is to vigorously move the patient's pelvis from side to side with your hands.

JAR TENDERNESS (MARKLE SIGN): The finding of jar tenderness may prove superior to rebound tenderness as a localizing sign of peritoneal irritation, especially in the pelvis. The sign is produced by the heel-drop jarring test. With the examiner demonstrating, the patient stands on the floor with straightened knees. The patient raises her body on her toes, then drops on her heels, which jars the whole body when the heels hit the floor. The location of any pain is noted. False-positive signs are uncommon. The sign may be elicited when rigid abdominal muscles prevent the palpation necessary to elicit rebound tenderness. Abdominal pain on walking is probably an equivalent sign.

✓ *REBOUND TENDERNESS—CLINICAL OCCURRENCE:* *Congenital* familial Mediterranean fever, acute intermittent and variegate porphyria; *Endocrine* ectopic or tubal pregnancy; *Inflammatory/Immune* peritonitis of any cause, appendicitis; cholecystitis, regional enteritis (Crohn disease) familial Mediterranean fever, acute intermittent and variegate porphyria; *Infectious* pelvic inflammatory disease, intraabdominal abscess; diverticulitis; *Mechanical/Trauma* intraabdominal bleeding; *Vascular* infarction of abdominal organs.

KEY SIGN

Direct Tenderness: *Pathophysiology:* tenderness may be caused by inflammation of the abdominal wall, the peritoneum, or a viscus. A solid organ may be tender when its capsule is distended. Ask your supine patient to raise her head from the pillow while you palpate for abdominal tenderness. If the tenderness diminishes, an intraabdominal process is more likely. If the tenderness is unchanged or worsens, a disorder of the abdominal wall is more likely.

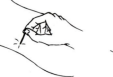 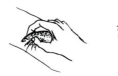

A. Testing Cutaneous Hyperesthesia

B. Testing Subcutaneous Crepitus

Fig. 9-25 Testing for Hyperesthesia, Allodynia, and Subcutaneous Crepitus. ***A. Hyperesthesia and Allodynia.*** *In one method, the skin is stroked lightly with the point of a sterile pin; in another, a fold of skin is pulled gently away from the underlying layers.* ***B. Subcutaneous Crepitus.***

KEY SIGN

Cutaneous Hyperesthesia and Allodynia: See Chapter 14, page 844. In one method, the skin is stroked *lightly* with the point of a sterile pin (Fig. 9-25A). The patient is asked to indicate if the sensation of pain is elicited. Observe the patient's facial expression for signs of discomfort. In another method, a fold of skin is plucked lightly between thumb and index finger, pulling the fold of skin away from the underlying layers (Fig. 9-25A); care should be taken not to pinch the skin painfully. The sensation is more intense, but not painful in areas of cutaneous *hyperesthesia*. DDX: *Allodynia* (pain with normally nonpainful stimuli) indicates damage to sensory nerves (e.g., after herpes zoster or with diabetic radiculopathy). In acute appendicitis, an area of hyperesthesia is frequently found in the right lower quadrant; it precedes perforation.

KEY SIGN

► **Subcutaneous Crepitus:** *Pathophysiology:* Subcutaneous crepitus is the tactile sensation of gas bubbles in the subcutaneous tissue. It is a sign of subcutaneous emphysema or infection with a gas-forming organism. When bubbles of air or other gas are present in the subcutaneous tissues or underlying muscle, pressure on the skin produces a peculiar sensation caused by the sliding of bubbles from under the fingers or, in some cases, the bursting of bubbles (see Fig. 9-25B). Occasionally this may be accompanied by a crackling sound. The bubbles feel like small fluctuant nodules that move freely with palpation. They are not painful or tender. DDX: The presence of subcutaneous crepitus is pathognomonic of subcutaneous emphysema or gas gangrene. In subcutaneous emphysema, the bubbles contain air that has entered the tissues through operative wounds or from trauma, such as a fractured rib piercing the lung. Infection with anaerobic and microaerophilic microorganisms may produce gas by fermentation; the signs of severe local infection with systemic toxicity distinguish it from subcutaneous emphysema.

KEY SIGN

Resistance to Palpation: Voluntary Rigidity of Muscle: Increased abdominal wall muscle tone can result from an unrelaxed posture, a cold room or examining hands, and anxiety. The rigidity interferes with effective deep palpation. It is distinguished from involuntary rigidity by being abolished with suitable maneuvers (see page 517).

KEY SIGN

Resistance to Palpation: Involuntary Rigidity of Muscle: *Pathophysiology:*   Reflex muscle spasm is caused by peritoneal irritation. Persistence of rigidity despite relaxing maneuvers suggest it to be involuntary. Pain is elicited when the patient attempts a sit-up without using the arms. Involuntarily rigid muscles are not necessarily tender and must be distinguished from abdominal wall masses. Rigidity of this type may be unilateral, while voluntary rigidity is symmetrical. When asymmetry is suspected, compare right to left in upper and lower quadrants by placing your hands symmetrically on the patient's abdomen and evaluating muscle tenseness on each side.

UPPER ABDOMINAL TENDERNESS: SUBPHRENIC ABSCESS: *Pathophysiology:*   Pus may collect in the spaces under either diaphragm secondary to suppurative lesions elsewhere in the abdomen, such as a perforated appendix. The patient has unexplained fever or anorexia following infection elsewhere in the abdomen; there may be no symptoms to direct attention to the subphrenic region. Learn to suspect abscesses under the diaphragm and search for the local signs. Elevation of either hemidiaphragm may be demonstrated by percussion and confirmed by x-ray. Pleural effusion, evidenced by percussion dullness, decreased breath sounds, and decreased fremitus, may occur on the affected side. Gas under the right diaphragm should be suspected when percussion over the normal area of hepatic dullness in the right axilla yields tympany. Further localization in the involved subphrenic spaces may be obtained by palpation for tenderness and edema in specific locations, as follows (Fig. 9-26).   *Right Anterior Superior Space:*   under the right costal margin in front of the liver, between the sixth and tenth right intercostal spaces anteriorly.   *Right Anterior Inferior Space:*   below the right anterior costal margin behind the liver.   *Left Anterior Superior Space:*   under the left costal margin anteriorly, between the sixth and tenth left interspaces in the midclavicular line.   *Left Anterior Inferior Space:*   under the left costal margin in the midaxillary line.   *Left Posterior Inferior Space:*   over the left twelfth rib.

KEY SIGN

Resistance to Palpation: Abdominal Masses: See *Abdominal Masses*, page 594ff.   *Pathophysiology:*   If sufficiently large or close to the abdominal wall, masses cause increased resistance to light palpation. Intraabdominal mass must be distinguished from muscle spasm and abdominal wall mass. Note the pattern of resistance, and whether it corresponds to abdominal muscles or resembles the shape of a viscus. When a mass is demonstrated, determine whether it

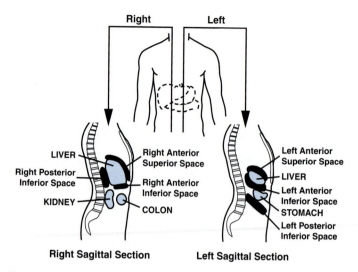

Fig. 9-26 Locations of Subphrenic Abscesses. *The loci are in the right midclavicular line, behind the costal margin, and the left upper quadrant. Posteriorly, the region of the right kidney should be examined.*

is in the wall or in the abdominal cavity. Failure to consider an intramural location results in the erroneous conclusion that all masses are intraabdominal. Intramural masses are palpable when the abdominal muscles are tensed; masses in the cavity are shielded from palpation in this situation (Fig. 9-27). Light palpation can determine only the pres-

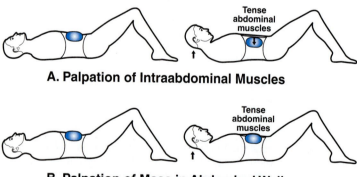

Fig. 9-27 Distinguishing Between Intramural and Intraabdominal Masses. *Palpate the mass while the patient raises his head from the pillow. When the abdominal muscles tense, the intraabdominal mass moves away from the palpating hand, while the intramural mass remains accessible.*

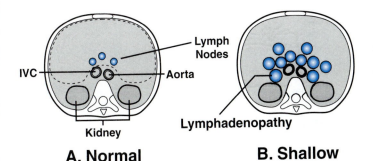

A. Normal   **B. Shallow**

Fig. 9-28 Shallow Abdominal Cavity. A. Normal small paraaortic lymph nodes are not palpable. B. Massive enlargement of prevertebral and preaortic lymph nodes cannot be distinguished from other retroperitoneal masses by palpation. These conditions merely give an impression that the abdomen is shallower than normal. IVC = inferior vena cava.

ence of a mass and its location; further information must be sought by deep palpation and other procedures. DDX: A frequently misdiagnosed mass is hematoma of the rectus muscle.

KEY SIGN

Shallow Abdominal Cavity: *Pathophysiology:* Enlargement of the paraaortic and/or mesenteric lymph nodes (retroperitoneal lymphadenopathy) fills the retroperitoneal space. The hyperplastic nodes are covered with fascia and abdominal viscera, so the floor of the abdominal cavity seems more accessible than normal; discrete nodes cannot be felt. With deep palpation the abdominal cavity is shallower than normal, but without definite masses (Fig. 9-28). The retroperitoneal nodes are best visualized by CT or MRI; lymphoma, metastatic germ cell tumors, and granulomatous diseases are most common.

KEY SIGN

Abdominal Wall Mass: Nodular Umbilicus (Sister Mary Joseph Nodule): Abdominal carcinoma, especially gastric, may metastasize to the navel [Moll S. Images in clinical medicine. Sister Joseph's node in carcinoma of the cecum [picture, *N Engl J Med* 1996;335:1568].

KEY SIGN

Pulseless Femoral Artery (Leriche Syndrome): Always palpate the femoral arteries during examination of the abdomen. See page 487 for further discussion.

Perineal, Anal, and Rectal Signs

Inspection

KEY SIGN

Pruritus Ani: See symptoms page 537.

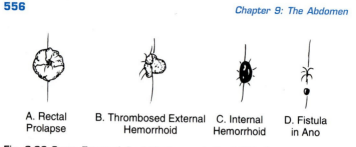

A. Rectal   B. Thrombosed External   C. Internal   D. Fistula
Prolapse   Hemorrhoid   Hemorrhoid   in Ano

Fig. 9-29 Some External Anal Findings. *A. Rectal Prolapse appears as a red doughnut of most rectal mucosa protruding through the anus. B. Thrombosed External Hemorrhoids are semispheric masses of erythematous skin at the mucocutaneous junction with the anus. C. Internal Hemorrhoids are mucosal masses sometimes seen through the retracted anus. D. Fistulous Opening in the skin is accompanied by a papule of hypertrophied skin on the margin of the orifice.*

KEY SIGN

Prolapsed Rectal Polyp: When pedunculated, polyps in the lower rectum may prolapse from the anus as spherical masses.

KEY SIGN

Hemorrhoids: *Pathophysiology:*   Large submucosal hemorrhoidal veins are normal anal cushions. They may dilate in normal people to form hemorrhoids; they are more common and severe with portal hypertension or obstruction of the IVC.   *Internal Hemorrhoids* (see Fig. 9-3) are irregular globular masses which arise above the pectinate line so are covered with rectal mucosa; they may prolapse into the anal canal.   *External Hemorrhoids*   arise below the pectinate line and are covered with skin. When thrombosed, they are purple-red, firm, and very painful (see Fig. 9-29). With edema of the overlying skin, they may be white.

KEY SIGN

Fistula in Ano: *Pathophysiology:*   Most fistulae in ano arise from abscesses in the anal crypts (crypts of Morgagni) and track to the perianal skin. Look for a small sinus track opening in the perianal skin (see Fig. 9-29). The internal orifices of their tracks can be found just above the pectinate line, where they may be probed (see Fig. 9-3A); fistulas should not be probed from the exterior. Gentle palpation around the orifice of the fistula may reveal the course of the track as a subcutaneous cord. DDX: Chronic lesions stimulate hypertrophy of an anal papilla *(sentinel pile)*. Multiple fistulas suggest Crohn disease or tuberculous proctitis.

KEY SIGN

Fissure in Ano: The extreme pain associated with fissures results from anal sphincter spasm. If the patient presents with pain, do not attempt a digital examination before inspecting the mucosa by re-

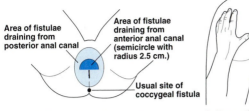
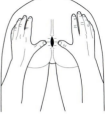

Area of fistulae draining from posterior anal canal

Area of fistulae draining from anterior anal canal (semicircle with radius 2.5 cm.)

Usual site of coccygeal fistula

A. Fistulae in the Perineum

B. Retraction of the Anus

*Fig. 9-30 Examination of the Perineum.   **A. Fistulae in the Perineum:** The dark blue semicircular area anterior to the anus, with a radius of 2.5 cm, indicates the location of fistulae sinuses that drain from the anterior surface of the anal canal (Salmon's law). Anal fistulae draining to the skin in the light blue area arise in abscesses from the posterior surface of the canal. A coccygeal fistula (pilonidal) is usually in the midline, near coccyx or sacrum. **B. Retraction of the Anus:** This is a method of stretching the anal orifice to inspect for fissure in ano, external hemorrhoids, or prolapsing internal hemorrhoids or polyps.*

tracting the skin on both sides and looking for the fissure posteriorly (Fig. 9-30B). It is an extreme unkindness to the patient to attempt further examination without giving either local anesthetics or analgesics. The fissure is a slit-like separation of the superficial anal mucosa, suggesting a longitudinal tear, rarely becoming an ulcerating crater.

KEY SIGN
Sentinel Pile: Various authors seem to apply this term to two structures. More commonly, it refers to a hyperplastic tag of skin frequently found external to a fissure in ano, resembling an external hemorrhoidal tag; it is also called a fibrous anal polyp. The name has been applied to a hypertrophied anal papilla internal to a fissure in ano (see Fig. 9-3). This lesion arises from the pectinate line, while an internal hemorrhoid arises above it.

KEY SIGN
Rectal Prolapse: When the patient strains, as if to defecate, the rectal mucosa may evert below the sphincter (see Fig. 9-29). When symptoms suggest prolapse, but the procedure fails to demonstrate it, have the patient squat and strain in the position for defecation. The prolapse may be either mucosal or complete; in the latter case, the sphincters are included.

Palpation

KEY SIGN
Anal Stricture: Benign: A congenital stricture is occasionally encountered as a narrow crescentic fold at the rectal entrance

to the anal canal. A fibrous stricture in the same region is usually the result of surgery for internal hemorrhoids. A sharply delimited stricture is usually the result of radiation therapy.

KEY SIGN

▶ **Anal Stricture: Carcinoma of the Anus:** *Pathophysiology:* Squamous cell carcinoma of the anal skin is related to human papillomavirus infection and is most common in homosexual men practicing anal-receptive intercourse; its incidence is greatly increased in HIV-infected men. The tumor presents as an exophytic or ulcerating mass narrowing the anal canal.

KEY SIGN

▶ **Anal Stricture: Carcinoma of the Rectum:** Cancer may cause plateau-like, nodular, annular, or cauliflower mass in the rectum. Endoscopic visualization and biopsy are essential.

KEY SIGN

Tight Sphincter: Apprehension: The most common cause of a tight anal sphincter is apprehension. Preliminary assurance should be combined with a gentle and slow exam. When you feel the sphincter tighten, stop advancing your finger until the sphincter is felt to relax, then advance a little further. Even though the procedure may be uncomfortable, it should not be painful.

KEY SIGN

Tight Sphincter: Fissure in Ano: When the sphincter is in spasm that cannot be relaxed by gentleness, suspect a fissure.

Tight Sphincter: Fibrosis of Anal Sphincter Muscles: The entire canal is narrowed so the finger feels encased in a rigid tube. This is caused by fibrosis of the anal muscles, frequently producing fecal impaction.

KEY SIGN

Relaxed Sphincter: Lacerated Anal Muscles: *Pathophysiology:* Damage to the anal sphincter is the result of childbirth or of sphincter injury during surgery for fistula in ano. When the anus is retracted by pulling the skin from each side, a dimple is visible in the posterior part of the anal ring. The sphincter feels weak when the finger is inserted. Ultrasonography of the sphincter will reveal the defect.

Relaxed Anal Sphincter: Atony of the Muscles: *Pathophysiology:* Damage to the peripheral and central sensory and motor control of the sphincters can produce decreased tone. The finding should prompt a careful neurologic examination.

Rectal Polyps: Some polyps can be palpated, especially if sessile. Because they are soft and, if pedunculated, mobile, they are easily missed.

Coccygeal Tenderness: When a patient complains of pain in the region of the coccyx exacerbated by sitting or defecation, you should test for tenderness in the sacrococcygeal joint during digital rectal exam: place the index finger in the rectum on the anterior surface of the coccyx and press the posterior surface of the bone with the thumb on the skin outside. The bone is moved backward and forward to elicit pain in the joint. The coccyx may be displaced from previous injury.

KEY SIGN
Fecal Impaction: The examining finger in the rectum discovers the lumen to be filled with hard, dry masses of feces. These must be removed by breaking up and extracting the pieces with the finger. The symptoms leading to this finding may be vague. The patient may complain of constipation or obstipation; but sometimes there is diarrhea, the fecal stream passing around the impaction to produce incontinence. In debilitated or postoperative conditions, the patient may be merely restless or have fever or anorexia. Barium suspensions administered for x-ray examination commonly cause impaction.

KEY SIGN
Coccygeal Sinus (Pilonidal Sinus):   *Pathophysiology:*   A congenital track extends from the coccyx or sacrum to the perineum, where it drains to the exterior, usually in the midline posterior to the anus (see Fig. 9-30A). The sinus is lined with epithelium and hairs, hence the alternate name pilonidal. When blocked, it may form a tender dimple or bulge just below the coccyx or on one side, usually the left.

Ischiorectal Abscess: *Pathophysiology:*   Abscess forms within the pelvic floor muscles and tissue spaces between the rectum and the ischium. This may not have visible signs because it is deep-seated. Tenderness on deep palpation between anus and ischial tuberosity locates the site. It must be considered as a source of neutropenic fever.

Anal Intermuscular Abscess: Abscesses between the muscles of the anus cause agonizing pain during defecation and discomfort during sitting. In high abscesses, a tender mass is felt just above the anorectal junction. Low abscesses are most frequently found with bidigital palpation near the distal end of the anal canal.

Abdominal, Perineal and Anorectal Syndromes

Gastrointestinal, Hepatobiliary and Pancreatic Syndromes

S KEY SYNDROME

Acute Illness after Dining: Chinese Restaurant Syndrome: *Pathophysiology:* This has been attributed to monosodium glutamate, a seasoning used in Asian cooking. It is characterized by onset, 10–20 minutes after eating, of severe headache, burning sensations, and feelings of pressure about the face. Occasionally, chest pain, prostration, gastric distress, and pain in the axillae, neck, and shoulders develop.

S KEY SYNDROME

Acute Hepatic Vein Thrombosis: Budd-Chiari Syndrome: *Pathophysiology:* Hepatic vein thrombosis from cirrhosis, suppuration, malignancy, trauma, polycythemia vera, or thrombophlebitis results in hepatic sinusoidal congestion, obstruction to portal flow through the liver, and development of signs of portal hypertension. The onset may be abrupt, with pain in the abdomen and vomiting. The liver enlarges rapidly and is tender. Mild jaundice may be present. Ascites rapidly accumulates. Shock may ensue, with death in a few days. If the initial stage is survived, the chronic findings may appear.

CHRONIC HEPATIC VEIN OCCLUSION: This is one phase of the Budd-Chiari syndrome. The findings very closely resemble those of hepatic cirrhosis, so the condition may be difficult to diagnose. Signs of portal hypertension are present, together with ascites, hepatomegaly, and evidence of secondary hepatocellular failure. Sudden onset and lack of alcoholic intake or hepatitis suggests the correct diagnosis.

S KEY SYNDROME

Obstruction of the Portal System: When occlusion occurs rapidly, symptoms are more likely to bring the patient to the physician before signs of portal hypertension or liver damage have developed. Slowly developing obstruction more commonly presents as ascites or symptoms and signs of bleeding from vessels forming the portosystemic shunts.

S KEY SYNDROME

Chronic Portal Vein Obstruction: Portal Hypertension: *Pathophysiology:* Any obstruction to the blood flow in the portal vein, the liver (presinusoidal, sinusoidal, postsinusoidal) or the hepatic vein produces portal hypertension. Increased pressure in the portal system (Fig. 9-31) produces splenic congestion with splenomegaly, development of venous collaterals about the esophagus, the rectum, and the abdominal wall, and the development of ascites be-

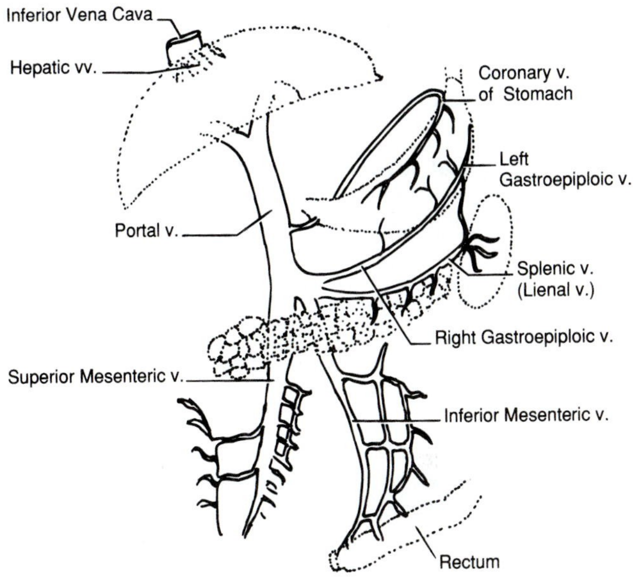

Fig. 9-31 The Portal Venous System.

cause of increased hydrostatic pressure in the mesenteric veins. Three physical signs are common: splenomegaly, visible collateral veins, and ascites. Collaterals are accessible to examination in the anus, the abdominal wall, and the esophagus. Hemorrhoids may be portal collaterals, but their occurrence from local causes is so common that their presence is rarely diagnostic. Dilatation of the paraumbilical vein can produce a venous rosette around the navel, a *caput medusae,* but it is rare. The common demonstrable collaterals are dilated superficial veins in the abdominal wall between the umbilicus and the lower thorax containing blood flowing upward, in the normal direction. When the veins are greatly dilated a venous hum with systolic accentuation may be heard below the xiphoid process, over the epigastric surface of the liver, or around the navel. Formerly, this hum was attributed to a patent umbilical vein in the *Cruveilhier-Baumgarten syndrome;* now it is recognized as coming from varices in the falciform ligament. Dilated veins in the lower esophagus and gastric cardia produce esophageal varices and portal gastropathy visible during endoscopy. Ascites is painless and may be mild, moderate, or severe. DDX: Portal obstruction with ascites and edema of the ankles is frequently mistaken for heart failure. Both conditions may produce pleural effusions, hepatomegaly, ascites, and ankle edema. Often, the first clue that one is not dealing with cardiac failure is the absence of orthopnea. Engorged neck veins are frequently apparent with congestive heart failure but absent with portal hypertension.

✓ *PORTAL HYPERTENSION—CLINICAL OCCURRENCE:* Thrombosis of the hepatic veins, cirrhosis of the liver, intrahepatic tumors and cysts, granulomatous diseases of the liver, portal vein thrombosis, septic thrombosis of the portal vein.

S KEY SYNDROME

Acute Portal Vein Thrombosis: Occlusion occurs after surgical manipulation of the portal vein, septic thrombophlebitis of the portal vein (*pylephlebitis*), trauma, polycythemia vera, neoplastic invasion of the vein lumen, or prolonged debilitating illness. At the onset, there is abdominal pain and tenderness, abdominal distention, ileus, diarrhea, and vomiting. Ascites and splenomegaly rapidly follow. Infarctions of the upper gastrointestinal tract may occur. Clinical suspicion should lead to imaging studies [Cohen J, Edelman RR, Chopra S. Portal vein thrombosis: A review. *Am J Med* 1992;92:173–181].

Acute Abdominal Pain Syndromes

S KEY SYNDROME

Acute Abdominal Pain: See general symptoms, page 529.

✓ *CLINICAL OCCURRENCE:* *Congenital* Meckel diverticulum, sickle cell crisis, pancreas divisum, angioedema; familial Mediterranean fever, acute intermittent porphyria (AIP), and variegate porphyria; *Endocrine* gastrinoma, multiple endocrine abnormalities; *Idiopathic* diverticulosis, abdominal aortic aneurysm, aortic dissection, endometriosis; *Inflammatory/Immune* pancreatitis, gastritis, esophagitis, autoimmune hepatitis, peritonitis, serositis, mesenteric lymphadenitis, systemic lupus erythematosus, vasculitis, inflammatory bowel disease (Crohn disease, ulcerative colitis), familial Mediterranean fever, AIP, and variegate porphyria; *Infection* typhoid fever and enteritis; *Clostridium difficile* enterocolitis; viral gastroenteritis; visceral larval migrans; varicella-zoster virus; cytomegalovirus; viral autoimmune hepatitis; tuberculous peritonitis and lymphadenitis; bovine tuberculosis; purulent peritonitis (spontaneous or secondary to perforation or penetration); *Metabolic/Toxic* ingestions, acute intermittent and variegate porphyria, heavy metal poisoning (lead, cadmium, arsenic, mercury), nonsteroidal antiinflammatory drug gastroduodenitis, macrolide antibiotics; *Mechanical/Trauma* fracture of a solid organ, perforation of bowel, bladder, or gallbladder, obstruction of the cystic, common bile, pancreatic ducts, ureter, ureteropelvic junction, or bowel by stones, masses, parasites, or bezoars; volvulus or strangulation of bowel in internal or abdominal wall hernias; penetrating and blunt trauma; *Neoplastic* mass effect of tumors pressing on other structures or causing traction on bowel or mesentery, hemorrhage into tumor, ischemia and necrosis of tumor, erosion into or metastasis to blood vessels, nerves or adjacent organs; *Neurologic* herpes zoster; diabetic radiculopathy, mononeuritis multiplex, abdominal cutaneous nerve entrapment, transverse myelitis; *Psychosocial* history of physical, emotional or sexual abuse in childhood or as an adult; poisoning, substance abuse with drug seeking, drug withdrawal; *Vascular* arterial dissection, leaking aneurysm, ischemic bowel, infarction of bowel or solid organs, vasculitis, mesenteric venous thrombosis, emboli (bland, septic, or atheroembolic), Henoch Schönlein purpura, strangulation of hernias, rectus sheath hemorrhage, retroperitoneal hemorrhage.

S KEY SYNDROME

▼ **Six-Dermatome Pain:** For a discussion of the six-dermatome pain pathophysiology and differential diagnosis, see Chapter 8, page 373 and Fig. 8-25.

S KEY SYNDROME

▼ **Six-Dermatome Pain: Esophageal Discomfort:** *Pathophysiology:* Esophageal spasm consists of uncoordinated contractions of the esophagus and is often associated with dysphagia (a sensation of food sticking retrosternally). Hypertensive or nutcracker esophagus consists of coordinated but prolonged high-pressure contractions (probably with decreased compliance of the esophageal muscle). In achalasia, the lower esophageal sphincter fails to relax, causing dysphagia and retrosternal chest pain. Esophageal spasm consists of uncoordinated contractions of the esophagus and is often associated with dysphagia (a sensation of food sticking retrosternally). Disorders of esophageal motility often cause chest discomfort identical in character and location to that found with angina or myocardial infarction. Gastroesophageal reflux may cause pyrosis (heartburn), a burning or constricting lower retrosternal discomfort. The key to distinguishing the pain of ischemic myocardium from esophageal spasm is a careful history. For example, association with dysphagia or meals or the ingestion of cold liquids in the absence of exercise, precipitation by reclining or bending over, or relief with antacids all favor esophageal origin. Because nitroglycerin relaxes smooth muscle, whether in arteries, veins, or esophagus, it may relieve discomfort from both disorders. An ECG recorded during intense pain is useful; a normal tracing favors esophageal pain, although it does not exclude cardiac ischemia. *The presence of a hiatal hernia has no diagnostic significance in the differential diagnosis of chest pain.*

S KEY SYNDROME

▼ **Esophageal Achalasia (Cardiospasm):** *Pathophysiology:* Tonic increased contraction of the lower esophageal sphincter of unknown cause results in functional obstruction at the gastroesophageal junction with proximal dilation of the esophagus. Symptoms include dysphagia and regurgitation of food, saliva, and esophageal secretions. Chest pain may be present and cough, especially after meals or with recumbency, suggests aspiration. Weight loss may occur.

S KEY SYNDROME

▼ **Esophageal Laceration: Mallory-Weiss Tear:** *Pathophysiology:* Esophageal laceration occurs near the esophagogastric junction following severe retching and vomiting. Hematemesis occurs after retching and vomiting. If bleeding is severe, hypotension may occur. Bleeding is usually self-limited.

**Six-Dermatome Pain with Dysphagia: Divertic-
ulum of the Esophagus:** Although pouches may form
anywhere in the gullet, only Zenker diverticulum regularly produces
symptoms. This is an outpouching in the posterior hypopharynx protruding downward between spine and esophagus. It fills with food,
causing dysphagia and regurgitation of putrefied food. Occasionally,
there is retrosternal pain. The esophagram visualizes the pouch.

**Six-Dermatome Pain with Dysphagia: Plummer-
Vinson Syndrome:** This occurs with severe iron deficiency.
A postcricoid web-like formation in the esophagus may be found to explain the dysphagia in some, although no anatomic basis can be discovered in many. The obstruction may be demonstrated by esophagram.

S KEY SYNDROME
**Six-Dermatome Pain with Dysphagia: Acute
Esophagitis:** There is retrosternal pain intensified by swallowing. This occurs after prolonged vomiting, nasogastric tubes, pill
esophagitis, esophageal burns from corrosive substances, acute infections (herpes simplex, *Candida spp.*, cytomegalovirus), and reflux of acid
or bile.

S KEY SYNDROME
**Six-Dermatome Pain with Dysphagia:
Chronic Esophagitis:** Pain and dysphagia are similar in
quality to those in the acute lesions, but the duration covers weeks or
months. It may be complicated by peptic ulceration and/or intestinal
metaplasia (Barrett esophagus), a premalignant lesion of the esophagus.
Esophageal stricture may occur secondary to the esophagitis. Gastroe-
sophageal reflux is the most common cause. Irradiation, infections (HIV,
Candida, herpes, and cytomegalovirus) are less common [Spechler SJ.
Barrett's esophagus. *N Engl J Med* 2002;346:836–842].

S KEY SYNDROME
**Six-Dermatome Pain with Dysphagia: Can-
cer of the Esophagus and Gastric Cardia:** The
early symptom is dysphagia; weeks or months later, pain retrosternally
may be added. The pain sometimes radiates to the neck or back. Chronic
esophagitis with metaplasia (Barrett esophagus) increases the risk.

S KEY SYNDROME
**Six-Dermatome Pain with Dysphagia: For-
eign Body:** Swallowed rigid objects may lodge at the level of the
aortic arch or diaphragm, causing pain and dysphagia. Esophagoscopy
is indicated.

S KEY SYNDROME
Abdominal Pain and Pallor: Abdominal pain accompanied by pallor is an ominous presentation requiring expeditious

evaluation. Of greatest concern is major hemorrhage from rupture of a major vessel or organ. Intense sympathetic activation, even without hemorrhage, may cause pallor and diaphoresis.

S KEY SYNDROME
Abdominal Pain and Pallor: Rupture and Hemorrhage from Tubal Pregnancy: See Chapter 11, page 644.

S KEY SYNDROME
Abdominal Pain and Pallor: Corpus Luteum Hemorrhage: See Chapter 11, page 644.

S KEY SYNDROME
Abdominal Pain and Pallor: Ruptured Aortic or Iliac Aneurysm: See page 569.

S KEY SYNDROME
Abdominal Pain and Pallor: Peptic Ulcer with Hemorrhage: See pages 566ff. *Pathophysiology:* Erosion of an ulcer into a major vessel can lead to life-threatening hemorrhage. Although bleeding may be proceeded by the typical symptoms of ulcer disease, it is not uncommon, especially for nonsteroidal antiinflammatory drug-induced ulcers, to present with painless hemorrhage and/or perforation. Blood should be sought in the stools and a nasogastric aspirate.

S KEY SYNDROME
Abdominal Pain and Pallor: Hemorrhagic Pancreatitis: *Pathophysiology:* Pancreatic inflammation erodes blood vessels in the retroperitoneum, leading to hemorrhage into the necrotic pancreas and dissection of hemorrhage into the retroperitoneal spaces. (See page 568 for complete discussion.)

S KEY SYNDROME
Acute Abdominal Pain: Rupture of Solid Organs: *Pathophysiology:* Blunt trauma to the lower thorax, back, and abdomen may fracture kidneys, liver, or spleen. The fracture and hemorrhage may be contained by the surrounding capsule. Rupture of the capsule resulting in severe hemorrhage may occur acutely or be delayed by hours or days. Upper quadrant and flank pain are present and tenderness may be present anteriorly or posteriorly. Renal fracture results in gross hematuria unless the ureter is obstructed. Fracture of solid organs must be sought emergently; CT scan is the diagnostic method of choice.

KEY SIGN
Acute Abdominal Pain: Volvulus: See also page 593. *Pathophysiology:* Volvulus most commonly occurs in the sigmoid colon (90%) or the cecum (10%) where the gut is suspended by a

lengthy mesentery. Twisting causes vascular compromise, distention of the involved segment, and formation of a closed loop, leading to ischemic perforation. Early diagnosis and treatment are imperative. A vague, tender mass may be felt, but frequently the only findings are a distended bowel that produces tympany, pain, violent peristalsis, and vomiting.

S KEY SYNDROME

Acute Epigastric Pain: Visceral pain arising in the intestine from the stomach to the transverse colon is carried by the vagus nerve and projects to the epigastrium. In addition, somatic pain from the upper abdominal peritoneum and retroperitoneal structures will be well localized to the epigastrium.

KEY SYMPTOM

▶ **Acute Epigastric Pain: Acute Appendicitis (Early):** See *Acute RLQ Pain: Appendicitis*, page 573.

KEY SIGN

▶ **Acute Epigastric Pain: Perforation of Peptic Ulcer Progressing to Peritonitis and Shock:** *Pathophysiology:* Perforation causes leakage of acid, digestive enzymes, blood, bacteria, and bowel contents into the peritoneal cavity, lesser sac, or retroperitoneum. With free perforation, sterile peritonitis is followed by purulent peritonitis, septicemia, shock, and death. The patient may give a history of chronic or subacute dull epigastric pain occurring 3 or 4 hours after meals and relieved by food or antacids. Occasionally, there are no antecedent symptoms; this is particularly common in elderly patients taking nonsteroidal antiinflammatory drugs. Three stages of symptoms may be seen:

1. *Stage of Prostration (Primary Shock).* The patient experiences a sudden, excruciating pain in the epigastrium and frequently collapses. Soon the pain spreads over the entire abdomen; sometimes it intensifies in the suprapubic region because of the downward flow of gastric contents (see Fig. 9-32). The patient is anxious and pale, and the body is diaphoretic. The respiratory movements are shallow because of pain with diaphragmatic breathing. Retching or vomiting occurs. Hypothermia and hypotension are common. This initial stage may last from a few minutes to several hours.
2. *Stage of Reaction (Masked Peritonitis).* This stage is a brief respite for the patient, but it may deceive the inexperienced physician. Although the blood pressure rises and the skin becomes warmer, the generalized abdominal pain and tenderness persist, although lessened in intensity. The patient moves cautiously because of pain; the thighs are flexed for comfort. Board-like involuntary rigidity results from contraction of abdominal muscles and shallow respiratory movements. The pelvic peritoneum is tender when examined rectally. Free fluid may rarely be demonstrated in the abdominal cavity. Gas under the diaphragm may be suggested by a diminished

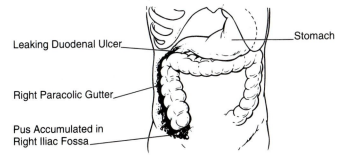

Fig. 9-32 Iliac Abscess from a Leaking Duodenal Ulcer. *The drainage of a duodenal ulcer is down the right paracolic gutter into the right iliac fossa, as indicated by stippling.*

area of liver dullness in the RUQ. Pain on the top of either shoulder results from irritation of the diaphragm and suggests anterior perforation of the stomach; pain on only the right shoulder points more to perforation of the pylorus or duodenum. Pain in the back can result from posterior perforation and pancreatitis.

3. *Stage of Frank Peritonitis.* The classic signs of advanced peritonitis appear. Ileus distends the abdomen, vomiting resumes and persists with increased violence, and the temperature again declines to subnormal levels. The entire abdomen is tender, but rigidity may lessen in the late stage. Dehydration and pain produce the classic facies hippocratica, with hollow features and anxious expression. Death usually ensues within 3 days.

▶ **ACUTE EPIGASTRIC PAIN: LIMITED PERFORATION OF PEPTIC ULCER:** *Pathophysiology:* When the perforation is into a closed space, the released gastric contents are walled off to produce a local abscess. The stage of prostration is mild, with the pain limited to the epigastrium or flank. The abscess may form in the subphrenic space or lesser peritoneal sac.

S KEY SYNDROME
▼ **Acute Epigastric Pain: Acute Gastritis:** *Pathophysiology:* Inflammation of the gastric mucosa is gastritis. It can occur as a result of infection, chemical irritation, autoimmune injury, or drug-induced injury. Frequently, the cause is unknown. Symptoms of gastritis are anorexia, nausea, and vomiting, sometimes with hematemesis. Signs include epigastric pain or discomfort with tenderness. Upper endoscopy is diagnostic revealing mucosal inflammation, erosions, and submucosal hemorrhage. Common causes are ingestion of aspirin, nonsteroidal antiinflammatory drugs, alcohol, or contaminated food, uremia, infection with *Helicobacter pylori*, cytomegalovirus, herpes simplex, or enteroviruses, and autoimmune gastritis.

Acute Epigastric Pain: Acute Pancreatitis:

Pathophysiology: Release of pancreatic enzymes into the parenchyma of the gland as a consequence of ductal obstruction, inflammation, ischemia, and the like, starts autodigestion of the tissue, which incites an intense sterile inflammatory response. Dissection of the expanding inflammatory mass within the retroperitoneum and occasional decompression intraperitoneally lead to spread of the process, hypotension, and shock. Secondary infection of necrotic tissue is common after the first few days. Without warning, the patient develops excruciating epigastric pain often with radiation to the back or flank. Irritation of the left hemidiaphragm causes pain radiation to the left shoulder via the phrenic nerve afferents. Occasionally, the pain spreads over the entire abdomen (generalized peritonitis) or primarily to the right lower quadrant. The pain is knife-like with a boring quality, going directly through to the back. Because pain is aggravated when supine, the patient may assume a sitting or fetal position, leaning forward or curled up. Nearly always, retching and vomiting are severe. The symptoms are more intense and prolonged than in perforation of the stomach and shock can occur. Frequently, one is impressed with the disparity between the severity of the symptoms and the paucity of abdominal findings. Epigastric tenderness is always present. Muscle rigidity is usually absent; when present, it is confined to the epigastrium. Occasionally, one can feel a tender transverse mass deep in the epigastrium. Slight jaundice may be evident in 1 or 2 days. Two or 3 days after onset, blue or green ecchymoses occasionally appear in the flank (*Turner sign*) or the umbilicus (*Cullen sign*) from extravasation of hemolyzed blood. Late complications include pseudocysts that are an accumulation of blood, necrotic debris, and fluid in the retroperitoneum; they are rarely palpable. Acute pancreatitis may be an isolated episode or an acute exacerbation of chronic, relapsing pancreatitis. Common causes of acute pancreatitis are alcohol and gallstones. Other causes include hypertriglyceridemia, pancreatic ductal obstruction and stricture, pancreas divisum, perforated peptic ulcer, ampulla of Vater dysfunction, mumps, and drugs.

Acute Epigastric Pain: Occlusions of Mesenteric Vessels:

Pathophysiology: The superior mesenteric artery or vein is most commonly involved, by either embolism or thrombosis. Arterial occlusion is more likely to produce the typical clinical picture; venous thrombosis is often atypical. Predisposing conditions for venous thrombosis include thrombophilic states. The onset is sudden with acute agonizing pain between the xiphoid and the umbilicus; slight if any relief is afforded by narcotics. A history of recurrent postprandial abdominal pain suggestive of abdominal angina is reported in up to 50% of those with arterial thrombosis. This presentation in an individual with rheumatic or atherosclerotic heart disease suggests the possibility of an arterial embolism. Usually, there are few localizing signs, but occasionally, a tender mass is palpable in the epigastrium. These events are soon followed by the signs of intestinal obstruction: abdominal distention, ileus, and vomiting. Blood may be passed per rectum. There is a severe metabolic acidosis as endotoxemia and shock supervene. Common causes are atherosclerosis, thrombophilia, atheroembolism, acute bacterial or fungal endocarditis, embolism of mural cardiac thrombus, and nonbacterial thrombotic (marantic) endocarditis [Kumar S, Sarr MG, Kamath PS. Mesenteric vein thrombosis. *N Engl J Med* 2001;345:1683–1688].

S KEY SYNDROME

Acute Epigastric Pain: Aortic Dissection: *Pathophysiology:* See Chapter 8, page 462. Dissections extending into the abdominal aorta may produce abdominal and back pain, pain in the groins, and occlusion of the abdominal branches of the aorta leading to ischemia of the downstream tissues. In some instances, abdominal pain is the initial complaint. This is agonizing to the extent that narcotics do not provide relief. The pain is usually in the epigastrium, causing intense involuntary rigidity of the abdominal muscles. The blood pressure is not affected early. Branches of the abdominal aorta may be progressively occluded, and ischemia of the spinal cord may cause paraplegia. A disparity in the pulses may be the most important clue to the diagnosis. Occasionally, dissection is slow and symptomless. Causes to consider are hypertensive vascular disease, giant cell arteritis, arteriosclerosis, Marfan syndrome, and pseudoxanthoma elasticum.

S KEY SYNDROME

Acute Epigastric Pain: Leak and Rupture of Abdominal Aortic Aneurysm: *Pathophysiology:* Abdominal aortic aneurysm (AAA) is often painless until it begins to rupture with leakage of blood into the adventitia and retroperitoneal space. Pain is moderate to severe, usually well localized, and often accompanied by nausea. Pain may radiate to one or both groins. Pain in the back and flank may dominate the presentation. Gentle palpation and urgent diagnosis are necessary [Lederle FA, Simel DL. The rational clinical examination. Does this patient have abdominal aortic aneurysm? *JAMA* 1999;281:77–82].

S KEY SYNDROME

Acute RUQ Pain: The liver, gallbladder, duodenum, head of the pancreas, right kidney, and pleural reflections of the right lung are the leading causes of pain located in the right upper quadrant. Failure to consider pneumonia with pleural involvement or myocardial infarction in the differential diagnosis of acute RUQ abdominal pain has led to inappropriate surgical exploration of the abdomen.

S KEY SYNDROME

Acute RUQ Pain: Cholelithiasis, Biliary Colic: *Pathophysiology:* Gallstones are made predominately of cholesterol, bile pigments, or a mixture. They rarely cause symptoms unless a stone perforates the gallbladder wall or obstructs the cystic duct, the common bile duct, or the pancreatic duct, producing colic because of forceful peristaltic contraction against the impacted stone. An attack

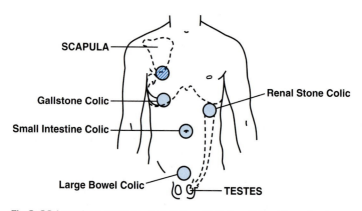

Fig. 9–33 Locations of Abdominal Colic. *Colic is a distinct type of pain, notable for its paroxysmal occurrence, severity and crescendo–decrescendo cycling. It occurs when a hollow viscus is obstructed; pain results from smooth-muscle contractions trying to overcome the obstruction. Note the radiation of gallstone colic from the right upper quadrant to the angle of the right scapula posteriorly. The colic of renal calculus frequently radiates to the testis on the same side.*

of biliary colic may be uncomplicated, or it may be associated with acute cholecystitis, obstructive jaundice, or gallstone pancreatitis. Onset of biliary colic is sudden, with pain in the epigastrium or right upper quadrant that radiates to the inferior border of the right scapula (Fig. 9-33). The pain is severe, recurring in cyclic paroxysms, and is associated with nausea and vomiting. During the attack, the right upper quadrant is rigid. Calcified gallstones can be seen on plain x-ray films, but ultrasonography is the preferred diagnostic exam. Gallstones are common in patients with hemolytic anemias and in certain racial groups, for example, Native Americans. Stones are more prevalent with obesity, female sex, multiparity, diabetes, and some drugs.

S KEY SYNDROME

▼ **Acute RUQ Pain: Acute Cholecystitis:** *Pathophysiology:* Obstruction of the cystic duct, usually by gallstone impaction, results in distention and sterile inflammation of the gallbladder wall. Acalculous cholecystitis is a complication of surgical or medical illness, with progressive gallbladder enlargement, ischemia, and rupture; it has a high mortality. The onset is acute and frequently preceded by episodes of more mild RUQ postprandial pain. Poorly localized pain develops in the right upper quadrant, which may radiate to top of the right shoulder. Nausea and anorexia are usual, and vomiting is less common but may be severe. Tenderness over the gallbladder at the inferior margin of the liver is constant. When the tips of the fingers are held under the right costal margin and the patient is asked to inspire, there is inspiratory arrest (*Murphy sign*). Fist percussion over the liver produces pain, but this sign also occurs in acute hepatitis. The abdominal muscles do not become rigid unless peritonitis is present. In some patients, the gallbladder is palpable as an exquisitely tender globular mass behind the lower border of the liver [Trowbridge RL, Rutkowski NK, Shojania KG. The rational clinical examination. Does this patient have cholecystitis? *JAMA* 2003;289:80–86]. Rarely, the distended gallbladder in cholecystitis reaches the right lower quadrant. Moderate fever is usually present, but high fever or chills suggest ascending cholangitis or suppurative cholecystitis. Ultrasonography demonstrates a thickened, edematous gallbladder wall with sludge or stones in the lumen. The most common cause is gallstone disease, including microlithiasis with sludge. Uncommonly, parasites, bacterial infection, and primary biliary cancer can precipitate attacks. The diagnosis may be confirmed with a radionuclide scan showing obstruction of the cystic duct. False-positive radionucleotide studies may occur in hospitalized patients who have been fasting for many days, because the fluid-filled gallbladder is distended and does not easily contract.

ACALCULOUS CHOLECYSTITIS: HYDROPS OF THE GALLBLADDER: *Pathophysiology:* Obstruction of the cystic duct, usually by stone, leads to gallbladder dilation with a tense, thin edematous wall that occasionally ruptures. This is an infrequent but serious complication of other medical and surgical illnesses. It is either asymptomatic or accompanied by epigastric pain, nausea, and vomiting. There is fever and RUQ abdominal tenderness, and a palpable tender RUQ mass may be appreciated.

ACUTE RUQ PAIN: RUPTURE OF THE GALLBLADDER, BILE PERITONITIS: *Pathophysiology:* Bile is extremely irritating to the peritoneum, producing a severe chemical peritonitis. Perforation of the gallbladder from erosion of a stone, infection, or ischemic necrosis are most common. The initial picture may be that of acute cholecystitis or gallstone colic, but the RUQ pain gradually spreads throughout the abdomen with signs of generalized peritonitis progressing to prostration and shock. Bile leak following cholecystectomy produces the same picture.

▼ KEY SYMPTOM
✔ **Acute RUQ Pain: Leaking Duodenal Ulcer:** *Pathophysiology:* A small duodenal perforation causes limited retroperitoneal leakage of duodenal contents into the right abdominal gutter leading to localized inflammation. The presentation is pain, tenderness, and rigidity in the right upper quadrant; pain may radiate through to the back. A history of peptic ulcer disease may be present. There is tenderness in the midline of the epigastrium, but no peritoneal signs. The gastric and duodenal contents can track down into the right lower quadrant and lead to pain and a mass in the RLQ (see Fig. 9-32).

▼ KEY SYMPTOM
✔ **Acute RUQ Pain: Ureteral Colic:** *Pathophysiology:* Acute ureteral obstruction induces vigorous peristaltic ureteral smooth muscle contractions that are intensely painful, but localize poorly and can radiate to similarly innervated regions, for example, the

testicle, vulva, or groin. Excruciating upper quadrant pain begins and radiates to the flank (see Fig. 9-33). The patient changes position frequently seeking comfort; this is uncommon with pancreatitis or dissecting aneurysm. Frequently, the pain radiates to the right testis, vulva, or groin. Anorexia is constant, nausea and vomiting can be severe. Microscopic hematuria is expected and sometimes gross hematuria occurs. A calcium-containing stone may be seen on plain x-ray films.

KEY SYMPTOM

Acute RUQ Pain: Right Pyelonephritis: *Pathophysiology:* Infection in the kidney produces inflammation and swelling, which distends the capsule, producing pain. Acute pyelonephritis produces upper quadrant and flank pain that is initially poorly localized and exacerbated by fist percussion over the kidney at the costovertebral angle posteriorly. The pain may be severe and accompanied by nausea. In the RUQ, the tenderness is deeper and less severe than with acute cholecystitis. Urinalysis and culture are diagnostic in most cases. Pyelonephritis results from ascending infection from a cystitis or septic emboli. In women with recurrent infections or men with a first infection, suspect congenital or acquired anatomic abnormalities in the urinary tract (stones, tumor, diverticulum, etc.).

ACUTE RUQ PAIN: RENAL OR PERIRENAL ABSCESS: *Pathophysiology:* Progressive necrotizing infection occurs, especially in the setting of infection complicating obstruction. Spread to the perinephritic space can lead to tracking into the pelvis. The patient experiences abdominal pain radiating into the groin with costovertebral angle tenderness and fever. If the cortex, but not the medulla, has been seeded by bacteremia, pyuria may be absent.

S KEY SYNDROME

Acute RUQ Pain: Acute Hepatitis: *Pathophysiology:* Acute inflammation of the liver results from infections, alcohol, or drugs producing hepatocyte injury and secondary inflammation. Pain results when acute parenchymal swelling creates distention of the Glisson capsule. Fever, malaise, and anorexia are usually present. Smokers may lose their taste for cigarettes. If palpable, the entire liver is tender, the edge blunt and smooth. Fist percussion over the liver produces a dull aching pain. Jaundice appears after several days.

S KEY SYNDROME

Acute RUQ Pain: Right-Sided Pleurisy: *Pathophysiology:* Right lower lobe pneumonia can present primarily with pain referred to the RUQ. The patient has pain in the RUQ, but there are no findings on abdominal exam. Deep breathing may accentuate the pain, so the patient takes shallow breaths. A pleural rub and signs of pneumonia should be sought. A chest x-ray is mandatory in the evaluation of any patient with upper abdominal pain.

S KEY SYNDROME

Acute LUQ Pain: The spleen, stomach, left kidney, splenic flexure of the colon, and pleural reflections of the left lung base are the most likely sources of LUQ pain.

S KEY SYNDROME

Acute LUQ Pain: Splenic Infarction: *Pathophysiology:* The spleen is highly vascular, and the sinusoidal structure creates a low redox environment that is susceptible to ischemic injury. Severe, sharp pain develops in the left upper quadrant accompanied with splinting of the abdominal muscles. Frequently the pain radiates to the top of the left shoulder. Fever and leukocytosis may be present. A splenic friction rub may develop. A CT scan will identify splenic infarction. Infarction results from emboli (e.g., endocarditis), vasculitis, or in situ vascular occlusion (as with sickle cell disease). Splenomegaly from hematologic disorders, such as polycythemia vera, chronic myelocytic leukemia, or myelofibrosis may also lead to infarction.

S KEY SYNDROME

Acute LUQ Pain: Ruptured Spleen: Rarely, the spleen ruptures spontaneously or with minimal trauma when it is enlarged from infectious mononucleosis, sepsis, or infarction. Large, soft spleens have been ruptured during palpation. Intense pain occurs in the left upper quadrant, radiating to the top of the left shoulder (*Kehr sign*). The pain may be accentuated by elevating the foot of the bed, increasing contact between peritoneal blood and the diaphragm. Abdominal CT scan is diagnostic.

S KEY SYNDROME

Acute LUQ Pain: Left Pyelonephritis, Left Ureteral Colic, Abscess of the Left Kidney: See discussion on pages 571–572 and 621.

S KEY SYNDROME

Acute LUQ Pain: Pleurisy: See page 444.

S KEY SYNDROME

Acute RLQ Pain: The RLQ is the usual anatomic site of the cecum, appendix, and terminal ilium, each of which is the site of unique inflammatory disorders.

S KEY SYNDROME

► **Acute RLQ Pain: Acute Appendicitis:** *Pathophysiology:* Obstruction of the appendix leads sequentially to appendiceal inflammation, transmural inflammation involving the peritoneum, ischemia, perforation of the wall, and localized or generalized peritonitis. Appendicitis usually results from impaction of fecal material or foreign matter in the appendiceal lumen. Less commonly, carcinoid tumors, vasculitis, or lymphoma may be implicated. Initial pain is mediated by vagal afferents, is poorly localized, accompanied by nausea and vomiting, and referred to the epigastrium. Local peritonitis is sensed by peritoneal somatic afferent nerves, is sharper, and locates to the appendix, commonly the RLQ; generalized peritonitis is diffuse sharp and accompanied by generalized abdominal and systemic signs. Epigastric pain is usually the first in a predictable sequence of symptoms and signs. The pain is poorly localized in the midline between the xiphoid and the umbilicus, is not accompanied by tenderness in the same area, but nausea or vomiting may occur. As the pain worsens, it shifts to the right lower quadrant accompanied by fever and leukocytosis. Until this localization occurs, the diagnosis of appendicitis cannot be made, and often it is not even considered. If the patient presents a different sequence of events, the diagnosis of appendicitis should be questioned. Deep tenderness is first demonstrated just below the midpoint of a line between the anterior superior iliac spine and the umbilicus, where the appendix is typically placed. When the appendix lies behind the ileum or ascends behind the cecum, the deep RLQ tenderness is less. When it is in the true pelvis, the right lower quadrant is not tender, but rectal palpation may elicit tenderness in the peritoneal pouches [Paulson EK, Kalady MF, Pappas TN. Suspected appendicitis. *N Engl J Med* 2003;348: 236–242; Wagner JM, MKinney P, Carpenter JL. Does this patient have appendicitis. *JAMA* 1996;276:1589–1594].

▶ **ACUTE RLQ PAIN: ACUTE APPENDICITIS WITH PERFORATION:** When the appendix ruptures, pain may transiently decrease, only to accentuate again over the next couple of hours. Generalized peritonitis may occur, or the perforation may be contained to form a local abscess identified as a tender mass. This finding may also be caused by edema and inflammation of the cecum without abscess, a phlegmon. Other signs depend on the location of the appendix.

Extrapelvic Appendix. When perforation is retrocecal, the back muscles are inflamed with tenderness below the twelfth rib on the right. If the appendix is lateral to the cecum, a mass may be felt, guarded by intense involuntary rigidity of the abdominal muscles. Irritation of the psoas muscle causes the patient to flex the right thigh or hold it rigidly extended. The iliopsoas test elicits pain when the supine patient tries to flex the thigh against the resistance of the examiner's hand (see Fig. 9-13A). When the appendix is medial and behind the ileum, an abscess may involve the right ureter, causing pain on urination and white cells in the urine.

Intrapelvic Appendix. When the appendix lies within the true pelvis, diffuse suprapubic pain occurs. There is no rigidity of the abdominal muscles. Irritation of the bladder and rectum produces painful urination and tenesmus. A key diagnostic sign is palpation of a tender mass in the peritoneal pouch by rectal examination. The abscess may lie in contact with the obturator muscle; the obturator test produces suprapubic pain by flexing the thigh and rotating the femur internally and externally (see Fig. 9-13B). Typhlitis, Crohn disease, pelvic inflammatory disease, ovarian disease, and ectopic pregnancy are frequently in the differential.

▶ **Acute RLQ Pain: Typhlitis (Neutropenic Enterocolitis, Cecitis):** *Pathophysiology:* Neutropenia of any cause, particularly following chemotherapy for malignancy or acute leukemia, is associated with acute inflammation of the cecum, progressing rapidly to ischemia with bloody diarrhea and perforation. Aerobic gram-negative bacteria play a role and mortality is significant despite antibiotics and surgery. Symptoms and signs are similar to acute appendicitis, although the patient may be more toxic initially. CT reveals thickening of the cecal wall.

▶ **Acute RLQ Pain: Regional Ileitis (Terminal Ileitis, Crohn Disease):** *Pathophysiology:* Granulomatous transmural inflammation of the terminal ileum of unknown cause leads to thickening of the bowel wall, obstructive symptoms, and localized perforation with abscess and fistula formation. A first attack of ileitis may be clinically indistinguishable from acute appendicitis. The single clue favoring ileitis is that diarrhea usually precedes the attack and a RLQ mass may be appreciated early in the course. If similar prior episodes have occurred, the probability is strong for chronic ileitis with an exacerbation [Podolsky DK. Inflammatory bowel disease. *N Engl J Med* 2002;347:417–429].

▶ **Acute RLQ Pain: Perforated Duodenal Ulcer:** See page 566. *Pathophysiology:* A perforated ulcer drains down the right paracolic gutter into the right iliac fossa (see Fig. 9-32). RLQ pain, tenderness, and rigidity may be pronounced, suggesting acute appendicitis. Some pain and tenderness are likely to persist in the epigastrium, directing attention to the possibility of peptic ulcer and a search for prior symptoms.

▶ **Acute LLQ Pain:** The left lower quadrant is filled with colon; consequently, most LLQ pain will be caused by colonic disorders.

▶ **Acute LLQ Pain: Colonic Diverticulitis:** *Pathophysiology:* Diverticulosis is common and usually asymptomatic. Obstruction of a diverticulum by feces can lead to local inflammation, abscess, and perforation. Typically, LLQ pain and tenderness are distinct from appendicitis. With a pelvic location, diverticulitis cannot be clinically distinguished from pelvic appendicitis. Known diverticulosis or a history of prior diverticulitis or appendectomy suggest diverticulitis. CT scans are the preferred diagnostic modality. Clinical differentiation between perforation from a right-sided diverticulum or colonic neoplasm and a ruptured appendix is exceedingly difficult. CT scans are very helpful, but surgical exploration is usually required. The absence of the typical sequence of events in acute appendicitis favors other causes of perforation.

S KEY SYNDROME

Acute Suprapubic Pain: *Pathophysiology:* Acute suprapubic pain is most often the result of pathology in the pelvis. Visceral pain from the pelvic organs is poorly localized until the process involves the peritoneum.

S KEY SYNDROME

▶ **Acute Suprapubic Pain: Rupture of Urinary Bladder:** *Pathophysiology:* When the bladder is full of urine, blunt abdominal trauma may cause it to burst; pelvic fractures can directly lacerate the bladder. Perforation may be into the peritoneal cavity or retroperitoneum. Deceleration injuries from motor vehicle accidents, especially with improperly worn lap seat belts, may include injury to the urinary bladder, bowel, mesentery, and intraabdominal vessels. Leakage of urine into the peritoneal cavity produces mild peritonitis with pain and tenderness in the suprapubic region. The usual bladder fullness cannot be felt above the prostate in the rectal examination or through the vagina in the female. When the rupture is retroperitoneal, urine extravasation dissects to the perineum, producing palpable bogginess about the rectum and vagina on rectal exam. Scrotal swelling may occur, but it is not as consistent or considerable as from extravasation of urine from a severed ureter.

S KEY SYNDROME

▶ **Acute Suprapubic Pain: Acute Salpingitis (Pelvic Inflammatory Disease):** See Chapter 11, page 642.

S KEY SYNDROME

▶ **Acute Suprapubic Pain: Ovarian Torsion:** *Pathophysiology:* Ovarian cyst or mass increases the risk of twisting of the ovary on its mesentery producing strangulation. The cyst may have been noted previously. Sudden pain in the region, accompanied by vomiting and the development of tenderness over the mass suggests a twisted pedicle.

S KEY SYNDROME

▶ **Acute Suprapubic Pain: Ectopic Pregnancy:** See Chapter 11, page 643.

Chronic Abdominal Pain Syndromes

S KEY SYNDROME

Chronic Abdominal Pain: See page 530. Pain is the presenting symptom for many chronic abdominal disorders. Chronic disease of a viscus usually produces pain in the same location as that from acute processes (see Fig. 9-19), but chronic pain is usually less severe.

✓ *CHRONIC ABDOMINAL PAIN—CLINICAL OCCURRENCE:* Congenital malrotation, familial pancreatitis, pancreas divisum, polycystic kidney disease, porphyrias, familial Mediterranean fever, sickle cell anemia,

Meckel diverticulum, cystic fibrosis, hereditary angioedema; *Endocrine* adrenal insufficiency, hypothyroidism; *Idiopathic* diverticulosis, diverticulitis, gastroesophageal reflux disease (GERD), gastritis, pancreatitis, ovarian cysts, arthritis of axial skeleton, abdominal aortic aneurysm, gastric ulcer, endometriosis; *Inflammatory/Immune* ulcerative colitis, Crohn disease, gastritis, chronic pancreatitis, autoimmune hepatitis, chronic cholecystitis, sclerosing cholangitis, primary biliary cirrhosis, pancreatic pseudocyst, celiac disease, adhesions, peritonitis, systemic lupus erythematosus (SLE), sarcoidosis, retroperitoneal and mesenteric fibrosis; *Infectious* Whipple disease, viral hepatitis (B, C), tuberculosis, *Giardia*, duodenal and gastric ulcers, diverticulitis, chronic malaria, schistosomiasis, visceral larval migrans, leishmaniasis, hookworm, roundworms, bartonellosis (peliosis hepatitis), HIV, syphilis with tabes; *Metabolic/Toxic* heavy metal poisoning, porphyrias, ketoacidosis, uremia, nonsteroidal antiinflammatory drug gastropathy and gastric ulcer; *Mechanical/Trauma* partial bowel obstruction and strictures, cholelithiasis, nephrolithiasis, pancreatic duct stricture, sphincter of Oddi spasm and stricture, biliary stricture, dumping syndromes; adhesions; ureteral obstruction, ureteropelvic junction obstruction, chronic hydrosalpinx; *Neoplastic* splenic and retroperitoneal lymphoma, primary carcinomas of the esophagus, stomach, colon, pancreas, liver, bile ducts, gallbladder, ovary; metastatic cancer to the liver (especially from pancreas, colon, lung, breast, pancreatic islets, carcinoid), spleen (lymphoma), retroperitoneal lymph nodes (cervix, testis, lymphoma, melanoma, bladder), and peritoneal surface (especially ovary); *Neurologic* postspinal cord injury, postherpetic neuralgia, diabetic radiculopathy, diabetic autonomic neuropathy, abdominal cutaneous nerve entrapment; *Psychosocial* history of domestic, sexual, or child abuse, substance abuse, opiate withdrawal; *Vascular* intestinal ischemia, vasculitis, atheroemboli, abdominal aortic or iliac aneurysm.

Abdominal Discomfort After Milk Drinking: Lactase Deficiency: See page 585.

S KEY SYNDROME

Chronic Abdominal Pain: Diabetic Radiculopathy: *Pathophysiology:* acute abdominal and/or thoracic pain accompanies ischemic or inflammatory radiculopathy of one or more thoracic and/or lumbar nerves. Pain and allodynia in the dermatomes and weakness of the muscles supplied by affected nerves are demonstrable by careful clinical exam. The acuity and severity of the pain is often mistaken for an acute intraabdominal event. It is unrelated to the duration or control of the diabetes, and usually resolves over 8–16 months. EMG is diagnostic.

S KEY SYNDROME

Chronic Abdominal Pain: Abdominal Angina (Visceral Ischemia, Intestinal Ischemia): *Pathophysiology:* Increased intestinal oxygen consumption required for di-

gestion and absorption of food following a meal exceeds the supply available because of obstruction of the mesenteric arteries. The bowel perfused by inferior mesenteric artery is most vulnerable because of limited collaterals. Visceral ischemia is characterized by the triad of postprandial pain, anorexia from fear of eating, and weight loss. Usually the pain is in the upper abdomen or the periumbilical region; sometimes it radiates to the back. It is typically intermittent, often coming on 30 minutes after eating, and persisting from 20 minutes to 3 hours, but many persons notice no relationship between the pain and the meals. Diarrhea, occasionally bloody, is fairly frequent. Sometimes a short systolic bruit is audible in the epigastrium or the umbilical regions. Similar symptoms are seen with mesenteric vein occlusions; in addition, these patients develop gastric and esophageal varices.

S KEY SYNDROME

Chronic Epigastric Pain: See the discussion of acute epigastric pain, page 566.

S KEY SYNDROME

Chronic Epigastric Pain: Xiphisternal Arthritis: The patient complains of epigastric or retrosternal pain that radiates to the back. Palpation elicits tenderness in the xiphoid-sternal joint that reproduces the complaint. Injection of cortisone and lidocaine into the joint gives complete relief. When the xiphoid cartilage is not palpated, the pain may be mistaken for that of angina pectoris, peptic ulcer, hiatal hernia, biliary colic, or chronic pancreatitis.

S KEY SYNDROME

Chronic Epigastric Pain: Peptic Ulcer: *Pathophysiology:* Peptic ulcer is caused by infection with *Helicobacter pylori,* nonsteroidal antiinflammatory drugs, or gastrin-secreting islet cell tumor (Zollinger-Ellison syndrome). Ulcer pain results from gastric acid irritation of exposed nerves. Epigastric pain occurs predictably 1 to 4 hours postprandially, and is relieved by food, H_2 blockers, and antacids. The symptoms are similar regardless of whether the ulcer is gastric, pyloric, duodenal, or stomal (anastomotic, marginal). Ulcer pain is aggravated by fasting, drinking alcohol, or coffee. The pain is described as gnawing, aching, burning, or hunger and is felt in the epigastrium near the xiphoid, sometimes radiating to the back. The pain varies from mild discomfort to severe and may awaken the patient from sleep. Untreated, ulcer symptoms may recur with periods of pain lasting from a few days to several months. Frequently there is moderate tenderness localized to the epigastrium. Diagnosis is by endoscopy [Suerbaum S, Michetti P. *Helicobacter pylori* infection. *N Engl J Med* 2002;347:1175–1186].

S KEY SYNDROME

Chronic Epigastric Pain: Pyloric Obstruction: *Pathophysiology:* Usually obstruction results from scarring of the pylorus from peptic ulceration. Pain is not an invariable accompaniment; if present, it ranges from vague discomfort to colicky epigastric pain, usually soon after eating. Emesis of undigested food eaten many hours or days before may be observed. Palpation of the abdomen may elicit a succussion splash. Occasionally, the condition is practically symptomless and is found incidentally on abdominal x-ray. When gastric retention is demonstrated, fixed outlet obstruction must be distinguished from diabetic gastroparesis and acute pylorospasm that will subside with treatment of peptic ulcer.

S KEY SYNDROME

Chronic Epigastric Discomfort: Postgastrectomy Syndrome: *Pathophysiology:* Loss of gastric storage capacity and pyloric sphincter function from subtotal gastrectomy often results in the uncontrolled dumping of hypertonic gastric contents into the small intestine. The large fluid shifts into the small bowel and the increased intestinal motility contribute to the symptoms. Gastric stapling procedures create a defunctionalized pouch which can develop inflammation (pouchitis) and the small remnant stomach can be a source of post prandial discomfort. *Early Dumping Syndrome* occurs shortly after eating; the patient experiences epigastric discomfort (not pain), weakness, sweating, nausea (but not vomiting), tachycardia, palpitation, and a feeling of epigastric fullness. Reclining may relieve the symptoms. Foods with high osmotic loads elicit the symptoms. *Late Dumping Syndrome* occurs more than 2 hours after eating with symptoms of sweating, trembling, weakness, hunger, nausea, vomiting, and, rarely, syncope.

S KEY SYNDROME

Chronic Epigastric Pain: Chronic Pancreatitis: *Pathophysiology:* Chronic pancreatitis results from alcohol, drugs, or ductal strictures. There are repeated attacks of pain which are identical with those of acute pancreatitis. Extensive loss of pancreatic tissue leads to inadequate endocrine and exocrine function producing diabetes and steatorrhea. A palpable pancreatic pseudocyst may develop [Steer ML, Waxman I, Freedman S. Chronic pancreatitis. *N Engl J Med* 1995;332:1482–1490].

S KEY SYNDROME

Chronic Epigastric Pain: Gastric Carcinoma: Pain is usually preceded by anorexia, loss of weight, and weakness. The pain may be a steady, unremitting ache in the epigastrium, sometimes radiating to the back, or it may resemble that of peptic ulcer.

S KEY SYNDROME

Chronic RUQ Pain: See the discussion of RUQ pain, page 569.

S KEY SYNDROME

Chronic RUQ Pain: Chronic Cholecystitis with or without Calculi: The RUQ pain varies from continual, ill-defined distress to recurring attacks of biliary colic with paroxysms of colicky pain radiating to the right scapula. Tenderness is localized to the right lower margin of the liver. Fist percussion tenderness is usually present during the attack and for several days afterward.

▶ **S KEY SYNDROME**
Chronic RUQ Pain: Hepatocellular Carcinoma: *Pathophysiology:* Hepatocellular carcinoma arises in a cirrhotic liver from any cause, particularly following chronic viral hepatitis B and C. Abdominal pain is the most common symptom. A hard, nodular, localized mass in the liver with centrifugal extension may be detected by palpation, sometimes with an overlying peritoneal friction rub. A bruit may be heard.

▶ **S KEY SYNDROME**
Chronic RUQ Pain: Metastatic Carcinoma: *Pathophysiology:* Hematogenous metastases via the portal vein are frequent in colon, and pancreatic cancer. Metastases from lung and breast cancer are also common. Poorly localized upper abdominal pain or discomfort may be the presenting symptom. Seldom does the patient have abdominal distention or mass. The diagnosis is suggested by palpation of a mass in the liver. The liver is often stony hard. When a single discrete hepatic mass is felt, hepatocellular carcinoma or abscess should be suspected. A peritoneal friction rub or a bruit may rarely be present.

D KEY DISEASE
Chronic Upper Abdominal Pain: Carcinoma of the Pancreas: *Pathophysiology:* Pain may occur as a result of acute or chronic pancreatitis, or invasion of the retroperitoneal structures and nerves. Retroperitoneal invasion causes constant, dull, poorly localized pain in the midepigastrium, flank, or back. When the head of the pancreas is involved, early, painless, persistent jaundice is the rule. As the tumor enlarges, the nearly universal triad of pain, weight loss, and jaundice is seen. The first sign of pancreatic carcinoma may be superficial migrating thrombophlebitis.

S KEY SYNDROME
Recurrent Abdominal Pain: Recurrent pain suggests an intermittent mechanical problem, a partially treated inflammatory disorder, or an episodic metabolic/toxic syndrome.

✓ *RECURRENT ABDOMINAL PAIN—CLINICAL OCCURRENCE:* *Congenital* porphyria, sickle cell disease, familial Mediterranean fever, other familial fever syndromes; *Idiopathic* chronic pancreatitis, sphincter of Oddi dysfunction; endometriosis; *Infection* chronic hepatitis, schistosomiasis, *Helicobacter pylori* ulcers and gastritis; *Inflammatory/Immune* systemic lupus erythematosus, autoimmune gastritis; *Metabolic/Toxic* lead poisoning; *Mechanical/Trauma* biliary colic, ureteral colic, adhesions, and partial bowel obstruction; *Neoplastic* partial bowel obstruction from luminal masses; *Psychosocial* domestic, sexual, and child abuse; *Vascular* mesenteric ischemia.

Abdominal Wall Pain Syndromes: Specific signs to be looked for are point tenderness (trigger points) not abolished by contraction of the abdominal muscles; superficial tenderness from clothing; hyperesthesia and allodynia of the skin; abdominal wall defects, with or without hernia; masses; surgical and varicella-zoster scars; and weakness or asymmetry of the abdominal wall. Injection of trigger points with local anesthetic frequently answers the diagnostic question without further testing. Be sure to fully examine the spine for evidence of problems referring pain to the abdomen.

Abdominal Wall Pain: Abdominal Cutaneous Nerve Entrapment (Rectus Abdominis Nerve Entrapment Syndrome): *Pathophysiology:* Anterior cutaneous nerve branches from T7 to L1 may be entrapped as they pass through the rectus sheath. Entrapment may occur from overuse of the rectus muscles or weight gain by putting increased traction on the nerve. The pain usually occurs laterally to the entrapment site and is increased when the patient tenses the rectus muscles. Pressure over the exit site in the fascia, felt as a small fascial defect, reproduces the pain. The pain is relieved by injection of local anesthetic into the trigger point.

Pain and Paramedial Mass: Hematoma of Rectus Abdominis Muscle: *Pathophysiology:* The epigastric artery and vein run vertically within the rectus sheath; hemorrhage within the sheath above the arcuate line is confined to the sheath, but dissects into the lateral abdominal wall below the arcuate line. It is often mistaken for such an intraabdominal mass. If one considers it, the diagnosis is easy; the mass remains palpable when the abdominal wall is tensed, a maneuver that obscures intraabdominal masses (see Fig. 9-27, page 554). The mass may be tender and painful. The diagnosis is readily proved by ultrasonography or CT. The usual setting is trauma, either direct or as a result of coughing, paracentesis and operative injury, especially in a debilitated or anticoagulated patient.

Bloating and Distention Syndromes

Bloating and Distention Syndromes: These are common complaints that can be the presenting signs for mechanical or functional bowel obstruction or abnormalities of digestion. Often, the sensations described by the patient are not matched by any finding on physical exam of abdominal distention or obstruction. The syndrome of visceral hyperalgesia may underlie this presentation.

Bloating and Distention Syndromes: Gastric Distention: *Pathophysiology:* Gastroparesis with gastric distention can result from reflex loss of gastric tone following abdominal surgery or upper intestinal inflammation, autonomic neuropathy as in diabetes, vagotomy, or with the decreased bowel motility associated with chronic illness and bed rest. In the most acute and severe cases, the patient, bedridden from some other disorder, becomes acutely more ill with an anxious or apathetic appearance, often accompanied by vomiting, with distention of the upper abdomen, and hypotension with a thready pulse. Inspection shows a greatly dilated stomach filling the epigastrium, rarely reaching to the pelvis. The mass is tympanitic and may have a succussion splash. Early, visible peristalsis may be present; later, peristaltic sounds are weak or absent, indicating ileus. The diagnosis is confirmed when nasogastric aspiration yields a large volume of fluid and the distention resolves. Less dramatic and more chronic gastroparesis is frequent and more difficult to diagnose. Difficult to control glucose in diabetics (because of the irregular gastric emptying) or presentation with nausea and emesis of undigested food several hours after meals should suggest the diagnosis. The major provocative factors are pain, abdominal trauma, and immobilization; postoperative cases are common. Many conditions may precipitate this syndrome, but gastroparesis associated with diabetes mellitus is the most frequent cause. Other causes of visceral autonomic neuropathy should be considered [Bityutskiy LP, Soykan I, McCallum RW. Viral gastroparesis: A subgroup of idiopathic gastroparesis—Clinical characteristics and long-term outcomes. *Am J Gastroenterol* 1997;92:1501–1504].

S KEY SYNDROME

Bloating and Distention Syndromes: Ascites: See page 542.

S KEY SYNDROME

Bloating and Distention Syndromes: Irritable Bowel Syndrome: See page 590.

S KEY SYNDROME

Bloating and Distention Syndromes: Lactose and Fructose Intolerance: See page 585.

Diarrhea Syndromes

S KEY SYNDROME

Acute Nonbloody Diarrhea: See page 534. Diarrhea lasting less than 2 weeks, and not preceded by a history of recurrent or relapsing diarrhea, qualifies as acute diarrhea. Infectious and toxic causes are by far the most common.

✓ *ACUTE NONBLOODY DIARRHEA—CLINICAL OCCURRENCE:* *Infectious* enteroviruses, Rotavirus, Norwalk agent, enterotoxigenic *Escherichia coli*, salmonella, shigella, *Campylobacter, Giardia,* cryptosporidium, microspora, amebiasis, *Clostridium difficile, Vibrio cholerae;* *Metabolic/Toxic* food poisoning (*Bacillus cereus,* staphylococcal, *Clostridium perfringens*), antibiotic-associated diarrhea, alcohol, osmotic laxatives, sugar-free candy and foods, drug withdrawal; *Vascular* ischemic colitis [Bartlett JG. Antibiotic-associated diarrhea. *N Engl J Med* 2002;346:334–339].

S KEY SYNDROME

Acute Nonbloody Diarrhea: Traveler's Diarrhea: *Pathophysiology:* Travelers ingest the colonic flora of their host country via contaminated food and water. Within 1 week of arrival in a tropical, underdeveloped area, temperate zone travelers may experience watery diarrhea, abdominal cramping, and anorexia which is self-limited to 1 to 5 days. The most common organism is enterotoxigenic *Escherichia coli*, while *Shigella, Salmonella, Campylobacter, Vibrio cholerae, Giardia, Cryptosporidium*, and viruses also occur.

S KEY SYNDROME

Acute Nonbloody Diarrhea: Viral Gastroenteritis: *Pathophysiology:* Infection of the bowel epithelium with loss of absorptive function. Systemic signs vary from none to mild (Norwalk) to severe (rotavirus). This is a common epidemic illness with sudden onset of nausea, vomiting, and explosive diarrhea, with or without abdominal cramps. Myalgia, malaise, and anorexia, usually without fever, are common. The diarrhea and vomiting subside within 48 hours; lassitude may persist for several days. The stools consist of water and fecal remnants; blood, pus, and mucus are absent. Common causes are rotavirus, Norwalk virus, noravirus, adenovirus, caliciviruses, enterovirus, and coronavirus. Specific diagnosis is not required.

S KEY SYNDROME

Acute Nonbloody Diarrhea: Food Intolerance: *Pathophysiology*: Local and systemic allergic response to specific food allergens. Ingestion of food allergens may cause nausea, vomiting, abdominal cramping, and diarrhea. Angioedema may occur. The history usually reveals the diagnosis, although first episodes present a challenge in identification of the allergen. Shellfish, peanuts, cow's milk, and cereals are common culprits.

S KEY SYNDROME

Acute Nonbloody Diarrhea: Cholera: *Pathophysiology:* Cholera toxin inhibits gut Na^+ absorption and activates Cl^- excretion, producing severe secretory diarrhea. Waterborne infection with *Vibrio cholerae* is locally endemic in some countries, and epidemic and pandemic disease occurs. There is sudden abdominal cramping, vomiting, and voluminous watery stools containing flecks of mucus ("rice-water stools") progressing to dehydration, electrolyte imbalances, prostration, shock, and death.

S KEY SYNDROME

Acute Nonbloody Diarrhea: Food Poisoning: *Pathophysiology:* Ingestion of preformed bacterial exotoxins in contaminated food. *Bacillus cereus* also causes a longer incubation diarrhea probably from exotoxin production in the gut. Severe cramping abdominal pain, nausea, vomiting, diarrhea, and prostration begin 1 to 6 hours after a meal. The symptoms resolve within hours. Frequently large groups of diners are affected. The type of food is a clue to the etiology: potato salad, mayonnaise, and cream pastries—*Staphylococcus aureus;* meat, poultry, legumes—*Clostridium perfringens;* fried rice—*Bacillus cereus.*

S KEY SYNDROME

▶ ▼ **Acute Bloody Diarrhea:** *Pathophysiology:* Acute diarrhea with blood indicates that the mucosa of the bowel, usually the colon, is being compromised. Infections that invade the mucosa or that cause toxic epithelial necrosis are most likely. Chronic inflammatory diseases can present as diarrhea initially, or with relapse. Patients may present with abdominal pain and tenesmus (dysentery syndrome) or without pain. Fever and leukocytosis suggest an enteroinvasive organism with the risk of systemic spread or local complications. Painless bleeding in otherwise healthy individuals suggest bleeding from a structural abnormality (Meckel diverticulum, polyp, or cancer).

✔ *ACUTE BLOODY DIARRHEA—CLINICAL OCCURRENCE:* Congenital Meckel diverticulum; *Inflammatory/Immune* ulcerative colitis, Crohn disease; *Infectious* bacteria (*Campylobacter jejuni, Salmonella spp., Shigella spp.,* enterohemorrhagic *Escherichia coli* [0157:H7]), protozoa (*Entamoeba histolytica, Balantidium coli),* cytomegalovirus; *Metabolic/Toxic* heavy-metal poisoning (arsenic, mercury, cadmium, copper, iron); *Mechanical/Trauma* rectal foreign body; *Neoplastic* villous adenoma with malignant change; *Vascular* ischemic colitis.

S KEY SYNDROME

▼ **Acute Bloody Diarrhea: Poisoning with Heavy Metals or Drugs:** The heavy metals (such as arsenic, cadmium, copper, or mercury) may be ingested accidentally or with suicidal or homicidal intent. Nausea, vomiting, cramping abdominal pains, and bloody diarrhea begin soon after ingestion.

S KEY SYNDROME

▼ **Acute Bloody Diarrhea: Infectious Dysentery:** *Pathophysiology:* Infectious diarrhea in which the stools contain pus and blood, indicating intestinal inflammation, often with invasion and ulceration. Bloody stools with mucous, fever, and tenesmus are distinct from simple gastroenteritis. Stool culture and examination for ova and parasites is required; sigmoidoscopy may be useful. Common etiologies are bacterial (*Campylobacter jejuni, Salmonella spp., Shigella spp.,* enterohemorrhagic *Escherichia coli* including 0157:H7) and protozoa (*Entamoeba histolytica, Balantidium coli, strongyloidiasis*).

D KEY DISEASE

▼ **Amebiasis:** *Pathophysiology:* Colon infection with *Entamoeba histolytica* occurs after ingestion of contaminated water, leading to ulcerations of the colon and terminal ilium and liver abscess. Onset may be acute and fulminant with cramping abdominal pain, bloody diarrhea, and tenesmus; exam reveals fever, diffuse abdominal tenderness, dehydration, and weight loss. Subacute infection is manifest by milder abdominal cramps, diarrheal stools containing mucus or blood, often alternating with intervals of normal function; exam may show fever and RLQ tenderness. Liver abscess is marked by spiking fevers, prostration and RUQ pain with mildly abnormal liver function tests.

S KEY SYNDROME

Acute Bloody Diarrhea: Ulcerative Colitis:

See *Chronic Constant Diarrhea: Ulcerative Colitis*, page 587. Although a chronic disease, its onset may be sudden, resembling acute dysentery. The absence of organisms in the stools and the subsequent course suggest the diagnosis, which is confirmed by colonoscopy and biopsy.

S KEY SYNDROME

Chronic Intermittent Diarrhea: *Pathophysiology:*

Diarrhea lasting more than 2 weeks is chronic and is less likely to be infectious. Intermittent diarrhea implies a disease with a relapsing–remittent course (e.g., Crohn disease) or an interaction of the host and the environment, particularly the diet (e.g., lactase deficiency). Most of the causes of chronic persistent diarrhea can present as chronic intermittent diarrhea.

S KEY SYNDROME

Chronic Intermittent Diarrhea: Irritable Bowel Syndrome: See page 590.

S KEY SYNDROME

Chronic Intermittent Diarrhea: Lactase Deficiency: *Pathophysiology:* Deficiency of small bowel mucosal

lactase in many blacks, Asians, and a few whites leads to incomplete digestion of lactose, the disaccharide in milk. The lactose is then fermented by colonic bacteria, producing gas and diarrhea. Eating milk products produces a watery diarrhea, gas, and often abdominal cramps. Patients are often unaware of the association because of the ubiquitous presence of milk products in the diet. Avoidance of milk products leads to prompt resolution and is the treatment of choice. Malabsorption of other disaccharides, such as sorbitol, used in sugarless candies, and fructose, may cause a similar picture.

S KEY SYNDROME

Chronic Intermittent Diarrhea: Fructose Intolerance: *Pathophysiology:* Some individuals are unable to

absorb fructose in the quantities ingested, especially those who consume large amounts of sugared soft drinks in their diets. The unabsorbed fructose creates an osmotic diarrhea and increased intestinal gas when fermented by colonic bacteria. Symptoms and signs are those of lactose intolerance.

S KEY SYNDROME

Chronic Intermittent Diarrhea: Regional Enteritis (Crohn Disease, Terminal Ileitis): *Pathophysiology:* Transmural granulomatous inflammation of the small and large intestine with perianal and enteroenteral fistula formation interferes with gut motility and absorption while producing chronic inflammation and blood loss. Extraintestinal manifestations may be the presenting complaint. Attacks of colicky pain occur in the right lower abdominal quadrant, commonly accompanied by diarrhea. Weight loss may be severe. An acute attack can resemble appendicitis so closely that operation is necessary. Perforations, strictures, and fistulas are common complications including perianal fistulas and anal stricture. Colon involvement is segmental with skip areas. Barium in the small bowel may show strictures, fistulas, loss of mucosal detail, and tubular thickening of the submucosa. Diagnosis is by endoscopic biopsy with gross and microscopic examination of resected tissue. Infections need to be in the differential diagnosis including *Yersinia, Salmonella, Shigella*, tuberculosis, amebiasis, and cytomegalovirus.

S KEY SYNDROME

Chronic Intermittent Diarrhea: Ulcerative Colitis: See page 587.

S KEY SYNDROME

Chronic Constant Diarrhea: Chronic constant diarrhea suggests an unremitting underlying structural or functional process involving digestion, absorption, bowel motility, or metabolism. The history (age of onset, exacerbating or palliative maneuvers), comorbid conditions, and characteristics of the stools are critical to a parsimonious differential diagnosis [Donowitz M, Kokke FT, Saidi R. Evaluation of patients with chronic diarrhea. *N Engl J Med* 1995;332:725–729].

✔ *CHRONIC DIARRHEA—CLINICAL OCCURRENCE: Congenital* cystic fibrosis, lactase deficiency, celiac disease; *Endocrine* hyperthyroidism, adrenal insufficiency, carcinoid syndrome, pheochromocytoma; *Idiopathic* irritable bowel syndrome, chronic pancreatitis, diverticulitis; *Inflammatory/Immune* ulcerative colitis, Crohn disease, microscopic colitis, mastocytosis, chronic pancreatitis, celiac disease, amyloidosis; *Infectious* Giardia, HIV/AIDS and opportunistic infections, microsporidiosis, cyclosporiasis, Whipple disease, bacterial overgrowth in the small bowel, intestinal parasites; *Metabolic/Toxic* hyperthyroidism, lactase deficiency, drugs (metformin, proton pump inhibitors, misoprostol, colchicine, digitalis, antacids), bile salt-induced, laxative abuse, nonsteroidal antiinflammatory drugs, alcohol; *Mechanical/Trauma* short-bowel syndrome, enterocolic fistulas, radiation enteritis; *Neoplastic* mastocytosis, villous adenoma, pancreatic islet cell tumors (producing vasoactive intestinal peptide, gastrin, glucagon, etc.), small-bowel lymphoma; *Neurologic* autonomic neuropathies; *Psychosocial* laxative abuse; *Vascular* vasculitis.

▼ Chronic Constant Diarrhea: Gluten-Sensitive Enteropathy (Celiac Disease, Nontropical Sprue): *Pathophysiology:* In persons with specific HLA-DQ2 alleles, ingestion of gluten (gliadin) from wheat flour induces chronic mucosal and submucosal inflammation, which produces characteristic flattening of the villi and chronic malabsorption. Patients present with fatigue, cramping, diarrhea, steatorrhea, and weight loss without anorexia. A family history may be present and dietary modifications may already have been made by the patient. The stools are soft, frothy, and malodorous from unabsorbed fat. Patients may present with unexplained iron deficiency, hypocalcemia, neuropathy, dermatitis herpetiformis, or weight loss without complaints of diarrhea [Farrell RJ, Kelly CP. Celiac sprue. *N Engl J Med* 2002;346:180–188].

▼ Chronic Constant Diarrhea: Ulcerative Colitis: *Pathophysiology:* Intense chronic mucosal inflammation and ulceration with crypt abscess formation. The clinical picture varies from acute dysentery, with fever, abdominal pain, tenesmus, bloody diarrhea, and weight loss, to mild abdominal discomfort with mostly formed stools and little blood. Inflammation is always present in the rectum and extends proximally in continuity. The extent of the disease varies from rectal involvement only to pancolitis. In long-standing disease, the lumen is contracted and irregular because of pseudopolyp formation. The terminal ileum may be inflamed and dilated, in contrast to the constriction found in regional enteritis. The diagnosis is made by endoscopic inspection and biopsy of the mucosa which is red, edematous, and friable, with the slightest touch causing bleeding; often the entire rectosigmoid is covered by purulent exudate obscuring the multiple ulcers. Disease duration greater than 10 years and pancolitis, but not the severity of symptoms, are associated with an increased risk for colon cancer. Ulcerative colitis must be distinguished from Crohn colitis, ischemic colitis, amebiasis, and bacillary infections [Podolsky DK. Inflammatory bowel disease. *N Engl J Med* 2002;347:417–429].

Chronic Diarrhea: Colonic Amyloidosis: *Pathophysiology:* Deposition of amyloid proteins in the bowel progressively impairs motility and absorptive capacity. Amyloidosis is classified by the specific amyloid protein (e.g., immunoglobulin light chains-AL, amyloid A protein-AA) and the presence of specific associated diseases, predominately hematologic cancer (e.g., multiple myeloma, chronic lymphatic leukemia) or chronic inflammatory disease (e.g., regional enteritis and ulcerative colitis). Amyloidosis may produce a chronic diarrhea, hypomotility, obstructive symptoms, ulceration, hemorrhage, and a protein-losing enteropathy.

Chronic Diarrhea: Zollinger-Ellison Syndrome: *Pathophysiology:* A pancreatic gastrinoma or adenomatous hyperpla-

sia of nonislet cells produces excess gastrin that stimulates high HCl secretion in the stomach, leading to diarrhea and ulcers in esophagus, duodenum, and jejunum. There are recurrent attacks of epigastric pain, nausea, vomiting, and diarrhea. Malabsorption and weight loss may occur.
The diagnosis is suspected when finding severe ulcer disease, absence
of *Helicobacter pylori,* and diarrhea.

Chronic Diarrhea: Carcinoid Syndrome: *Patho-physiology:*

Metastases from a carcinoid tumor of the gastrointestinal
tract produce large amounts of serotonin. Symptoms include intermittent flushing of skin, recurrent diarrhea, nausea and vomiting, and abdominal pain. Intermittent migratory flushing of face and neck occur
with rapid color changes between red, white, and violet. Right-sided
heart failure may develop from endomyocardial fibrosis with tricuspid
insufficiency.

Chronic Diarrhea: Whipple Disease (Intestinal Lipodystrophy): *Pathophysiology:*

Invasion of the intestinal
mucosa and lamina propria with *Tropheryma whippelii* produces foamy
macrophages filled with glycoprotein and produces lymphatic obstruction with malabsorption. Dissemination produces arthritis, lymphadenopathy, and an indolent meningitis. This can occur at any age,
most commonly in the fourth and fifth decades in white men. Migratory polyarthralgias and polyarthritis may precede the intestinal symptoms of abdominal cramping and episodic diarrhea of fatty, foul-
smelling stools and weight loss. There is generalized malaise and
weakness with cough and dyspnea. The fever is intermittent and may
be accompanied by hypotension, edema, lymphadenopathy, and emaciation. Central nervous system infection causes slowly progressive
chronic meningitis.

Chronic Diarrhea: Enteroenteric Fistula: *Patho-physiology:*

A fistula between the proximal and distal bowel produces
diarrhea with undigested food in the feces and/or fecal emesis. The diarrhea may be intermittent and results, in part, from bacteria overgrowth
in the proximal gut. The malabsorption of nutrients, fluids and electrolytes causes weight loss, hypoproteinemia, and dehydration. Fecal belching and vomiting suggests gastrocolic fistula.

S KEY SYNDROME

Chronic Diarrhea and Malabsorption (Maldigestion–Malabsorption Syndrome): *Patho-physiology:*

Maldigestion results from failure to deliver sufficient pancreatic enzymes and bile salts into the duodenum, inadequate mixing
of luminal contents, or insufficient time in the small bowel for digestion
to occur. **Malabsorbtion** results from damage to the small-bowel absorptive machinery or bypass of or loss of absorptive surface. **Steatorrhea** occurs when triglycerides are not digested or absorbed because of

a lack of micelle formation or insufficient pancreatic lipase secretion. Fat appears in the stool as triglycerides. Steatorrhea is suggested when the stools are frothy, greasy, and foul smelling. Weight loss is common despite a good appetite. Fat-soluble vitamins (A, D, E, and K) are malabsorbed and deficiency syndromes of each may be present or be the presenting complaint. Microscopic stool exam shows fat globules when stained with Sudan III; 72-hour fecal fat on a 100 g of fat per day diet is the diagnostic test.

S KEY SYNDROME

Chronic Diarrhea and Malabsorption: Blind-Loop Syndrome: *Pathophysiology:* Either decreased small intestinal motility leading to stasis or loss of protective gastric acid or decreased ileocecal valve function increases the risk of bacterial overgrowth, the blind- or stagnant-loop syndrome. Bacteria consume nutrients, including vitamins, leading to malnutrition and vitamin deficiency, particularly vitamin B_{12}. The patient presents with diarrhea, steatorrhea, weight loss, macrocytic anemia, and sometimes feculent belching. Because the bacterial overgrowth is responsible for the malabsorption, a short course of antibiotics should lead to demonstrable improvement. Common antecedent conditions include surgically created blind pouches, enteroenterostomies, a long afferent loop, strictures, fistulous communications, and small bowel diverticula. Tape worms can produce a similar picture.

S KEY SYNDROME

Chronic Diarrhea with Weight Loss: Chronic Pancreatitis: This is characterized by episodes of abdominal pain and loose, fatty stools. The stools are soft, frothy, and malodorous; they frequently float on water. When present, pancreatic calcification is diagnostic. Alcohol abuse and mild forms of cystic fibrosis are common causes.

Chronic Diarrhea with Weight Loss: Cystic Fibrosis: An autosomal recessive disease usually diagnosed in childhood. Patients with mild disease may present in adult life with pancreatic insufficiency.

S KEY SYNDROME

Chronic Diarrhea with Weight Loss: Celiac Disease: See page 587.

S KEY SYNDROME

Chronic Diarrhea with Weight Loss: Giardiasis: *Pathophysiology:* *Giardia* organisms adhere to the brush-border of enterocytes in the duodenum and upper small bowel, impairing absorption of nutrients, leading to diarrhea and weight loss. A travel history and exposure to surface water potentially contaminated by livestock and wildlife is useful. Stool antigen testing is available.

Constipation Syndromes

S KEY SYNDROME

▼ Acute Constipation: Intestinal Obstruction:
See page 591.

S KEY SYNDROME

▼ Subacute Constipation: Obstruction in the Distal Colon:
Pathophysiology: The colon narrows distally, especially in the descending and sigmoid regions, making them most susceptible to obstruction by mass or luminal narrowing. The recent onset of constipation associated with cramping abdominal pain after lifelong regular bowel habits suggests obstruction in the descending colon. Complete colonoscopy is required. Differential diagnosis includes colon cancer, diverticulosis or diverticulitis with stricture, and large benign polyps.

S KEY SYNDROME

▼ Acute Constipation: Fecal Impaction:
There may be no discomfort or the patient may complain of constipation, tenesmus, and inability to defecate. Frequently, diarrhea is the complaint, because of liquid stool passing around the impacted mass, leading to inappropriate treatment. A digital examination of the rectum reveals hard fecal masses that must be removed manually. Common inciting factors are immobilization, bedrest, dehydration, anticholinergic medications, dementia, and barium for GI contrast x-rays.

S KEY SYNDROME

▼ Chronic Constipation: Irritable Bowel Syndrome (Spastic Colon):
This common cause of constipation is characterized by periods of constipation alternating with bouts of diarrhea. Either symptom may be the main complaint. The triad of symptoms is long-standing intermittent constipation, scybalous stools, and abdominal pain relieved by defecation. The cause is uncertain though many patients have increased sensitivity to visceral discomfort (visceral hyperalgesia) [Talley NJ, Spiller R. Irritable bowel syndrome: A little understood organic bowel disease? *Lancet* 2002;360:555–564; Horwitz BJ, Fisher RS. The irritable bowel syndrome. *N Engl J Med* 2001;344:1846–1850].

S KEY SYNDROME

▼ Chronic Constipation: Atonic Colon, Laxative Abuse:
The patient has a long history of constipation, fancied or real. The stools may be alternately voluminous and scanty. Palpation of the abdomen often reveals large fecal masses; stools may be felt in the rectum during digital examination.

S KEY SYNDROME

▼ Chronic Constipation: Megacolon:
Lifelong constipation with occasional passage of an enormous formed stool suggests

megacolon. Causes are congenital (Hirschsprung disease) or acquired defects in the intrinsic myenteric innervation of the colon, for example, idiopathic intestinal pseudoobstruction.

> **S KEY SYNDROME**
> ▼ **Chronic Constipation: Drugs:** *Pathophysiology:* Many drugs slow bowel motility, including opiates, anticholinergic drugs, antihistamines, chronic laxative use, and overuse of bulk laxatives. Pill bezoars have been described. Medication history with particular inquiry into the use of laxatives and enemas is key. Ophthalmologic medications are systemically absorbed and can effect gut function.

Bowel Obstruction Syndromes

> **S KEY SYNDROME**
> ▼ **Noisy Tympanites with Colic and Vomiting: Mechanical Obstruction:** *Pathophysiology:* This pattern suggests localized bowel obstruction causing an increased force of peristaltic contraction proximal to the obstruction, producing colic and proximal bowel distension by retained luminal contents leading to decompression by vomiting. Mechanical obstruction is probable. Tympanites is present when the obstruction is distal to the mid jejunum. Increased peristalsis proximal to an obstruction is indicated by frequent, loud peristaltic sounds *(borborygmi)* accompanied by cramping, colicky pain. With partial obstructions, high-pitched high-pressure-to-low-pressure sounds ("rushes") accompanying the pain may be appreciated. Vomiting appears earlier and is more intense the more proximal the obstruction. Distal obstruction may result in feculent emesis which classically indicates colonic obstruction in a person with an incompetent ileocecal valve or a cologastric or coloenteric fistula [Bohner H, Yang Q, Franke C, et al. Simple data from history and physical examination help to exclude bowel obstruction and to avoid radiographic studies in patients with acute abdominal pain. *Eur J Surg* 1998;164:777–784].

ACUTE INTESTINAL OBSTRUCTION. Colicky pain is almost invariably present from the onset. In general, the more proximal the obstruction, the more severe the symptoms. *Proximal Small Intestine.* Epigastric pain is intense and vomiting is early and severe. If the vomitus contains bile, the obstruction is beyond the second portion of the duodenum. Abdominal distention appears late, and then is limited to the epigastrium. *Distal Small Intestine.* Symptoms are less severe, vomiting is delayed, but the vomitus may have become feculent. Diffuse abdominal distention gradually develops. *Colon.* The pain is less than from obstruction of the small intestine. Vomiting is late and may be fecal. Constipation is invariable, but the bowel must first empty its contents below the obstruction, delaying recognition. An empty rectal ampulla, void of gas, is strong presumptive evidence of colonic obstruction.

✓ *MECHANICAL BOWEL OBSTRUCTION—CLINICAL OCCURRENCE:* *Inflammatory/Immune* Crohn disease; *Infectious* parasites; *Mechanical/ Trauma* adhesions (most common), gallstone impaction, bezoars, foreign body, pyloric stenosis, volvulus, hernias (internal and abdominal wall), intussusception, external compression from intraabdominal cysts and neoplasms; *Neoplastic* benign and malignant tumors.

Bezoars: These are concretions of hair (trichobezoar), plant fibers (phytobezoar), or medicines (aluminum hydroxide gel or polystyrene sodium sulfonate) formed in the gastrointestinal tract. They may present with obstructive symptoms when they lodge at the pylorus (gastric outlet obstruction) or ileocecal valve (small-bowel obstruction). They may cause mechanical erosion of the bowel wall, leading to ulceration with bleeding and pain.

S KEY SYNDROME

▶ ▼ **Strangulated Hernia:** See page 602.

S KEY SYNDROME

▶ ▼ **Intussusception:** *Pathophysiology:* Intussusception is the invagination of bowel into the lumen of adjacent bowel. The enfolded portion always points down the fecal stream. There are four types: ileum into ileum, ileum into ileocecal valve, ileocecal valve into colon, and colon into colon (Fig. 9-34). This is the most common cause

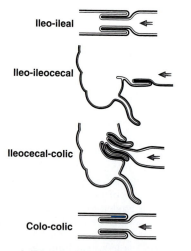

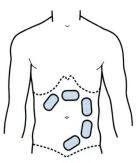

A. Types of Intussusception   **B. Location of Intussusception**

Fig. 9-34 Intussusception. *This is the prolapse of one segment of intestine into an adjoining segment.* ***A. The Four Types of Intussusception****: The enfolding of the lumen is in the direction of fecal flow, as shown by the arrows. In the intracolic type, the stippling indicates a neoplasm that is usually the cause of the telescoping.* ***B. Locations****: The usual sites of palpable masses are shown as sausage-shaped outlines; these are usually in the colon.*

of intestinal obstruction in infants. It is frequently preceded by a viral infection in children; in adults neoplasm in the intestinal wall is usually the cause. In addition to obstructive symptoms, mucus, and sometimes blood, are passed from the rectum. The pathognomonic sign is an oblong mass in the right or upper mid-abdomen and absence of bowel in the right lower quadrant (*Dance sign*) [Case records of the Massachusetts General Hospital. Case 26–2002. *N Engl J Med* 2002;347:601–606].

S KEY SYNDROME

▶ ▼ **Colon Cancer:** This is the second most common cause of intestinal obstruction in persons older than 50 years of age. Gradually increasing constipation culminates in the onset of low intestinal obstruction. Right colon obstruction distends the cecum, which forms a painful, rounded mass in the RLQ. Distal cancers cause gradual distention of the sigmoid and/or descending colon which is readily palpated in the LLQ [Ransohoff DF, Sandler RS. Screening for colorectal cancer. *N Engl J Med* 2002;346:40–44].

S KEY SYNDROME

▶ ▼ **Volvulus:** *Pathophysiology:* The gut twists upon itself, which results in a closed-loop obstruction. The cecum and sigmoid colon are most at risk because their longer mesenteries allow rotation. Diagnosis depends on identification of a distended loop of large bowel, often to enormous proportion, rotating up and out of the pelvis. A bird beak cutoff is noted in the colonic gas on noncontrast x-rays. Colonoscopy may be both diagnostic and therapeutic.

S KEY SYNDROME

▼ **Silent Tympanites without Colic or Vomiting: Ileus:** *Pathophysiology:* This pattern suggests a diffuse decrease in bowel motility and muscular tone, producing a silent abdomen with distended bowel. Nonmechanical, diffuse ileus is probable. Abdominal tympany is always present and the peristaltic sounds are diminished or absent. When present, abdominal pain is mild and colic is absent; vomiting is uncommon, but anorexia and nausea are to be expected.

✔ *ILEUS—CLINICAL OCCURRENCE: Inflammatory/Immune* Sterile peritonitis: perforated viscus—HCl and gastric contents from perforated stomach or duodenum, bile peritonitis, ruptured bladder; miscellaneous: enzymes released by acute pancreatitis, ruptured ovarian cyst, blood (e.g., bleeding from follicular cyst), recurrent serositis syndromes (e.g., systemic lupus erythematosus, familial Mediterranean fever, familial Hibernian fever), inflammatory bowel disease (ulcerative colitis, Crohn disease), toxic megacolon; *Infectious* infectious peritonitis (spontaneous bacterial peritonitis in cirrhosis, perforated bowel, perforating neoplasm, ruptured colonic diverticulum or diverticular abscess, tuberculosis, penetrating abdominal trauma, surgical wound dehiscence), *Clostridium difficile* colitis, amebic colitis, typhoid fever, *Giardia*, Whipple disease; *Metabolic/Toxic* hypokalemia, hypothyroidism, acidemia or alkalemia, diabetic ketoacidosis, uremia, heavy metal poisoning, porphyria, toxic megacolon or any major metabolic disorder, drugs (opiates, anticholinergics, vinca alkaloids, ganglionic blocking agents); *Mechanical/Trauma* manipulation of the gut (abdominal surgical procedures, trauma to the abdomen), adhesions, tumors, volvulus, intussusception, parasites; *Neurologic* trauma to the axial skeleton, compression fracture, herpes zoster, urinary retention, fecal impaction, aerophagia; *Vascular* Mesenteric arterial embolism or thrombosis, mesenteric venous thrombosis, hypotension, ischemic bowel.

Abdominal Masses

S KEY SYNDROME
Abdominal Wall Mass: Rectus Sheath Hematoma: See page 581.

S KEY SYNDROME
Abdominal Mass: Visceral Enlargement: A careful history and physical exam will identify the specific enlarged organs(s), and when combined with a judicious selection of laboratory and imaging studies, the probable pathophysiology can be identified. The liver, spleen, adrenals and kidneys are the parenchymal organs susceptible to enlargement.

✓*ENLARGED VISCERA—CLINICAL OCCURRENCE: Congenital* horseshoe kidney; infiltration by cells of the reticuloendothelial system (e.g., lipopolysaccharidases); *Idiopathic* single or multiple cysts; *Inflammatory/Immune* infiltration by cells of the reticuloendothelial system (e.g., histiocytosis syndromes), granulomatous diseases (sarcoid), deposition of extracellular proteins (amyloidosis); *Infectious* granulomatous diseases (fungal infections, tuberculosis), chronic infection and parasitosis (amebiasis, hydatid disease); *Metabolic/Toxic* hypertrophy of normal tissue as a consequence of increased functional demands (e.g., splenomegaly in hemolytic anemias), accumulation of intracellular inclusions (steatosis, glycogen storage diseases and lipopolysaccharidases); *Mechanical/Trauma* obstruction of normal effluent systems (hydronephrosis, hepatic vein obstruction), enlargement of fluid-containing hollow organs as a consequence of outflow obstruction (e.g., urinary retention and gallbladder hydrops); *Neoplastic* primary neoplasms, infiltration by metastatic neoplasm either diffusely or focally, extramedullary hematopoiesis; *Vascular* renal and hepatic vein obstruction.

S KEY SYNDROME
Abdominal Mass: Ptotic and Transplanted Kidney: *Pathophysiology:* The kidneys are only loosely constrained in their superior retroperitoneal location by the surrounding fascia, and inferior displacement is not rare. A displaced normal-sized kidney offers little difficulty in recognition by its shape and size, if it is considered. It may occur in the pelvis. Transplanted kidneys are placed in the pelvis where they are easily palpable above the inguinal ligament.

S KEY SYNDROME
Upper Abdominal Mass: Enlarged Kidney:

See page 512, for a description of the anatomic relationships of the kidneys. *Pathophysiology:* When the kidney enlarges, it is contained posteriorly by the psoas and the twelfth rib, and the overriding liver and spleen prevent extension superiorly. Therefore, the enlarged kidney pushes forward and downward into a position similar to that of an enlarged spleen or liver. Palpable renal masses extend posteriorly farther than the spleen. The kidney always lacks the sharp edge the spleen and liver may present. A lobulation of the kidney may be mistaken for the splenic notch. The surface of an enlarged kidney may be more often irregular than the spleen. Renal masses do not move with deep inspiratory effort because, unlike the spleen and liver, they are fixed in the retroperitoneum.

✓*ENLARGED KIDNEY—CLINICAL OCCURRENCE: Congenital:* polycystic kidney disease, horseshoe kidney, compensatory hypertrophy opposite absent kidney; *Idiopathic:* cysts; *Inflammatory/Immune:* amyloidosis; *Mechanical/Trauma:* hydronephrosis, hematoma; *Neoplastic:* renal cell carcinoma and renal sarcoma, transitional cell carcinoma of renal pelvis and ureter.

S KEY SYNDROME
Upper Abdominal Mass: Liver: See page 596.

S KEY SYNDROME
Other Abdominal Masses:

The masses previously described involve tissues more or less localized to a certain abdominal region. However, the gut may develop a localized lesion anywhere in its length, forming a palpable mass. **Volvulus** (page 593) is usually in the sigmoid colon or the cecum but may occur elsewhere. **Intussusception** (page 592) occurs primarily in children and is preceded by a viral syndrome. Intermittent colicky pain is common; the site is painful and tender. **Abscesses** may be present as palpable masses in any part of the peritoneal cavity. They should be suspected when a mass is palpated in a region normally devoid of solid organs. With the exception of intussusception, none of these conditions has distinctive physical findings.

S KEY SYNDROME
LUQ Mass: Splenomegaly: *Pathophysiology:* With

rare exceptions, the enlarged spleen retains its characteristic shape and the characteristic splenic notch persists on the medial edge near the lower pole. Because extension superiorly is blocked by the diaphragm, enlargement displaces the lower pole downward from behind the thoracic cage and along its oblique axis toward the left iliac fossa. Although it seldom crosses the midline, the lower pole may reach the pelvis. Many acute infections produce moderately enlarged soft spleens with blunted edges; chronic disorders cause firm or hard spleens and sharp edges. The enlarged spleen is not tender except when the peritoneum is inflamed from infection or infarction. The examiner must examine for splenomegaly with circumspection; although uncommon, the spleen has been ruptured during the over-vigorous attempt to identify enlargement. This has occurred most often in the patient with infectious mononucleosis. A common problem is distinguishing an enlarged spleen and left kidney; both organs have the same general shape. Renal tumors are deeper, rounded posteriorly, and never have a distinct edge. A medial border fissure might seem to identify spleen, but renal lobulation can closely mimic the splenic notch. Ultrasonography or CT may can make the distinction [Grover SA, Barkun AN, Sackett DL. The rational clinical examination. Does this patient have splenomegaly? *JAMA* 1993;270:2218–2221; Tamayo SG, Rickman LS, Mathews WC, et al. Examiner dependence on physical diagnostic tests for the detection of splenomegaly: A prospective study with multiple observers. *J Gen Intern Med* 1993;8:69–75].

✓ *SPLENOMEGALY—CLINICAL OCCURRENCE:* *Congenital* thalassemia minor and major, lipopolysaccharidases (Gaucher disease, Niemann-Pick disease); *Inflammatory/Immune* hemolytic anemia, systemic lupus erythematosus, rheumatoid arthritis, pernicious anemia, amyloidosis; *Infectious* acute and chronic malaria, typhoid fever, subacute bacterial endocarditis, abscess, schistosomiasis, congenital syphilis, leishmaniasis; *Metabolic/Toxic* pernicious anemia; *Mechanical/Trauma* chronic congestive heart failure, portal hypertension, hematoma; *Neoplastic* acute lymphatic leukemia, lymphoma, chronic myelocytic leukemia, chronic lymphocytic leukemia; *Vascular* infarcts, vasculitis, hematoma.

S KEY SYNDROME

RUQ Mass: The liver, gallbladder, and right kidney are most likely to present as masses in the RUQ. Pancreatic pseudocysts may present here, as can colon masses.

S KEY SYNDROME

RUQ Mass: Liver: *Pathophysiology:* The liver occupies the entire anterior RUQ behind the ribs while the left lobe extends to the left midclavicular line. It has convex and concave surfaces and the plane of the concave inferior surface is tipped backward and downward. Although the anterior-inferior edge of the normal liver extends across the midline, the left third is rarely felt. The liver is heavy, but its suspension is relatively meager. The coronal ligaments that attach it to the diaphragm arise posterior to the liver dome (Fig. 9-35). The diaphragm needs the aid of negative intrathoracic pressure, support of the hilar vessels, and the pressure of the abdominal viscera and abdominal wall muscles to support the liver's weight. There are two axes of liver rotation: a transverse axis near the attachment of the coronary ligaments and an anteroposterior axis near the hilum, to the left of the center of mass. Downward rotation through the transverse axis causes a normal-sized liver to present more of its anterior surface below the costal margin. Downward rotation about the anteroposterior axis results in a tongue of liver appearing in the right flank (Fig. 9-35A). Rotation may be expected in any condition that lowers the dome of the diaphragm, de-

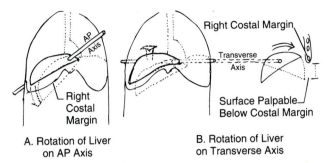

Fig. 9-35 Rotations of the Normal-Sized Liver Making it Palpable Beneath the Costal Margin. *Normally the liver is suspended, by its coronary ligaments and the fixation to the prevertebral fascia by its hilar blood vessels, behind the right costal margin inaccessible to palpation. The muscles of the diaphragm could not hold a 1500-g liver if they were not assisted by the negative intrapleural pressure above and the positive pressure of abdominal contents below. Depression of the diaphragm or relaxation of the intraabdominal pressure permits the normal-sized liver to fall beneath the costal margin and become palpable (ptosis). With the diaphragm fixed, the liver may rotate on one or two axes to become palpable; depression of the diaphragm increases the amount of palpable surface permitted by rotation. **A. The Liver May Rotate on an Anteroposterior Axis Near Its Left Side:** With this counterclockwise rotation the lower border appears below the costal margin, forming an angle with the costal margin. **B. The Normal-Sized Liver May Rotate on a Transverse Axis:** The edge presents below and approximately parallel to the costal margin. This is distinguished from enlargement of the liver only by the inward curve of the anterior surface.*

creases the normal amount of abdominal fat, or decreases abdominal muscle tone. Many clinical diagnoses of hepatomegaly are not confirmed with imaging or autopsy because the rotation of the normal liver is not appreciated. The liver of some normal persons is readily palpable just below the costal margin. The palpable margin should be roughly parallel to the costal margin rather than descending almost vertically in the flank (Fig. 9-35A). To evaluate for hepatomegaly, the upper border of hepatic dullness must be percussed, the lower border of the liver should be palpated, usually well below the costal margin, and the span determined. Only a tentative diagnosis of hepatomegaly is justified if the lower border is not definitely felt. A conclusion based solely on percussion is hazardous [Naylor CD. Physical examination of the liver. *JAMA* 1994;271:1859–1865]. The palpable surface should be examined for consistency and nodularity. Tenderness can be elicited by direct palpation or by fist percussion. Percussion tenderness occurs in acute cholecystitis and hepatitis. Palpate over the liver for friction rubs and auscultate for bruits. The coincidence of these two signs indicates a high probability of hepatic carcinoma.

✔ *HEPATOMEGALY—CLINICAL OCCURRENCE:* *Congenital* polycystic kidney disease, glycogen storage disease, lipopolysaccharidases, hemochromatosis; *Inflammatory/Immune* amyloidosis; *Infectious* liver abscess (bacterial or amebiasis), echinococcal cyst, viral hepatitis, schistosomiasis, leishmaniasis; *Metabolic/Toxic* steatohepatitis, rickets; *Mechanical/Trauma*hematoma, congestive heart failure, tricuspid insufficiency, pulmonary hypertension, cor pulmonale, constrictive pericarditis, hepatic vein thrombosis (Budd-Chiari); *Neoplastic* hepatocellular carcinoma, metastatic carcinoma (especially colon, pancreas, lung, breast), islet cell carcinoma and carcinoid, biliary carcinoma, histiocytosis syndromes, leukemic infiltration, lymphoma, myelofibrosis/ extramedullary hematopoiesis; *Vascular* hemangioma, infarction, hematoma.

S KEY SYNDROME

▼ RUQ Mass: Pulsatile Liver: *Pathophysiology:* The liver may move with arterial pulsation. This may occur by transmission of the abdominal aortic pulse, or by retrograde flow of blood in the central veins during ventricular systole, leading to expansion and contraction of the liver parenchyma. Expansile pulsation is demonstrated by placing the hands on opposite sides of the liver and observing that the surfaces move apart in systole. Tricuspid insufficiency is the usual cause.

S KEY SYNDROME

▼ Fatty Liver and Nonalcoholic Steatohepatitis (NASH): *Pathophysiology:* There is increased accumulation of fat in hepatocytes, often associated with obesity, hypertriglyceridemia, diabetes, and older age. Initially there is no inflammation, but with inflammation (NASH) fibrosis can occur, which leads to cirrhosis in some patients. The condition is asymptomatic until cirrhosis and signs and symptoms of portal hypertension and hepatic insufficiency appear. Transaminases may or may not be elevated during the course of the disease [Clark JM, Diehl AM. Nonalcoholic fatty liver disease: An underrecognized cause of cryptogenic cirrhosis. *JAMA* 2003;289:3000–3004; Angulo P. Nonalcoholic fatty liver disease. *N Engl J Med* 2002;346:1221–1231].

S KEY SYNDROME

▼ Hemochromatosis: *Pathophysiology:* Homozygous or compound heterozygous autosomal recessive mutations lead to excessive absorption of iron from the gut and leads to deposition of iron producing injury to the liver (cirrhosis), heart (failure), pancreas (diabetes mellitus), joints (arthritis), and pituitary (pituitary insufficiency). The patient is asymptomatic until progressive organ damage occurs. The penetrance of the disease is much higher in men; women are relatively protected during childbearing years by regular menstrual blood loss. With organ damage, lassitude, weight loss, darkening of skin, joint pain, abdominal pain, and loss of libido may occur. Signs are diffuse bronze pigmentation of skin (melanin), hepatomegaly, splenomegaly, spider angiomas, loss of body hair, edema, ascites, peripheral neuritis, arthropathy, and testicular atrophy. Early diagnosis and therapeutic phlebotomy avoids organ damage. Iron overload as a result of hypertransfusion in refractory amenia produces a similar syndrome.

S KEY SYNDROME
RUQ Mass: Enlarged Tender Gallbladder: See *Cholecystitis*, page 570.

S KEY SYNDROME
RUQ Mass: Enlarged Nontender Gallbladder: *Pathophysiology:* Obstruction of the common bile duct can lead to progressive enlargement of the gallbladder. A palpable nontender gallbladder may also result from distention with stones, acalculous cholecystitis, and gallbladder hydrops, in which mucous cells continue to secrete in the face of obstruction of the cystic duct. Chronic cystic duct obstruction usually produces a contracted gallbladder. *Courvoisier sign* states that dilatation of the gallbladder occurs with carcinoma of the head of the pancreas but not with a common duct stone because of a scared gallbladder wall from chronic cholelithiasis in the latter, but not the former, condition. There are many exceptions. Carcinoma of the gallbladder produces a hard, irregular mass that is moderately tender.

S KEY SYNDROME
RUQ Mass: Enlarged Right Kidney: *Pathophysiology:* The right kidney lies 1 or 2 cm lower than the left. In thin persons, the lower pole of the right kidney may be palpable while the left is not. Because the shapes of the kidney and liver are so dissimilar, there is usually no difficulty in distinguishing them with bimanual palpation. Rarely, a protruding renal mass may be confused with hydrops of the gallbladder or pancreatic pseudocyst. See page 595 for a discussion of renal enlargement.

S KEY SYNDROME
Epigastric Masses: *Pathophysiology:* Smooth epigastric masses suggest enlargement or distention of the normal organs in this region, without infection, hemorrhage, or active inflammation; irregular masses suggest neoplasm or a polycystic organ; tender masses suggest hemorrhage, infection, and/or inflammation. Acute gastric dilatation produces a visible enlargement of the epigastrium and LUQ. A smooth mass in the epigastrium of a person not acutely ill suggests a pancreatic cyst or pseudocyst. If the mass pulsates, consider aortic aneurysm. The profile of the abdomen may offer a clue (see Fig. 9-20). Enlargement of the left lobe of the liver will also present in the epigastrium. These liver and retroperitoneal masses are not mobile. Infections or neoplasms cause masses in the omentum, stomach, pancreas, left lobe of the liver, and transverse colon. A polycystic or horseshoe kidney sometimes presents as a midline epigastric mass. Periaortic lymph node enlargement may be palpable in lymphomas. Ultrasonography or CT are usually necessary for definition of the involved structure(s).

S KEY SYNDROME

RLQ Masses: Occasionally, the normal cecum can be felt as an indistinct soft mass, slightly tender, usually fluctuant. A firmer mass may be felt from involvement by tuberculous granuloma, pericecal or appendiceal abscess, Crohn disease involving the distal ileum, or carcinoma.

S KEY SYNDROME

LLQ Masses: Irregular plastic masses of feces may be palpated in sigmoid; they are occasionally mistaken for neoplasm until movement or disappearance is demonstrated in 1 or 2 days. A spastic sigmoid colon feels like a cord about the diameter of the little finger, lying vertically about 5 cm medial to the left superior anterior iliac spine; the cord can be rolled under the fingers and is slightly or moderately tender. A tender LLQ mass is frequently palpated with diverticulitis complicated by phlegmon or abscess.

S KEY SYNDROME

Suprapubic Mass: Masses presenting in the suprapubic location most often arise from the pelvis. Pelvic and rectal exams are necessary to define their extent and characteristics.

S KEY SYNDROME

Suprapubic Mass: Pregnancy: All women who have ever menstruated, but who have not gone through the menopause, and who present with a pelvic or suprapubic mass should be assumed to be pregnant until proven otherwise.

S KEY SYNDROME

Suprapubic Mass: Distended Urinary Bladder: *Pathophysiology:* A chronically obstructed urinary bladder may reach the umbilicus, usually in the midline. The patient may have minimal urinary symptoms, or complain of incontinence (because of overflow). The mass is dull to percussion, fluctuant, painless, and disappears with catheterization. It is sometimes mistaken for other tumors because of its extreme size or because a lateral diverticulum destroys its symmetry. It must be distinguished from ovarian cyst and pregnancy in the female.

S KEY SYNDROME

Suprapubic Mass: Ovarian Cyst: The largest cysts simulate ascites; they are discussed elsewhere (page 544). Those that extend just above the pelvic brim are in the midline and resemble a distended bladder. Often the cyst cannot be palpated vaginally because it is too high. Persistence of the fluctuant mass after catheterization suggests ovarian cyst or gravid uterus. Ultrasonography is diagnostic.

Suprapubic Mass: Uterine Fibroid: A markedly enlarged uterus with leiomyomas may be felt above the symphysis pubis as a hard, multinodular mass. Vaginal examination readily demonstrates that the masses move with the cervix and hence are attached to the uterine fundus.

S KEY SYNDROME

▼ **Pelvic Mass:** Pelvic masses arise from the colon, from the gravitational accumulation of neoplastic or inflammatory debris at the pelvic floor, or from infection or neoplastic change in the female or male pelvic organs.

S KEY SYNDROME

▼ **Pelvic Mass: Pelvic Abscess:** *Pathophysiology:* Pelvic abscesses result from suppurative disease of pelvic organs, perforation of pelvic or abdominal organs, dissection of abdominal wall infections, and lymphatic extension of regional infections. Knowledge of the specific anatomy of the male and female pelvis is necessary for interpretation of the exam. In the male, a tender, rounded mass, felt through the anterior rectal wall, superior to the prostate gland, is likely to be a pelvic abscess in the rectovesical pouch. Similarly in the female, a mass felt through the anterior rectal wall, superior to the cervix uteri, is probably an abscess in the rectouterine pouch. These abscesses result from perforation of the appendix or a colonic diverticulum, salpingitis, or prostatitis.

S KEY SYNDROME

▶ ▼ **Pelvic Mass: Colonic Neoplasm:** A carcinoma of the colon on a long mesocolon may prolapse into the rectovesical or rectouterine pouch and be palpated as a firm mass.

S KEY SYNDROME

▼ **Pelvic Mass: Redundant Bowel:** Occasionally, a loop of normal colon can be felt in the pelvic pouches. The mass is quite soft and freely movable; the sensation is distinctive and the mass will not be confused with cancer.

S KEY SYNDROME

▶ ▼ **Pelvic Mass: Rectal Shelf (Blumer Shelf):** Metastatic peritoneal seeding from a primary carcinoma high in the abdomen, for example, the stomach, may accumulate in the pelvis. This is felt through the anterior rectal wall as a hard shelf in the rectovesical or rectouterine pouch. Although usually caused by neoplasm, it can also occur from inflammation in female pelvic inflammatory disease and prostatic abscess in the male.

S KEY SYNDROME

▶ ▼ **Pelvic Mass: Mistaken Normal Structures:** If a vaginal examination has not been performed, the unwary examiner may interpret the hard mass of the cervix felt through the anterior rectal wall as a neoplasm. When the uterus is retroverted, the normal fundus has been mistaken for cancer. A vaginal tampon or pessary may similarly mislead when felt through the rectal wall.

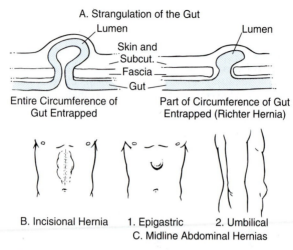

Fig. 9-36 Some Hernias and Complications. ***A. Strangulation of the Gut***: *A loop of gut protrudes through a fascial and the edges of the opening impinge upon the blood supply of the entire circumference of the lumen. If only a part of the circumference of the gut is pinched in the opening, it is called a Richter hernia.* ***B. Incisional Hernia***: *A bulge near an operative scar usually indicates an incisional hernia. The lack of fascial support can be readily palpated.* ***C. Midline Abdominal Hernias***: *In the adult-type umbilical hernia, the fascial ring is incomplete, so the bulge is superior to the umbilicus. An epigastric hernia is a small bulge of fat protruding from the deep layers through an opening in the linea alba. It may not be detected unless the patient is examined in the standing position and the examining finger is run down the linea alba.*

Abdominal, Inguinal, and Other Hernias

S KEY SYNDROME

Abdominal Hernia: Incisional Hernia: When an operative scar is present on the abdomen, palpate for a defect in the abdominal wall, then have the patient perform the Valsalva maneuver or raise their head from the pillow while supine. If present, herniation occurs adjacent to the scar (Fig. 9-36B).

S KEY SYNDROME

Strangulated Hernia: *Pathophysiology:* Impingement on a hernial ring occludes the venous return of herniating gut or omentum. Swelling and edema prevent reduction and gradually increase the pressure until capillary and arterial flow are occluded. When the blood supply of incarcerated contents is interrupted, the hernia is strangulated, and gangrene and perforation may quickly ensue (see Fig. 9-36A). The patient usually has a known hernia that becomes painful and tender. In addition to intestinal obstruction, one finds a tender, painful mass at the hernial site. Pinching and strangulation of only a partial circumference of the gut wall produces a *Richter hernia* (Fig. 9-36A). Strangulated bowel is painful, feels firm, but is usually not tender. Do not forcefully reduce a hernia because the result may be rupture of strangulated gut or reduction en masse, a condition where the sac accompanies the loop but the strangulation is not relieved.

S KEY SYNDROME

▼ **Abdominal Hernia: Epigastric Hernia (Fatty Hernia of the Linea Alba):** *Pathophysiology:* The hernia consists of preperitoneal fat protruding outward between the fibers of the linea alba (see Fig. 9-36C1). The patient can have pain in the midline of the epigastrium. If the bulge cannot be seen, the patient should stand while the examiner runs a finger down the midline to discover a small nodule that is occasionally reducible. Usually this hernia does not have a peritoneal sac.

S KEY SYNDROME

▼ **Abdominal Hernia: Umbilical Hernia:** *Pathophysiology:* A defect in the abdominal fascia occurs normally where the umbilical vessels and urachus exit the abdomen into the umbilical cord. The navel may protrude during relaxation or when intraabdominal pressure is increased by standing or Valsalva maneuver. The congenital type is distinguished by protrusion through the umbilical scar; palpation of the ring reveals a complete fibrous collar continuous with the linea alba. In the adult type of hernia, the collar is lacking; the upper part of the hernia is covered only by skin (see Fig. 9-36C2). It is properly termed a paraumbilical hernia. These are soft except when chronic inflammation has caused thickening. Umbilical hernias are very common in infants and tend to resolve spontaneously by about 4 years of age. The adult type frequently develops during pregnancy, in longstanding ascites, or when intrathoracic pressure is repeatedly increased as in asthma, chronic bronchitis, and bronchiectasis.

S KEY SYNDROME

▼ **Abdominal Hernia: Inguinal Hernias:** See *Physical Exam*, page 525.

S KEY SYNDROME

▼ **Indirect Inguinal Hernia:** *Pathophysiology:* The lateral end of the inguinal canal is the internal inguinal ring, lying just above the midpoint of the inguinal ligament. The spermatic cord of the male emerges through this ring from the abdominal cavity into the canal. The cord courses medially in the canal, emerging from the subcutaneous (external) ring, just lateral to the pubis, then droops over the brim of the bony pelvis into the scrotum. In the male, a hernia follows the course of the cord. From the abdominal cavity, it may enter the canal for only a slight distance, or it may descend to the bottom of the scrotal sac. In the female, the hernia follows a similar course in the canal that contains the round ligament, corresponding to the spermatic cord. In either sex, a small, indirect inguinal hernia may produce a bulge over the midpoint of the inguinal ligament, at the abdominal (internal) inguinal ring (Fig. 9-37). To palpate the male inguinal canal, place the fingertip at the most dependent part of the scrotum and invaginate the slack scrotal wall to insert the finger gently into the subcutaneous (external) inguinal ring (see Fig. 12-5). If the ring is sufficiently relaxed, guide the finger laterally and cephalad through the canal and have the patient cough or strain. A small hernia causes an impulse felt on the end of the fingertip. A larger hernia may feel like a mass in the canal. In the female, palpation of the inguinal canal is usually unsatisfactory, lacking the slack tissue of the male.

S KEY SYNDROME
Abdominal Hernia: Direct Inguinal Hernia: *Pathophysiology:* A hernia through the posterior wall of the inguinal canal is termed direct. The site of the weakness is the Hesselbach triangle, bounded laterally by the inferior epigastric artery and medially by the lateral border of the rectus muscle and the inguinal ligament; thus, it lies nearly directly behind the subcutaneous (external) inguinal ring. A bulge is produced close to the pubic tubercle, just above the inguinal ligament; this is medial to the site of the bulge for an indirect hernia (see Fig. 9-37). With the finger in the inguinal canal, coughing or straining causes an impulse to be felt not at the tip or end of the finger, but rather on the pad of the distal phalanx. A direct hernia seldom causes pain. It is always acquired and usually occurs in the male.

S KEY SYNDROME
Abdominal Hernia: Scrotal Hernia: An indirect hernia may enter the scrotum; there is doubt whether a direct hernia may do so. The two are said to be distinguished by palpating the lumen of the inguinal canal and following the hernial sac to the point of its emergence from the abdominal cavity, either close to the pubis in the direct, or at the midpoint of the inguinal ligament in the indirect.

S KEY SYNDROME
Abdominal Hernia: Femoral Hernia: *Pathophysiology:* The femoral nerve, artery, and vein lie lateral to medial just inferior to the midpoint of the inguinal ligament. Immediately medial to the vein is the femoral canal, a continuation of the femoral sheath, through which a hernia may bulge when intraabdominal pressure is increased (see Fig. 9-37). Large femoral hernias become irreducible and may push upward in front of the inguinal ligament where they must be distinguished from inguinal hernias. When the neck of the hernial sac can be palpated just lateral to and below the pubic tubercle, a femoral hernia is demonstrated; the neck of an inguinal hernia's sac is found above the inguinal ligament.

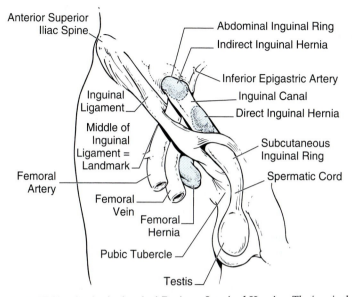

Anterior Superior Iliac Spine

Abdominal Inguinal Ring

Indirect Inguinal Hernia

Inferior Epigastric Artery

Inguinal Ligament

Inguinal Canal

Direct Inguinal Hernia

Middle of Inguinal Ligament = Landmark

Subcutaneous Inguinal Ring

Femoral Artery

Spermatic Cord

Femoral Vein

Femoral Hernia

Pubic Tubercle

Testis

*Fig. 9-37 Hernias in the Inguinal Region. **Inguinal Hernias:** The inguinal ligament stretches from the anterior superior spine of the ilium to the pubic tubercle. The flattened tube of the inguinal canal lies just above and parallel to it, between the superficial and deep layers of abdominal muscles. The lateral end of the canal opens posteriorly into the abdominal cavity through the abdominal inguinal ring (internal ring). The internal ring is not palpable, but it is just above the midpoint of the inguinal ligament. The medial end of the canal opens anteriorly into the subcutaneous tissue through the subcutaneous inguinal ring (external ring). In the male, this is where the spermatic cord emerges from the abdominal muscles. A hernia is indirect when it enters the canal from the abdominal cavity through the abdominal inguinal ring; a hernia entering medial to this ring is direct. In small hernias the relation of the bulge to the midpoint of the inguinal ligament is diagnostic of direct or indirect. If the hernia is large, palpation of the inguinal canal through the scrotum may determine its site of entrance into the canal. The direct hernia is represented as an anterior bulging of the posterior wall of the inguinal canal. **Femoral Hernia:** The femoral artery and vein emerge from the abdomen beneath the midpoint of the inguinal ligament, where the artery is palpable. The impalpable femoral vein is immediately medial to it. The femoral canal lies medial to the vein, so the canal is approximately 2 cm medial to the pulsating artery. A bulge in the region of the femoral canal is produced by a femoral hernia, especially on coughing or straining. The diagram shows a femoral hernia protruding upward in front of the inguinal ligament, where it may be confused with an inguinal hernia. Careful palpation will demonstrate that the inguinal canal is empty.*

▼ **Mass in Femoral Triangle: Obturator Hernia:** *Pathophysiology:* A peritoneal sac protrudes through the obturator foramen of the pelvis, causing a fullness or mass in the femoral triangle. The fullness is not sharply defined because the sac is covered by the pectineus muscle. This rare lesion occurs almost always in emaciated women over age 60 with a history of weight loss. On the affected side, the thigh is usually held in semiflexion; all hip motion is painful. Pain extends down the medial thigh to the knee and is increased by hip extension, abduction, and external rotation. Palpation through the rectum or vagina may reveal a soft, tender mass in the region of the obturator foramen. This condition must be distinguished from the far more common femoral hernia. The hernia is rarely diagnosed before it has caused intestinal obstruction. When only a portion of the circumference of the bowel is strangulated (Richter type) so obstruction does not occur, the presenting pain may occur late after perforation or sepsis has occurred. In almost half the cases of strangulation, the genicular branch of the obturator nerve is compressed, producing pain down the medial aspect of the thigh to the knee (*Romberg-Howship sign*).

▼ **Mass Above the Inguinal Ligament: Spigelian Hernia:** *Pathophysiology:* A peritoneal sac with considerable extraperitoneal fat perforates the linea semilunaris to lie within the abdominal wall; it is covered only by skin, subcutaneous fat, and the aponeurosis of the external abdominal oblique muscle. Usually asymptomatic until it strangulates, it produces a tender mass within the abdominal wall approximately 3–5 cm above the inguinal ligament. This should be inspected and palpated while the patient stands.

Other Inguinal Masses

Among the structures to be considered when a mass is found in the groin are lymph nodes, lymphoma, hernia, varix, lipoma, ectopic testis, ectopic spleen, and inguinal endometriosis.

Inguinal Mass: Saphenous Vein Varix: A bulge just below the femoral canal may be caused by a varix of the saphenous vein; this fills upon standing and empties in the supine position; palpation of the filled varix yields a distinctive thrill.

▼ **Inguinal Mass: Lymphadenopathy:** *Pathophysiology:* Inflammation, infection, or neoplastic involvement of lymph nodes causes enlargement with or without tenderness. Inflammation and fluctuant swelling of inguinal lymph nodes in the area of the femoral vessels below the inguinal ligament is a so-called bubo. It occurs commonly in chancroid, syphilis, and lymphogranuloma venereum. Neoplastic enlargement is felt as nontender rubbery or hard, nonfluctuant nodes. See Chapter 5, page 114.

Perineal, Anal, and Rectal Syndromes

S KEY SYNDROME

Brief Intense Perineal Pain: Proctalgia Fugax: The cause is unknown, but men are more often affected than women. The patient is awakened from sleep with intense, poorly localized pain in the perineum or rectum. The paroxysm reaches an agonizing maximum in 1–2 minutes, and then subsides rapidly and completely in about 5 minutes. During the pain the patient may arise and walk about or attempt defecation. Relief has been reported from pressure on the perineum, nitroglycerin, or an enema of warm water. Occasionally, the paroxysm is initiated by straining at stool, prolonged sitting on a hard surface, or ejaculation.

S KEY SYNDROME

Fecal Incontinence: See page 536.

Occult Gastrointestinal Blood Loss

KEY SIGN

Normally Colored Stools with Positive Guaiac Test ("Occult Blood"): Bleeding of small volume from any site in the alimentary tract or the upper respiratory tract may give a positive test for blood without coloring the stool. The source should be sought by endoscopy. Because colonic neoplasms may bleed intermittently or not at all, the stool guaiac test has a low sensitivity for detecting colon cancer and should be reserved for evaluating patients whose clinical circumstances provide a reason for testing [Gomez JA, Diehl AK. Admission stool guaiac test: Use and impact on patient management. Am J Med 1992;92:603–606]. Most cases of occult gastrointestinal blood loss are caused by duodenal ulcer, gastritis, malignancy, angiodysplasia, diverticulosis, or esophageal varices.

S KEY SYNDROME

Gastrointestinal Bleeding Associated with Dermal Lesions: *Pathophysiology:* In some patients, gastrointestinal blood loss is associated with dermal lesions having their counterparts in the gastrointestinal tract. We are indebted to Bluefarb and Carr for most of the following list of dermal lesions.

Peutz-Jeghers Syndrome: melanin spots on lips, buccal mucosa, and tongue suggest bleeding polypoid lesions in the small intestine.
Hereditary Hemorrhagic Telangiectasia (Rendu-Osler-Weber Disease): telangiectases on the face, buccal mucosa, and extremities suggest similar lesions in the gastrointestinal tract.
Blue Rubber-Bleb Nevus Syndrome: cavernous hemangiomas of the skin, especially on the trunk or extremities, suggest similar lesions of the small intestine.
Ehlers-Danlos Syndrome (Cutis Elastica): hyperelastic skin, hyperflexible joints, petechiae, and easy bleeding of the skin. They also may have intestinal hemorrhage from deficiency of factor IX.

Pseudoxanthoma Elastica: lax elastic tissue of skin, eye, cardiovascular system, and gastrointestinal tract. The skin contains small, soft yellow-orange papules running parallel to natural skin folds. Angioid streaks are seen in retina. Disintegration of arteries in the gastrointestinal tract causes hemorrhages.

Neurofibromatosis (von Recklinghausen Disease): café au lait pigmentation with sessile, pedunculated, or subcutaneous skin fibromas. Fibromas in gastrointestinal tract may bleed.

Amyloidosis (Either Primary or Secondary): wax-colored papules, nodules, or tumors about the face, lips, ears, and upper chest. Macroglossia may be seen. Deposits about blood vessels and in mucosa cause bleeding.

Malignant Atrophic Papulosis (Degos Disease): vasculitis of the skin and mucosa. Small, red papules on the skin become umbilicated, with porcelain-white depressed centers and dry scale. The border disappears, leaving a white patch. Patients may have acute abdominal pain with vomiting and bleeding which can progress to peritonitis and gangrene.

Dermatomyositis: nonpitting edema of the face, heliotrope discoloration of the eyelids, cutaneous erythematous rash and erythema over the extensor aspects of the interphalangeal joints. Skeletal muscles have local and general inflammation.

Schönlein-Henoch Purpura: symmetrical purpura on the buttocks, extensor surfaces of the limbs, angioneurotic edema, gastrointestinal pain with mucosal ulcers and bleeding.

Drug Eruptions: aspirin causes macular and purpuric lesions of lower limbs. Erosive lesions cause bleeding from gastrointestinal tract. Warfarin may cause petechiae, ecchymoses, and bleeding in the gastrointestinal tract.

Scurvy: perifollicular hemorrhages, ecchymoses of legs, bleeding gums, loose teeth, and gastrointestinal bleeding.

Polycythemia Vera: purplish red color of skin and mucosa with hemorrhages, spider nevi, rosacea, and peptic ulcer.

Kaposi Sarcoma: endemic Kaposi sarcoma is usually on the feet with dark-blue nodules and plaques. HIV-associated Kaposi sarcoma frequently involves the mucous membranes of the mouth and gastrointestinal and genitourinary tracts.

Mastocytosis: brown-red macules on the skin with urticaria. Hepatic cirrhosis of with esophageal varices may occur.

ADDITIONAL READING

Silen, W. *Cope's Early Diagnosis of the Acute Abdomen.* New York, Oxford University Press, 1991.

Urinary System: Overview of Anatomy and Physiology

The urinary system consists of the kidneys, collecting systems of the renal pelvis, ureters, urinary bladder, and urethra. Important sphincters are found at the ureterovesical junction, as the ureter passes obliquely through the bladder wall, and at the proximal urethra, as it passes through the urogenital septum. The urethral sphincter has an involuntary smooth muscle portion under parasympathetic and sympathetic control, and a voluntary striated muscle sphincter innervated via the lumbosacral plexus. The urinary system is designed to filter the blood at the glomerulus and to reabsorb and to secrete solutes and fluid across the renal tubules, and then to concentrate the urine in the medullary collecting ducts. The urine passes down the ureters to the bladder by gravity and by peristaltic contractions. The bladder is a hollow muscular structure that actively relaxes with urinary distention keeping intravesical pressures low until capacity is reached. Further filling occurs by stretching of the bladder wall at rapidly increasing pressures. Continence is maintained by tonic contraction of the smooth muscle sphincter and active inhibition of detrusor muscle contraction as the bladder fills. Voiding is a complex process involving simultaneous, coordinated relaxation of the urethral sphincters and contraction of the previously relaxed detrusor muscle. In males, the proximal urethra is surrounded by the prostate gland and receives prostatic secretions from the prostate and seminal vesicles. In the female the urethra is quite short.

The kidneys lie posteriorly partially under the eleventh and twelfth ribs and lateral to L1-4 (see Fig. 9-2). They are enclosed in a tight capsule and lie retroperitoneally, surrounded by Gerota fascia. The ureters course retroperitoneally, and descend over the psoas muscle and into the pelvis, where they run laterally and then anteriorly to enter the inferior portion of the bladder on either side of the midline. The bladder lies anteriorly in the pelvis behind and below the symphysis pubis. The urethra exits the bladder and runs through the urogenital diaphragm of the pelvic floor muscles to enter the male prostate and penis or the female perineum. Only the urethral meatus is visible on physical examination and normally the deeper structures cannot be identified by palpation.

Physical Examination of the Urinary System

See also Chapter 9: *The Abdomen;* Chapter 11: *The Female Genitalia and Reproductive System;* and Chapter 12: *The Male Genitalia and Reproductive System.*

DETERMINATION OF THE POSTVOID RESIDUAL URINE VOLUME.　The adequacy of bladder emptying is measured by determining the volume of urine remaining in the bladder after a full voluntary voiding: the residual volume. First, have the patient empty his or her bladder completely. Residual volume can be estimated by ultrasonography devices or measured directly by passing a sterile urethral catheter into the bladder to collect the residual urine. The risk of infection increases sharply with residual volumes of greater than 100 cc.

Urinary Symptoms

KEY SYMPTOM

Discolored Urine:　See *Urinary Signs: Discolored Urine,* page 613.

KEY SYMPTOM

Urethral Discharge:　See *Urinary Signs: Urethral Discharge,* page 616.

KEY SYMPTOM

Renal Colic:　See *Abdominal Pain,* pages 529 and 562ff. *Pathophysiology:*　Vigorous contraction of visceral smooth muscle in the ureters against an obstruction is intensely painful. Obstructing stones in the renal pelvis, ureter, or bladder produce acute, often extremely intense pain, whose location is dependent upon the site of obstruction. Obstruction at the renal pelvis gives flank and upper abdominal pain. Ureteral obstruction produces pain in the upper abdomen, lower abdomen, pelvis, testicles, and perineum. Bladder outlet obstruction leads to pain in the pelvis. The diagnosis is supported by an acute onset, absence of systemic symptoms other than nausea and anorexia, a previous or family history of urolithiasis, and the presence of microscopic hematuria without pyuria.

KEY SYMPTOM

Frequent Urination without Polyuria:　*Pathophysiology:*　Although the average adult urinates about five or six times daily, frequency depends upon fluid balance, renal function, individual habits, and the presence or absence of irritation in the genitourinary tract. Frequent urination can be caused by increased total urinary volume (polyuria; see *Frequent Urination, With Polyuria*, below), decreased bladder capacity, or increased stimulation of the micturition reflexes caused by irritation of the genitourinary tract. The history, physical examination, and measurement of 24-hour fluid intake and urine volume, volume of each voiding, and postvoid residual bladder volume will usually lead to the correct assessment.

✓ **URINARY FREQUENCY—CLINICAL OCCURRENCE:** *Congenital* small bladder capacity; ureterovesical reflux; urethral and meatal stricture; *Endocrine* atrophic vaginitis; *Idiopathic* benign prostatic hyperplasia, pelvic floor relaxation, cystocele, urethrocele; *Inflammatory/Immune* interstitial and chemical cystitis, prostatitis, appendicitis; *Infectious* bacterial and viral pyelitis, cystitis, urethritis, vaginitis, salpingitis; *Metabolic/Toxic* chemical cystitis, highly acidic urine; *Mechanical/ Traumatic* pelvic floor relaxation, cystocele, urethrocele, bladder stone, extrinsic compression of the bladder or urethra, bladder wall fibrosis, urethral stricture, bladder neck obstruction; *Neoplastic* bladder cancer, prostate cancer, locally invasive cervical and rectal cancer; *Neurologic* spinal cord, cauda equina and sacral plexus lesions, autonomic neuropathy, detrusor instability; *Psychosocial* untrained bladder, voiding habits.

◢ KEY SYMPTOM
◤**Frequent Urination, With Polyuria:** *Pathophysiology:* The adult male bladder holds about 500 mL; the adult female's bladder holds somewhat less. An average output of urine in 24 hours is 1200–1500 mL, but this volume is dependent upon the type and volume of fluid intake, sensible (vomiting, diarrhea) and insensible (sweating, respiratory) fluid losses, and the renal concentrating ability. Increased urinary volume (polyuria) can result from an increased osmotic load (e.g., diabetes mellitus), increased intake of fluids, medications, dietary exposures, and decreased renal concentrating ability. The history, physical examination, and urinalysis are able to establish the cause in most cases.

✓ **POLYURIA—CLINICAL OCCURRENCE:** *Congenital* renal tubular defects (e.g., renal tubular acidosis type 1); *Endocrine* diabetes mellitus, central or renal diabetes insipidus; *Idiopathic* chronic renal failure of any cause; *Inflammatory/Immune* interstitial nephritis; *Metabolic/ Toxic* diuretic use, hypercalcemia, hypokalemia; *Mechanical/Traumatic* postobstructive diuresis; *Psychosocial* excessive fluid intake, psychogenic polydipsia, alcohol and caffeine ingestion.

◢ KEY SYMPTOM
◤**Nocturia:** *Pathophysiology:* Urine production declines during sleep and sleep is usually not interrupted to urinate. Some people have habitual nocturia, which is aggravated by high fluid intakes, especially of caffeinated or alcoholic beverages taken in the evening. Nocturia also occurs with most disorders causing increased frequency of urination or polyuria. Edematous states (congestive heart failure, hepatic insufficiency, nephrotic syndrome, and chronic renal failure) are associated with nocturia caused by mobilization of dependent fluid from the

lower extremities and abdomen during recumbency. Reclining can also lead to loss of bladder support, particularly in women with pelvic floor relaxation or a history of hysterectomy, leading to increased frequency of urination at night.

KEY SYMPTOM

Urinary Incontinence: Involuntary loss of urine by children at night is referred to as *enuresis.* Urinary incontinence in the adult should initiate an evaluation for a specific cause, most of which are treatable. See *Urinary Syndromes: Incontinence,* page 617, for further discussion.

KEY SYMPTOM

Difficult Urination: *Pathophysiology:* Normal urination occurs with the effortless relaxation of the bladder sphincters coordinated with contraction of the detrusor muscle. Difficulty initiating or maintaining the urinary stream indicates an obstruction to flow or a decrease in detrusor strength. The patient may complain of hesitancy in starting the urinary stream, decreased force of urination, and/or dribbling at termination of urination. Occasionally, straining is required to maintain the stream.

✓ *CLINICAL OCCURRENCE:* *Idiopathic* prostatic hyperplasia, chronic sterile prostatitis; *Infectious* tabes dorsalis, prostatitis; *Mechanical/ Traumatic* urethral stricture or valve, bladder neck obstruction, bladder stone or clot, pregnancy, hematoma; *Neoplastic* urethral carcinoma, prostate cancer, uterine fibroid, vaginal cancer, cervical cancer; *Neurologic* detrusor weakness, multiple sclerosis, spinal cord injury or epidural compression, myelitis, syringomyelia.

KEY SYMPTOM

Painful Urination (Dysuria): *Pathophysiology:* Inflammation of or breaks in the urethral epithelium (exposing the submucosa to the acidic urine) results in pain located in the penis or the female urethra with urination. This is usually the result of infection or trauma. Ask whether the pain is greater on initiation or on termination of voiding. Pain during urination occurs with urethral obstruction, urethritis, cystitis, vulvitis and meatal ulcers. Pain after urination is more typical of bladder calculus, cystitis, prostatitis and seminal vesiculitis.

Urinary Signs

See also Chapter 9: *Abdominal Signs;* Chapter 11: *Female Genital and Reproductive Signs;* and Chapter 12: *Male Genital and Reproductive Signs.*

KEY SIGN

Urinary Retention: See *Urinary Syndromes: Urinary Retention,* page 617.

KEY SIGN

Anuria and Oliguria: *Pathophysiology:* Obstruction of the bladder outlet is the most common cause of anuria and oliguria as measured by voided urine volumes. Decreased urine production measured in the bladder is a result of a profound decline in glomerular filtration from a decrease in renal blood flow and/or intrarenal or ureteral obstruction. The process must involve both kidneys or obstruct both ureters. In oliguria, the 24-hour urinary output is between 50 and 400 mL (4–25 mL/h). The output is 0–50 mL in anuria. Even with dehydration, normal kidneys continue to excrete more than 500 mL daily. Therefore, oliguria and anuria indicate advanced degrees of renal dysfunction requiring immediate treatment. Acute renal failure may occur unexpectedly during the care of patients for another disorder. Usually patients do not complain of a lack of urine, thus delaying recognition. Often, the cause may be suspected from knowledge of the preexisting disease, but postrenal obstruction with hydronephrosis must always be excluded.

✓ **CLINICAL OCCURRENCE:** See *Urinary Syndromes: Acute Renal Failure*, page 618.

KEY SIGN

Discolored Urine: *Pathophysiology:* Urine is normally clear and colored yellow because of urea. Dilution and concentration of the urine will change the intensity, but not the color, of the urine. A true color change results from the presence of colored substances in the urine, either filtered from the blood or arising in the urinary tract itself. Increased opacity of the urine arises with the precipitation of solutes or the addition of cellular material or mucous. A complaint of abnormal urine color requires further history. First, determine if the change is one of intensity of the normal yellow color or a true change in color. Also, determine if the change is persistent or episodic and whether there is an association with activities, intake of foods, medications, or other symptoms. Inspection and analysis of a freshly voided urine specimen to confirm the patient's observation should precede any further investigation. Note that patients will describe any red discoloration of the urine as blood, a conclusion you must avoid until it is proven. Often discoloration of the urine is discovered by someone handling specimens for examination.

✓ *DISCOLORED URINE—CLINICAL OCCURRENCE:* *Colorless* urine of low concentration from excessive fluid intake, chronic glomerulonephritis, diabetes mellitus, diabetes insipidus; *Cloudy White* phosphates in an alkaline urine (the cloud disappears with the addition of acid), epithelial cells from the lower genitourinary tract, bacteria, pus, chyle (when the urine is centrifuged, chyle remains homogeneously distributed; milk fat added for malingering floats to the top); *Yellow* Highly concentrated normal urine, tetracycline, pyridine; *Orange* urobilinogen, pyridium (antispasmodic that is orange in acid urine and red in alkaline urine), rhubarb (food and purgative), cathartics (senna aloes), anthracyclines; *Red* beets, blackberries, aniline dyes from candy, freshly voided hemoglobin or myoglobin, pyridine, porphyrin, phenolphthalein (a cathartic, red in alkaline urine, colorless in acid urine), cascara (cathartic), rifampin, doxorubicin; *Blue-Green* bilirubin (urine with yellow froth), methylene blue, pseudomonas infection; *Black-Brown* highly concentrated normal urine, bilirubin (with yellow froth), acid hematin (hemoglobin standing in acid urine), methemoglobin, porphyrin, phenol (black in large quantities), cresol, homogentisic acid, tyrosine; *Brown-Black After Standing* porphyrin (changed from exposure to sunlight), melanin (changed from exposure to sunlight), homogentisic acid (changed from bacterial alkalinization of the urine).

KEY SIGN

▶ **Hematuria:** *Pathophysiology:* Microscopic hematuria is defined as >4 erythrocytes per high-powered field (HPF) on a spun urine specimen and gross hematuria indicates sufficient red blood cells to discolor the urine. Microscopic hematuria is detected by chemical or microscopic examination of the urine. Gross hematuria is frequently noticed by the male during micturition. Hematuria is distinguished from hemoglobinuria and myoglobinuria by finding erythrocytes in freshly voided urine collected within 1 hour after complete bladder emptying. In all three cases, chemical tests of the urine are positive for heme. Spectroscopic examination distinguishes myoglobin from hemoglobin, but it does not differentiate intracellular from extracellular hemoglobin. The pattern of gross hematuria observed by the patient may indicate the source of blood: *initial hematuria*—the urethra; *terminal hematuria*—a small hemorrhage from the trigone region of the bladder; *total hematuria*—hemorrhage from the kidney or profuse bleeding from the bladder; the presence of erythrocyte casts in the urine proves a renal source [Cohen RA, Brown RS. Microscopic hematuria. *N Engl J Med* 2003;348: 2330–2338].

In most instances, the occurrence of hematuria demands a complete investigation of the genitourinary tract, including upper tract imaging and cystoscopy. Bedside observations must suffice when instrumentation is contraindicated, as in urethral infection or hemorrhagic disorders.

✔ *HEMATURIA—CLINICAL OCCURRENCE:* *Congenital* hemophilia, sickle cell disease, polycystic kidney disease; *Endocrine* menstruation; *Idiopathic* bladder diverticulum, polyps, prostatic hyperplasia, endometriosis, uremia, thrombocytopenia; *Inflammatory/Immune* interstitial cystitis, fever, glomerulonephritis, polyarteritis, microscopic polyangiitis, Goodpasture syndrome, Wegener syndrome; *Infectious* urethritis, bacterial and viral (adenovirus 11) cystitis, prostatitis, pyelitis, schistosomiasis, malaria, yellow fever; *Metabolic/Toxic* chemical cystitis (e.g., cyclophosphamide or ifosfamide), analgesic nephropathy, anticoagulants, scurvy, vitamin K deficiency; *Mechanical/Traumatic* blunt or penetrating trauma, urethral stricture, instrumentation, postsurgical, decompression of a distended bladder, heavy exercise (e.g., marathon runners), foreign body, stones, rupture, radiation, medullary necrosis; *Neoplastic* kidney, ureter, bladder, prostate cancers; *Psychosocial* factitious; *Vascular* bladder and prostatic varices, renal infarction, vasculitis, arteriovenous malformation.

Hemoglobinuria: *Pathophysiology:* Hemoglobinuria is extracellular hemoglobin in the urine resulting from filtration of plasma-free hemoglobin or lysis of red blood cells present in the urine. Sufficient concentrations produce a red color identical to myoglobinuria and hematuria. When hemoglobin enters the plasma by the intravascular hemolysis, it binds to plasma haptoglobin and the large hemoglobin–haptoglobin complex is not filtered by the normal glomerulus. When the binding capacity of haptoglobin is exceeded, free hemoglobin passes through the glomerular basement membrane and a freshly voided urine specimen usually contains hemoglobin casts. Their presence excludes the possibility that hemolysis occurred in the bladder. Hemoglobin gives positive chemical tests whether intracellular or extracellular, so hemoglobinuria must be distinguished from hematuria by the absence of erythrocytes in freshly voided urine. Although myoglobin (molecular weight [MW] 17,500) can be differentiated from hemoglobin (MW 68,000) by spectroscopic examination, look for a concomitant red coloration of the blood plasma, which suggests hemoglobinuria because the smaller myoglobin molecules are cleared more rapidly from the blood. Hematuria and hemoglobinuria from hemolysis in the bladder occur when the urine is so dilute as to hemolyze the erythrocytes (specific gravity less than 1.006). Transfusion of improperly stored or frozen blood results in the direct infusion of hemoglobin from the lyzed red blood cells.

✓ *HEMOGLOBINURIA—CLINICAL OCCURRENCE:* *Congenital* G-6-PD (glucose-6-phosphate dehydrogenase) deficiency; *Endocrine* pregnancy and the puerperium; *Idiopathic* paroxysmal nocturnal hemoglobinuria (PNH); *Inflammatory/Immune* major transfusion reaction, autoimmune hemolytic anemia, hapten-associated hemolysis (quinine, sulfonamides), high-titer cold-agglutinin disease; *Infectious* malaria, blackwater fever, typhus, gas gangrene, generalized anthrax, yellow fever; *Metabolic/Toxic* oxidant drugs or fava beans in persons with G-6-PD deficiency (sulfonamides, sulfones, primaquine), envenomation by snake or spider bites, infusion of outdated, frozen, or improperly stored blood; *Mechanical/Traumatic* march hemoglobinuria, mechanical heart valves, severe aortic and paraprosthetic mitral regurgitation, extracorporeal circulation, major burns, intravascular devices; *Psychosocial* injection of distilled water; *Vascular* microangiopathic hemolytic anemia-thrombotic thrombocytopenic purpura (TTP), hemolytic-uremic syndrome (HUS), and malignant hypertension; renal infarction.

► **Myoglobinuria:** *Pathophysiology:* Excretion of myoglobin released from damaged muscle colors the urine red and gives chemical tests for heme (see *Signs: Hemoglobinuria* above). Muscle pain and a history of crush injury or prolonged muscle ischemia are usual although loss of consciousness associated with severe injury may obscure the findings.

✓ *MYOGLOBINURIA—CLINICAL OCCURRENCE:* *Congenital* McArdle disease; *Inflammatory/Immune* autoimmune hemolytic anemia, transfusion of incompatible blood; *Metabolic/Toxic* severe hypokalemia, ingestion of quail (idiosyncratic), opiate and sedative abuse, Haff disease (an epidemic myoglobinuria encountered in Königsberg, Germany, caused by the ingestion of fish feeding in a lagoon polluted with industrial wastes); *Mechanical/Traumatic* crush injuries, compression injuries caused by prolonged immobilization or impaired consciousness, electrical shock, compartment syndromes, intravascular hemolysis.

Urethral Signs

KEY SIGN

Urethral Discharge: *Pathophysiology:* Inflammation in the urethra and/or its exocrine glands distal to the urogenital septum leads to an increase in purulent secretions, which leak from the urethral orifice between times of urination. Men may complain specifically about discharge from the penis accompanied by staining of the underwear with pus or blood. Determine whether the discharge is clear or purulent, accompanied by painful and/or frequent urination and whether the patient has had any new sexual partners. Ask specifically about same-sex contacts and the use of condoms. In women, urethral discharge is confounded with vulvovaginitis.

✓ *URETHRAL DISCHARGE—CLINICAL OCCURRENCE:* *Inflammatory/Immune* Reiter syndrome, Behçet syndrome; *Infectious* Chlamydia trachomatis, Neisseria gonorrhoeae, Ureaplasma urealyticum, Trichomonas vaginalis, other sexually transmitted diseases; *Mechanical/Traumatic* urethral catheter and foreign bodies.

Urinary System Syndromes

S KEY SYNDROME

▶ **Hematuria:** See *Urinary Signs: Hematuria*, page 614.

S KEY SYNDROME

Loin Pain-Hematuria Syndrome: IgA Nephropathy: *Pathophysiology:* For unknown reasons, there are deposits of IgA in the mesangial region of the glomerulus. Patients present with painless hematuria or hematuria and loin pain, often following a mild viral infection. Progression is unpredictable, but a significant minority develop end-stage renal disease [Donanio JV, Grande JP. IgA nephropathy. *N Engl J Med* 2002;347:738–748].

S KEY SYNDROME

▼ **Urinary Incontinence:** *Pathophysiology:* Loss of bladder control results from abnormalities of genitourinary sensation and/or smooth muscle function (detrusor instability, urge incontinence), inadequate sphincter function (stress incontinence), urinary retention leading to overflow incontinence, combinations of these (mixed incontinence), abnormalities of cognition, and inability to respond in a timely fashion to reach a toilet. Urinary incontinence in the adult should initiate an evaluation for a specific cause, most of which are treatable. The onset, pattern, precipitating factors, fluid intake, and measures taken by the patient to reduce the incontinence are essential historical information. A detailed review of all prescription and nonprescription medications and dietary supplements is mandatory. It is especially important to identify whether the patient feels an urge to void prior to the episode and the volume of urine lost at each episode. Completion of a bladder journal by the patient for at least 2 weeks will greatly facilitate the evaluation.

✔ **URINARY INCONTINENCE—CLINICAL OCCURRENCE:** *Idiopathic* benign prostatic hyperplasia, cystocele urethrocele; *Infectious* cystitis, urethritis; *Mechanical/Traumatic* pelvic floor relaxation, sphincter injury from childbirth; *Neoplastic* prostate, bladder, cervix, and rectal cancers, especially with sacral plexus involvement, epidural cord compression, cauda equina syndrome; *Neurologic* stoke, spinal cord injury, dementia, autonomic and peripheral neuropathies, normal pressure hydrocephalus, multiple sclerosis, paralysis, muscular weakness and limited mobility.

S KEY SYNDROME

▼ **Urinary Retention:** *Pathophysiology:* The bladder is unable to empty because of mechanical obstruction of bladder outflow and/or loss of detrusor strength. Rapid increase in bladder volume leads to high wall tension, whereas slow increases lead to increased bladder compliance and flaccidity of the wall. Retention is more common in men than in women. Acute urinary retention in the bladder is usually painful, distinguishing it from painless anuria or oliguria. Seriously ill patients may be unable to communicate discomfort. Chronic retention develops gradually and is painless. The only symptoms may be frequent urination of small amounts or incontinence (overflow). The patient may have a sensation of fullness in the bladder, but often this is absent. Examination shows a suprapubic swelling of the distended bladder. Have the patient void, then measure the postvoid residual urine volume by catheterization or bladder ultrasonography.

✔ **URINARY RETENTION—CLINICAL OCCURRENCE:** *Congenital* urethral valves; *Inflammatory/Immune* prostatitis (nonbacterial); *Infectious* prostatitis (bacterial) and prostate abscess; *Mechanical/Traumatic* prostate, hyperplasia, bladder stone, occluded catheter, urethral stricture or calculus, ruptured urethral; *Neoplastic* prostate and bladder cancer, locally invasive cervical or rectal cancer; *Neurologic* spinal cord injury, autonomic neuropathy, tabes dorsalis.

S KEY SYNDROME

▶ ▼ **Acute Renal Failure:** *Pathophysiology:* Acute loss of renal function results from disorders which can be classified as *prerenal* (decreased effective renal blood flow), *renal* (glomerulonephritis, mesangial proliferation, tubular dysfunction, or interstitial inflammation), or *postrenal* obstruction of the ureters or bladder. Acute renal failure may occur unexpectedly during the care of patients for another disorder. Usually patients do not complain of lack of urine, delaying recognition. Often the cause may be suspected from knowledge of the preexisting disease. The physical exam, including assessment of intravascular volume status, cardiac output, and the presence of severe hepatic disease, will identify prerenal causes. Obstruction must be excluded in all patients by ultrasonographic imaging. Urinalysis helps to distinguish between glomerular causes (microscopic hematuria, red blood cell casts, proteinuria) and tubular disease (cellular and granular casts, decreased concentrating ability, salt wasting). Medications commonly cause or contribute substantially to acute renal failure. Congenital solitary kidney or the prior nonfunctioning of one kidney may precipitate acute renal failure from unilateral events that would not normally be associated with a sudden and dramatic loss of renal function. The following is a clinical classification of causes that is more diagnostically useful than pathologic categorizations.

✔ *ACUTE RENAL FAILURE—CLINICAL OCCURRENCE:* *Congenital* sickle cell crisis; *Endocrine* hyperparathyroidism (severe hypercalcemia), thyroid storm; *Idiopathic* advanced chronic renal failure of any cause; *Inflammatory/Immune* vasculitis (Wegener, polyarteritis, microscopic polyangiitis, hypersensitivity vasculitis), antibasement glomerular membrane disease (Goodpasture syndrome), systemic lupus erythematosus (SLE), progressive systemic sclerosis (PSS, scleroderma), serum sickness, retroperitoneal fibrosis; *Infectious* pyelonephritis, septicemia, hemorrhagic fevers, blackwater fever (malaria), bacterial endocarditis; *Metabolic/Toxic* *Medications:* antibiotics (aminoglycosides, amphotericin-B, sulfonamides), nonsteroidal antiinflammatory drugs, and hypersensitivity to any medication; *Toxins*: myoglobin, radiologic contrast material, heavy metals (mercury, bismuth, copper, uranium, arsenic), organic solvents (carbon tetrachloride), inorganic phosphorus, carbon monoxide, paraldehyde, ethylene glycol, heroin, biologics (mushrooms, rattlesnake venom), methemoglobinemia; *Blood Transfusion*: hemolysis from mishandled or incompatible blood; *Mechanical/Traumatic* *Major Trauma:* Hypovolemic shock, crush syndrome, burns, heat prostration, hematoma, ruptured kidneys, myoglobinemia; *Instrumentation*: retrograde pyelography and catheterization of ureters; *Postrenal Obstruction* (especially if one kidney is absent or poorly functioning): renal calculi, cysts, tumor or mass obstructing the ureters, obstruction by crystals of uric acid, oxalic acid, cystine, or calcium; *Neoplastic* lymphoma, extensive cervical cancer causing bilateral ureteral obstruction, tumor lysis syndrome; *Vascular* hypotension of any cause (sepsis, hemorrhage, obstetrical complications), postoperative (especially with major vascular procedures—aortic resection, cardiotomy, repair of injuries to blood vessels, etc.—or hemorrhage), vasculitis (polyarteritis nodosa, microscopic polyangiitis, Goodpasture syndrome, Wegener granulomatosis, hypersensitivity angiitis), or vasculopathy (hemolytic uremic syndrome, thrombotic thrombocytopenic purpura, malignant and accelerated hypertension, abdominal aortic dissection, atheroemboli).

S KEY SYNDROME

▼ **Chronic Renal Failure:** *Pathophysiology:* Chronic loss of renal function can occur from prerenal, renal, or postrenal causes. It may be the long-term result of an episode of acute renal failure or result from a slowly progressive process that gradually reduces function. When functioning nephron mass falls below a critical level, the increased filtration required of the remaining nephrons to maintain adequate solute clearance results in progressive failure of these remaining nephrons. This vicious cycle leads to end-stage kidney disease. Weakness, anorexia, fatigue, and nausea are common symptoms, while pruritus and dyspnea are late findings. The slow progression leads to adaptive metabolic and hemodynamic changes that may be apparent on physical exam. Hypertension, expansion of the extracellular fluid volume causing edema, muscle wasting, and anemia are common. Less frequently, pericarditis or soft-tissue calcifications may be found.

✓ *CHRONIC RENAL FAILURE—CLINICAL OCCURRENCE:* *NOTE:* **The causes of acute renal failure are not repeated here.** *Congenital* polycystic kidney disease, Alport syndrome; *Endocrine* diabetes mellitus the metabolic syndrome; *Inflammatory/Immune* glomerulonephritis, systemic lupus erythe-matosus; *Infectious* chronic pyelonephritis, renal tuberculosis; *Metabolic/Toxic* nonsteroidal antiinflammatory drugs, acetaminophen; *Mechanical/ Traumatic* bladder neck obstruction; *Vascular* hypertension, atherosclerotic renal artery stenosis, atheroemboli, vasculitis.

S KEY SYNDROME

▼ **Polycystic Kidney Disease:** *Pathophysiology:* An autosomal dominant defect of renal tubular development produces massive enlargement of the kidneys and progressive renal failure. Presenting symptoms are flank pain, nausea, malaise, renal colic, and hematuria. Hypertension is common and bilateral enlargement of the kidneys is often detected on abdominal palpation.

S KEY SYNDROME

▼ **Uremia:** *Pathophysiology:* A clinical picture associated with renal failure, it includes azotemia, although the symptoms do not necessarily parallel the degree of azotemia. Symptoms include increased fatigability, headache, anorexia, dyspnea, nausea and vomiting, diarrhea, hiccup, restlessness, and depression. Signs on physical exam include Cheyne-Stokes breathing, fetid breath, dehydration, pericardial friction rub, muscle twitching, convulsions, delirium, coma.

S KEY SYNDROME

► ▼ **Glomerulonephritis (Nephritic Syndrome):** *Pathophysiology:* Damage to the glomerular capillary endothelium, basement membrane, mesangium, and/or epithelial podocytes results in inflammation with destruction of normal glomerular architecture. Proteinuria and hematuria with red blood cell casts result from loss of the integrity of the glomerulus. If the glomerulonephritis is the consequence of a systemic disease, the signs and symptoms of the particular disease will be the clues leading to the diagnosis. Processes limited to the kidney will often only present with the onset of end-stage renal disease with oliguria, edema, severe hypertension, and electrolyte disorders.

S KEY SYNDROME

Nephrotic Syndrome: *Pathophysiology:* Damage to the glomerular basement membrane increases the filtration of low-molecular-weight proteins, particularly albumin. When the capacity of the tubules to reabsorb this protein is exceeded, proteinuria, sometimes massive, occurs. Albuminuria of >3.5 g/24 h is diagnostic; hypertension, edema, hypoalbuminemia, and elevated serum cholesterol are frequently present. Complications include protein malnutrition and increased risk of thrombosis, particularly in the renal vein. Renal function as measured by the creatinine and blood urea nitrogen (BUN) may remain normal. Nephrotic syndrome may complicate many forms of glomerular injury and is particularly common in diabetic nephropathy.

S KEY SYNDROME

Urolithiasis: *Pathophysiology:* Stones form either from solutes (usually calcium oxalate, but also uric acid) that accrete upon a nidus or as a result of chronic urinary tract infections with urea-splitting organisms (struvite stones). Stones are usually asymptomatic until they lodge at a narrowing in the ureter or bladder outlet. Pain is the presenting symptom, the site depending upon the location of the impacted stone (See *Renal Colic*, page 610). Microscopic or gross hematuria may be present intermittently during the asymptomatic phase.

S KEY SYNDROME

▶ **Uroepithelial Cancer (Bladder, Ureters, Renal Pelvis):** *Pathophysiology:* The transitional cell epithelium becomes neoplastic under the influence of substances excreted in the urine. Risk factors include the combination of alcohol and tobacco, industrial chemicals and certain chemotherapy agents (cyclophosphamide, ifosfamide). Hematuria, either gross or microscopic, is the only early sign. Advanced disease presents with direct extension to other pelvic and retroperitoneal organs causing pain, fistulas, and obstructions.

S KEY SYNDROME

▶ **Kidney Cancer:** *Pathophysiology:* Most renal cancers arise from the epithelium and have mutations of the von Hippel-Lindau gene, either inherited (von Hippel-Lindau syndrome) or acquired. Tobacco smoke is a major risk factor for acquired renal cell carcinoma. Renal cancers may invade the renal vein and inferior vena cava. They metastasize to the lungs and invade local retroperitoneal structures, including bone and CNS, causing pain. Microscopic hematuria may be present. The presenting flank pain is often mild and felt as a fullness or pressure prior to the onset of pain.

S KEY SYNDROME

▼ **Urinary Tract Infection: Urethritis and Urethral Syndrome:** *Pathophysiology:* Infection in the urethra causing pain and purulent discharge is caused by sexually transmitted diseases or complicates prolonged catheterization. Urethritis is usually caused by infection with *Neisseria gonorrhoea, Chlamydia trachomatis,* genital mycoplasmas, or herpes simplex. Burning dysuria is uniform and pus may be milked from the meatus by urethral stripping. Mixed infections are not unusual. Untreated, progression to upper tract infection is possible. Dysuria, urgency, and frequency with negative cultures for bacteria and lack of response to antibiotics defines the *urethral syndrome.* The etiology is poorly understood and may result from viral infection or sterile inflammation.

S KEY SYNDROME

▼ **Urinary Tract Infection: Cystitis:** *Pathophysiology:* Ascending infection with enteric flora (usually *Escherichia coli*) is common in normal women because of urethral colonization with fecal and vaginal flora and a short urethra. Cystitis in men suggests an anatomic, usually obstructing, abnormality. Residual urine volume >100 cc is associated with increased risk of infection. Inflammation of the bladder wall and trigone elicits urinary frequency, urgency, dysuria, and a sensation of incomplete voiding. Untreated, infection can ascend to the kidneys [Bent S, Nallamothu BK, Simel DL, et al. Does this woman have an acute uncomplicated urinary tract infection? *JAMA* 2002;287:2701–2710].

S KEY SYNDROME

▼ **Urinary Tract Infection: Acute Pyelonephritis:** *Pathophysiology:* Bacteria ascend from the bladder or, less commonly, reach the kidney via the bloodstream. Infection involves primarily the renal medulla and collecting system, but may extend to the cortex or perinephritic tissue with abscess formation. Symptoms are fever, chills, and flank pain. Physical exam reveals percussion tenderness at the costovertebral angle. Prompt diagnosis and treatment prevents bacteremia, urosepsis, and local suppurative complications.

S KEY SYNDROME

▼ **Urinary Tract Infection: Chronic Pyelonephritis:** *Pathophysiology:* Chronic kidney infection is caused by non-pyogenic bacteria, including slowly growing, often intracellular organisms, such as tuberculosis and brucellosis. **Vesicoureteral reflux** is associated with recurrent infections in addition to producing pressure induced renal injury. This condition may be asymptomatic with abnormalities on urinalysis (pyuria, cellular casts, and proteinuria) and declining renal function the only clues.

S KEY SYNDROME

▼ **Interstitial Nephritis:** *Pathophysiology:* Inflammation of the cortical and medullary renal interstitium (as distinct from the glomerular and vascular injury of glomerulonephritis) results in scarring, decreased tubular function, and progressive renal insufficiency. Injury may be acute (infection, drug induced) or chronic (toxins, drugs, infection, obstruction). This condition may be asymptomatic with abnormalities on urinalysis (pyuria, cellular casts, and proteinuria) and declining renal function the only clues.

✓ *INTERSTITIAL NEPHRITIS—CLINICAL OCCURRENCE:* *Congenital* polycystic kidney disease, medullary cystic and sponge kidney, sickle cell disease, vesicoureteral reflux; *Inflammatory/Immune* drug allergy (penicillins, sulfonamides, etc.), Sjögren syndrome, Goodpasture syndrome, transplant rejection; *Infectious* acute and chronic pyelonephritis, viral infection (Epstein-Barr virus, cytomegalovirus, HIV, hantavirus), brucellosis, yersinia, tuberculosis, leptospirosis, rickettsia, mycoplasma; *Metabolic/Toxic* drugs (nonsteroidal antiinflammatory drugs, diuretics, anticonvulsants, cyclosporin, and others), toxins (heavy metals, lithium, herbals, and others), hypercalcemia, hyperuricemia, prolonged hypokalemia; *Mechanical/Traumatic* chronic obstruction, ureterovesical reflux, radiation; *Neoplastic* multiple myeloma, lymphoma, leukemia; *Vascular* accompanying glomerulonephritis and vasculitis.

Interstitial Cystitis: *Pathophysiology:* A condition of unknown cause results in often painful inflammation of the bladder wall leading to fibrosis and decreased bladder capacity. This condition is most common in women who present with urinary frequency and bladder pain, but negative cultures for infection. Diagnosis is by exclusion of other causes of bladder pain and frequency and complete urologic evaluation.

11 The Female Genitalia and Reproductive System

Overview of Female Reproductive Physiology

Male and female external genitalia arise from identical embryologic anlage depending on the presence or absence of testosterone. Lack of the SRY gene (typically found on the Y chromosome) leads to development of ovaries, with subsequent maturation of female sex organs. The labia majora is a cognate of the scrotum and the clitoris and penis are similarly derived. Ambiguous genitalia occur when development and maturation occurs with a mixed hormonal environment or genetic substrate.

The female reproductive system consists of the ovaries on their suspensory ligaments, the fallopian tubes, the uterine corpus and cervix, the vagina with its muscular wall, the vaginal and introital glands of Cowper and Bartholin, the labia minora and majora, and the clitoris with its covering prepuce.

The ovary cyclically matures one ovum within a follicle under the stimulation of follicle-stimulating hormone (FSH) from the pituitary. The developing follicle produces estrogen, which causes proliferation of the endometrium. When the serum estrogen level reaches a threshold, a luteinizing hormone (LH) surge is triggered from the pituitary, effecting ovulation and formation of the corpus luteum that secretes increased levels of progesterone, inducing transformation of the endometrium from its proliferative to its secretory phase. The released ovum is captured by the fimbriated end of the fallopian tube down which it travels to the uterine corpus. If fertilized in the tube or uterine cavity, the ovum may implant into the receptive endometrium establishing a pregnancy. If not, implantation does not occur and the corpus luteum involutes. With the cessation of estrogen and progesterone production, the endometrium is sloughed as menstrual bleeding, FSH rises again to stimulate development of another follicle initiating another reproductive cycle. Implantation of a fertilized ovum leads to the development of the placenta which secretes beta-human chorionic gonadotropin (beta-hCG)–suppressing pituitary FSH and LH, leading to cessation of ovulation and menstruation.

Anatomy of the Female Genitalia and Reproductive System

The symphysis pubis is surmounted anteriorly by a fat pad, the mons pubis (see Fig. 11-1). At puberty, the eminence becomes covered with hair that extends onto the skin of the abdomen to form a transverse borderline, the base of an inverted triangle called the *female escutcheon*. This hair distribution contrasts with that of the male escutcheon, which describes an upright triangle with the apex near the umbilicus.

THE VULVA.   The vulva or pudendum comprises the external genitalia of the female (Fig. 11-2B). The *labia majora* are elevated ridges extending inferiorly and posteriorly from the mons pubis nearly to the anus, forming the sides of a lens-shaped figure. They contain fat, blood vessels, nerves, and tissue that resemble the dartos tunic in the scrotum. Between the two labia majora are two smaller skin folds, the *labia minora*, which extend posteriorly from the clitoris to unite in front of the anus by a transverse fold, the *fourchette*. The *clitoris* is the erectile homologue of the penis, composed of two small corpora cavernosa and surrounded superiorly by the *prepuce* and inferiorly by folds of the labia minora, the *frenulum*. The cleft posterior to the clitoris, between the two labia minora, is called the *vestibule*. It is pierced by the *urethral meatus*, approximately 2.5 cm posterior to the clitoris, and the *vaginal orifice*, immediately posterior to the meatus. The vaginal opening is a median slit, varying inversely with the size of the hymen. The *hymen* is a thin membrane covering part of the vaginal orifice. Commonly a perforate ring, widest posteriorly, the hymen may be cribriform, fringed, or even imperforate. After rupture, the hymenal remnants heal as irregular folds of mucosa. Two paired glands open onto the vestibular surface: just inferior to the urethra are the openings of the *paraurethral (Skene) glands*, and at the posterior edge of the vaginal orifice are found the openings of the *greater vestibular (Bartholin) glands*.

THE VAGINA, UTERUS, AND ADNEXA.   From its orifice, the *vagina* extends posteriorly into the pelvis (Fig. 11-1). It is a collapsed tube with a posterior wall approximately 9 cm long and a shorter anterior vaginal wall (6–7.5 cm), which reflect onto the *uterine cervix* located most commonly at its anterior apex. The recess of the vagina behind the cervix is termed the *posterior fornix*; recesses on either side of the cervix are called *lateral fornices*. The vaginal mucosa is thrown into transverse rugae, separated by furrows of variable depths. Through the vagina, the nulliparous cervix appears as a smooth button with its face rounded and pierced by a hole or slit, the cervical os. The parous cervix may be somewhat irregular. The anterior and posterior lips of the os are usually in contact with the posterior vaginal wall. Dorsal to the posterior vaginal wall lies the *rectum*; ventral to the anterior vaginal wall are the *urethra* and *bladder*. The peritoneal cavity extends inferiorly behind the posterior fornix to form the *rectovaginal pouch (cul-de-sac of Douglas)*; its lower part is interposed between the rectum and the cervix. The *uterus* is a muscular organ, shaped like an inverted pear flattened anteroposteriorly. From

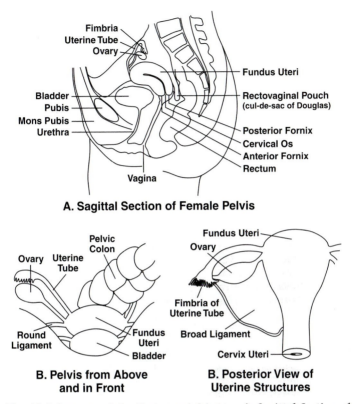

A. Sagittal Section of Female Pelvis

B. Pelvis from Above and in Front

B. Posterior View of Uterine Structures

Fig. 11-1 Anatomy of the Uterus and Adnexa. A. Sagittal Section of the Female Pelvis: Note the angle of the vagina with the vertical axis of the body, and the axis of the uterus perpendicular to the vaginal axis. The lips of the cervix uteri are shown to be in the same plane as the anterior vaginal wall, which is shorter than the posterior wall. The rectovaginal pouch (cul-de-sac of Douglas) lies anterior to the rectal wall; hence, it can be palpated during the rectal exam. The uterine fundus in the usual position is inaccessibile to the rectal examining finger, but very close to palpation from the lower abdomen. *B. View of the Pelvis from Above and in Front:* Note how the round ligament curves anteriorly and the uterine tubes curve posteriorly. *C. Posterior View of the Uterus and Broad Ligaments, Spread Out:* Note the suspension of the ovary near the fimbriated end of the uterine tube. The uterine tube forms the upper border of the broad ligament.

each side of the broad uterine fundus the *fallopian tubes* extend for approximately 10 cm, curving laterally and posteriorly in the pelvis. The tubes, suspended by the mesosalpinges, form the upper borders of the *broad ligaments* that spread from the lateral margins of the uterus to the pelvic wall. The uterus with the two wings of broad ligament forms a transverse septum dividing the pelvis into an anterior and posterior fossa. On the posterior surface of the broad ligaments the *ovaries* are suspended medial to and below the fimbriated ends of the fallopian tubes by ligaments which attact to the uterus (*ovarian ligament*) and the pelvic wall (*suspensory ligament*).

Physical Exam of the Female Genitalia Reproductive System

Inspection and palpation of the female pelvis can reveal many disorders of the reproductive organs, the lower urinary tract, and the lower abdomen. The pelvic examination is an extension of abdominal palpation and is mandatory for every female. Neglect of the pelvic examination often leads to serious errors in diagnosis. Routine Papanicolaou smear is effective in detecting early cancer.

The Female Pelvic Examination

The pelvic examination should be at the end of the physical examination because it requires special positioning, equipment, and attendance of a female chaperone to assist. After emptying her bladder, the patient is placed in the lithotomy position on the examination table. Cover her body with a sheet, place her feet in stirrups attached to the table, and wrap the lower corners of the sheet around her legs, leaving considerable slack for the cloth to envelope the thighs and lower abdomen (Fig. 11-2A). When the patient is too weak to be examined on the table, have her assume the lithotomy position in bed. Elevate her pelvis on an inverted bedpan.

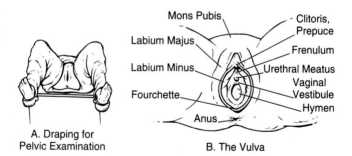

A. Draping for
Pelvic Examination

B. The Vulva

Fig. 11-2 Examination of the Vulva.   A. Draping for Pelvic Examination: The patient assumes the lithotomy position with feet in stirrups projecting from the end of the examining table. A sheet is spread over the patient so the two lower corners are wrapped about the thighs and legs. The middle of the lower edge of the sheet is slackly draped over the lower abdomen. B. Topographic Anatomy of the Vulva: The recessed vestibule contains a relatively small vaginal orifice, surrounded by one of the usual patterns of unruptured hymen. Bordering the vestibule are the two projecting folds of often deeply pigmented skin, the labia minora. Anteriorly, accessory folds of the labia form the prepuce that encloses the clitoris. Lateral to the labia minora are two parallel ridges of skin and fat that form the labium majus on either side of the labia minora.

Sit on a low stool within reach of a side table that holds specula, forceps, gauze, rubber gloves, lubricating jelly, and the materials for making the Pap smear and bacteriologic cultures. Shine a bright light onto the perineum. *For a complete examination, the following sequence is suggested:* (a) inspection of the vulva; (b) insertion of the vaginal speculum; (c) gathering of specimens for cytologic examination and bacteriologic tests; (d) inspection of the vaginal walls and cervix; (e) digital bimanual examination of the uterus and adnexa; (f) rectovaginal examination.

Inspection and Palpation of the Vulva (see Fig. 11-2B).   Observe the skin of the perineum for swelling, ulcers, and changes in color. Separate the labia with the gloved thumb and forefinger to inspect the clitoris and vestibule. Examine the urethral meatus for developmental anomalies, discharge, caruncle, neoplasm, and Skene abscess. Inspect the vaginal orifice for discharge, gaping of the edges, and protrusion of the vaginal walls. Palpate posteriorly and laterally to the hymen for enlargement of the Bartholin gland and for vestibular tenderness. Have the patient strain as if to defecate and look for bulging of the anterior or posterior vaginal wall through the introitus or leaking of urine.

Vaginal Speculum Exam (Fig. 11-3).   Unlubricated vaginal speculum exam should precede digital examination because lubricating jelly interferes with the Papanicolaou smear. Separating the vaginal walls by a speculum permits inspection of the vagina and cervix, and sample collection for cytologic and bacteriologic tests and for biopsies when indicted. Select a clean bivalve speculum of suitable size and ensure its proper temperature by storing it in a heated drawer or by immersing it in warm water.

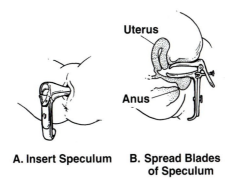

**A. Insert Speculum   B. Spread Blades
of Speculum**

Fig. 11-3 Using the Vaginal Speculum.   *The labia minora are retracted laterally with the gloved index and middle fingers. The closed blades of the vaginal speculum are inserted in the vagina with the widths of the blades almost horizontal.* ***A.*** *The closed blades of the speculum have been well inserted at a 30- to 45-degree angle posteriorly and the blades separated and locked open.* ***B.*** *A sagittal section shows the open blades of the speculum in proper position with the upper shorter blade lifting the vault of the vagina to expose the cervix uteri on the anterior vaginal wall.*

With one hand grasp the handle and close the blades of the speculum while separating the labia minora at the level of the posterior fourchette with the other hand. Insert the closed blades into the vaginal orifice with slight downward pressure to avoid pinching the urethra against the symphysis pubis. When the speculum tips reach the upper vagina, separate the blades and illuminate the vaginal cavity with a suitable light. Move the speculum handle so the blade tips expose the *cervix*, then lock the blades open with the set screw. Obtain specimens from the cervix for the *Pap test*. If the cervical os is obscured by discharge, gently sponge it with a large, sterile cotton swab. The cervical sample is obtained by gently scraping the cervix with a wooden spatula and turning a cytobrush in the cervical canal, or by using a special brush for liquid Pap preparation. When indicated, inoculate gonorrheal and chlamydial *cultures* from a swabbing of the cervical canal. *Inspect the cervix* for color, lacerations, ulcers, and new growths. Inspect the cervical os for size, shape, color, discharge, and polyps. Loosen the set screw and *inspect the vaginal walls* by rotating the speculum to expose all the cavity. Look for abnormal redness or blueness of the mucosa and loss of rugation. If present, determine whether a discharge exudes from the cervical os or the vagina. When indicated, obtain a sample of discharge from the lateral and anterior vaginal walls for microscopic examination. Finally, carefully withdraw the speculum while inspecting the mucosa.

Bɪᴍᴀɴᴜᴀʟ Pᴇʟᴠɪᴄ Exᴀᴍ. Always use the same hand for vaginal palpation, which, the right or the left, is a matter of personal preference. Many gynecologists palpate the vagina with the left hand and handle instruments with the right. The invariable use of the same hand in the bimanual examination permits each hand to become accustomed to its role, and the sense of touch is educated for the findings encountered. In the following directions, the right hand is arbitrarily assigned to the vagina and the left hand is employed to palpate the abdomen. If obstruction from a persistent hymen or a constricted vagina does not interfere, use two fingers for vaginal examination.

Place the gloved right hand in the gynecologic position: index and middle fingers straight and close together, thumb widely abducted, fourth and fifth fingers folded into the palm. Lubricate the straight fingers, spread the labia with the left thumb and forefinger to avoid the discomfort of pulling pubic hair into the vagina. Insert the two lubricated fingers in the vaginal cavity with the finger pads facing the anterior vaginal wall (Fig. 11-4A). Examine each structure systematically forming a mental picture of your observations.

The *greater vestibular glands* (vulvovaginal glands or Bartholin glands) are examined with the forefinger inside the vagina and the thumb opposite and outside on the posterior part of the labium majus feeling the inner wall for abscess or tenderness (see Fig. 11-4B). Evert that part of the vaginal mucosa to look for a red spot or pus marking the opening of an inflamed duct. The normal glands and ducts cannot be seen or felt. The *urethra* is palpated in the midline of the anterior vaginal wall near the introitus for tenderness or induration. The *base of bladder* is palpated in the midline of the anterior vaginal wall, halfway between the introitus and the cervix, for tenderness or induration produced by cystitis or

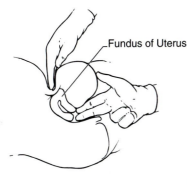
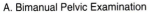
Fundus of Uterus

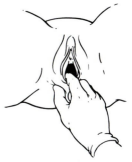

A. Bimanual Pelvic Examination

B. Palpating Bartholin's Gland
(vulvovaginal gland)

Fig. 11-4 Bimanual Pelvic Examination. *A. Palpation of the Uterus: The index and middle fingers of the gloved right hand are inserted in the vagina with the tips of the fingers facing anteriorly and touching the cervix. The fingers of the left hand are pressed deep into the abdomen above the mons pubis, pushing the uterine fundus downward and forward toward the two vaginal fingers. The adnexa are examined similarly, except the vaginal fingers are placed to the side of the uterus and the abdominal fingers are pushed into the belly at a point 2–3 cm medial to the anterior superior iliac spine. Attempt to approximate the fingertips of the two examining hands. The abdominal fingers are pulled inferiorly to push the tube and ovary onto the tips of the vaginal fingers. B. Palpation of the Greater Vestibular Gland (Bartholin Gland): The index finger is inserted in the vagina near the posterior introitus. The thumb is pressed outside on the labium majus and the finger and thumb are approximated.*

neoplasm of the bladder. Palpate the *vaginal wall* for tenderness, induration (from scars, granulomas, or neoplasm), strictures, septa, and adhesions (not to be confused with the normal transverse rugae). Next examine the *cervix*, which normally feels like a button, with a convex face and a central depression, the consistency of the tip of the nose. Feel for nodules and ulcers and note any abnormality of shape, size, or consistency. Determine the axis of the cervix; normally it faces posteriorly in the same plane as the anterior vaginal wall. Examine the *uterine corpus and fundus* bimanually by pushing the cervix anteriorly while the fingers of the left hand press into the abdomen posteriorly just above the mons pubis. Estimate the size of the uterus, its axis, tenderness, mobility, and characterize any nodules that may be present. To examine the *adnexa*, place the vaginal fingers on one side of the cervix and push their tips superiorly and posteriorly as far as possible. With the fingers of the left hand, locate a point on the same side of the abdomen 2–3 cm medially from the anterior superior iliac spine. Push the abdominal fingers deep so their tips approach the vaginal fingers. This should bring the approximated hands back to the uterine tubes and ovaries. If the structures are not felt at that point, move the fingertips of both hands inferiorly toward the pubis, so that the adnexa pass between the two hands. Exert abdominal pressure gently, but deeply, pressing the two hands a little closer each time the patient expires to avoid abdominal guarding. The role of the abdominal hand should be to displace the structures, while the vaginal hand feels them. The normal ovary and tube are usually not palpable. When the normal *fallopian tube* is felt, it is approximately 4 mm in diameter, about half the size of a common pencil. It has the consistency of a piece of rubber tubing. The normal *ovary* is approximately 3 cm by 2 cm by 2 cm; the lateral face is, therefore, about the size of the distal phalanx of the examiner's thumb, but the thickness of the ovary is about half that of the digit. The ovary is soft and naturally tender to palpation. Look for enlargement or asymmetry of the adnexa, unusual tenderness, decreased mobility, and other masses or induration. Examine the *pelvic floor*, noting the size of the introitus, and, with the examining fingers facing posteriorly, press the pelvic floor inferiorly and posteriorly to determine the resistance or relaxation.

RECTOVAGINAL EXAM.   Conclude the pelvic exam with a rectal and rectovaginal examination. Ordinarily, the female genitalia are felt much more satisfactorily through the vagina than the rectum. In the virgin, however, vaginal palpation may not be feasible, and enough may be learned by rectal examination to make or exclude diagnoses.

First note any distortion or defects in the circular *anal sphincter muscle*, a common consequence of vaginal delivery. Next, palpate the *anal canal* for intrinsic lesions (see page 526). Palpate the anterior *rectal wall* (posterior vaginal wall) for tenderness and masses then systematically examine the lateral and posterior rectum and ampulla. While using the left hand to press on the lower abdomen as in the bimanual vaginal examination, palpate the pelvis through the rectum and vagina. Through the anterior rectal wall, locate the *cervix*, attempt to feel the *body and fundus of the uterus*. This may be the only route by which a retroverted uterus is palpable. Insert your finger fully and palpate the anterior rectal wall in the region of the peritoneal *rectovaginal pouch* (cul-de-sac of Douglas; see Fig. 11-1). After changing gloves, insert the middle finger of the gloved right hand into the anal canal with the forefinger in the vagina palpating the *rectovaginal wall* between the two fingers. Thickening of the rectovaginal septum or parametrium occurs from spread of cervical carcinoma, puerperal infection, and pelvic inflammatory disease.

Female Genital and Reproductive Symptoms

General Symptoms

KEY SYMPTOM

Pelvic Pain: *Pathophysiology:* Pain in the pelvis is common. Pain arises from inflammation, usually as the result of infection, from distention of tubular structures or cysts, traction on serosal surfaces by masses or adhesions, hemorrhage, and invasion of sensitive structures by neoplasms or implantation of endometrial tissue. Visceral pain is poorly localized whereas serosal pain is usually well localized by the patient. It is essential to obtain a complete history of the patient's pain pattern, its relationship to menses, ovulation, bowel movements, urination, and physical and sexual activity. Describe the pain quality using the patient's words. The pelvic exam must be gentle and the patient relaxed for the examiner to localize the pain to a specific area or structure.

✔ *PELVIC PAIN—CLINICAL OCCURRENCE: Congenital* imperforate hymen, porphyria; *Endocrine* ectopic pregnancy, functional ovarian cysts; *Idiopathic* ovarian cysts, especially with hemorrhage or rupture, endometriosis, diverticulosis; *Inflammatory/Immune* inflammatory bowel disease, appendicitis; *Infectious* cervicitis, endometritis, salpingitis, tuboovarian abscess, cystitis, diverticulitis and diverticular abscess, appendicitis; *Mechanical/Traumatic* ovarian torsion, tubal pregnancy; *Neoplastic* any locally invasive cancer (e.g., cervical, endometrial, rectal, bladder), metastases, degenerating leiomyoma; *Psychosocial* physical, emotional, and sexual abuse; *Vascular* ovarian infarction (torsion), bleeding following ovulation (mittelschmerz).

KEY SYMPTOM
Painful Menstruation (Dysmenorrhea): *Pathophysiology:* Primary dysmenorrhea results from uterine ischemia caused by myometrial contraction under the influence of prostaglandins released during menstruation. Pain accompanying menses but arising from disease in the pelvis is secondary dysmenorrhea. The most prominent and most frequent complaint is severe abdominal cramps in the suprapubic region. Less severe are accompanying backache and headache. Dysmenorrhea may disappear after a pregnancy. Prostaglandin inhibitors can be quite helpful and may be used prophylactically. Secondary dysmenorrhea may result from endometriosis, pelvic neoplasms, and pelvic inflammations.

KEY SYMPTOM
Painful Intercourse: Dyspareunia: *Pathophysiology:* Physical stimulation of pelvic structures during vaginal intercourse can lead to pain preventing sexual enjoyment. Anxiety and fear increase perception of all forms of pain. Inquire whether the pain is felt superficially or deeply after penetration. Ask specifically whether the patient has sufficient stimulation to become sexually aroused, about the sufficiency of vaginal lubrication, whether the partner is so aggressive as to cause trauma, and any bleeding after intercourse. Inquire about sexual practices, including the use of foreign bodies as stimulants, rectal intercourse, and whether previous experiences have occurred that can produce a fear of intercourse, for example, rape, incest, molestation, and physical and emotional abuse.

✔ *DYSPAREUNIA—CLINICAL OCCURRENCE:* Insufficient foreplay, inadequate lubrication, postmenopausal estrogen deficiency with dryness of vaginal mucosa, vaginismus (reflex spasm of muscles around the lower vaginal opening), vulvar vestibulitis, lichen planus, perineal trauma and lacerations, pelvic and perineal infections, pelvic tumors.

KEY SYMPTOM

Menstrual Disorders: See *Female Reproductive Syndromes: Menstrual Disorders*, page 644ff.

Vulvar and Vaginal Symptoms

KEY SYMPTOM

Vulvar Pain: *Pathophysiology:* The vulva is somatically innervated and pain perception and localization are good. Infection, inflammation, and local trauma are the most common identifiable causes of pain. Dysesthetic vulvodynia may be neuropathic and vulvar vestibulitis may have an inflammatory basis.

VAGINAL PAIN: VAGINISMUS: *Pathophysiology:* Painful contraction of the pubococcygeus muscle around the lower third of the vagina results in severe pain that can be persistent or intermittent. The cause is unknown and treatment is difficult. Intercourse is painful or impossible.

KEY SYMPTOM

Vulvar Pruritus: Itching of the vulva is usually the result of obvious disease or chemical irritation of the vulvar skin. Candida infection and lichen sclerosis are common etiologies.

KEY SYMPTOM

► **Vaginal Bleeding:** See *Female Reproductive Tract Syndromes: Menstrual Disorders*, page 644ff.

Female Genital and Reproductive Signs

Vulvar Signs

KEY SIGN

Ambiguous Genitalia: Intersexuality: Refer to special works on this subject.

KEY SIGN

Genital Ulcer: *Pathophysiology:* Trauma and sexually transmitted diseases are the most common causes of genital ulceration. Painless ulcers are most typical of syphilis. Ulcers increase the risk of transmitting and acquiring sexually transmitted diseases (STDs) including HIV. Ulcers may be both more painful and slower healing in women than in men because of persistent warmth and moisture. See also pages 660–661.

✓ *GENITAL ULCER—CLINICAL OCCURRENCE: Idiopathic* lichen sclerosis; *Inflammatory/Immune* Behçet syndrome, vulvar vestibulitis, fixed drug reaction, lichen planus; *Infectious* herpes simplex types 1 and 2, chlamydia, syphilis, chancroid, lymphogranuloma venereum, HIV, cytomegalovirus, Epstein-Barr virus, granuloma inguinale; *Mechanical/Traumatic* inadequate lubrication during intercourse; *Neoplastic* squamous cell cancer.

KEY SIGN

Vulvar Rash: Determine if the rash is acute or chronic, pruritic, weeping or scaling, associated with bleeding or pain, or with the use of topical and systemic medications, creams, and lotions.

✓ *VULVAR RASH—CLINICAL OCCURRENCE:* See also *Vulvar Inflammation: Vulvitis,* below. *Endocrine* atrophic vulvovaginitis; *Idiopathic* lichen sclerosis; *Inflammatory/Immune* contact dermatitis; *Infectious* candidiasis, dermatophytes, cellulitis, abscess of skin and mucosal glands; *Metabolic/Toxic* diabetes mellitus; *Mechanical/Traumatic* abrasions and lacerations, tight-fitting clothing with poor ventilation; *Neoplastic* Bowen disease, vulvar carcinoma; *Psychosocial* pruritis vulvae, pruritis ani.

KEY SIGN

Vulvar Inflammation: Vulvitis: The skin is often red, warm, and variably edematous and tender. The condition may be associated with vaginitis and discharge, or occur alone. Alternatively, the skin may appear thinned, atrophic or opaque, and white. The latter changes are more common in lichen sclerosis and lichen planus.

✓ *VULVITIS—CLINICAL OCCURRENCE: Inflammatory/Immune* contact dermatitis, vulvar vestibulitis, lichen planus, lichen sclerosis; *Infectious* cellulitis, *Candida,* dermatophyte; *Metabolic/Toxic* topical irritants; *Mechanical/Traumatic* tight-fitting clothing; *Neoplastic* diffuse Bowen disease.

KEY SIGN

Atrophic Vulvovaginitis: *Pathophysiology:* Withdrawal of estrogen leads to skin which is thinned, inelastic, and easily irritated and inflammed. A careful history focusing on menstrul pattern and symptoms of estrogen insufficiency, especially hot flushes, point to the diagnosis. Exam shows absent rugae and a thin dry mucosa (see page 636).

KEY SIGN

Vulvar Swelling, Masses, and Growths: *Pathophysiology:* All the normal vulvar structures are susceptible to neoplastic change. Infection with human papilloma virus (HPV) or syphilis can produce condylomas. Evaluation is identical to other skin growths with special respect for the sensitivity of the tissues and the need to maintain cosmesis.

✔ *VULVAR MASSES—CLINICAL OCCURRENCE:* *Inflammatory/Immune* granulomatous disease; *Infectious* condyloma latum (syphilis), condyloma acuminatum (HPV), histoplasmosis; *Mechanical/Traumatic* obstructed mucosal glands and Bartholin and Skene glands; *Neoplastic* Bowen disease, melanoma, invasive squamous cell cancer.

DIFFUSE SWELLING OF THE VULVA: *Pathophysiology:* Obstruction of the lymphatic channels from any cause may produce lymphedema of the labia and surrounding tissues. Likewise, the labia will be edematous when systemic venous pressure is very high and dependent edema reaches above the inguinal ligaments, for example, advanced right ventricular failure or constrictive pericarditis. Irritation may produce hypertrophy of the labia. Look for local irritation and history and physical finding for systemic disease affecting the lymphatics or venous system.

SWELLING OF A LABIUM MAJUS: HEMATOMA: A large, painful, bluish swelling of the labium may occur within a few hours after local trauma. Without a history of trauma, the condition may be confused with cellulitis of the vulva.

SWELLING OF A LABIUM MAJUS: LABIOINGUINAL HERNIA: *Pathophysiology:* Failure of the peritoneal pouch to obliterate in the fetus may permit a hernia to descend from the abdomen into the labium majus. It is analagous to the scrotal hernia in the male and presents with visible swelling.

KEY SIGN
Swelling of a Labium Majus: Abscess of the Greater Vestibular Gland (Bartholin Gland Abscess): *Pathophysiology:* Bartholin gland cysts are common and asymptomatic. Infection of the cyst leads to abcess formation, which may tract to the skin or toward the ischiorectal fossa. The normal glands are not palpable and their ducts are not visible. Epidermal inclusion cysts are a common cause of swelling. Cysts and smaller abscesses are found only by vaginal examination (Fig. 8-11B). Inflammation causes a red spot in the mucosa at the site of the ductal orifice, and pus may be expressed from it. If the abscess is large, the posterior portion of the labium is swollen and fluctuant and the overlying skin is tender, hot, and red.

KEY SIGN
Urethral Meatus Abnormalities: Urethritis: See also Chapter 10, *Urinary Syndromes, Urinary Tract Infections: Urethritis,* page 621. A purulent discharge issues from the meatus. This is usually caused by the inflammation from *Neisseria gonorrhoea, Chlamydia trachomatis,* genital mycoplasmas or herpes simplex. Palpation of the anterior vaginal wall, beginning at the cervix and stroking toward the meatus, reveals tenderness and induration along the course of the urethra. Pus may be squeezed from the meatus in this manner. A urethral diverticulum may also produce pus.

KEY SIGN

Urethral Meatus Abnormalities: Inflammation of the Periurethral (Skene) Gland and Duct: The periurethral gland (the Skene gland) lies on either side of, and posterior to, the female urethra, just inside the meatus. Often it becomes the site of chronic infection. If inflamed, the mouth of the duct is visible and red, when reviewed on spreading of the meatus.

Urethral Meatus Abnormalities: Urethral Caruncle: This papilloma appears as a small red mass in the meatus or the visible portion of the urethra. It usually occurs as a complication of urethritis. It may be tender and painful on urination.

Urethral Meatus Abnormalities: Prolapse of the Urethra: Slight gaping of the meatus is common in the multipara. When more severe, the urethral mucosa may protrude from the meatus and become tender and inflamed.

Vaginal Signs

KEY SIGN

Vaginal Ulcers: The same types that occur on the vulva may involve the vaginal mucosa; see page 632.

KEY SIGN

Vaginal Discharge: *Pathophysiology:* A clear to slightly white vaginal discharge containing mucous, epithelial cells, and commensal bacteria (particularly lactobacilli) at a pH of 4.0 is normal. Infection and/or inflammation lead to increased mucous production and exudation of white blood cells from the mucosa, producing vaginal discharges. Depending upon etiology, discharges vary from thick white to thin, frothy, and bloody with variable odor, pH, and accompanying pruritis. (For a review of vaginitis, see [Sobel JD. Vaginitis. *N Engl J Med* 1998;337:1896–1903].)

✔ *VAGINAL DISCHARGE—CLINICAL OCCURRENCE: Endocrine* atrophic vaginitis; *Inflammatory/Immune* contact dermatitis; *Infectious* bacterial vaginosis, *Candida, Trichomonas; Metabolic/Toxic* cytolytic vaginosis; *Mechanical/Traumatic* retained tampons, pessary, foreign body; *Neoplastic* vaginal and cervical cancers (often bloody).

KEY SIGN

Reddened Vaginal Mucosa: Vaginitis: *Pathophysiology:* Inflammation of the vaginal mucosa from infection, allergy, or irritants leads to erythema. History and examination of the vaginal secretions, which are frequently increased to a discharge, will usually yield a diagnosis.

✔ *VAGINITIS—CLINICAL OCCURRENCE: Inflammatory/Immune* contact dermatitis, Behçet disease; Infectious: *Candida, Trichomonas,* bacterial vaginosis, viral enanthems;   *Metabolic/Toxic*   cytolytic vaginosis;   *Mechanical/Traumatic*   retained foreign bodies, inadequate lubrication during intercourse;   *Neoplastic*   diffuse Bowen disease.

REDDENED VAGINA: VULVOVAGINAL CANDIDIASIS: Itching, pain, dyspareunia, with erythema and edema characterize infection with *Candida albicans.* The discharge has a normal vaginal pH ($\leq$4.5) and pseudohyphae and many neutrophils can be identified in a 10% KOH preparation. Culture may be needed to confirm the diagnosis and distinguish it from less-common noninfectious causes.

REDDENED VAGINA: TRICHOMONAS VAGINITIS: *Trichomonas vaginalis* produces a tender, reddened mucosa, studded with small hemorrhagic spots. The resulting malodorous discharge is yellow-green to gray and is frequently frothy, with a pH of 5.0–6.0. In a more chronic stage, the vaginal mucosa contains scattered red papules, giving a granular appearance. Rapid diagnosis may be made by suspending a bit of discharge in isotonic saline solution and finding many neutrophils and mobile trichomonads by microscopic examination.

REDDENED VAGINA: ATROPHIC VAGINITIS: *Pathophysiology:*   The vaginal mucosa is estrogen dependent and following menopause becomes thin, dry, and smooth without rugae. The thin and tender mucosa contains abraded patches and adhesions that bleed easily. Frequently, a serosanguinous discharge with a pH greater than 6.0 results.

REDDENED VAGINA: BACTERIAL VAGINOSIS: This is one of the most common causes of vaginitis in women of childbearing age. They present with a thick, off-white, malodorous discharge with a "fishy smell" and a pH greater than 4.5. Diagnosis is confirmed by finding clue cells (exfoliated vaginal epithelial cells to which *Gardnerella vaginalis* adhere) in vaginal secretions. Cultures are of no value because *G. vaginalis* is present in 50–60% of healthy women.

REDDENED VAGINA: CYTOLYTIC VAGINOSIS: *Pathophysiology:*   Overgrowth of *Lactobacillus spp.* produces a low vaginal pH leading to breakdown of epithelial cells and inflammation. The vaginal pH is between 3.5 and 4.5, and microscopic exam shows few polymorphonuclear cells, cytolytic changes in the epithelial cells, and no evidence of *Candida, Trichomonas*, or bacterial vaginosis.

Bluish Vagina: Cyanosis: The mucosa becomes cyanotic as a result of local venous engorgement in pregnancy or a pelvic tumor. The generalized cyanosis of congestive cardiac failure is also visible in the mucosal lining.

Vaginal Tenderness: Vaginitis: Tenderness of the walls and a discharge from the introitus may be the first signs of vaginitis encountered, before a speculum examination has been performed.

▶ **Vaginal Mass: Neoplasm:** Neoplasms in the vaginal mucosa may be primary or secondary to carcinoma of the uterus, rectum, bladder, or external genitalia.

Vaginal Mass: Vaginal Polyp: Polyps can arise from the vaginal wall or extend from the cervix. Polypoid deformities of the vaginal apex following hysterectomy are common.

KEY SIGN
Masses in the Rectovaginal Pouch: *Pathophysiology:* Because the rectovaginal pouch is the most dependent portion of the abdominal cavity, it collects fluid, exfoliated cells, and mobile masses from within the abdomen. Masses include prolapsed ovary, bowel loops, carcinoma of the colon, implants of endometriosis or ovarian carcinoma, a rectal shelf formed by other intraabdominal cancer, or an accumulation of pus, fluid, or blood from abdominal lesions.

KEY SIGN
Rectovaginal Fistula: *Pathophysiology:* Breakdown of the rectovaginal wall occurs after extensive radiation, obstetrical trauma, surgery, Crohn disease, and malignancy. A fistula from rectum to vagina is usually suggested by the history of fecal contamination of the vagina. The mouth of the fistula may be palpable as a small patch of induration in the posterior wall of the vagina. The opening may be identified through the vaginal speculum. The rectal wall may be indurated from scar tissue.

KEY SIGN
Pelvic Floor: Relaxation: *Pathophysiology:* the muscular pelvic floor is pierced by the rectum, vagina, and urethra. It is subject to extensive trauma during vaginal delivery which stretches and may tear the muscles. Tearing of the urethral and anal sphincters may also occur. Inadequate support of the pelvic organs leads to loss of sphincter functions and prolapse of tissues. Patients complain of incontinence, feelings of pressure and fullness, and the occurrence of visible or palpable prolapsing tissues.

Pelvic Floor: Enlarged Introitus: When the hymen is ruptured, the vaginal orifice normally admits the examiner's two fingers. When three fingers are accommodated, the introitus is definitely enlarged, usually indicating some degree of pelvic relaxation from childbirth.

KEY SIGN
Pelvic Floor: Cystocele (Bladder Prolapse): When the patient stands or strains, the anterior vaginal wall containing a portion of the bladder, bulges into the vagina and may emerge from the introitus as a soft, spheric tumor (Fig. 11-5B). This finding usually indicates pelvic floor laceration during childbirth.

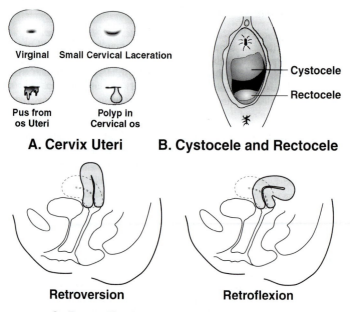

Virginal   Small Cervical Laceration

Pus from
os Uteri

Polyp in
Cervical os

A. Cervix Uteri

Cystocele

Rectocele

B. Cystocele and Rectocele

Retroversion

Retroflexion

C. Retrodisplacements of the Uterus

Fig. 11-5 Some Pelvic Signs.   A. Lesions of the Cervix: The lacerations of childbirth leave various scars. Pus or a polyp may be seen coming out from the os. B. Cystocele and Rectocele: When the patient is asked to strain as if to defecate, the introitus widens and bulging may develop anteriorly (cystocele) or posteriorly (rectocele). C. Uterine Displacements: If the axis of the uterus remains straight and the whole organ is tilted, it is called retroversion. If the axis of the uterus is bent, the condition is called retroflexion.

KEY SIGN

Pelvic Floor: Rectocele (Rectal Prolapse): When the patient stands or strains, the posterior vaginal wall, containing a portion of the rectum, protrudes into the vagina and may emerge from the introitus (see Fig. 11-5B). This is also evidence of pelvic floor laceration during childbirth. Examination in the left decubitus position may be better able to detect larger rectoceles than exam with the patient supine [Delemarre JB, Kruyt RH, Doornboss J, et al. Anterior rectocele: Assessment with radiographic defecography, dynamic magnetic resonance imaging, and physical examination. *Dis Colon Rectum* 1994;37:249–259].

KEY SIGN

Pelvic Floor: Uterine Prolapse: When the patient stands or strains, the cervix may protrude from the introitus. This results from loss of the normal ligamentous support for the uterus.

Cervical Signs

KEY SIGN
Cervix: Cyanosis: Bluish discoloration of the cervix is a sign of early pregnancy (Chadwick sign). It also occurs in tumors of the pelvis and in congestive cardiac failure. (See *Hegar Sign,* page 640.)

Cervix: Softening: An early sign of pregnancy is softening of the cervix in the first trimester.

KEY SIGN
Cervix: Lacerations: *Pathophysiology:*   During vaginal delivery, the cervix nearly always sustains some laceration (see Fig. 11-5A). Commonly, the tear is transverse and bilateral; occasionally, the laceration is unilateral, or multiple tears produce a stellate lesion. Recently torn edges appear raw. In a few weeks, healing leaves scarred fissures or notches. The cleft lips of the cervix may become everted; healing may be incomplete, causing an area of erosion. Healed lacerations of the cervix leave notches or fissures in the surface of the cervix that can be felt with the finger.

KEY SIGN
Cervical Discharge: Endocervicitis: *Pathophysiology:*   While the vagina is quite resistant, the columnar epithelium of the endocervix is particularly susceptible to infection with gonorrhea, chlamydia, herpes, and genital mycoplasmas. A mucopurulent or purulent discharge emerges from the cervix os (see Fig. 11-5A). The cervical lips are usually inflamed and eroded. The absence of tenderness on palpation of the uterine fundus suggests that the infection is limited to the cervical canal. Cervicitis is acute and is usually caused by gonorrhea or chlamydial infection. Extension into the uterine cavity and tubes produces endometritis and pelvic inflammatory disease, which can lead to tuboovarian abcess and sterility.

KEY SIGN
Cervical Discharge: Endometritis: See *Uterine Signs: Endometritis,* below.

Cervical Eversion: Velvety red mucosa, without ulceration, extending outward from the cervical os is usually the result of migration of the endocervical tissue onto the visible portions of the cervix.

KEY SIGN
Cervical Ulcer: There is a loss of epithelium and sloughing of underlying tissue. Specific causes are herpes simplex, chancroid, syphilis, tuberculosis, and carcinoma. Biopsy is indicated when tests for microbial diseases are negative. This may result from the abrasion of a pessary.

Cervical Mass: Hypertrophy: The lips of the cervix may enlarge and elongate. This most frequently occurs in parous women. In hypertrophy the fundus retains its normal position. The cervix is also more visible, but not enlarged, in uterine prolapse; however, the fundus descends toward the vaginal orifice. The cervix retains its normal contour in hypertrophy, whereas neoplasm distorts the proportions.

KEY SIGN

Cervical Mass: Polyp: A soft, bright-red, benign tumor, usually pedunculated, often emerges from the cervical os (see Fig. 11-5A). It may cause discharge and bleeding.

Cervical Mass: Cysts: Occlusion of glands in the cervical mucosa causes 1–3 mm clear or white retention cysts, called nabothian cysts, that are visible on speculum exam.

KEY SIGN

► **Cervical Mass: Cervical Carcinoma:** Frequently, a bloody discharge follows straining or coitus. Whereas a cervical polyp is small and soft, a hard mass in the cervix suggests a neoplasm, which should prompt Pap smear and cervical biopsy. A chronic ulcer of the cervix with induration is a late sign of carcinoma. In the later stages, extensive ulceration, induration, and nodularity make the diagnosis obvious [Sawaya GF, Brown AD, Washington AE, Garber AM. Current approaches to cervical-cancer screening. *N Engl J Med* 2001;344:1603–1607].

Uterine Signs

Uterus: Softening (Hegar Sign): During the first trimester of pregnancy, the fundus uteri softens at the junction of the cervix with the body. This change in consistency is easily palpable; sometimes the contrast between fundus and isthmus is so pronounced that the cervix seems to separate from the fundus [Bastian LA, Piscitelli JT. The rational clinical examination. Is this patient pregnant? Can you reliably rule in or rule out early pregnancy by clinical examination? *JAMA* 1997;278:586–591].

KEY SIGN

► **Uterine Tenderness: Endometritis:** The appearance of the cervix is similar to that in endocervicitis, but tenderness of the uterine body or fundus indicates involvement of the endometrium. Endometritis is caused by sexually transmitted diseases (gonorrhea, chlamydia, and mycoplasmas) or by infection following childbirth or abortion.

Uterus: Displacement: (See Fig. 11-5C.) The most common position of the uterine body is anteriorly in the same axis as the cervix. *Retroversion* is displacement of both fundus and cervix in a common axis and is present in 25% of normal women. The axis of the fundus and cervix is in the direction of the spine and the plane of the cervix faces the anterior wall of the vagina. The fundus encroaches upon the rectum. The uterine fundus may be felt through the anterior rectal wall when it cannot be palpated per vagina. When freely movable, it is symptomless; when fixed, it suggests endometriosis. *Retroflexion* is posterior displacement of the fundus. The plane of the cervix is in the normal position but the fundus is palpable through the posterior fornix and rectum (Fig. 11-5C). *Lateral displacement* of the uterus is frequently caused by adhesions or masses in the adnexa.

KEY SIGN

Uterine Enlargement: Pregnancy: Generalized uterine enlargement in a woman of childbearing age should be considered a pregnancy until proven otherwise. In the first few months of pregnancy, the gravid uterus becomes globular or more rounded in shape. Other symptoms and signs of pregnancy are morning sickness, tenderness of the breasts, amenorrhea, cyanosis of the vaginal and cervical mucosa (*Chadwick sign*), softening of the cervix, and softening of the uterine fundus (*Hegar sign*). Urine pregnancy testing is mandatory. The gravid uterus may be distinguished from large ovarian cysts by hearing the fetal heartbeat, remembering that concurrence of ovarian cysts with pregnancy is common. The height of the uterus reflects the stages of pregnancy: 3 months, at the pubis; 4.5 months, at the umbilicus; 9 months, at the xiphoid.

KEY SIGN

Uterine Enlargement: Leiomyoma (Fibroid): Hard, often painless nodules, frequently multiple, are firmly attached to the uterus. The nodules and the fundus move freely together. An asymmetric gravid uterus is sometimes mistaken for a uterine fibroid in a woman of childbearing age. Fibroids are three to five times more common in blacks than in whites.

KEY SIGN

► **Uterine Enlargement: Neoplasm of the Uterus:** Carcinoma and sarcoma of the uterus produce more- or less-generalized enlargement, which may be associated with bloody discharge. Evaluate with ultrasonography and seek gynecology evaluation.

Adnexal Signs

KEY SIGN

Pelvic Mass: Endometriosis: See *Female Genital and Reproductive Syndromes, Endometriosis*, page 648.

KEY SIGN

► **Adnexal Tenderness:** *Pathophysiology:* Pain arises from inflammation of structures, usually as the result of infection, and from distention of tubular structures or cysts, traction on serosal surfaces by masses or adhesions, hemorrhage, and invasion of sensitive structures by neoplasms or implantation of endometrial tissue. It is essential to obtain a complete history of the patient's pain pattern, its relationship to menses, ovulation, bowel movements, urination, and physical and sexual activity. The pelvic exam must be gentle and the patient relaxed for the examiner to localize the pain to a specific area or structure.

✓ *ADNEXAL TENDERNESS—CLINICAL OCCURRENCE:* *Congenital* imperforate hymen, porphyria; *Idiopathic* ovarian cysts, especially with hemorrhage or rupture, endometriosis, diverticulosis; *Inflammatory/Immune* inflammatory bowel disease, appendicitis; *Infectious* cervicitis, endometritis, salpingitis, tuboovarian abscess, cystitis, diverticulitis and diverticular abscess, appendicitis; *Mechanical/Traumatic* ovarian torsion, tubal pregnancy; *Neoplastic* any locally invasive cancer, for example, cervical, endometrial, rectal, bladder, metastatic, appendicitis; *Vascular* ovarian infarction (torsion), bleeding following ovulation (mittelschmerz).

KEY SIGN

► **Adnexal Mass: Pelvic Inflammatory Disease (Salpingitis, Hydrosalpinx, Pyosalpinx, Tuboovarian Abscess):** *Pathophysiology:* Infection ascends from the cervix via the endometrium. Sexually transmitted organisms (gonorrhea, chlamydia, mycoplasmas) initiate infection, but aerobic and anaerobic enteric florae are frequent secondary complications in the advanced stages of infection. With acute infections, the fallopian tubes are tender and swollen, which frequently obscures the separate structures in the adnexa. Movement of the uterus and cervix is extremely painful. In more chronic stages, the exudate and fibrosis around the tubes feel like an unyielding mass, termed a frozen pelvis. When adhesions or inflammation seal a tube at both ends it may become filled with fluid or pus, felt as a sausage-shaped mass, termed a *hydrosalpinx* and *pyosalpinx*, respectively. When the ovary and broad ligament become involved a tuboovarian abscess is formed. See also page 648, STDs.

KEY SIGN

► **Tubal Mass: Ectopic Pregnancy:** See page 643. Irregular vaginal bleeding and pelvic pain during childbearing years indicates ectopic pregnancy until proven otherwise. Thickening, or a mass, may or may not be appreciated in the adnexa. Softening of the cervix and fundus occurs with tubal pregnancy, as well as with intrauterine pregnancy. Movement of the uterus and cervix is painful. Occasionally, a bulging mass is felt in the rectovaginal pouch from a pelvic hematoma.

Ovarian Mass: Oophoritis: Although inflammation of an ovary causes it to enlarge, the change in size is usually not detected by palpation because the same inflammatory process involves the uterine tubes, so that the component structures in the mass cannot be recognized.

Ovarian Mass: Neoplasm: A variety of benign and malignant neoplasms may involve the ovaries which can be specifically diagnosed only by operation. The sensitivity of physical examination, even in experienced hands, is not good for detection of adnexal masses [Padilla LA, Radosevich DM, Milad MP. Accuracy of the pelvic examination in detecting adnexal masses. *Obstet Gynecol* 2000;96:593–598].

Ovarian Mass: Endometriosis: Enlargement of the ovaries is frequently encountered in endometriosis (page 648).

Ovarian Mass: Cyst: See *Female Genital and Reproductive Syndromes: Ovarian Cysts*, page 647. An often fluctuant, nontender spheroidal mass is felt in the region of the ovary. When the mass is relatively small, palpation is diagnostic. When the cyst enlarges such that it emerges from the pelvis and into the abdomen, no distinctive pelvic signs are present and the mass must be distinguished from other abdominal masses (see Chapter 9, page 544).

Rectal Signs

Healed Anal Laceration: *Pathophysiolgy:* This is usually the result of childbirth, but it may be evidence of sexual abuse. If the laceration extended through the anal canal it is evidenced by the appearance of the anus, whose edges are either not approximated or form an irregular line rather than a depression with puckered borders. Palpation reveals weakness of the sphincter. When the sphincter ani is severed, the condition is termed a third-degree laceration. Partial sphincter lacerations are common and may be palpable on rectal exam. See *Fecal Incontinence*, Chapter 9, page 536.

Female Genital and Reproductive Syndromes

Ectopic Pregnancy: *Pathophysiology:* Implantation of the fertilized ovum normally occurs in the endometrium. Implantation can occur in the fallopian tubes, ovary, or peritoneum. Presentation depends upon the site of implantation. Pain and bleeding are frequent. These pregnancies are not viable to term and must be aborted surgically or pharmacologically to protect the woman from life threatening hemorrhage [Dart RG, Kaplan B, Varaklis K. Predictive value of history and physical examination in patients with suspected ectopic pregnancy. *Ann Emerg Med* 1999;33:283–290].

▶ **Abdominal Pain and Pallor: Rupture and Hemorrhage from Tubal Pregnancy:** *Pathophysiology:* Failure of the fertized ovum to pass the fallopian tube with implantation in the tube results in tubal pregnancy. The gestational tissue stretches and finally ruptures the tubal wall, which has become very vascular, resulting in a sudden, large-volume hemorrhage into the peritoneal cavity. A previously healthy young woman presents with agonizing abdominal and pelvic pain that may be poorly localized. Sometimes the pain begins in the suprapubic or pelvic region, probably from serosal inflammation and premonatory small volume bleeding prior to frank rupture. The abdomen is quiet, increasingly tender, and rigidity develops progressively. The abdomen becomes distended and evidence of free fluid may appear. Signs of hemorrhagic shock quickly develop. Uterine bleeding or spotting is common. Because rupture of tubal pregnancy usually occurs in the first 8 weeks of gestation, menstrual irregularities may have been slight or unnoticed. With subacute hemorrhage, the symptoms are not so severe. The patient may be seen after the first episode has subsided, when hemorrhage has ceased. Blood in the pelvis gives a sense of fullness when palpating the fornices. A definite mass of clot or liquid blood may be present in the rectouterine pouch, where it can be identified by ultrasonography. *Urine pregnancy tests must be obtained in all women of childbearing age with abdominal pain.* Transvaginal ultrasonography is diagnostic. The severe attack must be distinguished from most other causes of acute abdominal pain. One must suspect ectopic pregnancy in any fertile woman with acute abdominal pain. Tubal pregnancy occurs most commonly as the result of previous pelvic inflammatory disease with tubal scarring or previous tubal surgery. Ectopic pregnancy in other locations (ovary, broad ligament, abdomen) can also present with pain and abdominal bleeding.

Abdominal Pain and Pallor: Follicular and Corpus Luteum Hemorrhage: *Pathophysiology:* Rupture of the ovarian surface to release the ovum into the fallopian tube can result in pain associated with minor bleeding from the follicle *(mittelschmerz).* Persistant bleeding, especially in women on anticoagulants, can occur. The corpus luteum matures over 7–10 days and rupture of a corpus luteum cyst usually occurs around the onset of menses. Minor bleeding may be symptomless, but, when heavy, the classic signs of intraabdominal hemorrhage result (see discussion of tubal pregnancy above). Sonography will show free fluid (blood) in the peritoneal cavity and may demonstrate the follicular or corpus luteum cyst.

Menstrual Disorders: *Normal Physiology:* Menstruation usually begins *(menarche)* between the ages of 12 and 15 years in temperate climates and at 9 or 10 years in the tropics. The anterior pituitary gland produces follicle-stimulating hormone (FSH) and luteinizing hormone (LH), in response to pulsitile hypothalamic secretion of gonadotropin-releasing hormone (GnRH). FSH causes the maturation of an ovarian graafian follicle by growth of its granulosa cells and the formation of follicular fluid. In combination with FSH, LH causes the theca interna to secrete estrogen. The mature follicle ruptures through the ovarian surface, releasing the ovum. It enters the fimbriated end of the fallopian tube passing down the tube, and if fertilized, implants in the endometrium. The ruptured ovarian follicle becomes the corpus luteum, whose cells secrete both estrogen and progesterone under the influence of LH and FSH. If the ovum is not fertilized, the corpus luteum gradually degenerates and scarifies. Ovulation occurs about 2 weeks before menstruation. During the time when estrogen is the primary secretion (follicular phase), the uterine endometrium undergoes proliferation. Later, when the secretion of progesterone predominates (luteal phase), the endometrium differentiates into secretory endometrium. With involution of the corpus luteum and decline in estrogen and progesterone, the endometrium degenerates and sloughs as menstrual blood. The menstrual cycle usually recurs in periods of 27–32 days, although great variability exists. The menstrual flow lasts about 5 days. During the entire menses, the average blood loss is from 60 to 250 mL, most during the first and second days. A menstrual pad is considered filled when it contains 30–50 mL of blood. The menopause may occur between the ages of 40 and 55 years. Menstrual disturbances may be caused by disorders of the anterior pituitary gland, the hypothalamus, the thyroid gland, the ovary, or the uterus.

It is first necessary to establish the woman's normal menstrual pattern starting at menarche, including the menstrual cycle length, the amount and duration of normal flow, and her history of conception, live births, abortions, stillbirths, and contraception. Determine the time of the last normal cycle and then seek specific information about the current problem. It is important to differentiate problems of cycle length (early or delayed menses), duration of flow (protracted or short), quantity of flow (too much or too little) and associated symptoms, for example, pain (dysmenorrhea). The terminology for these disorders can be confusing so use clear descriptions, avoiding Greek and Latin obscurations. Evaluation of menstrual abnormalities requires a thorough history, complete pelvic examination, and evaluation of the woman's hormonal status, frequently combined with imaging of the pelvis and/or endometrial sampling. Remember that pregnancy and menopause are the most common causes of menstrual disorder.

PROFUSE MENSTRUATION: MENORRHAGIA: Menorrhagia is the condition in which menstruation persists longer or the daily volume of flow is greater than normal. Excessive blood loss with menorrhagia is a common cause of iron-deficiency with or without anemia.

✓ *MENORRHAGIA—CLINICAL OCCURRENCE: Congenital* von Willebrand disease, hemophilia; *Endocrine* persistence of the corpus luteum, anovulation, perimenopause, hypothyroidism; *Idiopathic* endocervical and endometrial polyps, endometriosis; *Inflammatory/ Immune* systemic lupus erythematosus; *Infectious* endometritis, salpingitis; *Metabolic/Toxic* scurvy; *Neoplastic* uterine leiomyoma, endometrial hyperplasia or carcinoma, leukemia; *Vascular* coagulation defects (thrombocytopenia, von Willebrand disease, hemophilia).

INTERMENSTRUAL AND IRREGULAR BLEEDING: METRORRHAGIA: Irregular and intermenstrual bleeding suggests an abnormality of the endometrium. Although metrorrhagia is commonly synonymous with intermenstrual bleeding, it also refers to irregular bleeding. Some causes of heavy bleeding, in more severe form, produce irrregular bleeding as well. The most common causes are endometritis, uterine leiomyoma, endometrial polyp, cervical polyps, cervical and endometrial cancer, pregnancy, ectopic pregnancy, threatened abortion, and retained products of conception.

ABSENT MENSTRUATION: PRIMARY AMENORRHEA: *Pathophysiology:* Primary amenorrhea is failure to initiate regular menstrual cycles at a chronologically appropriate age. It results from genetic, endocrinologic, or anatomic abnormalities of sex chromatin, sexual differentiation, and/or sexual maturation. Severe psychologic stress can result in amenorrhea in otherwise normal individuals. The examination should focus upon the correlation of sexual and somatic maturation with chronological age and, if necessary, bone age. Obtain growth records from birth to identify long-standing growth problems. Estimate the stage of secondary sexual development by using the Tanner system of classification. In addition to confirming normal external genitalia by physical exam, imaging studies may be needed to confirm the presence of a normal vagina, uterus, and ovaries.

✓ *PRIMARY AMENORRHEA—CLINICAL OCCURRENCE:* *Congenital* delayed puberty, uterine agenesis, imperforate hymen (cryptomenorrhea), ovarian agenesis or dysgenesis (Turner syndrome), and other disorders of sex chromosomes; *Endocrine* hypo- and hyperthyroidism, hypopituitarism, androgens; *Metabolic/Toxic* lead, mercury, morphine, alcohol, malnutrition, chemotherapy, excessive exercise, obesity, debilitating diseases; *Mechanical/Traumatic* hysterectomy, oophorectomy, pelvic irradiation; *Neoplastic* androgen-producing tumors, prolactinoma, craniopharyngioma; *Psychosocial* anorexia nervosa, depression.

GONADAL DYSGENESIS: TURNER SYNDROME, OVARIAN AGENESIS: *Pathophysiology:* There is an inherited deficiency of one X chromosome. The karyotype is XO with no Y and a diploid number of 45 in 80% of cases. Only congenitally fibrotic ovarian anlagen is associated with negative (male pattern) sex chromatin of buccal mucosal cells and neutrophils. There is short stature, webbed neck, a shield-like chest, cubitus valgus, short metacarpals, lymphedema, and infantile female genitalia and breasts. Sexual maturation is delayed with primary amenorrhea and delayed growth of axillary and pubic hair.

ABSENT MENSTRUATION: SECONDARY AMENORRHEA: *Pathophysiology:* Secondary amenorrhea is the cessation of menstrual cycles after previous menstrual bleeding. It results from endocrinologic or anatomic abnormalities. Severe psychologic stress can result in amenorrhea in genetically, endocrinologically, and anatomically normal individuals.

Evaluation of secondary amenorrhea requires a detailed personal medical, psychologic and menstrual history, a family history, and physical examination wth attention to signs of endocrine disease. Secondary amenorrhea is expected in midlife, associated with ovarian aging (menopause). Pregnancy is the most common cause of secondary amenorrhea in women of childbearing age.

✓ *SECONDARY AMENORRHEA—CLINICAL OCCURRENCE:* *Congenital* polycystic ovary syndrome, adrenal hyperplasia; *Endocrine* pregnancy, menopause, hyper- and hypothyroidism, hypopituitarism (Sheehan syndrome, after irradiation or surgery, primary), primary ovarian failure, hormonal contraceptives (oral, injectable, and implanted), elevated prolactin (normal lactation, prolactinoma), diabetes mellitus; *Inflammatory/Immune* systemic lupus erythematosus, vasculitis; *Infectious* HIV, tuberculosis; *Metabolic/Toxic* lead, mercury, morphine, alcohol, malnutrition, chemotherapy, excessive exercise, obesity, debilitating diseases; *Mechanical/Traumatic* hysterectomy, oophorectomy, pelvic irradiation, after uterine curettage; *Neoplastic* androgen-producing tumors, prolactinoma; *Psychosocial* anorexia nervosa, depression.

POLYCYSTIC OVARY SYNDROME: *Pathophysiology:* Increased production of androgenic steroids by the ovary, or, less commonly, the adrenal, is associated with insulin resistance and impaired fertility because of anovulation. Genetic factors are important, although the genes and mode of inheritance are unknown. Patients may present in adolescence or more commonly the third or fourth decade of life with oligomenorrhea, amenorrhea, infertility, obesity, and excessive hair growth. About half the women with the metabolic abnormality have polycystic ovaries. There is an increased risk for diabetes [Franks S. Polycystic ovary syndrome. *N Engl J Med* 1995;333:853–861].

S KEY SYNDROME
▼ **Ovarian Cysts:** See also *Female Reproductive Tract Signs: Ovarian Cysts*, page 643. *Pathophysiology:* Cystic change in the ovary can result from the follicles, the corpus luteum, the stroma, and the ovarian epithelium. Cysts can be degenerative or neoplastic (benign and malignant) or teratomas. Specific diagnosis can only be made pathologically.

S KEY SYNDROME
▼ **Ovarian Cancer:** *Pathophysiology:* Malignant tumors arise predominantly from the epithelium, although germ cell and stromal tumors are not rare. BRCA-1 and BRCA-2 genotypes increase the risk for ovarian cancer. Screening for ovarian cancer is not currently effective and the disease often presents after generalized peritoneal spread as ascites.

S KEY SYNDROME
▶ ▼ **Endometrial Cancer:** *Pathophysiology:* It is more common in women with increased levels of estrogen in the absence of progesterone-induced cycling. This is a disease predominately of post-

menopausal women who present with vaginal spotting or bleeding. Diagnosis is by endometrial biopsy. Obesity, unopposed estrogen therapy, a positive family history, and atypical endometrial hyperplasia are risk factors.

Vaginal Cancer: This is a rare disease. Clear-cell vaginal cancer was associated with the exposure of female fetuses to maternal diethylstilbestrol (DES), given in an attempt to prevent spontaneous abortion.

S KEY SYNDROME
▶ **Sexually Transmitted Diseases (STDs):** STDs can present locally as ulcers or inflammation, systemically, or be asymptomatic. All sexually active women, especially those with new or multiple partners, should be screened for STDs. The presence of one STD increases the risk of acquiring or transmitting others. Barrier contraceptives (condoms) are somewhat effective at decreasing the risk of acquiring an STD. All persons with an STD must be screened for other treatable STDs, including HIV and syphilis, which are often acquired asymptomatically. Extension of infection to the tubes, ovaries and broad ligament results in pelvic inflammatory disease (see page 642), a frequent cause of female infertility. In addition, several infectious diseases, not usually defined as STDs, can be acquired sexually, for example, hepatitis B.

S KEY SYNDROME
▼ **Infertility:** *Pathophysiology:* The capacity to become pregnant with a viable fetus requires the coordinated functioning of complex physiologic systems in an anatomically normal woman. Failure of any component of this system can result in infertility. Initial examination should focus on an assessment of general health and nutrition, the menstrual history, and a physical exam to confirm normal sexual development and anatomy. Evaluation of the sexual partner is also required. The etiology and evaluation of infertility is a complex subject. See specialized texts for further information.

S KEY SYNDROME
▼ **Endometriosis:** *Pathophysiology:* Normal-appearing endometrial tissue forms implants in ectopic sites including the ovaries, posterior surface of uterus, sigmoid colon, uterosacral ligaments, and, less often, distant sites such as pleura. Cyclical bleeding is associated with pain and the development of adhesions. The cause is unknown. Patients present with dysmenorrhea and abdominal or pelvic pain that is often cyclical. Tender nodular masses surrounded with fibrosis may be felt. Frequently, the ovaries are enlarged. The uterus may be fixed or painful with movement. Infertility is common and diagnosis usually requires laparoscopy.

12 Male Genitalia and Reproductive Tract

Overview of Male Reproductive Physiology

Male and female external genitalia arise from identical embryologic anlage depending on the presence or absence of testosterone. Lack of the SRY gene (typically found on the Y chromosome) leads to development of ovaries, with subsequent maturation of female sex organs. Conversely, the presence of this gene leads to testicular development, with masculinization of the reproductive tract. The scrotum is a cognate of the labia majora and the penis and clitoris are similarly derived. Ambiguous genitalia occur when development and maturation occurs with a mixed hormonal environment or genetic substrate.

The male reproductive organs are the testes, epididymis, vas deferens, seminal vesicles, prostate, and penis. The testes arise intraabdominally and descend through the inguinal canal into the scrotum, usually by birth. The scrotal location is more conducive to spermatogenesis being slightly cooler than body temperature. Leydig cells in the testes produce testosterone under the control of luteinizing hormone production by the pituitary gland and spermatogenesis takes place in the seminiferous tubules under the control of follicle-stimulating hormone (FSH) and local paracrine testosterone production. Sperm are collected in the epididymis and travel up the vas deferens in the spermatic cord, which includes the testicular artery and vein and the lymphatics, to reach the prostate and seminal vesicles. Ejaculate contains sperm, prostatic, and seminal vesicle secretions.

Anatomy of the Male Reproductive System

At puberty, the pubes becomes covered with hair that extends onto the skin of the abdomen to form the *male escutcheon*, which describes an upright triangle with the apex near the umbilicus.

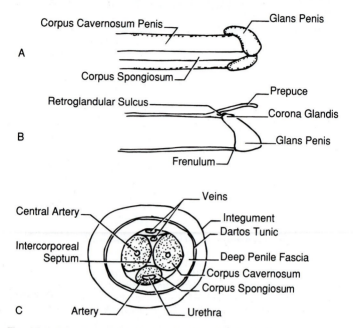

Fig. 12-1 Structure of the Penis.   A. The Shaft in its Ventrolateral Aspect, with Integument Removed. B. A Sagittal Section of the Shaft with Integument Included. C. A Cross-section of the Shaft.

The Penis

The shaft of the penis is formed by three columns of erectile tissue, the two dorsolateral *corpora cavernosa* and the ventral smaller *corpus spongiosum* containing the urethra (Fig. 12-1). Fibrous tissue binds the three columns into a cylinder. The end of the shaft is an obtuse cone of erectile tissue, the *glans penis,* containing the urethral meatus. The glans has a corona at its junction with the shaft. A flap of skin, the *prepuce* or foreskin, covers the glans. The *frenulum* is a fold of the prepuce that extends ventrally into the ventral notch in the glans. Penile erection and ejaculation are complex physiologic and hemodynamic processes that can be disrupted by vascular disease, drugs, injury to nerves, endocrine abnormalities, and anxiety. The male reproductive system is designed to produce and store sperm cells, which can be deposited at the entrance to the female cervix with forceful ejaculation of the sperm and spermatic fluids via the erect, penetrating penis. Successful reproduction is dependent upon the coordinated functioning of this system.

The Scrotum

This pouch is formed by a layer of thin, rugous skin overlying the tightly adherent dartos tunic consisting of muscle and fascia (Fig. 12-2C). The sac hangs from the root of the penis. The scrotal skin is bisected by a

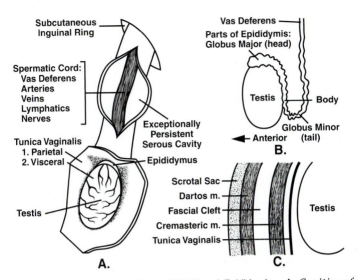

Fig. 12-2 Anatomy of the Scrotal Wall and Epididymis. A. Cavities of the Tunica Vaginalis Are Opened Anteriorly to Show Testis and Cord. B. Parts of the Epididymis and Cord. C. Layers of the Scrotum.

median raphe. Internally, the two halves of the pouch are separated by a septal fold of dartos tunic. Each half contains a testis with its epididymis and spermatic cord. The scrotal contents slide easily in a fascial cleft between the scrotal wall and the covering of the testis and cords. The skin of the scrotum is deeply pigmented and contains large, sebaceous follicles that have a tendency to form cysts. The dartos muscle tone determines scrotal size, with exposure to cold shrinking the sac and heat enlarging the pouch. In advanced age, the dartos muscle becomes relatively atonic. The action of the dartos muscles is independent of contractions of the cremasteric muscles that elevate the testes. The arterial, venous and lymphatic drainage of the scrotal contents arises intraabdominally and reaches its scrotal location via the inguinal canal and spermatic cord. Lymphatics from the scrotal contents drain to the pelvic lymph nodes. The scrotal vascular and lymphatic supply is in continuity with the perineum and its lymphatics drain to the inguinal lymph nodes.

Testis, Epididymis, Vas Deferens, and Spermatic Cord

Toward the end of fetal development, the testis begins its descent from the abdomen to the scrotum. The peritoneum covering the testis becomes the processus vaginalis, and the gubernaculum leads the testis into its scrotal position. Normally, the spermatic cord portion of the peritoneal pouch is obliterated, leaving a cavity surrounding the testis and epididymis, except for their posterior aspect (see Fig. 12-2A). This serous membrane is the *tunica vaginalis.* Abnormal persistence of this peritoneal connection leads to congenital hernias or funicular hydroceles. The *testis*

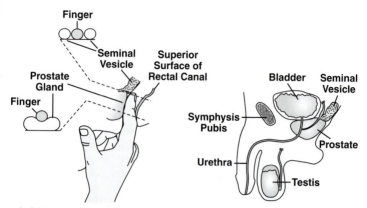

A. Digital Examination of Prostate   **B. Sagittal Section of Male Pelvis**

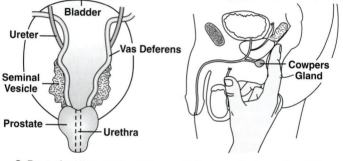

C. Posterior View of Prostate   **D. Cowper Bulbourethral Gland**

Fig. 12-3 Rectal Examination of the Male Genitalia. A. Relationship of the Examining Finger to the Prostate and Seminal Vesicles: The lower section shows the finger at the prostate gland; the higher section shows the finger between the two seminal vesicles. B. A Sagittal Section of the Male Penis and Pelvic Organs. C. A Posterior View of the Prostate, Seminal Vesicles, and Vasa Deferentia. D. Palpation of the Cowper Bulbourethral Gland: There is one gland on each side of the urethra. The diagram shows a sagittal section of the male pelvis. The tip of the index finger is in the rectum with the pad facing the anterior rectal wall, between the inferior border of the prostate and the inner edge of the anal canal. The thumb is outside the rectum, pressing the perineum on the medial raphe toward the fingertip. A normal gland is not palpable, but an inflamed gland is tender. If it contains pus, it forms a palpable mass, from pea to hazelnut size (the round black spot).

is a smooth, solid ovoid, compressed laterally, and roughly 4 cm × 2 cm. The spermatic cord suspends the testis in the scrotum with the long axis nearly vertical. The head of the *epididymis* caps the upper pole of the testis. The body of the epididymis forms an elongated inverted cone attached vertically to the posterior surface of the testis. The apex of the cone, or tail of the epididymis, approaches the lower pole of the testis (see Fig. 12-2B). The epididymis is continuous with the *vas deferens*, which joins other vessels to form the spermatic cord. The *spermatic cord* consists of the vas deferens, arteries, veins, nerves, and lymphatic vessels, all held together by the spermatic fascia. From the testis, the cord extends upward, entering the external inguinal ring and coursing through the inguinal canal to the internal inguinal ring, where its components diverge. In the abdominal cavity, the vas deferens continues backward and downward behind the peritoneum until it lies behind the bladder and anterior to the rectum, joining the duct of the seminal vesicle to become the ejaculatory duct.

The Prostate and Seminal Vesicles

The prostate contains glands dispersed in a stroma of smooth muscle and fibrous tissue. It is shaped roughly like a truncated cone the size of a chestnut and is prone to hyperplasia with age. It lies in the pelvis approximately 2 cm posterior to the symphysis pubis; the cone is inverted so the base is superior and the apex inferior (Fig. 12-3B and C). The anterior and posterior surfaces are somewhat flattened. The basal surface is directed superiorly and is overlaid by the bladder; the apical surface faces inferiorly and rests on the urogenital diaphragm. The prostatic urethra pierces the basal or superior surface, slightly anterior to the center, and runs inferiorly in a vertical axis to emerge through the apical or inferior surface. The only palpable portion of the prostate is the slightly vertically convex posterior prostatic surface, which is in close contact with the rectal wall. A shallow median furrow divides all except the upper portion of the posterior surface into a right and left lobe. Near the superior edge of the posterior surface is a transverse depression made by the ejaculatory ducts which enter the prostate and converge to enter the urethra. The paired ampullae of the vas deferens and the seminal vesicles diverge superiorly from the prostate base. The ampulla of the vas is superior and medial to the seminal vesicles and both contact the posterior wall of the bladder. The bulbourethral glands of Cowper lie on each side of the midline just inferior to the caudal border of the prostate.

Physical Examination of the Male Genitalia and Reproductive System

Inspection and palpation reveal many disorders of the external and internal male reproductive organs and the lower urinary tract. Familiarity with the genital disorders demonstrated by inspection and palpation is necessary for any physician performing a physical examination.

Examination of the Penis

Wearing gloves, view the penis in its usual state, then have the patient retract the prepuce revealing the size of the foreskin orifice and the glans. Observe any superficial lesions of the corona or retroglandular sulcus. Palpate lesions for induration and tenderness. Palpate the length of the shaft, ventrally along the corpus spongiosum, and laterally over both corpora cavernosa, feeling for nodules and plaques. Compress the glans anteroposteriorly between the thumb and forefinger to open and inspect the meatus and terminal urethra. If urethral symptoms are present, strip the ventral penis from its base to the glans to collect a drop of urethral discharge for microscopic examination.

Examination of the Scrotum

The scrotum is examined by inspection and palpation. Because rugae are produced by contractions of dartos muscle, the walls should be inspected by spreading the layers between gloved fingers. Transillumination is readily performed, but it is most informative for examining the scrotal contents.

Examination of Scrotal Contents

Palpation and transillumination identify most structures within the scrotal sac. Examine the scrotum systematically in the following sequence: (a) testes, (b) tunica vaginalis, (c) epididymis (head, body, and tail), (d) spermatic cord, and (e) inguinal lymph nodes. The complete sequence should be followed in every routine physical examination. If the scrotum is swollen, first exclude an inguinal hernia descending into the scrotum, then examine for the structures normally in the scrotum.

Examination for Scrotal Hernia

Palpate the root of the scrotum to determine if the mass extends that high. If the fingers can get above the mass, a hernia is excluded. Insert a finger into the external inguinal ring and feel for a cough impulse from hernia. Inguinal hernias always descend in front of the spermatic cord and testes, so identify these structures and their anatomic relations to the mass. A swollen scrotum should be transilluminated by using a cool light source in a darkened room. With the thumb and forefinger, pull the scrotal wall tightly over the mass. Place the light in contact with the posterior wall of the scrotum, shining the light anteriorly through the mass to determine whether the structure is translucent or opaque. Most hernia contents are opaque, although occasionally a gas-filled loop of gut will transmit light. Listen with a stethoscope for peristaltic sounds.

Examination of the Testes

Examine the testes simultaneously by grasping one with each gloved hand, using thumb and forefinger. Determine their size, shape, consistency, and sensitivity to light pressure. Transilluminate each, even if they feel normal; one may be atrophied and the normal size attained by a hydrocele. Use scrotal ultrasonography to help distinguish between intra- and extratesticular masses or lesions [Junnila J, Lassen P. Testicular masses. *Am Fam Physician* 1998;59:685–692].

Examination of the Epididymis

Locate each epididymis by palpating the smooth testis to find a vertical ridge of soft nodular tissue beginning at the upper pole and extending to the lower pole. Usually the epididymis is behind the testis, but in approximately 7% of males, the structure develops anterior to the testis, anteversion of the epididymis. Recognizing the anteversion, the examiner will expect the cavity of the tunica vaginalis to be posterior to the testis. Compare the findings from palpation in both epididymides, in their component segments of head, body, and tail.

Examination of the Spermatic Cord

Palpation of varicoceles is best done in the upright position, while it is easiest to examine the scrotal contents in the supine position. Compare the spermatic cords by simultaneously grasping each at the neck of the scrotum. With the thumb in front and the forefinger behind the scrotum, gently compress the cord (Fig. 12-4). The normal vas deferens is felt as a distinct hard cord, which can be separated from other cord structures. The other, less-definable strands are nerves, arteries, and fibers of cremasteric muscle. The vas may be congenitally absent. Trace the cords down to the testes.

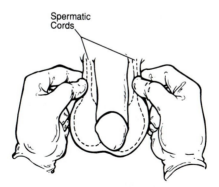

Spermatic Cords

Fig. 12-4 Palpation of the Spermatic Cords. *Each gloved hand simultaneously grasps a cord between thumb and index finger, comparing the two structures. Normally, the vasa deferentia feel like distinct whipcords. The other components of the cord, arteries, veins, vessels, and nerves, feel like indefinite strands.*

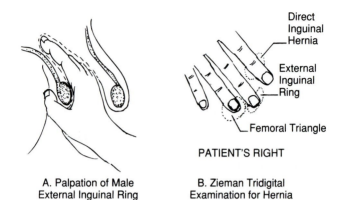

A. Palpation of Male
External Inguinal Ring

B. Zieman Tridigital
Examination for Hernia

Fig. 12-5 Examination of the Inguinal Regions for Hernia. A. Palpation of the Inguinal Ring in the Male. B. Zieman Tridigital Examination for Hernia: The left side of the patient is examined from his left and with the examiner's left hand.

Examination of the Inguinal Regions for Hernia

The tip of the index finger is placed at the most dependent part of the scrotum and directed into the subcutaneous inguinal ring by invaginating the slack scrotum with it (see Fig. 12-5A). The patient coughs or strains so an impulse from the hernial sac may be felt on the fingertip.

ZIEMAN INGUINAL EXAMINATION.   This procedure reveals direct and indirect inguinal hernias, and hernias of the femoral triangle. With the patient standing, stand at the patient's right side and place the palm of your right hand against the right lower abdomen. Spread your fingers slightly so your long finger lies along the inguinal ligament with its pulp in the external inguinal ring, your index finger is over the internal inguinal ring, and your ring finger palpates the region of the femoral canal and the opening of the saphenous vein (see Fig. 12-5B). Have the patient take a deep breath, hold it, and bear down, as if to have a bowel movement. Then repeat the maneuver, standing at the patient's left side and palpating his left groin with your left hand. A hernia in any of the three sites is perceived either as a gliding motion of the walls of the empty sac or as a protrusion of a viscus into the sac. When the internal ring is closed by the palpating finger, any herniating mass cannot be an indirect inguinal hernia.

PALPATION OF PROSTATE AND SEMINAL VESICLES   Place the patient in the lithotomy position, the knee–chest position, the left-lateral-prone position (Sims), or bent-over-the-table position. Three of these have been considered elsewhere (see Fig. 9-16, page 526). In the bent-over-the table position, the patient stands with legs apart, the trunk flexed on the thighs, and the elbows resting on the knees or the examining table. Whatever the position, the details of the procedure are the same. Cover the examining hand with a rubber glove and generously lubricate the forefinger. Place the pad or pulp of the forefinger on the anal orifice with light pressure while the patient bears down gently until the sphincter relaxes, admitting the curve of the pad. Then incline the finger until the tip is also inserted. Gradually ease the tip past the anal canal and into the rectal ampulla. Keep the pad of the finger facing the anterior rectal wall.

As the finger moves cephalad from the anal canal, it encounters the elastic bulging surface of the *prostate* (see Fig. 12-3A). Feel the median furrow that separates the lateral lobes. When the fingertip reaches the superior edge of the prostate, the median furrow thins out to the flat middle lobe. Superior to the prostate, the fingertip reaches the seminal vesicles on either side of the midline. Determine whether the prostatic surface is smooth or nodular; whether the consistency is elastic, hard, boggy, soft, or fluctuant; whether the shape is rounded or flat; whether the size is normal, enlarged, or atrophied; whether sensitivity to pressure is abnormal; whether there is normal mobility or fixation.

Normally, the *seminal vesicles* are not palpable because they are too soft; only diseased structures can be felt. The seminal vesicles are approximately 7.5 cm long, so only their lower portions can be reached. Examine each seminal vesicle for distention, sensitivity, size, consistency, induration, and nodules. Palpate in the region of the bulbourethral glands, they are normally not palpable. When enlarged, they are felt as rounded masses in the anterior rectal wall.

On completion of the exam, either clean the patient or provide tissue to the patient for this purpose.

Male Genital and Reproductive Symptoms

KEY SYMPTOM

Scrotal Pruritus: *Pathophysiology:* Scrotal skin is thin, rugated, and susceptible to irritation and infection because it is usually warm and often moist. Pruritus often indicates inflammatory or infectious dermatitis, but sometimes exists and persists without skin changes or evident cause.

KEY SYMPTOM

Pain in the Testis and Epididymis: *Pathophysiology:* Innervation of the testis and epididymis is somatic and sympathetic arising in the lower thoracic roots. Pain arising from these structures frequently radiates to the epigastrium and/or hypogastrium. If the scrotal wall or tunica vaginalis is involved, the pain is well localized. Pain arising in the testis may be mild or excruciating and is frequently accompanied by nausea. Look for a relationship to activities, sexual activities, and signs of systemic or sexually transmitted disease. A complete sexual history is essential.

✓ *TESTICULAR PAIN—CLINICAL OCCURRENCE:* *Congenital* very large hydrocele; *Idiopathic* inguinal hernia, large varicocele; *Infectious* acute orchitis (mumps, echovirus, lymphocytic choriomeningitis virus, arbovirus group B), chronic orchitis (leprosy, tuberculosis), acute epididymitis (gonorrhea, chlamydia, *Escherichia coli*, mycoplasma), and chronic epididymitis (leprosy, tuberculosis, syphilis, brucellosis); *Mechanical/Traumatic* blunt and penetrating trauma, testicular rupture, torsion, ureteral stone; *Neoplastic* testicular carcinoma, leukemia; *Neurologic* neuropathy; *Vascular* testicular infarction and hemorrhage.

KEY SYMPTOM

Penile Curvature: See *Male Genitourinary Signs: Plastic Induration of the Penis*, page 663.

KEY SYMPTOM

Erectile Dysfunction and Impotence: See *Syndromes: Erectile Dysfunction and Impotence,* page 673. Many patients do not volunteer information about their inability to sustain an erection of sufficient rigidity or duration satisfactory for intercourse, although they may acknowledge the problem on a questionnaire. Commonly, however, this problem will not be identified unless you ask specifically about sexual performance. Awakening with early morning erections argues against neurologic, vascular, or endocrinologic causes, and suggests a functional problem.

Male Genital and Reproductive System Signs

Penis Signs

Ambiguous Genitalia: Intersexuality: See page 632.

KEY SIGN

Condyloma Acuminatum (Venereal Wart, Papilloma): *Pathophysiology:* Infection with human papillomavirus (HPV) produces the lesion. The condyloma is a villous projection (acuminata means pointed) that may be single or conglomerate (Fig. 12-6E). It can occur on the corona, in the retroglandular sulcus, and on the shaft, and frequently it is found about the anus. In the presence of moisture, secondary infection produces ulceration. In its uncomplicated form, the verrucous appearance is quite distinctive. An exuberant growth with much ulceration must be distinguished from carcinoma by biopsy.

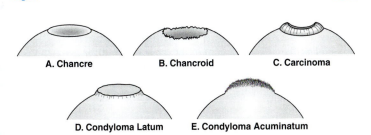

Fig. 12-6 Penile Lesions. **A. Chancre**: *The border is smooth; there is no necrosis or suppuration. Induration surrounds the lesion so it can be picked up like a disk.* **B. Chancroid**: *The border is irregular without induration and the center is necrotic. There is profuse suppuration.* **C. Ulcerating Carcinoma**: *The necrotic ulcer may resemble chancroid, but soon the process is surrounded by induration and nodulation.* **D. Condyloma Latum**: *This is the flat, nonsuppurating nodule of secondary syphilis.* **E. Condyloma Acuminatum**: *The lesions are moist, villous growths that protrude above the skin and undergo secondary ulceration.*

KEY SIGN
Condyloma Latum: As the name implies, the growth is flat and warty (see Fig. 12-6D). It may occur about the genitalia or anus. It is a secondary syphilid. The flat appearance is diagnostic. When the lesion has an exuberant growth, it must be distinguished from the acuminate condyloma and carcinoma.

KEY SIGN
Urethral Discharge: See *Urinary System Signs: Urethral Discharge*, page 616, and Male Genital and Reproductive Syndromes: Urethritis, page 672.

Penis: Hyperplasia: This is usually evident only before the age of normal puberty, when a discrepancy between size of the organ and age is evident. The causes of hyperplasia are tumors of the pineal gland or hypothalamus, tumors arising from the Leydig cells of the testis, or tumors of the adrenal gland.

Penis: Hypoplasia: Wide variation occurs in the normal size of the penis. The normal range is learned only by the examination of many individuals. Striking discrepancies between the penile size and the age of the patient lead to the inference of hypoplasia. Penile hypoplasia is either a manifestation of eunuchoidism occurring before puberty or is a feature of intersexuality. In the latter condition, distinction between a hypoplastic penis with hypospadias and a hyperplastic clitoris may be difficult or impossible without histologic examination of the gonads.

Generalized Penile Swelling: Edema: *Pathophysiology:* Fluid accumulates in the loose tissue of the penis in generalized edematous states from any cause and with obstruction of the penile veins or lymphatics. The penis, and usually scrotum, are diffusely swollen without erythema, warmth, or tenderness.

Generalized Penile Swelling: Contusion: Especially during erection, trauma to the penis may cause extravasation of blood that is usually painless. In a few days, the skin of the penis and scrotum may be stained blue from degraded hemoglobin.

Generalized Penile Swelling: Fracture of the Shaft: *Pathophysiology:* Trauma during erection may rupture one or both corpora cavernosa penis. Severe pain occurs at the time of injury, with immediate subsidence of the erection and temporary relief of pain. Subsequent engorgement from extravasation of blood produces recurrence of pain. This is a urologic emergency. Rupture may not be distinguishable from contusion unless an operation is performed.

Genital Ulcer: *Pathophysiology:* Ulceration of the penile shaft, glans, or foreskin occurs at the site of trauma or inoculation of sexually transmitted infectious organisms. The character of the ulcer is useful diagnostically (see Fig. 12-6). Inspect the base and edges, looking for vesicles preceding ulceration, noting especially the presence of pain, which may have antedated the visible lesion in herpes simplex. Palpate for induration of the surrounding tissue and base of the ulcer, and carefully feel for regional lymphadenopathy. Because these are usually sexually transmitted diseases, serologic evaluation for syphilis and HIV are indicated, as are counseling on safe sexual practices and use of condoms.

✓ *GENITAL ULCER—CLINICAL OCCURRENCE:* Inflammatory/Immune Behçet syndrome; *Infectious* herpes simplex, syphilis, chancroid, lymphogranuloma venereum; *Mechanical/Traumatic* traumatic sex, tight-fitting clothing; *Neoplastic* penile cancer.

GENITAL ULCER: SYPHILITIC CHANCRE (HARD CHANCRE): This is the primary lesion of syphilis, the first manifestation of disease. It commonly occurs on the glans or the inner leaves of the foreskin but is occasionally on the shaft or scrotum. Rarely, it is extragenital, usually on the lips. The chancre begins as a silvery papule that gradually erodes to form a superficial ulcer with a serous discharge containing *Treponema pallidum* (see Fig. 12-6A). Because the organisms penetrate the unbroken skin, the examiner must always wear gloves. Early in the evolution, the regional superficial inguinal lymph nodes undergo painless moderate enlargement. The chancre is painless, usually single, round or oval, with a smooth, slightly raised border. The underlying induration permits the superficial lesion to be lifted as a small disk between the thumb and forefinger. Neither the ulcer nor the lymph nodes suppurate. Physical signs are not conclusive and because the lesion appears before serologic tests for syphilis become positive, the diagnosis must be confirmed by demonstrating the *T. pallidum* in the serous exudate with the dark-field microscope.

GENITAL ULCER: CHANCROID (SOFT CHANCRE): A suppurative infection caused by the bacillus *Haemophilus ducreyi,* it usually involves the genitalia, although it may be extragenital. The lesion begins as a small red papule that quickly becomes pustular and enlarges to form a punched-out ulcer with undetermined edges (see Fig. 12-6B). The base is covered with a gray slough, discharging pus profusely. Extensive necrosis ensues and multiple ulcers form. The lesions are quite painful. In one-third of the cases, the regional lymph nodes become swollen and tender (the bubo). These frequently suppurate. While the clinical appearance is quite typical, mixed infections must be excluded by examination of the exudate with the dark-field microscope for *Treponema pallidum.*

GENITAL ULCER: LYMPHOGRANULOMA VENEREUM (LYMPHOGRANULOMA INGUINALE, LGV): *Pathophysiology:* LGV is caused by *Chlamydia trachomatis,* a rickettsia-like organism, and primarily involves the lymphatic system. The painless and evanescent initial lesion, an erosion less than 1 mm in diameter, is frequently overlooked. Occasionally, the penile lesion becomes vesicular, papular, or nodular. One or 2 weeks after infection, the inguinal lymph nodes become swollen and tender, matting together with areas of softening and reddening of the overlying skin. Multiple small fistulas form, discharging creamy pus or serosanguineous exudate. Healing with much fibrosis occurs over many months. A cicatrizing proctitis may be a late complication. The late clinical appearance is fairly distinctive. In the early stages, syphilis, chancroid, and herpes simplex need to be excluded. Diagnosis is confirmed by culture and polymerase chain reaction (PCR).

GENITAL ULCER: HERPES SIMPLEX: A small group of vesicles surrounded by erythema frequently occurs on the glans or prepuce. The vesicles rupture, producing painful superficial ulcers that heal in 5 to 7 days. The ulcers may serve as portals of entry for other organisms. The grouped vesicles or ulcers are fairly characteristic. Recurrent relapsing painful vesiculation and ulceration is characteristic.

GENITAL ULCERATION: BEHÇET SYNDROME: Painful aphthous ulcers with yellowish necrotic bases occur singly or in crops lasting 1 to 2 weeks, and resemble those seen in the oral mucosa.

KEY SIGN

Prepuce: Phimosis: The orifice of the prepuce is too small for the foreskin to be retracted from the glans (Fig. 12-7A). The congenital form results from malformation; the acquired type may be caused by preputial adhesions to the glans as the result of infection. The lips of the prepuce are pallid, striated, and thickened. The narrow orifice may actually obstruct urination. Retained smegma and dirt lead to inflammation and even calculus formation. Circumcision is curative.

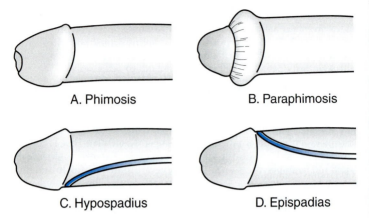

A. Phimosis   B. Paraphimosis

C. Hypospadius   D. Epispadias

Fig. 12-7 Structural Abnormalities of the Prepuce (Foreskin). A. Phimosis: The preputial orifice is too tight to permit retraction of the foreskin over the glans penis. B. Paraphimosis: A prepuce with small orifice has been retracted over the glans and the lips have impinged on the retroglandular sulcus, preventing return to the normal position. Edema occurs in the prepuce, the skin of the shaft, and the glans. C. Hypospadias: This is a developmental anomaly in which the urethral meatus opens on the underside of the shaft. D. Epispadias: A developmental anomaly in which the urethral meatus is on the dorsal side of the penis.

KEY SIGN

Prepuce: Paraphimosis: A tight foreskin, once retracted, may become edematous, so that it cannot resume its normal position over the glans (see Fig. 12-7B). The edema impedes the venous drainage of the glans causing swelling. Manual replacement of the prepuce may be attempted. Surgical incision may be necessary.

KEY SIGN

Glans: Carcinoma of the Penis: This lesion occurs in areas of irritation or inflammation of the foreskin or glans. Commonly, the primary lesion involves the dorsal corona or the inner lip of the foreskin. A warty growth develops, ulcerates, and discharges watery pus. Parts of the tumor undergo necrosis and slough (see Fig. 12-6C). Metastasis occurs, most often to the inguinal lymph nodes. Often the clinical appearance is not sufficiently typical to distinguish this from condyloma, so a biopsy is necessary.

KEY SIGN

Glans: Erosive Balanitis: The skin of the glans undergoes desquamation and erosion; small ulcers form and become confluent, involving the entire glans. Rarely, this results in gangrene. The identity of the infective organism is unknown.

Dorsal Shaft: Thrombosis of the Dorsal Vein:
A thrombus in the dorsal vein of the penis causes a palpable cord, approximately 1 mm in diameter, in the midline dorsally. This condition is usually secondary to inflammation of the glans.

Dorsal Shaft: Varicose Veins: Varicosities of the dorsal veins of the penis may be visible and palpable. They may be sufficiently large to require surgical treatment.

Lateral Shaft: Cavernositis: An irregular hard mass may occur in the lateral or ventral cavernous corpora from inflammation. Priapism and edema usually accompany this condition. Suppuration may occur, with drainage through the skin or the urethra.

KEY SIGN
Lateral Shaft: Plastic Induration of the Penis (Peyronie Disease): *Pathophysiology:* This is a chronic disease of unknown cause, characterized by irregular fibrosis of the septum or sheath of the corpus cavernosum penis, extending into the tunica albuginea. It never affects the corpus spongiosom. It is considered a component of Dupuytren diathesis along with palmar and solar fibrosis. Firm, nontender plaques may be felt laterally in the corpora cavernosa penis or dorsally over the intercorporeal septum. The plaques may be single or multiple; they are not necessarily symmetrical. The patient may complain of curvature of the penis during erection. The findings may resemble those in gumma, scars from trauma, cavernositis, subcutaneous gouty tophi, fibromas, chondromas, and carcinoma.

KEY SIGN
Priapism: *Pathophysiology:*   Erection is sustained by reflex or central nerve stimulation, or by local mechanical causes, such as thrombosis, hemorrhage, neoplasm, injection of vasoactive agents, and inflammation in the penis. Prolonged, persistent, penile erection occurs without sexual desire. The condition is usually painful. It may complicate leukemia and sickle cell anemia. Urgent surgical manipulation is usually required.

Urethral Signs

KEY SIGN
Meatus: Stricture: Narrowing of the urethral meatus may be observed with anteroposterior pressure on the glans. It is usually a congenital malformation. Strictures in other portions of the urethra must be demonstrated by the passage of catheters or sounds.

Meatus: Hypospadias: The urethral meatus appears on the ventral surface of the glans, the shaft, or at the penoscrotal junction (see Fig. 12-7C).

Meatus: Epispadias:　Maldevelopment results in the meatus opening dorsally on the glans, shaft, or at the penoscrotal junction (see Fig. 12-7D). This anomaly is often associated with exstrophy of the bladder.

Meatus: Morgagni Folliculitis:　The follicles of Morgagni open into the urethra laterally, immediately behind the meatal lips. When the urethral mucosa is inflamed, the mouths of these ducts become prominent, and pus can be seen exuding when the follicles are involved.

Meatus: Papilloma:　A benign tumor in the meatus may be visible when the orifice gapes from pressure on the glans.

KEY SIGN
Ventral Penile Shaft: Acute Urethritis:　See also, *Male Genital and Reproductive Syndromes: Urethritis*, page 672. An acute indurating urethritis, especially as the result of infection from an indwelling catheter, may cause a palpable cord that extends the entire length of the ventral midline of the penis.

KEY SIGN
Ventral Penile Shaft: Urethral Stricture:　A tunnel stricture of the urethra may cause a palpable, cord-like mass in the corpus cavernosum urethrae at the penoscrotal junction. Strictures in other parts of the penile urethra are usually not palpable.

Ventral Penile Shaft: Urethral Diverticulum:　When located at the penoscrotal junction, a diverticulum frequently produces a visible swelling, felt as a soft midline mass.

Ventral Penile Shaft: Periurethral Abscess:　An accumulation of pus in the midportion of the penile urethra in the Littre follicle will produce visible swelling.

► **Ventral Penile Shaft: Urethral Carcinoma:**　Occasionally, a neoplasm may be felt in an indurated mass in the corpus spongiosum.

Scrotum Signs

KEY SIGN
Blue Papules: Scrotal Venous Angioma (Fordyce Lesion):　Frequently, venous angiomas develop in the superficial veins of the scrotum in men older than 50 years of age. The papules are usually multiple, 3–4 mm in diameter, and filled with venous blood that colors them dark red, blue, or almost black (see Fig. 6-14B, page 165). They are of no significance.

Scrotal Swelling: Edema: *Pathophysiology:* Extra-cellular fluid collects in the dependent scrotum when venous or lymphatic outflow is obstructed and when urine extravasates from a ruptured ure-thra below the urogenital diaphragm. Acute obstruction of the lymphat-ics from any cause may produce lymphedema that pits on pressure; when long-standing, it can be nonpitting. Pitting edema will occur when sys-temic venous pressure is very high and dependent edema reaches above the inguinal ligaments (e.g., advanced right ventricular failure or con-strictive pericarditis, thrombosis of the pelvic veins or inferior vena cava, nephrotic syndrome) and often in the setting of tense ascites.

Scrotal Swelling: Hematoma and Laceration: The conditions are usually evident and cause no difficulty in diagnosis.

Scrotal Gangrene: *Pathophysiology:* This necrotizing perineal infection (Fournier gangrene) is caused by polymicrobial mixed aerobic and anaerobic, gram-positive and gram-negative organisms, of-ten with gas production. The rapid progression results from subcuta-neous vascular thrombosis leading to gangrene of the overlying dermis. It is most common in diabetic patients beyond the sixth decade who present clinically with fever, a toxic appearance, and evidence of sepsis, and who have necrotic, foul-smelling, rapidly advancing lesions of scro-tum with crepitus. The condition is life-threatening unless antibiotics and wide surgical debridement of all nonviable tissues are instituted promptly.

Scrotal Cysts: Sebaceous Cysts: This is the most common nodular lesion of the wall and is benign. It may be single or multiple. The white content of the cyst may show through the skin.

Scrotal Carcinoma: The neoplasm is similar to those in other areas of skin. It is particularly common in workers with occupa-tional exposure to tar and oil.

Testis, Epididymis, and Other Intrascrotal Signs

Maldescended Testis: Cryptorchidism: *Patho-physiology:* During fetal development, the descent of the testis may be arrested in the abdomen, in the inguinal canal, or at the puboscrotal junction. Either or both testes may be affected. When the testis remains in the abdomen, it cannot be palpated. In the inguinal canal or at the puboscrotal junction, the testis is palpable, but frequently it is atrophied, so the mass is smaller than might be expected. More complicated anom-alies of development result in the testis lodging in the perineum near the median raphe of the scrotum, in the femoral canal, or anteriorly and dorsally at the root of the penis. Testicular maldescent may result in decreased fertility. A maldescended testis is frequently associated with a congenital inguinal hernia on the same side as a result of persistence of part of the saccus vaginalis. Maldescended testis carries an increased risk of testicular cancer.

KEY SIGN
Small Testes: Atrophy: The testis may be smaller than normal from maldevelopment. Atrophy may occur after infarction, trauma, mumps orchitis, cirrhosis, Klinefelter syndrome, Prader-Willi syndrome, syphilis, filariasis, or surgical repair of an inguinal hernia.

KEY SIGN
► **Nontender Testicular Swelling: Neoplasm:** Testicular cancer is most common in young men who may present with regional or disseminated disease. It is aggressive, yet curable. The mass is indistinguishable from gumma or tuberculoma and biopsy by the transinguinal (never transscrotal) approach is required for diagnosis. The testis is usually enlarged and harder than normal, and it frequently contains softer cystic regions (Fig. 12-8D and H). A carcinomatous testis is heavier than that with orchitis or hydrocele. The presence of metastatic lesions elsewhere is presumptive evidence that a nodule in the testis is neoplastic.

KEY SIGN
► **Tender Testicular Swelling: Testicular Torsion:**   *Pathophysiology:*   The testicle is suspended on the spermatic cord within the scrotum. It is normally anchored at its distal pole. When the spermatic cord becomes twisted, venous and lymphatic obstruction occur first because of the nature of the vessel walls and lower pressures, as contrasted with arterial wall thickness and arterial pressure. This produces engorgement of the testicle, worsening circulation and leading to arterial, as well as venous and lymphatic, occlusion. The condition is painful and urgent. It is frequently confused with acute epididymoorchitis and strangulated scrotal hernia. Palpation reveals a tender, irregular, edematous mass in the scrotum. The testicle lies in a horizontal position and the epididymis lies in an anterior location. The pain may be referred to the right lower quadrant (RLQ) of the abdomen, mimicking appendicitis. Occasionally, the twist in the cord can be felt. Five distinguishing features are commonly noted: (a) The testis on the affected side lies higher than normal from the twisting of the cord and the spasm of the cremasteric muscles. (b) Palpation cannot distinguish between the testis and the epididymis. In acute epididymoorchitis, the epididymis can usually be felt separately from the testis. (c) Elevation and support of the scrotum for an hour usually relieves the pain of epididymoorchitis; it does not ameliorate the pain in torsion *(Prehn sign)*. (d) In torsion, the leg of the involved side is often held in flexion. (e) When a secondary hydrocele is present, the aspirated contents yield serosanguineous fluid from torsion, serous fluid in epididymoorchitis. Sometimes strangulated hernia cannot be distinguished from torsion without operation.

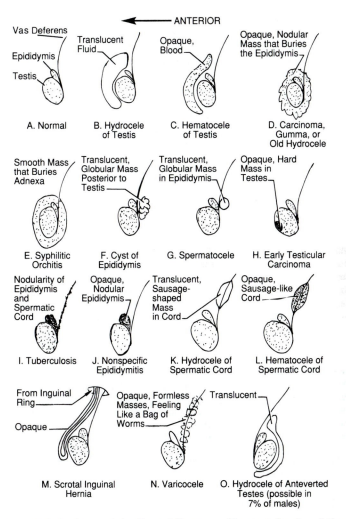

Fig. 12-8 Swellings of the Scrotal Contents. [See text for descriptions of A-O.]

Tender Testicular Swelling: Acute Orchitis:
Pathophysiology: Inflammation of one or both testes occurs frequently in mumps, and occasionally in other infectious diseases. The gland is swollen, tender, and usually extremely painful. Frequently, the inflammation causes acute hydrocele, but the inflammatory edema and the pain of palpation prevent accurate distinction. Often, primary or secondary epididymitis is associated. Orchitis is sometimes confused with torsion of the spermatic cord.

Non-tender Intra-scrotal Swelling: Hydro-cele: *Pathophysiology:* Serous fluid accumulates in the cavity of the tunica vaginalis congenitally or from infection or trauma. Palpation reveals a pear-shaped mass with the smaller pole upward. Pinching the root of the scrotum indicates that the mass does not extend that high. The mass feels smooth and resilient. The testis and epididymis are usu-ally behind the mass (see Fig. 12-8B), except when anteversion is pres-ent and the structures are then anterior (see Fig. 12-8O). Transillumina-tion shows the mass to be translucent; it also reveals the opaque shadow of the testis. The translucency of the hydrocele distinguishes it from the opaque hematocele. Except in anteversion of the testis, the location of the mass in front of the testis distinguishes it from spermatocele that arises from the epididymis and is behind the testis. Hydrocele of the spermatic cord occurs above the testis.

Non-tender Intra-Scrotal Swelling: Hydro-cele of the Spermatic Cord: *Pathophysiology:* When the saccus vaginalis fails to be obliterated around the spermatic cord, a serous cavity persists. This cavity may become filled with fluid to form a hydrocele. Typically, the resulting mass is smooth, resilient, and sausage-shaped; it is located above the testis and transilluminates (see Fig. 12-8K). When no other abnormalities are present, the diagnosis is made by palpation and transillumination. When associated with a her-nia, spermatocele, or testicular hydrocele, the distinction may be diffi-cult or impossible without operation. Occasionally, there exists a com-munication between the hydrocele and the peritoneal cavity, so-called communicating hydrocele. This is characteristically identified by the variation in size from large to nonexistent, depending on the quantity of fluid contained.

Non-tender Intra-scrotal Swelling: Hematocele: The cavity of the tunica vaginalis is filled with blood. The swelling re-sembles that of a hydrocele, but blood is opaque to transillumination (see Fig. 12-8C). A history of recent trauma suggests hematocele.

Non-tender Intra-scrotal Swelling: Hematoma of the Cord: When trauma causes bleeding around the sper-matic cord, a boggy mass may be felt in the region. The mass is opaque to transillumination (see Fig. 12-8L). The history of trauma should as-sist in diagnosis.

Non-tender Intra-scrotal Swelling: Chylocele: In filariasis, opalescent lymph may accumulate in the cavity of the tu-nica vaginalis. The mass is translucent and distinction from hydrocele can be made only by aspiration of the fluid.

KEY SIGN

Non-tender Intra-scrotal Swelling: Varicocele: *Pathophysiology:* Varicosities of the pampiniform plexus of veins form a soft, irregular mass in the scrotum. The condition occurs predominantly on the left side; occasionally it is bilateral; almost never is the right side involved exclusively. Palpation gives a sensation likened to feeling a bag of worms that is rarely mistaken for anything else (see Fig. 12-8N). To distinguish the condition from an indirect inguinal hernia containing omentum, have the patient lie down; place your gloved finger over the subcutaneous inguinal ring. When the patient stands, with your finger in place, the veins refill but the hernia will be held back.

KEY SIGN

Non-tender Epididymal Swelling: Spermatocele: Retention cysts of the epididymis, especially in the globus major, contain fluid that may be milky or clear. Spermatozoa may be present microscopically. The cysts are usually small but may attain a diameter of 8 or 10 cm. The cyst is usually translucent when transilluminated (see Fig. 12-8G).

▶ **Non-tender Epididymal Swelling: Solid Tumor:** Opaque masses of the epididymis are rare; when present, they are usually neoplasms. They should be biopsied because they are frequently malignant.

Non-tender Epididymal Swelling with Nodularity: Syphilis: The globus major is usually first involved; then the process extends to the body of the epididymis (see Fig. 12-8J). The organ is usually not tender. The cause is inferred from positive serologic tests for syphilis and the presence of syphilitic lesions elsewhere.

Non-tender Epididymal Swelling with Nodularity: Tuberculosis: The body of the epididymis is usually first involved. The hard nodules are not tender. The epididymis becomes adherent to the scrotum, and sinuses may form (Fig. 12-8I). The cause is usually inferred from the presence of tuberculosis in other structures.

KEY SIGN

Tender Epididymal Swelling: Acute Epididymitis: *Pathophysiology:* Infection of the epididymis occurs by extension from infections in the urethra, prostate, or seminal vesicles. Indwelling urethral catheters increase the risk of epididymitis. The painful, tender swelling of the epididymis may be accompanied by fever, leukocytosis, and pyuria. In young, sexually active men with multiple or new sexual partners, sexually transmitted organisms are expected; in men over age 40 and in those with catheters, enteric organisms are common.

Thickening of the Vas Deferens: Deferentitis:
This is inflammation of the vas deferens. In acute diseases, the vas is tender and swollen. The inflammation is usually an extension from other structures. With chronic inflammation the vas may be thickened and indurated, with some nodularity (see Fig. 12-8I), suggesting either tuberculous or syphilitic extension from other parts of the genitourinary tract.

Prostate and Seminal Vesicle Signs

KEY SIGN
► **Non-tender Prostate Enlargement: Benign Prostatic Hyperplasia (BPH):** BPH affects a majority of men in their seventies, but only a minority experience urethral obstruction with symptoms of straining at urination, weak urinary stream, nocturia, and dribbling. When the lateral lobes are involved, they are symmetrically enlarged, elastic to rubbery or firm, and the rectal mucosa can be made to slide over them readily. Hyperplasia of the median lobe may be difficult to detect because the bulk of the lobe may protrude anteriorly to produce urethral obstruction without being palpable, so size cannot be used to judge propensity for obstruction.

KEY SIGN
► **Non-tender Prostatic Enlargement: Prostate Cancer:** This is usually asymptomatic; dysuria and symptoms of obstruction may occur in advanced disease. A discrete nodule may be palpated on the posterior surface of the prostate or the gland my feel diffusely enlarged. The entire gland may become stony hard, or there may be several hard nodules. The median furrow becomes obliterated. Early spread is often in the direction of the seminal vesicles. It is important to note the size of the mass, whether it involves one or both lobes, whether normal anatomic landmarks are preserved or obliterated, and whether there is extension beyond the prostate. Extension is palpable or inferred from fixation of the rectal mucosa to the posterior surface of the prostate. If the digital rectal exam is positive, ultrasound-guided needle biopsy is indicated.

KEY SIGN
Non-tender Prostate Enlargement: Chronic Prostatitis: Palpation of the prostate may not reveal distinctive findings. A history suggesting chronic urinary tract infection prompts the finding of large mucous shreds in the urine specimen. Prostatic massage is accomplished by repeatedly and firmly stroking the posterior surface of the prostate from the lateral margins toward the midline, sometimes a painful procedure. The fluid is milked from the urethra and examined under the microscope. In prostatitis, the fluid contains many leukocytes. Chronic prostatitis may be either infective or noninfective, a distinction sometimes difficult to make.

KEY SIGN

Tender Prostatic Enlargement: Acute Prostatitis: In sexually active young men, chlamydia and gonorrhea are most likely, whereas in men over age 40 or those men with an indwelling urethral catheter, enteric organisms (*Escherichia coli* or *Klebsiella*) are the cause. It may begin with dysuria, chills, and fever. Gentle palpation reveals an enlarged, tense or boggy and tender prostate, surrounded by edematous tissue. The urine specimen contains large mucous shreds. Vigorous massage of the prostate to obtain fluid for examination is contraindicated because it may induce bacteremia, and a urine specimen containing bacteria and white blood cells will be adequate for culture.

Palpable Seminal Vesicle: Vesiculitis: The normal seminal vesicle is not palpable. When the structure can be felt as a dilated or indurated mass, it is the site of acute or chronic infection or obstruction. The finger in the rectum may procure fluid for examination by massaging the vesicle toward the prostate, then milking the urethra to extrude the seminal fluid.

Palpable Cowper Gland: Inflammation of Bulbourethral Gland (Cowperitis): Normally the bulbourethral glands are not palpable. When they are inflamed, they are exquisitely tender. In chronic inflammation, they enlarge from the size of a pea to that of a hazelnut. The tenderness or mass is readily demonstrated if the condition is considered and searched for in the proper place. One gland lies on each side of the membranous urethra between the inferior edge of the prostate and the inner border of the anal canal. With the gloved forefinger in the rectum, explore the anterior rectal wall inferior to the prostate and superior to the edge of the anal canal (see Fig. 12-3D). At the same time, the thumb is held outside on the median raphe of the scrotum just anterior to the anus. The tissue between the thumb and forefinger is compressed to detect tenderness or a mass.

Male Genital and Reproductive Syndromes

S KEY SYNDROME

Inguinal Hernia: See Chapter 9, *Hernias*, page 602ff.

S KEY SYNDROME

Sexually Transmitted Diseases (STDs): STDs can present locally as ulcers or inflammation, systemically, or be asymptomatic. All sexually active men, especially those with new or multiple partners, should be screened for a history of STDs. The presence of one STD increases the risk of acquiring and transmitting others. Barrier contraceptives (condoms) are somewhat effective at decreasing the risk of acquiring an STD. All persons with an STD must be screened for other treatable STDs, including HIV and syphilis, which are often acquired asymptomatically. In addition, several infectious diseases, not usually defined as STDs, can be acquired sexually, for example, hepatitis B.

S KEY SYNDROME

▼ **Syphilis (Lues):** *Pathophysiology:* Treponema pallidum acquired from sexual contact causes an acute ulcer (chancre) at the inoculation site followed by dissemination throughout the body. *Primary syphilis* presents as a chancre (see Fig. 12-6A), a single, firm, painless, punched-out ulcer on or near the genitalia or uncommonly on the lips, mouth, or woman's breast with regional lymphadenopathy. *Secondary syphilis* presents with headache, sort throat, myalgia, malaise, and itching. Physical exam reveals a maculopapular rash on the soles, palms, and extremities appearing about 6 weeks after the chancre. There may be lymphadenopathy, fever, and alopecia. *Tertiary syphilis* presents with various clinicopathologic pictures depending on tissues involved. Findings may include aortic insufficiency, tabes dorsalis, general paresis, or gumma formation.

S KEY SYNDROME

▼ **Meatus: Urethritis:** *Pathophysiology:* Infection, usually by sexually transmitted organisms, results in inflammation and purulent discharge from the urethral orifice accompanied by burning pain with urination. The edges of the meatus may be reddened, edematous, and everted. A variable amount of pus discharges from the urethra. The lymphatic channels in the dorsum of the penis may be tender and palpable. Tender, swollen, palpable lymph nodes develop in the inguinal regions. Micturition and erection may be painful. The diagnosis is usually obvious by direct inspection and the presence of mucous shreds and pus in the first part of the urine specimen. The challenge is to determine the causative agent. In young, sexually active men, chlamydia, gonorrhea, and the genital mycoplasmas are the most common pathogens. In men over age 40, enteric bacteria predominate. Prostatitis may complicate urethritis by extension of infection into the prostatic ducts. Urethritis may constitute a member of the triad, along with conjunctivitis and arthritis, in Reiter disease; the urethritis frequently appears before the other members.

S KEY SYNDROME

▼ **Erectile Dysfunction: Impotence:** *Pathophysiology:* Sexual arousal, rigid distention of the corpora cavernosum of the penis, orgasm, and effective ejaculation require a normal affect and intact endocrine, neurologic, and vascular function. Dysfunction anywhere in this complex and coordinated process can produce erectile dysfunction, the inability to sustain a penile erection of sufficient rigidity or duration to consummate satisfactory coitus. A thorough history focusing on the onset and progression of symptoms, libido, medications,

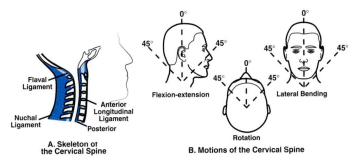

Fig. 13-1 Anatomy and Motions of the Cervical Spine. A. The Skeleton of the Cervical Spine. B. Motions of the Cervical Spine: Normal range of motion exceeds the angles, which are shown as points of reference.

ture. There are seven cervical vertebrae, three of which are specialized: C1 is the atlas (bearing a globe, like the Greek god after whom it is named); C2 is the axis about which the atlas rotates; and C-7 is the vertebra prominens. Nodding of the head occurs chiefly at the atlantooccipital joint. Flexion and extension involve the occiput—C1 and C3 to C7. All vertebrae permit lateral bending. Half of rotation occurs at the atlantoaxial joint, with the remainder distributed through the cervical spine. For measurements of cervical motion, see Fig. 13-1B.

Thoracolumbar Spine and Pelvis

Below the neck, the vertebral column has 12 thoracic (dorsal) vertebrae, 5 lumbar vertebrae, a fused mass of 5 sacral vertebrae articulated with the pelvic bones at the sacroiliac joint and 4 variously separated coccygeal vertebrae. Viewed laterally, the vertebral column presents four curves (Fig. 13-2A). Least pronounced is the cervical curve, which is concave backwards, beginning at C2 and ending at T2. The thoracic curve is convex backwards, beginning at T2 and ending at T12. The lumbar curve, more pronounced in the female, is concave backwards, from T12 to the lumbosacral joint. The pelvic curve, convex backwards and downward, extends from the lumbosacral joint to the tip of the coccyx. The spinal motions are flexion–extension, lateral bending, and rotation. For methods of measurement see Fig. 13-2B.

Appendicular Skeleton Including Joints, Ligaments, Tendons, and Soft Tissues

The Hand

The hand includes the carpal, metacarpal, and phalangeal bones, their joints, and the covering soft tissues. Abnormalities in size and disproportions in a part are usually caused by bone abnormalities. The *posture of the hand* results from the relative tone of the finger and wrist flexors, extensors, and intrinsic hand muscles and the presence or absence of joint disorders.

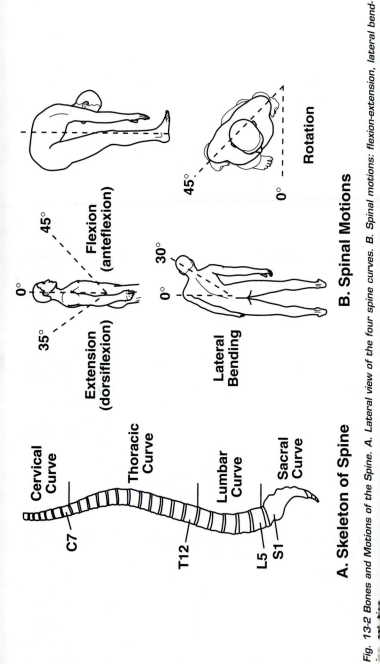

A. Skeleton of Spine

Cervical Curve

C7

Thoracic Curve

T12

Lumbar Curve

L5

S1

Sacral Curve

B. Spinal Motions

Extension (dorsiflexion)   Flexion (anteflexion)

35°   0°   45°

Lateral Bending

0°   30°

Rotation

45°   0°

Fig. 13-2 Bones and Motions of the Spine. A. Lateral view of the four spine curves. B. Spinal motions: flexion-extension, lateral bend-

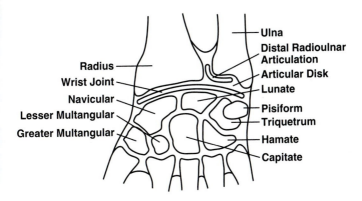

Fig. 13-3 Bones of the Wrist.

The Wrist

The wrist includes the radiocarpal joint, the eight carpal bones in two parallel rows, and the overlying tendons and tendon sheaths (Fig. 13-3). The radiocarpal joint is the articulation of a concave with a convex surface. The proximal concave surface is formed by the distal end of the radius and the adjacent triangular articular disk that caps the distal end of the ulna. The distal convex surface consists of the curving sides of three carpal bones of the proximal row, from the radial to the ulnar side, the navicular, the lunate, and the triquetrum. The pisiform does not participate because it lies on the volar aspect of the triquetrum. The navicular is most commonly fractured, because the radius has wider contact with it than with the lunate, and the forces transmitted from the ulna to the triquetrum are cushioned by the articular disk. The major synovial cavity lies between radius and the navicular. A minor cavity separates the distal end of the ulna and the articular disk, extending proximally between the radius and ulna.

Knowledge of the topography is necessary to examination of the wrist (Fig. 13-4). *Volar Aspect of the Wrist:* The pisiform bone can be palpated as a bony prominence on the ulnar side, just distal to the palmar crease and proximal to the base of the hypothenar eminence. Four tendons can be palpated and often seen. With the digits slightly flexed and muscles tensed, three tendons are apparent in most persons. From the ulnar to the radial side, they are the flexor carpi ulnaris, palmaris longus, and flexor carpi radialis. The palmaris longus is absent in approximately 10% of persons. With the fist clenched hard, the tendon of the flexor digitorum sublimis also appears between the flexor carpi ulnaris and the palmaris longus. *Dorsal Aspect of the Wrist:* The most conspicuous prominence is the ulnar styloid process. Extension of the thumb accentuates the borders of the anatomist's snuffbox, a recess formed by the more prominent lateral extensor pollicis longus and medially by the less pronounced extensor pollicis brevis. In the intervening hollow the radial artery and the radial styloid process can be felt. On the volar side

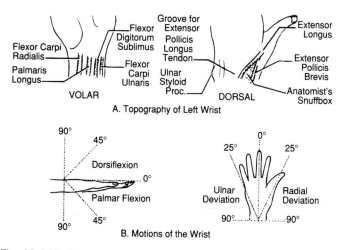

Fig. 13-4 The Wrist. *A. Topography of the Wrist Joint. B. Motions of the Wrist Joint.*

of the extensor pollicis longus tendon is a prominence formed by the articular margin of the radius, called the dorsal radial tubercle (Lister tubercle); this marks the lip of the tendon's groove.

The Forearm

The forearm extends from the elbow to the wrist. *Inspection* and *palpation* are used for examination. The radius and ulna articulate with the humerus proximally. They are connected by an interosseous membrane throughout most of their length. The radius and ulna are practically subcutaneous, so their entire length can be palpated. The dorsal muscle mass is formed by the wrist and finger extensor muscles which insert on the lateral epicondyle of the humerus. The volar mass is the finger and wrist flexors inserting on the medial epicondyle.

The Elbow

There are two articulations in the elbow. The hinged humeroulnar joint is formed by the semilunar notch of the ulnar olecranon process embracing and moving around the transverse drum of the spool-shaped trochlea of the distal humerus (Fig. 13-5A). When the elbow is in full extension, the olecranon process fits into the olecranon fossa of the humerus just above the trochlea. The trochlea forms the medial two-thirds of the lower humeral articulation. The lateral third is the rounded capitulum on which a cup-shaped depression in the radial head pivots and glides to form the humeroradial joint. The radial head is a squat cylinder whose sides rotate in the annular ligament during pronation and supination of the forearm.

Viewed from the back (Fig. 13-6), the flexed elbow presents three bony prominences of an inverted equilateral triangle: the two basal

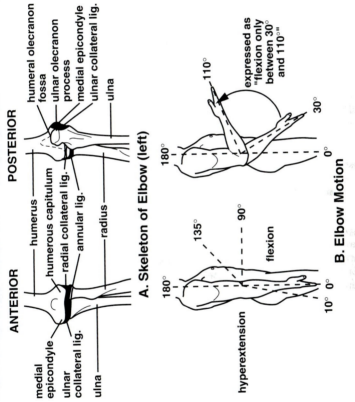

Fig. 13-5 Structure and Motions of the Elbow.

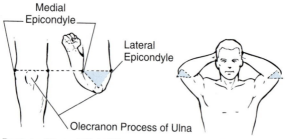

Fig. 13-6 Topographic Relations of the Elbow. *In extension, the ulnar ole-cranon process lies on a straight line between the medial and the lateral epi-condyles of the elbow. In flexion, the olecranon process moves downward to produce an inverted equilateral triangle between the three bony prominences. Any distortion of this triangle after trauma points to a fracture involving one or more of its points.*

points are the medial and lateral epicondyles of the humerus, the tip of the olecranon process forms the apex. During full extension, the three points form a straight transverse line.

The Shoulder

The shoulder girdle includes bones (humerus, scapula, clavicle, sternum), joints (glenohumeral, acromioclavicular, sternoclavicular, and scapulothoracic), their ligamentous connections, and the overlying muscles, tendons, and bursae. The shoulder joint is a ball-and-socket articulation with the hemispheric humeral head fitting into the shallow scapular glenoid cavity (Fig. 13-7). The articulating surfaces are enclosed by a short tube of joint capsule. The scapular coracoid process projects

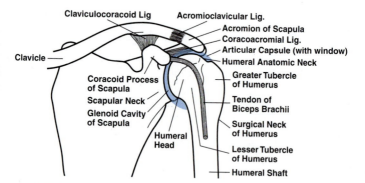

Fig. 13-7 Anatomy of the Shoulder Joint. *The anterior window in the joint capsule exposes the inner attachment of the biceps brachii muscle.*

anterior and medial to the joint and the acromion forms a rigid fender above the joint. They are connected by the coracoacromial ligament. The clavicle is connected to the acromion by the superior acromioclavicular ligament and to the underlying coracoid process by the coracoclavicular ligament. From its origin within the joint capsule, the tendon of the long head of the biceps emerges anteriorly through a capsular opening between the greater and lesser tubercles of the humeral head. The joint capsule is lined by a synovial membrane with a prolongation forming a tubular sheath for the biceps tendon which follows the tendon distally to the surgical neck of the humerus.

The joint capsule is loose, exerting little tension except in extreme positions. Therefore, shoulder stability is maintained by muscle pull. The shoulder joint enjoys great freedom of motion from the shallowness of the glenoid cavity and the lack of restraining ligaments, but this also makes it vulnerable to dislocation. The scapula is held to the thoracic wall entirely by its muscular attachments, its wing gliding freely over the thoracic muscles. Scapular movements add greatly to the mobility of the upper limb, so scapular motion must be distinguished from movements of the glenohumeral joint. The single ligament-bone connection of the shoulder girdle to the axial skeleton is via the acromioclavicular joint, the clavicle, and the sternoclavicular joint.

The principal bony landmarks of the shoulder form a right-angled triangle: the tip of the coracoid, the greater tubercle of the humeral head, and the acromion. The right angle is at the greater tubercle. The acromion is easily seen and felt beyond the end of the clavicle. The coracoid is palpated near the anterior border of the deltoid muscle on a horizontal line with the greater tubercle.

The Hip Joint and Thigh

In the diagnostic examination, the hip joint and thigh are considered together. The femoral axis slants medially toward the knee. The greater trochanter of the femur presents a lateral bony mass, palpable through the thigh muscles (Fig. 13-8A). On the medial side and a little distal is the lesser trochanter, smaller in size and inaccessible to palpation. Arising between the trochanters, the femoral neck slants proximally and medially, forming an angle with the femoral axis of 120–160 degrees. An increase in the angle produces lateral deviation of the femoral shaft, *coxa valga,* a decrease in the angle deviates the shaft medially, *coxa vara.* The neck is surmounted by the globular femoral head, which fits into the cupped acetabulum of the pelvis, forming a ball-and-socket joint. This joint permits flexion-extension, abduction-adduction, and internal-external rotation (Fig. 13-8C). An important topographic relationship is defined by the Nélaton line, extending from the anterosuperior iliac spine to the ischial tuberosity. With the thigh flexed, the line passes through the tip of the greater trochanter; an upward deviation of 1 cm is considered normal (Fig. 13-8B).

The Knee

The knee region includes the tibiofemoral and tibiofibular joints, the patella, the adjacent segments of the femur, tibia, and fibula, their liga-

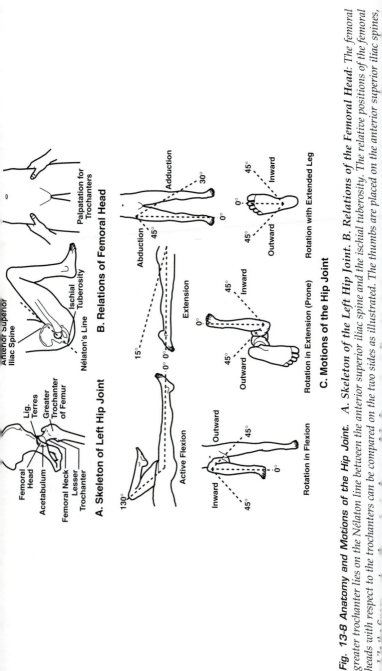

A. Skeleton of Left Hip Joint

B. Relations of Femoral Head

C. Motions of the Hip Joint

Fig. 13-8 Anatomy and Motions of the Hip Joint. A. Skeleton of the Left Hip Joint. B. Relations of the Femoral Head: The femoral greater trochanter lies on the Nélaton line between the anterior superior iliac spine and the ischial tuberosity. The relative positions of the femoral heads with respect to the trochanters can be compared on the two sides as illustrated. The thumbs are placed on the anterior superior iliac spines,

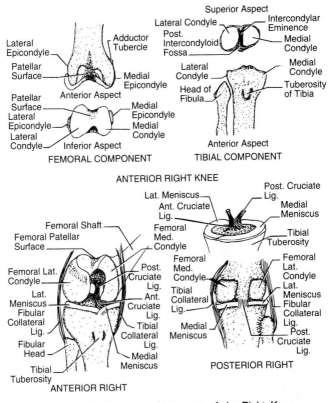

Fig. 13-9 Articular Surfaces and Ligaments of the Right Knee.

ments, menisci, and muscles. Viewed from below (Fig. 13-9), the articular surface of the femur is shaped like a horseshoe with its open end posterior. The two anteroposterior legs of the shoe are formed by nearly parallel lateral and medial femoral condyles, separated by the intercondylar fossa. The surface of the anterior bow is indented by a shallow median groove curving upward onto the anterior femur, the patellar articular surface. Superior to the articular surfaces of the condyles are the medial and lateral epicondyles. Viewed from above, the articular surface of the tibia presents two lateral almost flat, oval facets, the medial and lateral tibial condyles, separated by an intercondylar fossa with anterior and posterior segments. The lateral borders of the fossa are the raised rims of the condyles, the intercondylar eminences. On the central anterior tibia, slightly below the joint, is the tibial tuberosity.

The *knee joint has three articulations:* a medial and a lateral condylar articulation and an anterior joint where the patella glides over the femur (see Fig. 13-9). The femoral condyles may be likened to two thick disks with their edges resting on the almost flat tibial condyles. The small radius of curvature of the femoral condyles presents little apposing surface with the tibia in any position. The lateral and medial *menisci* are flattened crescents of fibrocartilage that rim the peripheral borders of the tibial condyles. Their cross-sections are wedge-shaped, with the thickest part outward. This arrangement deepens the articular surfaces of the tibial condyles and fills the space between the curved femoral condyles and the flatter tibial surface. The menisci are covered with smooth synovial membranes. The ends of their crescents are attached to the intercondylar fossa.

The principal internal ligaments are the *anterior and posterior cruciate ligaments*, named for the positions of their tibial attachments and their crossing arrangement (see Fig. 13-9). The anterior cruciate ligament begins in front of the anterior tibial intercondyloid eminence and passes upward, backward, and lateralward to the back of the lateral femoral condyle. The posterior cruciate ligament attaches to the posterior intercondyloid fossa, passes upward, forward, and medially, to the front of the medial femoral condyle. The *lateral (fibular) collateral ligament* is a strong fibrous cord ascending vertically from the lateral aspect of the fibular head to the back of the lateral femoral condyle. Its opposite is the *medial (tibial) collateral ligament* ascending from the medial aspect of the medial tibial condyle to the medial femoral condyle.

The flat triangular *patella*, a sesamoid bone, is embedded in the tendon of the quadriceps femoris. The distal extension of this tendon is the patellar ligament, attached distally to the tibial tuberosity. During extension of the knee, the patella rides loosely in front of the distal femur. In flexion, the patella opposes the lateral part of the medial femoral condyle (Fig. 13-10A), while with active extension it is often pulled against the lateral femoral condyle.

The head of the *fibula* articulates with the lateral tibial condyle by an arthrodial joint. This joint is inferior to the knee joint and entirely separated from it. The fibula is held to the tibia by the joint capsule and anterior and posterior ligaments.

The *joint capsule of the knee* is a complex of fibrous sheets reinforced by bands from the muscle tendons crossing the joint. It is a single synovial sac that envelops the articular surfaces of both pairs of condyles forming the largest joint cavity in the body. A large suprapatellar pouch of the sac ascends anteriorly, first between the patella and the anterior

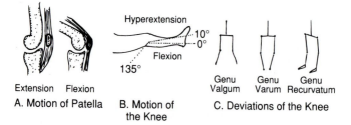

Extension   Flexion
A. Motion of Patella

Hyperextension
10°
0°
Flexion
135°
B. Motion of the Knee

Genu Valgum   Genu Varum   Genu Recurvatum
C. Deviations of the Knee

Fig. 13-10 Motions and Deviations of the Knee.

aspect of the femur, then into a bursa between the quadriceps tendon and a fat pad in front of the femur. A precise understanding of the extent of this sac is diagnostically important.

The *principal bursae of the knee* are of diagnostic importance: (a) a bursa lying between the skin and the patella, the prepatellar bursa; (b) a smaller bursa between the skin and the patellar ligament, the superficial infrapatellar bursa; (c) a bursa between the skin and the tibial tuberosity; (d) the anserine bursa medial and inferior to the knee joint between the tibia and the tendons of the semitendinosus, gracilis, and sartorius muscles. The suprapatellar pouch of the knee joint extending superiorly between the quadriceps tendon and the femur is not a true bursa, although it functions as such. It may be erroneously called the suprapatellar bursa.

The Ankle

The ankle joint is a hinged articulation between the tibia and the talus of the foot. The articular surface of the talus, the trochlea, is rounded superiorly with a transverse axis that is tipped slightly medially, and flattened on its medial and lateral faces (Fig. 13-11). The upper curvature articulates with the flat surface of the lower tibia. The proximal sides of the joint are flat, downward projections, the medial malleolus of the tibia and the lateral malleolus of the fibula. These serve as the sides of a mortise, articulating with the flat lateral surfaces of the talus and stabilizing the joint laterally and medially. During ankle flexion and extension, the tibial surface glides over the curved surface of the talus changing the angle between leg and foot and rotating the leg medially

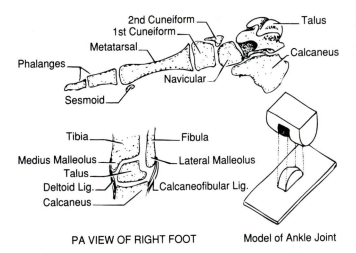

MEDIAL ASPECT OF RIGHT FOOT

2nd Cuneiform
1st Cuneiform
Metatarsal
Phalanges
Navicular
Sesmoid
Talus
Calcaneus

Tibia — Fibula
Medius Malleolus
Talus
Deltoid Lig.
Calcaneus
Lateral Malleolus
Calcaneofibular Lig.

PA VIEW OF RIGHT FOOT   Model of Ankle Joint

Fig. 13-11 Structure of the Ankle Joint and Foot.

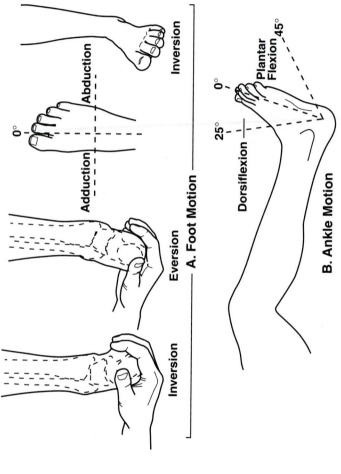

Fig. 13-12 Motions of the Ankle.

on the foot with increasing dorsiflexion helping to transfer weight toward the medial foot and great toe during stance and push-off phases of gait. The lower ends of the tibia and fibula are bound together by the anterior and posterior tibiofibular ligaments. The medial malleolus is attached to the talus and calcaneus by a triangular band, the *deltoid ligament.* The lateral malleolus is attached below to the talus and the calcaneus by the calcaneofibular ligament and the anterior and posterior talofibular ligaments. The joint capsule surrounds the articulation and is lined with synovial membrane.

The motions of the ankle joint are dorsiflexion (extension) and plantar flexion (flexion) (Fig. 13-12). The only bony landmarks are the lateral and medial malleoli; the lateral is lower than the medial.

The Foot

The foot is a complex structure designed to withstand the enormous forces transmitted from the body to the ground during walking, running, and jumping. It is both flexible and strong, and able to adapt to virtually any ground surface. It is divided into the *hindfoot* (talus and calcaneus), *midfoot* (navicular, cuboid and medial, intermediate and lateral cuneiforms), and the *forefoot* (metatarsals, phalanges, and sesamoids). The hindfoot and midfoot are separated by the transverse tarsal joint between the talus and the navicular and the calcaneus and the cuboid. The transverse tarsal joint is responsible for inversion and eversion. The midfoot is separated from the forefoot at the tarsometatarsal joint. The foot has two prominent arches: the longitudinal arch forms the instep medially from the tubercles of the calcaneus to the heads of the metatarsals; and the mediolateral metatarsal arch from the first to the fifth metatarsal heads. The calcaneus is palpable on all but its superior and distal surfaces. The bones of the midfoot and forefoot are best palpated dorsally where they are not covered by muscle. There is a bony prominence on the midlateral margin just above the sole formed by the tuberosity of the fifth metatarsal. The foot can be visualized anatomically as a series of triangles, each with an apex and a base. The first has its apex at the calcaneus and its base along the metatarsal heads. This tripod allows stable weight bearing on uneven ground. The second is the longitudinal arch with its apex at the transverse tarsal joint and its base the calcaneus and first metatarsal head. The third is the metatarsal arch, with its base the first and fifth metatarsal heads and its apex the third metatarsal head. Lastly, each toe forms a triangle with the apex at the proximal interphalangeal joint and the base at the pad of the toe and the metatarsal head.

Physical Examination of the Spine and Extremities

Because the examination overlaps the imprecise divisions between internal medicine, neurology, and orthopedics, most examiners follow a routine in which anatomic regions are examined in a sequence dictated by the mechanical convenience of the doctor and patient, rather than a logical exploration of physiological systems. Any attempt to present diagnostic findings as they are encountered in an anatomic region necessitates considerable cross-reference to the examination of the nervous and the peripheral vascular systems.

Examination of the Axial Skeleton: Spine and Pelvis

EXAMINATION OF THE CERVICAL SPINE

 Following trauma or suspected cervical injury, the cervical spine must ALWAYS be immediately IMMOBILIZED in a rigid collar PRIOR TO ANY MOVEMENT or examination of the patient.

Absent this situation, examine the patient in the seated position. View the neck from the front, sides, and back for deformities and unusual posture. Ask the patient to point to the site of pain. Test active motions of the neck with the instructions: "chin to chest," "chin to right and left shoulder," "ear to right and left shoulder," and "head back." With the flat of the hand, palpate the paravertebral muscles for the hardening of muscle spasm, and with the finger tip for tender points or trigger points. Test for tenderness of the spinous processes by palpation and by percussion with the finger or rubber hammer.

GENERAL EXAMINATION OF THE THORACOLUMBAR SPINE AND PELVIS

Following trauma or suspected spinal injury, the spine must ALWAYS be immediately immobilized on a back board PRIOR TO ANY MOVEMENT or examination of the patient.

A man should be undressed to his undershorts. A woman's clothes should be replaced by a short-sleeved examining gown that ties in back so it may be opened to reveal the spine. ***With the Patient Standing:*** Observe from behind and the side noting deformity, muscle atrophy, local swelling, abnormal curvature or lateral deviations of the spine. If the spinal processes are hidden by muscle or fat, palpate each and mark with a skin marker; the resulting broken line will disclose any deviations from the midline. When lateral deviation is present, have the patient lean forward observing whether the spine straightens. At the same time, examine the chest wall beside the spine. In structural scoliosis, one side will be higher than the other (Fig. 13-13) while with curvature from muscle spasm or disease of ligaments or joints, the lateral masses will be level. Have the patient tense the glutei to reveal atrophy. Percuss each spinous process with finger or rubber hammer to elicit tenderness. Have the patient walk and note the gait. Have the patient hop on each foot to find muscle weakness and pain. Direct the patient to flex, extend, and laterally bend the spine without assistance. Test rotation by grasping the hips while the patient turns first one shoulder, then the other. Palpate

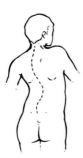

Scoliosis as Demonstrated
by Marking Spinous Processes

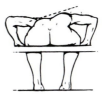

Scoliosis as Viewed
with Spine Hyperflexed

Fig. 13-13 Structural Scoliosis. *Inspection of the flexed spine from behind shows the unequal elevation of the two erector spinae muscle masses.*

for tenderness, for muscles spasm or tender or trigger points. **With the Patient Supine:** Have the patient lie face-upward on the examining table, the head pillowed and the knees slightly flexed for comfort. Do the *straight-leg-raising test* (Fig. 13-14A) by grasping the ankle, with the knee held in extension, and lifting the lower limb to its limit. Note the location of pain elicited, especially contralateral radiation indicating nerve root compression *(Lasèque sign).* With the straight leg elevated at a little-less-than-complete flexion, dorsiflex the foot for aggravation of pain. An alternative test is to gradually extend the flexed knee, with the finger pressing on the tibial nerve in the popliteal fossa; this produces pain if there is irritation of the lower lumbar nerve roots. **With the Patient Prone:** Ask the patient to turn from the supine to the prone position and note the amount of guarding as an indication of pain severity. For comfort, place a pillow between the table and the patient's pelvis. Notice if the muscle spasm and spinal deformity observed while erect persists in the prone position. Reexamine for areas of tenderness and deformity. A step deformity between L5 and S1 indicates spondylolisthesis. With the heel of the hand, press along the spinous processes. Pain from light pressure suggests approximating spines with an intervening bursa; pain from deep pressure arises from intervertebral facets or disks. **With the Patient Sitting:** Look for diminished tendon reflexes and atrophy of muscle masses in the lower limb as evidence of nerve injury in the back.

SCHOBER TEST FOR LUMBAR FLEXION. Have the patient stand erect with heels together. Mark the lumbosacral junction at the L5 spinous process or the point where a horizontal line between the posterior superior iliac spines intersects the spine. Place a mark on the spine 10 cm above and 5 cm below the lumbosacral junction. Have the patient bend forward trying to touch the fingers to the toes. Normally, the distance between those two marks increases by 5 cm or more with maximum flexion. If the distance increases less than 4 cm, mobility is restricted.

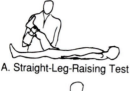

A. Straight-Leg-Raising Test

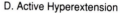
Push Upraised Knee Laterally

B. Patrick Test

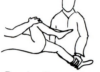

C. Passive Hyperextension

D. Active Hyperextension

Fig. 13-14 Tests at the Hip and Sacroiliac Joint. *A. Straight-Leg-Raising Test: The examiner lifts the supine patient's lower limb when the knee is held in extension. **B. Patrick Test**: Lateral rotation of the hip is assessed by having the knee flexed and the foot of that leg placed on the opposite patella. The examiner then pushes the flexed knee down and out to rotate the head of the femur. **C. Passive Hyperextension of the Thigh (Gaenslen Test)**: While supine, the patient flexes the knee and femur on the affected side and holds the knee with the hands to eliminate lumbar lordosis. The examiner then hyperextends the unaffected thigh by letting it sink over the side of the table. In disease of the sacroiliac joint, this maneuver evokes pain. **D. Active Hyperextension**: With the patient prone and the abdomen resting on a pillow, the patient lifts the spine against the resistance offered by the examiner's hand; sacroiliac disease causes pain.*

ADDITIONAL EXAMS FOR HERNIATED DISK. Test neurosensory function by assessing knee and ankle tendon reflexes, flexion and extension strength at the knee and ankle, great toe extension strength, and sensation to touch. *Crossed-Straight-Leg-Raising Test:* Have the patient lie supine and lift the unaffected limb with the knee held straight. In the presence of herniated disk, this maneuver will exacerbate the pain in the affected limb, and may cause sciatic pain in the hitherto unaffected limb. This is considered by some writers to be pathognomonic of herniated disk. *Reverse Straight-Leg-Raising Test for Intervertebral Disk:* With the patient lying prone and the knee flexed maximally on the thigh, the normal person complains of quadriceps tightness in the anterior thigh. With true disk disease, the pain is felt in the back or in the sciatic distribution on the affected side. This pain is evoked by the root tightening over the involved disk, while abdominal compression increases the pressure in the subarachnoid space.

TESTING THE SACROILIAC JOINT. Have the patient seated with the patient's back toward you. Locate the sacroiliac joints by the dimples in the overlying skin. If dimples are lacking, place your thumbs on the iliac crests with your hands around the patient's trunk (Fig. 13-15); fol-

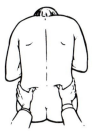

Fig. 13-15 Palpation of the Sacroiliac Joints.

low the crests medially with your thumbs to locate the posterosuperior iliac spines; move your thumbs one fingerbreadth medial to the spines for the area of the joints most accessible to palpation. With your thumbs in place, have the patient bend forward slowly, and press deeply along the joint clefts to elicit tenderness. In the *Gaenslen test of the sacroiliac joint* (see Fig. 13-14C), have the supine patient hold the knee of the affected side with both hands, flexing the knee and the hip to fix the lumbar spine against the table; then hyperextend the other thigh by pushing it downward over the side of the table. An affected sacroiliac joint will be painful with this maneuver. Active prone hyperextension of the spine (see Fig. 13-14D) may aggravate sacroiliac pain when the patient attempts to lift the spine against the resistance of the examiner's hand held in the lumbar region.

Low Back Pain: Pointing Test for Malingering. Low back pain is a favorite complaint of malingerers. One method of exposure is the *Magnuson test.* When the patient indicates a painful spot in the lower back, it is marked with a skin pencil. As a diversion, the examiner proceeds with tests elsewhere in the body; later, the examiner again palpates the back and elicits a different painful site. The patient with organic disease identifies the same point each time.

Examination of the Appendicular Skeleton Including Joints, Ligaments, Tendons, and Soft Tissues

GENERAL EXAMINATION OF JOINTS

Examine all joints systematically from head to foot or in reverse sequence. Place the patient so the joint to be examined is supported at rest with the least pain and muscle spasm. Compare joints, right and left, when one is involved. *Inspect* for normal bony landmarks, joint deformity from swelling, angulation, rotation, subluxation, contracture, or ankylosis. Note the size and contour of the joint, keeping in mind the location of the joint capsule, and the color of the overlying skin. *Palpate* gently for skin temperature and to locate areas of tenderness in the skin, muscles, bursae, ligaments, tendons, fat pads, and joint capsule. Palpate the joint capsule. The normal synovium is not palpable, while a thickened synovium feels "doughy" or "boggy." *Test the joint for effusion* by compressing laterally with the fingers of one hand while the fingers of the other hand rest on the opposite side of the joint; fluid in the joint cavity will displace the receiving fingers. Effusion may be in the joint cavity and/or in a bursa, the borders and other anatomic relations may distinguish them. *Test active range of motion* by directing the patient to move the joint through its full range. To *test passive range of motion*, anchor the joint proximally with one hand while the other hand moves the distal member gently to its full limits. Determine if the limitation of motion is from muscle spasm, gelling that improves with repeated movement, effusion in the joint, locking from loose bodies in the joint, fibrosis ("soft arrest"), or bony ankylosis ("hard arrest"). Palpate over the joint for crepitus on active motion. *Test for ligament integrity* by noting the resistance to joint displacement when anchoring the bone proximal to the joint while gently displacing the distal bone in the plane to be tested. The muscles must be relaxed when testing ligament stability. Always compare right and left since normal ligament tightness is quite variable, from tight to loose ("double jointed").

The Upper Limb

This anatomic region includes the structures of the neck, shoulder girdle, upper arm, forearm and hand. The examination usually begins with the hands and works upward, the sequence used here.

EXAMINATION OF THE HAND

The structures of the hand are relatively superficial and easily examined, comparing right to left. *Inspection:* The fingertips in extension form an arc with the apex at the middle finger. In men, the fourth finger is longer than the index; in women, the index finger is usually longer. With flexion the finger tips align at the base of the thenar eminence with the nails in the same plane; if there is shortening or crossing of the fingertips prior injury with shortening and/or rotation of the affected phalanges or metacarpal is present. Have the patient gently make a fist and observe the proximal knuckles, which are the distal metacarpal heads. There should be a smooth arc between the index and little fingers. Depression of one knuckle from its proper place in the arc indicates shortening of the metacarpal, either congenital or posttraumatic. Observe the dorsum of the hand and the web space between the thumb and index finger for the bulk of the intrinsic hand muscles. Prominence of the tendons and bones occurs with loss of muscle mass, usually resulting from an ulnar nerve lesion. Inspect the palmar aspect of the hand for normal skin creases, the bulk of the thenar and hypothenar muscle masses, callosities or thickening of the palmar fascia. Inspect the nails and finger tips for deformities, ulcers, and signs of previous trauma. *Palpation:* Examine each joint for bony prominences, synovial thickening, or effusion. Palpate the thenar, hypothenar and first web space muscles both relaxed and with contraction. If bone injury is suspected, palpate the entire length of the bone. Squeeze the palm from front to back and laterally across the knuckles to detect tenderness.

Functional Tests of Fingers

Complete functional examination of the hand requires an in-depth understanding of the anatomy of the bones, muscles, tendons, ligaments, and nerves of the hand and forearm. This is beyond the scope of this text. Here, we present a screening examination. The fingers are named thumb, index, long or middle, ring, and little, or they are numbered one through five. The phalangeal joints are termed distal interphalangeal (DIP), proximal interphalangeal (PIP), and metacarpophalangeal (MCP). The aspects of the fingers are dorsal (extensor surface) and volar (flexor or palmar surface). Figure 13-16 illustrates the functional assessment of the joints. The normal limits of motion are indicated by zones with indefinite borders to emphasize individual variation and changes from aging. The testing of muscles is described on page 805. Test active flexion and extension against resistance at the DIP and PIP joints. The superficial flexors attach on the middle phalanx assisting flexion of the MCP and PIP. Flexion at the DIP is performed solely by the deep flexors. Next, test abduction and adduction of the fingers; these movements are powered by the interosseus and lumbrical muscles innervated by the ulnar nerve. Last, test the thumb for flexion and extension power at the MCP and IP, as well as abduction and adduction. The latter movements are performed by the thenar muscles innervated by the median nerve.

EXAMINATION OF THE WRIST

Inspect and *palpate* the wrist for swelling, tenderness, and deformities. Assess weakness and atrophy in the muscles of the forearm that supply the hand. Palpate the moving wrist for crepitus. Listen with the stethoscope to the volar surface of the joint for a rub.   *Testing Wrist Motion:* The primary motions of the wrist are extension-flexion (dorsiflexion and palmar flexion) and radial-ulnar deviation. The diagrams in Fig. 13-4 depict the methods of measurement. When only one wrist is affected, compare it with the other, because average values vary between persons and with age.

EXAMINATION OF THE FOREARM

Inspect the muscle masses for symmetry; often the dominant arm is better muscled. Both the radial and ulnar arterial pulses are palpable proximal to the wrist. The motions of the forearm are pronation and supination (Fig. 13-17). Test for active and passive range of motion and power against resistance. Pain with resisted motion is especially important and the sites of pain should be palpated.

EXAMINATION OF THE ELBOW

Inspect and *palpate* the region for deformity, tenderness, and swelling. Swellings are more common on the extensor surface. Subcutaneous nod-

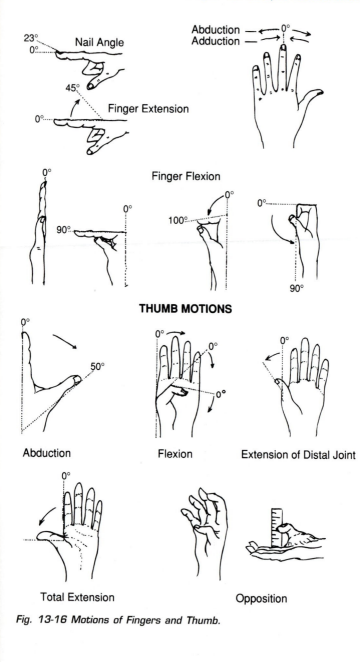

THUMB MOTIONS

Abduction   Flexion   Extension of Distal Joint

Total Extension   Opposition

Fig. 13-16 Motions of Fingers and Thumb.

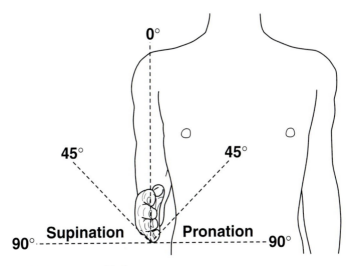

Fig. 13-17 Forearm Motions.

ules are often found in the olecranon bursa and distally in the ulnar region.

TESTING ELBOW MOTION. The movements of the humeroulnar joint are extension-flexion. Pronation-supination principally involves the humeroradial and the distal radioulnar joints. Measurements of these motions are indicated in Fig. 13-5B. Test passive and active motion and strength by resisting active motion.

INSPECTION AND PALPATION OF THE SHOULDER JOINT

Examine the disrobed patient, sitting with the arms relaxed, from front and back (Fig. 13-18). *Inspect* the shoulder anteriorly and the scapula posteriorly for deformities and muscle atrophy, realizing that nearly everyone carries one shoulder higher than the other. *Palpate* the scapular spine, following it forward to the acromion and palpate the acromioclavicular joint. Palpate the sternoclavicular joint for deformity or tenderness. Next palpate the subacromial space and the deltoid muscle and its subdeltoid bursa. Palpate the tendons of the rotator cuff for defects or tenderness and their insertions on the greater (supraspinatus, infraspinatus, and teres minor tendons) and lesser (subscapularis tendon) tuberosities of the humerus. Feel the bicipital groove between greater and lesser tuberosities for tenderness in the bicipital tendon sheath. Stand behind and to the side of the patient to palpate the supraspinatus tendon and the subacromial bursa. For the right shoulder, place your left hand over the shoulder so your index finger palpates the tendon just behind its attachment on the greater tubercle of the humeral head, and

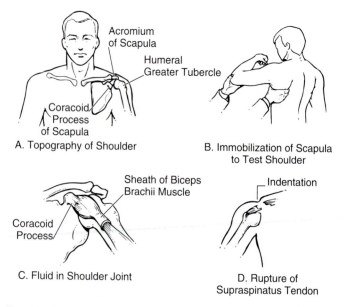

Acromium
of Scapula

Humeral
Greater Tubercle

Coracoid
Process
of Scapula

A. Topography of Shoulder

B. Immobilization of Scapula
to Test Shoulder

Sheath of Biceps
Brachii Muscle

Coracoid
Process

C. Fluid in Shoulder Joint

Indentation

D. Rupture of
Supraspinatus Tendon

Fig. 13-18 Examination of the Shoulder Joint. A. Topography of the Shoulder: The bony prominences of the humeral greater tubercle and the coracoid and acromial processes of the scapula form a right-angled triangle. B. Immobilization of the Scapula to Test Shoulder Motion. C. Fluid in the Shoulder Joint: The heavily stippled structures are the joint capsules distended with fluid. D. Rupture of Supraspinatus Tendon.

your middle finger palpates the subacromial bursa. With your right hand on the patient's flexed elbow, move the arm backward and forward a few times to detect crepitus or tenderness at either point. Finally, place your fingers in the axilla with the pulps facing laterally and palpate the humeral head and the lateral aspect of the glenoid synovial sac.

MEASUREMENTS OF SHOULDER MOTION. Imagine the shoulder joint as the center of a sphere, marked as a globe with a north and south pole and meridians (Fig. 13-19). Then an anterior-posterior (parasagittal) plane through the shoulder joint describes an anterior meridian on the sphere's surface that is *0 degrees of abduction-adduction*. Meridians lateral to it mark degrees of *abduction* and those medial to it are degrees of *adduction*. When the arm hangs at the patient's side, it is in *0 degrees of elevation and of abduction*. The arm can be lifted from the south pole to the north pole, or from *0 to 180 degrees of elevation*. While elevating, the arm must follow in a meridian that designates abduction or adduction. If the arm is raised directly forward to the horizontal, the position is *90 degrees of elevation with 0 degrees of abduction*; this is the cardinal motion of FLEXION. When the arm is raised laterally to the horizontal, the position is *90 degrees of elevation with 90 degrees of abduction*; this is the car-

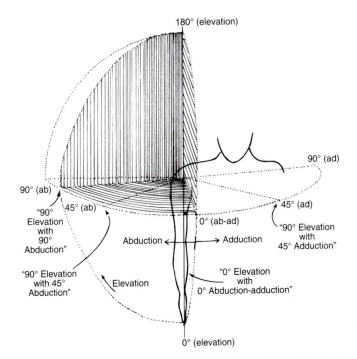

Fig. 13-19 Motions at the Shoulder. *There has been much confusion in terminology about shoulder motion. The system presented here leaves no room for misinterpretation. Elevation is a movement of the arm along any meridian, measured from position at the south pole. Elevation along the meridian in the parasagittal plane passing through the shoulder joint are flexion (forward) and extension (backwards). Movement medial to this is adduction; movement lateral to the plane is abduction. When the arm is elevated in any meridian other than the parasagittal one, the motion is expressed as "elevation in abduction" or "elevation in abduction." The amount of deviation from the parasagittal plane is noted in degrees, for example, "elevation in 70 degrees of abduction."*

dinal motion of ABDUCTION. When the arm is raised directly posteriorly, the position is *elevation with 180 degrees of abduction;* this is the cardinal motion of EXTENSION. If, however, the arm is raised to the horizontal in a meridian 20 degrees medial to 0 degrees, the position is *90 degrees of elevation with 20 degrees of adduction.*

TESTING MOBILITY OF THE SHOULDER. Shoulder mobility includes scapulothoracic and glenohumeral joint motions. Test the unaffected shoulder first and compare the affected side with it. The cardinal movements of the shoulder are abduction (*elevation at 90 degrees abduction*), adduction (*at 90 degrees elevation*), flexion (*elevation at 0 degrees abduction*), extension (*posterior elevation at 0 degrees abduction*) and internal and external rotation. Range of motion should be assessed both actively and passively. *Active motion* is accomplished by the patient and assesses joint mobility and muscle and tendon integrity and reveals limitations of motion as a result of pain. The examiner provides the power during *passive motion* while the patient relaxes, eliminating muscle and tendon limitations, to reveal the full range of motion available to each joint. *Elevation with abduction* involves both scapulothoracic and glenohumeral movement. Have the patient slowly raise the arm laterally from the side to straight overhead; the scapula should begin to move when elevation of the arm attains 60 degrees. *To test glenohumeral motion alone,* grasp the scapular wing and hold it fast to the thorax with one hand while the patient's arm is resting at his side (see Fig. 13-18B). Alternatively, place one hand on top of the acromion to stabilize the scapula. Have the patient raise the arm laterally (90 degrees of abduction) and let the patient complete the motion as far as possible, with the scapula fixed. For *adduction (at 90 degrees elevation)*, rest the fingers of one hand on the top of the patient's shoulder with your thumb behind, fixing the patient's scapula. Have the patient move the arm across the front of the patient's chest as far as the patient can, to place the patient's wrist over the opposite shoulder. *Flexion (elevation at 0 degrees abduction)* is tested by having the patient elevate the arm forward from rest to straight overhead in the anterior-posterior plane. For *extension (posterior elevation at 0 degrees abduction)* have the patient push the arm straight backward in the same plane to the limit of motion. Test *internal and external rotation* with the arm at 90 degrees of abduction and 90 degrees of elevation, starting with the elbow flexed at 90 degrees and the palm facing the floor. For *internal rotation,* ask the patient to lower the hand, palm down, as far as possible without moving the elbow. For *external rotation,* start from the neutral position and have the patient raise the hand, palm forward, as far as possible without moving the elbow. When there is a deficit in active motion, test passive range of motion by repeating the maneuver with the patient relaxed and the examiner supporting the arm and gently putting it through the motion. Test for abduction strength and pain by resisting abduction at 30 degrees (supraspinatus) and 90 degrees (deltoid).

AUSCULTATION OF BONY CONDUCTION THROUGH THE SHOULDER.   The olecranon–manubrium percussion sign is useful in evaluating patients with possible shoulder dislocations, clavicular fractures, or humeral fractures. Place the bell of the stethoscope over the manubrium with the patient's elbows flexed at 90 degrees and percuss the olecranon. Normally, with no disruption of bony conduction, percussion of both sides will produce equal crisp sounds. When dislocation or fracture disrupts bony conduction, the affected side will have decreased intensity and duller pitch.

The Lower Limb

This region includes the pelvis, buttocks, hip joint, thigh, knee, leg, ankle, foot, and toes. Its principal function is maintenance of an upright stance against gravity and providing locomotion.

EXAMINATION OF THE HIP AND THIGH

The patient should be disrobed from the waist down, covering the genitalia but not the buttocks.

SITES OF PAIN.   Have the patient point to the site of pain. An affected hip joint commonly causes pain in the inguinal region or in the buttocks posterior to the greater trochanter. *Pain from the hip joint may be felt only in the knee; this has led to many diagnostic errors.*

BEGIN THE EXAMINATION WITH THE PATIENT STANDING.   Have the patient walk looking for abnormalities of gait: swinging the leg from the lumbar spine suggests ankylosis; a waddling gait is typical of bilateral hip dislocation; the gluteal gait (*Trendelenburg gait*), with the trunk listing to the affected side with each step, suggests unilateral hip dislocation. With the patient standing still, look for a list to one side, asymmetry of the buttocks or other muscle masses, and scars or sinuses.

LATERAL TILTING OF THE PELVIS.   To determine if the pelvis is level, sit in front of the standing patient, with your thumbs on the anterior superior iliac spines; the interspinous line should be horizontal. Lateral tilting results either from adduction of one thigh or from shortening of the limb. Next, measure the distance between the greater trochanters and the anterior superior iliac spines: with your middle fingers, find the tips of the greater trochanters and palpate the distances to the spines. Small disparities can be detected in this manner (see Fig. 13-8B). If the pelvis is not horizontal, place books or blocks under the foot of the shorter limb until the pelvis becomes horizontal; this provides an accurate measurement of shortening.

Next, *have the patient lie on the examining table. All the following tests except that for extension are made in the supine position.*

TEST FOR ROTATION WITH EXTENSION.   This motion should be tested first because it is gentlest; if it is painful, all other maneuvers should be carried out cautiously. With the patient supine, place a hand on each side of the lower thigh and rock it from side to side, watching the patella or the foot for the range of rotation (Fig. 13-20A). Alternatively, the foot may be rocked from side to side.

TEST FOR ROTATION WITH FLEXION.   Flex the knee and hip to 90 degrees, then move the foot maximally both medially (external rotation) and laterally (internal rotation) (see Fig. 13-8C).

TEST FOR ABDUCTION.   Have the patient lie supine with the legs together. Place a hand on the iliac crest and grasp the ankle with your other hand; gradually abduct the patient's thigh until you feel the pelvis move, and note the angle attained (Fig. 13-8C).

TEST FOR ADDUCTION.   With each hand, grasp an ankle, holding one leg down in extension while you move the other thigh across it (see Fig. 13-8C). Note the angle attained from the neutral position. Normally, the thigh should cross the other at midthigh.

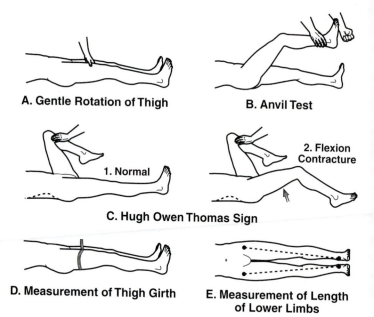

A. Gentle Rotation of Thigh

B. Anvil Test

1. Normal

2. Flexion Contracture

C. Hugh Owen Thomas Sign

D. Measurement of Thigh Girth

E. Measurement of Length of Lower Limbs

Fig. 13-20 Tests of the Hip Joint and Thigh. A. *Gentle Rotation of Thigh.* B. *Anvil Test.* C. *Hugh Owen Thomas Sign for Lumbar Lordosis: Flexion of the unaffected hip presses the lumbar spine against the table. If extension of the opposite hip is shown to be impaired when eliminating lumbar lordosis, it is a positive Hugh Owen Thomas sign.* D. *Measurement of the Girth of the Thigh: Mark similar levels on both limbs, measured down from the anterior superior iliac spines. Measure the girth at each level.* E. *Measurement of Length of Limbs: Have the two limbs approximated, or in the same relative positions from the midline. Measure from the anterior superior iliac spine to the medial malleolus, with the tape running medial to the patella.*

TEST FOR HIP FLEXION CONTRACTURE. *Pathophysiology:* Flexion contracture of the hip is compensated for by a lumbar lordosis, allowing an upright stance that masks the contracture. Place your hand under the lumbar spine flexing the unaffected thigh until the spine presses your hand against the table to indicate that the lumbar lordosis has been straightened. Now, extend the other thigh. It should be able to lie flat on the exam table. Lack of full extension reveals a flexion contracture on the affected side, a positive *Hugh Owen Thomas sign* (see Fig. 13-20C).

THE ANVIL TEST. If other maneuvers have not been painful, raise the leg from the table with the knee in extension and strike the calcaneus with your fist, using a moderate blow in the direction of the hip joint (see Fig. 13-20B). This may elicit pain in early disease of the joint.

DIRECTION PALPATION OF THE HIP JOINT. Facing the patient, examine the left hip with your right hand, and the right hip with your left hand. Hook your fingers about the greater trochanter with your thumb placed on the anterior superior iliac spine (see Fig. 13-8B). With your thumb, follow the inguinal ligament medially until you feel the femoral artery, then move your thumb just below the inguinal ligament and lateral to the artery; this should bring your thumb over the small portion of the femoral head that is extra acetabular. Exert increasingly firm pressure to elicit pain from arthritis. Rock the femur gently, to feel crepitus. If the head does not move, fracture of the neck is probable. If the head cannot be felt, dislocation is suggested.

PATRICK TEST. Passively flex the knee to a right angle and place the foot on the opposite patella. Push the flexed knee towards the table as far as the hip joint permits (see Fig. 13-14B). Painless and full external rotation (negative Patrick sign) excludes symptomatic disease of the hip joint.

TEST FOR EXTENSION. *With the patient prone,* steady the pelvis with one hand while you raise the limb posteriorly (see Fig. 13-8C). Normal extension is about 15 degrees.

MEASUREMENT OF THE LOWER LIMBS. The girth of the thighs and legs is ascertained by measuring the circumferences with a tape measure at symmetrical levels, determined by measuring distances from the anterior superior iliac spines and marking them with a skin pencil (see Fig. 13-20D). The length of the lower limbs is measured in straight lines from the anterior superior iliac spines to the medial malleoli of the tibiae (see Fig. 13-20E). Care should be taken to have the tape in a straight line running medial to the patellae. Both extremities should lie exactly equidistant from the midline. If one limb cannot be placed in normal position, its opposite should be measured in a similar position. A difference of >1.5 cm suggests hip deformity in the shorter leg.

EXAMINATION OF THE KNEE

The normal movements of the knee are flexion and extension. For measurements, see Fig. 13-10B.

GENERAL EXAMINATION OF THE KNEE. *Inspection:* Have the legs and thighs uncovered and the patient standing. Inspect the knee region for deformities, swelling, redness, and muscle atrophy. Note the position of the patella. *Palpation:* Test swellings for fluctuance, joint effusion, crepitation with motion, and points of localized tenderness in the ligaments, bones, and along the joint line. Palpate for doughy thickening of the synovium with obscuration of bony landmarks. With the patient supine, test the range of flexion and extension, test for abnormal anterior and posterior mobility of the tibia on the femur, and stress the medial and collateral ligaments for laxity or pain. Always compare right to left because considerable individual variation exists for joint stability.

With a history of pain in the knee or locking, test for internal disorders of the knee joint, as described on page 706ff.

EXAMINATION FOR KNEE EFFUSION.   *Inspection*   may reveal bulging on both sides of the patellar tendon and in the suprapatellar pouch, obliterating the natural hollows in these regions. The swelling may assume the shape of a horseshoe around the patella (Fig. 13-44A, page 758). *Palpate*   with the patient supine and the knees extended. Gently press the thumb and fingers of the right hand against the anterior femoral condyles at the medial and lateral sides of the knee slightly proximal to the joint line at the lower end of the patella. Slide the left hand down the distal thigh with constant pressure until the patella rests in the space between the thumb and first finger; you will be compressing the suprapatellar pouch. If effusion is present you will palpate and often see a bulge of fluid appear under the palpating right thumb and/or fingers as the fluid is mobilized out of the suprapatellar bursa by the left hand. Small amounts of fluid can be detected visually by compressing the swelling in one of the obliterated hollows beside the patella then watching for the hollow to slowly refill spontaneously or with compression of the suprapatellar pouch. Test for *patellar ballottement* (patellar tap or floating patella) by compressing the suprapatellar pouch, as described above, while the fingers of the other hand push the patella sharply against the femur (Fig. 9-44B, page 758). If fluid is present in sufficient quantity to elevate the patella from the femur, brisk pressure on the patella will force it down against the femoral condyles with a palpable tap, the *patellar ballottement sign.*

EXAMINATION OF THE KNEE LIGAMENTS.   This is part of the routine knee exam. Determine the degree of tightness or laxity of the anterior and posterior cruciates and both collateral ligaments.

Collateral Ligaments: With the patient supine, flex the knee to 10 degrees. Palpate the insertions proximally and distally and each ligament at the joint line. The rope-like lateral ligament is easily identified at the joint line posterolaterally. The broader medial ligament is more difficult to identify. Grasping the calf with one hand while the other hand supports and stabilizes the femur from behind with the thumb and fingertips on opposite joint margins overlying the collateral ligaments (Fig. 13-21). Stress first the lateral, then the medial collateral ligaments by exerting a varus then a valgus force on the calf while palpating over the ligaments at the joint margin. Feel for separation of the tibia from the femur while observing the amount of medial or lateral displacement of the tibia.

Cruciate Ligaments: Test the anterior cruciate with the *Lachman test* (Fig. 13-22A). Have the patient lie supine and flex the affected knee to an angle of 30 degrees. Sit on the patient's foot to fix it. Grasp the upper part of the leg with your fingers in the popliteal fossa and your thumbs on the anterior joint line. Pull the head of the tibia toward you so it glides on the femoral condyles. Forward movement of more than 1 cm is a positive Lachman test, indicating rupture of the anterior cruciate ligament. To test the posterior cruciate, start as in the Lachman test and observe for sagging of the tibia posteriorly. Then push the head of

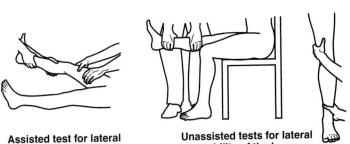

**Assisted test for lateral
stability of the knee**

**Unassisted tests for lateral
stability of the knee**

Fig. 13-21 Tests for Lateral Stability of the Knee Joint.

the tibia posteriorly. Displacement should be less than 5 mm. Always compare the two knees because considerable individual variability in ligament tightness is normal; a discrepancy between the two sides is a sign of previous injury.

EXAMINATION OF THE PAINFUL KNEE

Obtain a detailed account of previous trauma, including the exact mechanism of injury. This is essential to understanding which structures

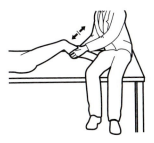

**A. Lachman Test for Torn
Cruciate Ligament**

**B. Examination for Ruptured
Achilles Tendon**

Fig. 13-22 Testing the Cruciate Ligaments and Achilles Tendon. **A.** *Lachman Test for Torn Cruciate Ligament: The patient is supine with the knee flexed at 30 degrees and the foot flat on the table. The examiner sits on the foot to anchor it, then pulls the head of the tibia toward himself to test the anterior cruciate ligament. Forward motion of more than 1 cm is positive. Pushing the knee backward with the knee flexed at 90 degrees tests the posterior cruciate ligament.* **B. Examination for Ruptured Achilles Tendon:** *The prone patient hangs the feet over the end of the table. Inspection shows less natural plantar flexion on the side of rupture.* **Simmonds Test:** *Squeeze the calf muscles transversely; a normal or partially ruptured tendon will produce plantar flexion; complete rupture will not respond.*

might have been injured. Ask which motions cause discomfort or locking, and ascertain whether unlocking is sudden or gradual (as in muscle spasm). Have the patient point to sites of pain and demonstrate the position of fixation if locking has occurred. *Inspection:* Examine the patient supine on the table. Note evidence of joint effusion and muscle atrophy. *Palpation:* Feel the knee carefully for point tenderness, especially over the quadriceps tendon, patellar tendon, collateral ligaments, anserine bursa, and along the joint line. Palpate the surface of the patella and under its edges, then push the patella aside and palpate the underlying femoral condyles. Feel for a click with pain while putting the knee through a full range of motion. A painless click is relatively unimportant as it may be caused normally by tendons moving over a bony prominence. Have the patient put the knee through a full range of active motion and compare with the range of passive motion by the examiner. Remember that joint effusion limits flexion and full extension. Immediately after injury, muscle spasm and swelling may make full examination impossible, in which case, immobilize the knee for a day or two and then reexamine it [Solomon DH, Simel DL, Bates DW, et al. The rational clinical examination. Does this patient have a torn meniscus or ligament of the knee? Value of the physical examination. *JAMA* 2001;286:1610–1620].

TESTING FOR MENISCUS INJURY. Several tests can be performed to identify meniscus injury.

McMurray Test (Fig. 13-23A): With the patient prone on the table, grasp the patient's knee with one hand so that your fingers press the medial and lateral aspects of the joint. Grasp the patient's heel with your other hand so that the plantar surface of the foot rests along your wrist and forearm. First, flex the knee until the heel nearly touches the buttock. To test the posterior half of the medial meniscus, rotate the foot laterally, and then slowly extend the knee fully. If a click is felt or heard during the extending motion, and the patient recognizes it as the sensation preceding pain or locking, the medial meniscus is torn. To test the lateral meniscus, repeat the maneuver with the foot rotated medially.

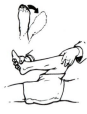
A. McMurray Test

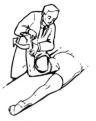

B. Apley Test

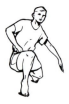
C. Childress Test

Fig. 13-23 Tests for Tear of the Medial Meniscus. A. McMurray Test. B. Apley Test. C. Childress Test.

Apley Grinding Test (See Fig. 13-23B):   Have the patient lie prone on a low couch, about 2 feet (60 cm) high, with the patient's affected limb toward you. Grasp the foot with both your hands, flex the knee to 90 degrees, and rotate the foot laterally. This should cause little discomfort. Now, rest your knee on the patient's hamstrings to fix the femur, and pull the leg to further flexion while the foot is held in lateral rotation; pain indicates a lesion of the medial collateral ligament. Next, compress the tibial condyles onto the femoral condyles by placing your body weight onto the plantar surface of the foot, still in lateral rotation. Pain from this maneuver indicates tear of the medial meniscus.

Childress Duck-Waddle Test (See Fig. 13-23C):   This test is strenuous and is reserved for athletes. Have the patient squat and waddle on the toes, swinging from side to side. With rupture of the posterior horn of the meniscus, complete flexion cannot be attained; the maneuver elicits pain or clicking in the posteromedial portion of the joint.

EXAMINATION OF THE ANKLE JOINT

With the patient supine, *inspect* and *palpate* the ankle for edema, effusion, or tenderness. Test dorsiflexion and plantarflexion by grasping the heel firmly with your left hand to immobilize the subtalar joints while your right hand grasps the midfoot and moves the ankle through the full range of flexion and extension. Test anterior stability (drawer test) by stabilizing the distal tibia with one hand while grasping the heel and pulling it directly forward with the other. Test inversion and eversion stability by stabilizing the tibia as above while alternately firmly inverting and everting the heel. Increased mobility with each test indicates injury to the ankle ligaments stabilizing that motion.

EXAMINATION OF THE FOOT

Inspect the shoes for uneven wear. Normal wear is on the lateral edge of heel and sole. Wear on the medial side of the heel and tilting of the vertical heel seam indicates abnormal foot mechanics. With the patient barefoot and standing inspect the heels from behind, the sides and the front. Always compare right to left. Look for the normal slight outward angulation of the heel which should rotate medial when standing on the toes. Note any deformities (e.g., hammertoes or bunion), the height of the pedal arches, and alignment (a plumb line hanging from the midpatella should point between the first and second metatarsal bones). Have the patient point to the site of pain and palpate the site for tenderness or crepitus. With the patient supine, inspect the sole for the position of callus formation and palpate the fat pads under the calcaneus and metatarsal heads. Test motion by supporting the heel with the supine hand and grasping the foot with the other hand, to move it in dorsiflexion, plantarflexion, eversion, and inversion (see Fig. 13-12A). When tendon inflammation is suspected, listen with the stethoscope for a rub over the painful site [Adler RH, Gertsch M. The stethoscope as a diagnostic aid in tenosynovitis. (letter) *N Engl J Med* 1999;340:156].

EXAMINATION FOR FLATFOOT: Have the patient stand with the feet parallel and separated by about 10 cm. Note the height of the medial longitudinal arch. If it is flattened, see if it resumes a normal height when weight is removed. Test strength of the anterior leg muscles by having the patient stand on the heels. Test for shortening of the Achilles and peroneal tendons by dorsiflexion and inversion, respectively, in the supine position. Test eversion, which is limited in rigid flatfoot.

MUSCLE EXAMINATION

See Chapter 14, *The Neurologic Examination*, page 805.

BRIEF EXAMINATION FOR SKELETAL INJURIES

> *If pain or other symptoms or signs lead you to suspect injury to the spine, IMMEDIATELY IMMOBILIZE the patient and obtain radiographic confirmation of stability before moving the neck or spine or proceeding with the exam. Trauma of sufficient force to cause injury to major skeletal structures is frequently accompanied by internal visceral injuries, which ALWAYS take precedence over the skeletal injuries.*

The following procedure is recommended for the rapid examination of injured but conscious persons to uncover skeletal lesions in the absence of specific complaints.

Head: Have the patient open and close his mouth and bite down when your fingertips are on the masseter muscles; if no pain is elicited, the facial bones are not affected. Palpate the zygomatic arch and nose for tenderness. Palpate the scalp for bruises and lumps. With your hands press from opposite sides of the patient's head for the pain of a skull fracture.

Neck: Palpate the spines of the cervical vertebrae with your fingers before moving the neck. Have the patient roll his head gently from side to side while your fingers palpate the neck muscles for tenderness or spasm. Ask the patient to lift his head while you place your hand under it. Ask the patient to push down with his head to estimate his strength and discomfort.

> *If PAIN is elicited with any of these maneuvers, IMMEDIATELY IMMOBILIZE the neck and cease further movement or examination until the neck is cleared by adequate radiologic exam.*

Chest: Ask the patient to take a deep breath; if this is painful, place your hands on opposite sides of the patient's chest and squeeze to locate the point of tenderness of a rib fracture. Palpate the length of each clavicle.

Spine: With the patient supine, slip your hand under the patient's back, lift the patient's chest slightly, and run your fingers over the spinous processes for tenderness and angulation. Determine if there is limitation of spinal motion.

 If PAIN is elicited with any of these maneuvers, IMMEDIATELY IMMOBILIZE the spine and cease further movement or examination until the spine is cleared by adequate radiologic exam.

Arms and Hands: Have the patient move his arms, hands, and fingers in succession and through a full range of motion. Palpate each finger for phalangeal and metacarpal injuries. Shake hands, both right and left, and ask the patient to twist his arm, with elbow both straight and flexed. Performance of these motions, with normal strength and painlessly, excludes injuries of hand, wrist, forearm, elbow, arm, shoulder, clavicle, and scapula.

Pelvis: Place downward pressure medially with a hand on each anterior ilium, then on the symphysis pubis. Place your clenched fist between the patient's knees and ask the patient to squeeze it; lack of pain excludes fractures of pelvis and femora.

Legs and Feet: Ask the patient to move first one leg, then the other, through a full range of motion. Palpate each toe. Have the patient stretch his legs flat on the table. Press his feet together and have him rotate them laterally against your resistance. If the patient employs normal strength without pain, you have excluded major injuries of legs and pelvis.

Musculoskeletal and Soft Tissue Symptoms

KEY SYMPTOM
Joint Pain: Arthralgia: Arthralgia means joint pain with or without objective signs of inflammation. The onset, location, severity, and temporal pattern of pain are important clues to the diagnosis. It is especially helpful to inquire whether activity makes the pain better or worse, and whether morning stiffness is present. In a patient with arthralgia and arthritis, the differential diagnosis is based upon the pattern of the arthritis. Recognize that early in the course of disease, arthralgias may precede arthritis by weeks or months.

KEY SYMPTOM
Bone Pain: *Pathophysiology:*   Pain in bone is caused by mechanical injury, inflammation, infarction, increased intraosseous pressure, or stretching of the periosteum. Somatic afferent nerves carry the pain fibers and the pain is well localized, especially when the periosteum or endosteum is involved. Bone pain is often the only symptom of disease in bone, although it may be accompanied by localized ten-

derness and swelling. Characteristically, bone pain is constant, well localized, worse at night and often intensified by movement or weight bearing. Bone pain may be referred to the nearest joint, but careful examination can usually distinguish between articular and bone pain. Squeezing the overlying muscles between thumb and index finger should exclude tender muscles as the source of pain. The occurrence of bone pain should prompt x-ray examination.

✓ **BONE PAIN—CLINICAL OCCURRENCE:** *Congenital* hemoglobin S and C (bone infarction), aseptic necrosis (Legg-Calvé-Perthes disease) of the femoral head; *Endocrine* hyperparathyroidism (osteitis fibrosa cystica); *Idiopathic* osteitis deformans (Paget disease of bone), hypertrophic osteoarthropathy, osteoarthritis; *Inflammatory/Immune* eosinophilic granuloma of bone; *Infectious* osteomyelitis, Brodie abscess (localized staphylococcal infection of the metaphysis of a long bone), untreated syphilis of more than 3 years, syphilitic osteoperiostitis, tuberculosis of bone; *Metabolic/Toxic* osteoporosis, osteomalacia, drugs (granulocyte colony-stimulating factor, erythropoietin; *Mechanical/ Traumatic* fractures (spontaneous or pathologic), tendon avulsions and ruptures, ligament avulsions, epiphyseal plate injuries (e.g., Osgood-Schlatter disease of the tibial tuberosity); *Neoplastic* osteosarcoma, multiple myeloma, giant cell tumor, large cell lymphoma, Ewing tumor, metastases to bone, fibrosarcoma, chondrosarcoma; *Vascular* avascular necrosis (with glucocorticoids, hemoglobin S and C diseases).

KEY SYMPTOM
Muscle Pain: Myalgia: *Pathophysiology:* Muscle pain is carried on somatic sensory neurons and is generally well localized. Pain can result from external trauma, repetitive or sustained contraction, inflammation, ischemia, and metabolic disturbances. Chronic myofascial pain is of unknown etiology, but probably represents alterations in the peripheral or central neural circuits. Pain is frequently referred from and to muscle from regional structures. History is the key to diagnosis noting the onset, duration, and character of the pain, its relationship to activity, rest, and symptomatic therapy. Myalgias frequently accompany systemic inflammatory illnesses with or without fever. In many chronic inflammatory disorders, the muscle pain is more severe at night or with prolonged inactivity. Neuromuscular exam is performed looking for signs of atrophy, hypertrophy, spasm, tenderness, trigger points, tender points, weakness, or fasciculations.

✓ **MYALGIA—CLINICAL OCCURRENCE:** *These are examples, only. Congenital* McArdle disease (paroxysmal myoglobinuria); *Endocrine* hyper-/hypoparathyroidism, hypothyroidism; *Idiopathic* osteoarthritis; *Inflammatory/Immune* rheumatic fever, rheumatoid arthritis, dermatomyositis, polymyositis, systemic lupus erythematosus, vasculitis, polymyalgia rheumatica; *Infectious* Any acute infection, for example, influenza, (uncommon but important to remember: malaria, rubella, dengue, rat-bite fever, trichinosis, leptospirosis, typhus, rickettsiosis, *Bartonella*), epidemic pleurodynia (Bornholm disease, devil's grip), pyomyositis; *Metabolic/Toxic* fever, acute hyponatremia, hypocalcemia, hypophosphatemia, hypomagnesemia, dehydration, diuresis, malabsorption, drugs (statins and others); *Mechanical/Traumatic* trauma, strain, hematoma, march myoglobinuria, tonic contractions (such as tension headaches), spinal stenosis; *Neoplastic* paraneoplastic myopathy and dermatomyositis; *Neurologic* fibromyalgia, neurogenic claudication; *Psychosocial* abuse; *Vascular* compartment syndromes, ischemia, atheroemboli, vasculitis.

TRICHINOSIS: *Pathophysiology:* Heavy infection with *Trichinella spiralis* after ingestion of incompletely cooked infected meat (pork, bear meat) may cause severe disease and, infrequently, death. The organisms localize in muscle. One to 4 days after ingestion, the patient complains of nausea and vomiting, diarrhea, and abdominal pain. Within 10 days there are fever, dyspnea, anorexia, myalgia, and asthenia. Physical findings include periorbital edema, scarlatiniform rash, splinter hemorrhages under nails, tremors, and involuntary movements.

KEY SYMPTOM

Back Pain: In common usage, backache refers to the spinal region inferior to the seventh cervical vertebra. Aching discomfort in the back may be acute and/or chronic. It is useful to think of backache in terms of the anatomic structures that cause back pain and pain radiating to the back. Acute pain is usually the result of mechanical trauma from excessive forces applied to the back or repetitive use injury. Chronic pain can be the consequence of any acute injury or repetitive use disorder. It is essential to remember that pain from internal organs can be referred to the back so disorders not of musculoskeletal orgin must be considered in patients with back pain [Deyo RA, Weinstein JN. Low back pain. *N Engl J Med* 2001;344:363–370; Deyo RA, Rainville J, Dent DL. The rational clinical examination. What can the history and physical examination tell us about low back pain? *JAMA* 1992;268:760–765].

✓ *BACK PAIN—CLINICAL OCCURRENCE:* *Acute* **Bones and Ligaments:** fractures, dislocations, torn or avulsed ligaments; *Cartilages:* herniated intervertebral disk, diskitis; *Joints:* reactive arthritis; *Muscles:* muscle strain, myositis, hematoma; *Nerves:* radiculopathy (disk compression, diabetes), epidural mass or abscess, after myelography, subarachnoid hemorrhage, poliomyelitis, tetanus; *Referred Pain:* dissecting aortic aneurysm, angina pectoris, retrocecal appendicitis, pancreatitis, cholecystitis, biliary colic, pneumothorax, pleurisy, nephrolithiasis, pyelonephritis.

Chronic **Bones and Ligaments:** osteoporosis, osteomalacia, osteomyelitis, diffuse idiopathic skeletal hyperostosis (DISH), spondyloarthritides (ankylosing spondylitis, reactive and psoriatic arthritis, etc.), Pott disease (tuberculous spondylitis), osteitis of syphilis, Paget disease (osteitis deformans), primary or secondary neoplasm of bone, spina bifida; *Cartilage:* herniated intervertebral disk; *Joints:* osteoarthritis; *Muscles:* chronic muscle strain, fibromyalgia, myositis;

Nerves: syringomyelia, Chiari malformation, arachnoiditis; *Referred Pain*: esophageal carcinoma, peptic ulcer, chronic pancreatitis, pancreatic carcinoma, renal cell carcinoma, retroperitoneal lymphoma, hepatomegaly from any cause, spinal cord tumor, aortic aneurysm.

KEY SYMPTOM
Pain in the Upper Arm, Forearm, and Hand: When pain is well localized to one part of an extremity, the diagnosis is relatively simple. However, often the pain is more or less diffuse throughout the upper limb, so an anatomic classification of causes is useful. Limb pain does not always arise in musculoskeletal sources, for example, pain may be referred to the upper arm from myocardial ischemia.

✓ *ARM, FOREARM, AND HAND PAIN—CLINICAL OCCURRENCE:* *Well-Localized Pain* arthritis, bursitis, bone fracture, tendon rupture, tenosynovitis, cellulitis, muscle strain, neoplasm, ischemia and claudication. *Diffuse Pain* herniated cervical intervertebral disk, polymyalgia rheumatica, spondylitis, Pott disease, neoplasm of bone, Pancoast tumor, syringomyelia, radiculitis, carpal tunnel syndrome, ulnar tunnel syndrome, complex regional pain syndrome (reflex sympathetic dystrophy).

KEY SYMPTOM
Pain in the Shoulder: Pain in the shoulder is a common complaint, which the patient may have difficulty localizing. Specific diagnosis depends upon identifying the provocative and palliative circumstances, the quality of the pain, the anatomic region of the pain, its severity, and timing. It is helpful to consider the common conditions arranged by anatomic location [Steinfeld R, Valente RM, Stuart MJ. A common sense approach to shoulder problems. *Mayo Clin Proc* 1999;74:785–794].

✓ *SHOULDER PAIN—CLINICAL OCCURRENCE:* *Shoulder Joints* arthritis of sternoclavicular, acromioclavicular, and glenohumeral joints; subluxations of humeral head, acromioclavicular joint, sternoclavicular joint; *Bursae* subacromial and subdeltoid bursitis. *Tendons* supraspinatus tendonitis, tear of supraspinatus tendon (partial or complete), other rotator cuff tears, rupture of long tendon of the biceps, bicipital tenosynovitis; *Muscles* muscle strain, fibromyalgia (tender points), myositis, hematoma, rupture of muscle (complete or incomplete), polymyalgia rheumatica; *Bones* fractures of humeral neck, scapular neck, clavicle; *Nerves* nerve compression by the scalenus anticus muscle (scalenus anticus syndrome), first rib and clavicle (costoclavicular syndrome); complex regional pain syndrome (shoulder–hand syndrome, reflex sympathetic dystrophy); *Vascular* aneurysm or thrombosis of the subclavian artery.

KEY SYMPTOM
Pain Referred to the Shoulder: *Pathophysiology:* Pain is referred to the shoulder from many sites in the chest,

especially those innervated by the phrenic or vagus nerves or cervical sympathetic chain. When the diaphragm is involved (phrenic nerve) patients present with aching or sharp pain usually felt over the top of the shoulder or in the trapezius at the base of the neck. Angina is most often referred to the inner arms, jaw, and shoulder. Pain from nerve involvement is often burning in quality and follows the appropriate dermatome. The following anatomic sites and conditions must be considered.

✓ *REFERRED SHOULDER PAIN—CLINICAL OCCURRENCE:* *Cardiovascular* angina pectoris (to either or both shoulders), aortic aneurysm or dissection; *Pleura* pleuritis of the central part of diaphragm, pneumonia, tuberculosis, pneumothorax, or carcinoma of the superior sulcus (Pancoast syndrome); *Spleen* (left shoulder only) infarction, rupture; *Diaphragm* subphrenic abscess, leaking peptic ulcer; *Stomach and Duodenum* gastritis, peptic ulcer, gastric carcinoma; *Liver and Gallbladder* cholelithiasis, cholecystitis, hepatitis, hepatic cirrhosis or carcinoma, hepatic abscess; *Pancreas* chronic pancreatitis, carcinoma, calculus, or pseudocyst; *Nerves* herpes zoster, brachial plexitis, neoplasm of cervicothoracic vertebrae, myelitis, spinal cord tumor.

KEY SYMPTOM
Pain in the Hip, Thigh, or Leg: Pain in the lower extremity frequently presents the problem of distinguishing between the primary lesion and pain resulting from redistribution of weight bearing to favor the original disorder. For example, limping on a chronically painful foot causes muscle strain in the back, pelvic girdle, and both lower limbs. Painful structures are identified by localization of palpable tenderness and accentuation of the pain with specific movements. Pain arising in somatic tissues (muscle, bone, tendon, ligament) is usually well localized by the patient. Pain also is frequently referred to regional structures innervated by the same spinal segment. As an example, lesions involving the hip joint frequently produce pain in the medial aspect of the knee. An anatomic organization for diagnostic purposes is useful.

✓ *HIP, THIGH, AND LEG PAIN—CLINICAL OCCURRENCE:* *Muscle* strains and tears, hematoma, polymyalgia rheumatica, fibromyalgia, ischemia and infarction, infection, tumors; *Soft Tissues* herniation of fat through muscle fascia, bursitis; *Tendons* tenosynovitis, tendon strain and rupture; *Joints* arthritis (inflammatory, septic, crystal-induced, osteoarthritis), dislocations, sprains; *Bones* fractures, neoplasms, osteomyelitis, osteoporosis, osteomalacia, aseptic necrosis, spondylolisthesis; *Arteries* thrombosis, embolism (thrombus, atheroma, fat, septic vegetations), vasculitis, aneurysm; *Veins* thrombosis, thrombophlebitis, venulitis, venous insufficiency; *Nerves* herniated intervertebral disk, epidural mass, contusion, vasculitis (mononeuritis multiplex), tabes dorsalis, neoplasms (especially neurofibromas), postherpetic neuralgia, peripheral neuropathies (e.g., diabetes and others).

Musculoskeletal and Soft Tissue Signs

Fractures are discussed in this section for the purpose of illustrating relatively common physical findings. This text should not be used as a guide for the definitive diagnosis of traumatic musculoskeletal injuries. Orthopedic texts should be consulted for details, differential diagnosis, and as a guide to diagnosis and management.

General Signs

KEY SIGN
Painless Nodules Near Joints or Tendons:
Several diseases produce painless nodules in joint capsules, tendons, ligaments, or the surrounding connective tissue. Subcutaneous nodules of *rheumatoid arthritis* are usually over bony prominences, where they are loosely attached to articular capsules. They are also found in the periosteum or the deeper layers of the skin. *Gouty tophi,* although usually in bursae, are also formed in the Achilles tendon and the pinna of the ear. Subcutaneous nodules of *rheumatic fever* are freely movable and occur especially over bony prominences or tendons. The diagnostic *xanthomas* of hypercholesterolemia occur in tendons of the hands and in the Achilles tendon and patellar tendon. Juxtaarticular nodes (Jeanselme nodules) occur near joints in syphilis, yaws, and other *treponemal diseases.* Periarticular **calcium deposits** occur in the CREST syndrome and tumoral calcinosis.

KEY SIGN
Nontender Fluctuant Swelling Near Joints and Tendons: Synovial Cyst, Mucoid Cyst:
Pathophysiology: These are either bursae or tendon sheaths distended by fluid or protrusion cysts herniated by hydrostatic pressure from joint capsules. They are usually nontender and fluctuant. The protrusion cysts may collapse under pressure. Synovial cysts occur in the course of *rheumatoid arthritis,* usually on the dorsal aspects of the proximal interphalangeal joints. In osteoarthritis, they commonly occur over the distal interphalangeal joints of the hands and feet. When cysts arise from the extensor sheaths of the wrists, they cause oval swellings on the dorsa of the hands. In this region, the synovial cysts are often called *ganglions.* The protrusion cyst of the knee is known as a *Baker* or *popliteal cyst.*

KEY SIGN
Bursitis: *Pathophysiology:* Bursae are synovial cavities under periarticular tendons or between the skin and bony prominences. Some periarticular bursae communicate with the joint space. Effusions occur as a result of repetitive use trauma, direct blunt or penetrating

trauma, crystal deposition, or infection. The history and exam combined with knowledge of the local anatomy is essential for diagnosis.

KEY SIGN

Crepitation: *Pathophysiology:* Normal joint surfaces produce a smooth, gliding motion without palpable or audible friction or noise. Inflammation, cartilage injury, and loose bodies are often associated with demonstrable friction and crepitation on movement. Moving joints may emit several types of sounds that prompt medical consultation. The knees or hips especially may produce creaking. Crepitus is a grating sound whose vibrations may also be palpated. It is produced by the roughened surfaces of cartilage rubbing together and indicates significant damage to the surface of the joint. Some persons have apparently normal joints that crackle or pop under certain conditions.

KEY SIGN

Muscle Tenderness: Pain in the muscles is distinguished from articular or neuritic pain by eliciting moderate tenderness when the muscle is squeezed between the examiner's thumb and fingers. Tonic muscle contraction is identified as palpable persistent firmness in the muscle. Both muscle and joint pain are intensified by movement. Neuritic pain is associated with tenderness over the nerve trunk and intensification of the pain in the distribution of its branches. Chronic neuritic pain may stimulate secondary tonic muscle contractions.

KEY SIGN

Increased Joint Mobility: *Pathophysiology:* Passive joint motion is restrained by the ligaments attaching the bones on either side of the joint. Active motion is also restrained by muscular contraction. Excessive motion implies disorders of the ligaments. Abnormalities can be congenital or acquired. Acquired laxity results from acute or chronic injury to the ligament(s) leading to disruption and loss of support. It is limited to the affected joint and involves only the motion usually restrained by the affected ligament. There is asymmetry between the affected and the unaffected side. Diffuse joint laxity results from congenital disorders of connective tissue in the Ehlers-Danlos syndromes. Increased laxity of the skin, easy bruising, and poor scar formation are among the more common manifestations of these syndromes.

Axial Musculoskeletal Signs

Neck Signs

KEY SIGN

Neck Pain: Nuchal Headache: Onset of dull pain is unilateral in the occipital region, progressing in a few hours to the back of the eye, where it may persist for hours to days and become throbbing. Palpation of the posterior cervical muscles may disclose one or more trigger points that reproduce the pain, although the muscle itself is not tender. The pain may be reproduced or accentuated by pressing on the vertex of the skull when the neck is bent laterally. Passive extension of the neck may relieve the pain. The physical signs in the neck distinguish the condition from migraine, occipital neuritis, trigeminal neuralgia, and brain tumor.

KEY SIGN

▶ **Pain in the Neck and Shoulder: Pancoast Syndrome (Superior Sulcus Syndrome):** *Pathophysiology:* Lung cancer at the thoracic apex invades locally to involve the pleura, thoracic muscles, and neurovascular bundles, including the brachial plexus and cervical sympathetic chain. Pain is felt in local structures and is referred in the distribution of the involved nerves. Severe pain is present in the posterior part of the shoulder and axilla, often shooting down the arm, with paresthesia of the arm and hand. Paresis or atrophy of arm muscles may occur. In addition to neck and shoulder pain, the complete syndrome includes Horner syndrome (unilateral miosis, ptosis, and absence of sweating on the ipsilateral face and neck). It may be confused with rupture of the supraspinatus tendon, cervical spondylosis, and peripheral neuritis.

KEY SIGN

Pain in the Neck and Shoulder: Cervical Spondylosis (Cervical Osteoarthritis): *Pathophysiology:* Spondylosis results from degeneration of the vertebrae and intervertebral disks. Osteophytes forming about the degenerating tissue may encroach on the intervertebral neural foramina or protrude into the spinal canal. Pain is usually present in the neck or scapula and frequently extends to the shoulder, the occiput, or down the arm with radiculopathy (see *Nuchal Rigidity with Arm Pain: Cervical Syndrome* below). Numbness and tingling of the hands are frequent, but muscle atrophy is rare. Active and passive motions of the neck are restricted and may be painless, but often produce subjective and objective crepitus. Coughing with the head held in extension may reproduce the pain. The biceps tendon reflex is frequently diminished or absent with a radiculopathy of C5 or C6. The triceps reflex is decreased with a radiculopathy of C7. Attribution of the symptoms to spondylosis depends on exclusion of other causes, such as incomplete rupture of the supraspinatus, Pancoast tumor, and peripheral neuropathy.

KEY SIGN

Nuchal Rigidity with Arm Pain: Cervical Syndrome: *Pathophysiology:* Contusion of a cervical root in the neural foramen produces severe pain and disability in the nerve distribution. Commonly, the cause is narrowing of intervertebral foramina or compression of nerve roots by osteophytes. Uncommonly, the lesion is caused by protrusion of an intervertebral disk or by C1-C2 instability from rheumatoid arthritis. Usually minor trauma precedes the onset of pain. Painful spasm of the neck muscles causes temporary torticollis, with the head tilted away from the painful side. Sharp, shooting pains spread slowly down the shoulder, the lateral aspect of the upper arm, and the radial aspect of the forearm, to the wrist. The neck muscles are rigid on the affected side. Tenderness is often present in the trapezius, brachioradialis, pectoralis major, and the forearm extensors. The biceps and triceps jerks are frequently diminished or absent. The hand is occasionally involved with tingling and numbness in the thumb, index and middle fingers. Symptoms remit gradually over days to weeks.

Stiff Neck, With or Without Pain: Tuberculous Spondylitis (Cervical Pott Diseases): *Pathophysiology:* Tuberculosis of the spine is an indolent osteomyelitis of the anterior vertebral endplates with extension to the paravertebral soft tissues. The neck is held stiffly and spontaneous rotation of the head is absent. There may be pain in the neck, but often the neck is painless. When seated, the patient may support her head with the hands (*Rust sign*). An abscess of the cervical vertebra may track to the retropharyngeal space.

 KEY SIGN

Post-traumatic Neck Pain:

Following trauma or suspected cervical injury, the cervical spine must ALWAYS be immediately IMMOBILIZED in a rigid collar PRIOR TO ANY MOVEMENT or examination of the patient.

POST-TRAUMATIC NECK PAIN AND HEADACHE: WHIPLASH CERVICAL INJURY: *Pathophysiology:* Sudden, forceful hyperextension of the neck with flexion recoil commonly occurs to a passenger in an automobile that is struck from behind (Fig. 13-24). Posterior neck pain develops slowly over hours or days. Nerve-root irritation produces spasm of the

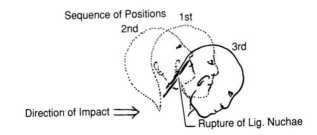

Fig. 13-24 Extension Injury (Whiplash) of the Cervical Spine. *Violent impact from behind produces rapid translation between three sequential positions, causing rupture of the ligamentum nuchae.*

neck muscles and torticollis. Occipital headache develops, sometimes with blurring of vision. The chin is turned toward the painful side of the neck. Palpation over the lower cervical spinous processes elicits tenderness. An effusion with soft crepitus can sometimes be felt over the lowest part of the ligamentum nuchae. The biceps reflex may be diminished or absent on one or both sides. Occasionally, the pupil is dilated on the affected side.

POST-TRAUMATIC NECK PAIN: FRACTURE OF A SPINOUS PROCESS: *Pathophysiology:* The long, thin, spinous process of vertebrae near the cervicothoracic junction break readily from a direct blow or from violent muscular contraction, such as raising a heavy load with a shovel. Sudden, severe pain extends from the neck to the shoulder, accentuated by flexion and rotation of the neck. Tenderness is exquisite over the fracture site. Sometimes the fractured process is mobile laterally and crepitus can be felt.

▶ POST-TRAUMATIC NECK PAIN: FLEXION FRACTURE OF THE NECK: *Pathophysiology:* The C5 vertebral body is most frequently fractured when there is forceful hyperflexion of the neck, for example, when a diver strikes his head on the bottom. The patient who escapes immediate death or quadriplegia may be unable to walk without supporting his head with his hands. Pain restricts all motions of the neck. The spinous process of the affected vertebra is tender and may be somewhat prominent.

▶ POST-TRAUMATIC NECK PAIN: PARTIAL DISLOCATION FROM HYPEREXTENSION: *Pathophysiology:* A fall or blow on the forehead may hyperextend the neck and rupture the anterior longitudinal ligament. There is intense pain in the neck. One spinous process may seem more prominent. Paraplegia frequently occurs.

▶ POST-TRAUMATIC NECK PAIN: FRACTURE OF THE ATLAS (C1) OR THE ODONTOID PROCESS (C2): *Pathophysiology:* Loss of integrity of the vertebral ring of bone and ligament restraining the odontoid process on fracture at the base of the odontoid produce instability of C1 on C2 leading to compression of the cervical spinal cord. If immediate death does not result, the patient supports his head with his hands; he is unwilling to nod his head. There is severe occipital headache. The patient cannot rotate the head. If the clinical diagnosis is not made immediately and the neck completely immobilized, sudden death may ensue. In rheumatoid arthritis, pannus may erode the transverse ligament of C1 that supports the posterior odontoid leading to C1-C2 instability with trivial trauma. A high index of suspicion is required to make the diagnosis.

Thoracolumbar Spine and Pelvis Signs

Dorsal Protrusion from the Spine: Spina Bifida Cystica: *Pathophysiology:* Failure in fusion of the neural arch of a vertebra is spina bifida. In spina bifida occulta, there is no protrusion of the meninges; the only external manifestation may

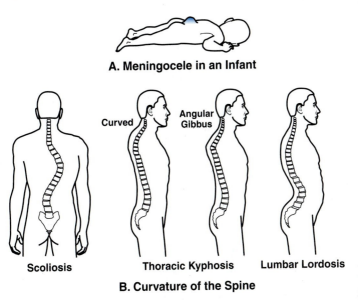

A. Meningocele in an Infant

Curved

Angular Gibbus

Scoliosis **Thoracic Kyphosis** **Lumbar Lordosis**

B. Curvature of the Spine

Fig. 13-25 Spinal Disorders. A. Meningocele. B. Curvatures of the Spine.

be a dimple in the skin, a patch of hair, or a lipomatous nevus. When the meninges form a sac protruding through the defective arch, it is a meningocele (Fig. 13-25A). When the sac contains spinal cord or cauda equina, it is termed a myelomeningocele. The sac is covered by healthy skin; the local swelling is filled with spinal fluid, so it is fluctuant and translucent. With myelomeningocele the overlying skin is frequently defective and transillumination may show cord or nerve fibers. Transmission of pressure from the open fontanelle to the meningocele shows the communication to be wide. Sometimes a sinus leads from a spina bifida occulta to the skin of the sacral region, a congenital sacrococcygeal sinus, often mistaken for a pilonidal sinus.

KEY SIGN

Spinal Deformity, Lateral Deviation: Scoliosis: *Pathophysiology:* Lateral curvature of the thoracic spine is usually accompanied by some rotation of the vertebral bodies, but only the lateral deviations of the spinous processes are visible. Minor functional scoliosis forms a single lateral curve, usually with convexity to the right. With structural changes, the lateral curve in the thorax produces an opposite compensatory curve inferiorly, so the line of spinous processes forms an S-shaped curve. The spinous processes always rotate toward the concave side. On the convex side, rotation of the vertebral bodies causes flattening of the ribs anteriorly and bulging of the chest posteriorly, elevation of the shoulder, and lowering of the hip. Viewed from the patient's back, the posterior bulge is augmented with anteflexion of the spine (see Fig. 13-2). Lateral deviation with a single curve is usually postural, as proved by its disappearance in extreme spinal flexion. An S-shaped or other complex curve may be compensatory or structural (Fig. 13-25B). Compensatory scoliosis occurs with torticollis, thoracoplasty, congenital dislocation of the hip, and shortened lower limb. Structural scoliosis occurs in congenital deformities and paralysis of back or abdominal muscles. It is most often idiopathic, occurring most commonly in adolescent girls.

KEY SIGN

Forward Spinal Curvature: Kyphosis: The forward concavity of the thoracic curve is accentuated, producing a hunchback (see Fig. 13-25B). A smooth curve results from faulty posture, rigid kyphosis of adolescence (Scheuermann disease), ankylosing spondylitis (Marie-Strümpell disease), Paget disease (osteitis deformans), osteoporosis (dowager's hump), acromegaly, and senile kyphosis (dorsum rotundum). Of these, only the curve of faulty posture disappears with spinal extension. In *Gibbus deformity,* an abrupt angular curve caused by the collapse of one or more contiguous vertebrae (see Fig. 13-25B), results from osteoporotic compression fracture, tuberculosis (Pott disease), neoplasm (e.g., multiple myeloma), trauma, or syphilis. In either curved or angular kyphosis, the spinal flexion may force the thorax to permanently assume the inspiratory position, with increased anteroposterior diameter and horizontal ribs. The thoracic distortion is identical with the barrel chest of pulmonary emphysema, but the auscultatory signs of emphysema are absent.

KEY SIGN

Spinal Deformity: Kyphoscoliosis: The thoracic deformity of scoliosis is accentuated and compounded when kyphosis is also present. The thoracic cavity may be so reduced as to compromise the heart and lungs.

KEY SIGN

Backward Spinal Curvature: Lordosis: The normal posterior concavity of the lumbar curve is accentuated (see Fig. 13-25B). Weakness of the anterior abdominal muscles is a common cause. This may occur to counterbalance a protuberant abdomen in pregnancy and obesity or complicate rickets. It compensates for other spinal deformities in spondylolisthesis, thoracic kyphosis, flexion contracture of the hip joint, congenital hip dislocation, coxa vara, and shortening of the Achilles tendons. Accentuation of the lumbar curve throws the thoracic spine backward and the thoracic cage becomes flattened from the pull of the abdomen, causing an expiratory position to be assumed.

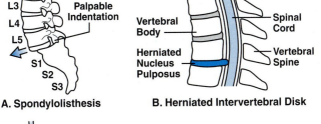

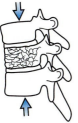 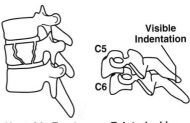

Fig. 13-26 Lesions of a Single Vertebra. A. Spondylolisthesis. B. Herniated Intervertebral Disk. C. Stable Compression Vertebral Fracture. D. Unstable Compression Vertebral Fracture. E. Interlocking or Subluxation of Vertebra.

KEY SIGN
Low Back Pain with Spinal Indentation: Spondylolisthesis: *Pathophysiology:* Usually L5 slips forward on S1 (Fig. 13-26A) because of fracture or degeneration of the articular processes of the neural arch; occasionally, a defect of the lamina may be inherited. If symptoms occur, there is low back pain, often referred to the coccyx or the lateral aspect of the leg (L5 dermatome). Inspection frequently discloses a transverse loin crease. Palpation of the lumbar spine reveals a deep recession of the spinous process of L5. There is restricted flexion of the lower spine.

KEY SIGN
Post-traumatic Mid-Back Pain: Stable Compression Fracture of Vertebral Body (with Intact Spinal Ligaments): *Pathophysiology:* The thoracic or lumbar vertebrae are fractured by trauma that crushes their bodies, such as forceful hyperflexion of the spine, falling and landing on the feet or buttocks, or a downward blow on the shoulders (see Fig. 13-26C). Pain and tenderness at the fracture site may be mild or even absent for weeks, so fracture may not be suspected until a radiograph is obtained. Occasionally, slight kyphosis is present.

▶
Post-traumatic Mid-Back Pain: Unstable Compression Fracture of Vertebral Body (with Torn Spinal Ligaments): *Pathophysiology:* Rupture of the interspinal and supraspinal ligaments, accompanying the compression fracture, permits the articular facets of two adjacent vertebrae to slide apart; on recoil, they may interlock (see Fig. 13-26E). This dangerous condition may be suggested clinically by palpating a gap between two spinous processes (see Fig. 13-26D).

▶
Post-traumatic Back Pain: Fracture–Dislocation of Vertebrae: *Pathophysiology:* Violent hyperflexion of the spine, in addition to fracturing the vertebrae, may tear the supporting ligaments, permitting vertebral dislocation and consequent damage to the spinal cord. This is a potentially unstable condition requiring immediate immobilization and evaluation. This should be suspected when the palpating finger finds a gap between two spinous processes.

Post-traumatic Low Back Pain: Fracture of a Transverse Process: *Pathophysiology:* Usually, the transverse process of a lumbar vertebra is fractured from violent contraction of the attached muscles. There is severe pain in the lumbar region, with intense muscle spasm. The spinous processes are not tender. If caused by a direct blow, look for blood in the urine to identify a concomitant kidney injury.

S
▼ **Chronic Back Pain: Ankylosing Spondylitis (Marie-Strümpell-Bechterew Syndrome):** Nonspecific symptoms often begin in adolescence and occur intermittently for 5 or 10 years. In the late teens or early twenties, pain and significant morning stiffness are felt in the lumbar region, buttocks, and sacroiliac region. The spine loses its flexibility: the normal lumbar lordosis is straightened with diminished anterior flexion and spinal rotation and lateral bending are impaired. Slowly the process ascends the lumbar and thoracic spine, the cervical region may be involved late. Fatigue, fever, and weight loss may occur. Episodes of acute or subacute arthritis may involve hip, knee, shoulder, sternoclavicular, or manubriosternal joints. Tenderness is found over the involved joints. Iridocyclitis occurs in one-fifth of the cases. Aortic regurgitation is a late complication in 3% of patients. DDX: Idiopathic ankylosing spondylitis needs to be distinguished from psoriatic arthritis and reactive spondyloarthritis (Crohn disease, ulcerative colitis, Reiter disease), Whipple disease, and diffuse idiopathic spinal hyperostosis (DISH).

Appendicular Skeleton, Joint, Ligament, Tendon, and Soft-Tissue Signs

Finger Signs

Some abnormalities of the fingers have been included in consideration of the entire hand; the more localized disorders are discussed here.

Malformation: Polydactyly (Supernumerary Fingers): The condition may be congenital, familial, or associated with certain syndromes. In the Lawrence-Moon-Biedl syndrome, polydactyly is associated with juvenile obesity, retinal degeneration, genital hypoplasia, and mental retardation; approximately 80% of the cases of this syndrome are familial.

Malformation: Syndactyly (Webbed Fingers): This congenital deformity may be hereditary. The web may be only soft tissue, or it may cover fused bones. Scar tissue from burns may form an acquired web.

Divergent Fingers: Trident Hands: A characteristic of achondroplasia, the fingers approach uniform length and radiate from the hand like the spokes in a wheel with a fat hub (Fig. 13-27D).

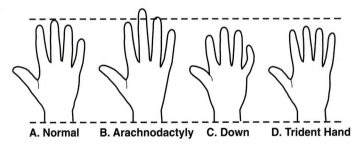

A. Normal   B. Arachnodactyly   C. Down   D. Trident Hand

Fig. 13-27 Congenitally Disproportionate Hands. A. A Normal Hand: In practically all normal male hands, the ring finger is longer than the index finger; most women have longer index fingers, although a few exceptions occur. B. Arachnodactyly: The fingers are remarkable for their length and slenderness; the joints are abnormally hyperextensible. This occurs in Marfan syndrome. C. Down Syndrome: The digits are short and the little finger often has a peculiar radialward curve. D. Trident Hand: This occurs in achondroplasia. The fingers are short and almost equal in length; the index and middle fingers are widely separated.

KEY SIGN

Thumb Pain Following a Fall: Ulnar Collateral Ligament Sprain:
There is a history of a fall onto the palm, often while grasping an object with the thumb. The patient complains of pain in the metacarpophalangeal (MCP) joint of the thumb and an inability to exert significant pressure on the pad of the thumb tip without pain or giving way. Exam shows tenderness and laxity of the ulnar collateral ligament.

KEY SIGN

Painless Nodules on the Interphalangeal Joints: Heberden and Bouchard Nodes:
Pathophysiology: These findings are a result of marginal osteophytes on the distal interphalangeal (DIP) and proximal interphalangeal (PIP) joints. Heberden nodes of the DIP joints are hard nodules, 2–3 mm in diameter, one on either side of the dorsal midline (Fig. 13-28K). They are usually painless, motion is slightly limited, and deformity is progressive, but function is preserved. They are more pronounced on the dominant hand. Involvement begins in several joints most commonly in peri- or postmenopausal women. The condition in women is usually hereditary and the process is a result of osteoarthritis. A single Heberden node may result from trauma. Nodules on the PIP joints are called Bouchard nodes. They occur together with Heberden nodes, but somewhat less frequently than the latter.

KEY SIGN

Clubbing of the Fingers:
Clubbing has intrigued physicians since Hippocrates because of its association with serious systemic disorders. The mechanism is unknown, but clubbing is reversible when the cause is removed. The three key observations are floating of the nail base, loss of the unguophalangeal angle, and increased longitudinal convexity of the nail plate. Clubbing is painless and usually bilateral. With long-standing clubbing, the soft tissue and terminal phalanx become thickened, the convexity of the nail plate is extreme, and the fingers are bulbous; appropriate terms are drumstick fingers or parrot's beak. In the literal sense, the term clubbing should be reserved for this late stage, but it is now applied to the general process in all stages, from the first sign of floating nail. The floating nails and alteration of the unguophalangeal angle distinguish clubbing from all other conditions. Convexity alone is seen in other conditions or as a normal variant (certain occupations, inherited forms).

DEMONSTRATING CLUBBING. *Obliteration of the Unguophalangeal Angle (Lovibond Angle):* Inspect the profile of the terminal digit. Normally, the nail makes an angle of 20 degrees or more with the projected line of the digit. With clubbing, this angle is diminished or may be obliterated or extend below the projected line of the digit (Fig. 13-29). *Floating Nail:* Palpate the proximal nail with the tip of your finger. You can feel and see the springy softness as the root of the nail is depressed (Fig. 13-29). This may be simulated as follows: with your right index finger

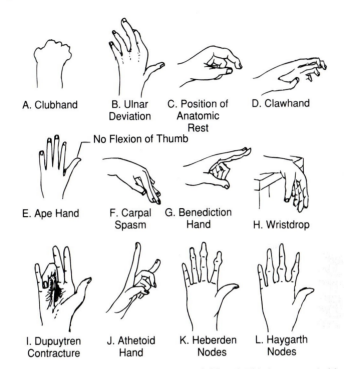

Fig. 13-28 Deformities of the Hand. *A. Clubhand: This is a congenital lesion in which the hand development is rudimentary; the stub may be surmounted by rudimentary or normal digits. B. Ulnar Deviation: Also called ulnar drift. C. Position of Anatomic Rest. D. Clawhand. E. Ape Hand. F. Carpal Spasm. G. Benediction Hand. H. Wrist-drop. I. Dupuytren Contracture. J. Athetoid Hand. K. Heberden Nodes. L. Haygarth Nodes: The spindle-shaped enlargements of the middle interphalangeal joints occur in rheumatoid arthritis.*

press the mantle of your left middle finger; the plate rests snugly against the bone without movement. Now depress the free edge of the nail with your left thumb and test the mantle again with your right index finger; the plate root now sinks with pressure and springs back when released. *Convexity of the Nail:* A month or so after the floating nail and nail angle changes occur, a transverse ridge appears in the plate from beneath the mantle. The ridge marks the change from the normal distal curve to a new curve of smaller radius in the proximal nail.

The floating nail and flattened angle occur rapidly, for example, within 10 days after a tonsillectomy complicated by lung abscess. With chronic illness of over 6 months the entire nail has abnormal convexity. The sequence of changes can occasionally be observed in a patient with subacute bacterial endocarditis. When first seen with a 3-month history

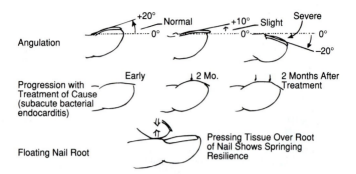

Fig. 13-29 Characteristics of Clubbed Fingers. *There are three principal signs of clubbing of the fingers: (1) angulation; (2) curvature of the nail; and (3) floating nail root.*

of illness, a transition ridge is visible (see Fig. 13-29). After treatment of the infection a second ridge appears, this one marking the transition between distal abnormal curvature and proximal normal profile.

✓ *CLUBBING—CLINICAL OCCURRENCE:* *Congenital* cyanotic congenital heart disease, familial, cystic fibrosis; *Endocrine* hypothyroidism; *Idiopathic* chronic obstructive lung disease, bronchiectasis; *Inflammatory/Immune* inflammatory bowel disease, biliary cirrhosis, alcoholic cirrhosis; *Infectious* infective endocarditis, lung abscess, pulmonary tuberculosis; *Neoplastic* lung cancer, metastatic cancer to lung, mesothelioma; *Vascular* hypertrophic osteoarthropathy, pulmonary arteriovenous malformations (including dialysis shunts).

CLUBBING WITH PERIOSTOSIS: HYPERTROPHIC PULMONARY OSTEOARTHROPATHY: Hypertrophic osteoarthropathy (HOA) is recognized by clubbing and periosteal new bone formation. Acquired HOA results from systemic disease (see page 792). Primary hereditary HOA (Marie-Bamberger syndrome) is an autosomal dominant syndrome, which is expressed much more commonly in males. It has clubbing, greasy thickening of the skin, especially noticeable on the face, and hyperhidrosis of the hands and feet.

● KEY SIGN

Swelling of the Fingers: Dactylitis, Sausage Digits: Inflammation of the entheses of one or more fingers produces fusiform swelling with or without joint effusion in patients with reactive and psoriatic arthritis. Dactylitis is also seen in the hand–foot syndrome of sickle cell or sickle–thalassemia disease.

Fusiform Monarticular Swelling: Sprain of an Interphalangeal Joint: A painful fusiform joint swelling may persist for several months. In most cases, there is a history of trauma.

Localized Swelling Over a Joint: Synovial or Mucous Cyst: A synovial cyst results from myxomatous degeneration of a joint capsule. A small, tense nodule appears over an interphalangeal joint; frequently it is mistaken for a sesamoid bone. It may be so tense that it feels bony hard; usually it is not fluctuant. Pressure may elicit slight tenderness. Often there is slight transverse mobility.

KEY SIGN

Flexion Deformity of Distal Finger Joint: Mallet Finger: *Pathophysiology:* This is caused by rupture of the extensor tendon that inserts on the terminal phalanx or avulsion fracture of the distal phalanx. The terminal phalanx of the finger is flexed at the distal interphalangeal (DIP) joint and cannot be voluntarily extended (Fig. 13-30A).

KEY SIGN

Extension Deformity of the PIP Joint: Swan Neck Deformity: *Pathophysiology:* Fixed extension of the proximal interphalangeal (PIP) joint occurs when the flexor tendons are injured or sublux to the dorsum of the joint, holding the joint in extension. This deformity is common in rheumatoid arthritis and systemic lupus erythematosus. In the latter, it is usually reducible, a *Jaccoud-type deformity.*

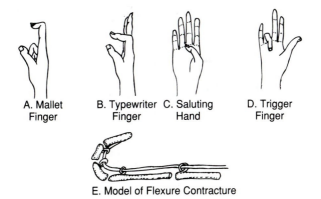

A. Mallet Finger B. Typewriter Finger C. Saluting Hand D. Trigger Finger

E. Model of Flexure Contracture

Fig. 13-30 Acquired Flexion Deformities of the Fingers. A. Mallet Finger. B. Boutonnière Deformity: There is permanent flexion of the proximal interphalangeal joint from rupture of the extensor tendon inserting on the middle phalanx, giving a position similar to that employed when using a typewriter or computer keyboard. C. Saluting Hand: The thumb is limply flexed in the palm and cannot be voluntarily extended. D. Trigger Finger: The fourth or ring finger moves into flexion painlessly, but attempted extension is temporarily impeded. Extension is accomplished with a palpable snap. E. Flexure Contractures of the Fingers: With sheath adhesions, passive motion of the tendon is nil, even with wrist flexion.

Flexion Deformity of the PIP Joint: Boutonnière Deformity, Typewriter Finger: *Pathophysiology:* This results from rupture of the central band of the extensor tendon that inserts on the middle phalanx. Volar subluxation of the intact lateral band to the distal phalanx holds the finger in flexion. The finger is flexed at its proximal interphalangeal (PIP) and lacks voluntary extension (see Fig. 13-30B). Extension followed by flexion of the PIP joint may produce a palpable or audible diagnostic click, as the lateral slips of the distal extensor tendons diverge and slip laterally over the head of the proximal phalanx, hence, buttonhole rupture.

Flexion Deformity of the Thumb: Saluting Hand: *Pathophysiology:* Extension at the thumb metacarpophalangeal (MCP) and interphalangeal joint is performed by the extensor pollicis longus tendon; rupture leads to loss of function. This is approximately the position of the hand in an American military salute (see Fig. 13-30C). The thumb is limply flexed in the palm and cannot be voluntarily extended. The tendon is often worn through by moving over the fragments of a Colles fracture; rupture may occur from 3 weeks to 4 months after the fracture has been reduced.

Snapping or Locking of Finger: Trigger Finger: *Pathophysiology:* A nodular thickening forms in the long flexor tendon just proximal to the metacarpal head as a result of inflammation or repetitive trauma. With finger extension, the nodule lies within the tendon sheath; during flexion, it is pulled without difficulty from the proximal end of the sheath by the flexor muscles. During finger extension by the weaker extensor muscles, the constricted mouth of the sheath resists reentry of the nodule. Entry is suddenly achieved with a noticeable click. Either the middle or ring finger is usually involved (see Fig. 13-30D). Flexion of the finger feels normal, but extension is accompanied by a snap that the patient sometimes refers to the region of the proximal interphalangeal (PIP) joint. The nodule can be palpated moving with the tendon on active or passive flexion-extension. Triggering may or may not be painful.

Contracture of a Flexor Tendon: Tendon Adhesions or Tendon Shortening: *Pathophysiology:* Adhesions between a tendon and its sheath are caused by tenosynovitis. Fibrotic shortening of the tendon without synovial adhesions occurs in Volkmann ischemic contracture (page 740). Distinction between the two mechanisms can be made with the wrist flexed. Grasp the tip of the flexed finger and pull it into extension. With the slack provided by wrist flexion, the shortened tendon permits partial extension; adhesions to the sheath or palmar fascia entirely prevent extension (see Fig. 13-30E).

KEY SIGN

Flexion Deformity from Tight Skin: Sclerodactyly: *Pathophysiology:* In scleroderma, the skin and underlying tissues become contracted and fibrosed. Movements of the digits are inhibited by the tight envelope, but there is no ankylosis or swelling of joint. All digits are usually involved, Raynaud phenomenon is nearly always present, and calcinosis of the skin may occur. Skin in other areas of the body is progressively involved in the sclerodermatous process with thickening, stiffening, hyperpigmentation, and limited motion. Opening the mouth, swallowing, and respiratory movements may be limited. With muscle contracture or tendon adhesions, the skin is normal.

KEY SIGN

Digital Infection: Deep tissue infections in the fingers are initially limited to specific tissue compartments giving characteristic signs.

Paronychia: The skin over the matrix of the nail and the lateral nail folds is swollen, reddened, painful, and tender (Fig. 13-31A). When infection is over the nail root, light palpation of the inflamed area provokes exquisite pain. Pain from pressure on the nail plate indicates subungual abscess, between nail plate and periosteum.

Digital Inflammation: Chronic Paronychia: *Candida* paronychia is minimally tender and does not drain. Chronic ulceration of the nail mantle and lateral folds occurs in occupations requiring fre-

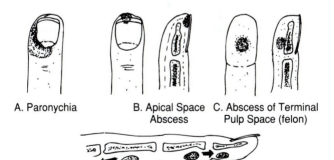

A. Paronychia   B. Apical Space Abscess   C. Abscess of Terminal Pulp Space (felon)

D. Abscess of Volar Spaces

Fig. 13-31 Common Locations for Finger Abscesses. A. Paronychia. B. Abscess of the Apical Spaces: The apical space is located in the nail bed near the free margin of the nail plate. C. Abscess of the Terminal Pulp Space (Felon): The stippled region on the volar surface represents the site of rupture through the skin. D. Abscess of the Volar Spaces: The stippled regions are the sites of abscesses; the arrows point in the direction of burrowing to reach the flexor creases of the finger.

quent immersion of the hands in water or contaminated oil. The ulcers are indolent; abscess formation is rare.

Digital Infection: Abscess of the Terminal Pulp Space (Felon): Inflammation of the terminal finger pad is confined within small fascial compartments attached to the periosteum (see Fig. 13-31C). The onset is heralded by swelling of the fingertip and dull pain. The pain gradually heightens and becomes intense and throbbing and the tip exquisitely tender. The presence of pus is indicated by induration of the pulp and loss of resilience. The great pressure in the confined space may cause the abscess to burst through the volar surface of the finger pad. Osteomyelitis may occur.

Digital Infection: Abscess of the Apical Space: Symptoms follow a puncture wound beneath the nail, as the distal quarter of nail bed becomes extremely painful without much swelling (Fig. 13-31B). The nail bed shows red through the plate. Maximum tenderness is proximal to the free edge of the plate, unlike a felon, which produces tenderness at the fingertip. When the abscess ruptures, drainage is at the free edge of the nail plate.

Digital Infection: Abscess of the Middle Volar Pulp Space: The finger is held in partial flexion to reduce the pain. A painful, tender swelling occurs on the volar aspect of the finger between the distal interphalangeal (DIP) and proximal interphalangeal (PIP) joints (see Fig. 13-31D). The symptoms resemble those of the felon. Osteomyelitis may occur or the abscess may burst after burrowing to the distal flexor crease.

Digital Infection: Abscess of the Proximal Volar Pulp Space: An abscess forms on the volar aspect between the middle and proximal joints (see Fig. 13-31D). The symptoms and signs are similar to those in the middle space, except the infection burrows proximally to involve the web space.

Nodules in the Finger Web: Barber's Pilonidal Sinus: Short hair shafts may penetrate the skin of the finger webs and produce inflammation. One or more nodules may be felt in the soft skin; they are drained by sinuses, which are seen as black dots between the fingers.

KEY SIGN
Nodules in Finger Pads: Osler's Nodes: *Pathophysiology:* Septic emboli from infective endocarditis lodge in the cutaneous vessels producing microscopic abscesses. These are pea-sized, tender bluish or pink nodules, sometimes with a blanched center, which occur on the pads of the fingers, palms of the hands, and soles of the feet in some patients with infective endocarditis.

Digital Fractures and Dislocations: Given an appropriate history, the physical signs of tenderness and deformity are sufficient to indicate the diagnosis.

Circulatory Disorders of the Fingers: See Chapter 8, pages 440–443 and 485–490.

Janeway Spots: Janeway spots are only a few millimeters in diameter. They appear over a few hours or days as crops of erythematous or hemorrhagic, macular or nodular lesions. They occur in the palms, soles, or distal finger pads. Although painless and nontender, they may ulcerate. Most writers consider them hallmarks of bacterial endocarditis or mycotic aneurysm. The causative organisms have been isolated from the lesions.

KEY SIGN
Fingernail Signs: See Chapter 6, pages 152–158.

Palm Signs

KEY SIGN
Yellow Palms: Carotenemia: *Pathophysiology:* The yellow skin color is imparted by fat-soluble carotene concentrated in the stratum corneum of the creases on the palms and soles. The pigment is excreted in the sebum by the sebaceous glands. The water-soluble pigments of bilirubinemia are more uniformly distributed, including coloration of the sclerae and thin skin. Excessive carotene excretion occurs from chronic ingestion of large quantities of carrots, squash, oranges, peaches, apricots, and leafy vegetables. Because carotene is converted to vitamin A in the liver with the assistance of thyroid hormone, carotenoderma is more common in hypothyroidism.

Granular Palms: Hyperkeratoses: Palpation with the fingertips discloses rough granular excrescences in the horny layer. The most common cause is chronic arsenic poisoning. A rare cause is *hyperkeratosis (tylosis) palmaris et plantaris,* an autosomal dominant disease.

KEY SIGN
Thenar Atrophy: *Pathophysiology:* The thenar eminence is formed by the bellies of *opponens pollicis, abductor pollicis brevis* and *flexor pollicis brevis* innervated by the median nerve; denervation leads to atrophy. Atrophy suggests a lesion of the median nerve, most commonly carpal tunnel syndrome, or severe osteoarthritis at the base of the thumb. Diminution in size of the eminence may accompany general atrophy of all intrinsic hand muscles (Fig. 13-32B).

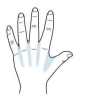

A. Interosseous Atrophy   **B. Thenar Atrophy**   **C. Hypothenar Atrophy**

Fig. 13-32 Atrophy of the Intrinsic Muscles of the Hand.   *Regions of atrophy are indicated by stippling.*

KEY SIGN

Hypothenar Atrophy: *Pathophysiology:* The hypothenar eminence is formed by the bellies of *palmaris brevis, abductor digiti quinti, flexor digiti quinti,* and *opponens digiti quinti* innervated by the ulnar nerve; denervation leads to atrophy. Atrophy suggests damage to the ulnar nerve (see Fig. 13-32C). If both thenar and hypothenar atrophy are present, consider cervical myelopathy.

KEY SIGN

Localized Thickening of Palmar Fascia: Dupuytren's Contracture: See page 738. An early finding, antedating the contracture, is the palpation of a thick, nontender, nodular thickening in the palmar fascia (see Fig. 13-28I).

KEY SIGN

Painful Palmar Swelling: Web Space Infection: Fever, malaise, and diffuse pain in the hand, with dorsal edema occur early. When localization has occurred, the two involved fingers are separated by swelling at their bases. The skin over the web, both back and front, is reddened. Maximal tenderness is located on the palmar surface near the base of the involved finger (Fig. 13-33A).

KEY SIGN

► **Painful Palmar Swelling: Infection of the Thenar Space:** The affected thenar eminence is swollen, tender, and may show erythema and warmth. The interphalangeal joint of the thumb may be flexed, but extension is not resisted as it is in tenosynovitis of the flexor pollicis longus.

KEY SIGN

► **Painful Palmar Swelling: Deep Abscess of the Palm:** In addition to severe dorsal edema, the concavity of the palm is obliterated, or even elevated; the raised area is tender.

KEY SIGN

► **Painful Palmar Swelling: Abscess of the Ulnar Bursa:** There is dorsal edema and fullness on the ulnar side of the palm (see Fig. 13-33A). The point of maximum tenderness is halfway between the lunate and the fifth metacarpophalangeal joint.

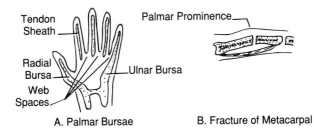

Tendon Sheath

Palmar Prominence

Radial Bursa

Ulnar Bursa

Web Spaces

A. Palmar Bursae

B. Fracture of Metacarpal

Fig. 13-33 Swellings of the Hand. A. Palmar Bursae: The locations of the bursae are indicated by stippling. Note the tendon sheaths ending proximally near the palmar crease; there is a connection between the radial and ulnar bursae. The radial bursa is continuous from the thumb to the region of the thenar eminence. The web spaces are indicated as sites of abscesses. B. Fracture of a Metacarpal Bone: Diagram shows displacement of the fragments into the palm, where an abnormal prominence may be noted.

○ KEY SIGN
Painful Palmar Swelling: Abscess of the Radial Bursa: The interphalangeal joint of the thumb is flexed and passive extension produces pain. There is tenderness and swelling over the sheath of the flexor pollicis longus.

○ KEY SIGN
Painful Palmar and Digital Swelling: Acute Suppurative Flexor Tenosynovitis: Throbbing pain may begin in a finger and progress toward the palm. Dorsal edema appears and the entire finger swells. The affected finger is held in the posture of rest, slightly flexed, and the patient will not move the finger. Gentle passive extension of adjacent fingers is painful, so the examiner should not attempt to test the affected finger. To find the point of maximum tenderness, have the patient rest the supinated hand on a table. Test for tenderness by gently palpating with the blunt end of an applicator or tongue depressor. If the point is located at the proximal end of the tendon sheath of the index, middle, or ring finger, involvement of the sheath is certain. If there is no localization, the sheath may have ruptured.

○ KEY SIGN
Painful Palmar Swelling: Fracture of a Metacarpal Bone: In a transverse fracture, the fragments of the metacarpal bone are bowed into the palm to produce a painful prominence (see Fig. 13-33B). The prominence may be obscured by soft-tissue swelling, but dorsal palpation will localize tenderness at the fracture site. In a spiral fracture, proximal slippage of the distal fragment produces shortening revealed by loss of prominence in the corresponding knuckle when the fist is closed. Rotation of the distal fragment is present if the affected finger is not aligned with the unaffected fingers when the tips are flexed onto the base of the thenar eminence. Bennett

fracture is an oblique break through the base of the first metacarpal, frequently with subluxation of the carpal–metacarpal joint. The thumb is semiflexed, and it cannot be opposed to the ring or little finger and the fist cannot be clenched.

Hand and Wrist Signs

KEY SIGN

Swelling of the Wrist: The anatomic location of swelling is identified by the physical signs. Periarticular edema in the subcutaneous tissues around the joint, but outside the synovium, pits with pressure. With thickening of the joint capsule and synovium the tissues feel boggy. When the synovial envelope is bulging and fluctuant, fluid is present. Effusion, pus, or blood are identified by aspiration. With bony enlargement, palpation may distinguish between osteophytes at the joint margins, local bone tumors, or acromegalic hyperplasia.

KEY SIGN

Painful Swelling or Limited Motion of the Wrist: Chronic Arthritis: With active inflammation, there is enlargement of the wrist joint, accompanied by variable degrees of pain and tenderness. The overlying skin may be warm and reddened. In rheumatoid arthritis, there is limited motion. The joint is swollen, red, hot, and tender with gout, pseudogout, and septic arthritis. Primary osteoarthritis does not affect the wrist.

KEY SIGN

Painful Swelling in the Anatomic Snuffbox: Acute Tenosynovitis: Pain is experienced in the region of the snuffbox. A sausage-like swelling, about 4 cm long (Fig. 13-34C), involves the tendon sheath of the extensor pollicis brevis and abductor pollicis longus at the radial border of the snuffbox. With thumb extension crepitus can be felt over the sheath. The cause is usually trauma, although inflammation can be produced by gout or gonococcal infection.

KEY SIGN

Chronic Pain in the Anatomic Snuffbox: Chronic Stenosing Tenosynovitis (De Quervain Tenosynovitis): The tendon sheath of the extensor pollicis brevis is maximally painful on palpation over the radial styloid. In longstanding cases, one or two swellings the size of orange seeds are palpable in the snuffbox near the radial styloid process. Chronic inflammation involves all layers of the tendon sheath. When the fist is clenched over the flexed thumb, gentle but firm ulnar deviation of the hand by the examiner elicits pain at the radial styloid process (*Finkelstein test,* see Fig. 13-34B). This pain may be transmitted down the thumb or toward the elbow. Passive extension of the thumb is painless.

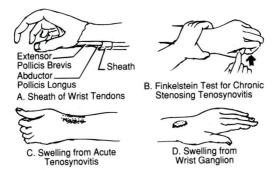

Extensor
Pollicis Brevis
Abductor � Sheath
Pollicis Longus
A. Sheath of Wrist Tendons

B. Finkelstein Test for Chronic
Stenosing Tenosynovitis

C. Swelling from Acute
Tenosynovitis

D. Swelling from
Wrist Ganglion

Fig. 13-34 Some Disorders of the Wrist. *A. Sheaths of the Wrist Tendons: This shows the sheath, which swells to obstruct the motion of the tendons of extensor pollicis brevis and abductor pollicis longus in chronic stenosing tenosynovitis. B. Finkelstein Test for Tenosynovitis: The patient clenches his fist on his thumb while the examiner pushes the fist toward the ulna. A positive test elicits pain at the radial styloid process. C. Swelling from Acute Nonsuppurative Tenosynovitis. D. Frequent Site of Ganglion of the Wrist: The swelling is painless and sometimes translucent.*

KEY SIGN

Localized Painless Swelling on the Dorsum: Ganglion: A cyst from myxomatous degeneration of the joint capsule usually occurs on the dorsum of the naviculolunate joint (see Fig. 13-34D). The swelling is round, sessile, tense, and translucent. Flexion of the wrist brings it into prominence, extension obscures it.

KEY SYNDROME

Numbness, Tingling, and Pain in the Hand: Carpal Tunnel Syndrome (Compression Neuropathy of the Median Nerve in the Carpal Tunnel): *Pathophysiology:* The median nerve is compressed in the channel beneath the volar transverse carpal ligament of the wrist (Fig. 13-35). Progressive compression of the nerve initially produces dysesthesia and pain, then loss of fine (two-point) sensation, and, finally, thenar muscle atrophy and weakness. The patient complains of numbness and tingling in the hand, particularly at night. There may be associated pain, limited to the hand or running up the forearm. Ultimately, there is progressive weakness and awkwardness in the finer movements of the fingers. It may be unilateral or bilateral. Although patients frequently describe tingling of the entire hand, hypoesthesia is distributed on the palmar aspects of the 3.5 radial digits and the distal two-thirds of the dorsal aspects of the same fingers. Light percussion on the radial side of the palmaris longus tendon may produce a tingling sensation (*Tinel sign*, Fig. 13-35). Flexion of the wrists at 90 degrees with the dorsal surfaces of the hands in apposition for 60 seconds (*Phalen test*) may reproduce the pain (Fig. 13-35). Neither maneuver is particularly sen-

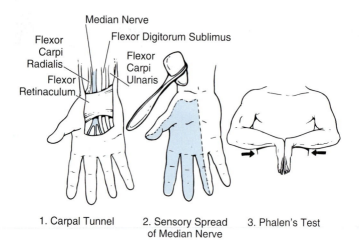

1. Carpal Tunnel   2. Sensory Spread   3. Phalen's Test
                             of Median Nerve

Fig. 13-35 Carpal Tunnel Syndrome. 1. The Carpal Tunnel: The flexor retinaculum in the wrist compresses the median nerve to produce hyperesthesia in the radial digits. 2. Tinel Sign: Percussion on the radial side of the palmaris longus tendon produces tingling in the digital region. 3. Phalen Test: Hyperflexion of the wrist for 60 seconds produces pain in the median nerve distribution, which is relieved by extension of the wrist.

sitive or specific for the finding of nerve injury by nerve conduction studies. The condition is most common with repetitive use injury, for example, meat-packing workers, grocery clerks, and keyboard operators [Katz JN, Simmons BP. Carpal tunnel syndrome. *N Engl J Med* 2002;346: 1807–1812; D'Arcy CA, McGee S. The rational clinical examination. Does this patient have carpal tunnel syndrome? *JAMA* 2000;283:3110–3117].

✔ *CARPAL TUNNEL SYNDROME—CLINICAL OCCURRENCE:* *Congenital* congenitally small carpal tunnel; *Endocrine* hypothyroidism, diabetes, acromegaly, pregnancy; *Idiopathic* osteoarthritis; *Inflammatory/ Immune* rheumatoid arthritis, amyloidosis, sarcoidosis; *Metabolic/ Toxic* gout, Paget disease; *Mechanical/Traumatic* repetitive wrist flexion and extension, posttraumatic arthritis; *Neoplastic* multiple myeloma, MGUS.

Abnormal Hand Posture: Position of Anatomic Rest: In inflammation of the hand, the parts are held in this position to ease the pain, with fingers and thumb flexed, the index finger less bent than the others (see Fig. 13-28C, page 725).

KEY SIGN

Abnormal Hand Posture: Ulnar Deviation or Drift of Fingers: Most common in rheumatoid arthritis, primarily as a result of muscle atrophy and the muscle pull on subluxated joints. The fingers deviate at the metacarpophalangeal joints toward the ulna. There may also be subluxations of the metacarpophalangeal (MCP) joint (see Fig. 13-28B, page 725).

KEY SIGN

Abnormal Hand Posture: Diabetic Hand, Diabetic Cheiropathy: In long-standing diabetes, the soft tissues of the hand become thick and contracted, bending the fingers into a slightly flexed position. Have the patient attempt to place the palms together; a space will remain between the palms and fingers in a "prayer sign."

KEY SIGN

Abnormal Hand Posture: Clawhand: *Pathophysiology:* This occurs from the predominant pull of the extensor communis digitorum and the flexor digitorum against weak or paralyzed interosseus and lumbrical muscles. The claw is caused by hyperextension of the metacarpophalangeal joints and flexion of the interphalangeal articulations (see Fig. 13-28D, page 725). Paralysis may result from brachial plexus, ulnar and median nerve injuries, syringomyelia, the muscular atrophies, or acute poliomyelitis.

Abnormal Hand Posture: Ape Hand: The thumb is held in extension by its inability to flex (see Fig. 13-28E). This may occur in syringomyelia, progressive muscular atrophy, or amyotrophic lateral sclerosis.

KEY SIGN

Abnormal Hand Posture: Carpal Spasm: The characteristic position occurs in tetany (Fig. 13-28F, page 725) and hand dystonia associated with repetitive hand activities. This is also called obstetrician's hand because it somewhat resembles the position of the physician's hand in performing a pelvic examination. The thumb is flexed on the palm, the wrist and metacarpophalangeal joints are flexed, while the interphalangeal joints are hyperextended and the fingers are adducted in the shape of a cone. All the hand muscles are rigid. The spasm is involuntary and usually painless. This posture occurs in tetany; when present, it is involuntary and cannot be altered by the patient.

Abnormal Hand Posture: Benediction Hand (Preacher's Hand): The ring and little fingers cannot be extended while the other digits move normally and may be extended to produce the posture (see Fig. 13-28G, page 725). This occurs in ulnar nerve palsy, syringomyelia, and extensor tendon rupture in rheumatoid arthritis. It is named from the ecclesiastical gesture of pronouncing benediction. Do not confuse with Dupuytren contracture of the palmar fascia.

Abnormal Hand Posture: Wrist-Drop: This results from weakness of the wrist extensors. When the pronated hand is held horizontally without support from beneath, it drops from the wrist because of weakness of the extensors (see Fig. 13-28H, page 725), which are unable to overcome gravity. Common causes are radial nerve palsy, poliomyelitis, neuropathy from lead or arsenic poisoning and radial nerve compression.

Abnormal Hand Posture: Dupuytren Contracture (Palmar Fibrosis): *Pathophysiology:* This disorder is a painless nodular thickening of the palmar aponeurosis from hyalinization of collagen fibers beginning near the base of the digit. It extends to form a plaque or band adhering to the palmar fascia and producing retraction and dimpling of the palmar skin and flexion contracture of the fingers. It usually begins after the age of 40 years as an inconspicuous nodule, which is often not noted by the patient until finger deformity occurs. One or both hands may be involved. The ring finger is most often affected, but others may be involved, in order of diminishing frequency, the little, long, index, and thumb. Retraction of the fascia forces the affected finger into partial flexion (see Fig. 13-28I, page 725). Palpation of the palm reveals a hard cord over the tendon. Passive extension of the finger raises the cord taut, where it can be readily seen. With progression, a painless contracture of the digit results that may require surgical correction. The contracture, named after the French surgeon Baron Guillaume Dupuytren, is considered by some writers as the prototypical manifestation of Dupuytren disease. Less-common manifestations, occurring singly or in combination, are plantar fibrosis (Lederhosen syndrome), knuckle pads, plastic induration of the penis (Peyronie disease), and fibrosis of the male breast (fibrosis mammae virilis). Approximately 40% of the patients have affected kin; only whites are susceptible. Men are affected twice as often as women. The manifestations are more common in persons with alcoholism, epilepsy, or diabetes mellitus; the cause for these associations is unknown.

Abnormal Hand Posture: Athetoid Hand: A grotesque pattern is seen in athetosis in which involuntary muscle contractions produce simultaneous flexion of some digits and hyperextension of others, resembling the writhing of a snake (see Fig. 13-28J, page 725).

Large Hands: Acromegaly and Gigantism: See page 774. The bones of the hands are perfectly proportioned, but soft-tissue overgrowth increases the finger girth, making them ponderous, a paw hand or spade hand. Acromegalic arthritis is frequently present.

Large Hands: Hypertrophic Osteoarthropathy: See page 792. All dimensions of the hands are increased, as in acromegaly, but the condition is invariably accompanied by clubbing of the fingers and parrot-beak nails.

Enlargement of One Hand: Hemihypertrophy and Local Gigantism: An entire side of the body may be enlarged in a congenital deformity known as hemihypertrophy. Local gigantism is often the result of a congenital arteriovenous fistula of the upper limb. In either case, the hand is perfectly proportioned.

Long, Slender Hands: Spider Fingers (Arachnodactyly, Marfan Syndrome): All the long bones of the hands are slender and elongated, often with hyperextensible joints (see Fig. 13-27B, page 723). The *wrist sign* is useful to distinguish elongated fingers from long, normal fingers of tall, thin individuals. The patient encircles his own wrist, with his thumb and little finger proximal to the styloid process of the ulna. In normal persons, the encircling digits scarcely touch, but in arachnodactyly they may overlap by 1–2 cm. The positive sign results from the combination of long digits and narrow wrist. The hands in Marfan syndrome may also show a positive thumb sign (*Steinberg sign*): when the fingers are clenched over the thumb, the end of the thumb protrudes beyond the ulnar margin of the hand [Falk RH. The "thumb sign" in Marfan's syndrome. *N Engl J Med* 1995; 333:430 (picture)]. Neither the thumb sign nor the wrist sign is proof of Marfan syndrome.

Long, Slender Hands: Eunuchoidism: These may be similar to the spider fingers in Marfan syndrome.

Short, Thick Hands: Congenital Hypothyroidism (Cretinism): The hands are short, thick, and fat. The radius may be shortened.

Short, Thick Hands: Trisomy 21 (Down Syndrome): The hands are short and thick; the thumb diverges from nearer the wrist than normal; the little finger is curved (see Fig. 13-27C, page 723).

Interosseous Atrophy: *Pathophysiology:* Wasting suggests injury to the ulnar nerve. The hands appear shrunken with prominence of the extensor tendons and metacarpals on the dorsum (see Fig. 13-32A, page 732). Palpation discloses lost of muscle mass, most easily detected in the first dorsal interosseous between the thumb and index finger. Adduction of the fingers is weak. Common causes are ulnar nerve entrapment at the elbow, rheumatoid arthritis, and diabetic neuropathy.

Painless Swelling of the Dorsum: *Pathophysiology:* Edema arising from the deep spaces of the hand accumulates in the loose subcutaneous tissue dorsally, rather than the palmar surface, because of the restricting palmar fascia. Causes include infection, obstruction of the superior vena cava, anasarca, and relapsing symmetrical seronegative synovitis with pitting edema (RS3PE). Unilateral edema may also occur from occlusion of the venous or lymphatic drainage of the upper arm.

KEY SIGN

Painful Dorsal Swelling: Infection and extensor tenosynovitis cause edema, erythema, and localized tenderness. Fluctuation may not be present with an abscess.

KEY SIGN

Pain in Ulnar Side of Hand: Ulnar Tunnel Syndrome: *Pathophysiology:* The ulnar nerve passes posterior to the medial humeral epicondyle in the ulnar groove, and then deep to the superficial flexors and above the deep flexors of the forearm, where it is stretched and compressed during vigorous muscular activity. Injury to the ulnar nerve at the elbow causes pain in the little finger, the ulnar half of the ring finger, and the ulnar side of the palm. Atrophy of the hypothenar eminence and interosseus muscles may result from prolonged compression. These findings should direct attention to the elbow. The ulnar nerve may be stretched or injured by a cubitus valgus deformity or an old elbow fracture. Other risk factors for ulnar entrapment include alcoholism and diabetes. Press on the ulnar nerve in its groove behind the median epicondyle; tingling in the ulnar distribution of the hand suggests ulnar tunnel syndrome.

Forearm and Elbow Signs

► KEY SIGN

Forearm Pain and Weakness: Flexor Compartment Syndrome and Volkmann Ischemic Contracture: *Pathophysiology:* Ischemic necrosis of muscle results from either primary arterial events (compression, vascular spasm, arterial injury or embolism) or secondary to hemorrhage or swelling within the confining fascia of the flexor muscle compartment (compartment syndrome, page 794). Volkmann contracture, the fibrosis and shortening of the muscles, is a late finding. Early recognition of the initial ischemic phase may prevent damage leading to contracture. The onset of ischemia is indicated by the five Ps: pain, puffiness, pallor, pulselessness, and paralysis. Passive extension of the fingers produces pain in the forearm. The fingers may be cyanotic and are often edematous. The radial pulse is absent, the skin over the hands is cool and median nerve sensation is diminished. Measure compartment pressures if signs of compartment syndrome appear. In Volkmann contracture, the fingers are held in flexion by shortening of the fibrotic bellies of the digital flexors in the forearm. Because the flexor tendons are free to move in their sheaths, slight extension of the fingers is permitted with passive motion when the wrist is held in flexion. This distinguishes it from adhesions of flexor tendons to their sheaths; both prevent any extension. Precipitating events are forearm and supracondylar fractures and circumferential bandages or casts applied shortly after trauma.

Smooth Forearm Curvature: Diseases of Osseous Growth: Smooth curves of the radius and ulna are usually attributable to syphilis, rickets, osteomalacia, or osteitis deformans.

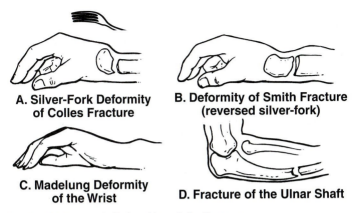

A. Silver-Fork Deformity
of Colles Fracture

B. Deformity of Smith Fracture
(reversed silver-fork)

C. Madelung Deformity
of the Wrist

D. Fracture of the Ulnar Shaft

Fig. 13-36 Traumatic Deformities of the Forearm.

KEY SIGN
Silver-Fork Deformity: Colles Fracture: The most common cause is a fall on the outstretched hand. The radius is fractured within 2.5 cm of its distal end (Fig. 13-36A). Fracture of the ulnar styloid process occurs in half the cases. When the pronated arm is laid on the table, its profile resembles a dinner fork lying horizontally with the tines pointing downward, so the base of the tines forms an upward curve. The corresponding hump in the fractured arm occurs from dorsal displacement of the distal radial fragment. To exclude a hump from soft-tissue swelling, palpate the volar aspect of the radius and compare it to the opposite side. The normal anterior convexity of the shaft is obliterated below the fracture.

KEY SIGN
Reversed Silver-Fork Deformity: Smith Fracture (Reversed Colles Fracture): Like the Colles fracture, this is a break of the distal end of the radius, but the distal fragment is displaced volarward, making a deformity somewhat resembling the silver fork with its tines pointing upward (see Fig. 13-36B). The fracture usually results from a blow or fall on the hyperflexed hand.

Dorsal Angulation of the Wrist: Madelung Deformity: The pronated hand presents a profile in which the wrist is deformed by a sharp protrusion upward (dorsally) of the lower ulna (see Fig. 13-36C). This is caused by a dorsal subluxation of the distal end of the ulna.

Pain and Tenderness in the Bony Shafts: Radial and Ulnar Fractures: In fractures of the ulnar shaft, the bone is well splinted by the radius, so displacement and deformity are rare (see Fig. 13-36D). The only physical signs are localized tenderness and swelling. Ulnar fractures accompanied by volar dislocation of the radial head (Monteggia fracture/dislocation), especially common in children, permit considerable bowing of the fractured ulna. A fractured radial shaft presents variable degrees of bowing, especially with concomitant dislocation of the lower radioulnar joint.

Painful Angular Deformity: Fractures of Both Forearm Bones: Greenstick fractures produce little deformity, but complete fractures of the radius and ulna present easily recognizable deformity.

KEY SIGN

Post-traumatic Elbow Pain: Fracture of the Coronoid Process of the Ulna: Fracture of the ulnar coronoid process, which forms the distal part elbow joint, is easily missed if not considered and searched for.

Post-traumatic Elbow Pain: Fracture of the Olecranon Process: Pronounced swelling results, particularly around the dorsum of the elbow. The olecranon process is tender. When the fracture is complete, the patient cannot extend the flexed forearm (Fig. 13-37A). The bony equilateral triangle may be flattened.

KEY SIGN

Post-traumatic Elbow Pain: Humeral Supracondylar Fracture: The injury is usually caused by falling on the outstretched hand in children younger than 10 years of age. The patient supports the forearm with the opposite hand. Usually the distal

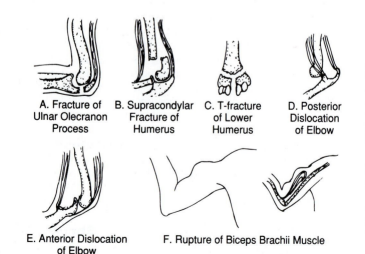

A. Fracture of Ulnar Olecranon Process

B. Supracondylar Fracture of Humerus

C. T-fracture of Lower Humerus

D. Posterior Dislocation of Elbow

E. Anterior Dislocation of Elbow

F. Rupture of Biceps Brachii Muscle

Fig. 13-37 Fractures and Dislocations about the Elbow.

fragment is displaced posteriorly, so elbow angulation is unusually prominent (see Fig. 13-37B). The elbow's bony equilateral triangle is intact. Tenderness and swelling are present at the fracture site. To prevent injury to the antecubital structures avoid moving the fragments. Seek the early signs of compartment syndrome (see above). In the uncommon anterior displacement of the distal fragment, the signs are less distinctive.

Post-traumatic Elbow Pain: Lower T-Shaped Humeral Fracture: A blow on the elbow may result in the humeral shaft being driven between the two condyles, producing widening of the elbow (see Fig. 13-37C). Crepitus of the fragments occurs with light palpation when the fragments are not separated. Swelling may obscure the distortion of the bony equilateral triangle, but blood in the joint cavity produces fluctuation and bulging on both sides of the olecranon process.

KEY SIGN
Post-traumatic Elbow Pain: Dislocation of the Elbow: Falling on the outstretched hand usually causes a posterior dislocation (see Fig. 13-37D). The olecranon process is unusually prominent. The arm is held in 40 degrees of flexion, and is immovable, actively or passively. The forearm is not supported by the opposite hand. The height of the bony triangle is shortened. The last two features distinguish it from supracondylar fracture.

Deformity of the Elbow: Cubitus Valgus and Varus: The carrying angle of the elbow is not normal, and differs more than 10 degrees between right and left. Because the normal angle is approximately 170 degrees as measured on the lateral side of the arm and forearm, an angle less than 165 degrees is a valgus deformity, and one greater than 175 degrees is a varus deformity (Fig. 13-38A).

KEY SIGN
Swelling of the Elbow: Effusion in the Elbow Joint: The synovial sac of the elbow joint is very loose. Fluid dis-

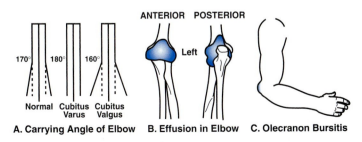

A. Carrying Angle of Elbow   B. Effusion in Elbow   C. Olecranon Bursitis

Fig. 13-38 Disorders of the Intact Elbow.

tention produces fluctuant bulging posteriorly, on both sides of the olecranon process and the attached triceps brachii tendon (see Fig. 13-38B).
It is most accessible to palpation laterally in the sulcus between the lateral epicondyle, radial head, and olecranon. The elbow is held in semiflexion to accommodate maximal fluid volume. Careful note of the borders of the sac in Fig. 13-38B will assist in distinguishing whether the
fluid is in the joint cavity or in the olecranon bursa. The joint may be
distended by synovial fluid, pus, or blood.

KEY SIGN

**Swelling of the Elbow: Olecranon Bursitis
(Miner's Elbow, Student's Elbow):** Trauma, inflam-
mation, infection or gout produces an accumulation of fluid in the olecranon bursa, a subcutaneous space overlying the olecranon process (see
Fig. 13-38C). The swelling is fluctuant. The location of the bulge readily distinguishes it from fluid in the joint.

S KEY SYNDROME

**Lateral Elbow Pain: Lateral and Medial Epi-
condylitis (Tennis Elbow):** *Pathophysiology:* Repetitive
forceful wrist and/or finger flexion and extension focus tension on the
common proximal tendon insertions at the lateral (extensors) and medial (flexors) humeral epicondyles. *Lateral Epicondylitis* causes pain
in the lateral aspect of the elbow, accentuated by use of the hand during a power grip (when the wrist extensors are also contracting), as in
lifting objects. Palpation discloses tenderness over the lateral epicondyle
and 1 cm distally. In the *Cozen test* (resisted wrist extension), the patient
is asked to keep the fist clenched while extending the wrist against resistance reproducing the patient's lateral epicondylar pain. In the *Mill
maneuver,* have the elbow held in extension with the wrist flexed; when
you pronate the forearm against the patient's resistance, epicondylar
pain is elicited. *Medial Epicondylitis* is less common. The pain is located just distal to the medial epicondyle in the flexor tendons and is
reproduced by maneuvers requiring wrist and finger flexion or arm
pronation against resistance.

Arthritis of the Elbow: Any type of arthritis may involve
the elbow joint. Suppurative arthritis produces painful swelling, with
pus in the joint. Rheumatic fever and rheumatoid arthritis cause painful
swelling; the chronic stage of rheumatoid arthritis often results in limited extension. A loose body in the joint is suggested by a history of
locking. An enlarged, painless joint, suggesting osteoarthritis but unilateral, may be neurogenic arthropathy (Charcot joint); when encountered in the elbow, syringomyelia is the most likely cause.

KEY SIGN

**Post-traumatic Elbow Pain: Subluxation of
the Radial Head:** This usually occurs in childhood (the "pulled
elbow"). There is no deformity of the elbow and tenderness is maximum

near the radial head. Flexion–extension elicits pain, but pronation and supination are painless.

Post-traumatic Elbow Pain: Fracture of the Radial Head: Usually this results from a fall on the outstretched hand. Swelling is minimal and there is no deformity; the bony equilateral triangle is normal. Flexion and extension are painless, but there is severe restriction of pronation-supination and the radial head is tender.

Upper Arm Signs

This region includes the shaft of the humerus and its covering muscles, principally the biceps brachii and the triceps brachii.

Pain in the Upper Arm: Bicipital Tenosynovitis: *Pathophysiology:* A day or so after excessive use of the biceps brachii, inflammation occurs in the tendon sheath of the biceps where it emerges anteriorly from the capsule of the shoulder joint. Pain is located near the insertion of the pectoralis major on the humerus and may shoot down the arm. Shoulder motions are somewhat limited, especially flexion of the arm (elevation at 0 degrees abduction). Tenderness is elicited by palpating the tendon in the bicipital groove. *Yergason Sign:* Have the patient flex the elbow to 90 degrees and pronate the forearm. Grasp the hand and ask the patient to supinate against your resistance. It is positive when this produces pain in the anteromedial aspect of the shoulder.

Bicipital Humps: Rupture of the Biceps Brachii: The usually smooth profile of the biceps is interrupted by one or two humps. One hump results with rupture of the tendon or muscle sheath (see Fig. 13-37F). Rupture of the belly causes two humps. Rupture occurs during lifting excessive weight and is usually painful. Absence of this history suggests degeneration of the bicipital long-head tendon in the shoulder joint, often associated with chronic impingement or shoulder synovitis. Rupture of the long-head tendon is most common, resulting in mild weakness. Rupture of the muscle may not greatly impair strength.

Painful Immobility of the Upper Arm: Fracture of the Humeral Shaft: These are painful injuries, and the arm is useless, being held in the opposite hand. Transverse fracture is usually caused by a direct blow and there is unmistakable deformity. Spiral fracture, commonly from a fall on the hand, may not cause deformity. Lacking deformity, gently palpate the lateral and medial aspects of the humerus for local tenderness and swelling. Shaft fractures can lacerate the radial nerve and distal brachial artery as they lie in contact with the posterior upper third of the humerus. In all cases of fractured humerus, feel the radial arterial pulse and test for radial nerve injury. Test the motor function of the nerve by having the patient flex the elbow with the forearm pronated and look for wrist-drop. Anesthesia on the radial dorsum of the hand is evidence of sensory loss of the radial nerve.

Shoulder Signs

KEY SIGN

Deficits of Arm Abduction: See Fig. 13-39. Full painless abduction effectively excludes serious injury to the shoulder. Pain with elevation or limited active range of motion suggest pathology in the shoulder. Pain between 60 degrees and 120 degrees of elevation, with the remainder of the arc painless, suggests partial rupture of the supraspinatus tendon, supraspinatus tendinitis, or subacromial bursitis. Minimal elevation and support of the arm with the opposite hand point to fracture, dislocation, or complete rupture of the supraspinatus; in the latter case, passive motions of the joint are normal. Pain throughout the range of elevation indicates arthritis. Descriptions of these conditions follow.

S KEY SYNDROME

PAIN BETWEEN 60 DEGREES AND 120 DEGREES OF ABDUCTION (PAINFUL ARC, IMPINGEMENT SIGN): PARTIAL RUPTURE OF THE SUPRASPINATUS TENDON, SUPRASPINATUS TENDINITIS, AND SUBACROMIAL BURSITIS: *Pathophysiology:* During arm abduction the supraspinatus tendon and its insertion on the proximal margin of the greater humeral tuberosity must pass beneath the acromion. The subacromial bursa is positioned to decrease the friction, or impingement, which occurs with this motion. Repetitive forceful motion causes mechanical irritation to the tissues eliciting inflammation of the tendon and bursa. Sudden or severe loading of the shoulder may result in incomplete or complete tears of the supraspinatus tendon. These three condi-

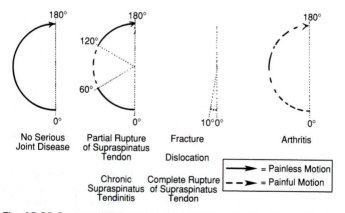

Fig. 13-39 Causes of Pain and Limited Motion with Elevation of the Arm in Abduction.

tions present with similar signs and symptoms. A history of sudden on-set favors partial tear of the tendon, whereas repetitive shoulder motion and subacute or chronic onset favor tendonitis or bursitis. All have painful abduction between 60 degrees and 120 degrees, often prohibiting full active range of motion. Passive range, though painful, is preserved. Precise distinction between the three is not possible with physical examination. *Partial Rupture of the Supraspinatus Tendon:* When the tendon is only incompletely torn, the rotator cuff is intact. Pain is referred to the humeral insertion of the deltoid muscle, but there is no tenderness at that point. Sometimes the pain extends down the arm to the elbow or beyond. Tenderness is elicited just beneath the acromial tip or in the notch between greater and lesser humeral tubercles. DDX: If weakness of the supraspinatus, weak external rotation and impingement signs are all present, a rotator cuff tear is likely [Murrell GA, Walton JR. Diagnosis of rotator cuff tears. *Lancet* 2001;357:769–770]. *Acute Supraspinatus Tendinitis:* This usually occurs in a person 25 to 45 years of age, with a dull ache developing in the shoulder without antecedent trauma. The pain steadily worsens and may be excruciating. The diagnostic test is abduction to 90 degrees and then full internal rotation, which reproduces pain. Tenderness is pronounced beneath the acromial tip. *Chronic Supraspinatus Tendinitis:* Dull shoulder pain develops in a patient who is usually between 45 and 60 years old and without preceding trauma. Abduction is painless to 60 degrees, where the patient feels a jerk with pain in the region of the deltoid muscle. Pronounced tenderness can be elicited in the notch between the greater and lesser tubercles of the humeral head or beneath the acromial tip. Crepitus may also be present. Lying on the shoulder produces pain that prevents sleeping on the affected side for months. *Subacromial Bursitis:* This can be acute or chronic and often accompanies supraspinatus tendonitis. The pain is constant and aggravated by elevation in abduction. There is often a history of heavy arm use.

MINIMAL ARM ELEVATION AND SUPPORT WITH THE OPPOSITE HAND: COMPLETE RUPTURE OF THE SUPRASPINATUS TENDON, TORN ROTATOR CUFF: *Pathophysiology:* The supraspinatus muscle initiates arm abduction from 0 to 45 degrees, where the deltoid becomes engaged. Inability to initiate elevation in 90° abduction indicates rupture of the supraspinatus tendon. This usually occurs after age 40. The patient cannot elevate the arm against minimal resistance at 30 degrees elevation and 90 degrees abduction, but passive motion is free and painless. Initial shoulder motion is mostly with the scapula. There is resistance to external rotation when the arm is held at the side with elbow flexed. As the arm is moved forward, one may palpate a jerk, fine crepitus, or an indentation in the subacromial region between the greater and lesser humeral tubercles (see Fig. 13-18D, page 698). After 3 weeks, atrophy of the supraspinatus and infraspinatus occurs.

MINIMAL ARM ELEVATION WITH SUPPORT OF OPPOSITE HAND: SHOULDER DISLOCATION: *Pathophysiology:* When the hand or arm are forcefully abducted and externally rotated, the humeral head dislocates out of the glenoid tearing through the anterior rotator cuff. The humeral head is usually displaced anteriorly and medially from its normal location im-

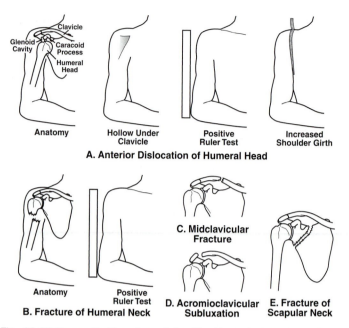

Anatomy   Hollow Under   Positive   Increased
                 Clavicle   Ruler Test   Shoulder Girth

A. Anterior Dislocation of Humeral Head

Anatomy   Positive   **C. Midclavicular**
                 Ruler Test   **Fracture**

B. Fracture of Humeral Neck   **D. Acromioclavicular**   **E. Fracture of**
                                    Subluxation   **Scapular Neck**

*Fig. 13-40 Traumatic Disorders of the Shoulder. A. Anterior Disloca-
tion of the Humeral Head. B. Fracture of the Humeral Neck. C. Midclavicular Fracture. D. Acromioclavicular Subluxation. E. Fracture of
the Scapular Neck.*

mediately below the acromial tip and lateral to the coracoid to a position under the coracoid process (Fig. 13-40A). The shoulder profile is
flattened and the bony triangle is disrupted. The bony hardness of the
humeral head can be palpated medially in the normally soft belly of the
upper third of the deltoid. With the *ruler test of Hamilton,* a straight edge
can rest simultaneously on the acromial tip and the lateral epicondyle
of the elbow; normally, the humeral head intervenes. The test is also
positive in fracture of the humeral neck. The *Calloway test,* useful in obese
patients, consists of measuring the girth of the two shoulder joints. A
tape measure is looped through the axilla and the girth measured at the
acromial tip; the girth of the affected joint is increased. In the *Dugas test,*
the patient cannot adduct the arm sufficiently to place the hand on the
opposite shoulder. Posterior dislocations are rare. The humeral head is
felt posteriorly under the spine of the scapula near the base of the acromial process. A common cause of this uncommon dislocation is a major motor (grand mal) seizure. Shoulder dislocation can be identified by
a scapular Y-view x-ray without manipulation of the shoulder. Dislocation of the humeral head can damage adjacent structures including the
labrum of the glenoid and the axillary nerve (causing paralysis and later
atrophy of the deltoid). Palpate the pulses of the arm to detect compression of the axillary vessels.

MINIMAL ARM ELEVATION AND SUPPORT WITH OPPOSITE HAND: HUMERAL NECK FRACTURE: Usually this results from a fall on the outstretched hand. Pain is present in the shoulder, with immobility of the arm, which is supported by the opposite hand. Viewed laterally, the profile may show an anterior angular deformity (see Fig. 13-40B). The axillary aspect of the arm and the chest wall may be ecchymotic. Rotate the arm gently, while palpating the humeral head; if the fracture is not impacted, the head will not move with the shaft, confirming the diagnosis. When displacement is present, the ruler test of Hamilton (see *Shoulder Dislocation* above) may be positive. If a break is not obvious, consider impacted fracture and measure the distance from acromial tip to epicondyle on the two sides; the impacted side should be shorter.

MINIMAL ARM ELEVATION AND SUPPORT WITH OPPOSITE HAND: CLAVICULAR FRACTURE: Fractures at the center of the shaft are most common. Because the fragments are usually displaced, diagnosis can be made by inspection and palpation (see Fig. 13-40C). Greenstick or impacted fractures may be detected by tenderness and swelling.

MINIMAL ARM ELEVATION AND SUPPORT WITH OPPOSITE HAND: ACROMIOCLAVICULAR SUBLUXATION: There is pain in the shoulder with reluctance to elevate the arm. Inspection may disclose elevation of the distal clavicular tip. Have the patient place the hand of the affected side on the opposite shoulder and press firmly on the distal end of the clavicle. The end of the clavicle moves downward and the maneuver is painful (see Fig. 13-40D). When the patient holds a weight in both arms, observe the downward displacement of the acromion relative to the end of the affected clavicle.

MINIMAL ARM ELEVATION AND SUPPORT WITH OPPOSITE HAND: STERNOCLAVICULAR SUBLUXATION: The more common injury is forward dislocation and subluxation, causing painful clicking in the joint with elevation of the arm in abduction. The deformity is usually obvious to inspection. The rarer backward dislocation is seen as a hollow where the normal clavicular head protrudes. If the mediastinum is invaded, dyspnea and cyanosis may occur.

MINIMAL ARM ELEVATION AND SUPPORT WITH OPPOSITE HAND: SCAPULAR FRACTURE: There is pain in the shoulder preventing elevation of the arm (see Fig. 13-40E). Sit at the patient's affected side supporting the forearm while palpating the shoulder. Abduct the forearm to 90 degrees; crepitus in the joint strongly suggests fracture of the scapular neck when the clavicle is intact.

KEY SIGN

Restriction of All Shoulder Motions: Trauma and Arthritis: All types of arthritis may involve the shoulder. In the early stages of inflammatory processes, motions are inhibited by pain; later, adhesions restrict motion. Osteoarthritis may be associated with crepitus in the joint, but effusions are relatively rare. Over time there is progressive loss of glenohumeral motion. With chronically limited motion, generalized muscle atrophy occurs. Joint effusion suggests rheumatoid arthritis, crystal arthritis (calcium pyrophosphate dihydrate deposition [CPPD]) or less-common disorders such as villonodular synovitis.

RESTRICTION OF ALL SHOULDER MOTIONS: ADHESIVE CAPSULITIS (FROZEN SHOULDER): *Pathophysiology:* Chronic inflammation of the rotator cuff and joint capsule leads to shortening of the usually loose tendinous cuff and to progressive loss of motion. This often follows unresolved subacromial bursitis or supraspinatus tendinitis. At onset, pain is that of the original injury. Progressive limitation of motion ensues until capsular contraction and fibrosis abate the pain with associated muscle atrophy.

Pain in the Shoulder: Coracoiditis: *Pathophysiology:* Repeated acute or chronic arm work may produce inflammation at the origin of the short head of the biceps and the coracobrachialis muscles on the tip of the coracoid process. There is a history of trauma with pain and tenderness at the tip of the coracoid process. The pain is reproduced by adduction and external rotation of the humerus, or having the patient perform against resistance either supination of the forearm with the elbow flexed, forward flexion of the shoulder, or adduction of the flexed shoulder.

Pain in Deltoid Muscle: Subdeltoid Bursitis (Subacromial Bursitis): Sometimes regarded as a single clinical entity, inflammation of the subdeltoid bursa usually occurs in association with inflammation or tears of the supraspinatus tendon.

Painful Nodules in Shoulder Muscles: Trigger Points: Pain is usually present on arising or after inactivity, while exercise diminishes or abolishes the pain. Small nodules may be palpated on the surface of the trapezius or other muscle. Pressure on the nodule reproduces the pain, often with radiation to the neck and upper arm.

Shoulder-Pad Sign: Amyloidosis: Bilateral anterolateral swelling of the shoulder joints is a conspicuous, although uncommon, sign of amyloid disease. The periarticular swellings feel hard and rubbery, suggesting the shoulder pads worn by American football players.

Winged Scapula: Paralysis of the Long Thoracic Nerve: *Pathophysiology:* Paralysis of the serratus anterior permits the scapula to be separated posteriorly from the thoracic wall, a winged scapula. Have the patient stand and push the hands against a wall while you observe the scapulae (Fig. 13-41A). Injury to

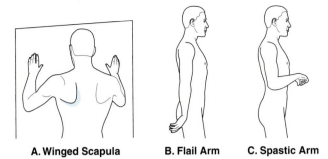

A. Winged Scapula   **B. Flail Arm**   **C. Spastic Arm**

Fig. 13-41 Disorders of the Intact Shoulder.   A. Winged Scapula: When the patient pushes the hands against a wall the involved scapula protrude posteriorly, forming a winged scapula. B. Flail Arm: The arm hangs limply at the side with palm posterior and fingers partially flexed. C. Spastic Arm: The arm assumes flexion at the elbow with the upper arm at elevation, flexion at the wrist and fingers, with slight adduction of the humerus; the forearm is in pronation.

the long thoracic nerve is caused by stretching during heavy lifting or surgical trauma.

Winged Scapula: Sprengel Deformity: This is a congenital condition with unilateral or bilateral winged scapulae. It is sometimes associated with a short, webbed neck.

Conditions of the Entire Upper Limb

Flail Arm: *Pathophysiology:* Lower motor neuron or peripheral nerve injuries produce muscular denervation with flaccid paralysis and muscular atrophy. After injuries to the brachial plexus or poliomyelitis, the arm may hang limply at the side with the flexed palm facing backward (see Fig. 13-41B).

KEY SIGN
Spastic Arm: *Pathophysiology:* Injury to upper motor neurons leads to uninhibited muscular contraction with the antigravity flexors overpowering the weaker extensors. With hemiplegia, the arm is carried in elevation with flexion of the elbow, wrist, and fingers (see Fig. 13-41C).

Hip, Buttock, and Thigh Signs

KEY SIGN
▶ **Sacral Pain: Lesions of the Cauda Equina:** *Pathophysiology:* Compression of the cauda equina ("horse's tail": the spinal roots below the level of the spinal cord termination, or conus), results in compromise of nerve function in one or more lumbar or spinal

nerves, often accompanied by pain. Pain is localized to the sacrum and inner thigh and the skin may be anesthetic. Bladder symptoms (including decreased urinary stream, hesitancy, and urinary retention), anal sphincter laxity, absent anal wink, and impotence are common. Compression occurs from a herniated intervertebral disk with posterior protrusion, epidural hematoma or abscess, and neoplasms.

KEY SIGN
Sacroiliac Pain: Sacroiliac Arthritis: On arising, there is painful stiffness in the upper medial buttocks, which improves with exercise. Pain may be referred to the upper outer quadrant of the buttock, or the posterolateral aspect of the thigh. Sometimes there is a limp. Spinal rotation accentuates pain. The joint is tender to palpation or percussion. Sacroiliac arthritis is characteristic of the spondyloarthropathies (see page 782).

KEY SIGN
Sacroiliac Pain: Sacroiliac Strain: *Pathophysiology:* Mechanical strain or postpartum relaxation of the ligaments about the joint is followed by inflammation. The patient complains of pain in the joint or in the upper inner quadrant of the buttock or the posterolateral aspect of the thigh (dermatomes L4, L5, S1). The joint is tender. The pain is accentuated by compressing the anterior iliac crests while the patient lies supine. The tendon reflexes in the lower limbs are normal.

Sacroiliac Pain: Tuberculous Arthritis: Frequently there is pain in the lower midline of the spine, in the inguinal region, or sometimes in the sciatic distribution. Although the abscess is extraarticular, joint pain and tenderness are intense. The abscess may burst and drain through the skin over the joint posteriorly or in the inguinal region along the iliopsoas.

KEY SIGN
Pain in the Buttock: Ischiogluteal Bursitis (Weaver Bottom): *Pathophysiology:* When standing, the gluteal muscles cover the ischial tuberosities; however, when sitting, the muscles slide upward, exposing the tuberosities to pressure, protected only by intervening skin, subcutaneous tissue, and the ischiogluteal bursa, which is not always present. Prolonged sitting on a hard surface with the thighs flexed may cause irritation of the bursa. Inflammation of the bursa may produce secondary irritation of the adjacent sciatic nerve. Certain occupations are associated with this disorder, as indicated by the ancient name derived from Chaucer's weaver [Buchan RF. Weaver's bottom. *JAMA* 1974;228:567–568]. The pain may be spontaneous or caused by sitting on a vibrating, poorly cushioned seat, for example, a tractor. The onset is sudden with exquisite, unrelenting pain in the buttock that persists throughout the night despite attempts to find a comfortable position. Mild analgesics give no relief and the pain is aggravated by sitting, although the patient prefers a hard seat to a soft one. Coughing induces pain down the posterior aspect of the thigh to

the knee. Often the patient needs assistance with dressing and undressing. The patient stands and walks with a list toward the affected side and the stride is shortened on the affected side with circumduction of the foot. Standing on tiptoe is painfully impossible. The patient sits on the exam table with his affected buttock carefully elevated and to lie down he supports his pelvis with the hand on the unaffected side, suggesting sciatic nerve irritation. Point tenderness in the region of the ischial tuberosity is a cardinal sign. When supine, the straight-leg-raising test causes pain (*Lasègue sign*). The *Patrick Fabere sign* is present and causes severe pain (the heel of the affected side is placed on the opposite patella and the knee is pushed downward to rotate the hip externally). On rectal examination a region of tender, bulging, doughy tissue may be palpated in the lateral rectal wall. DDX: Patients with herniated disk and lumbosacral disease lie quietly and lack the Patrick Fabere sign. The bursa may also be affected by gout.

KEY SIGN

Painless Limping: Hip Dislocation: *Pathophysiology:* Dislocation of the hip may be congenital or acquired. Acquired weakness of the supporting muscles (from nerve or muscle injury), hip joint infections, and trauma produce hip dislocation in adults. Screening by physical exam for congenital hip dislocation should begin at birth. A child who has not begun to walk by 18 months should be suspected of having congenital hip dislocation. The buttocks and perineum may be unusually broad and adductor folds may be present on the medial aspects of the thighs. Examination shows inability to abduct the thighs to 90 degrees in flexion. Pathognomonic for subluxation is the *Ortolani jerk sign,* which is elicited with the baby supine on the table. Stand at its head and grasp the thighs in your hands. Fix the opposite side of the pelvis to the table by encircling the thigh with your hand so that the thumb presses along the subcutaneous aspect of the tibia. On the side to be tested, grasp the thigh with your hand so that your thumb is on the medial aspect, just below the inguinal fold, and your fingers are over the trochanteric region. While slowly abducting the thigh, push downward on the flexed knee with your palm and pull upward with your fingers near the trochanter until you feel a click as the femoral head engages the acetabulum. Congenital hip dislocation is sometimes not noticed until a limp or other abnormal gait is noticed when the child starts walking. In childhood and adolescence, signs include a female contour to the pelvis (both sexes have a male contour at this age), and prominence of the buttocks and abdomen. A gluteal or Trendelenburg gait in which the hip lurches upward and the shoulder dips downward on the weight-bearing side is present. With the patient supine, observe the thigh length from the foot of the table with the knees and thighs flexed. The knee of the affected leg will be lower than the other in unilateral disease. Have the patient undressed and standing while you inspect the buttocks. Ask the patient to stand on one leg; normally, the free buttock is raised when the pelvis tilts (Fig. 13-42A). In the *Trendelenburg sign,* the free buttock falls because the muscles are not strong enough to sustain the position when the femur is not engaged in the acetabulum. The sign

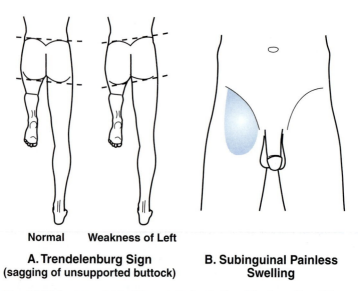

Normal   **Weakness of Left**

A. Trendelenburg Sign
(sagging of unsupported buttock)

B. Subinguinal Painless Swelling

Fig. 13-42 Lesions of the Hip and Groin. A. Trendelenburg Sign: When the patient stands on one foot, the buttock falls. B. Subinguinal Painless Swelling: Swelling below the inguinal ligament may be either a psoas abscess or an effusion in the psoas bursa.

is also positive with disease of the glutei, fracture of the femoral head, and in severe degrees of coxa vara. In adults, in addition to the childhood signs, there are hip pain and premature osteoarthritis of the affected joint.

KEY SIGN
Painless Limping: Osteonecrosis, Aseptic Hip Necrosis: *Pathophysiology:* Ischemia of the femoral head leads to necrosis of bone and to the collapse and mushrooming of the femoral head. It may be unilateral or bilateral. Although the cause may be unknown, use of corticosteroids, diabetes, obesity, and alcohol are each associated with an increased risk. Usually it begins with a painless limp and all motions of the hip are slightly impaired. Later, there is severe limitation of abduction and rotation. Muscle atrophy and shortening of the limb are common. The waddling gait suggests dislocation of the hip. Osteonecrosis of the epiphysis in childhood (Legg-Calvé-Perthes disease) is relatively painless, whereas osteonecrosis in adults may be painful.

KEY SIGN
Pain in the Hip: Septic Arthritis of the Hip: Usually, there is groin pain, fever, leukocytosis, and prostration. All motion of the hip is painful. Rarely, fluctuation can be felt in the joint. Be-

cause pain may be referred only to the knee, knee pain should always prompt examination of the hip. Early diagnosis is urgent because the joint cartilage may be irreparably damaged in a few hours without proper drainage and antibiotics.

Pain in the Hip: Tuberculous Arthritis: The onset is insidious, with the appearance of a limp. Pain in the hip or thigh may occur only after exertion, subsiding with rest. There is early flexion of the hip masked by lumbar lordosis, as detected by Hugh Owen Thomas sign (page 703). The thigh may be held in slight abduction and lateral rotation to best accommodate the joint effusion. When the fluid is absorbed, the posture changes to flexion, adduction, and inward rotation. Finally, erosion of the joint causes shortening of the limb.

KEY SIGN
Pain in the Hip: Slipped Capital Femoral Epiphysis: *Pathophysiology:* The femoral head dislocates on the femoral neck at the growth plate during rapid growth when this area is structurally weak. A limp with hip pain develops during adolescence, usually in boys who are either obese or unusually tall or thin. The distinguishing feature is painful limitation of internal rotation when thigh and knee are both flexed. This may be succeeded by shortening and outward rotation from anterosuperior displacement of the femoral neck.

KEY SIGN
Pain in the Hip: Osteoarthritis: *Pathophysiology:* Osteoarthritis is a disease of cartilage leading to desiccation, fibrillation of the surface, thinning of the joint space, and, ultimately, complete loss of the cartilage with bone-on-bone articulation. Occasionally painless, the chief symptom is usually boring pain in the joint, frequently felt in the groin and buttocks, sometimes with referral to the knee. Initially, there may be <30 minutes of stiffness after rest, which disappears with exercise. The patient may be unaware of a limp, but later, walking is limited by pain. Abduction and internal rotation are restricted by pain. In unilateral disease, the thigh is held in adduction, with eversion of the foot and the pelvis is tilted upward on the affected side. Passive motion is most commonly restricted in internal rotation and may be restricted in all directions. Capsular swelling from thickening and effusion is rarely palpable. Motion of the joint may cause palpable and audible crepitus.

KEY SIGN
► **Mass in the Femoral Triangle: Psoas Abscess:** Painless abscess is usually an extension of spinal tuberculosis. Painful abscess suggests purulent infection from an intraabdominal source. The mass appears beneath the inguinal ligament in a conical form (see Fig. 13-42B). DDX: Palpation discloses a similar swelling in the iliac fossa distinguishing it from effusion in the psoas bursa. Abscess must be distinguished from fluctuant lymphadenopathy.

Mass in the Femoral Triangle: Psoas Bursitis:
A painless effusion in the psoas bursa, occasionally associated with osteoarthritis of the hip, produces tense, nonfluctuant, immobile conical
swelling beneath the inguinal ligament (see Fig. 13-42B). The absence of
a mass in the iliac fossa excludes psoas abscess.

KEY SIGN
**Mass in the Femoral Triangle: Lym-
phadenopathy:** See Fig. 9-37, page 605.

KEY SIGN
**Mass in the Femoral Triangle: Femoral Her-
nia:** See pages 114 and 604.

KEY SIGN
**Post-traumatic Hip Pain: Traumatic Dislo-
cation of the Hip:** *Pathophysiology:* A blow on the knee
while a person is sitting drives the femoral head posteriorly out of its
socket, frequently fracturing the rim of the acetabulum (Fig. 13-43A).
The rare anterior traumatic dislocation occurs from landing on the feet
in a fall. *Posterior Dislocation:* Inguinal and thigh pain is severe and
constant. The thigh lies in extreme internal rotation, adduction, and
slight flexion (Fig. 13-43C, *right* panel) and only the foot can be actively
moved without pain. The greater trochanter is abnormally prominent,
while palpation for the femoral head beneath the inguinal ligament
yields an indentation. The limb is shortened and passive rotation of the
femur is absent. *Anterior Dislocation:* The joint is fixed in abduction,
outward rotation, and slight flexion (Fig. 13-43C, *left* panel). There is no
shortening of the limb, because the head is impaled anteriorly in the il-
iofemoral ligament.

KEY SIGN
**Post-traumatic Hip Pain: Fracture of the
Femoral Neck:** The femoral neck may be fractured below the

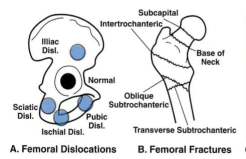

A. Femoral Dislocations   **B. Femoral Fractures**

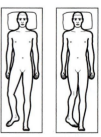

**C. Abnormal Rotations
of the Hip**

Fig. 13-43 Femoral Dislocations and Fractures.

capsule, a low fracture, or within the capsule, a high fracture (see Fig. 13-43A). In the *extracapsular fracture*, the femur is shortened and externally rotated in the supine position (see Fig. 13-43C, *left* panel). With an *intracapsular fracture* the tense joint capsule restrains rotation and swelling of the upper thigh is considerable. If the patient can lift the foot off the bed, the fracture is impacted. In *impacted fractures*, the patient can sometimes walk with little pain, so a fracture may not be suspected. However, passive rotation of the thigh will usually yield some pain.

Post-traumatic Hip Pain: Avulsion Fracture of the Lesser Trochanter: This usually occurs in muscular postpubertal men. The sitting patient cannot flex the thigh (*Ludloff sign*).

KEY SIGN

Post-traumatic Thigh Pain: Fracture of the Femoral Shaft: This may lead to shock because of blood loss, so careful observation is required. The thigh is rotated externally, often with obvious deformity and shortening as a consequence of muscle spasm and overlap of the proximal and distal femur.

Knee Signs

KEY SIGN

Painless Unilateral Knee Deformity: Neurogenic Arthropathy (Charcot Joint): See Fig. 13-44C and *Charcot Joint* on page 779.

Knee Deformity: Genu Varum (Bowleg): The legs deviate toward the midline so that the knees are farther apart than normal when the medial malleoli are approximated (see Fig. 13-9C). The deformity is measured between the knees when the patient is supine with the medial malleoli together. The feet are turned inward when walking. The most common cause is osteoarthritic narrowing of the medial knee compartment. Other causes are rickets affecting the upper tibial and lower femoral epiphyses, Paget disease, or occupational stress.

Knee Deformity: Genu Valgum (Knock-Knee): The legs deviate away from the midline, often bilaterally (see Fig. 13-9C). Congenital enlargement of the medial femoral condyles produces genu valgum in children. The most common cause is osteoarthritic narrowing of the lateral knee compartment. The deviation is measured between the medial malleoli with the patient standing and the knees together.

KEY SIGN

Knee Swelling: Fluid Within the Joint: *Pathophysiology:* An excess of synovial fluid in the knee joint is an *effusion*. Blood in the joint space is *hemarthrosis*. The presence of pus indicates suppurative arthritis. Fluid signs are independent of fluid type, so specific diagnosis can only be made by aspiration. Effusion is commonly caused by trauma, rheumatoid arthritis, osteoarthritis, gout, other crystalline arthritides (calcium pyrophosphate, basic calcium phosphate) or intermittent hydrarthrosis. Traumatic hemarthrosis suggests intracapsular fracture or ligament disruption. Nontraumatic hemarthrosis occurs with hemophilia and neoplasms.

KEY SIGN

Anterior Knee Swelling: Prepatellar Bursitis: A fluctuant subcutaneous swelling occurs anterior to the lower patella and patellar ligament, the distribution of the prepatellar bursa (Fig. 13-44D). It is often found associated with occupational trauma to the tissue overlying the patella. This differs from fluid in the joint cavity that produces swelling on the medial side of the patella.

KEY SIGN

Anterior Knee Swelling: Infrapatellar Bursitis: Swelling occurs in a bursa on both sides of the patellar ligament near the tibial tuberosity (see Fig. 13-44E). Fluctuation can be demonstrated from one side of the ligament to the other. This often results from occupations requiring kneeling, such as roofing and floor laying.

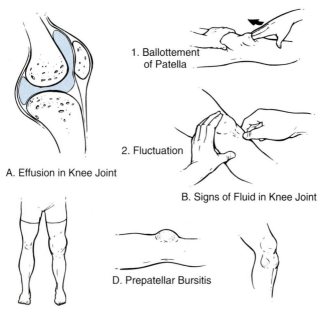

1. Ballottement of Patella

2. Fluctuation

A. Effusion in Knee Joint

B. Signs of Fluid in Knee Joint

D. Prepatellar Bursitis

C. Charcot Knee

E. Infrapatellar Bursitis

Fig. 13-44 Swellings of the Knee and their Diagnosis. *A. Knee Effusion. B. Signs of Knee Effusions. C. Charcot Knee. D. Prepatella Bursitis. E. Infrapatellar Bursitis.*

Anterior Knee Swelling: Infrapatellar Fat Pad:
The infrapatellar fat pad becomes inflamed, causing tenderness and swelling on both sides of the patellar ligament. The tenderness and lack of fluctuance distinguish it from bursitis and synovitis.

Popliteal Swelling: Semimembranosus Bursitis:
Fluid accumulates in the bursa between the head of the gastrocnemius and the tendon of the semimembranosus, forming the upper medial border of the diamond-shaped popliteal fossa (Fig. 13-45). Extension of the knee causes painful tensing of the bursa, while flexion relaxes it. Fluctuation is difficult to demonstrate.

KEY SIGN

Popliteal Swelling: Baker Cyst: The cyst is a pressure diverticulum of the synovial sac protruding through the posterior joint capsule of the knee. Sometimes dull pain is present. The cyst is best seen by inspection of the fossa when the patient is standing. In contrast to the semimembranosus bursitis, the swelling is in the midline at or below the tibiofemoral junction (see Fig. 13-45). The cyst protrudes when the knee is extended and, unless it is very large, is not visible with flexion. When the cyst freely communicates with the joint, gradual, steady pressure on the sac forces some fluid back into the joint cavity, temporarily reducing the swelling. The swelling may be translucent. Baker cysts often complicate rheumatoid arthritis and osteoarthritis. Large cysts can compress the popliteal vessels. If the artery is compressed, forced extension of the knee or strong dorsiflexion of the foot may obliterate the pedal pulse.

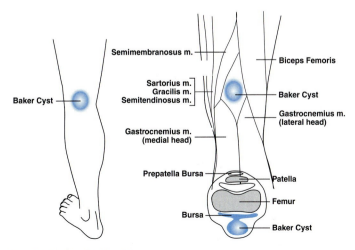

Fig. 13-45 The Popliteal Fossa.

Popliteal Swelling: Popliteal Abscess: There is tender induration in the popliteal fossa. Swelling may be minimal and fluctuation is a late occurrence. The knee is held in partial flexion to reduce the pain caused by extension. Examine the foot for the potential sources of infection.

KEY SIGN
► **Popliteal Cyst: Popliteal Aneurysm:** This feels like a cyst and only a conscious effort to detect pulsation will identify it.

KEY SIGN
Medial Knee Swelling: Anserine Bursitis: The anserine bursa lies superficial to the tibial collateral ligament and deep to the pes anserina (goose foot) formed by the tendons of the sartorius, gracilis, and semitendinosus (see Fig. 13-45). The patient complains of pain in the anterior medial aspect of the knee 2–3 cm distal to the joint line. Pain is aggravated by walking, especially up stairs. Tenderness, usually without swelling, is palpated on the medial aspect of the knee.

Medial Knee Swelling: Cyst of the Medial Meniscus: The cyst is a developmental anomaly of the medial meniscus, which protrudes medially. Dull pain may be present on standing. It is felt as a fluctuant joint line, swelling slightly above the anserine bursa. The oval, transversely elongated cyst may protrude either anterior or posterior to the tibial collateral ligament. Flexion of the knee makes it more prominent.

Lateral Knee Swelling: Cyst of the Lateral Meniscus: This congenital cyst occurs at the tibiofemoral junction, posterior to the fibular collateral ligament. Flexion accentuates the transverse fluctuant swelling. It may be painful and, occasionally, protrudes into the popliteal fossa.

KEY SIGN
Post-traumatic Pain Proximal to the Patella: Rupture of the Rectus Femoris Muscle: The muscle fibers of the rectus femoris attach to the tendon well above the patella. Traumatic muscular tears often occur at this musculotendinous junction. The injury is painful and the knee is held in semiflexion. Abnormal shortening of the torn fibers forms a lump that enlarges when the patient tenses the thigh muscles. A hollow is felt distal to the lump; the normal muscle mass is not felt in the suprapatellar region.

KEY SIGN
Post-traumatic Patellar Pain: Patellar Fracture: This results from a direct blow to the patella, usually from falling onto the flexed knee. Stellate fractures are often not displaced and are easily missed without proper radiologic examination. With nondisplaced fractures, active extension is preserved but painful. Trans-

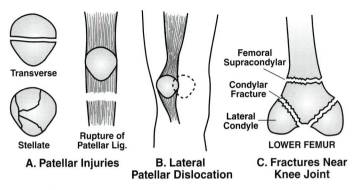

Fig. 13-46 Some Traumatic Injuries to the Anterior Knee.

verse fractures are most likely to be displaced. If there is separation of the bone fragments, the joint is semiflexed and active extension is impossible (Fig. 13-46A). To identify a separation, palpate down the surface of the patella feeling for a crevice. Hemarthrosis always occurs with displaced fractures.

KEY SIGN

Post-traumatic Patellar Pain: Rupture of the Patellar Ligament: The pathognomonic sign is an upward shift of the patella. After the swelling subsides, the ruptured ligament may be palpated (see Fig. 13-46A). Tenderness at the tibial tuberosity suggests concomitant avulsion of the tuberosity.

KEY SIGN

Anterior Knee Pain: Chondromalacia Patellae: Degeneration of the articular surface of the patella occurs from unknown cause. It is more common in women than men. Pain is felt anteriorly and is aggravated by prolonged sitting and walking down stairs. A small effusion may be present. Passive joint motion is painless. Rocking the patella in the femoral groove frequently elicits pain, often with palpable crepitation.

KEY SIGN

Sudden Collapse with Locking Knee: Patellar Dislocation: This is frequently a recurrent problem and the diagnosis may be made from the history. The patient complains that the knee abruptly gives way with pain and subsequent swelling. Acutely, the patella is displaced laterally (see Fig. 13-46B). Between episodes, there is increased lateral mobility of the patella and quadriceps atrophy may be seen.

KEY SIGN

Knee Pain and Recurrent Locking: Loose Body in the Joint: A history of intermittent joint pain with recurrent effusions or locking suggests a loose body in the joint. Crepitus may be present; rarely, the examiner may be able to palpate a mass. Loose bodies are usually a chip of bone resulting from previous injury.

KEY SIGN

Post-traumatic Knee Pain: The evaluation of patients with knee injuries starts with a detailed history of the mechanism of injury and the true cause of pain, swelling and disability. A complete knee exam should be attempted, but may be limited by pain. See page 706 and the following reference for further discussion. [Stiell IG, Greenberg GH, Wells GA, et al. Prospective validation of a decision rule for the use of radiography in acute knee injuries. *JAMA* 1996;275:611–615]

Post-traumatic Knee Pain: Femoral Supracondylar Fracture: A direct blow above the patella may produce a fracture 2.5–5 cm above the femoral condyles (see Fig. 13-46C). Active motion of the knee is impossible. Extreme tenderness with swelling is identified just above the patella. Displacement is usually absent. If displacement occurs, the distal fragment is pulled backward by the gastrocnemius. Always examine the distal pulses and sensation for evidence of neurovascular damage.

Post-traumatic Knee Pain: Femoral Condylar Fracture: The two condyles may be separated by a T fracture, with widening of the knee. Alternatively, only one condyle may be fractured (see Fig. 13-46C) with upward displacement of the affected condyle (see *Post-traumatic Knee Pain: Femoral Supracondylar Fracture* above).

Post-traumatic Knee Pain: Tibial Infracondylar Fracture: A fall with the knee extended and bent medially may cause fracture of one or both tibial condyles. Pain, swelling, and hemarthrosis occur. A valgus deformity may result. Occasionally, a concomitant fracture of the fibular head is found.

Post-traumatic Medial Knee Pain: Rupture of the Medial Meniscus: The meniscus is usually injured when the femur is twisted medially while the knee is flexed and the foot and tibia are fixed by bearing weight. The cartilage may be split longitudinally, or either the anterior or posterior horn may be torn. Most commonly, there is a bucket-handle tear in which the horns remain attached while the curved portion is torn from its fixation on the tibial surface, so the loop is free to move laterally into the joint. Locking may occur. The most constant sign is tenderness over the tibial collateral ligament at the joint line, when the knee is flexed. Tearing of the posterior horn causes tenderness posterior to the tibial collateral ligament. Tibial (medial) collateral ligament injuries are often coexistent.

Post-traumatic Medial Knee Pain: Rupture of the Medial (Tibial) Collateral Ligament: Injuries of the medial collateral ligament occur from valgus stress to the knee, such as a blow to the lateral side of the knee during weight bearing. Usually the femoral attachment is torn. The region of the ligament is tender and somewhat swollen. Because the medial meniscus attaches to the midportion of the ligament, medial collateral ligament injury often accompanies medial meniscus injury. With incomplete rupture, pain in the region is severe, but function is not completely lost and movement is resumed in a few hours; medial stability is present, although stress on the ligament elicits pain. When complete rupture occurs there is medial instability demonstrated when a valgus stress on the joint produces palpable separation of the tibia from the medial femoral condyle. In addition to pain and swelling, palpation of the ligament attachment may disclose a movable fragment of bone. Always compare the injured to the uninjured side because there is considerable individual variation in the baseline degree of joint stability.

Post-traumatic Lateral Knee Tenderness: Rupture of the Lateral Meniscus: The trauma may be so slight as to escape attention. Pain may be felt either laterally or medially. Tenderness is found in the lateral joint line. McMurray and Apley tests are positive when the procedures are modified by producing inward rotation of the foot instead of outward rotation. Locking of the joint is uncommon.

Post-traumatic Lateral Knee Tenderness: Rupture of the Lateral (Fibular) Collateral Ligament: This injury is produced by varus force on the knee with external rotation of the femur on the fixed tibia. Usually the fibular attachment is torn and the head of the fibula may be avulsed. Tenderness is found on the lateral aspect of the knee between the lateral femoral epicondyle and the fibular head. With a complete tear, the defect in the ligament may be palpable. Crepitus indicates avulsion of the fibular head. Stability is tested by placing a varus stress on the knee while palpating for opening of the lateral joint line. The common peroneal nerve may be injured simultaneously, so test the strength of the anterior and lateral muscles of the leg and the short extensors of the toes.

Post-traumatic Pain and Instability of the Knee Joint: Rupture of the Anterior Cruciate Ligament: Rupture of the anterior cruciate ligament occurs as the result of high-impact injury where the tibia is driven anterior relative to the femur. At the time of injury, there is severe pain and the joint is held in slight flexion. Physical examination of the ligament is difficult or impossible acutely because of pain and limited mobility secondary to tense hemarthrosis. After aspiration or resolution of the hemarthrosis, examination shows a positive Lachman test for anterior instability (see page 705).

Post-traumatic Pain and Instability of the Knee Joint: Rupture of the Posterior Cruciate Ligament: Posterior cruciate injury results from a direct blow on the head of the tibia while the knee is flexed. The tibia may sag posteriorly when compared to the uninjured knee while both knees are flexed at 90 degrees. The acute and late signs are similar to injury of the anterior cruciate ligament except that there is a positive *posterior* drawer sign. This is elicited by pushing the tibial head backward on the femoral condyles with the knee flexed at 90 degrees. Also, a sharp blow to the proximal anterior tibia, with the knee in 90 degrees of flexion, will elicit pain.

Leg Signs

KEY SIGN

Calf Pain: Intermittent Claudication: *Pathophysiology:* The arterial perfusion in the legs is sufficient at rest, but during walking the increased circulatory demands of the muscles cannot be met, lactate accumulates, and pain, as in angina pectoris, occurs in the affected muscles. The balance of arterial stenosis and collateral circulation determines the distance of asymptomatic walking. Anemia increases symptoms by loss of oxygen-carrying capacity, while polycythemia does so by increasing the blood viscosity, which slows the flow rate. The Latin *claudicatio* means limping or lameness. There are no symptoms at rest, but the patient begins to limp from pain or weakness in the calf or foot of one or both legs after walking a certain fixed distance. If the patient stops, symptoms subside within a few minutes, permitting walking for another similar distance before symptoms recur. With continued walking, despite symptoms, muscle cramps are likely to occur, although occasionally the pain subsides while walking. Pulses are diminished or absent in the popliteal, dorsalis pedis, and/or posterior tibial arteries of the affected leg. Common causes are atherosclerosis of the arteries in the legs, thrombosis, atheroembolism, thromboangiitis obliterans, and, rarely, premature calcification of arteries in pseudoxanthoma elasticum. Predisposing factors are tobacco use and diabetes.

UNILATERAL CLAUDICATION IN THE YOUNG: POPLITEAL ARTERY ENTRAPMENT SYNDROME: *Pathophysiology:* Entrapment of the popliteal artery by the medial head of the gastrocnemius muscle is a congenital anomaly. A young person develops unilateral claudication, with absence of or diminished pulses in the ipsilateral popliteal and dorsalis pedis arteries.

Post-traumatic Midcalf Pain: Soleus Tear: Trauma causing extreme dorsiflexion of the foot may tear the soleus muscle. This produces severe pain and tenderness in the midcalf.

KEY SIGN

Post-traumatic Achilles Pain: Rupture of the Achilles Tendon: The injury is most common in men over age 45 attempting unusual and vigorous activities requiring sudden accelerations or jumping. Complete rupture usually occurs about 5 cm above the calcaneal insertion. There is sudden excruciating pain and walking is not possible. Examine the patient in the prone position, with the feet hanging over the end of the table (see Fig. 13-22B, page 705). The affected foot is less plantar flexed and passive dorsiflexion is excessive. With incomplete rupture, squeezing the calf muscles transversely produces plantar flexion of the foot. This motion is absent when the tendon is severed completely (*Simmonds test*). In complete rupture, a gap can be felt in the tendon, the distal portion of the tendon is thicker and less taut, and the calf muscles are shortened into a visible lump.

Post-traumatic Anterior Leg Pain: Fracture of the Tibial Shaft: The injury may be a result of a fall on the leg or a direct blow to the anterior tibia. Pain is severe, and the leg cannot bear weight. Palpation discloses localized tenderness at the fracture site. Rolling a pencil over the subcutaneous aspect of the tibia will discover local tenderness.

Post-traumatic Anterior Leg Pain: Fracture of the Fibular Shaft: A direct blow on the anterolateral aspect of the leg is the most common cause. Fracture proximal to the ankle may also accompany severe inversion ankle injuries. There is pain at the site of injury, but, usually, the patient can walk. Compressing the tibia and fibula together causes pain at the fracture site.

Post-traumatic Leg Pain: Fracture of Both Tibia and Fibula: This injury is the most common cause of compound fracture. Frequently, the foot is turned outward in obvious deformity; manipulation should be avoided, but always palpate the dorsalis pedis pulse for evidence of arterial damage. When deformity is absent, ascertain if the normal straight line is present between the medial aspect of the great toe, the medial malleolus, and the medial patellar border.

KEY SIGN
Abrupt Calf Pain: Tear of Gastrocnemius (Tennis Leg): A violent combination of knee extension and dorsiflexion at the ankle causes a sensation like a blow to the posterior calf, sometimes accompanied by an audible snap. Unassisted walking is immediately intensely painful in the posteromedial midcalf. There is tenderness and a palpable defect in the medial belly of the gastrocnemius. After a few hours, swelling obscures the defect for a few days. The power of plantar flexion is diminished and muscle tone is absent in the medial head of the gastrocnemius for a few weeks. Ecchymoses develops over days extending from the medial calf to the heel, ankle and foot.

KEY SIGN

Post-exercise Tibial Pain: Stress Fracture of the Tibia: An incomplete cortical fracture of the tibia results from repeated strenuous use of the leg. Pain is gradual in onset; it is dull and aching. It occurs with progressively shortening intervals after exercise and persists for hours. There is localized tenderness over the tibia, frequently along the medial border. Pain at the fracture site may be elicited by springing the tibia: with the patient supine, place one hand on the knee and the other on the heel; pull the tibia laterally against your knee as a fulcrum.

KEY SIGN

► **Post-exercise Anterior Leg Pain: March Gangrene (Anterior Tibial Compartment Syndrome):** See page 794. Several hours after unusually strenuous leg exercise, stiffness followed by severe pain occurs in the anterior tibial muscular compartment. The region becomes swollen, tense, tender, and warm. Ischemic necrosis of the muscles may occur if the pressure is not relieved by fasciotomy.

KEY SIGN

Post-exercise Subpatellar Pain: Osteochondritis of Tibial Tubercle (Osgood-Schlatter Disease): Repetitive vigorous exercise during adolescence, before closure of the epiphysis of the tibial tubercle, produces chronic traction injury with partial avulsion of the tubercle. Pain occurs after exercise and a tender, hard swelling is seen and felt at the attachment of the patellar tendon.

Thickened Achilles Tendon: Thickening is most easily detected by inspection and palpation when the foot is dorsiflexed. Several diseases may produce inflammation (e.g., seronegative spondyloarthropathies, rheumatoid arthritis) or deposits in the tendon (e.g., xanthomas).

Ankle Signs

KEY SIGN

Swelling of the Ankle Joint: Joint Effusion: The foot is held in slight dorsiflexion and inversion. The distended joint produces bulging beneath the extensor tendons, near the talotibial junction and in front of the lateral and medial malleolar ligaments.

KEY SIGN

Post-traumatic Ankle Pain: Ankle trauma is common and the examiner needs a practical approach to the evaluation. The most common mechanism of injury is inversion injury of the flexed ankle while running or jumping. Ligament injuries are expected, but fractures may occur; this is the diagnostic dilemma. Careful prospective studies indicate that radiographs of the ankle are necessary only if there is pain near the malleoli and the patient is older than 55 years of age, is unable to bear weight immediately after the injury or take four steps when examined, or has bone tenderness at the posterior edge or tip of either malleolus [Stiell IG, Greenberg GH, McKnight RD, et al. Decisions rules for the use of radiography in acute ankle injuries. *JAMA* 1993;269: 1127–1132; Bachmann LM, Kolb E, Koller MT, et al. Accuracy of Ottawa ankle rules to exclude fractures of the ankle and mid-foot: Systematic review. *BMJ* 2003;326:417]. If these conditions are not met, fracture is very unlikely.

POST-TRAUMATIC LATERAL ANKLE PAIN: RUPTURE OF THE JOINT CAPSULE: Forceful plantarflexion with eversion of the foot may disrupt the anterolateral portion of the articular capsule. Pain and tenderness occur just anterior to the lateral malleolar ligaments (calcaneofibular and talofibular). A hematoma in the site rapidly appears, accompanied by some edema.

POST-TRAUMATIC LATERAL ANKLE PAIN: RUPTURE OF THE CALCANEO-FIBULAR LIGAMENT, COMMON ANKLE SPRAIN: This results from forced inversion of the foot. The tenderness is anterior and inferior to the lateral malleolus. With complete rupture, careful passive inversion of the foot demonstrates tilting of the talus. When the lateral malleolus is fractured, the posterior-lateral malleolus itself is tender.

POST-TRAUMATIC MEDIAL ANKLE PAIN: RUPTURE OF THE DELTOID LIGAMENT: This ligament is rarely injured in isolation. It may occur as part of severe fracture dislocation of the ankle.

Pain or Click During Dorsiflexion with Eversion: Recurrent Slipping of Peroneal Tendons:
The tendons of the peroneus longus and brevis curve behind and under the lateral malleolus, held in a groove by the a ligamentous band, the superior peroneal retinaculum. Relaxation of the retinaculum may permit slipping of the tendons during dorsiflexion with eversion. Pain or click occurs with the slipping. Physical examination at rest is normal but active motion may produce palpable tendon subluxation.

Pain on Inversion of the Foot: Chronic Stenosing Tenosynovitis of the Peroneal Tendon Sheath:
This causes pain only on inversion of the foot. Tenderness and swelling occur in the sheath behind and below the lateral malleolus.

Foot Signs

KEY SIGN
Deformed Foot: Talipes: The five principal varieties are talipes varus (inversion), talipes valgus (eversion), talipes equinus (plantar flexion), talipes calcaneus (dorsiflexion), and talipes or pes cavus (hollowing the instep) (Fig. 13-47). Combined deformities are

Talipes Equinus

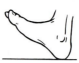

Talipes Calcaneus

Talipes Valgus

Talipes Varus

Pes Cavus

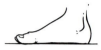

Pes Planus

Fig. 13-47 Deformities of the Foot.

talipes equinovarus (clubfoot), talipes equinovalgus, talipes calcaneo-varus, and talipes calcaneovalgus. The diagnosis is usually made by inspection.

KEY SIGN

Deformed Foot: Pes Planus (Flatfoot): (See Fig. 13-47.) One or more of the pedal arches are lowered. A functional classification includes relaxed flatfoot, in which the arch is lowered only while bearing weight; rigid flatfoot, caused by bony or fibrous ankylosis; spasmodic flatfoot, from contraction of the peronei; and transverse flatfoot, from flattening of the transverse arch.

KEY SIGN

Post-traumatic Heel Pain: Calcaneal Fracture: Landing on the heel during a fall may cause fracture of the calcaneus (os calcis) (Fig. 13-48A). The heel appears broader than normal from the back and the hollows beneath the malleoli are obliterated. Tenderness is maximal in the calcaneus near the insertion of the Achilles tendon. Palpation below the malleolus discloses the sides of the calcaneus to be flush with the malleolus, rather than indented. All motions of the ankle are restricted by pain. A hematoma forms in the sole of the heel. Signs of fracture may be subtle, so a high index of suspicion is required.

Pain in the Heel: Retrocalcaneal Bursitis: The bursa between the Achilles tendon and the calcaneus may be inflamed, causing pain, swelling, and tenderness near the tendon insertion (see Fig. 13-48B). The lesion is caused by pressure from footwear, especially high-heeled shoes or stiff-backed boots.

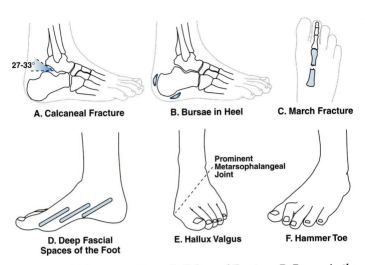

A. Calcaneal Fracture

B. Bursae in Heel

C. March Fracture

D. Deep Fascial Spaces of the Foot

E. Hallux Valgus

Prominent Metatarsophalangeal Joint

F. Hammer Toe

Fig. 13-48 Lesions of the Foot. A. Calcaneal Fracture. B. Bursae in the Heel. C. March Fracture of a Metatarsal Bone. D. Deep Fascial Spaces of the Foot. E. Hallux Valgus: This deformity shows lateral deviation of the great toe, with prominence of the 1st metatarsophalangeal joint. F. Hammer Toe: The second toe is always affected. There is permanent flexion of the proximal interphalangeal joint.

KEY SIGN

Pain in the Heel: Plantar Fasciitis: *Pathophysiology:* The plantar fascia is a thick band of fibrous tissue arising from the medial tuberosity of the calcaneus and spreading like a fan across the sole to insert on the proximal phalanges of the toes. Unusual or prolonged weight-bearing activity leads to microtrauma, which is concentrated at the calcaneal insertion. Pain is present in the plantar aspect of the heel and is usually worst with the first steps in the morning. Pain improves with activity, only to recur after rest. Tenderness is elicited at the insertion of the plantar fascia on the distal calcaneus somewhat medially.

Pain in the Heel: Inflammation of the Calcaneal Fat Pad: *Pathophysiology:* Fibrous bands extend from the calcaneal periosteum to the skin; their interstices are filled with fat. Infection or inflammation is compartmentalized by the fibrous bands leading to increased tissue pressure and intense pain. The region is too tender to permit weight bearing. Usually edema accumulates around the ankle; fluctuation occasionally is present.

KEY SIGN

Pain in the Heel: Tarsal Tunnel Syndrome: *Pathophysiology:* The tarsal tunnel is behind and inferior to the medial malleolus of the tibia. Its bony floor is roofed by the flexor retinaculum extending from the medial malleolus to the calcaneus. Through the tunnel pass several tendons and the posterior tibial nerve, which divides into the calcaneal nerve to the skin of the heel, the medial plantar nerve to the skin and muscles of the medial aspect of the sole, and the lateral plantar nerve to the lateral portion of the sole. Compression of the nerves in the tunnel causes numbness, burning pain, or paresthesias in portions of the sole. Paresis or paralysis of some small muscles of the foot may occur. Occasionally, a tender area is palpated at the posterior margin of the medial malleolus. The diagnosis is confirmed by nerve conduction studies. Precipitating conditions include fracture or dislocation of the bones near the tunnel, traumatic edema, tenosynovitis, chronic stasis of the posterior tibial vein and foot strain.

KEY SIGN

Metatarsal Pain: Metatarsalgia: *Pathophysiology:* Loss of the normal transverse metatarsal arch from the first to the fifth metatarsal heads leads to abnormal weight bearing on the second to fourth metatarsal heads, which are insufficiently padded to bear the weight. Ask the patient to point to the site of the pain. Pain occurs in the region of the distal metatarsal heads. Examination may show callus under the second to fourth metatarsals and decreased callus under the first and fifth. Pressure on the callus reproduces the pain. Symmetrical bilateral metatarsalgia may be an early symptom of rheumatoid arthritis. Fibroneuroma may also be the cause, so squeeze the foot transversely to see if the pain is reproduced.

KEY SIGN

Metatarsal Pain: Metatarsal Stress Fracture (March Fracture): Excessive walking or standing may cause a fracture of the metatarsal shaft (see Fig. 13-48C). Pain develops gradually. Muscle cramps and slight swelling may occur. Motion of the corresponding toe is painful. Pain is usually localized several centimeters proximal to the metatarsal head.

KEY SIGN

▶ **Metatarsal Pain: Infection in the Interdigital Space:** Puncture of the sole may cause infection of one of the four interdigital subcutaneous spaces. The resulting abscess may remain under the sole, or it may point between the two metatarsals to the dorsum of the foot, forming a collar-stud abscess. Walking produces pain between the metatarsals. Tenderness is localized to the interdigital space. Swelling of the dorsum occurs when the abscess has penetrated through the foot.

KEY SIGN

▶ **Pain in the Instep: Infection in the Deep Fascial Spaces:** The central plantar space has four compartments between the sole and the pedal arch (see Fig. 13-48D). Infection of the spaces occurs from direct puncture or backward extension from an interdigital space. There is tenderness in the instep (midfoot), dorsal edema, and the curve of the instep becomes obliterated.

Localized Swelling on the Dorsum: Ganglion: This is a cyst arising from a tarsal joint capsule or an extensor tendon.

Contracture of Plantar Fascia: Lederhosen Syndrome: The plantar fascia becomes thickened, but it is usually symptomless. Contracture may occur unilaterally or on both sides; occasionally, it is associated with Dupuytren contracture of the palms and Peyronie syndrome.

KEY SIGN
Lateral Deviation of the Great Toe: Hallux Valgus: Lateral deviation and rotation of the great toe produces abnormal prominence of the first metatarsophalangeal joint (see Fig. 13-48E). The second toe may overlap the first, or it may be a hammer toe. The great toe retains good motion. Pain is caused by accompanying hammer toe, an inflamed bursa over the prominent metatarsophalangeal joint (bunion), or metatarsalgia from transverse flatfoot (splay foot). The most common causes are improper shoes and primary osteoarthritis.

KEY SIGN
Stiffened Great Toe: Hallux Rigidus: *Pathophysiology:* Chronic arthritis or epiphysitis of the first metatarsophalangeal (MTP) joint from injury, or from wearing short shoes, may cause ankylosis, usually in extension; occasionally there is fixation in the more awkward flexion. A prominent osteophyte is usually present on the dorsal aspect of the joint. Pain in the joint occurs with walking and climbing. Extension of the MTP is severely limited and flexion is present mainly in the interphalangeal joint. Osteophytes may cause palpable irregularity on the joint edges.

KEY SIGN
Deformity of the Second to Fifth Toes: Hammer Toes: The proximal joint (metatarsophalangeal [MTP]) is fixed in dorsiflexion and the proximal interphalangeal (PIP) joint is fixed in plantarflexion, while the distal interphalangeal (DIP) joint is freely movable (see Fig. 13-48F). A corn or inflamed bursa frequently occurs over the PIP joint. Hammer toes are usually bilateral with several toes on each foot involved. It often accompanies hallux valgus.

Shortened Fifth Toe: Absence of Middle Phalanx: This is a frequent developmental anomaly.

Painful Swelling of a Toe: Fractured Phalanx: No matter how trivial the trauma seems, consider the possibility that the bone has been fractured.

KEY SIGN
Painful Swelling of the Metatarsal Pha-langeal Joint: Gout: This is the classic lesion (podagra) of early gout, described on page 776.

Toenail Signs

See Chapter 6, *The Skin and Nails*, page 157.

Muscle Signs

See also Chapter 14, *The Neurologic Examination.*

KEY SIGN
Muscular Atrophy: Loss of muscle substance occurs from disuse or from damage to muscle tissue or motor nerves. Fasciculation of the muscles indicates denervation, while the history will disclose injury and disuse.

KEY SIGN
Muscle Contracture: *Pathophysiology:* Prolonged disuse, immobilization, ischemia leading to muscle necrosis, or inflammatory processes, as in dermatomyositis, result in fibrosis of muscle with inelastic shortening. On palpation the muscle is firm to hard and atrophic. The shortened muscle does not permit full range of joint movement. The joints, however, are normal as distinct from joint contracture.

KEY SIGN
Muscle Hypertrophy: *Pathophysiology:* Increased muscle volume results from enlargement of normal muscles or infiltration of the muscle by cellular or extracellular material. Resistance exercise increases muscle bulk and power. Hypertrophy may also occur with anabolic steroid use, in hypothyroidism, congenital myotonia, Duchenne muscular dystrophy, and focal myositis.

KEY SIGN
Muscle Masses: To prove that a mass is intramuscular the mass must be freely movable transversely to the long axis, with the muscle relaxed. Tensing the muscle must limit the transverse mobility. A mass may result from rupture of a muscle, herniation of a muscle through its sheath, intramuscular hemorrhage, neoplasm, or localized myositis ossificans.

KEY SIGN
Trigger Points: Myofascial Pain: Painful firm nodules or bands occur in muscles under frequent tonic contraction. The patient complains of pain, often with projection of pain in a nondermatomal pattern around the area and distally into the arm from trigger points in the upper back and neck, or into the leg from trigger points in the pelvic girdle. The pain often has a burning quality. Motor strength and sensation are normal. Trigger points are characteristic of myofas-

cial pain syndromes. They occur most commonly in large muscles of the back and in proximal extremities. Injection of local anesthetic, heat, massage, and stretching, combined with avoidance or changes in precipitating postural activities, is effective therapy. Left untreated, changes may occur in central and peripheral pain pathways leading to chronic persistent pain syndromes.

KEY SIGN

Tender Points: Fibromyalgia: Persistent reproducible pain is elicited by palpation of specific muscles. The patient does not complain specifically of pain in these sites, unlike trigger points. Eighteen symmetrically located sites in the neck, back, and extremities have been standardized for the diagnosis of fibromyalgia (see page 793) [Bennett RM. Emerging concepts in the neurobiology of chronic pain: Evidence of abnormal sensory processing in fibromyalgia. *Mayo Clin Proc* 1999:74:385–398].

Musculoskeletal and Soft-Tissue Syndromes

General Syndromes

S KEY SYNDROME

Complex Regional Pain Syndrome: Reflex Sympathetic Dystrophy: *Pathophysiology:* Minor injury, usually to an extremity, initiates a complex series of spinal and central nervous system responses that result in altered autonomic function and pain perception. The patient initially complains of pain, often burning or throbbing in quality, disproportionate to visible injury. Examination may reveal hyperalgesia, hyperesthesia, edema, erythema, and changes in skin temperature. Progression leads to vascular changes, including cyanosis and mottling, atrophy of skin, muscle and subcutaneous tissue, contractures, and altered sweating. The affected part is cool and painful at rest and with any activity. Early recognition and treatment is essential to avoid long-term disability. (See Chapter 4, page 97).

S KEY SYNDROME

Necrotizing Soft-Tissue Infection: *Pathophysiology:* Rapid expansion of infection in subcutaneous tissue planes produces ischemia of fat, connective tissue, skin, and underlying muscle as a consequence of local vascular thrombosis. The infection spreads proximally and distally along tissue planes and invades deeper structures along neurovascular bundles that penetrate these planes. When the muscular fascia is involved the term *necrotizing fasciitis* is applied. Pain and fever accompanied by signs of inflammation (erythema, warmth, tenderness) result from infection with group A streptococci or polymicrobial (mixed aerobic/anaerobic) soft-tissue infections. Systemic hypotension, tachycardia, and delirium develop rapidly, and outcome is fatal without complete surgical debridement. Predisposing factors include diabetes mellitus, immunosuppression, and trauma (often minor).

 Urgent surgical debridement is mandatory to save limb and life.

CT and MRI help to assess the extent of involved tissues [Hoadley DJ, Mark EJ. Weekly clincopathological exercises: Case 28-2002: A 35-year-old long-term traveler to the Caribbean with a rapidly progressive soft-tissue infection. *N Engl J Med* 2002;347:831–837].

S KEY SYNDROME

Acromegaly and Gigantism: *Pathophysiology:* The hands enlarge from overgrowth of bone and soft tissues, stimulated by an excess of growth hormone, usually from an adenoma of the anterior pituitary gland. When the condition occurs before the epiphyses close, the enlarged skeleton is well proportioned and the condition is termed gigantism. When growth occurs after epiphyseal closure, the skeletal pattern is called acromegaly, in which the hands, feet, face, head, and soft tissues are enlarged. Patients often have diffuse muscular or joint stiffness and may complain of headaches and back pain. Examination shows thickening of the soft tissues, particularly apparent in the face, hands, and feet. Widening without lengthening of the bones leads to prominence of the jaw, wide spacing of the teeth, prominent supraorbital ridge, and enlarged hands and feet. Osteoarthritis is common. In advanced disease with suprasellar extension of the tumor, signs of hypopituitarism and bitemporal hemianopsia may be present.

S KEY SYNDROME

Marfan Syndrome: *Pathophysiology:* This is a congenital disease, frequently inherited as an autosomal dominant, but sporadic cases do occur. It affects the development of bone, ligaments, tendons, arterial walls, and supporting structures in the heart and eyes. Many persons show only a few stigmas, while the complete syndrome presents a striking portrait. The long, slender phalanges, spider fingers, have given the name arachnodactyly to the disease, although some patients with Marfan syndrome lack this sign. The skull is long and narrow, and the palate is high and arched. The long bones are thin and elongated, so the finger-to-finger span with the outspread arms exceeds the body height. Thoracic deformities may be either pectus excavatum (funnel breast) or pectus carinatum (pigeon breast). The spine may exhibit fused vertebrae or spina bifida. Joint laxity permits hyperextension (double-jointedness), dislocations, kyphoscoliosis, pes planus, or pes cavus. The ears may be long and pointed, satyr ear. Weakness of the supporting structures of the eye produces elongation of the globe (myopia), retinal detachment, lenticular dislocation, and blue sclerae. Degeneration of the vascular elastic media leads to aneurysmal dilatation of the aorta or pulmonary artery. Subsequent dissection or rupture are common causes of early death. Deformities of the cardiac valve cusps are sites for bacterial endocarditis. The foramen ovale may remain patent.

Conditions Primarily Affecting Joints

S KEY SYNDROME

Arthritis: Inflammatory and Noninflammatory Joint Disease:

The diagnosis of *arthritis* requires the examiner to confirm signs of acute or chronic joint inflammation: redness, warmth, tenderness, synovial thickening, effusion, bony enlargement, or erosive changes on x-ray. The most diagnostically useful descriptive classification of joint diseases is based upon the history and physical findings. First, the number of joints actively involved is assessed as *monarticular* (1 joint), *oligoarticular* (2–4 joints) or *polyarticular* (>4 joints). For patients with oligo- or polyarthritis, note the pattern of joint involvement: (a) large more proximal joints or distal small joints; (b) axial joints and/or peripheral joints; and (c) whether involvement is *symmetric* or *asymmetric*. Widespread and symmetrical joint involvement increases the likelihood of a systemic inflammatory disease primarily involving the joints (e.g., rheumatoid arthritis, systemic lupus erythematosus).

Careful attention during the physical exam is necessary to distinguish involvement of the joint (synovium and articular cartilage: *arthritis*) from inflammation of the periarticular tendon and ligament insertions into bone (the enthesis: *enthesitis*), the tendons and their sheaths (*tendonitis* and *tenosynovitis*) or the underlying bone (*osteitis*).

No classification system is perfect and the examiner must always be alert to evolution of the pattern over periods ranging from days to weeks or years. Remember that polyarthritic diseases may initially present with single joint involvement. Correct rheumatologic diagnosis requires patience and an open mind.

S KEY SYNDROME

Monarticular Arthritis:

Arthritis involving a single joint is likely caused by local mechanical, inflammatory, or infectious factors. Less commonly, it is the initial manifestation of a systemic process that will involve other joints. Sequential involvement of single joints with intervening remissions suggest an underlying systemic disorder (congenital or acquired) with superimposed local precipitating events, for example, trauma in hemophilia.

✓ *MONOARTHRITIS—CLINICAL OCCURRENCE:* *Congenital* hemophilia; *Endocrine* hyperparathyroidism, hypothyroidism; *Idiopathic* osteoarthritis; *Inflammatory/Immune* postinfectious reactive arthritis (e.g., Reiter syndrome, viral exanthems), psoriasis, rheumatoid arthritis (initial presentation), systemic lupus erythematosus (SLE), amyloidosis; *Infectious* acute septic arthritis (*Staphylococcus aureus*, gonococcemia, others), Lyme disease, mycobacteria, osteomyelitis, viral (e.g., HIV, parvovirus, others); *Metabolic/Toxic* crystal-induced diseases (e.g., gout, calcium pyrophosphate deposition, calcium hydroxyapatite, calcium oxalate), scurvy; *Mechanical/Traumatic* blunt trauma, hemarthrosis, fracture, repetitive use/overuse; *Neoplastic* sarcoma (bone, synovium, or cartilage), metastases to bone, benign tumors (e.g., osteochondroma, osteoid osteoma, pigmented villonodular synovitis), leukemia; *Neurologic* neuropathy producing a Charcot joint; *Vascular* osteonecrosis.

▶

ACUTE MONARTHRITIS: SUPPURATIVE ARTHRITIS: *Pathophysiology:* Bacterial infection, most commonly with *Staphylococcus aureus,* results from direct extension (from skin, soft tissue, or periarticular bone) or from hematogenous spread (e.g., bacterial endocarditis, gonorrhea bacteremia). Release of lysosomal enzymes can rapidly destroy the joint. Usually one joint is involved, often the knee, but in gonococcal arthritis, three-fourths of the patients have an initial transient (2–4 days) migratory oligoarthritis and/or tenosynovitis. Symptoms often begin suddenly with chills and fever. The joint swells rapidly, the overlying skin is red and warm, and the joint is painful and tender to touch. The swelling becomes fluctuant, indicating fluid in the synovial cavity. Signs of infection in immunosuppressed patients are frequently absent. Joint aspiration discloses purulent fluid that must be cultured and gram stained to identify the causative organism.

✔ *SEPTIC ARTHRITIS—CLINICAL OCCURRENCE:* In addition to *S. aureus* and gonorrhea, less-common organisms to consider are streptococci, meningococci, *Haemophilus influenzae* (especially in unimmunized infants and children), and, rarely, brucellosis, typhoid fever, glanders, blastomycosis, granuloma inguinale, tuberculosis, and fungi, as well as others.

ACUTE MONARTHRITIS: GOUT: *Pathophysiology:* Uric acid accumulates in tissue and extracellular fluid as a result of genetic (primary gout) or acquired (secondary gout) causes of uric acid overproduction or underexcretion. When the fluid becomes supersaturated, crystals form in the tissue. When crystals are shed into the joint fluid and phagocytosed by polymorphonuclear neutrophils (PMNs), acute inflammation results. Large tissue deposits of uric acid (tophi) occurring around joints over bony prominences are not usually inflamed. The initial attack presents the chief diagnostic problem because a history of recurrent stereotypic episodes is very suggestive of gout. Frequently, the patient is awakened from sleep by severe burning pain, tingling, numbness, or warmth in a joint. The joint rapidly swells and becomes excruciatingly tender, intolerant to the pressure of the bedclothes. Typically, the overlying skin becomes red or violaceous. There may be malaise, headache, fever, and tachycardia. Untreated, the attack lasts for 1–2 weeks. In more than half the cases, the metatarsophalangeal joint of the great toe is affected initially (podagra). Other sites are the midfoot (instep), ankle, knee, elbow, or wrist. Acute gout in the midfoot resembles cellulitis. The attacks may be triggered by trauma, surgery, acidosis, infection, exposure to cold, changes in atmospheric pressure, overindulgence in alcoholic beverages, or any acute illness.

ACUTE MONARTHRITIS: CALCIUM PYROPHOSPHATE DIHYDRATE DEPOSITION DISEASE (CPPDD, PSEUDOGOUT, CHONDROCALCINOSIS): *Pathophysiology:* Calcium pyrophosphate dihydrate, shed from articular cartilage, crystalizes within the joint into small, rhomboidal, weakly positive birefringent crystals that trigger the inflammation. Articular fibro-cartilage may calcify and be detected by x-ray *(chondrocalcinosis)* in the knee or wrist. This disorder is quite similar to true gout in both its acute and chronic forms. The attack begins abruptly with painful swelling and heat, usually in a single joint, occasionally in two or more joints. The knee, ankle, and wrist are most commonly affected. Untreated, the pain and tenderness are intense for 2–4 days, then they gradually subside during the next 1–2 weeks. It is commonly associated with increasing age and osteoarthritis and may be a clue to hyperparathyroidism or hemochromatosis (approximately 5% of CPPDD).

CHRONIC MONARTHRITIS: TUBERCULOSIS: There is chronic swelling of a single joint with only moderate pain. Joint effusion may be present with thickening of the synovium. Most commonly affected are the hips, knees, and spine. Previous intraarticular or oral corticosteroids and immunosuppressive drugs are major risk factors. Cultures of aspirated joint fluid or synovial biopsy yield *Mycobacterium tuberculosis.*

CHRONIC MONARTHRITIS: SYPHILIS: Clinically, this may be identical to tuberculous arthritis. Negative cultures and positive serologic tests for syphilis make the distinction.

MONARTHRITIS: EPISODIC PAINLESS EFFUSIONS OF THE KNEES: The patient experiences episodes of painless swelling and joint effusion in one or both knees, with no constitutional symptoms over a number of years, with an average duration of 3–5 days. The cause is unknown, though, occasionally, the condition presages the onset of rheumatoid arthritis.

MONARTHRITIS: TRAUMA: *Pathophysiology:* Mechanical trauma as a result of falls, sports, or other activities causes bleeding (hemarthrosis) or effusion with pain as a consequence of damage to the joint capsule, intra- or periarticular ligaments, cartilage, or bone. The knee and ankle are commonly affected, but any joint can be injured. The exact mechanism of injury, time course of pain (immediate versus delayed), and physical examination will assist in suggesting the type and degree of injury. Guidelines for the proper use of radiologic exam for injuries to the ankle and knee have been developed.

MONARTHRITIS: CHARCOT JOINT: See page 779.

S KEY SYNDROME

Oligoarthritis and Polyarthritis: Arthritis involving several joints, either simultaneously or sequentially, is termed oligoarthritis and polyarthritis. The pattern of involvement can be useful in helping to identify the exact diagnosis. Generally, oligoarthritis involves larger joints and is *asymmetric* while the classic polyarthritis syndromes (rheumatoid arthritis [RA], systemic lupus erythematosus [SLE]) involve *symmetric* joints, including the small joints of the hands and feet. These are only guidelines and must not be interpreted as hard-and-fast rules.

✓ *OLIGO- AND POLYARTHRITIS—CLINICAL OCCURRENCE:* *Congenital* hemophilia, familial Mediterranean fever, hemochromatosis, sickle cell disease; *Endocrine* hyperparathyroidism, hypothyroidism, acromegaly;

Idiopathic inflammatory osteoarthritis; *Inflammatory/Immune* postinfectious reactive arthritis (e.g., Reiter syndrome, viral exanthems, inflammatory bowel disease), psoriasis, rheumatoid arthritis, SLE, rheumatic fever, ankylosing spondylitis, systemic sclerosis (scleroderma), polymyositis/dermatomyositis, Still disease, Behçet syndrome, relapsing polychondritis, amyloidosis, sarcoidosis, erythema multiforme, erythema nodosum, drug reactions, serum sickness; *Infectious* septic arthritis (bacterial endocarditis, *Staphylococcus aureus*, gonococcemia, others), Lyme disease, viral (e.g., HIV, parvovirus, rubella, mumps, others), Whipple disease, mycoses (coccidioidomycosis, histoplasmosis, blastomycosis, cryptococcosis), actinomycosis, secondary syphilis, brucellosis, typhoid fever; *Metabolic/Toxic* crystal-induced diseases (e.g., gout, calcium pyrophosphate deposition, calcium hydroxyapatite, calcium oxalate), scurvy; *Neoplastic* sarcoma (bone, synovium, or cartilage), metastases to bone, benign tumors (e.g., osteochondroma, osteoid osteoma, pigmented villonodular synovitis); *Vascular* osteonecrosis, systemic vasculitis, hypertrophic osteoarthropathy.

D   KEY DISEASE

MIGRATORY OLIGOARTHRITIS: GONOCOCCAL ARTHRITIS: *Pathophysiology: Neisseria gonorrhoeae* infects the urethra or uterine cervix and then disseminates hematogenously to synovial membranes and skin, causing local inflammation. Infectious arthritis, tenosynovitis, and skin lesions are the most common extragenital complications of gonorrhea. One to 4 weeks after the onset of urethritis, inflammation may suddenly occur in the knees, wrists, and ankles, although other joints may be affected. The most common pattern is a migratory oligoarthritis and tenosynovitis. Small amounts of thin fluid may accumulate in joint cavities, from which organisms are difficult to isolate. In other cases, suppurative arthritis develops, with inflammation of a single joint and production of purulent exudate in which the gonococcus can be identified. Tenosynovitis in the hands, wrists, or ankle is more common in gonorrhea than in arthritis from any other cause. The diagnosis may not be easy because the gonococcus is difficult to culture from the joints. Pustular skin lesions on an erythematous base are seen with gonococcal bacteremia and help to distinguish gonococcal arthritis from other conditions. Genital, rectal and throat specimens for culture or polymerase chain reaction (PCR) testing of urine for gonococcus and chlamydia should be obtained. Reiter syndrome (nonspecific urethritis, arthritis, and conjunctivitis) following nongonococcal urethritis may cause confusion, because conjunctival infection is present in up to 10% of patients with gonorrhea.

OLIGOARTHRITIS: ANKYLOSING SPONDYLITIS: See page 722.

S   KEY SYNDROME

OLIGOARTHRITIS: REACTIVE ARTHRITIS (REITER SYNDROME): Following infection of the urethra (chlamydia) or gut (*Shigella, Salmonella, Yersinia, Campylobacter*) an oligoarthritis, predominately of the lower extremities, develops. It may be accompanied by enthesitis of the hands, ankles, and feet, conjunctivitis, urethritis, and rash on the glans penis (circinate balanitis) and feet (keratoderma blenorrhagica). Sacroiliitis and spine involvement may occur. In addition, 85% of patients are HLA-B27–positive.

OLIGOARTHRITIS: ENTEROPATHIC ARTHRITIS: Inflammatory asymmetric arthritis predominately of the ankles and knees may occur in association with inflammatory bowel disease (ulcerative colitis and Crohn disease). *Enthesitis* is common, especially at the Achilles tendon insertion, and symmetrical sacroiliac and spinal involvement occurs. The arthritis may precede clinical manifestations of the inflammatory bowel disease.

D KEY DISEASE

OLIGOARTHRITIS: PSORIATIC ARTHRITIS: The joint disease is usually an asymmetrical oligo- or polyarthritis of small and large joints. It is occasionally a symmetrical polyarthritis resembling rheumatoid arthritis (RA). Destructive arthritis of the distal interphalangeal joints is seen in psoriatic arthritis but not in RA. Spondylitis and sacroiliitis occur in up to 25% of patients with psoriatic arthritis, especially those with HLA-B27. Enthesitis may predominate in some patients. The arthritis may precede, accompany, or follow onset of the skin rash. Physical examination should include a careful skin examination, especially of the scalp (the rash may be hidden by hair or dismissed as seborrhea) and fingernails (looking for pits and onycholysis).

OLIGOARTHRITIS: TOPHACEOUS GOUT: See page 776. *Pathophysiology:* Tophi are masses of sodium urate crystals deposited in the tissues often over bony prominences and around joints where they erode bone. Acting as foreign bodies, they stimulate low-grade inflammation that may extrude the tophi through the skin. The asymmetrical nodular swellings and cartilage degeneration may impair joint function. Clinical signs of inflammation are variable, from mild to moderately severe. The olecranon, bunion and prepatellar bursae, and hands are most frequently affected.

S KEY SYNDROME

OLIGOARTHRITIS: CHARCOT JOINT: *Pathophysiology:* Absence of pain or proprioceptive sensation in a joint leads to loss of joint integrity. Repeated injuries cause successively three stages of articular damage: swelling, joint degeneration, and formation of new bone. In the initial stage, erythema and swelling are the only findings. The course is progressive with hypermobility, traumatic osteophyte formation, and subluxation leading to painless deformities and crepitus on movement. In any stage, the diagnostic clue is the absence of the expected pain with movement and loss of pain sensation and proprioception in the involved limb. A single joint may be affected, or, commonly, all the joints in an anatomic region (e.g., the midfoot joints) are involved. Physical exam should try to determine if the neuropathy is part of a local or systemic neuropathic process. Classic clinical conditions causing Charcot joints include tabes dorsalis (knee most commonly involved [Fig. 13-44C]; hip, ankle, lower spine, less frequently involved), diabetes mellitus (tarsal and metatarsal joints most commonly, ankle occasionally, knee rarely), syringomyelia (usually joints of the upper limbs), and leprosy [Hartemann-Heurtier A, Van GH, Grimaldi A. The Charcot foot. *Lancet* 2002;360:1776–1779].

D   KEY DISEASE

SYMMETRIC INFLAMMATORY POLYARTHRITIS: RHEUMATOID ARTHRITIS (RA): *Pathophysiology:* RA is characterized by proliferation of inflamed synovial tissue (pannus) that enters the joint cavity in tongue-like projections. The pannus erodes cartilage, periarticular bone, and soft tissues, including tendons and ligaments. Untreated, the result is destruction of the joint surfaces and supporting structures producing subluxation, deformity, and loss of joint function. The onset may be insidious with morning stiffness and pain followed by swelling and tenderness of the joints, proceeding over weeks to months into a small and large joint polyarthritis. Less commonly, the onset is sudden with pain and swelling occurring simultaneously in several joints accompanied by fever and prostration. Smaller joints of the hands (metacarpophalangeal [MCP], proximal interphalangeal [PIP]), feet (metatarsophalangeal [MTP]), wrists, and ankles are typically involved early and symmetrically, although onset in a single larger joint, usually a knee, is not rare. Interphalangeal joints become fusiform from joint effusion (fluctuant) or thickening of the joint capsule (palpable as thickening of tissue over the joint). Distal interphalangeal joints are invariably spared. Tenderness is confined to the region of the capsule. Early, joint motion is limited by pain or fluid; later, it is limited by fibrosis or muscle shortening. Muscle weakness and atrophy may be rapid and disproportionate to the degree of disuse. Although remissions may occur, the disease is usually progressive over a period of years. Joint contracture and subluxations are frequent, with subluxation of the metacarpophalangeal joints producing characteristic ulnar deviation of the fingers. Tenosynovitis is manifest as swelling of the tendon sheaths. In 20–35% of cases, subcutaneous *rheumatoid nodules* develop over bony prominences and tendon sheaths. They are painless, firm, and freely movable over bones, similar to those in rheumatic fever (RF). A serious late complication is instability of the cervical spine as a consequence of subluxation of C1 on C2, which may present as neck pain or upper motor neuron signs. There is no specific diagnostic test and diagnosis is based upon clinical and laboratory criteria. Although rheumatoid factor can be demonstrated in 80% of cases, it is neither sensitive nor specific. Frequently, the patient must be observed for many months before the diagnosis is secure. DDX: RA frequently involves the temporomandibular joint unlike RF. In rheumatic fever, the arthritis is migratory, while it is persistent in RA. Reactive arthritis (Reiter syndrome, postdysentery, or urethritis) is usually oligoarticular and mainly affects large joints, especially ankles and knees. An initial monarthritis may suggest an infectious or crystalline arthritis; however, aspiration of joint fluid excludes these possibilities.

VARIANTS OF RHEUMATOID ARTHRITIS. *Felty's syndrome* is the triad of rheumatoid arthritis, splenomegaly, and leukopenia. *Palindromic rheumatism* presents as multiple afebrile attacks of polyarthritis lasting for only 2 or 3 days, leaving no residua. Secondary *Sjögren's syndrome* is diagnosed when keratoconjunctivitis sicca and xerostomia accompany rheumatoid arthritis. *Vasculitis* may accompany RA and involve the skin (necrosis and nodules) and lung. *Juvenile rheumatoid arthritis* is a group of disorders which may overlap with the adult disease. See pediatric texts for descriptions and details.

D KEY DISEASE

▼ **INFLAMMATORY POLYARTHRITIS: SYSTEMIC LUPUS ERYTHEMATOSUS (SLE):** *Pathophysiology:* The cause is unknown, but the disease involves inflammation of multiple tissues and organs accompanied by antibodies to specific nuclear antigens that are detectable in the serum. The role of these antibodies in the pathogenesis of the syndrome is unclear. This is a chronic inflammatory multisystem disease, more common in women than men. Lupus, the Latin word for wolf, was applied because the malar erythema on the cheeks resembled a wolf's face. No one symptom or sign is pathognomonic of SLE; rather, the diagnosis is established by clinical criteria. The most common symptoms and signs are fatigue, malaise, or fever (90% of cases), arthritis or arthralgias (90%), and skin rashes (50–60%). The arthralgias, myalgias, and joint inflammation resemble mild rheumatoid arthritis, but without the deformities and subluxations seen in RA. The malar ("butterfly") rash is a macular to maculopapular, sometimes scaly, erythematous process forming the "wings" of the butterfly on each malar prominence, with the "trunk" of the insect on the bridge of the nose. It may be more intense after exposure to sunlight. In addition, there may be skin atrophy, telangiectasia, and mucosal ulcers. Serositis is common, presenting as pleurisy (with effusion and/or pleural rubs), abdominal pain, or pericarditis. Nonbacterial endocarditis with valvular insufficiency (usually mitral), CNS disease (with personality change, psychosis, or seizures) and glomerulonephritis can occur at any time in the course of the disease, and may be the presenting syndromes. Other signs are recurrent urticaria, mononeuritis multiplex and lymphadenopathy. Fetal wastage and thromboembolic disease are associated with antiphospholipid antibodies.

D KEY DISEASE

▼ **NONINFLAMMATORY POLYARTHRITIS: OSTEOARTHRITIS (DEGENERATIVE JOINT DISEASE):** *Pathophysiology:* This is a disease of articular cartilage with degradation of the proteoglycan matrix leading to fissuring, thinning, and loss of articular cartilage, and secondary thickening of subchondral bone. In late stages, the bone ends rub directly on each other so their surfaces become worn and polished. The joint capsules are little affected, so adhesions are not formed, and although joint motion is restricted, ankylosis does not result. The bony margins proliferate to form spurs, lipping, and exostoses. Genetic and acquired factors (trauma, surgery, obesity, excessive use) contribute to the pathogenesis. Symptoms are usually first noticed in the weight-bearing joints after age 40 and signs of inflammation are relatively slight. Symptoms correlate poorly with the objective extent of joint disease. The most common symptom is pain with use that disappears with rest. The patient may note grating during motion. Initially, the range of motion is normal, with a gradual decrease occurring as the disease progresses. Enlargement of the distal and proximal interphalangeal joints of the fingers (Heberden and Bouchard nodes, respectively), is frequently encountered. Painless knee effusion is frequent as is asymmetric loss of knee cartilage leading to valgus or varus deformity.

NONINFLAMMATORY POLYARTHRITIS: HEMOCHROMATOSIS: The second and third metacarpal phalangeal joints and the radiocarpal joint of the wrist are most commonly affected. Chondrocalcinosis is present. Symmetric noninflammatory arthritis of the metacarpophalangeal joints should initiate a search for an iron-storage disorder.

D KEY DISEASE

MIGRATORY POLYARTHRITIS: RHEUMATIC FEVER: *Pathophysiology:* This disease is a delayed inflammatory reaction following infection with specific Lancefield groups of group A beta-hemolytic streptococci. Tissues affected include the heart, joints, skin, and central nervous system. The disease is protean in its clinical manifestations. The classic presentation begins from 1 to 4 weeks after streptococcal pharyngitis, with gradual onset of malaise, fatigue, anorexia, and fever. A single large joint becomes painful, tender, and swollen, and the overlying skin is red and hot. An effusion forms that is turbid and sterile. While the fever and other signs of illness persist, the joint inflammation spontaneously subsides in a few days, only to reappear in another joint, and later in another joint—a *migratory polyarthritis*. Joint involvement may be so mild that pain is unaccompanied by physical signs of inflammation. Months of observation may be required to distinguish it from rheumatoid arthritis; involvement of the temporomandibular joint often occurs in rheumatoid arthritis, practically never in rheumatic fever. Rheumatic fever leaves no residual joint deformity. At onset, the inflammation of a single joint with effusion requires distinction from suppurative arthritis. *Carditis* is manifest as tachycardia, muffled heart sounds, heart enlargement, valvular insufficiency murmurs, pericardial friction rub, or gallop rhythm on examination. The electrocardiogram may show PR prolongation. Two distinct types of *skin lesions* may be associated with rheumatic fever, although neither is pathognomonic. Erythema marginatum or circinatum is characterized by coalescing circular erythematous areas over the trunk and extremities, migratory and transitory, changing within the hour. With chronic disease, subcutaneous rheumatic nodules may appear as firm, nontender masses over the joint prominences and tendon sheaths of the limbs, scalp, and spine. They are loosely attached to the underlying tissue; when numerous, their distribution tends to be symmetrical. *Sydenham chorea* may appear several months after onset. There are no diagnostic laboratory tests, but the full clinical picture is fairly distinctive. Diagnosis is based upon the Jones criteria of major and minor manifestations.

POLYARTHRITIS: RELAPSING SYMMETRICAL SERONEGATIVE SYNOVITIS WITH PITTING EDEMA (RS3PE): This condition of unknown cause presents with recurrent episodes of symmetrical synovitis of the hands and wrists with pitting edema and erythema of the dorsum of the hands. Pain is relatively mild and the condition remits after several days to a couple of weeks.

S KEY SYNDROME

▼ **Spondyloarthritis:** *Pathophysiology:* Inflammation at the insertion of ligaments and tendons into bone (the enthesis, enthesitis) leads to joint and tendon sheath effusions and calcification of periarticular structures. Genes (HLA-B27) and acquired illness (inflammatory bowel disease, infectious colitis, nongonococcal urethritis, psoriasis) predispose to these disorders. Asymmetric oligoarthritides of the large joints with prominent involvement of the spine and sacroiliac joints and negative tests for rheumatoid factor are described as the *seronegative spondyloarthritides.* Patients present with back pain and stiffness, and occasionally with fever, malaise, and weight loss. Look for extraarticular disease, such as genitourinary or gut symptoms, eye involvement (uveitis), and skin disease.

✓ *SPONDYLOARTHRITIS—CLINICAL OCCURRENCE:* *Congenital* ochronosis; *Idiopathic* disk disease, diffuse idiopathic skeletal hyperostosis (DISH); *Inflammatory/Immune* ankylosing spondylitis, reactive arthritis (e.g., Reiter), enteropathic arthritis (inflammatory bowel disease), psoriasis; *Infectious* after diarrheal and genitourinary infections (see reactive arthritis, Reiter syndrome).

SPONDYLOARTHRITIS: ANKYLOSING SPONDYLITIS: See page 722. This is a chronic, progressive arthritis of the spine often leading to severe ankylosis. It begins with sacroiliac involvement and progresses proximally. Decreased lumbar spinal motion is an early sign. In 20% of cases, there is an accompanying large joint oligoarthritis of hips and shoulders.

SPONDYLOARTHRITIS: REACTIVE ARTHRITIS (REITER SYNDROME): See page 778.

SPONDYLOARTHRITIS: PSORIATIC ARTHRITIS: See page 779.

SPONDYLOARTHRITIS: DIFFUSE IDIOPATHIC SKELETAL HYPEROSTOSIS (DISH): A condition of unknown cause that affects women more often than men. Asymmetric osteophytes develop at multiple levels of the spine leading to bridging of multiple intervertebral spaces and irregular ankylosis with decreased spinal motion, especially in the cervical and lumbar regions. The disk spaces are preserved.

Conditions Primarily Affecting Bone

S KEY SYNDROME

▼ **Osteoporosis:** *Pathophysiology:* Bone resorption exceeds bone formation, leading to decreased bone mass and decreased mechanical strength. Trabecular bone is affected more than cortical bone. Increased resorption of bone results from immobilization, inflammation, multiple myeloma, and hyperparathyroidism. Decreased bone formation results from gonadal hormone deficiency and glucocorticoid steroid excess, and with advanced age. Trabecular bone deficiency is especially important in the vertebrae and pelvic bones, while cortical bone loss is predominant in long bones. Osteoporosis is asymptomatic until insufficiency fractures occur, usually in the thoracic or lumbar spine and pelvis. Thoracic kyphosis results from anterior wedging of thoracic vertebrae. Bone mineral density is assessed by dual x-ray absorptiometry (DEXA) scan.

✓ *OSTEOPOROSIS—CLINICAL OCCURRENCE:* *Congenital* vitamin D-resistant rickets, Marfan syndrome, hemochromatosis, Ehlers-Danlos syndrome, hemophilia, thalassemia, positive family history; *Endocrine* postmenopausal estrogen deficiency, premature menopause, hypogonadism, hyperthyroidism, hyperparathyroidism, Cushing syndrome, glucocorticoid use, diabetes mellitus, pregnancy, adrenal insufficiency, acromegaly, hyperprolactinemia; *Idiopathic* advanced age; *Inflammatory/Immune* sarcoidosis, amyloidosis, rheumatoid arthritis, ankylosing spondylitis; *Metabolic/Toxic* vitamin D deficiency, malnutrition, chronic renal insufficiency, heparin, cirrhosis, postgastrectomy, parenteral nutrition, cigarette smoking, low body weight; *Mechanical/Traumatic* immobilization, disuse, and nonweight bearing; *Neoplastic* multiple myeloma, paraneoplastic (parathyroid hormone-related protein secretion), lymphoma, prolactinoma; *Neurologic* paralysis, stroke, multiple sclerosis; *Psychosocial* anorexia nervosa; *Vascular* hyperemia of bone.

S KEY SYNDROME
Osteogenesis Imperfecta (Brittle Bones):
Pathophysiology: Decreased mechanical strength of all bones caused by an inherited disorder of type I collagen results in pathologic fractures during the first decade of life. Autosomal dominant inheritance occurs in 60% of cases, but four different types have been recognized. The bones are harder and more brittle than normal, so spontaneous or pathologic fractures are common. The fractures are sometimes painless. Blue sclerae may be observed. Short stature is usual and skull deformity is often present. Hypermobility of joints is common.

S KEY SYNDROME
Osteomalacia: *Pathophysiology:* Vitamin D deficiency, hypocalcemia, or hypophosphatemia after the epiphyses are closed prevents calcification of newly formed bony matrix. Early there are no symptoms or signs, while later, bone pain and tenderness occur. Low back pain and striking muscle weakness are common. Low serum calcium levels may produce spontaneous carpopedal spasm with the Chvostek and Trousseau signs. Insufficiency (stress) fractures are common and pseudofractures may be seen by x-ray.

✓ *OSTEOMALACIA—CLINICAL OCCURRENCE:* *Congenital* vitamin D-resistant rickets; *Endocrine* hyperparathyroidism, rapid deposition of calcium and phosphorus in the tissues after ablation of the parathyroid glands in osteitis fibrosa cystica, hypoparathyroidism; *Inflammatory/*

Immune celiac disease; *Metabolic/Toxic* vitamin D deficiency, hypocalcemia, hypophosphatemia, malabsorption, pancreatic insufficiency, malnutrition, chronic renal insufficiency, renal tubular acidosis, Fanconi syndrome, ureterosigmoidostomy, essential hypercalciuria, drugs (anticonvulsants, e.g., phenytoin, glucocorticoids, etidronate), fluoride and aluminum intoxication.

RICKETS: *Pathophysiology:* vitamin D deficiency in childhood before epiphyseal closure results in inadequate calcification of cartilage and new bone. See Chapter 8, Fig. 8-28, page 385. Softening of bone produces widening of the cranial sutures and fontanelles (craniotabes), Parrot bosses, rachitic rosary, Harrison grooves, thoracic kyphosis or lordosis, genu valgum or varum, and a contracted pelvis. With the sole exception of the rosary, all deformities are permanent stigmas of childhood disease.

S KEY SYNDROME

Paget Disease of Bone: Osteitis Deformans:

Pathophysiology: Increased resorption of bone combines with rapid growth of new bone with disordered architecture with decreased mechanical strength. The cause is unknown. Bone pain is inconstant and seldom severe. With the exception of the hands and feet, any bones may be involved. The skin over affected bones may be warm. The classic osseous deformities are increased girth of the calvarium, thoracic kyphosis, genu varum, and shortening of the spine by flattening of the vertebrae, giving the appearance of disproportionately long arms (Fig. 13-49).

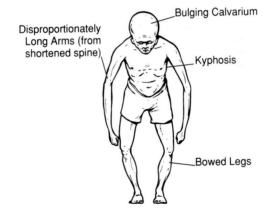

Fig. 13-49 Bony Signs of Osteitis Deformans (Paget Disease of Bone) . *The chief features of Paget disease are the enlarged calvarium (contrasting with the normal-sized face underneath), kyphosis and shortening of the spine, shortening of the spine so the arms look proportionately longer than the trunk, and bowed legs. The figure represents a collection of features, which are unlikely to occur together in the same person.*

Spontaneous or stress fractures can occur and rarely osteogenic sarcoma develops. Increased blood flow through the spongy bone may produce an arteriovenous fistula leading to high-output cardiac failure.

KEY SYNDROME

Hyperparathyroidism, Primary: Osteitis Fibrosa Cystica Generalisata, Recklinghausen Disease: *Pathophysiology:* Increased production of parathyroid hormone (PTH) causes bone resorption to exceed new bone formation, leading to hypercalcemia, hypercalciuria, hyperphosphaturia, and hypophosphatemia. The disease may be asymptomatic, although diffuse musculoskeletal aching and fatigue is seen in many patients. Late findings are bone tenderness, muscle weakness, and waddling gait. Subperiosteal cysts in the skull and long bones can cause visible and palpable swellings. Peptic ulcer and urolithiasis should prompt a search for hyperparathyroidism.

HYPERPARATHYROIDISM, SECONDARY AND TERTIARY: *Pathophysiology:* Hyperphosphatemia and hypocalcemia combined with disordered vitamin D metabolism in chronic renal failure (renal osteodystrophy), or osteomalacia from other causes, leads to increased production of parathyroid hormone (PTH), hyperplasia of the parathyroid glands, and progressive bone disease. Combinations of dietary, hormonal, and renal replacement therapies can help control the disorder. When PTH production is not suppressible with appropriate treatment, it is termed tertiary hyperparathyroidism.

Fibrous Dysplasia of Bone: Osteitis Fibrosa Cystica Disseminata: *Pathophysiology:* The cause of this disease is unknown. The architecture of one or more bones is distorted by fibrosis; the cranium and long bones are especially involved. There is asymptomatic bowing of the affected long bones. The skin often contains melanotic spots with jagged borders. In young girls, precocious puberty may occur.

Hereditary Multiple Exostoses: Osteochondromatosis: *Pathophysiology:* The autosomal dominant disease is characterized by exostoses arising from the bony cortex, deforming the metaphyseal region of some long bones. Involvement is usually bilateral but not symmetrical. The ulna may be shortened, producing ulnar deviation of the hand. Valgus deformities of the ankle are common. The only symptom may be mechanical interference with normal joint function.

Achondroplasia: Chondrodystrophia Foetalis: *Pathophysiology:* There is a disturbance in the epiphyseal cartilage and enchondral bone formation that produces short limbs, a large head, and a spine of normal length—classic achondroplastic dwarfism. An autosomal dominant inherited or spontaneous mutation in fibroblast growth factor receptor 3 is the cause. The stature is foreshortened, with the short lower limbs supporting a relatively large trunk, so the central point of the figure is near the xiphoid process, rather than the symphysis pubis. The humeri and femora are relatively shorter than the forearms and legs. The head is brachycephalic and exam may show a saddle nose, thick lips, protruding tongue, high-arched palate, trident hands (short, thick fingers diverging from the bases like spokes of a wheel), restricted extension of the elbows, thoracic kyphosis, and lumbar lordosis with a tilted pelvis.

D KEY DISEASE

Multiple Myeloma: *Pathophysiology:* This malignant clonal proliferation of immunoglobulin-producing plasma cells (terminally differentiated B cells) in the bone marrow causes destruction of bone by activation of osteoclasts leading to hypercalcemia. Normal immunoglobulin production is suppressed, there is production of monoclonal plasma proteins (heavy chains, light chains, and intact immunoglobulin), and anemia and thrombocytopenia develop. Renal insufficiency results from tubular toxicity of light chains (Bence-Jones proteins), hyperuricemia, and hypercalcemia. This is the most common malignant tumor primarily affecting bone. Fatigue or generalized aching discomfort may be the only early symptoms. The most common specific symptom is bone pain. With spinal compression fractures, localized pain in the back with radicular distribution occurs. The presenting complaints may be referable to anemia, renal failure, or a pathologic fracture. Multiple myeloma should be considered in patients over age 45 with back pain and anemia.

S KEY SYNDROME

Metastasis to Bone: Metastatic disease presents as a localized swelling or pain in a bone, a pathologic fracture, or is found incidentally on radiographs taken for another reason. The most frequent primary lesions are carcinomas of the breast, lung, and prostate.

S KEY SYNDROME

Fractures: *Pathophysiology:* Fractures are mechanical disruptions of the mineralized bone and its collagenous matrix. Forceful localized trauma fractures the entire bone. Fracture of the mineralized bone leaving the collagenous matrix intact results from trauma in children (*greenstick fracture*) and repetitive activities in adults (*stress fracture*). If the bone is inherently weak because of local destructive disease, it may fracture at usual loads (*pathological fracture*). When fracture fragments penetrate the skin, it is an *open fracture*. When fracture is suspected, immobilize the part and assess neurovascular function distal to the injury. Inspection and unavoidable movement often reveals deformity, abnormal mobility, and bone crepitus, two distinctive signs of fracture (signs one does not deliberately try to elicit). Muscle contraction attempting to splint the fracture often aggravates pain. Localized bone tenderness indicates the site of the fracture. Shortening of a long bone may be the crucial sign of an impacted fracture.

SPONTANEOUS OR PATHOLOGIC FRACTURE: This is a fracture that occurs with trauma insufficient to break a normal bone. Judging the amount of trauma is difficult and diseased bone may be subjected to much trauma, hence spontaneous fractures are easily mistaken for traumatic fractures and a high index of suspicion is warranted. X-ray signs of generalized or local bone disease should be sought if pathologic fracture is suspected. Sometimes spontaneous fractures are less painful than those of healthy bone. Osteomalacia, osteoporosis, osteitis deformans, osteitis fibrosa cystica generalisata, multiple myeloma, osteogenesis imperfecta, and primary and metastatic neoplasms in bone are common underlying conditions.

FRACTURES: FAT EMBOLISM: *Pathophysiology:*   After trauma to large bones, and especially after fractures, fat globules embolize via the veins to the lungs, brain, and other tissues. The pathogenesis remains controversial. The onset of fat embolism is sudden, with restlessness and vague pain in the chest. Symptoms reach a maximum in about 48 hours. Dyspnea and cyanosis are common and purulent sputum occasionally containing diagnostic fat droplets may be produced. Fever occurs with a disproportionately high pulse rate. Cerebral symptoms and signs are extremely variable; delirium and coma indicate a grave prognosis. Fat droplets may be seen in retinal or conjunctival vessels. On the second or third day, petechiae appear over the shoulders and chest as well as in the conjunctivae and retinae. Fat embolism should be considered in acutely ill patients with trauma to long bones or skull, insertion of prostheses, chronic alcoholism, diabetes mellitus, and sickle cell disease.

S KEY SYNDROME

▼ **Acute Osteomyelitis:** *Pathophysiology:*   Bloodborne bacteria from superficial infections are carried to the terminal capillary loops of the metaphyseal cortex, causing a necrosing infection that erodes to the periosteum. The initial infection is in the metaphysis, near but not involving the epiphysis. *Staphylococcus aureus* is the most common organism. Osteomyelitis is most common in children. The onset is usually sudden, with fever and pain. Older children may be able to point to the painful site, although the pain may be referred to the nearest joint where sympathetic effusion may be noted. Inspection frequently discloses localized swelling and redness of the overlying skin with increased warmth. Light percussion on the bone with the fingertips frequently discovers the site of tenderness. Localize the affected area with firm forefinger pressure on the bone, beginning in a normal region and moving toward the suspected site until the point of maximum tenderness is found. The proximal femoral metaphysis is within the hip joint in children, so they present with a septic hip. Sometimes deep cellulitis cannot be distinguished clinically from osteomyelitis.

Chronic Osteomyelitis:
Pathogenesis: After the acute phase, the purulent discharge from the necrosing bone breaks through the periosteum and drains through sinuses in the skin. The circulation of the cortex becomes impaired, producing islands of dead bone, sequestra. A sequestrum may be absorbed or discharged through the sinus or surrounded by new bone, the involucrum. Continuing necrosis of bone and retention of sequestra cause persistence of the infection.

Bony Swellings:
Swelling is detected by inspection and palpation, but the signs are rarely diagnostic. The location of the swelling in a long bone may be distinctive. Hamilton Bailey formulated the following diagnostic aids: (a) Swelling in all diameters of the bulbous end of a long bone is most likely caused by *giant cell tumor.* (b) Swelling on one aspect of a bone, near the epiphyseal line, is most likely an *epiphyseal exostosis.* (c) Swelling in all diameters, beginning at the metaphysis and extending toward the center of gravity, may be *Brodie abscess, osteoid osteoma,* or *osteosarcoma.* (d) Swelling in all diameters, at the center of gravity, may be *Ewing tumor, eosinophilic granuloma,* or *bone cyst.* (e) Consider that any localized bone tumor may be *metastatic from a distant primary,* so complete examination is indicated. X-ray findings may be distinctive, but biopsy is often indicated.

Bony Nodules (Occupational):
Repeated trauma to a limited region of soft tissue and underlying bone during work or sport may cause bosses of the bones with overlying calluses. Examples are *surfer's nodules* on the dorsa of the feet (from pressure on the surfboard as the surfer sits cross-legged) and *painter's bosses* on the subcutaneous surface of the tibia at the junction of the upper and middle thirds (from standing on a ladder and resting the tibiae against the next higher rung).

Axial Skeleton: Spine and Pelvis Syndromes

► ## Infectious Spondylitis:
Pathophysiology: Spinal infection most commonly affects the disks (diskitis) and anterior endplates of the vertebrae. Untreated the infection may extend anteriorly into the psoas or posteriorly into the epidural space leading to spinal cord compression. At the site of the lesion, pain and tenderness of the spinous vertebral processes are usually present, although not invariably in tuberculosis, often with spasm of the sacrospinalis. The pain may be referred along a spinal nerve to be mistaken for appendicitis, pleurisy, or sciatica, if the back is not examined. Collapse of the vertebral body causes a gibbus and paraplegia may result. Psoas abscess, classic in tuberculosis, may form along the sheath of the psoas and point beneath the inguinal ligament. Pain in the spine may be localized by the *heel-drop test*: have the patient rise onto tiptoes, and then drop onto the heels.

✓*INFECTIOUS SPONDYLITIS—CLINICAL OCCURRENCE:* Infections with pyogenic organisms, such as *Staphylococcus aureus*, are most common. Tuberculosis, typhoid fever, brucellosis, coccidioidomycosis, and actinomycosis are rare causes.

TUBERCULOSIS OF THE SPINE: POTT DISEASE: *Pathophysiology:* Infection involves the vertebral bodies with spread to the epidural space or prevertebral space. There is progressive destruction of the vertebrae leading to pathologic fracture. Patients present with fever, night sweats, and back pain, and may have signs of spinal cord compression with epidural extension. Rarely, cold abscess may present as an inguinal mass from prevertebral extension.

S KEY SYNDROME

► **Epidural Spinal Cord Compression:** *Pathophysiology:* Tumor masses in the closed epidural space may erode bone, compress spinal nerves, and compress the spinal cord. Most epidural masses extend from the adjacent vertebrae or from retroperitoneal malignancy to press on the anterior or anterolateral cord. Progressive axial, radicular, or referred back pain, unrelieved by recumbency, should prompt an immediate search for spinal cord compression by metastatic epidural neoplasm. Pain is the most common presenting symptom followed by leg weakness, constipation, incontinence, and sensory disturbances. The latter indicate advancing cord compression, from which there is less chance for complete recovery. Paraplegia may occur in a matter of hours after the onset of neurologic signs. The pain may occur at any level and is increased by straight-leg raising, Valsalva maneuver, neck flexion, and movement. MRI of the entire vertebral column and cord is the most sensitive and specific test.

✓*EPIDURAL SPINAL CORD COMPRESSION—CLINICAL OCCURRENCE:* Breast, prostate, or lung cancer are the most frequent causes. Other cancers in adults include multiple myeloma, malignant lymphoma, renal carcinoma, sarcoma, and melanoma. In children, consider lymphoma, sarcoma, and neuroblastoma. Epidural abcess complicates infectious spondylitis.

S KEY SYNDROME

▼ **Sciatica:** *Pathophysiology:* Compression or direct injury to the sciatic nerve produces pain, altered sensation (dermatomes L4-S3), loss of muscle reflexes (ankle jerk), and, if severe, muscle power and in the distribution of the nerve (e.g., ankle flexion, extension, inversion and eversion, great toe extension). Sciatica is pain in the distribution of the sciatic nerve. Pain is initially felt in the buttock and posterior thigh, and may extend to involve the posterolateral aspect of the leg to the lateral malleolus, the lateral dorsum of the foot and the entire sole. When nerve function is compromised, paresthesias are felt in the same distribution. Pain and paresthesias are intensified by coughing or straining at defecation. The nerve trunk is tender when palpated at the sciatic notch. Pain is also elicited by stretching the nerve when the leg is extended while the thigh is flexed (Lasègue sign or straight-leg raising). Rectal examination should always be done to look for pelvic masses. A pulsating rectal mass associated with sciatica suggests aneurysm of the internal iliac or common iliac artery compressing the nerve. The great majority of the cases are attributable to herniated intervertebral disk, spondylosis, or sacroiliac disease.

S KEY SYNDROME

Lumbosacral Strain: *Pathophysiology:* Mechanical injury commonly occurs to the soft tissues (muscles, tendons, and ligaments) of the low back where the mobile lumbar spine meets the fixed sacrum, concentrating mechanical forces at the transition zone. Injury can be the result of a single, large loading force or of a repetitive loading with lesser forces. Usually the patient is between 25 and 50 years of age and complains of aching pain near L5 or S1. The pain may radiate laterally or to the lateral aspect of the thigh. There is an increased lumbar lordosis and attempted spinal motion is accompanied by muscle spasm. Spinal flexion is limited and painful. The patient cannot lie flat without flexing the knees and hips to relieve pain. The straight-leg-raising test is negative except that lumbosacral pain occurs at extreme flexion. Have the patient lie prone with the pelvis resting on four pillows to separate the spinous processes. In this position, palpation of the supraspinous ligament may reveal tenderness above or below the spine of L5; sometimes a depression is found at that site.

S KEY SYNDROME

Herniated Intervertebral Disk: *Pathophysiology:* Herniation of a desiccated nucleus pulposus through tears in the annulose fibrosa may produce pressure on nerve roots in the neural foramina laterally or directly on the cauda equina, conus or spinal cord if the extrusion is directly posterior (Fig. 13-26B, page 721). The onset of low back pain may be gradual or sudden and is partially relieved in recumbency. *Sciatica* may be the presenting symptom with pain in the buttock radiating to the thigh. In severe cases, the pain involves the leg, usually the lateral aspect, and some or all of the toes (dermatomes L4 to S3). Coughing, sneezing, or the Valsalva maneuver accentuates the pain. Chronic herniated disk is attended by symptom-free periods; continuous back pain is usually caused by some other lesion. On examination, the spine may be flexed, frequently with a lateral deviation toward the affected side. Active flexion and extension of the spine are limited, more so than lateral bending and rotation. Muscle spasm is most severe over the ipsilateral sacrospinalis with local deep tenderness, most pronounced on the affected side, present 5 cm lateral to the midline. Palpate for muscle rigidity, areas of tenderness, tender fibrositic points, and trigger points. Look for weakness by having the patient heel-and-toe walk, and extend the great toe against resistance. With the straight-leg-raising test, record the angle at which pain is experienced, then repeat the maneuver, dorsiflexing the foot sharply, as the painful angle is approached, to stretch the sciatic nerve and test its irritability. Pain often occurs at less than 40 degrees when there is actual impingement of a prolapsed disk;

when pain occurs only at much greater angles, the nerve sensitivity may be from other causes. Check sensation noting the dermatome involved [Vroomen PC, de Krom MC, Knottnerus JA. Diagnostic value of history and physical examination in patients suspected of sciatica due to disc herniation. *J Neurol* 1999;246:899–906; Vroomen PC, de Krom MC, Knottnerus JA. Consistency of history taking and physical examination in patients with suspected lumbar nerve root involvement. *Spine* 2000;25:91–96].

S KEY SYNDROME

Spinal Stenosis: *Pathophysiology:* Compression of the lower lumbar and sacral roots occurs from overgrowth of bony tissue from congenital narrowing or degenerative disk disease that narrows the spinal canal. *Pseudoclaudication* is pain in the buttocks, bilateral posterior thighs, and calves while standing or walking upright, which is relieved by sitting or bending forward (reversing the lumbar lordosis and decreasing the degree of stenosis). Unlike intermittent claudication from vascular insufficiency, pain occurs while standing without walking, that is, leg exertion is not required. Sitting gives relief, in contrast to lumbar disk disease. Osteoporosis, spondylolisthesis, trauma, laminectomy, spinal fusion, spondylosis, scoliosis, acromegaly, and Paget disease are all potential contributors. Congenital narrowing of the canal also occurs.

Appendicular Skeletal Syndromes (Including Joints, Tendons, Ligaments, and Soft Tissues)

S KEY SYNDROME

Hypertrophic Osteoarthropathy: *Pathophysiology:* This syndrome, beginning as a periostitis of unknown cause, consists of (a) clubbing of the fingers, (b) new subperiosteal bone in the long bones, (c) swelling and pains in the joints, and (d) autonomic disturbances of the hands and feet, such as flushing, sweating, and blanching. The earliest sign is clubbing of the fingers. With progression, bone pain occurs while swelling and pain in the joints may become severe and tenderness is elicited by palpation over the distal forearms and legs. In advanced cases, sweating and flushing of the hands and feet may alternate with the Raynaud phenomenon. The condition may be congenital, with signs appearing in childhood, or acquired. Onset of hypertrophic osteoarthropathy in the adult should initiate a search for an underlying disease.

✓ *HYPERTROPHIC OSTEOARTHROPATHY—CLINICAL OCCURRENCE:* *Congenital* familial, cyanotic congenital heart disease, cystic fibrosis; *Endocrine* Grave disease, pregnancy; *Idiopathic* emphysema, cirrhosis; *Inflammatory/Immune* ulcerative colitis, Crohn disease, chronic interstitial pneumonitis, sarcoidosis, dysproteinemia; *Infectious* lung or liver abscess, bronchiectasis, tuberculosis, bacterial endocarditis, dysentery; *Metabolic/Toxic* malabsorption, chronic hypoxemia; *Neoplastic* lung, pleural, and gastrointestinal cancer, metastatic disease to lung; *Vascular* aortic aneurysm.

S KEY SYNDROME
▼ **Chronic Painless Enlargement of the Legs:**
Several causes must be distinguished.

Adiposity. Although some evidence of obesity is present elsewhere in the body, the fat about the ankles may be disproportionately great, but the feet are spared. The tissue has the consistency of fat, and pitting edema is absent.

Chronic deep venous obstruction usually is preceded by a history suggesting thrombophlebitis. The venous deficit may produce pain in the legs. Some pitting edema is usually present, although it may be obscured by thickening of the skin from chronic inflammation *(dermatoliposclerosis)*. The skin is hemosiderin stained- and cyanotic. Superficial veins may be dilated.

Postphlebitic syndrome results from previous occlusion of the deep veins either without recanalization or resulting in destruction of the valves with persistent venous incompetence. One-third of patients with acute deep vein thrombosis will develop postphlebitic syndrome. The leg is persistently enlarged, usually with pitting edema. Sensations of fullness and pain occur with prolonged sitting or standing and chronic stasis changes are common. Early treatment decreases long-term disability.

Varicose veins are readily recognized when they are associated with edema.

Lymphedema causes a firm, nonpitting swelling with no venous engorgement or cyanosis.

Muscle Syndromes

See also Chapter 14, *The Neurologic Examination.*

S KEY SYNDROME
▼ **Fibromyalgia:** See *Tender Points*, page 773. Fibromyalgia is more common in women than men. It is characterized by widespread, diffuse, aching musculoskeletal pain, stiffness, nonrestorative sleep, and fatigue. Although the cause and pathogenesis are unknown, it has been associated with antecedent trauma, surgery, medical illness, and emotional stress. The diagnosis is based upon clinical criteria; laboratory studies are normal. The American College of Rheumatology criteria for diagnosis include a history of pain in the all four body quadrants for at least 3 months with at least 11 of 18 paired, bilateral tender points elicited on physical examination: suboccipital muscle insertion, low cervical, trapezius, supraspinatus, second rib, lateral epicondyle, gluteal, greater trochanter, and knee (Fig. 13-50).

S KEY SYNDROME
▼ **Myofascial Pain Syndrome:** *Pathophysiology:* Afferent signals from the trigger areas are believed to remodel spinal and possibly thalamic pain pathways to cause reflex muscle spasms and diminished blood flow, which, in turn, increase the sensitivity of the trig-

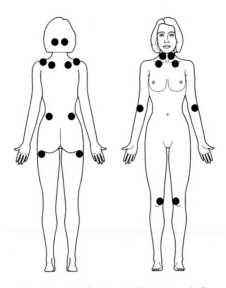

**Tender Points of Fibromyalgia
in at Least 11 of 18 Sites**

Fig. 13-50 The Tender Points of Fibromyalgia. There should be tenderness in at least 11 of the 18 points to diagnose fibromyalgia.

ger area. See *Trigger Points*, page 772. Chronic recurrent pain occurs roughly in the distribution of one or more muscles and their distribution of referred pain. The pain may be lancinating, aching, boring, or a feeling of muscular stiffness. Often, the patient relates the onset to some specific trauma or activity. The distinguishing feature is the presence of one or more trigger points, with or without palpable muscle spasm. The examiner should palpate the entire region carefully with firm pressure of the fingertips. Often, the trigger point is discovered some distance from the referred pain area. The diagnosis is confirmed when the pain is relieved by injection of the primary trigger point with a local anesthetic.

S KEY SYNDROME
▼ **Polymyalgia Rheumatica (PMR):** *Pathophysiology*:   This inflammatory disease of unknown origin is characterized by pain in proximal muscle groups, with inflammation demonstrable by MRI in the shoulder girdle tendon sheaths and bursae, and less commonly the shoulder joint itself. It usually occurs after the sixth decade of life and is most common in women. Pronounced morning stiffness of the neck, shoulder, and upper back muscles usually begins gradually. Some patients have rather sudden onset and can note the day and time of their first symptoms. Muscles of the low back, pelvic girdle and thighs

are less prominently involved and/or may develop later. It is common in patients with temporal arteritis, but only 15% of patients presenting with PMR develop temporal arteritis. Although spontaneously painful, the muscles are seldom very tender, trigger points are not characteristic, and the stiffness is improved by activity. The erythrocyte sedimentation rate (ESR) is usually >80 and symptoms are promptly relieved by low-dose corticosteroids.

S KEY SYNDROME

Compartment Syndrome: *Pathophysiology:* Injury to muscle enclosed within constricting fascial compartments leads to swelling from edema, hemorrhage and inflammation. When the pressure within the compartment exceeds 30 cm of water, progressive ischemia ensues leading to further injury. A high index of suspicion is required to recognize this serious disorder before irreversible muscle injury occurs. The patient complains of severe pain often disproportionate to apparent injury. Palpation of the affected muscle compartment reveals tense distention of the fascia with severe pain. If major arteries or nerves pass through the compartment, distal pulses may be diminished and sensation impaired. Without relief of pressure, muscle necrosis leads to chronic fibrosis, shortening, and loss of function. Diagnosis is made by measuring compartment pressure and treatment is surgical fasciotomy.

ADDITIONAL READING

1. Mense S, Simons DG. *Muscle Pain*. Philadelphia, Lippincott Williams & Wilkins, 2001.
2. Sheon RP, Moskowitz RW, Goldberg VM. *Soft Tissue Rheumatic Pain. Recognition, Management and Prevention*. 3rd ed. Baltimore, William and Wilkins, 1996.
3. Walter B. Greene (ed.). *Essentials of Musculoskeletal Care,* 2nd edition. Rosemont, IL, American Academy of Orthopedic Surgeons, 2001.
4. *Primer of the Rheumatic Diseases*. Atlanta, GA, The Arthritis Foundation, 2001.
5. Travell JG, Simons DG. *Myofascial Pain and Dysfunction. The Trigger Point Manual.* Baltimore, Williams & Wilkins, 1983.

Diagnostic testing of the nervous system is based upon specific tests of its functional characteristics, not on the traditional physical examination modalities of inspection, palpation, percussion, and auscultation.

In the routine physical examination, most clinicians test the components of the nervous system as they elicit the history and examine the body by regions. The patient's speech and behavior may indicate abnormalities of cerebral function. When examining the head, some, if not all, of the cranial nerves are tested. Muscular strength is assessed by inspection of gait and movement. Tendon reflexes are elicited during examination of the extremities. When evidence of nervous system malfunction is encountered, a more complete and systematic neurologic examination is required.

The first objective of the systematic neurologic examination is to discover all cognitive, sensory, motor, and coordination deficits. From a complete inventory, the clinician deduces the site of the lesion from knowledge of nervous system anatomy and physiology. Several general principles help to organize an approach to localizing the problem:

1. *Deficits of intellect, memory, or higher brain function* imply lesions of the cerebral hemispheres.
2. *Deficits of consciousness* indicate lesions of the brainstem reticular activating system or bilateral cerebral damage.
3. *Paralysis with loss of deep tendon reflexes* indicates a lower motor neuron lesion interrupting the reflex arc. This can be at the spinal cord, spinal root, plexus or peripheral nerve level. Acute upper motor neuron lesions can be associated with decreased reflexes initially, but produce increased reflexes after hours to days.
4. *Paralysis with an accentuated deep tendon reflexes* (spasticity) indicates an upper motor neuron lesion. This may reflect disease of the hemisphere, brainstem, or spinal cord.
5. *Unilateral loss of touch and position sensation and contralateral loss of temperature and pain sensation* indicate a unilateral lesion of the spinal cord ipsilateral to the loss of touch and position. This happens because the ascending tracts for touch and position sensation decussate in the medulla, while the ascending tracts for pain and temperature sensation cross near where they enter the spinal cord.

6. *Paralysis is contralateral to lesions above the medulla and ipsilateral below.* This is because the descending motor tracts, like the tracts for discriminative sense, decussate in the medulla.
7. *A lower motor neuron paralysis accompanied by anesthesia in an appropriate distribution usually indicates a peripheral nerve lesion,* because many nerves carry both motor and sensory fibers. Sometimes spinal root or segmental cord lesions cause similar signs.
8. *Muscle atrophy with fasciculation results from a lower motor neuron lesion;* without fasciculation, atrophy is often attributable to intrinsic muscle disease.

Overview of the Major Neurologic System Components and their Function

An accurate diagnostic neurologic examination requires comprehensive understanding of nervous system anatomic and functional organization. A full understanding of the relationships between the anatomy and the functional components of the nervous system is beyond the scope of this book. The reader should consult anatomy and neurology texts for detailed discussions of neuroanatomy and functional physiology.

Anatomic Organization

For diagnostic purposes, the nervous system is divided anatomically into the brain, the spinal cord and the peripheral nerves.

THE CENTRAL NERVOUS SYSTEM (CNS).   The **brain** consists of the cerebrum, the brainstem, and the cerebellum. The *cerebrum* performs cognitive functions, is the site of emotion and mood formation and determines personality and behavior. The deep cerebral structures modulate motor and sensory function and control endocrine and appetitive functions. The *brainstem* consists of the midbrain, the pons and the medulla and contains nuclei of cranial nerves III to XII. The *cerebellum* is involved in many motor and sensory pathways and controls the coordination of complex motor activities.

The **spinal cord** contains the ascending sensory tracts, the descending motor and autonomic tracts and the lower motor neurons which activate skeletal muscles. The dorsal and ventral *spinal roots* contain the sensory and motor tracts respectively. The *dorsal root ganglia* contain the cell bodies of afferent sensory nerves.

THE PERIPHERAL NERVOUS SYSTEM.   The **peripheral nervous system** is equally complex. Cranial and spinal nerves come together to form *ganglia* and *plexuses* (brachial, lumbar, sacral) where the sensory and motor components of the cranial and spinal segments are redistributed into peripheral nerves which serve specific anatomic areas of the periphery.

Functional Organization of the Nervous System

It is also necessary to have an understanding of the functional organization of the nervous system. Function can be systematically described as follows: *cognition* (intellect, language, registration, memory, attention, orientation, spatial discrimination); *mood and affect*; *special sensory* (sight, hearing, balance, taste, smell); *somatic and visceral sensation* (touch, position, pain, temperature, vibration, pressure, two-point discrimination); *motor function* (pyramidal tracts and extrapyramidal system); *posture, balance, and coordination* (cerebellar, vestibular, and basal ganglia function); and *autonomic function*. The autonomic nervous system is divided into the *parasympathetic* and *sympathetic* systems. The parasympathetic outflow is from the cranial, cervical, and sacral roots, with ganglia close to the organs they innervate. The sympathetic outflow is from the thoracic and lumbar roots via the sympathetic spinal ganglia.

Superficial Anatomy of the Nervous System

The brain is encased within the rigid skull and the spinal cord within the spinal canal of the vertebral column. The segmental organization of the nervous system is most evident in the chest and abdomen, much less so in the head and extremities. The ganglia, plexuses, and nerve trunks are inaccessible to physical examination lying deep to the muscles and bones of the spine, chest, abdomen, and pelvis. The peripheral nerves, however, are distributed in the neurovascular bundles, along with their corresponding arteries and veins, and may be accessible to palpation where they exit the trunk and in the extremities.

The Neurologic Examination

CRANIAL NERVE EXAMINATION

The 12 pairs of cranial nerves (CN) emerge from the brain and pass through foramina in the base of the skull. They are designated by Roman numerals I to XII. The physical examination of several of the cranial nerves is contained in the discussion of the head and neck in Chapter 7.

Olfactory Nerve (Cranial Nerve I)

The olfactory mucosa lining the upper third of the nasal septum and the superior nasal concha contains the receptors and ganglion cells. Their fibers converge into about 20 branches that pierce the cribriform plate of the ethmoid bone and consolidate to form the olfactory tract.

TESTING SMELL.   Ensure the patency of the nasal passages. Have the patient close her eyes; test each nostril separately while the other is occluded. Ask the patient to identify familiar odors, such as coffee, cloves, and peppermint. Noxious substances, such as ammonia or alcohol, should not be used because they also stimulate receptors of the trigeminal nerve and give a false-positive response.

Optic Nerve (Cranial Nerve II)

The examination and structure of the optic nerve, chiasm, and tract is discussed in Chapter 7, on pages 213 and 259ff.

TESTING THE RETINA.   Use suitable tests for vision, depending on the patient's acuity and ability to cooperate (page 219). Examine the fundi with the ophthalmoscope (page 217). Test the visual fields by the confrontation method (page 213); perimetry is required if more accurate and detailed information is needed.

Oculomotor Nerve (Cranial Nerve III)

This is the motor nerve to five extrinsic eye muscles: the levator palpebrae superioris, medial rectus, superior rectus, inferior rectus, and inferior oblique. Its nucleus lies in the posterior midbrain, subdivided into a part for each muscle. After emergence from the brain, the nerve proceeds between the superior cerebellar and posterior cerebral arteries, then lateral and forward past the posterior clinoid process, and then along the lateral wall of the cavernous sinus, to enter the orbit through the superior orbital fissure.

TESTING FOR OCULOMOTOR PARALYSIS.   See Chapter 7, pages 212–214 and 266.

Trochlear Nerve (Cranial Nerve IV)

CN-IV innervates the superior oblique muscle. The trochlear nucleus also lies in the posterior midbrain, inferior to the third nerve nucleus. It follows a circuitous course around the superior cerebellar and cerebral peduncles to pierce the free border of the tentorium cerebelli near the posterior clinoid process. It proceeds forward in the lateral wall of the cavernous sinus and passes through the superior orbital fissure to enter the substance of the superior oblique muscle.

TESTING FOR TROCHLEAR PARALYSIS.   See Chapter 7, page 212.

Trigeminal Nerve (Cranial Nerve V)

CN-V is the largest cranial nerve; its sensory root supplies the superficial and deep structures of the face and the deep structures of the head and its motor root innervates the muscles of mastication. Its nucleus has a pontine locus and another portion descends through the pons and medulla to the substantia gelatinosa. After leaving the pons the nerve enters the trigeminal ganglion, lying at the petrous apex of the temporal bone. The first trigeminal division, or ophthalmic branch (CN-V1), emerges from the trigeminal ganglion, giving fibers to the cornea, ciliary body, conjunctiva, nasal cavity and sinuses, and skin of the eyebrows, forehead, and nose. The second division, or maxillary branch

(CN-V2), supplies sensory fibers to the skin of the side of the nose, the upper and lower eyelids, the palate, and maxillary gums. The third division, or mandibular branch (CN-V3), is mixed. Its sensory fibers supply the temporal region, the auricula, lower lip, lower face, mucosa of anterior two-thirds of the tongue, mandibular gums, and teeth. The motor root of CN-V3 innervates the muscles of mastication: masseter, temporalis, and internal and external pterygoid.

TESTING THE TRIGEMINAL NERVE. *Motor Division:* Inspect for tremor of the jaw, involuntary chewing movements, and trismus (spasm of the masticatory muscles). Test the paired temporal and masseter muscles by palpating symmetrical regions while the patient clenches the teeth; compare muscle tension on the two sides (Fig. 14-1A); disparity in tension of the two muscles indicates paralysis on the weak side if and when the teeth are aligned naturally or a tongue blade is inserted to correct a malalignment. The mouth cannot be closed tightly in bilateral paralysis. If there is malalignment of the incisors when the mouth is opened, paralysis of the pterygoid muscle on the weak side is indicated. *Sensory Division:* With the patient's eyes closed, test tactile perception of the facial skin by asking the patient to indicate when you touch him with a shred of gauze (Fig. 14-1B). Test pain sensibility of the skin and mucosa with sterile pinpricks. When pain sensibility is lost, one can also test for temperature perception by touching the patient with test tubes of warm and cold water. In each test, compare symmetrical points; map out areas of abnormal sensation in detail. The jaw jerk tests both the motor and sensory components of the trigeminal nerve. Test the corneal reflex by having the patient look upward while you gently touch the cornea (not the sclera) with a small shred of sterile gauze; this normally induces blinking. The corneal reflex is a bilateral reflex testing the fifth and seventh cranial nerves on the side stimulated and the seventh consensually. With an afferent (CN-V) lesion, the response from both sides will be depressed. With an ipsilateral efferent (CN-VII) lesion, the direct reflex is lost, but the consensual is preserved.

Abducens Nerve (Cranial VI)

The abducens is the motor nerve to the lateral rectus. Its nucleus lies beneath the facial colliculus. The nerve runs below the posterior clinoid process, through the cavernous sinus and the superior orbital fissure, to enter the substance of the lateral rectus muscle.

TESTING FOR ABDUCENS PARALYSIS. See Chapter 7, page 212.

Facial Nerve (Cranial Nerve VII)

The facial nerve contains motor, autonomic, and sensory fibers. It supplies motor fibers to the muscles of the scalp, face, and auricula as well as to the buccinator, platysma, stapedius, stylohyoideus, and the posterior belly of the digastricus. Autonomic motor fibers run through the chorda tympani nerve, a branch of CN-VII, to cause vasodilatation and secretion in the submaxillary and sublingual salivary glands. Sensory fibers furnish the organs of taste on the anterior two-thirds of the tongue and sensation to the ear canal and behind the ear.

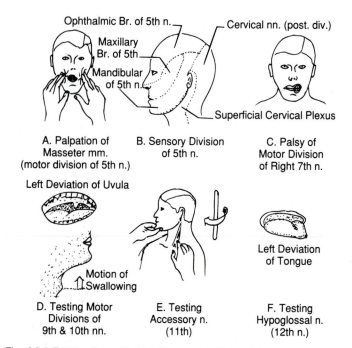

A. Palpation of
Masseter mm.
(motor division of 5th n.)

B. Sensory Division
of 5th n.

C. Palsy of
Motor Division
of Right 7th n.

Left Deviation of Uvula

Motion of
Swallowing

Left Deviation
of Tongue

D. Testing Motor
Divisions of
9th & 10th nn.

E. Testing
Accessory n.
(11th)

F. Testing
Hypoglossal n.
(12th n.)

Fig. 14-1 Testing Some Cranial Nerves.   A. Motor Division of the Fifth (Trigeminal) Nerve: See text. B. Sensory Division of the Fifth (Trigeminal): The three branches of the sensory trigeminal are ophthalmic, maxillary, and mandibular, as indicated by the areas. C. Motor Division of the Seventh (Facial): When the patient opens the mouth to show clenched teeth, only the unparalyzed side of the face retracts; the cheek muscles form creases on the normal side; the eyelid fissures are increased. The paralyzed side remains smooth with eyelid open. D. Motor Division of the Ninth (Glossopharyngeal) and Tenth (Vagus) Nerves: When the patient opens the mouth and says "ah," the uvula deviates toward the strong side. Upon swallowing, the larynx normally elevates, as indicated by the motion of the thyroid cartilage in the neck (Adam's apple); it does not rise in bilateral paralysis. E. The Accessory (Eleventh Nerve): The patient is asked to rotate the head toward the midline against the resistance of the examiner's hand while the other hand palpates the tension in the sternocleidomastoid muscle. The trapezius can likewise be tested for paralysis. F. The Twelfth (Hypoglossal) Nerve: The protruding tongue deviates to the paralyzed side; muscle atrophy may also be present.

TESTING THE FACIAL NERVE.   *Motor:* Inspect the face in repose for evidence of flaccid paralysis. Have the patient perform these seven motions to demonstrate asymmetry indicating unilateral paralysis and to determine whether the cause is a lower motor neuron (LMN) or an upper motor neuron (UMN) lesion. Because the LMNs of the lids and forehead are innervated bilaterally from the UMNs, UMN lesions do not affect the upper lid or forehead. (a) Face in repose: shallow nasolabial folds in both UMN and LMN; palpebral fissure widened in LMN. (b) Elevation of an eyebrow and wrinkling of the forehead is absent in LMN, but present in UMN. (c) Frowning: lowering of the eyebrow is absent in LMN, present in UMN. (d) Tight closing of an eye is absent in LMN, with an associated upturning of the unclosed eye (*Bell phenomenon*). The lids close normally in UMN. When the eyes are tightly closed, weakness of one upper lid can be detected by forcing the lids open with the thumb. (e) Showing teeth: the lips do not retract fully in either UMN or LMN (see Fig. 14-1C). (f) Whistling and puffing cheeks are absent or diminished in both UMN and LMN. (g) A natural smile: the lips and corners of the mouth do not fully elevate with LMN lesions. The paralysis of the mouth is overcome by motions responding to emotion, so a symmetrical smile may occur in UMN disease. *Sensory (Taste):* Test with sugar, vinegar (dilute acetic acid), quinine, and table salt. Write the words sweet, sour, bitter, and salty on a piece of paper so the patient can point out her sensations. Hold the protruded tongue in gauze and touch successively one side of the anterior two-thirds of the lingual dorsum with the test substance on an applicator; after the patient has responded, apply a substance to the other side. Remember, sweet receptors are located on the tip of the tongue. Have the patient rinse the tongue well with water between tests.

Acoustic Nerve (Cranial Nerve VIII)

The eighth nerve is a relatively short trunk consisting of the cochlear and vestibular sensory nerves. They are morphologically and functionally distinct. Beginning in different nuclei, the two sets of fibers join a single trunk entering the internal auditory meatus. The cochlear nerve supplies the organ of Corti, while the vestibular nerve furnishes sensory endings for the semicircular ducts.

TESTING THE ACOUSTIC NERVE. *Cochlear Portion:* The tests for hearing are described in Chapter 7 on pages 209–210. *Vestibular Portion:* Note spontaneous nystagmus; use the labyrinthine tests described in Chapter 7 on pages 210–211.

Glossopharyngeal Nerve (Cranial Nerve IX)

CN-IX contains sensory, motor, and autonomic fibers. It supplies the sensory organs for pain, touch, and temperature in the mucosa of the pharynx, fauces, and palatine tonsil; in addition, it is the nerve of taste for the posterior third of the tongue. Somatic motor fibers travel through both the glossopharyngeal and vagus to innervate the muscles of the pharynx. The nerve trunk emerges from the medulla and passes through the jugular foramen of the skull with the vagus and accessory nerves. It follows the internal carotid artery and curves under the styloid process, then goes forward to the pharynx.

TESTING THE GLOSSOPHARYNGEAL NERVE. This is tested with the vagus nerve.

Vagus Nerve (Cranial Nerve X)

Most extensive of the cranial nerves, the vagus carries motor, sensory, and autonomic fibers to the neck, thorax, and abdomen. It exits the skull in the jugular fossa. Its cervical branches are the pharyngeal, superior laryngeal, recurrent laryngeal, and superior cardiac nerves. The thoracic branches are the inferior cardiac, anterior and posterior bronchials, and esophageal nerves. In the abdomen, its major branches are the gastric and hepatic nerves and the celiac and superior mesenteric ganglia.

TESTING OF THE GLOSSOPHARYNGEAL AND VAGUS NERVES.   *Pharynx:* While inspecting the pharynx, have the patient open his mouth and say "ah," noting elevation of the uvula. Absence of elevation indicates bilateral paralysis while unilateral elevation deviates the uvula toward the strong side (see Fig. 14-1D). Note whether the faucial pillars converge equally. Test the gag reflex by touching the back of the tongue with a tongue blade. Test the pharyngeal mucosa for areas of anesthesia by touching with an applicator.   *Larynx:*   Watch the laryngeal contours in the neck to ascertain if they rise with swallowing (see Fig. 14-1D). Test further by having the patient swallow some water; paralysis may cause coughing or reflux into the posterior nose. Hoarseness may indicate unilateral vocal cord paralysis, while dyspnea and inspiratory stridor are associated with bilateral involvement. Make an indirect examination of the vocal cords, as described in Chapter 7 on page 225.

Accessory Nerve (Cranial Nerve XI)

The accessory nerve (formerly the spinal accessory) is the motor nerve to the trapezius and sternocleidomastoid. It arises in the medulla and the upper cervical cord and passes upward through the foramen magnum and emerges from the skull through the jugular foramen. It runs backward near the internal jugular vein and descends before branching. One branch enters the upper part of the sternocleidomastoid, and the other enters the posterior triangle of the neck to supply the upper portion of the trapezius.

TESTING OF THE ACCESSORY NERVE.   Palpate the upper borders of the trapezii while the patient raises his shoulders against the resistance of your hands. Look for scapular "winging" as the patient leans against a wall with palms and arms extended. Test the sternocleidomastoid by having the patient turn his head to one side and attempt to bring his chin back to the midline against the resistance of your hand (see Fig. 14-1E). Note the strength of rotation and the prominence of the tensed muscles in the neck.

Hypoglossal Nerve (Cranial Nerve XII)

The hypoglossal is the motor nerve to the tongue. It arises in the medulla, passes through the hypoglossal canal beside the foramen magnum, courses downward with the internal carotid artery, jugular vein, and vagus nerve, then curves forward behind the mandible to the root of the tongue.

TESTING OF THE HYPOGLOSSAL NERVE.   When the tongue protrudes, look for tremors, atrophy of one lateral muscle mass, and fasciculations. When one side is paralyzed, the tongue deviates toward the weak side (see Fig. 14-1F). Occasionally, deviation of the tongue results from an upper motor neuron lesion. Test muscle strength by having the patient push the tongue against the cheek while your hand resists from the outside. Test lingual speech by having the patient repeat "La, La, La" (linguals; see Chapter 7, page 226 for K, L, M test).

MOTOR EXAMINATION

Motor system function requires a normal and intact skeleton, normal muscle mass and function and normal function of the pyramidal and extrapyramidal motor nerve systems. Joint motion must be tested to assess muscle movements, so orthopedic, rheumatologic, and neurologic examinations overlap and are interdependent.

Inspecting for Muscle Atrophy

Whenever possible, compare the masses of symmetrical muscles at the same level. When bilateral atrophy is suspected, the examiner must evaluate the findings from knowledge of normal anatomy and the individual variations encountered in experience with many persons.

Testing Muscle Tone

The patient is asked to relax while muscle tone is assessed by resistance to passive joint motion through a normal range. The examiner must learn the feel of normal resistance with which to compare the patient's findings. Relaxation is difficult for some patients, so learn to test tone when the patient's attention is diverted. Gently rocking or lifting a limb from the bed and watching it fall discloses its tone. When the patient sits on the edge of the examining table, the freedom with which the legs swing indicates their tone.

Testing Muscle Strength

First, have the patient actively move the muscle (Fig. 14-2). When motion is accomplished, have the patient contract the muscle or move against your resistance while palpating the contracting muscle. If the

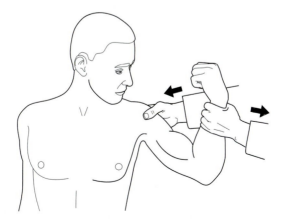

Fig. 14-2 Testing Muscle Strength. *The patient is required to act against the resistance of the examiner.*

patient cannot move a limb in the usual manner, lay the extremity on the table or bed and have the patient move it in a direction unaffected by gravity. An arbitrary scale is used for grading muscle strength.

Grading of Muscle Strength (Oxford Scale)

Grade 0	No muscle movement
Grade 1	A trace of muscle movement without joint motion
Grade 2	Body part moves with gravity eliminated
Grade 3	Body part moves against gravity but not resistance
Grade 4	Body part moves against gravity and some resistance
Grade 5	Normal

Muscle strength in the lower extremities normally exceeds upper arm strength in the examiner, so mild degrees of weakness are easily missed with resisted motion. To test lower extremity strength, the following tests are useful: (a) Observe the patient arise after sitting on the floor. Use of both arms to assist rising and raising the buttocks, first by work-ing the hands on the floor toward the feet and then up the legs, indi-cates proximal muscle weakness (*Gowers sign*). (b) Have the patient hop on both feet, then on each foot independently. Normally, the heel will not strike the ground. Having the patient hop on a piece of paper will accentuate the sound of the heel strike (creating a "gallop" rhythm), in-dicating gastrocnemius and soleus muscle weakness.

EXAMINATION OF REFLEXES

The stretch reflex is a simple reflex arc of a muscle cell, a sensory, and a motor neuron. The afferent limb is the sensory neuron whose cell body is in the dorsal root ganglion, sensory dendrite in the muscle and whose axon penetrates the gray matter of the cord. The dendrite inner-vates the muscle spindle, a specialized receptor organ within the mus-cle. Stretching the muscle evokes an afferent impulse through the dor-sal root ganglion to the cord's gray matter, where it synapses with the axon and the dendrite of the LMN in the anterior horn. The efferent limb of the arc consists of the LMN, the muscle synapse, and the muscle fibers of the motor unit.

Most reflex arcs are more complex but are extensions of the basic two-neuron unit (Fig. 14-3). The afferent and efferent neurons may be separated by intervening connector neurons at the same spinal level or at widely different levels, so afferent and efferent impulses travel up and down the cord for considerable distances.

The integrity of the reflex arc is broken by malfunction of any of its elements: receptor organ, sensory nerve, dorsal root ganglion, spinal gray matter, anterior spinal root, motor nerve, motor endplate, or ef-fector organ. The physical sign of an interrupted reflex arc is a dimin-ished or absent reflex. When a descending motor pathway (the pyra-midal tract) in the cord is injured at a level higher than the reflex arc, normal inhibition from higher centers is lost, producing a hyperactive reflex.

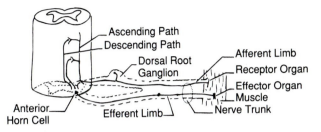

Fig. 14-3 Components of a Spinal Reflex Arc.

Inferences are made from assessment of reflex arcs at known levels of the brainstem and spinal cord. A normal reflex (a) attests the integrity of every element in the reflex arc and (b) indicates the proper functioning of the descending motor tracts. A diminished or absent reflex indicates malfunction of one or more components of the arc or absence of facilitatory influences from above. A lesion may be localized from the known levels of the reflex centers.

In the routine examination, the clinician usually tests a few reflex arcs, representative of various levels in the cord and brainstem. When an abnormality is encountered, its lesion may be pinpointed by testing specific reflex arcs.

Brainstem Reflexes

Many of these are tested in the routine examination of the cranial nerves. The findings are valuable only when the level of the reflex center is known. The cranial nerve innervation of the afferent and efferent limbs are shown in parentheses.

DIRECT PUPILLARY REACTION TO LIGHT. The iris constricts when bright light is shone upon the retina (afferent CN-II; efferent ipsilateral CN-III).

CONSENSUAL PUPILLARY REACTION TO LIGHT. Stimulation of one retina with light causes contralateral constriction of the pupil as well as a homolateral response (afferent CN-II; efferent contralateral CN-III).

CILIOSPINAL REFLEX. Pinching the skin of the back of the neck causes pupillary dilatation (afferent cervical somatic nerves; efferent-cervical sympathetic chain).

CORNEAL REFLEX. Touching the cornea causes blinking of the eyelids (afferent CN-V; efferent CN-VII).

JAW REFLEX. When the mouth is partially opened and the muscles relaxed, tapping the chin causes the jaw to close. The reflex center is in the mid-pons (afferent CN-V; efferent CN-V).

GAG REFLEX. Gagging occurs when the pharynx is stroked. The reflex center is in the medulla (afferent CN-IX, -X; efferent CN-IX, -X).

The Muscle Stretch Reflexes

These muscle stretch reflexes are misnamed deep tendon reflexes (DTRs). They are elicited by a sudden tap on the tendon, which stretches the muscle.

GENERAL PRINCIPLES FOR ELICITING MUSCLE STRETCH REFLEXES. The limb should be relaxed. Identify the tendon of insertion of the muscle to be tested. Stretch the muscle slightly by limb positioning or thumb pressure on the tendon. Strike a brisk blow on the tendon with the finger or reflex hammer. If no reflex is present, reinforcement can be used. This is accomplished by having the patient concentrate on a voluntary act such as pulling on interlocked fingers or clenching the fists.

There is considerable variability in normal reflexes, from absent to brisk. Significant asymmetry between right and left at the same level is abnormal. Clonus, the sustained repetitive maintenance of the reflex arc with tonic stretch of the muscle is always abnormal. A four-point scale, denoted by numbers or pluses, is commonly used to grade the reflex response.

0, 0	No response
1, +	Detectable, but weak
2, ++	Easily detectable
3, +++	Brisk with at most a few beats of clonus
4, ++++	Sustained clonus

REFLEX CENTER AT C5 TO T1: PECTORALIS REFLEX (MEDIAL AND LATERAL ANTERIOR THORACIC NERVES). Have the patient elevate the arm about 10 degrees in 90 degrees of abduction (Fig. 14-4A). Place the fingers of your left hand on the patient's shoulder with your thumb extended downward to press firmly on the tendon of the pectoralis major. With the rubber hammer, strike your thumb a blow directed slightly upward toward the patient's axilla. The muscle contraction can be seen or felt.

REFLEX CENTER AT C5 TO C6: BICEPS REFLEX (MUSCULOCUTANEOUS NERVE). Place the elbow at 90 degrees of flexion with the arm slightly pronated. Grasp the elbow with your left hand so that the fingers are behind and your thumb presses the biceps brachii tendon (see Fig. 14-4B). Strike a series of blows on your thumb with the rubber hammer, varying your thumb pressure with each blow until the most satisfactory response is obtained. The normal reflex is elbow flexion.

REFLEX CENTER AT C5 TO C6: BRACHIORADIALIS REFLEX (RADIAL NERVE). Hold the patient's wrist with your left hand with the forearm relaxed in pronation (see Fig. 14-4C). With a vertical stroke, tap the forearm directly, just above the radial styloid process. The normal response is elbow flexion and supination of the forearm.

REFLEX CENTER AT C6 TO C7: PRONATOR REFLEX (MEDIAN NERVE). Hold the patient's hand vertically so the wrist is suspended (see Fig. 14-4D). From the medial side, strike the distal end of the radius directly with a horizontal blow. The normal response is pronation of the forearm. An alternate method is to strike the distal end of the ulna directly with a blow mediad.

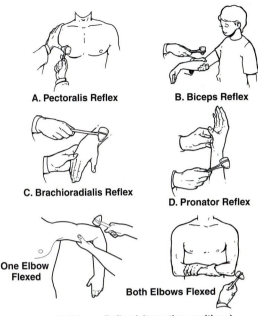

A. Pectoralis Reflex

B. Biceps Reflex

C. Brachioradialis Reflex

D. Pronator Reflex

One Elbow Flexed

Both Elbows Flexed

E. Triceps Reflex (alternative positions)

Fig. 14-4 Deep Reflexes I. A. Pectoralis Reflex. B. Biceps Brachii Reflex. C. Brachioradialis Reflex. D. Pronator Reflex. E. Triceps Brachii Reflex: There are two alternative positions: Hold the patient's arm at 90 degrees abduction, allowing the relaxed forearm to dangle with the elbow at flexion, or have the patient fold the arms and grasp the forearms with the hands (reinforcement can be obtained by having the patient tighten the grasp on the arms).

REFLEX CENTER AT C7 TO C8: TRICEPS REFLEX (RADIAL NERVE). Hold the patient's arm at 90 degrees abduction and elevation, allowing the relaxed forearm to dangle with the elbow at 90 degrees flexion (see Fig. 14-4E). Tap the triceps brachii tendon just above the olecranon process. The normal response is elbow extension. Alternatively, have the patient flex both elbows, bringing the arms parallel across the chest (see Fig. 14-4E). Have each hand grasp the other forearm. Reinforcement can be obtained by having the patient grasp harder and extending the elbow slightly.

REFLEX CENTER AT T8 TO T9: UPPER ABDOMINAL MUSCLE REFLEX. Tap the muscles directly near their insertions on the costal margins and xiphoid process (Fig. 14-5A).

REFLEX CENTER AT T9 TO T10: MIDDLE ABDOMINAL MUSCLE REFLEX. Stimulate the muscles of the mid-abdomen by tapping an overlaid finger or doubled-tongue blades (see Fig. 14-5B).

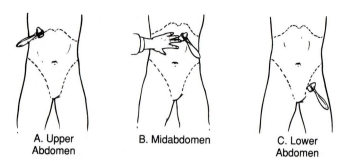

A. Upper Abdomen

B. Midabdomen

C. Lower Abdomen

Fig. 14-5 Abdominal Muscle Reflexes. A. Upper Abdomen: Tap the abdominal muscles directly with the reflex hammer, near their attachments to the costal margin. B. Mid-Abdomen: Place your finger or a double-tongue blade on the muscles and tap the pleximeter. C. Lower Abdomen: Tap the lower abdominal muscles directly at their attachments near the symphysis pubis.

REFLEX CENTER AT T11 TO T12: LOWER ABDOMINAL MUSCLES.   Tap the muscle insertions directly, near the symphysis pubis (see Fig. 14-5C).

REFLEX CENTER AT L2 TO L4: QUADRICEPS REFLEX (FEMORAL NERVE). Several methods are available. In each, a normal response is extension of the knee and contraction of the quadriceps femoris can be palpated. *Legs Dangling (Fig. 14-6A):*   Grasp the lower thigh with your left hand

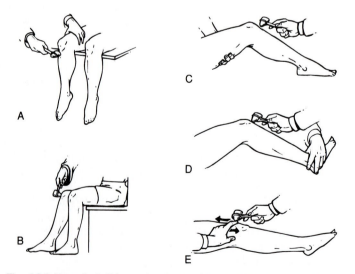

Fig. 14-6 Knee Jerk (Alternative Positions). A. With the Patient's Legs Dangling. B. Sitting. C. With the Patient Supine, Method 1. D. With the Patient Supine, Method 2. E. With the Patient Supine and Knee Extended, Method 3.

while your right delivers a hammer tap on the patellar tendon, just below the patella. *Sitting, Feet on the Floor (Fig. 14-6B):* The patient sits on a chair or low bed. Have the patient's toes curled in plantarflexion and knee slightly extended from a right angle by moving the foot forward on the floor. Tap the patellar tendon directly. *Lying Supine (Three Methods):* *Method 1* With your hand under the popliteal fossa, lift the patient's knee from the table. Tap the patellar tendon directly (see Fig. 14-6C). *Method 2* Grasp the patient's foot, flexing the hip and knee, and rotate the knee outward and dorsiflex the foot. Tap the patellar tendon directly (see Fig. 14-6D). *Method 3* With the knee extended and the limb lying on the table, push the patellar tendon distad with your index finger on the insertion of the quadriceps tendon. Tap downward on the index finger (see Fig. 14-6E). The muscle contraction pulls the patella proximally.

REFLEX CENTER AT L2 TO L4: ADDUCTOR REFLEX (OBTURATOR NERVE). With the patient supine, place the lower limb in slight abduction (Fig. 14-7A). Directly tap the adductor magnus tendon just proximal to its insertion on the medial epicondyle of the femur. Normally, the thigh adducts. If the quadriceps reflex is absent and the adductor reflex is present, this indicates a lesion of the femoral nerve.

REFLEX CENTER AT L4 TO S2: HAMSTRING REFLEX (SCIATIC NERVE). Have the patient supine with hips and knees flexed at about 90 degrees and the thighs rotated slightly outward. Place your left hand under the popliteal fossa so the index finger compresses the medial hamstring tendon (a bundle of tendons from semitendinosus, semimembranosus, gracilis, sartorius) (see Fig. 14-7B). Tap your finger. The normal response is flexion of the knee and contraction of the medial mass of hamstring muscles. Test the lateral hamstrings in a similar manner: with your finger

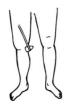

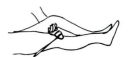

B. Hamstring Reflex

A. Adductor Magnus Reflex

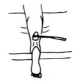

Dangling   Kneeling   Supine
C. Achilles Reflex (three ways)

Fig. 14-7 Deep Reflexes II. A. Adductor Magnus Reflex. B. Hamstring Reflex. C. Achilles Reflex (Three Ways): Leg dangling, kneeling, and supine.

compress the lateral hamstring tendon just proximal to the fibular head and tap your finger. The normal response is contraction of the lateral hamstring mass (biceps femoris) and flexion of the knee.

REFLEX CENTER AT L5 TO S2: ACHILLES REFLEX (TIBIAL NERVE).   The normal response is contraction of the gastrocnemius and plantarflexion of the foot.   *Legs Dangling (see Fig. 14-7C):*   With your left hand, grasp the patient's foot and pull it into dorsiflexion to find the degree Achilles stretch that produces the optimal response. Tap the tendon directly. *Kneeling (see Fig. 14-7C):*   Have the patient kneel with the feet hanging over the edge of a chair, table, or bed. With your left hand dorsiflexing the foot, tap the tendon directly. Assess both the contraction and relaxation of the muscle; delayed relaxation (hung-up reflex) is characteristic of hypothyroidism.   *Supine (see Fig. 14-7C):*   Partially flex the patient's hip and knee while rotating the knee outward as far as comfort permits. With your left hand, grasp the foot and pull it into dorsiflexion, then tap the Achilles tendon directly.

The Superficial (Skin) Reflexes

These reflex arcs have receptor organs in the skin rather than in muscle fibers. Their adequate stimulus is stroking, scratching, or touching. If there is no response, a painful stimulus should be tried. The superficial reflexes are lost in disease of the pyramidal tract.

REFLEX CENTER AT T5 TO T8: UPPER ABDOMINAL SKIN REFLEX.   Have the patient supine and relaxed, with the arms at the sides and knees slightly flexed. Use a fresh (previously unused) pin to stroke the skin over the lower thoracic cage from the midaxillary line toward the midline (Fig. 14-8A). Watch for ipsilateral contraction of the muscles in the epigastric abdominal wall. When the muscle contractions cannot be seen, observe for umbilical deviation toward the stimulated side. In very obese persons, retract the umbilicus toward the opposite side to feel it pull toward the side of stimulation.

REFLEX CENTER AT T9 TO T11: MID-ABDOMINAL SKIN REFLEX.   Make similar strokes from the flank toward the midline at the umbilical level.

REFLEX CENTER AT T11 TO T12: LOWER ABDOMINAL SKIN REFLEX.   Make similar strokes from the iliac crests toward the midline of the hypogastrium.

REFLEX CENTER AT L1 TO L2: CREMASTERIC REFLEX.   In males, stroke the inner aspect of the thigh from the inguinal crease down (see Fig. 14-8B). Normally, this causes contraction of the cremaster with prompt elevation of the testis on the ipsilateral side. A slow and irregular rise of the testis results from muscular contraction in the dartos tunic and is not the reflex response.

REFLEX CENTER AT L4 TO S2: PLANTAR REFLEX.   Grasp the patient's ankle with your left hand. With a blunt point and moderate pressure, stroke the sole near its *lateral* border, from the heel toward the ball, where the course should curve medial to follow the bases of the toes (see Fig. 14-8D). For the blunt point, use a wooden-tip applicator, the end of a

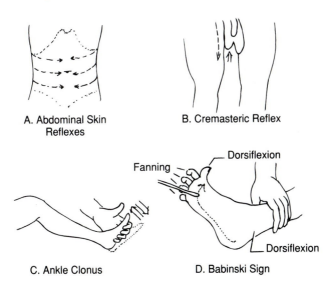

A. Abdominal Skin Reflexes

B. Cremasteric Reflex

Fanning — Dorsiflexion

C. Ankle Clonus

D. Babinski Sign

Dorsiflexion

Fig. 14-8 Skin Reflexes and Pyramidal Tract Signs. A. Abdominal Skin Reflexes. B. Cremasteric Reflex. C. Ankle Clonus: With the patient supine, lift the knee in slight flexion with the muscles relaxed. Grasp the foot and jerk it into dorsiflexion, then hold it under slight tension in that direction. In a positive response, the foot reacts with a number of cycles of alternating dorsiflexion and plantarflexion. The motion may die in a few cycles (unsustained clonus), or it may persist as long as the tension is held (sustained clonus). D. Babinski Sign.

split wooden tongue blade, or the dull handle end on a reflex hammer. If no response is observed, a pin should be used as this is a nociceptive reflex. Normally, this produces plantarflexion of the toes and, often, the entire foot responds with plantarflexion. The presence of an extensor plantar response is called a *Babinski sign*; it should be noted as present or absent. In disease of the pyramidal tract, this reflex results, with some or all of four components: dorsiflexion of the great toe, fanning of all toes, dorsiflexion of the ankle, and flexion of the knee and thigh.

REFLEX CENTER AT S1 TO S2: SUPERFICIAL ANAL REFLEX. Stroke the skin or mucosa of the perianal region. Normally, the anal sphincters contract.

POSTURE, BALANCE, AND COORDINATION: THE CEREBELLAR EXAM

Precise voluntary movement requires graded contraction of the agonist, or prime mover, with a corresponding graded relaxation of the antagonist about each joint. Other muscles act to fix the joint with proper tension. The total integration of these movements, called *coordination*, is partially mediated through efferent and afferent tracts of the cerebellum. The vestibular apparatus and the cerebral cortex also participate. Maintenance of posture and balance requires sensory input from the joints, muscles, tendons, and vestibular system, and coordinated motor outputs mediated by the cerebral cortex and basal ganglia.

Testing Station (Equilibratory Coordination)

Ask the patient to stand comfortably with the hands at the sides. Observe the position of the feet. Normally, the feet will be just a few centimeters apart and the knees opposed. A wide stance suggests an accommodation to instability of stance. Next have the patient put the feet together and observe for stability. Note swaying of the trunk or elevation of the arms to maintain balance. Now have the patient close her eyes while again observing for loss of balance. Be ready to support her should she lose her balance and reassure her you will protect her. Falling during the test is the *Romberg sign.* If she remains stable, tell her you are going to tap her gently to assess her stability. Gently push her laterally on each upper arm, forward on the upper back and, last, backward on the chest. With normal proprioception, vestibular mechanism, cerebellum and motor pathways she will remain stable throughout. Have her open her eyes, and, after fair warning, push more firmly on her chest to check for maximal stability.

Testing of Diadochokinesia

Normal coordination includes the ability to arrest one motor impulse and substitute its opposite. Loss of this ability (*dysdiadochokinesia*) is characteristic of cerebellar disease. Many simple tests may be employed to test for dysdiadochokinesis. *Alternating Movements (Fig. 14-9A):* (a) Have the patient hold his forearms vertically and alternate pronation and supination in rapid succession. In cerebellar disease, the movements overshoot, undershoot, or are irregular and inaccurate; the motions may be slowed or incomplete in disease of the pyramidal tract. (b) Have the patient rapidly tap his fingers on the table, or close and open the fists. (c) Holding the arms at 90 degrees elevation and 0 degrees abduction may show the affected arm deviating in abduction. (d) *Stewart-Holmes Rebound Sign* (Fig. 14-9A): While the patient clenches his fist, with elbow flexed and forearm pronated, grasp his fist from above and pull strongly attempting to extend his elbow against his resistance; suddenly release your grip and observe for rapid control of rebound. The examiner must guard against injury to the patient. With cerebellar disease the forearm may rebound in several cycles of extension–flexion, or the patient may strike himself if not guarded.

Testing for Dyssynergia and Dysmetria

Finger-to-Nose Test: With the patient's eyes open, have the patient fully extend his elbow and, in a wide arc, rapidly bring the tip of the index finger to the tip of his nose (see Fig. 14-9B). In cerebellar disease, this action is attended by an action tremor. When the maneuver is performed with the eyes closed, the sense of position in the shoulder and

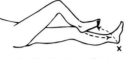

Pronator-supinator

Stewart-Holmes
Rebound Sign

A. Tests for Diadochokinesia

B. Finger-to-nose Test

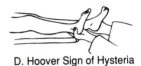

C. Heel-to-knee Test

D. Hoover Sign of Hysteria

Fig. 14-9 Test for Cerebellar Disease. *See text for full descriptions. **A.*** *Tests for Diadochokinesia: The ability to perform alternating movements may be tested by having the patient hold the forearms vertically; then ask the patient to quickly alternate pronation and supination in the vertical position. Another method is the Stewart-Holmes rebound test, in which the patient is requested to flex the biceps brachii muscle by pulling against the wrist held by the examiner. While at full strength, the examiner suddenly releases the wrist and observes for control of the rebound. **B.** Finger-to-Nose Test. **C.** Heel-to-Knee Tests. **D.** Hoover Sign of Hysteria: This distinguishes hysterical paralysis of the lower limb from paralysis with an organic cause. Take a position at the foot of the supine patient. Cradle each of the patient's heels in one of your palms and rest your hands on the table. Have the patient attempt to raise the affected limb. In organic disease, the associated movement causes the unaffected heel to press downward; in hysteria, the associated movement is absent.*

elbow is tested. In a variant of this maneuver, have the patient make wide arcs with both arms to approximate the tips of his index fingers in front of him.   *Heel-to-Shin Test:*   With the patient supine and the lower limbs resting in extension, ask the patient to raise one heel and place it on the opposite knee, then slide the heel down the shin (see Fig. 14-9C). The moving foot should be dorsiflexed, and the motion should be performed slowly and accurately. In cerebellar disease, the arc of the heel to the knee is jerky and wavering, the knee is frequently overshot, and the slide down the shin is accompanied by an action tremor. With the eyes closed, the motions are inaccurate in posterior spinal column disease. Frequently, the heel slides off the shin, but action tremor is absent.

Testing Skilled Acts

To inspect handwriting, ask the patient to write sentences on paper. Test the patient's skill at buttoning and unbuttoning a coat or shirt. Let the patient pick up pins or thread a needle. Test the patient's skill at cutting figures out of paper with scissors.

Testing the Vestibular Apparatus

Past pointing and other tests are described in Chapter 7 on page 211.

The Gait

The gait is influenced by the rate, rhythm, and the character of the movements employed in walking. In assessing the neurologic contribution to gait, painful and restrictive conditions of the joints, muscles, and other structures must be excluded. Observe the patient's usual gait in a well-lighted hallway. Note the posture of the head, neck and trunk, swing of each arm, leg swing, width of stance, size of steps and clearance of the toe from the floor. Be sure to observe all three phases of gait: touch down, which should occur with the lateral heel; stance, which should be centered; and push-off which should come off the great toe. Foot strikes are normally in a nearly straight line. Also observe the turn for loss of balance or multiple small steps to get turned around. Next, have the patient walk away from you on the toes, observing from behind, turn and walk toward you on the heels observing from the front; note how far the heels and toes, respectively, are held off the ground. Examine the wear on the patient's shoes; abnormal wear pattern is a good clue to disorders of the foot and gait.

SENSORY EXAMINATION

A complete assessment of sensory functions is not made in the routine physical examination, with the exception of patients with diabetes. But a history of localized pain, numbness, or tingling, or the finding of motor deficits, calls for a detailed sensory examination.

The prerequisites for sensory assessment are (a) detailed knowledge of segmental and peripheral nerve distribution in the skin by reference to such charts as Figs. 14-10 and 14-11, (b) a lucid sensorium and adequate attention on the part of the patient to secure cooperation, and (c) a graphic record of the distribution of sensory deficits. The diagram may be used for immediate comparison on retesting, because several examinations for sensation should always be performed. Disparities in two examinations may point to deception by the patient, so you should confuse the patient by varying the order.

The detailed examination of the cranial nerves includes testing of the special senses and the cutaneous sensibility of the head. For the remainder of the body, the distribution of sensibility for cutaneous pain, touch, pressure, position, and vibration should be evaluated. When a deficit in the pain sense is encountered, the sensibility for temperature should also be tested. When an area of altered cutaneous sensibility is found, the borders should be marked with a skin pencil, and a diagram should be made in the patient's record.

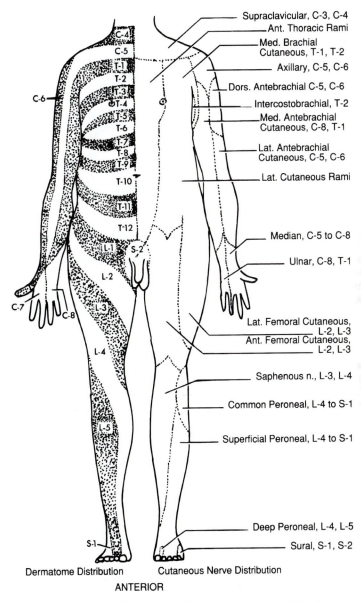

Supraclavicular, C-3, C-4
Ant. Thoracic Rami
Med. Brachial Cutaneous, T-1, T-2
Axillary, C-5, C-6
Dors. Antebrachial C-5, C-6
Intercostobrachial, T-2
Med. Antebrachial Cutaneous, C-8, T-1
Lat. Antebrachial Cutaneous, C-5, C-6
Lat. Cutaneous Rami
Median, C-5 to C-8
Ulnar, C-8, T-1
Lat. Femoral Cutaneous, L-2, L-3
Ant. Femoral Cutaneous, L-2, L-3
Saphenous n., L-3, L-4
Common Peroneal, L-4 to S-1
Superficial Peroneal, L-4 to S-1
Deep Peroneal, L-4, L-5
Sural, S-1, S-2

C-4, C-5, T-1, T-2, T-3, T-4, T-5, T-6, T-7, T-8, T-9, T-10, T-11, T-12, L-1, S-2, L-2, L-3, L-4, L-5, S-1

C-6, C-7, C-8

Dermatome Distribution   Cutaneous Nerve Distribution

ANTERIOR

Fig. 14-10 Cutaneous Sensation in the Anterior Aspect of the Body.

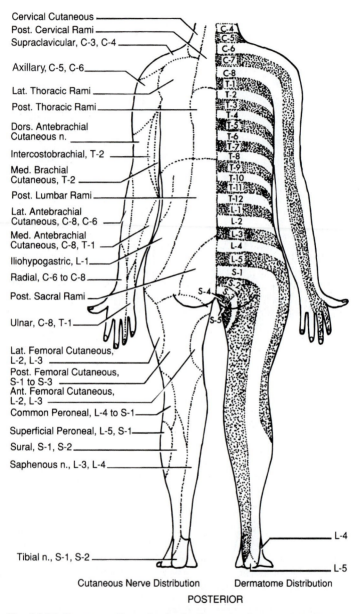

Cervical Cutaneous

Post. Cervical Rami

Supraclavicular, C-3, C-4

Axillary, C-5, C-6

Lat. Thoracic Rami

Post. Thoracic Rami

Dors. Antebrachial Cutaneous n.

Intercostobrachial, T-2

Med. Brachial Cutaneous, T-2

Post. Lumbar Rami

Lat. Antebrachial Cutaneous, C-8, C-6

Med. Antebrachial Cutaneous, C-8, T-1

Iliohypogastric, L-1

Radial, C-6 to C-8

Post. Sacral Rami

Ulnar, C-8, T-1

Lat. Femoral Cutaneous, L-2, L-3

Post. Femoral Cutaneous, S-1 to S-3

Ant. Femoral Cutaneous, L-2, L-3

Common Peroneal, L-4 to S-1

Superficial Peroneal, L-5, S-1

Sural, S-1, S-2

Saphenous n., L-3, L-4

Tibial n., S-1, S-2

C-4
C-5
C-6
C-7
C-8
T-1
T-2
T-3
T-4
T-5
T-6
T-7
T-8
T-9
T-10
T-11
T-12
L-1
L-2
L-3
L-4
L-5
S-1
S-2
S-3
S-4
S-5

L-4

L-5

Cutaneous Nerve Distribution   Dermatome Distribution

POSTERIOR

Fig. 14-11 Cutaneous Sensation in the Posterior Aspect of the Body.

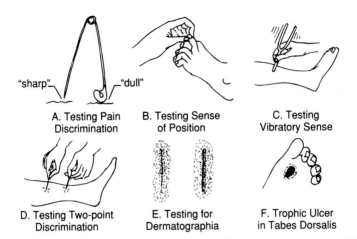

A. Testing Pain Discrimination

B. Testing Sense of Position

C. Testing Vibratory Sense

D. Testing Two-point Discrimination

E. Testing for Dermatographia

F. Trophic Ulcer in Tabes Dorsalis

Fig. 14-12 Sensory Testing and Other Phenomena. *See text for descriptions.* ***A. Testing "Sharp-Dull" with a Safety Pin. B. Testing Position Sense in the Toes. C. Testing Vibratory Sense. D. Testing Two-Point Discrimination. E. Testing for Dermatographism:*** *Stroke the skin with a blunt object; the normal response is a pale line along the path of stimulation, the "white line." The abnormal responses are a "red line" in which the area becomes bright red and then extends with red mottling, and, with more exaggerated response, the line develops a wheal that becomes raised, edematous, and pale.* ***F. Trophic Plantar Ulcer in Tabes Dorsalis.***

Basic Sensory Modalities

TESTING PAIN AND TOUCH SENSE. *Superficial Pain (Sharp-Dull):* Have the patient close his eyes and ask, "What do you feel?" Use the point and the dull guard end of a sterile open safety pin as a stimulus (Fig. 14-12A). Hold it lightly between your thumb and index finger so that the pin slides slightly with each application. If there is doubt about the response, mix sharp and dull stimuli from the point and head of the pin. Compare side-to-side with the same degree of pressure and ask, "Is it the same"; it is more objective if the patient reports differences than if you suggest them. In mapping deficit borders, slowly stimulate the skin from nonsensitive to sensitive skin, having the patient indicate where the sensation changes. Sensibility to pain may be normal, reduced (*hypalgesia*), absent (*analgesia*), or increased (*hyperalgesia*). *Deep Pain:* Test for deep or protopathic pain by pressure on the nerve trunks, and tendons. For example, in the *Abadie sign* for tabes dorsalis, the normal pressure tenderness of the Achilles tendon is lost.

TESTING TEMPERATURE SENSE. When pain sense is impaired, test for temperature sensibility because the pathways are closely associated. Have the patient close the eyes. Use glass tubes of hot and cold water or test for cold perception with a cold tuning fork and warm perception by exhaling on the skin through your widespread lips. Ask the patient to distinguish between warm and cold.

TESTING TACTILE SENSE.   With the patient's eyes closed, compare sensation right to left by stroking the skin with a shred of sterile gauze and having the patient indicate when and where you touch him. If you suspect that he is using his eyes, make sham tests near but without touching the skin. Grade the results as normal, *anesthetic, hypesthetic,* and *hyperesthetic.*

TESTING PROPRIOCEPTION: POSITION SENSE.   With the patient's eyes closed, grasp a finger on the sides (avoid grasping on the top and bottom or touching adjacent fingers because that provides touch cues). Extend or flex the finger at one joint and ask the patient to state its position (see Fig. 14-12B). Similarly, test the sense of position in the distal joint of the patient's great toe. Normal young patients discriminate 1–2 degrees of movement in their distal finger joints and 3–5 degrees of the great toe. Test position sense in the leg or arm with the eyes closed. Place one limb in a position and ask the patient to place its counterpart in a symmetrical position.

VIBRATORY SENSE: PALLESTHESIA.   Place the handle of a vibrating 128-Hz tuning fork over bony prominences, such as the styloid processes of the radii, the subcutaneous aspects of the tibiae, the malleoli of the ankles, or the interphalangeal joint of the great toe, and time how long the patient feels the vibration (see Fig. 14-12C). Compare symmetrical points. When the patient indicates that the vibration of the fork has ceased, place the handle on your own wrist to detect any persistence of vibration. Young patients feel vibration for about 15 seconds in the great toe and 25 seconds in the distal joint of the finger, whereas 70-year-olds feel it for 10 and 15 seconds, respectively. Make sham tests by setting the fork in vibration and unobtrusively stopping it with your finger before applying the handle to the patient.

PRESSURE SENSE.   Standardized monofilaments are available to precisely check for protective pressure sensation. Anesthesia to a 10-g monofilament is a sensitive test for loss of protective sensation to pressure injury. All diabetics should be tested at least once a year with this technique [Caputo GM, Cavanagh PR, Ulbrecht JS, et al. Assessment and management of foot disease in patients with diabetes. *N Engl J Med* 1994;331:854–860].Test the patient's ability to discriminate between objects of different weights by placing them in the patient's palms. Test the ability to distinguish between pressures from the head of a pin and the tip of your finger. Press over the joints and subcutaneous aspects of bones for perception of pressure.

Testing Higher Integrative Functions

STEREOGNOSIS.   Simple sensory perception should have been previously demonstrated as normal. Test the patient's ability to distinguish forms by placing objects in the patient's hands while the patient's eyes are

Sensation Intact in Index
and Little Fingers

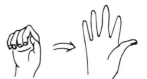

Normal Extension of Digits

Fig. 14-13 Exclusion Test for Major Nerve Injury in the Upper Limb. *Sensation is intact in the palmar tips of the index and little fingers; extension of the digits of the hand is unimpaired.*

closed. Use coins, pencils, glass, wood, metal, cloth, and other familiar articles.

TWO-POINT DISCRIMINATION. Test the ability to distinguish the separation of two simultaneous sterile pinpricks (see Fig. 14-12D). By separating two pinpoints at various distances, find the distance at which the patient perceives them as two points rather than as one. Test and compare symmetric regions. The normal distance varies in different parts of the body, from 1 mm on the tongue, to 2–8 mm on the fingertip, 40 mm on the chest and forearm, and 75 mm on the upper thigh and upper arm.

PERCEPTION OF FIGURES ON THE SKIN (GRAPHESTHESIA). Tell the patient whether you will write numerals or letters "right-side up." Then, with the patient's eyes closed, use a blunt point to trace a figure 1 cm high on the distal pad of the index finger. The figures should be at least 2 cm high on other body parts. Ask the patient to identify them.

TESTING SPECIFIC PERIPHERAL NERVES

Exclusion Test for Major Nerve Injury in the Upper Limb

Normal sensibility to a sterile pinprick in the tips of the index and little fingers excludes major injury to the median and ulnar nerves. Normal ability to extend the thumb and fingers excludes injury of the radial nerve (Fig. 14-13).

TESTING THE MEDIAN NERVE. *Motor Function: Ochsner Test (Fig. 14-14A).* Have the patient clasp the hands firmly together; the index finger cannot flex when the innervation of the flexor digitorum sublimis has been injured anywhere below the antecubital fossa. *Flexion of the Thumb (Fig. 14-14B).* Hold the patient's first metacarpophalangeal joint with your thumb and index fingers so that the metacarpal bone is extended and ask the patient to bend the interphalangeal joint; failure indicates paralysis of the flexor pollicis longus, innervated by the volar interosseus that branches from the median nerve in the middle third of the forearm. *Abduction of Thumb.* Test the action of the abductor pol-

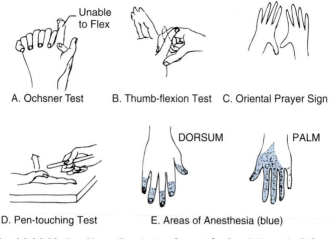

A. Ochsner Test   B. Thumb-flexion Test   C. Oriental Prayer Sign

D. Pen-touching Test   E. Areas of Anesthesia (blue)

*Fig. 14-14 Median Nerve Paralysis. See text for descriptions. **A. Ochsner Test:** The patient cannot flex the index finger on the paralyzed side. **B. Thumb Flexion Test:** The patient cannot flex the distal joint of the thumb. **C. Wartenberg Oriental Prayer Sign:** Paralysis prevents extension of the thumb so its tip cannot reach its mate. **D. Pen-Touching Test:** The thumb cannot abduct to touch the object when the median nerve is paralyzed. **E. The Area of Anesthesia:** This includes the radial three digits of the palmar aspect and folds over the tips to the dorsal aspect where it covers the distal phalanges of the same digits (blue).*

licis brevis, innervated exclusively by the median nerve, to distinguish it from low-level paralysis of the ulnar nerve. (a) *Wartenberg Oriental Prayer Position* (Fig. 14-14C). Have the patient extend and adduct the four fingers of each hand, with thumbs extended, then raise the two hands in front of the face so they are side by side in the same plane, with thumbs and index fingers touching tip to tip. Paralysis of the abductor pollicis brevis prevents full range of thumb abduction, so thumbs do not coincide when index fingers touch. (b) *Pen-Touching Test* (Fig. 14-14D). Have the patient rest the supinated hand on the table holding the patient's fingers flat. Hold a pen or pencil horizontal above the thumb and ask the patient to raise his thumb to touch the object in a plane of 90 degrees with the table. This tests the patient's ability to abduct the thumb. ***Sensory Function:*** *Phalen test* is performed by having the patient press the backs of the hands together with the wrists flexed at 90 degrees for a minute. Numbness and tingling of the thumb, index, middle, and half of the ring finger indicate compression of the median nerve, as in the carpal tunnel syndrome (Fig. 14-14E). The *Tinel sign* (page 735) is often useful. When the nerve lesion is in the wrist, the sensory loss on the palmar surface is restricted to the distal two-thirds of the radial digits.

TESTING THE ULNAR NERVE. ***Motor Function:*** Weakness in adduction of the fingers results from paralysis of the interosseus palmaris. This is

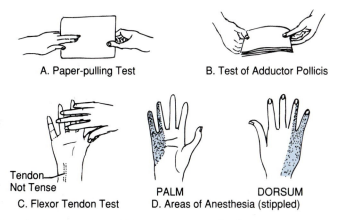

A. Paper-pulling Test

B. Test of Adductor Pollicis

Tendon
Not Tense

C. Flexor Tendon Test

PALM

DORSUM

D. Areas of Anesthesia (stippled)

Fig. 14-15 Ulnar Nerve Paralysis. See text for descriptions. *A. Paper-Pulling Test:* This tests the adductors of the fingers by having the patient hold a piece of paper between two adducted fingers; the examiner pulls the paper to test the strength of compression exerted by the adductors. *B. Adductor Pollicis Test:* In ulnar paralysis, the thumb cannot exert enough pressure in adduction, so it flexes involuntarily from action of the flexor pollicis longus. *C. Test of Flexor Carpi Ulnaris:* The patient attempts to flex the free finger, but the paralyzed tendon in the wrist does not tense. *D. Area of Anesthesia:* The ulnar 1.5 digits on both aspects of the hand (blue).

demonstrated by pulling a sheet of paper from between the patient's extended and adducted fingers to assess the pressure exerted by the sides of the fingers (Fig. 14-15A). Paralysis of the adductor pollicis can be tested by asking the patient to grip each end of a folded paper between thumbs on top and index fingers underneath. Have the patient pull the hands apart while gripping the paper. The thumb with an inadequate adductor becomes flexed at its interphalangeal joint from involuntary action of the flexor pollicis longus, innervated by the median nerve (Fig. 14-15B). In lesions at or below the elbow, test for paralysis of the flexor carpi ulnaris by having the patient's supinated hand lie on the table. Hold all digits but the little finger flat against the table. Have the patient abduct the little finger maximally; if there is no paralysis, the tensed tendon may be seen or palpated at the wrist (Fig. 14-15C). *Sensory Function:* An area of anesthesia covers the ulnar digits and the corresponding region of the palm. A similar distribution occurs on the dorsal aspect, except when the nerve lesion is at the wrist so the area is constricted to the distal half of the little finger (Fig. 14-15D).

Movements of Specific Muscles and Nerves

It is frequently desirable to identify the muscles and nerves involved in a deficit of bodily movement. The following is a compilation of the principal muscle movements, their causative muscles, and their innervation (in parentheses). Our survey starts with cranial nerves and proceeds distally identifying movements served by cervical, thoracic, lumbar, and

sacral roots sequentially. The reader can use the list in several ways: an
abnormal movement can be traced to the peripheral nerve and spinal
roots; abnormal movements can be predicted for each peripheral nerve
or spinal segment.

Eyebrow, elevation. Frontalis (CN-VII from inferior pons).

**Eyebrow, depression downward and inward, wrinkling of the fore-
head**. Corrugator (CN-VII from inferior pons).

Upper eyelid, elevations. Levator palpebrae superioris (CN-III from
upper midbrain).

Eyelids, closing, wrinkling of forehead, compression of lacrimal sac.
Orbicularis oculi (CN-VII from inferior pons).

*****Eyeball, elevation and adduction**. Superior rectus (CN-III from upper
midbrain).

*****Eyeball, elevation and outward rotation**. Inferior oblique (CN-III from
upper midbrain).

*****Eyeball, depression and rotation downward and inward**. Inferior rec-
tus (CN-III from upper midbrain).

*****Eyeball, depression and rotation downward and outward**. Superior
oblique (CN-IV from midbrain) or primary downward rotation, secondary inward (intorsion) rotation, and tertiary weak outward rotation.

*****Eyeball, adduction**. Medial rectus (CN-III from upper midbrain).

*****Eyeball, abduction**. Lateral rectus (CN-VI from inferior pons).

Pupil, constriction. Ciliary (CN-III and parasympathetic from upper
midbrain).

Lips, retraction. Zygomatic (CN-VII from inferior pons).

Lips, protrusion. Orbicularis oris (CN-VII from inferior pons).

Mouth, opening. Mylohyoid (CN-V from pons), digastricus (CN-VII
from pons).

Mandible, elevation and retraction. Masseter and temporalis (CN-V
from mid-pons).

Mandible, elevation and protrusion. Pterygoid (CN-V from mid-pons).

Pharynx, palatine elevation and pharyngeal constriction. Levator veli
palatini and pharyngeal constrictor (CN-IX and X from medulla).

Tongue, depression and protrusion. Genioglossus (CN-XII from
medulla).

Neck, rotation of the head. Sternocleidomastoid and trapezius (CN-XI
from medulla and upper cervical cord).

Neck, flexion. Rectus capitis anterior (C1 to C3).

Neck, extension, and rotation of the head. Splenius capitis et cervicis
(C1 to C4).

*****Ophthalmologic Interpretation of Muscle Action.** The items marked with asterisks
constitute the actions of the oculorotatory muscles, as assigned by the anatomists and
some neurologists. Sharply divergent interpretations are furnished by the ophthalmol-
ogists on the basis of clinical findings. The direction of movement of the eyes is a result of the actions of synergists and antagonists producing six cardinal positions of gaze,
corresponding to the six extraocular muscles. Paralysis of a single muscle results in the
inability of the eye to attain its cardinal position, which, in four of the six muscles, does
not correspond to the prediction of the anatomists.

Neck, lateral bending. Rectus capitis lateralis (C1 to C4 and suboccipital nerve).

Spine, flexion. Rectus abdominis (T8 to T12).

Spine, extension. Thoracic and lumbar intercostals (thoracic nerves from T2 to L1).

Spine, extension and rotation. Semispinalis (thoracic nerves from T2 to T12).

Spine, extension and lateral bending. Quadratus lumborum (lumbar plexus from T10 to L2).

Ribs, elevation and depression. Scaleni and intercostal (cervical and thoracic nerves from C4 to T12).

Ribs, elevation. Serratus posterior superior (from T1 to T4).

Diaphragm, elevation and depression. The diaphragmatic muscles (phrenic nerve from C3 to C5). Remember diaphragmatic innervation by the phrenic nerve with the rhyme, "C3, 4, and 5 to keep the man alive."

Scapula, rotation and extension of neck. Upper trapezius (CN-XI from C3 to C4).

Scapula, retraction with shoulder elevation. Middle and lower trapezius (CN-XI from C3 to C4).

Scapula, elevation and retraction. Rhomboids (dorsal scapular nerve from C5).

Arm, elevation. Supraspinatus (suprascapular nerve from C5 to C6), upper trapezius (CN-XI from C3 to C4).

Arm, elevation and rotation. Deltoid (axillary nerve from C5 to C6).

Arm, depression and adduction. Middle pectoralis major (anterior thoracic nerve from C5 to T1).

Arm, depression and medial rotation. Subscapularis (subscapular nerve from C5 to C7), teres major (thoracodorsal nerves from C5 to C7).

Arm, depression and lateral rotation. Infraspinatus (suprascapular nerve from C5 to C6).

Elbow, flexion. Biceps brachii, brachialis (musculocutaneous nerve from C5 to C6).

Elbow, extension. Triceps brachii (radial nerve from C7 to T1).

Elbow, supination. Biceps brachii (musculocutaneous nerve from C5 to C6), brachioradialis (radial nerve from C5 to C6).

Elbow, supination and elbow flexion. Brachioradialis (radial nerve from C5 to C6).

Elbow, pronation. Pronator teres (median nerve from C6 to C7).

Wrist, extension and adduction. Extensor carpi ulnaris (radial nerve from C7 to C8).

Wrist, extension and abduction of hand. Extensor carpi radialis longus (radial nerve from C6 to C7).

Wrist, extension of the hand. Extensor digitorum communis (radial nerve from C7 to C8).

Wrist, flexion and abduction. Flexor carpi radialis (median nerve from C7 to C8).

Wrist, flexion and adduction. Flexor carpi ulnaris (ulnar nerve from C7 to C8).

Thumb, adduction and opposition. Adductor pollicis longus (ulnar nerve C8 to T1).

Thumb, abduction and extension. Abductor pollicis longus and brevis (median and radial and [posterior interosseous nerves] from C7 to C8).

Thumb, extension of distal phalanx. Extensor pollicis longus (radial nerve from C7 to C8).

Thumb, extension of proximal phalanx. Extensor pollicis brevis (radial nerve from C7 to C8).

Thumb, flexion of distal phalanx. Flexor pollicis longus (median nerve from C7 to T1).

Thumb, flexion of proximal phalanx. Flexor pollicis longus and brevis (median nerve from C7 to T1).

Thumb, flexion and opposition. Opponens pollicis (median nerve from C8 to T1).

Fingers, flexion and adduction of little finger. Opponens digiti minimi (ulnar nerve from C8 to T1).

Fingers, adduction of four fingers. Palmar interossei (ulnar nerve from C8 to T1).

Fingers, abduction of four fingers. Dorsal interossei (ulnar nerve from C8 to T1).

Fingers, extension of hand. Extensor digitorum communis (radial nerve from C7 to C8).

Fingers, flexion of hand. Palmar interossei (interosseous nerves from C7 to T1), lumbricales (ulnar and median nerves from C7 to T1).

Fingers, extension of interphalangeal joints. Interossei palmaris and lumbricales (interosseous nerve; median and ulnar nerves from C7 to T1).

Fingers, flexion of the distal phalanges. Flexor digitorum profundus (median and ulnar nerves from C7 to T1).

Fingers, flexion of middle phalanges. Flexor digitorum sublimis (median nerve from C7 to T1).

Abdomen, compression with flexion of trunk. Rectus abdominis (lower thoracic nerves from T6 to L1).

Abdomen, flexion of abdominal wall obliquely. Obliquus abdominis externus (lower thoracic nerves from T6 to L1).

Hip, flexion. Iliacus (femoral nerve), psoas (L2 to L3), sartorius (femoral nerve from L2 to L3).

Hip, extension. Gluteus maximus (inferior gluteal nerve from L4 or S2), adductor magnus (sciatic nerve and obturator nerve from L5 to S2).

Hip, abduction. Gluteus medius (superior gluteal nerve from L4 to S1), gluteus maximus (inferior gluteal nerve from L4 to S2).

Hip, adduction. Adductor magnus (sciatic and obturator nerves from L5 to S2).

Hip, outward rotation. Gluteus maximus (inferior gluteal nerve from L4 to S2), obturator internus (branches from S1 to S3).

Hip, inward rotation. Psoas (branches from L2 to L3).

Knee, flexion. Biceps femoris, semitendinosus, semimembranosus, gastrocnemius (all through sciatic nerve from L5 to S2).

Knee, extension. Quadriceps femoris (femoral nerve from L2 to L4).

Ankle, plantar flexion. Gastrocnemius (tibial nerve from L5 to S2).

Ankle, dorsiflexion. Anterior tibial (deep peroneal nerve from L4 to S1).

Ankle, inversion. Posterior tibial (tibial nerve from L5 to S1).

TABLE 14–1   Mini-Mental State Examination

		Points
Orientation		
_____	What is the (time) (date) (day) (month) (year)?	(5)
_____	Where are we (state) (county) (city) (hospital) (ward)?	(5)
Registration		
_____	Name three objects and ask the patient to repeat them until all three are learned. Record the number of trials.	(3)
Attention and Calculation		
_____	Ask the patient to subtract serial 7s for five times.	(5)
Recall		
_____	Ask the patient to recall the three objects named above.	(3)
Language		
_____	*Naming*: Pencil and watch.	(2)
_____	*Repetition*: "No ifs, ands, or buts."	(1)
_____	*Three-stage command*: "Take paper in your right hand, fold it in half, and put it on the floor."	(3)
_____	*Reading*: Obey instruction given in writing: "Close your eyes."	(1)
_____	*Writing*: "Write a sentence."	
_____	"Copying: Construct a pair of intersecting pentagons and ask the patient to copy them.	(1)

SOURCE: Crum RM, Anthony JC, Bassett SS, Folstein MF. Population-based norms for the Mini-Mental State Examination by age and educational level. *JAMA* 1993;269:2386–2391.

Ankle, eversion. Peroneus longus (superficial peroneal nerve from L4 to S1).

Great toe, dorsiflexion. Extensor hallucis longus and brevis (superficial peroneal nerve from L4 to S1).

MENTAL STATUS SCREENING EXAMINATION

During the history and physical examination, the alert physician forms an impression of the patient's mental status. We are indebted to Folstein and colleagues for devising and validating the Mini-Mental State Exam (MMSE, Table 14-1), an efficient inventory of cognitive function [Folstein MF, Folstein SE, McHugh PR. Mini-mental state—A practical method for grading the cognitive state of patients for the clinician. *J Psychiatr Res* 1975;12:189–198]. Scores of less than 20 may indicate dementia, delirium, schizophrenia, or affective disorder.

The Mini-Cog is a validated screening test that uses the registration and recall questions from the Mini-Mental State Examination and the clock drawing exercise. The latter is performed by drawing a circle and placing the numeral "12" in its proper clock position. Then ask the patient to fill in the remaining numerals followed by indicating a particular time such as "4:35" [Scanlan J, Borson S. The Mini-Cog: Receiver operating characteristics with expert and naive raters. *Int J Geriatr Psychiatry* 2001;16:216–222]. Errors in either task indicate the need for detailed evaluation of cognitive function (see Chapter 15).

Neurologic Symptoms

General Symptoms

KEY SYMPTOM
Headache: See page 805ff.

KEY SYMPTOM
Memory Loss: Patients often complain of forgetfulness, especially of people's names. Paradoxically, it is rarely the patient who is concerned about memory loss who has a serious problem. Changes in behavior, failure to complete expected tasks, difficulty with instrumental activities of daily living, especially managing finances, are more likely to be clues to significant impairments in memory and cognition. Always formally screen for cognitive impairment if there is any concern.

Cranial Nerve Symptoms

KEY SYMPTOM
Visual Loss: See Chapter 7, page 232.

KEY SYMPTOM
Absent or Abnormal Taste and Smell: Ageusia, Dysgeusia, Anosmia: See Chapter 7, page 232.

KEY SYMPTOM
Ringing in the Ears: Tinnitus: See Chapter 7, page 230.

KEY SYMPTOM
Hearing Loss: See Chapter 7, page 322.

KEY SYMPTOM
Vertigo: See Chapter 7, page 322.

KEY SYMPTOM
Double Vision: Diplopia: See Chapter 7, page 231.

KEY SYMPTOM
Difficulty Swallowing: Dysphagia: See Chapter 7, pages 233 and 327, and Chapter 8, pages 533 and 563–564.

KEY SYMPTOM

Difficulty Speaking: Dysarthria: See Chapter 7, page 330ff and page 875.

KEY SYMPTOM

Difficulty Speaking: Aphasia: See page 875.

KEY SYMPTOM

Pain in the Face: See Chapter 7, page 229.

KEY SYMPTOM

Asymmetrical Face or Smile: See page 832, Facial Nerve Signs.

KEY SYMPTOM

Hoarseness: See Chapter 7, page 304.

KEY SYMPTOM

Neck and Shoulder Weakness: See Chapter 13, pages 716ff and 746ff.

Motor Symptoms

KEY SYMPTOM

Weakness: See page 833. *Pathophysiology:* Weakness may arise from lesions in the brain, spinal cord, peripheral nerves, motor endplate, or muscle, either primary or as a result of generalized metabolic abnormalities. Weakness is a common complaint that requires a complete evaluation. A careful history is required to identify the specific activities that are impaired. Difficulty with rising from a chair or climbing stairs suggests proximal muscle weakness, whereas difficulty writing, opening jars and doors, and catching the toes while walking suggest distal weakness. Global weakness can be seen with generalized muscle diseases, myasthenia gravis, and polyneuropathies (e.g. Guillain-Barré syndrome). During physical examination, observe for fasciculations, assess muscle mass, tone, and strength, and evaluate the reflexes. Hysterical weakness is not rare and malingering is perhaps more common; these diagnoses can only be made after organic disease is excluded by a thorough evaluation, including laboratory tests.

KEY SYMPTOM

Acute Episodic Weakness: Cataplexy: Episodic loss of motor and postural control is precipitated by laughter or strong emotions. There is momentary loss of voluntary motor power including speech, without loss of consciousness or postural tone. Cataplexy is seen in patients with narcolepsy.

KEY SYMPTOM

Muscle Pain: Myalgia: See also Chapter 13, page 710. This is a common, but nonspecific finding. Generalized myalgias, especially in the back and proximal limb muscles frequently accompany febrile illness of any cause. Severe myalgias are common in several infectious diseases (e.g., Lyme disease, trichinosis, and dengue); other elements of the history are of more use than the presence of myalgia in making the specific diagnosis. Drugs (e.g., statins) also cause myalgias so a complete medication and herbal therapy history is mandatory. In persons older than 50 years of age, abrupt onset of myalgias in the proximal muscles (shoulders > pelvic girdle) suggests polymyalgia rheumatica.

KEY SYMPTOM

Muscle Stiffness: *Pathophysiology:* Overuse of skeletal muscle induces a damage–repair cycle that is felt by the patient as pain and stiffness. Underuse leads to muscle atrophy, which may be accompanied by stiffness. The unconditioned patient often complains of sore, stiff muscles 1–2 days following unaccustomed exercise (weekend athlete syndrome). Examination shows no abnormalities other than tenderness and occasionally mild spasm in the affected muscles. Patients with inherited disorders of muscle metabolism or electrolyte disorders can develop severe myonecrosis with exercise. DDX: Abrupt onset of proximal muscles stiffness in a person older than 50 years of age without a clear-cut precipitating event suggests polymyalgia rheumatica. Generalized cramps with tetany are seen with hypocalcemia.

KEY SYMPTOM

Twitches and Tics: See page 842.

KEY SYMPTOM

Irresistible Leg Movements: Restless Legs Syndrome: See page 878.

KEY SYMPTOM

Muscle Spasm: Cramps, Dystonias: See page 873.

Reflex Symptoms

KEY SYMPTOM

Muscle Spasm: Spasticity: See page 834.

Posture, Balance, and Coordination Symptoms

KEY SYMPTOM

Loss of Balance: Falling: See page 850.

KEY SYMPTOM

Difficulty Walking: See page 840.

KEY SYMPTOM

Vertigo: See Chapter 7, page 322.

KEY SYMPTOM

Shaking: Tremors: See page 841.

Sensory Symptoms

KEY SYMPTOM

✔️ **Altered Sensation: Tingling and Numbness, Paresthesias:** *Pathophysiology:* Tingling and numbness of a body part indicate impairment of the normal pressure, pain, and/or touch sensory function. The pattern of the symptoms gives a good indication of the anatomic level of the nerve injury: symptoms on one side of the entire body indicate a problem in the thalamus or cortex; loss on one side of the body below a specific level suggests spinal cord injury; symptoms in a peripheral nerve distribution implies injury to that nerve; and symmetrical distal paresthesia (stocking-glove distribution) suggests a generalized sensory (with or without motor) neuropathy. Test for the specific modalities of sensation are required.

KEY SYMPTOM

✔️ **Pain with Non-painful Stimuli: Allodynia:** See page 844.

KEY SYMPTOM

✔️ **Altered Sensation: Pain:** See page 844.

Neurologic Signs

Cranial Nerve Signs

Because the signs of cranial nerve dysfunction can be mimicked by non-neurologic end-organ disease, these signs are discussed in Chapter 7, *The Head and Neck Examination*. Signs of cranial nerve dysfunction are the absence of normal functions as demonstrated by the physical exam. Once end-organ disease is excluded, the challenge is to decide whether the lesion is central (brain) or peripheral (nerve). The following is a brief list of some specific cranial nerve signs.

KEY SIGN

📥 **Olfactory Nerve (CN-I): Anosmia:** See Chapter 7, page 281.

KEY SIGN

📥 **Optic Nerve Signs: Visual Field Cuts:** See Chapter 7, page 258.

KEY SIGN

📥 **Oculomotor (CN-III) Paralysis:** See *Eye Movement Signs*, page 252, Abnormalities of Gaze, page 253, and *Pupil Signs*, page 266 (Fig. 14-16). Unilateral complete paralysis is usually caused by direct pressure from tumor, aneurysm, or herniating brain. Less common are cavernous sinus thrombosis and granulomatous process at the base of the brain, for example, tuberculous meningitis and Tolosa-Hunt syn-

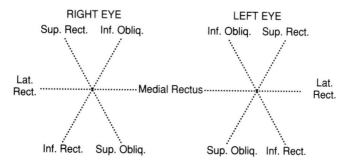

Fig. 14-16 The Cardinal Positions of Gaze. *Each of the six positions is the result of synergists and antagonists acting with a specific muscle. Paralysis of the specific muscle prevents the eye from attaining the cardinal position for the muscle.*

drome. Pupillary-sparing oculomotor nerve palsy may be a complication of diabetes mellitus.

KEY SIGN

Trochlear Nerve (CN-IV) Paralysis: See *Eye Movement Signs*, page 252, and *Abnormalities of Gaze*, page 253 (see Fig. 14-16). CN-IV may be involved with CN-III and CN-VI in the cavernous sinus.

KEY SIGN

Trigeminal Nerve (CN-V) Signs: The corneal reflex may be absent and the jaw closure weak and/or asymmetric. Irritative lesions of the motor root may cause spasm or trismus. Irritation of the sensory root results in tic douloureux.

KEY SIGN

Abducens Nerve (CN-VI) Signs: See *Eye Movement Signs*, page 252, and *Abnormalities of Gaze*, page 253 (see Fig. 14-16). Diabetic mononeuropathy is also common. CN-VI may be involved with CN-III and CN-IV in the cavernous sinus.

KEY SIGN

Facial Nerve (CN-VII) Signs: Irritation of the cornea (*keratitis*) and conjunctivae (*keratoconjunctivitis sicca*) may occur as a result of inadequate lid closing. Weakness may be manifest by pocketing of food in the cheeks and difficulty with efficient mastication. *Facial spasm,* clonic contractions of the facial muscles, may occur because of denervation. The cause of peripheral palsies of the facial nerve is usually unknown. They occasionally occur in sarcoidosis, tumors of the temporal bone and cerebellopontine angle, poliomyelitis, neoplasms, infectious polyneuritis (Guillain-Barré syndrome), Lyme disease, AIDS, and syphilis. The face is expressionless, the mask-like facies, in Parkinson disease. In the *Ramsay-Hunt syndrome,* herpes zoster virus infects the geniculate ganglion of the sensory branch of the facial nerve to produce a facial palsy, loss of taste on the anterior two-thirds of the tongue, and pain and vesicles in the external auditory canal on the same side. Herpetic lesions in the ear canal is the clue to diagnosis. Idiopathic facial nerve paralysis is *Bell palsy.*

KEY SIGN

Auditory Nerve (CN-VIII) Signs: Abnormal Hearing and/or Balance: See pages 245 and 246, respectively.

KEY SIGN

Glossopharyngeal Nerve (CN-IX) and Vagus Nerve (CN-X) Signs: Patients will have difficulty with articulation and the pharyngeal phase of swallowing. Exam shows poor and/or asymmetric elevation of the soft palate and uvula.

KEY SIGN

Accessory Nerve (CN-XI) Signs: Weakness of the Sternocleidomastoid and Trapezius Muscles: Patients will have weakness of head rotation and shoulder shrug.

KEY SIGN

Hypoglossal Nerve (CN-XII) Signs: Tongue Deviation and Atrophy: See pages 297–298.

Motor Signs

Most abnormal movements of muscle are responses of normal contractile tissue to abnormal nervous stimuli, so they are properly included in the neurologic examination. The signs are frequently encountered in an appraisal of the musculoskeletal system by anatomic regions.

KEY SIGN

Weakness: Muscle Paralysis, Paresis, and Palsy: *Paralysis* is defined as complete loss and *paresis* as diminution of muscle power from abnormalities of the upper motor neuron (UMN), lower motor neuron (LMN), peripheral nerve or muscle fibers. *Palsy* is a nonspecific descriptive term that indicates paralysis and/or paresis. Increased tone and uninhibited reflexes (*spasticity*) occur with UMN lesions, whereas LMN and peripheral nerve lesions result in flaccid paralysis and muscle atrophy. Primary disease of muscle is associated with flaccid paralysis and variable changes in muscle bulk. It is essential to take a careful history to assess the onset of paralysis: acute, subacute, or chronic.

✓ *MUSCLE PARALYSIS—CLINICAL OCCURRENCE:* *Congenital* porphyria, muscular dystrophy, familial periodic paralysis, paramyotonia congenita, cerebral palsy; *Endocrine* hyperthyroidism; *Idiopathic* noninflammatory myopathies; *Inflammatory/Immune* Guillain-Barré syndrome, myasthenia gravis, polymyositis, dermatomyositis, multiple sclerosis, vasculitis; *Infectious* poliomyelitis; *Metabolic/Toxic* electrolyte disturbances (high or low potassium, magnesium, calcium), drugs (muscle relaxants, anesthetics, aminoglycosides-rarely), heavy metal poisoning, hyperthyroid myopathy, beriberi, anemia, pernicious anemia, amyloidosis; *Mechanical/Trauma* brain and spinal cord trauma, epidural hematoma, peripheral nerve trauma; *Neoplastic* epidural metastases; *Neurologic* polyneuropathy, transverse myelitis; *Psychosocial* hysteria, malingering; *Vascular* stroke, spinal cord infarction, subdural and epidural bleeding, vasculitis.

KEY SIGN

Muscle Atrophy: *Pathophysiology:* Severe muscle atrophy occurs with LMN and peripheral nerve injury as a result of loss of the trophic effect of motor nerves on muscle fibers; much less atrophy occurs with UMN lesions. Atrophy only becomes apparent after weeks to months following the nerve injury. *Fasciculations* (see *Fasciculations* below) are seen with LMN lesions, but are absent with UMN lesions. Generalized weakness and atrophy accompanied by fasciculations, often most evident in the tongue and small muscles of the hands, along with upper motor neuron signs, suggest primary motor neuron disease, for example, amyotrophic lateral sclerosis. Segmental disease is characteristic of poliomyelitis and diseases of the spinal cord and nerve plexuses.

KEY SIGN

Hypotonia: Decreased resting muscle tone occurs with lower motor neuron injury, such as poliomyelitis, a root syndrome, and peripheral neuropathy. It is also encountered in cerebellar and other central lesions.

KEY SIGN

Hypertonia: Extrapyramidal lesions, such as parkinsonism, produce increased resting muscle tone.

KEY SIGN

Cogwheel Rigidity: On passive motion of a limb, the examiner feels muscular resistance as a series of stepwise relaxation–arrest cycles, rather than a smooth giving way. This phenomenon is an expression of the increased muscle tone in Parkinson disease. It disappears during sleep.

KEY SIGN

Spasticity: *Pathophysiology:* In upper motor neuron paralysis, tone of the stretched muscles is increased, and uninhibited stretch reflexes produce continuous clonic contraction (spasticity). When a limb is moved against spastic muscles, the resistance may suddenly cease, giving a *clasp-knife* effect. Long, continued spasticity results in muscle fibrosis and shortening, known as *contracture*.

KEY SIGN

Myoclonus: A single, sudden jerk, or a short series, occurring in slow or rapid succession, may be so powerful as to throw the patient to the floor. Unlike tremor, myoclonus may not disappear with sleep and is frequent at sleep onset. It is a common complication of chronic meperidine use and other metabolic encephalopathies.

Myotonia: The muscles continue in contraction after a voluntary or reflex act has ceased. Recovery from contraction induced by tapping the muscle belly with a reflex hammer is prolonged. After shaking hands, the fingers reluctantly relax. When the fingers are flexed on the supinated palm, attempted extension is slow and difficult. The movement is typical of myotonia congenita and myotonic dystrophy.

KEY SIGN

Tetany: *Pathophysiology:* The threshold for muscular excitability is lowered such that involuntary sustained contractions occur, either painless or painful. Any cause of a low ionized serum calcium can result in tetany, including hypoparathyroidism, acute hyperventilation, and hypomagnesemia. The contracting muscles feel rigid and unyielding. Spasm may be preceded by numbness and tingling in the lips and limbs. Contractions of the hands and feet are termed collectively *carpopedal spasm.* In carpal spasm, the wrist is flexed and flexion at the metacarpophalangeal joints is combined with extension of the interphalangeal joints. The hyperextended fingers are also adducted to form a cone and the thumb is flexed on the palm. This presents a diagnostic posture called obstetrician's hand. In latent tetany, carpal spasm may be induced by occluding the brachial artery for 3 minutes with an inflated sphygmomanometer cuff; tetany induced by this maneuver is called the *Trousseau sign.* Tapping the facial nerve against the bone just anterior to the ear produces ipsilateral contraction of facial muscles; this is *Chvostek sign.* It is uniformly present in latent tetany, but some contraction occurs in some normal persons.

KEY SIGN

Fasciculations: *Pathophysiology:* Damage to the nerve supplying a muscle results in spontaneous motor unit firing that is visible as a twitching of muscle fibers. Coarse twitches are often caused by exposure to cold, fatigue, or other conditions, and are not serious. Fasciculations must be carefully sought when the muscle is relaxed because they are not powerful enough to move a joint or a part. In the presence of muscle atrophy or weakness, their presence is attributable to progressive denervation of the muscle. *Fibrillations* are twitches of individual muscle fibers; they are invisible, but can be demonstrated by electromyography.

Reflex Signs

Abnormal Reflexes in Pyramidal Tract Disease

ALTERED NORMAL REFLEXES. A lesion of the pyramidal tract almost invariably causes complete suppression of the normal superficial reflexes caudal to the level of the lesion. On the contrary, the muscle stretch reflexes are hyperactive except during the acute stage of damage, as in spinal shock, when they are absent.

Increased Reflexes: Clonus, Spasticity:
Pathophysiology: Normally central inhibition of the spinal cord limits the stretch reflex to a single beat. Loss of inhibition allows the reflex to become self-perpetuating. Spasticity occurs with complete loss of cortical inhibition, leading to sustained contractions of opposing muscle groups, the flexors dominating in the arms, and the extensors in the back and legs. A hyperactive reflex may produce clonus, a rhythmic contraction of muscles initiated by stretching. Clonus may be unsustained, lasting for only a few jerks despite continued stretching, or it may be sustained (more than seven beats), persisting as long as stretching is applied.

ANKLE CLONUS (GASTROCNEMIUS CLONUS): With the patient's knee flexed, grasp the foot and briskly dorsiflex it. Rhythmic contractions of the gastrocnemius and soleus cause the foot to alternate between dorsiflexion and plantar flexion (see Fig. 14-8C).

PATELLAR CLONUS (QUADRICEPS CLONUS): With the patient supine and the relaxed lower limb extended, grasp the patella and push it quickly distal. The patella will jerk up and down from the rhythmic contractions of the quadriceps femoris.

WRIST CLONUS (FINGER FLEXOR CLONUS): Grasp the patient's fingers and forcibly hyperextend the wrist. The wrist will alternate rhythmically between flexion and extension.

Babinski Sign: Perform the test for the plantar reflex, page 812. Alternate methods of eliciting Babinski reflex have been described as eponymic signs. In the *Oppenheim sign*, great toe dorsiflexion is elicited with pressure applied by the thumb and index finger or knuckles to the anterior tibia. The pressure stroke should begin at the upper two-thirds of the bone and be continued to the ankle. In *Chaddock sign*, the stimulus is a scratch with a dull point. The path of stimulation should curve around the lateral malleolus of the ankle, then along the lateral aspect of the dorsum of the foot. The normal response is plantar flexion of the toes and foot. The complete Babinski sign is (a) dorsiflexion of the great toe, (b) fanning of all toes, (c) dorsiflexion of the ankle, and (d) flexion and withdrawal of the knee and hip. All of these signs are pathologic responses to noxious stimuli in or spreading to the S1 dermatome. Partial responses include only dorsiflexion of the great toe, failure of the small toes to abduct or fan, and fanning of small toes without great toe dorsiflexion. Complete and partial responses are all indicative of different degrees of pyramidal disease, so the details of response should be accurately recorded.

Hoffmann Sign: Finger Flexor Reflex: This is also called the finger flexor reflex and has the same significance as other muscle stretch reflexes. Hold the patient's pronated hand in your hand, with fingers extended and relaxed. Support the patient's extended middle fin-

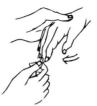

A. Grasp Reflex   B. Hoffman Sign   C. Mayer Reflex

Fig. 14-17 Some Pathologic Reflexes. See text for descriptions. *A. Grasp Reflex: In lesions of the premotor cortex, the patient may be unable to release her grasp. B. Hoffmann Sign: In pyramidal tract disease, the patient's thumb may flex and adduct asymmetrically. C. Mayer Reflex: Have the patient present her relaxed supinated hand to you. Firmly flex the ring finger at the metacarpophalangeal joint. The normal response is adduction and flexion of the thumb. Absence of this occurs in pyramidal tract disease.*

ger by your right index finger held transversely under the distal interphalangeal joint crease (Fig. 14-17B). With your thumb, press the patient's fingernail to flex the terminal digit. The abnormal reflex is flexion and adduction of the thumb. The other fingers may also flex. When the reflex is present bilaterally, it may be a normal variant.

Primitive Reflexes (Release Signs)

All of these signs may indicate diffuse cerebral disease, but are sometimes present in normal individuals.

Grasp Reflex: Place your index and middle fingers between the patient's thumb and index finger, laying them across the patient's palm. Gently pull them across the palm with a stroking motion. Grasping with the thumb and index finger is a positive response (see Fig. 14-17A). When the grasp reflex is present, the patient cannot release the fingers at will. This is a normal response in infants. Later in life, lesions of the premotor cortex may uncover the reflex as a pathologic finding.

Palmomental (Radovici Sign): Scratching or pricking of the thenar eminence causes ipsilateral contraction of the muscles of the chin. This occurs in diffuse cerebral disease.

Snout/Suck Reflexes: Scratching or gentle percussion of the upper lip may induce a puckering or sucking movement.

Spinal Automatisms

Spinal automatisms occur when the central inhibitions of reflexes are lost in severe disease of the spinal cord or brain.

Spinal Reflex Reactions: In extensive lesions of the cord or midbrain, painful stimulation of a limb may produce ipsilateral flexion of both upper and lower extremities, called ipsilateral mass flexion reflex, spinal withdrawal, or shortening reflex.

KEY SIGN

Mass Reflex: A transverse lesion of the cord may produce flexion followed by extension of the limbs below the level of lesion. In complete transection, only flexion occurs, accompanied by contractions of the abdominal wall, incontinence of urine and feces, and autonomic responses, such as sweating, flushing, and pilomotor activity. This complex is termed *mass reflex*. Involuntary urination may be stimulated by stroking the skin of the thighs and abdomen, an automatic bladder. Priapism and seminal ejaculation may be induced by similar mechanisms. In the crossed extensor reflex, flexion of one limb may be associated with extension of its counterpart. In some cases, the extensor thrust reaction is encountered: pressure on the sole causes extension of the leg. When the leg is placed in flexion, scratching on the skin of the thigh induces extension of the leg. Painful stimulation of the arm or chest may result in abduction and outward rotation of the shoulder.

KEY SIGN

► **Signs of Meningeal Irritation:** Irritation of the meninges by meningitis, subarachnoid hemorrhage, drugs, and increased intracranial pressure cause abnormal contraction of various muscle groups, which are identified on physical examination.

► **NUCHAL RIGIDITY:** The patient cannot place the chin on the chest. Passive flexion of the neck is limited by involuntary muscle spasm, while passive extension and rotation are normal.

► **KERNIG SIGN:** With the patient supine, passively flex the hip to 90 degrees while the knee is flexed at about 90 degrees (Fig. 14-18A). With the hip kept in flexion, attempts to extend the knee produce pain in the

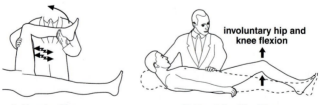

A. Kernig Sign   **B. Brudzinski Sign**

Fig. 14-18 Two Signs of Meningeal Irritation. A. Kernig Sign: With the patient supine, flex the hip and knee, each to about 90 degrees. With the hip immobile, attempt to extend the knee. In meningeal irritation, this attempt is resisted and causes pain in the hamstring muscles. B. Brudzinski Sign: Place the patient supine and hold the thorax down on the bed. Attempt to flex the neck. With meningeal irritation this causes involuntary flexion of the hips.

hamstrings and resistance to further extension. This is a reliable sign of meningeal irritation, which may occur with meningitis, herniated disk, or tumors of the cauda equina.

BRUDZINSKI SIGN: With the patient supine and the limbs extended, passively flex the neck. Flexion of the hips, a sign of meningeal irritation, is a positive Brudzinski sign (see Fig. 14-18B).

▶ SPINAL RIGIDITY: Movements of the spine are limited by spasms of the erector spinae. In extreme cases, the spinal muscles are in tetanic contraction, producing rigid hyperextension of the entire spine with the head forced backward and the trunk thrust forward. The condition is termed *opisthotonos.*

Paradoxical Reflexes

Inversion of the Brachioradialis Reflex: This occurs when the head of the radius is tapped and there is flexion of the fingers with no elbow flexion and forearm supination. It indicates a lesion of the C5 nerve root coupled with spinal cord damage at that level, usually because of cervical spondylosis.

Paradoxical Triceps Reflex: With lesions at C7 to C8, the elbow may not extend; instead, flexion may occur from the higher innervation of the forearm flexors, a *paradoxical reflex.*

Posture, Balance, and Coordination Signs: Cerebellar Signs

The perfect execution of skilled acts is *eupraxia;* loss of previous ability in performance is *apraxia.* This reflects a brain disturbance in converting an idea into a skilled act. Maintenance of postural equilibrium at rest and with movement requires the proper function of proprioceptive mechanisms, the vestibular apparatus, and the cerebellum. Loss of coordination in maintaining proper posture is *ataxia.* The patient who is incoordinate lying down has *static ataxia;* if the condition is only evident on standing or moving, it is *kinetic ataxia.*

KEY SIGN
Dysdiadochokinesis: Loss of the ability to arrest one motor impulse and substitute its opposite, *dysdiadochokinesia,* is characteristic of cerebellar disease.

KEY SIGN
Dyssynergia and Dysmetria: Failure to properly coordinate the contraction of synergistic muscle during a movement is *dyssynergia.* Inability to control the distance, power and speed of a movement is *dysmetria.   Finger-to-Nose Test:*   In cerebellar disease, this action is attended by an action tremor. When the maneuver is performed with the eyes closed, the sense of position in the shoulder and elbow is

tested. *Heel-to-Shin Test:* In cerebellar disease, the arc of the heel to the knee is jerky and wavering, the knee is frequently overshot, and the slide down the shin is accompanied by an action tremor. In posterior column disease, the heel may have difficulty finding the knee, and the ride down the shin weaves from side to side, or the heel may fall off altogether.

KEY SIGN

Wide Stance: Ataxia from proprioceptive, vestibular, or cerebellar disease is less when the patient stands on a broad base, the feet widely apart.

KEY SIGN

Instability of Station: *Visual Compensation:* Cerebellar ataxia is not ameliorated by visual orientation, while the ataxia from posterior column disease involves disordered proprioception and only appears or is worsened when the eyes are closed (*Romberg sign*). *Direction of Falling:* In disease of the lateral cerebellar lobes, falling is toward the affected side. Lesions of the cerebellar midline or vermis may cause falling indiscriminately, depending entirely on the initial stance of the patient.

KEY SIGN

Gait Ataxia: *Pathophysiology:* Gait is a complex activity requiring normal sensory input from the feet, spinal cord, and vestibular system, and normal motor and cerebellar function. Impairments in any of these systems leads to characteristic changes in the gait. Careful inspection of gait can greatly aid identification of the site of the lesion.

GAIT ATAXIA: CEREBELLAR DISEASE: The ataxia produces a staggering, wavering, and lurching walk that is not visually compensated. With a lesion in the mid-cerebellum, movements are in all directions. When a cerebellar lobe is involved, staggering and falling are toward the affected side. The ataxia is somewhat steadied by standing or walking on a wide base; that is, with the legs far apart. Ataxia secondary to vestibular disease may appear similar.

GAIT ATAXIA: POSTERIOR COLUMN DISEASE: In tabes dorsalis, the posterior column of the cord is affected, so proprioceptive impulses are defective. The ataxia is much greater with the eyes closed. The feet are lifted too high, and frequently they are set down with excessive force. The patient fixes his eyes where he is walking to compensate for loss of proprioception. Ataxia caused by peripheral nerve sensory loss may look similar.

GAIT ATAXIA: DEMENTIA: Ataxia of gait in patients without dementia predicts a significantly increased risk for the development of non-Alzheimer dementia during a follow-up of over 6 years [Verghese J, Lipton RB, Hall CB, et al. Abnormality of gait as a predictor of non-Alzheimer's dementia. *N Engl J Med* 2002;347:1761–1768].

GAIT ATAXIA: STEPPAGE GAIT, FOOT DROP: When the dorsiflexors of the foot are paralyzed, the foot slaps down onto the floor. To compensate for the toe drop, the patient must raise the thigh excessively, as if walking upstairs. Unilateral toe drop usually results from injury of the peroneal nerve. Bilateral paralysis may occur from polyneuropathies, poliomyelitis, lesions of the cauda equina, or peroneal atrophy in Charcot-Marie-Tooth disease.

PERONEAL MUSCULAR ATROPHY: CHARCOT-MARIE-TOOTH DISEASE: This is a hereditary disease of unknown cause. Presenting symptoms are foot drop, pain, weakness, numbness and paresthesias of the lower legs. The syndrome is slowly progressive with clawfoot and foot drop, from weak peronei, tibialis anterior, and extensor longus digitorum. Muscle stretch reflexes are absent and there is cutaneous hypesthesia and the slapping gait. The forearm may be affected.

GAIT ATAXIA: HEMIPLEGIC GAIT: The patient walks with the affected lower limb extended at the hip, knee, and ankle, and the foot inverted. The thigh may swing in a lateral arc *(circumduction)* or the patient may push the inverted foot along the floor.

GAIT ATAXIA: SPASTIC GAIT, SCISSORS GAIT: In paraparesis with adductor spasm, the knees are pulled together so the body must sway laterally away from the stepping limb to allow it to clear the floor. The feet may overstep each other laterally, alternately crossing across the line of travel with each step.

GAIT ATAXIA: FESTINATING GAIT, PARKINSONIAN GAIT: The trunk and neck are rigid and flexed. The arm swing is diminished or lost unilaterally or bilaterally. The steps are short and shuffling and become faster in an attempt to avoid falling forward (chasing the center of gravity: *festination*). Turns are slow and in-block, without evident turning of the head on the trunk or the trunk on the pelvis.

GAIT ATAXIA: MAGNETIC GAIT: The stance is wide and the steps are short and shuffling. The feet are not lifted from the floor, as if held down by magnets. This indicates diffuse cerebral disease.

GAIT ATAXIA: CLOWNISH GAIT, HUNTINGTON CHOREA: Walking is attended by grotesque movements caused by the interposition of purposeless involuntary chorea on gait movements.

GAIT ATAXIA: WADDLING GAIT, MUSCULAR DYSTROPHY: The patient walks with a broad base. The thighs are thrown forward by twisting the pelvis to compensate for the weak quadriceps muscles. A similar gait is employed by those with bilateral dislocations of the hips.

KEY SIGN

Tremors: *Pathophysiology:* Coarse, poorly coordinated, contractions of opposing muscle groups are unable to maintain stable posture and so produce oscillating movements at one or more joints. The amplitude may be either fine or coarse, and the rate either rapid or slow. Movements may be rhythmic or irregular. All tremors disappear during sleep. Examine the affected part at rest with the muscles relaxed, with maintenance of posture against gravity and with movement.

ESSENTIAL TREMOR: *Pathophysiology:* This is an accentuation of the normal fine motor movements made to maintain posture. It is accentuated with increased adrenergic stimulation of muscle and may be a familial trait. All persons have this type of tremor, but it is usually at an amplitude below the limit of visible detection. It is accentuated with anxiety and is characteristic of hyperthyroidism and alcohol withdrawal. The tremor is rapid and fine. It is absent is repose and accentuated by trying to maintain a posture [Louis ED. Essential tremor. *N Engl J Med* 2001;345:887–891].

PARKINSON TREMOR: *Pathophysiology:* This is a result of damage to the extrapyramidal motor system of the substantia nigra in Parkinson disease. The tremor is present at rest and diminished or absent with movement. It is slow and coarse and often described as "pill-rolling" from the characteristic movements of the fingers and wrist. Parkinson tremor is usually asymmetric at onset [Utti RJ. Tremor: How to determine if the patient has Parkinson's disease. *Geriatrics* 1998;53:30–36].

CEREBELLAR TREMOR: *Pathophysiology:* Poor cerebellar coordination of muscle contraction associated with movement leads to limb oscillation, often accentuated with attempts at fine control. Action or intention tremor occurs in multiple sclerosis and cerebellar disease in which voluntary movements initiate and sustain a slow oscillation of wide amplitude.

KEY SIGN

Tics: Normal movements of muscle groups, such as grimacing, winking, or shoulder shrugging, are repeated at inappropriate times. The reaction is stereotyped for the individual. Tics may be acquired behavioral habits or a sign of organic disease, for example, Tourette syndrome. They may be abolished by diverting the patient's attention and they disappear during sleep [Jankovic J. Tourette's syndrome. *N Engl J Med* 2001;345:1184–1192].

KEY SIGN

Dyskinesia: Dyskinesias are complex abnormalities of muscle movement. They are centrally mediated. Several characteristic patterns are recognized:

CHOREIFORM MOVEMENTS: Rapid, purposeless, jerky, asynchronous movements involve various parts of the body. Although some are spontaneous, many are initiated and all are accentuated by voluntary acts, as in extending the arms or walking. They commonly occur in both Sydenham and Huntington chorea; in the latter, the movements are coarser and more bizarre. They disappear with sleep.

ATHETOID MOVEMENTS: In contrast to choreiform movements, these are slower and writhing, resembling the actions of a worm or snake. The distal parts of the limb are more active than the proximal. Grimaces are more deliberate than in chorea. The grotesque athetoid hand is produced by flexion of some digits with others extended. They disappear with sleep. The mechanism is not understood, but the movements are frequently associated with diseases of the basal ganglia and levodopa therapy of Parkinson disease.

HEMIBALLISMUS: One side of the body is affected by sustained, violent, involuntary flinging movements of the limbs. These result from a lesion in the contralateral subthalamic nucleus of Luys, usually secondary to stroke. They disappear with sleep.

KEY SIGN
Episodic Loss of Extensor Tone: Asterixis (Liver Flap):   Ask the patient to elevate his or her arms to 90 degrees in 0 degree abduction, with fingers and wrists extended and fingers spread. There is sudden relaxation of tone followed by restoration at the wrists and interphalangeal joints. This occurs because extensor tone is lost and regained, resembling a flapping motion. The fingers deviate laterally and exhibit a fine tremor. When the leg of the supine patient is elevated and the foot dorsiflexed, a similar flap occurs at the ankle. An alternate test for an obtunded patient is to induce the patient to squeeze two of the examiner's fingers; asterixis is felt as an alternately clenching and unclenching grip. Asterixis occurs in any form of metabolic encephalopathy including liver failure, uremia, and hypercapnia as a consequence of respiratory failure.

KEY SIGN
Muscle Cramps: Dystonias: See page 873.

KEY SIGN
Associated Movements: Synkinesia: Associated movements, or synkinesias, are involuntary motor patterns, more complex than reflexes, that normally accompany voluntary acts, such as swinging the arms while walking, facial movements of expression, and motions accompanying coughing and yawning. Frequently, these are lost in disease of the pyramidal tract or the basal ganglia; for example, the patient with parkinsonism walks without swinging the arms. An early sign of corticospinal tract damage may be loss of synkinetic movements. Knowledge of normal and abnormal patterns of synkinesis can assist in the identification of the patient with factitious neurologic illness. The detailed testing of synkinesis is beyond the scope of this text. The reader should consult textbooks of neurologic diagnosis.

Sensory Signs

Loss of normal sensation can result from injury to either the peripheral or central nervous system. The distribution of the sensory loss, the modalities involved and the presence or absence of motor involvement are useful in distinguishing peripheral nerve from plexus, root, and central injury.

KEY SIGN

Abnormal Pain Sensation: Changes in pain sensation can result from injury to any portion of the pain pathway (peripheral nerve, spinal cord, or brain). Sensibility to pain may be normal, reduced (*hypalgesia*), absent (*analgesia*), or increased (*hyperalgesia*).

ALLODYNIA: *Pathophysiology:* Allodynia indicates damage to the sensory pathways, usually in the dorsal root or spinal cord; it is not a sign of peripheral nerve injury. Allodynia (*allo* = differing from normal; *dynia* = pain) is the perception of pain with stimuli that are normally not painful such as light touch or vibration. Patients complain of pain with the touch of clothing or bedding and with weight bearing on the feet. Lightly touch and stroke the skin over the suspected area and apply a tuning fork to look for allodynia. Use a mildly uncomfortable stimulus like the sharp end of a broken tongue depressor to elicit hyperesthesia. Allodynia is found in postherpetic neuralgia, diabetic radiculopathies, and complex regional pain syndrome and other chronic pain syndromes.

Hysterical Anesthesia: Hysteria may be revealed in outlining the borders of an area of "anesthesia" by stimulating from the center to the border in a zigzagging line, which seems to confuse the patient and results in disparities between successive tests.

KEY SIGN

Loss of Pain and Temperature Senses: *Pathophysiology:* Pain and temperature fibers cross near their entry into the cord. Disruption of the crossing fibers leads to loss of these modalities with preservation of other regional sensation. Ask the patient to distinguish between hot and cold. Temperature and pain discrimination is lost in syringomyelia while tactile sense is retained.

KEY SIGN

Tactile Extinction Test: In parietal lobe disease, the patient may perceive touch accurately when the stimulation is applied to the right and left consecutively; if the points are stimulated simultaneously, the patient no longer perceives, or *extinguishes,* the affected side.

KEY SIGN

Loss of Position and Vibration Sense: *Pathophysiology:* Position and vibration sense are carried in the posterior columns of the spinal cord. Damage to the posterior columns results in impaired proprioception leading to abnormalities in stance and gait. Posterior column diseases include vitamin B_{12} deficiency and tabes dorsalis.

KEY SIGN

Loss of Integrative Function: Astereognosis: Inability to recognize familiar objects by touch is astereognosis. Assuming the primary sensory modalities are intact, it is a sign of cortical disease, an inability to integrate the multiple inputs.

Autonomic Nervous System Signs

Temperature Regulation: See Chapter 4, page 59. Some instances of hyperthermia occur from lesions of the hypothalamus or high cervical cord. Hypothermia is encountered in insulin shock and myxedema, although the role of the autonomics in the latter condition is doubtful.

Perspiration: Localized areas of sweating may occur in syringomyelia, peripheral nerve injury, or neuropathy. Anhidrosis is a component of Horner syndrome and autonomic insufficiency (severe combined degeneration).

KEY SIGN
Trophic Disturbances: *Pathophysiology:* Loss of innervation leads to functional deficiencies of the sweat and oil glands of the skin. Combined with decreased sensation, the skin is more vulnerable to injury and infection. The skin becomes shiny, smooth, thin, and dry. Painless ulcers may develop over bony prominences of the feet in peripheral neuropathy from diabetes or tabes dorsalis, and syringomyelia (see Fig. 14-12F). Charcot joints (Chapter 13, page 799) are a neuropathic arthropathy caused by loss of proprioception and protective sensation required to maintain joint alignment.

Pilomotor Reactions: Scratching the midaxillary skin produces pilomotor erection (gooseflesh). The normal response is abolished below the level of a transverse cord lesion. An exaggerated reaction may occur on the affected side in hemiplegia.

KEY SIGN
Blood Pressure Regulation: See Chapter 4, page 86. Orthostatic hypotension without tachycardia is common with autonomic nervous system diseases.

KEY SIGN
Bladder/Bowel Function: Patients with autonomic nervous system diseases often lose control of bladder and bowel function producing incontinence and/or urinary and fecal retention.

Some Peripheral Nerve Signs

KEY SIGN
Sciatica: See Chapter 13, page 790.

Acquired Calcaneovalgus: Tibial Nerve Palsy (A Sciatic Component): The tibial nerve is the motor nerve to the gastrocnemius group and intrinsic muscles in the sole of the foot; it is sensory to the skin of the sole. Paralysis of the tibial nerve causes a calcaneovalgus deformity by the unopposed action of the dorsiflexors and evertors of the foot (Fig. 14-19A). Plantar flexion and inversion of

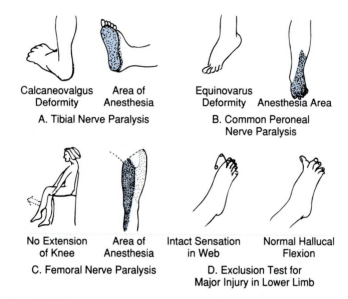

Calcaneovalgus   Area of
Deformity   Anesthesia

A. Tibial Nerve Paralysis

Equinovarus   Anesthesia Area
Deformity

**B. Common Peroneal
Nerve Paralysis**

No Extension   Area of
of Knee   Anesthesia

C. Femoral Nerve Paralysis

Intact Sensation   Normal Hallucal
in Web   Flexion

**D. Exclusion Test for
Major Injury in Lower Limb**

Fig. 14-19 Nerve Lesions of the Lower Limb. *A. Tibial Nerve Paralysis:* *The foot assumes the posture of calcaneovalgus from paralysis of the plantar flexors. The sole of the foot is anesthetic (blue).* **B. Common Peroneal Nerve Paralysis:** *The foot assumes the position of equinovarus; it cannot be dorsiflexed—a foot drop. The dorsum of the foot, and frequently the lateral aspect of the leg, are anesthetic (blue).* **C. Femoral Nerve Paralysis:** *The knee cannot be extended when sitting. The region of anesthesia covers the major portion of the anterior thigh and medial aspect of the leg.* **D. Exclusion Test for Major Nerve Injury in Lower Limb:** *Sensation is intact in the web between the great toe and second toe; extension (dorsiflexion) of the great toe is normally performed.*

the foot are weak and the ankle jerk is absent. The sole is anesthetic, thus vulnerable to trophic ulcers.

Acquired Equinovarus: Common Peroneal Nerve Palsy [A Sciatic Component]: The common peroneal nerve is the motor nerve to the muscles of the anterior and lateral compartments of the leg and the short extensors of the toes; it is sensory to the dorsum of the foot and ankle. Peroneal paralysis causes an equinovarus deformity with inability to dorsiflex the foot and toes—a foot drop (see Fig. 14-19B). An area of anesthesia covers the dorsum of the foot and sometimes extends up the lateral side of the leg. The nerve may be rolled under the fingers where it winds around the fibular head; this maneuver elicits extreme tenderness when neuritis is present while there is little tenderness in tabes. Pressure injury to the nerve at the fibular head may occur in coma and from constricting casts.

Complete Paralysis of the Foot: Combined Tibial and Common Peroneal Palsy (Complete Sciatic Paralysis): All muscles below the knee are paralyzed. An area of anesthesia extends over the sole and dorsum of the foot and up the lateral aspect of the leg.

Lack of Knee Extension: Femoral Nerve Palsy: The femoral nerve is the motor nerve for the quadriceps femoris. When the nerve is injured, patients cannot walk and standing is unstable. Extension of the knee is impossible (see Fig. 14-19C). Anesthesia is widespread over the anteromedial aspect of the thigh, knee, leg, and the medial aspect of the foot.

Shoulder Weakness: Dorsal Scapular Nerve Paralysis: The nerve supplies the rhomboids that elevate and retract the scapula. These muscles ascend obliquely from the medial border of the scapula to the spinous processes of the upper thoracic vertebrae. Although covered by the trapezius, they may be palpated through this superficial muscle when the shoulders are drawn backward; comparison of the two sides may disclose unilateral palsy.

Shoulder Weakness: Suprascapular Nerve Paralysis: The nerve supplies the supraspinatus and the infraspinatus. Paralysis prevents (a) scratching of the back of the head, (b) turning a doorknob with the arm outstretched, and (c) completing a line of writing without moving the paper to the left (when the patient is right-handed). Atrophy of these muscles may be palpated as depressions above and below the scapular spine.

Shoulder Weakness: Long Thoracic Nerve Paralysis: The nerve supplies the serratus anterior that holds the scapula to the thorax. Paralysis produces a winged scapula (see Fig. 13-41A, page 751) when the patient pushes the hand forward against a wall.

Weak Abduction of the Arm: Axillary Nerve Paralysis: This may be caused by neuritis, fracture of the humeral neck, dislocation of the shoulder, or occasionally by scapular fracture. The deltoid is paralyzed and atrophied. Elevation of the arm in 90 degrees of abduction is impossible. A patch of sensory loss on the lateral aspect of the shoulder is often found.

Weak Adduction and Depression of the Arm: Anterior Thoracic Nerve Paralysis: This nerve supplies the pectoralis major and minor. Inspection discloses paralysis when the patient presses the hand down on the hip (Fig. 14-20B).

Weak Adduction and Depression of the Arm: Thoracodorsal Nerve Paralysis: The latissimus dorsi

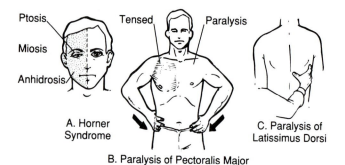

Fig. 14-20 Nerve Lesions of the Upper Trunk. ***A. Horner Syndrome:*** *In-jury to the superior cervical sympathetic ganglion on one side causes ipsilat-eral ptosis of the eyelid, miosis, and anhidrosis of the face.* ***B. Paralysis of the Pectoralis Major Muscle:*** *Injury to the anterior thoracic nerve causes paral-ysis of the pectoralis major and minor muscles. When the patient is asked to press the hands down on the hips, the normal pectoralis muscle is tensed but the paralyzed one is not.* ***C. Paralysis of the Latissimus Dorsi Muscle:*** *The examiner grasps the latissimus muscles in his hands and asks the patient to cough. A paralyzed muscle does not tense with coughing.*

is supplied by this nerve. To demonstrate palsy, grasp the posterior ax-illary fold of muscle, just below the scapular angle, and have the patient cough; the normal muscle tenses (see Fig. 14-20C).

Flail Arm: Erb-Duchenne Paralysis: Lower motor neuron paralysis of the brachial plexus may occur from forceful de-pression of the shoulder during birth or a blow on the shoulder later in life. The arm hangs limply with the fingers flexed and turned posteri-orly, a flail arm (see Fig. 13-41B, page 751). With partial recovery, mo-tions of the elbow and hand may be regained. The biceps reflex is lost and there is muscle wasting.

Weak Elbow Flexion: Musculocutaneous Nerve Paralysis: The biceps brachii and brachialis are supplied by this nerve. Paralysis can usually be demonstrated by inspection of the arm when the elbow is flexed against resistance. A small area of anesthesia occurs on the volar surface of the forearm.

KEY SIGN
Incomplete Extension of Wrist and Fingers: Radial Nerve Paralysis: *Pathophysiology:*   In its spiral course around the humerus, this nerve is exposed to injury from frac-ture of the shaft. The radial nerve is often compressed during its course around the spiral groove of the humerus (Saturday night palsy). Motor deficits depend upon the level of injury. Injury in the axilla causes paral-ysis of the triceps brachii, anconeus, brachioradialis, and extensor carpi

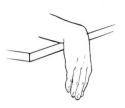
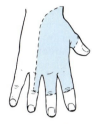

Wrist drop

Area of Anesthesia

Fig. 14-21 Radial Nerve Paralysis. *The extensors of the wrist are paralyzed, so the hand droops when it is placed at the end of the table with no support; this sign is called wrist-drop. The region of anesthesia includes the dorsal aspect of the radial three digits (blue shading).*

radialis longus. A lesion at the level of the upper third of the humerus spares the triceps while damage between the humeral upper third and 5 cm above the elbow also spares the brachioradialis. Innervation of the wrist extensors may be injured at a lower level. Any lesion involving the extensor carpi radialis longus prevents fixation at the wrist in grasping, producing a wrist-drop (Fig. 14-21A). Paralysis of the extensor digitorum communis prevents extension of the wrist and fingers with thumb and finger drop. When the deep branch of the radial nerve is injured, radial deviation of the wrist may occur without wrist-drop. Sensory loss on the dorsum of the hand extends from the radial border to the dorsum of the fifth metacarpal; the dorsum of the thumb is involved (Fig. 14-21B). The distribution of anesthesia is quite irregular, but it usually includes dorsum of thumb to first phalanx and web.

KEY SIGN

Incomplete Flexion of Thumb and Fingers: Median Nerve Paralysis: The nerve is exposed to trauma in the antecubital fossa. It supplies the flexors of the wrists, digits, and pronators of the forearm: pronator teres, pronator quadratus, flexor carpi radialis, flexor digitorum sublimis, flexor digitorum profundus (except the fourth and fifth digits), flexor pollicis brevis, flexor pollicis longus, opponens pollicis, lumbrical, abductor pollicis longus, and brevis. All these muscles are innervated below the elbow. The most common site of median nerve entrapment is at the carpal tunnel (see *Carpal Tunnel Syndrome*, Chapter 13, page 735).

KEY SIGN

Adductor Weakness of Fingers: Ulnar Nerve Paralysis: The ulnar nerve is most vulnerable near the elbow where it curves posteriorly around the medial epicondyle. The chief motor disability from palsy is loss of the finer intrinsic motions of the hand, as may be inferred from a list of innervated muscles: adductor pollicis, flexor carpi ulnaris, interosseus palmaris and dorsalis, flexor pollicis brevis, opponens digiti minimi, flexor digitorum profundus (in part). With injury to the nerve, inspection will show an abduction deformity of the little finger from paralysis of the interossei, interosseous muscle atrophy, and partial clawhand from flexion deformity of the middle and distal interphalangeal joints of the ring and little fingers.

Clawhand: Klumpke Paralysis: A lower motor neuron lesion at the brachial plexus or ulnar nerve produces paralysis of the intrinsic hand muscles results in the clawhand (see Fig. 13-28D, page 725). Sensation on the ulnar aspect of the arm, forearm, and hand may be lost.

Neurologic Syndromes

Falling

S KEY SYNDROME

Loss of Balance and Falls: Falls are a common problem, especially over age 75. Many patients will not volunteer this information unless specifically asked. Maintenance of normal balance requires the complex interaction of many parts of the nervous system: proprioceptive sensory nerves and tracts, vestibular system, motor tracts and nerves, muscles, cerebellum, and basal ganglia. Abnormalities in any of these structures can produce falls. When proprioceptive function is impaired, patients compensate with their eyes to locate themselves in space; visual impairment (including use of bi- and trifocal lenses) are a frequent contributor to falls. Skeletal abnormalities, especially of the joints, are a common precipitant. Decreased mentation and reaction times because of drugs (e.g., benzodiazepines, anticholinergics) or aging frequently contribute to a risk of falling. A complete neurologic examination is required to identify all the contributing abnormalities. Prevention of falls is a major focus of the geriatric assessment [Tibbitts GM. Patients who fall: How to predict and prevent injuries. *Geriatrics* 1996;51: 24–28, 31; Studenski S, Rigler SK. Clinical overview of instability in the elderly. *Clin Geriatr Med* 1996;12:679–688; Tinetti ME, Inouye SK, Gill TM, Doucette JT. Shared risk factors for falls, incontinence, and functional dependence: Unifying the approach to geriatric syndromes. *JAMA* 1995;273:1348–1353].

Headache

S KEY SYNDROME

Headache: *Pathophysiology:* The head contains many pain-sensitive structures. Mechanisms of headache include inflammation, infection, arterial dilation, hemorrhage, changes of pressure within closed spaces, expanding mass lesions producing traction or compression of structures, trauma, tissue ischemia, and tissue destruction. The common extracranial cause of headache is sustained contraction of the muscles of the head, neck, and shoulders. Headache refers to pain perceived more than momentarily in the cranial vault, the orbits, and the nape of the neck; pain elsewhere in the face is not included. An urgent intensive search for serious pathology is required if your patient describes a severe headache unlike any experienced in the past [Steiner TJ, Fontebasso M. Headache. *BMJ* 2002;325:881–886]. See also pages 316–317.

✓ *HEADACHE—CLINICAL OCCURRENCE:* *Congenital* arteriovenous malformations, hydrocephalus; *Endocrine* pheochromocytoma; *Idiopathic* idiopathic intracranial hypertension; *Inflammatory/Immune* giant cell arteritis, sarcoidosis; *Infectious* meningitis (bacterial, viral, mycobacterial, fungal, drugs), encephalitis (viral, e.g., herpes simplex, HIV, West Nile fever, eastern and western equine encephalitis, St. Louis encephalitis, California encephalitis, LaCrosse encephalitis, and dengue), rickettsial infections, sinusitis, otitis, mastoiditis, non-CNS viral infections (e.g., influenza, cytomegalovirus, varicella), parasites (e.g., malaria, neurocysticercosis), protozoa (e.g., toxoplasmosis); *Metabolic/Toxic* analgesic rebound headache, hypoxia, hypercapnia, hypoglycemia, alcohol and illicit drug withdrawal, carbon monoxide poisoning, caffeine abstinence; *Mechanical/Trauma* accelerated and malignant hypertension, trauma, head trauma, concussion, muscular tension, temporomandibular joint disease, increased intracranial pressure, glaucoma, decreased intracranial pressure (CSF leak); *Neoplastic* primary and metastatic brain tumors, tumors in the sinuses, pituitary tumors; *Neurologic* migraine, cluster headache, paroxysmal hemicrania, trigeminal neuralgia, occipital neuralgia; *Psychosocial* stress; *Vascular* migraine, intracranial aneurysm, hemorrhage (intracerebral, subdural, epidural, and subarachnoid), venous sinus thrombosis, stoke, cerebral vasculitis.

History: Inquire carefully for the attributes of pain (PQRST): *Provocative and Palliative Factors* trauma, medications, substance abuse, position of the head and body, coughing, straining, emotional tension, relief with massage, and resolution with sleep; *Quality* whether burning, aching, deep or superficial, lancinating, throbbing, or continuous; *Region Involved* cranial, facial, orbital, unilateral, bilateral; *Severity* use the 1–10 scale; and *Timing* when headaches began, frequency, time of day, duration, pattern of intensity. Inquire about family members with a headache history. Identify associated symptoms, for example, fever, stiff neck, nausea and vomiting, constipation or diarrhea, diuresis, rhinorrhea, visual disturbances (e.g., photophobia, scotomata, tearing, diplopia), cerebral symptoms (e.g., confusion, slurred speech, aura, paresthesias, anesthesias, motor paralysis, vertigo, mood, and sleep disturbances). *Physical Exam:* Inspect the skin and scalp for bulges and areas of erythema. With deep pressure palpate and percuss the bones of the cranium and face for tenderness and irregularities of contour. Palpate the neck muscles and the upper borders of the trapezii for unusual tenderness. Palpate the carotid and temporal arteries for pulsations and tenderness. Examine the eyes for pupillary irregularities, conjunctival injection or abnormal extraocular motion; use the confrontation test (page 213) to detect gross defects in the visual fields. Examine the fundus for choked disks and retinal hemorrhages. Auscultate the cranium for bruits. Perform a thorough neurologic examination with special attention to the cranial nerves and the deep tendon reflexes.

S KEY SYNDROME

▼ **Muscular Contraction Headache: Tension-Type Headache:** *Pathophysiology:* Sustained contraction of the neck, head, and shoulder muscles causes fatigue and pain. Chronic intermittent headaches occur in the occiput and temporal regions, often with tenderness in the neck and trapezii. Usually the pain has recurred irregularly for many years, without periodicity. The sensation is described as mild or moderate discomfort, vise-like, a heavy feeling, a sense of pressure, a tight band, cramping, aching, or soreness; it is steady rather than throbbing. The pain is not augmented by coughing, straining at stool, or shaking the head. It usually begins in the occiput and extends upward to the temporal regions and down the nape of the neck to the shoulders. It may last for a few hours, with intensification near the day's end; or it may persist for many days, waxing and waning throughout. The onset of an episode is often related to emotional tension or to occupational activity. The pain is relieved by external support of the head, the application of hot packs or massage to the neck and mild analgesics. *Physical Signs.* Tenderness may be found in the upper border of the trapezii or the intrinsic neck muscles. DDX: The symptoms and signs are characteristic. Tension-type headaches are the only type not intensified by coughing or straining at stool; they are also the only type ameliorated by shaking the head. It common to have features of both tension type and migraine headache.

S KEY SYNDROME

▼ **Migraine:** *Pathophysiology:* The exact pathogenesis of migraine is uncertain, but genetic factors are important. Some patterns have a defined genetic basis, for example, 50% of patients with familial hemiplegic migraine have an identified genetic abnormality. Spreading cortical neurologic depression is characteristic, perhaps initiated in the trigeminal projection system of the brainstem. Vascular constriction and dilation occur in many, but not all patients; constriction can rarely lead to ischemic cerebral events. Release of substance P and neurogenic inflammation may play a role. Serotonin, dopamine, and noradrenaline are all important in the migrainous process and their receptor blockers are used in treatment. This is heritable disorder with periodic unilateral headache frequently preceded by an aura (*classic migraine*). Generalized throbbing headache associated with nausea, light and sound sensitivity is even more common. The prevalence of migraine is estimated to be 25% (more common in women than in men) in the United States. Patients with migraine have an increased incidence of Raynaud phenomenon. Onset is usually in adolescence, but may occur at any age; many have experienced motion sickness in childhood. The attacks occur from a few times a year to several times per week. Periods of frequent headache attacks may be separated by periods of none or few attacks. Often, migraine is coincident with some phase of the menstrual cycle. The clinical pattern varies so much among individuals that each individual must be considered separately. Persons with recurrent "sick" or "sinus" headaches, without definite documentation of infection, most likely have migraine [Goadsby PJ, Lipton RB, Ferrari MD. Migraine—Current understanding and treatment. *N Engl J Med* 2002;346:257–270; Cady R, Dodick DW. Diagnosis and treatment of migraine. *Mayo Clin Proc* 2002;77:255–261].

MIGRAINE WITH AURA: CLASSIC MIGRAINE: The paroxysm of classic migraine has four phases. *The Prodrome:* An attack is often triggered by a period of anxiety, tension, or sluggishness. Other triggers include bright lights, loud noise, strong odors, skipped meals, various foods and beverages, and changes in sleep patterns. A day or so before the attack, the patient may feel depressed or feel a sense of unusual well-being; occasionally, hunger is noted. *The Aura:* Migrainous phenomena are typically unilateral, but are occasionally bilateral; the side may vary in different attacks. Patients tend to repeat their distinctive aura in successive attacks. *Visual Disturbances:* A *scintillating scotoma*, usually involving both eyes, presents as flashing lights; sometimes there are black and white wavy lines, like the shimmering made by heat waves rising from pavement. *Fortification spectra* may be exhibited, with zigzag colored patterns with dark centers moving across the visual field. Distinct patterns of the aura are associated with migraine variant syndromes (see *Classic Migraine Variants* below). *Other Neurologic Events:* Neurologic symptoms occurring during the aura define special migraine syndromes discussed below. *The Headache:* The attack may begin any time of the day or night; the headache is frequently present on awakening. Some patients have a typical aura without succeeding headache. Usually, as the aura diminishes, unilateral headache appears on the side opposite to unilateral visual or somatosensory symptoms during the aura. The pain may start above one orbit and spread over the entire side of the head to the occiput and neck, or it may begin in the back of the head and move forward. Rarely, the site of pain is below the eye, in front of the ear, behind the mandibular angle, in the nape of the neck, or in the shoulders. The pain spreads and intensifies to a severe throbbing, boring, aching headache over about an hour. Constant nonthrobbing pain occurs in 50% of patients. The pain is often augmented in the reclining position, lessened when sitting or standing. Shaking the head, coughing, or straining at stool intensifies the pain. Although the pain may be severe, it usually does not disrupt sleep; in fact, the headache is usually lessened by lying in a dark, quiet room. Nausea and, less commonly, vomiting often accompany the headache. Photophobia, phonophobia, and annoyance from odors (*hyperosmia*) are common during the headache. *Physical Signs During Headache:* The patient may appear normal or be incapacitated with cold limbs and pale skin. The duration of the paroxysm is usually from 2 to 6 hours and is relieved by sleep. *The Recovery:* When an attack terminates with sleep, the patient awakens without headache and experiences a sense of buoyancy and well-being. DDX: The diagnosis is easy in a long-established case with relatively typical symptoms. When the onset is recent and the symptoms unusual, other intracranial disorders must be excluded. Ophthalmoplegic migraine can simulate a leaking aneurysm in the circle of Willis. Although hemiplegia can be a migrainous phenomenon, more serious causes should be sought.

Classic Migraine Variants: These variant forms of classic migraine are distinguished by the particular pattern of the aura.

Ophthalmic Migraine: The scotomata may be succeeded by momentary blindness, *anopsia,* in the entire field, or in the lower or upper quadrants; or the pattern may be bitemporal or homonymous hemianopsia.

Ophthalmoplegic Migraine: Transient unilateral paralysis of CN-III (oculomotor) produces lateral deviation and ptosis. This occurs in young girls.

Dysphagic Migraine: Unilateral paresthesias or anesthesias may occur in the face, the arm, or the foot. When the right side is involved, expressive dysphasia and homonymous hemianopsia may be present.

Basilar Artery Migraine: The scotomata and anesthesias of the face and limbs are bilateral, and vertigo or cranial nerve palsies may be present from brainstem nuclear ischemia. The transition from aura to headache may be accompanied by momentary loss of consciousness or light sleep.

Hemiplegic Migraine: This is spectacular but rare. The paralysis is most likely to occur in migrainous patients experiencing paresthesias. The right side is more often involved. The patient complains of numbness or "woodenness" of the affected limbs. Although weakness may be the complaint, it may only be manifest by exaggeration of the deep tendon reflexes and Babinski sign. The paralysis lasts for 10–40 minutes, but may persist for 2–3 days; usually there are no permanent sequelae. Many neurologists are reluctant to make this diagnosis without excluding more serious and irreversible disorders. The diagnosis is strongly supported by a family history of hemiplegic migraine.

MIGRAINE WITHOUT AURA: COMMON MIGRAINE: The onset is slower than classic migraine and the duration is often longer, 4–72 hours. It may persist through sleep. The headache is unilateral or bilateral. In other respects, common and classic migraine are similar.

S KEY SYNDROME

▼ **Cluster Headache: Histamine Headache, Histamine Cephalgia:** *Pathophysiology:* The headache is produced by dilatation of branches of the internal carotid artery, especially those supplying the meninges innervated by the trigeminal nerve. Although the syndrome can be simulated by the injection of histamine into the internal carotid artery, there is no conclusive evidence that histamine plays a role in the natural disorder. This is five to six times more common in men; onset is typically in the third to fourth decades of life. A family history of migraine or cluster headaches is not uncommon. Cluster headache are most commonly episodic (occurring several times a day or week for several weeks, with long intermissions between episodes), but may be chronic (headaches persisting for more than a year without intermission). The headache begins without aura and lasts 15–120 minutes (average 40 minutes). It is unilateral, severe, boring, and throbbing. It recurs consistently on the same side. It is usually maximal just inferior to the medial canthus of the orbit, but may occur in the temple or in the side of the face, and it may spread to the neck and shoulder. Flushing, edema and sweating of the skin, lacrimation, conjunctival injection, nasal congestion, rhinorrhea, partial Horner syndrome, and temporal artery dilatation may occur on the affected side. DDX: Paroxysmal hemicrania is briefer and more common in women; in Raeder syndrome, the pain is identical in quality but is persistent without discreet attacks.

Paroxysmal Hemicrania: The cause is unknown; women are more commonly affected than men. It is more often chronic than episodic. The headache is indistinguishable from cluster headache, but the pattern is distinct. Headaches are short, lasting on average 15 minutes, more frequent, up to 40 times per day, and uniformly abolished by indomethacin.

S KEY SYNDROME
Chronic Daily Headache: Transformed Migraine, Rebound Headache: *Pathophysiology:* Regular daily use of mild and/or opiate analgesics leads to rebound headaches when the patient goes without the medication for a few hours. Often these are patients with a history of tension-type or migraine headache who have developed daily persistent headache relieved only temporarily by medication. A history of regular daily use of prescription or over-the-counter analgesics and the absence of aura, neurologic findings, or other causes of headache are the keys to diagnosis. Overuse of caffeine in migraineurs will also precipitate chronic daily, rebound headaches. The treatment is complete abstinence from analgesics for 2 weeks. Migraineurs should not use analgesics more than 2 days a week. If this proves inadequate, prophylactic therapy should be instituted.

Ice Cream Headache: See Chapter 7, page 317.

Hypertensive Headache: *Pathophysiology:* The evidence points to segmental dilatation of branches of the external carotid artery. Digital compression abolishes the headache when applied to the external carotid, frontal, supraorbital, postauricular, or occipital arteries. In patients with mild hypertension, the incidence and types of headache are no different than in normotensive persons. Headache occurs in half the patients with accelerated hypertension without encephalopathy. The diastolic pressure must exceed 120 mmHg to cause headache. The headaches are often occipital, although other regions may be involved. They are not necessarily unilateral and there is no aura.

Headache from Fever: See Chapter 4, page 61.

S KEY SYNDROME
▼ **Headache: Giant Cell Arteritis, Temporal Arteritis:**   See Chapter 8, page 471.

Headache: Occipital Neuritis: See page 317.

S KEY SYNDROME
▼ **Headache: Traction, Displacement, Inflammation Causing Intracranial Headaches:** *Pathophysiology:* The pain-sensitive intracranial structures are the dura and the arteries at the base of the brain, the cerebral arteries in the same region, the great venous sinuses, and certain nerves (CN-V, -IX, -X, and C1–3). The greater portion of the dura and cranium is insensitive. Mechanisms producing headaches from intracranial disorders include (a) traction on the superficial cerebral veins and venous sinuses, (b) traction on the middle meningeal arteries, (c) traction on the basilar arteries and their branches, (d) distention and dilatation of the intracranial arteries, (e) inflammation near any pain-sensitive region, and (f) direct pressure or traction by tumors on cranial and cervical nerves. The resulting headaches may be throbbing when arteries are involved; otherwise the pain is steady. Headaches are often intensified by movements of the head, certain postures, and rapid changes in cerebrospinal fluid pressure.

▶ TRACTION-DISPLACEMENT: BRAIN TUMOR: *Pathophysiology:* Benign and malignant intracranial neoplasms compress and place traction on surrounding structures. Headache may be the first symptom. It can be intermittent or constant. The pain may be mild or excruciating and occur anywhere in the cranium. The headaches are not characteristic of any defined headache syndrome. A symptom that occurs with increased intracranial pressure, *pulse synchronous tinnitus,* identifies the headache as caused by raised intracranial pressure. DDX: Brain tumor should be suspected whenever the onset is recent, a recent change in the customary headache pattern has occurred, or an apparent migraine aura persists after the headache subsides.

▶ TRACTION-DISPLACEMENT: BRAIN ABSCESS: *Pathophysiology:* A localized region in the brain parenchyma becomes infected and encapsulated, enclosing liquefied brain and pus. Infection is either hematogenous or from local extension. Symptoms and signs of brain mass appear coincident with or after infection in the ears, paranasal sinuses, lungs or, rarely, osteomyelitis or other source. When the primary infection has not been recognized, the distinction from brain tumor may not be evident until imaging is obtained. Less than half the patients with brain abscess exhibit the classic triad of fever, headache, and focal deficit.

✓ *BRAIN ABSCESS—CLINICAL OCCURRENCE:* *Direct Extension* from otitis or sinusitis; *Hematogenous* pneumonia, endocarditis (especially *Staphylococcus aureus*), osteomyelitis, other bacteremias (patients with cyanotic congenital heart disease and right-to-left shunts are particularly susceptible), toxoplasmosis in HIV-infected patients; *Penetrating Trauma* after neurosurgery, gunshot wounds, open skull fractures.

S KEY SYNDROME

▶ **TRACTION-DISPLACEMENT: SUBDURAL HEMATOMA:** *Pathophysiology:* Trauma leads to tearing of the smaller veins between the fixed dura and the mobile arachnoid and brain, producing low-pressure bleeding and slowly accumulating hematoma. Symptoms and signs of expanding intracranial mass occur some time following head trauma. After a severe head injury, the immediate accumulation of blood in the subdural space is not unexpected and offers no diagnostic difficulty. However, minor head trauma may be followed by a latent period of days, weeks, or months before the onset of headaches or other neurologic symptoms. The progression, timing, and attributes of the pain are similar to those of a brain tumor with relatively rapid expansion. Often no physical signs are present initially; later, localizing signs of an expanding intracranial mass become evident. Drowsiness, mental confusion, or coma may appear without headache or other signs, especially with bilateral frontal subdurals. The diagnosis is confirmed by CT or MRI imaging.

S KEY SYNDROME

▶ **TRACTION-DISPLACEMENT: INTRACEREBRAL HEMORRHAGE:** *Pathophysiology:* The mechanism of arterial rupture in hypertension is unknown; bleeding is usually from deep striatal vessels. The site is usually intracerebral; rarely is it subarachnoid. Cerebral amyloid angiopathy weakens vessel walls; it is associated with intracerebral hemorrhage without preceding hypertension. In about half the patients, the onset is marked by a sudden, severe, generalized headache, followed by rapidly evolving neurologic signs. Frequently, the patient vomits; often, there is nuchal rigidity. Seizures and/or coma may supervene. The sequence of events and the neurologic manifestations vary with the site and volume of hemorrhage. *Putamen:* A sensation of intracranial discomfort is followed in 30 minutes by dysphagia, hemiplegia, and sometimes anesthesias. *Thalamus:* Hemiplegia and hemianesthesias with dysphasia, homonymous hemianopsia, and extraocular paralyses are common. *Cerebellum:* Slowly developing, with repeated vomiting, occipital headaches, vertigo, paralysis of conjugate lateral gaze, and other ocular disorders. *Pons:* Prompt unconsciousness and death within a few hours.

✓ *INTRACEREBRAL HEMORRHAGE—CLINICAL OCCURRENCE:* Hypertension, aneurysm (traumatic, inflammatory, saccular or mycotic), angiomas, cerebral amyloid angiopathy, erosion from neoplasm, complicating cerebral infarction (embolism, thrombosis), hemorrhagic disorders, and coagulation defects.

S KEY SYNDROME

TRACTION-DISPLACEMENT: SUBARACHNOID HEMORRHAGE: *Pathophysiology:* Subarachnoid hemorrhage usually results from rupture of a saccular (berry) aneurysm of the circle of Willis. Often, rupture is preceded by leakage, in contrast to the rupture of an artery from hypertension. New onset of severe headache between age 14 and 50 should suggest a ruptured aneurysm; prompt diagnosis and therapy may be lifesaving. CN-III signs may be seen and should always suggest a ruptured aneurysm; stiff neck may be present, but its absence does not exclude a ruptured aneurysm. The patient usually reports having the worst headache of his life. Excruciating generalized headache may be succeeded by nuchal rigidity, coma, and often death.

TRACTION-DISPLACEMENT: LUMBAR PUNCTURE HEADACHE: *Pathophysiology:* CSF is lost through the puncture hole in the dura, decreasing the CSF volume. A few hours or days after a lumbar puncture, the patient develops a constant or throbbing, usually bifrontal or suboccipital, deep headache. Moderate neck stiffness may occur. The pain is intensified when standing, shaking the head, or with bilateral jugular vein compression. It is lessened by the horizontal posture and flexion or extension of the neck.

TRACTION-DISPLACEMENT: IDIOPATHIC INTRACRANIAL HYPERTENSION: Symptoms resemble those of a brain tumor. Elevated cerebrospinal fluid pressure is found, with no structural abnormality. The typical patient is a young obese woman with recent rapid weight gain. Funduscopic exam reveals papilledema; if long-standing, the disks may be pale. Transient visual observations are common. Prevention of visual loss requires prompt diagnosis and therapy. The headache is much like common migraine except that it is often daily. If present, pulse synchronous tinnitus identifies increased intracranial pressure.

S KEY SYNDROME

INFLAMMATORY: BACTERIAL MENINGITIS: Headache is a prominent early symptom of meningitis. It is generalized, throbbing or constant, and accompanied by fever and stiff neck. Because the meninges are inflamed, the headache is intensified by sudden movements of the head. The headache may be accompanied or followed by drowsiness or coma. Signs of meningeal irritation are nuchal rigidity and Kernig and Brudzinski signs. Although many febrile illnesses are accompanied by some degree of head pain, the headache of meningitis is especially severe. When headache is associated with stiff neck, a lumbar puncture is indicated [Attia J, Hatala R, Cook DJ, Wong JG. Does this adult patient have acute meningitis? *JAMA* 1999;282:175–181].

S KEY SYNDROME

Headache Present on Awakening: Headaches present on awakening should suggest migraine, carbon monoxide poisoning, sleep apnea, and analgesic rebound headache. Tension headaches are not present on first awakening.

CARBON MONOXIDE POISONING: *Pathophysiology:* Excessive amounts of carboxyhemoglobin are formed from inhalation of carbon monoxide gas leading to decreased oxygenation. This results from inhalation of products of combustion in poorly ventilated spaces, for example, cars with malfunctioning exhaust systems, homes with malfunctioning gas furnaces, and burning charcoal in an enclosed space. Symptoms consist of headache, dizziness, nausea and vomiting, mental confusion, and visual disturbances progressing to obtundation, coma and death. The key sign is cherry-red skin and mucosa accompanied by a bounding pulse, hypertension, muscular twitching, stertorous breathing, and dilated pupils.

Localized Headache: Paranasal Sinusitis: See page 325.

Seizures

S KEY SYNDROME
Seizures: *Pathophysiology:* Seizures are caused by disordered electrical activity in the brain that may be focal, focal in onset with generalization, or generalized at the onset. Seizures are classified as generalized or partial. Partial seizures are defined as those with a focal onset, regardless of whether they generalize later in their course [Chabolla DR. Characteristics of the epilepsies. *Mayo Clin Proc* 2002;77:981–990].

✓ *SEIZURES—CLINICAL OCCURRENCE:* *Congenital* congenital brain injury; *Endocrine* hypoglycemia; *Idiopathic* idiopathic epilepsy; *Inflammatory/Immune* vasculitis; *Infectious* meningitis, encephalitis, brain abscess, neurocysticercosis; *Metabolic/Toxic* fever, drug withdrawal (alcohol, barbiturates, benzodiazepines, anticonvulsant medications), amphetamines, cocaine, phencyclidine, theophylline, hypoglycemia, hypocalcemia, uremia, liver failure, hypoxia, penicillins and other beta-lactams; *Mechanical/Trauma* head trauma; *Neoplastic* primary or metastatic cancer, insulinoma; *Neurologic* epilepsy, degenerative diseases of the CNS; *Psychosocial* drug abuse, physical abuse; *Vascular* stroke, vasculitis, hemorrhage.

When the patient has a seizure the immediate approach is to prevent injury and support cardiorespiratory function if necessary. However, the physician rarely observes the event, so a thorough history and examination are essential to identify the cause and to exclude other causes of impaired consciousness. In a patient treated for seizures, look for causes of relapse and evaluate adequacy of therapy. For patients with new onset of seizures, seek the cause, supplementing your neurologic examination with appropriate imaging and laboratory studies.

S KEY SYNDROME
Partial Seizures: *Pathophysiology:* Partial seizures begin within a specific region of the brain identified by the initial symp-

toms of the seizures. They may remain localized, spread to a larger but limited area of the cortex, or progress to a generalized seizure involving both cerebral hemispheres. Partial seizures are classified as simple if the event is limited to a small portion of one cortex and consciousness is not altered. Complex partial seizures involve larger areas of the cortex and consciousness is impaired, although not lost.

PARTIAL SEIZURE: PARTIAL MOTOR, JACKSONIAN SEIZURE: This is an episodic disorder. An attack often begins with twitching of the muscles in a single region of the body. The twitches become more violent with increasing amplitude. The disturbance spreads to contiguous muscle groups until the entire ipsilateral side may be involved in clonic contractions. The seizure may stop at any stage of its spread, or the contralateral side may be affected to produce a generalized motor seizure. Consciousness is usually retained except when the attack is generalized. Usually the seizures are caused by a focal lesion in the motor cortex supplying the muscles initially involved in the progression.

PARTIAL SEIZURE: PARTIAL-COMPLEX, PSYCHOMOTOR: These are often accompanied by an aura of an abnormal psychic event. These can be olfactory, visual, or gustatory disturbances, or even a phenomenon such as déjà vu. The attack may last from a few minutes to a few hours. Sudden but subtle loss of higher levels of consciousness occurs in which the patient is unaware of what transpires but retains motor functions and ability to react in an automatic fashion. The patient may respond to questions, but the answers disclose lack of understanding. This may be the only objective clue. Repetitive aimless movements, which are often stereotyped, may be reported. Patients generally do not become violent or assaultive during an attack. Only occasionally are there tonic muscle spasms of the limbs. Amnesia for the attack is partial or complete. This condition should prompt a search for a focal lesion in the temporal lobe.

S KEY SYNDROME

Secondary Generalized Seizure: Tonic–Clonic, Major Motor, Grand Mal: *Pathophysiology:* Most major motor seizures begin from a unilateral small focus in one hemisphere then progress to involve the ipsilateral hemisphere and cross the corpus callosum to involve the contralateral hemisphere, producing a secondary generalized seizure. There may or may not be a warning or aura. Several hours or days before the attack, prodromata may be noted, with feelings of strangeness, dreamy states, increased irritability, lethargy or euphoria, ravenous appetite, feeling of impending disaster, headaches, or other symptoms. The aura is a partial seizure, and the patient learns its significance. The patient may experience vague epigastric sensations such as nausea or hunger and palpitation, vertigo, or sensations in the head. Any aura or focal seizure reflects focal brain disease. Consciousness is lost suddenly and simultaneously with the epileptic cry from sudden expulsion of air through the glottis. The patient is helpless and falls, often incurring injuries. Tonic spasm of all muscles occurs which may be so violent as to fracture bones. Breathing ceases from spasm of the thoracic muscles and cyanosis may be deep. Suddenly, the tonic state subsides, followed by clonic movements that increase in strength with repetition then cease. Foaming at the mouth results from forced expulsion of air and saliva. Clonic movements of the jaws cause biting of the tongue, cheeks and lips. Frequently, there is involuntary defecation and urination. Unconsciousness usually lasts a few minutes, but may last hours. On return of consciousness patients are often confused and amnestic for the seizure and preceding events and complain of headache, stiffness, and sore muscles. Seizures are frequently followed by a deep sleep.

S KEY SYNDROME

Generalized Seizure: *Pathophysiology:* Generalized seizures involve the entire cerebral cortex at onset so they do not have an aura. History obtained from bystanders is critical in determining whether a seizure was generalized or focal at onset.

GENERALIZED SEIZURE: ABSENCE, PETIT MAL: An episode consists of a sudden transitory diminution or loss of consciousness with no abnormal muscle movements. The attack usually lasts from several to 90 seconds, during which time the patient's eyes are wide open and staring. Full consciousness is rapidly and completely restored. Injuries may result from the momentary lapse, but not from falls because there is no loss of postural tone. The patient is vaguely aware of having "missed something."

GENERALIZED SEIZURE: MAJOR MOTOR, GRAND MAL: This seizure is identical to the secondary generalized seizure except for the absence of an aura or any evidence of focal onset of the event. Consciousness is lost without warning and the patient is amnestic for the event.

Impaired Consciousness

Disturbances of consciousness may be classified partially according to degree. *Lethargy* is drowsiness caused by a condition other than normal sleep. In *confusion*, attention is dulled, perception is impaired, memory is defective, and the general awareness of surroundings is limited. In *delirium,* confusion is accompanied by hallucinations. Although delirium is sometimes accompanied by agitation and violent emotional responses, the patient may be quiet and withdrawn. *Stupor* is a somnolent state during which the patient may be momentarily aroused by questions or painful stimuli. *Coma* is the deepest state of unconsciousness in which the patient is motionless and unresponsive to stimuli. A brief loss of consciousness is *syncope* and presents a different group of diagnostic problems from those suggested by coma.

Episodic Impaired Consciousness

S KEY SYNDROME

Narcolepsy: *Pathophysiology:* This disorder is idiopathic or occurs secondary to brain injury. There is impaired ability to voluntarily maintain wakefulness associated with immediate onset of REM (rapid eye movement) sleep. The idiopathic form usually occurs in young adults and may be associated with sudden loss of motor tone without loss of consciousness (*cataplexy*), inability to move upon awakening (*sleep paralysis*), and visual or auditory hallucinations at sleep onset (*hypnagogic hallucinations*) or on awakening (*hypnopompic hallucinations*). The patient experiences unexpected, inappropriate, and irresistible short spells of sleep. There may be several attacks per day of brief somnolent periods with no deterioration of mentation.

S KEY SYNDROME

Syncope: *Pathophysiology:* Syncope occurs during transient diminution of the cerebral circulation or changes in the composition of the blood, as in hypoglycemia or hypocapnea. Impaired circulation of the brain may occur from ineffective cardiac action (myocardial insufficiency or dysrhythmias), loss of peripheral resistance in the vascular tree producing hypotension, or from vascular reflexes. In the erect position, consciousness is lost when the mean arterial pressure declines to 20–30 mmHg or when the heart stops for 4–5 seconds. In the horizontal position, more extreme conditions can be tolerated. The patient may complain of "weak spells," "light-headedness," or "blackouts." A careful history must be obtained from both the patient and witnesses. The history and initial physical exam are of the greatest usefulness in establishing a specific etiology. Extensive investigations are unlikely to be useful, unless the history or exam direct you to a specific diagnosis [Kapoor WN. Syncope. *N Engl J Med* 2000;343:1856–1862]. The most common cause of syncope is the vasovagal, or vasodepressor, faint. Other considerations are cardiac dysrhythmias (Adams-Stokes attacks—either tachy- or bradycardia), seizure, anaphylaxis, autonomic dysfunction with orthostatic hypotension, pulmonary embolism, aortic stenosis, and cerebrovascular disease.

SYNCOPE: VASOVAGAL SYNCOPE, FAINTING: *Pathophysiology:* Sudden vasodilation leads to decreased cardiac filling and forceful myocardial contraction on an underfilled ventricle triggers myocardial receptors, which reflexively cause strong vagal outflow, leading to bradycardia, further hypotension, and syncope. With recumbency, the venous return improves and recovery ensues. The attack is induced in healthy persons by fear, anxiety, or pain. A hot environment facilitates the onset by producing vasodilatation. Fatigue, illness, alcohol consumption, or hunger increases susceptibility. The patient can usually supply a history of the prodrome that is diagnostic. Recovery follows assumption of the horizontal position. The vasovagal (neurocardiogenic) attack has three stages. The prodrome is brief and usually begins in the erect position. The patient feels light-headed and unsteady. Yawning, dimming of vision (as a consequence of the intraocular pressure collapsing arterioles), nausea and vomiting, and sweating are common. The face becomes pale or ashen gray. If the patient reclines promptly the attack may be aborted. The syncopal stage consists of muscle weakness and impaired consciousness. The patient falls to the floor either slowly or abruptly, usually avoiding injury. The patient may be mentally confused but still hear

voices and dimly see the surroundings, or, there is complete unconsciousness. Unconsciousness may last for a few seconds to at most a few
minutes. Usually the muscles are utterly flaccid and motionless, although sometimes there are a few clonic jerks of arms and legs (*convulsive syncope*) but seldom a full tonic–clonic convulsion. Urinary or fecal
incontinence is rare. The skin appears strikingly pale or cyanotic and
the pulse is weak or absent. Bradycardia is accompanied by arterial hypotension and extremely shallow, quiet breathing. During recovery the
patient remains weak, but is awake and lucid. In the horizontal position, the face gradually suffuses with pink, the blood pressure rises, the
pulse becomes palpable and accelerated, the breathing deepens and
quickens, the eyelids may flutter. The patient awakens with immediate
awareness of the surroundings and memory for the prodrome. The muscle weakness persists for some time, so attempts to rise prematurely may
induce another attack [Fenton AM, Hammill SC, Rea FR, et al. Vasovagal syncope. *Ann Intern Med* 2000;133;714–725].

SYNCOPE: AKINETIC EPILEPSY: Common features in akinetic epilepsy,
but rare in syncope, are lack of pallor, sudden onset without prodrome,
injury from falling, tonic convulsions with upturned eyes, urinary or fecal incontinence, and postictal mental confusion with headache and
drowsiness. Most of these features occur occasionally with syncope.

SYNCOPE: ORTHOSTATIC OR POSTURAL SYNCOPE: See Chapter 4, page
86. *Pathophysiology:* Normally in the erect position, pooling of the
blood in the lower limbs is prevented by vasoconstriction mediated
through the autonomic nervous system. When there is decreased intravascular volume or the compensatory mechanism is blocked, blood
is pooled in the legs and arterial hypotension results. Distinctive features of autonomic insufficiency are normal heart rate, and absence of
pallor and sweating. Recovery occurs in the horizontal position.

SYNCOPE: HYSTERICAL SYNCOPE: This was the swoon of young nine-
teenth-century women with strong emotions. It usually occurred in the
presence of witnesses. The fall was graceful and harmless. The skin color,
heart rate, and blood pressure were all normal. Either the patient lay
motionless or made uninhibited resisting movements.

SYNCOPE: ADAMS-STOKES SYNDROME: *Pathophysiology:* The attacks
of unconsciousness occur when cardiac asystole lasts more than 5 seconds in the vertical position or 10 seconds in the horizontal. Usually,
asystole results during the transition from a partial to a complete heart
block or from the onset of paroxysmal tachycardia or ventricular fibrillation. When the heart rhythm is regular and the rate less than 40 per
minute, heart block can be distinguished from sinus bradycardia by
the variation in intensity of the first heart sounds. An ECG is required
for confirmation. This form of syncope occurs in any position without
a prodrome.

SYNCOPE: SYNCOPE WITH VALVULAR HEART DISEASE: *Pathophysiology:*
Muscular vasodilation with exercise in patients with a fixed cardiac out-

put leads to cerebral hypoperfusion and syncope. Exertion may induce typical syncope in a patient with aortic stenosis or, less commonly, aortic regurgitation or pulmonary hypertension.

▶ **SYNCOPE: CAROTID SINUS SYNCOPE:** *Pathophysiology:* Usually this occurs in patients older than age 60 years with hypertension or occlusion of one carotid artery. Rotation of the head or wearing a tight collar puts pressure on the carotid bulb, inducing syncope. The vagal stimulation may result in one of three responses: (a) sinoatrial block, (b) hypotension without bradycardia, or (c) syncope with normal pulse rate and blood pressure. Syncope related to specific motions of the neck suggest carotid sinus syncope. Circumstantial proof is furnished when an attack is reproduced by massaging the carotid sinus. Before stimulation is attempted, determine that both carotid arteries are pulsating and patent. The maneuver is dangerous when one artery is occluded. Both carotids should never be stimulated simultaneously. Continuous ECG monitoring is performed while the carotid sinus is gently massaged; *do not to occlude the vessel.* Occlusion during the maneuver has produced cerebral infarction and death.

SYNCOPE: HYPERVENTILATION: *Pathophysiology:* Hyperventilation results in hypocapnea; this induces diminished cerebral blood flow. Before the attack, the patient is anxious or emotionally upset. The patient is not conscious of hyperventilation but feels tightness in the chest or suffocation. The prodrome is usually attended by numbness and tingling of arms and face, sometimes carpopedal spasms occur. Loss of consciousness may be prolonged compared with most other types of syncope. The symptoms are reproduced by having the patient overventilate. Rebreathing into a paper bag will arrest the attack and demonstrate a method of self-treatment.

SYNCOPE: COUGH SYNCOPE (TUSSIVE SYNCOPE): Severe paroxysms of coughing, laughing, or vomiting may induce an attack of syncope, usually in men, rarely in women. The history of the onset is usually diagnostic. The mechanism is disputed: either compression of the cerebrum by transmission of increased intrathoracic pressure to the cerebrospinal fluid or reduction of cardiac output by the Valsalva maneuver.

SYNCOPE: MICTURITION SYNCOPE: Particularly in a patient with peripheral vasodilatation from a warm bed, voiding of a large volume may cause syncope. Similarly, the rapid decompression of an overfilled bladder by catheterization or the removal of large volumes of ascitic fluid may also cause syncope.

▶ **SYNCOPE: HYPOGLYCEMIC SYNCOPE:** The prodrome may resemble a vasovagal spell but confusion is prominent. The syncopal stage is frequently prolonged and loss of consciousness is usually incomplete. Instead, there is muscle weakness with mental confusion. The blood sugar is usually below 30 mg/100 mL; the symptoms are relieved by the intravenous administration of glucose or injection of glucagon.

Coma

▼ **Coma:**   *Pathophysiology:*   Coma results from serious disruption of brain function that impairs the reticular activating system such that consciousness is lost. Coma is a state of prolonged unconsciousness. The examination requires a special approach because the patient cannot give a history, and cooperation is absent. The medical student or house officer who is first confronted with this situation may well be baffled and disconcerted, but experience demonstrates that the correct diagnosis will be rapidly established in most cases by a structured complete physical and neurologic examination and use of radiologic and laboratory testing. In formulating a diagnosis, two axioms should be followed. (a) Finding one clue to the cause of coma does not prove the cause. For instance, a comatose patient with the odor of alcohol on the breath may have sustained a head injury while intoxicated; a person injured in an automobile accident may have had an antecedent stroke that led to the accident; or an unconscious patient with a few sedative tablets at the bedside may have taken the drug for symptoms of meningitis or brain tumor. (b) A complete neurologic examination is insufficient, the other systems of the body must also be assessed: finding atrial fibrillation raises the possibility of cerebral embolism; the retinae may contain signs of diabetes; demonstration of a consolidated lung suggests lobar pneumonia or pneumococcal meningitis; examination of the abdomen has discovered a distended bladder, leading to a diagnosis of uremia from prostatic obstruction. The differential diagnosis and management of coma is beyond the scope of this text. The reader should consult textbooks of medicine, neurology, and emergency medicine.

HISTORY OF THE COMATOSE PATIENT: Interview the relatives, acquaintances, attendants, or police officers who discovered the patient.   *Circumstances of Discovery:*   How was the patient found? Were there any drugs or poisons nearby? Were the surroundings such as to suggest poisoning from carbon monoxide or gasoline fumes? Was there evidence of trauma? What was known about the patient's antecedent intake of food and fluids? Who prepared the food? What were the symptoms and actions before the onset of coma? Did the patient have pain, diarrhea, or vomiting?   *Past History:*   Was the patient known to have epilepsy, diabetes, hypertension, or alcohol or drug addiction? Did the patient have suicidal thoughts? Was the patient ever hospitalized in a mental institution? Was the patient known to be taking medicines? Had there ever been operations for malignancy? Has this happened before?

Assess patency of the airway and the presence of adequate respirations and pulse.   *Vital Signs:*   Note any abnormalities.   *General Inspection:*   Note posture; look for tremors or muscle jerks; inspect the respiratory movements for bradypnea, tachypnea, Kussmaul breathing,

Cheyne-Stokes breathing. *Color:* Look for pallor, icterus, the cyanosis of methemoglobinemia, the cherry-red color of carbon monoxide hemoglobin. *Scalp and Skull:* Look for contusions, lacerations, gunshot wounds; palpate for depressed skull fractures and inspect the mastoid for hematoma of basilar skull fracture (*Battle sign*). *Eyes:* Inspect for periorbital bruising (*raccoon sign*) of basilar skull fracture. Lift the eyelids and let them close; lagging of one lid suggests hemiplegia. The patient with hysteria resists opening by closing the lids tighter. In coma, the eyes remain fixed or oscillate slowly from side to side; oscillation is lacking in hysteria in which the eyes may wander but fix momentarily. Conjugate deviation of the eyeballs is toward the affected side in destructive lesions of the frontal lobe, away from the affected side in irritative lesions. The presence of extraocular muscle palsies assists in localizing an intracranial lesion. After confirming the absence of neck injury, open the eyelids and quickly turn the head from side to side. The eyes of the comatose patient with cerebral damage turn in the opposite direction in a conjugate movement if the brainstem is intact (doll's eyes). This oculocephalic reflex is lost with lesions of the pons or midbrain. Caloric studies, in which you test an oculovestibular reflex, provide information of similar significance. These are performed by irrigating the ear canal with 30–50 mL of ice water and noting that, with cerebral dysfunction and an intact brainstem, a tonic conjugate deviation of the eyes toward the cold ear lasts for 30–120 seconds. Bilateral, widely dilated pupils occur in profound posttraumatic shock, massive cerebral hemorrhage, encephalitis, poisoning with atropine-like drugs, and the end stages of brain tumor. Bilateral pinpoint pupils suggest opiate poisoning or a pontine hemorrhage. A unilateral unreactive pupil indicates a rapidly expanding lesion on the ipsilateral side, as in subdural or middle meningeal epidural hemorrhage or brain tumor. Examine the ocular fundi for the exudates and hemorrhages of diabetes and nephritis, and the choked disks of increased intracranial pressure. *Facial Muscles:* Asymmetry of the face may indicate hemiplegia. The mouth droops on the affected side; the cheek puffs out with each expiration. Painful pressure on the supraorbital notch causes the mouth to grimace in an asymmetric pattern to reveal the weak side. *Oral Cavity:* Examine the tongue for lacerations from biting during a seizure. Look for a diphtheritic membrane, other signs of pharyngitis, or ulceration or discoloration from poisons. *Breath:* Smell the breath for acetone, ammonia, alcohol or its successor aldehydes, paraldehyde, and other odors. *Ears:* Look for pus, spinal fluid, or blood emerging from the external acoustic meatus or blood behind the drum from basilar skull fracture. *Neck:* Test for nuchal rigidity, Kernig sign, and Brudzinski sign, looking for evidence of meningeal irritation. *Chest:* Percuss and auscultate the chest for pneumothorax, consolidation, wheezing, or crepitation. *Heart:* Auscultate for rhythm, rate, and strength of the heart sounds and any abnormal sounds. *Abdomen:* Auscultate for bruits and palpate for masses or rigidity suggesting peritonitis or fluid. *Limbs:* Test each limb successively for flaccidity by lifting it and letting it fall to the bed. If any muscle tone is retained, a difference in the two sides indicates a hemiplegia. The reflexes on the paralyzed side are absent during the stage of spinal shock, but in deep coma, all reflexes are lost. In deep coma, the Babinski reflex is present bilaterally, so it cannot be employed to localize a lesion. If some reflexes are retained, a difference in the two sides is significant. **Sensory Examination:** In semicoma, only the responses to painful stimuli can be evaluated. The patient will show defensive reactions when pricked in sensitive areas, but no response is forthcoming when analgesic regions are stimulated. If the stimulated region is sensitive but paralyzed, a defense or withdrawal movement may occur on the opposite side; the facial expression will indicate pain. Deep pressure sense should be tested by compression of the Achilles tendon, the testis, and the supraorbital notch.

Classify the seriousness of cerebral dysfunction by using the Glasgow Coma Scale (Table 14-2) in which mild is 13 through 15, moderate is 9 through 12, and severe is 3 through 8 points. Patients with scores less than 8 are in coma.

DIFFERENTIAL DIAGNOSIS OF COMA: The multiple etiologies of coma can be conveniently divided into three categories, which may be suggested by findings from the history and physical examination.

METABOLIC ENCEPHALOPATHY: *Pathophysiology:* Metabolic derangements or toxin exposure impairs brain function and leads to coma. Coma occurs with normal pupillary responses, normal brainstem reflexes and

TABLE 14–2 Glasgow Coma Scale

Response		Score
Eyes Open		
_____	Spontaneous	4
_____	To speech	3
_____	To pain	2
_____	Absent	1
Verbal		
_____	Converses/oriented	5
_____	Converses/disoriented	4
_____	Inappropriate	3
_____	Incomprehensible	2
_____	Absent	1
Motor		
_____	Obeys	6
_____	Localizes pain	5
_____	Withdraws (flexion)	4
_____	Decorticate (flexion) rigidity	3
_____	Decerebrate (extension) rigidity	2
_____	Absent	1

no focal neurologic deficits. Asterixis, myoclonus, and Cheyne-Stokes respiration co-occur. No neuroimaging is needed. Treatment is correction of the metabolic disturbance. See Delirium, page 890.

✓ *METABOLIC ENCEPHALOPATHY—CLINICAL OCCURRENCE:* Hypoglycemia, hypoxia, hypercarbia, hyponatremia, intoxications (e.g., alcohol, benzodiazepines, barbiturates, opiates), severe hypothyroidism, and many others.

TRANSTENTORIAL HERNIATION: *Pathophysiology:* An expanding mass in a supratentorial compartment moves tissue to another compartment. Typically, the uncus of the temporal lobe compresses the third nerve and then the midbrain initially producing focal deficits. Progression from the focal deficits to coma and death can be rapid.

✓ *CLINICAL OCCURRENCE:* Brain tumor (primary or metastatic), bleeding (intracerebral, subdural, epidural), cerebral edema associated with infarction (arterial or venous), abscess, encephalitis, or massive liver necrosis.

BRAINSTEM INJURY: *Pathophysiology:* Direct damage occurs to the brainstem reticular activating system that runs from the upper pons to the lower diencephalon and is responsible for maintaining consciousness. The onset is usually abrupt, either following trauma or acute severe headache. Emergent neuroimaging is required.

✓ *CLINICAL OCCURRENCE:* Trauma and spontaneous hemorrhage are the most common etiologies.

Cerebrovascular Syndromes

S KEY SYNDROME

▶ **Transient Ischemic Attack (TIA):** *Pathophysiology:* TIA results from a failure of perfusion due to hemodynamic causes or microembolism. Less common causes are in situ arterial thrombosis, arterial dissection and venous sinus thrombosis. The symptoms reflect the area of ischemia. TIA is, by definition, the acute onset of a focal neurologic deficit in a specific vascular distribution with full recovery within 24 hours of onset. Events usually last 5–20 minutes. The differential diagnosis of TIA includes convulsions, syncope, migraine, focal cerebral masses, such as subdural hematomas, cardiac diseases, and labyrinthine disorders. Diplopia, syncope, transient confusion, and paraparesis are uncommon symptoms of TIA. Neurologic signs are usually absent between attacks. The correct diagnosis and prompt evaluation of TIA are important because it is an indication of impending serious cerebral infarction; up to 25% of patients with a new TIA will have a stroke within 24 hours [Johnston SC. Transient ischemic attack. *N Engl J Med* 2002;347:1687–1692].

TRANSIENT ISCHEMIC ATTACK (TIA): CAROTID ARTERY TIA: Symptoms and signs are related to the ipsilateral cerebral hemisphere and/or retina. Findings include contralateral weakness, clumsiness, numbness of the hand, hand and face, or entire half of the body, dysarthria, aphasia, and ipsilateral amaurosis fugax with monocular visual loss (which can be complete blindness sector visual loss), usually described as a shade coming down. Carotid bruits or retinal emboli may be found.

AMAUROSIS FUGAX: *Pathophysiology:* Cholesterol emboli from ruptured atherosclerotic plaques in the common or internal carotid artery transiently occlude flow to the retinal artery. There is sudden onset of monocular blindness, often described as a shade being pulled down, which lasts a few minutes and resolves spontaneously. It is a transient ischemic attack (TIA) of the ipsilateral carotid circulation and carries a 25% risk of stroke in the next 48 hours.

TRANSIENT ISCHEMIC ATTACK (TIA): VERTEBROBASILAR ARTERY TIA: Symptoms and signs are related to the posterior circulation and may affect vision and cranial nerve function. Frequent complaints are combinations of binocular visual disturbance or loss, vertigo, dysarthria, ataxia, unilateral or bilateral weakness or numbness and drop attacks (sudden loss of postural tone and collapse without loss of consciousness).

S KEY SYNDROME

▶ **Hemiparesis (Hemiplegia): Stroke:** *Pathophysiology:* Paresis of either the right or left side of the body indicates contralateral disease of the brain or ipsilateral high spinal disease. The most common cause is vascular occlusion of the middle cerebral artery. Consciousness is not impaired and the patient is sometimes unaware of the deficit. If the visual pathways are affected, a homonymous hemianopsia will be found. With middle cerebral occlusions, the arm is more severely affected than the leg; with anterior cerebral artery stroke, the leg is more affected than the arm. Cerebral venous sinus thrombosis presents with symptoms and signs of cerebral vascular disease with less discrete evidence of focal lesions.

Hemiparesis: Conversion Reaction: In patients with complaints of unilateral weakness or paralysis of the legs but confusing findings, try to elicit the *Hoover sign,* which depends on the absence of a normal associated movement *(synkinesia).* Place the patient supine, stand at the foot of the table, and place a palm under each heel. Ask the patient to raise the affected limb (see Fig. 14-9D). Normally, the unaffected limb will press downward in the effort to raise the affected limb. In neither organic disease nor hysteria will the leg be normally raised, but in organic disease, the associated movement of pressing down with the unaffected heel will still be present. It is absent in conversion reaction. The sign is helpful only when the patient has, or claims to have, paralysis of one leg. Paraplegia must be excluded.

S KEY SYNDROME

▶ **Cavernous Sinus Thrombosis:** *Pathophysiology:* Thrombosis with occlusion of the cavernous sinus results from bacterial infection of the upper lip, tooth socket, eyes, or face. Patients present with pain in the eye and forehead, chills, fever, and impaired vision. Physical findings include chemosis, edema of the eyelids, exophthalmos, hyperemia, papilledema, orbital tenderness, and cranial nerve palsies of CN-III, -IV, and -VI. Progression leads to leptomeningitis, blindness, intracerebral abscess, septicemia, and death.

Other Motor and Sensory Syndromes

S KEY SYNDROME

Trigeminal Neuralgia: Tic Douloureux: The cause is unknown. Paroxysms of excruciating pain occur in the distribution of a branch of the fifth cranial nerve, often triggered by cold air on the face, sneezing, shaving, chewing, or other movements. Muscle spasms, flushing of the face, lacrimation, and salivation, may occur during an attack.

S KEY SYNDROME

▶ **Paraparesis:** *Pathophysiology:* Loss of motor power to both legs indicates a transverse lesion of the spinal cord. The level is determined by the sensory findings. Frequent causes of paraparesis are trauma and transverse myelitis, which may follow several different types of viral infection. Extrinsic cord compression by herniated disk or epidural abcess or neoplasm are less common but potentially treatable.

S KEY SYNDROME

Quadriparesis: *Pathophysiology:* Paresis or paralysis of all limbs without changes in consciousness indicates impairment of the descending corticospinal (pyramidal) tracts. The most common cause is traumatic injury to the cervical spine; in this case the bulbar muscles are spared. Less common, but not rare, causes, usually with some bulbar involvement, are multiple sclerosis, primary motor system disease (e.g., amyotrophic lateral sclerosis), and botulism. Onset of nontraumatic generalized weakness or paralysis over a few hours or days suggests an electrolyte disturbance (most commonly severe hypokalemia). In the hospital, other causes to be considered are inadvertently high spinal anesthesia, paralytic drugs, and the polyneuropathy of severe illness.

S KEY SYNDROME

Multiple Sclerosis: *Pathophysiology:* Multifocal demyelinization occurs in the nervous system presumed to be mediated by autoimmune mechanisms. The onset is usually fairly abrupt over hours to a few days, with remissions occurring over weeks, if at all. Acute optic neuritis with transient visual loss is a common presenting symptom. Other symptoms include incoordination, paresthesias, weakness and loss of sphincter control. The signs depend upon the location of the demyelinating lesion(s): ataxia, dysarthria, intention tremor, ocular palsies, visual loss, hyperactive deep reflexes, diminished abdominal reflexes, and trophic changes in skin. The *Charcot triad* of signs is intention tremor, nystagmus, and scanning speech. The disease may be progressive from onset with inexorable loss of function, or relapsing-remitting with complete resolution of the symptoms and signs between relapses. Many patients with initially relapsing–remitting disease will progress to chronic progressive disease with incomplete remissions of each relapse [Compston A, Coles A. Multiple sclerosis. *Lancet* 2002;1221–1231].

S KEY SYNDROME

▼ **Amyotrophic Lateral Sclerosis:** *Pathophysiology:* Degeneration of upper and lower motor neurons leads to progressive weakness and muscle wasting. The disease begins gradually, proceeds progressively, and ends fatally in 2 to 3 years. Muscle aches and cramps are accompanied by weakness of distal upper limbs, spreading to the lower extremities; dysarthria, dysphagia, and drooling indicate bulbar involvement. Muscle fasciculation and atrophy are seen, especially in upper limbs. Fasciculations may be evident in the tongue. Hyperreflexia and spasticity of lower limbs indicate upper motor neuron involvement [Rowland LP, Shneider NA. Amyotrophic lateral sclerosis. *N Engl J Med* 2001;344:1688–1700].

Poliomyelitis: *Pathophysiology:* Infection of the spinal cord by poliomyelitis virus types I, II, or III leads to destruction of lower motor neurons. Polio still occurs outside the Western Hemisphere, despite efforts to eradicate it through vaccination. Fever, headache, sore throat, stiff neck, and pain in the back and limbs is followed by inability to move one or more muscle groups. Signs are varying deep reflexes, weakness, fasciculations, hyperesthesia, paresthesias, and lymphadenopathy. Kernig and Brudzinski signs may be present. Healing may lead to complete return of function or be followed by muscular atrophy. Bulbar involvement leads to weakness of the pharyngeal muscles and diaphragm. Many years after recovery, insidious weakness may recur in the affected muscles, *postpolio syndrome.*

S KEY SYNDROME

▼ **Syringomyelia and Chiari Malformations:** *Pathophysiology:* There is cavitary expansion within the cervical spinal cord that damages the centrally crossing sensory tracts and the pyramidal tracts. Syringomyelia (*syrinx*—to become hollow; *myelia*—marrow) is of unknown cause. Syringomyelia is frequently associated with hindbrain malformations—herniation of the cerebellar tonsils through the foramen magnum (Chiari type 1). Patients present with decreased pain and temperature sensation in the arms and shoulders, lower motor neuron weakness in the arms and upper motor neuron weakness with spasticity in the legs. Chiari type 2 malformation (incomplete closure of the spinal canal) is always accompanied by myelomeningocele.

Tabes Dorsalis: Neurosyphilis of the Spinal Cord: *Pathophysiology:* Chronic infection with *Treponema pal-*

lidum produces degeneration of the spinal cord posterior columns, dorsal roots, and dorsal root ganglia. Symptoms include lightning-like pains in the trunk and lower limbs, paresthesias, urinary incontinence, and impotence. There is loss of position sense, ataxic wide-based gait, footdrop, and loss of reflexes. Loss of position sense leads to joint destruction with Charcot deformities. *Tabetic crisis* is abdominal pain and vomiting with a relaxed abdominal wall.

General Paresis: Neurosyphilis of the Brain:
Pathophysiology: Brain infection with *Treponema pallidum* produces a tertiary syphilis syndrome of degenerative brain disease. The finding can be recalled using the pneumonic PARESIS: personality, affect, loss of reflexes, eye findings (Argyll-Robinson pupil), sensory changes, intellectual deterioration (*dementia precox*), and speech changes. Other signs of tertiary syphilis may be present, such as aortitis with aortic insufficiency and gumma formation.

S KEY SYNDROME
Hemisection of the Spinal Cord: Brown Sequard Syndrome: *Pathophysiology:* Hemisection of the cord damages the ipsilateral descending motor pathways and ascending proprioceptive pathways (cross in the brainstem), and the contralateral sensory pathways for pain and temperature (cross at their spinal root levels). Patients have motor paralysis with spasticity and loss of proprioception on the side of the lesion and absent pain and temperature sensation on the opposite side, below the level of the injury.

S KEY SYNDROME
Botulism: *Pathophysiology:* Neurotoxins produced by *Clostridium botulinum* may be ingested or absorbed from contaminated wounds. Symptoms onset is over hours with variable combinations of weakness, headache, dizziness, dysphagia, abdominal pain, nausea and vomiting, diarrhea, and diplopia. Physical findings include fixed and dilated pupils, nystagmus, ptosis, irregular respiration, swollen tongue, hyporeflexia, and incoordination. Improperly canned foods prepared in the home are the most common cause.

S KEY SYNDROME
Myasthenia Gravis: *Pathophysiology:* An autoantibody binds to the acetylcholine receptor at the neuromuscular junction blocking neuromuscular transmission, especially with repetitive excitation. Affected individuals complain of increased fatigability, transient muscle weakness, diplopia, ptosis, easy fatigue with chewing and talking, regurgitation, and dysphagia. During an attack there may be lack of facial expression, abnormal speech or aphonia, disconjugate gaze. In extreme cases, the patient sometimes cannot lift his head from the pillow without hand support. There is an association with thymoma.

Tetanus: Tetanus is caused by the toxin of *Clostridium tetani* acting on myoneural junctions. A single muscle or many groups become rigid with sustained tonic spasm. The masseter is frequently involved early, hence the term lockjaw *(trismus)*. Loud noises, bright lights, or pain induce superimposed violent generalized spasms. The condition should not be confused with tetany, which it resembles only in name.

D KEY DISEASE

Rabies: *Pathophysiology:* Infection by a neurotropic virus is transmitted by the bite of infected mammals. Onset is marked by local dysthesia radiating from the site of entry, malaise, nausea, and sore throat. Later, restlessness and hallucinations occur. There is hyperesthesia of the wound and later, dysarthria, dysphagia for fluids, convulsions, delirium, and opisthotonos stimulated by lights or noises. Breathing becomes shallow and irregular with hoarseness or aphonia. The stretch reflexes are hyperactive and there is nuchal rigidity, Babinski sign followed by flaccid paralysis, and death. A high index of suspicion is required to make the diagnosis and to protect contacts to body fluids. Many patients diagnosed in the United States do not have an identified source of infection; bats are the most common source when one is identified.

S KEY SYNDROME

Dystonias: Dystonias are abnormally prolonged tonic contractions of a muscle or muscle group. Dystonias are often associated with certain activities and can become disabling. The patient will refer to them as a cramp. Examples are writer's cramp, torticollis, and dystonias associated with playing musical instruments.

S KEY SYNDROME

Acute Demyelinating Polyneuropathy: Guillain-Barré Syndrome: *Pathophysiology:* This is an immune-mediated demyelinating disorder occurring 1–3 weeks after viral infection, *Campylobacter jejuni* gastroenteritis, or, rarely, after surgery or with malignant lymphoma. There is usually rapidly progressive ascending motor weakness with pain in back and limbs, headache, and distal numbness and tingling. Nausea and vomiting can occur. There is ascending flaccid paralysis with diminished deep and superficial reflexes. Cranial nerve involvement causes dysphasia, dysphagia and dysarthria. With chest wall involvement, respiratory failure supervenes.

S KEY SYNDROME

Peripheral Neuropathy: *Pathophysiology:* Peripheral nerve dysfunction in the absence of central nervous system disease is common. Diffuse lesions are classified as axonal if the nerve cell axon is primarily involved, or demyelinating if the lesion is in the myelin coating of the nerve. Single nerve trunk lesions may be traumatic, ischemic, or inflammatory. Patients present with complaints of numbness, burning, unsteadiness (often described as dizziness), falling, or weakness. Physical exam may show sensory impairment (pressure, vibration, position, pain and temperature or simple touch depending on the size of nerves involved), muscle weakness and atrophy with fasciculations, and/or diminished reflexes. Release signs are not present and plantar response is flexor if present. Diffuse symmetrical neuropathies are usually sensory at onset and later involve motor nerves; they are primarily distal and progress proximally affecting the feet before the hands. Isolated nontraumatic involvement of all components of a single nerve is called *mononeuritis multiplex,* usually resulting from an inflammatory lesion causing ischemia; recovery is common and complete [Hughes RAC. Peripheral neuropathy. *BMJ* 2002;324:466–469; Poncelet AN. An algorithm for the evaluation of peripheral neuropathy. *Am Fam Physician* 1998;57:755–764].

✓ PERIPHERAL NEUROPATHY—CLINICAL OCCURRENCE: *Congenital* Charcot-Marie-Tooth disease, porphyria, familial neuropathy; *Endocrine* diabetes; *Idiopathic* ICU polyneuropathy, idiopathic polyneuropathy; *Infectious* leprosy, rabies (early at inoculation site), postherpetic neuralgia; *Inflammatory/Immune* acute and chronic inflammatory polyneuropathy, vasculitis, systemic lupus erythematosus, amyloidosis, celiac disease; *Mechanical/Trauma* contusion and laceration, repetitive use, vibration (e.g., jackhammers, pneumatic drills), cold injury (chilblains and frostbite), electrical injury; *Metabolic/Toxic* amyloidosis, porphyria, diabetes, poisoning (arsenic, other heavy metals, pyridoxine), drugs (e.g., vincristine), nutritional deficiency (vitamins B_{12} and B_6); *Neoplastic* paraneoplastic syndromes, metastatic invasion of nerves; *Psychosocial* substance abuse producing unconsciousness with pressure-induced ischemia; *Vascular* vasculitis.

PERIPHERAL NEUROPATHY: DIABETES: *Pathophysiology:* Diabetes types 1 and 2 are associated with peripheral nerve injury with a latency of about 15 years from onset for type 1. Damage is thought to be metabolic in most forms, and ischemic in the acute reversible forms. Several forms of diabetic neuropathy are recognized. *Distal sensorimotor neuropathy* is most common, presenting as numbness or burning pain in the feet and progressing proximally with loss of protective sensation, trophic skin changes, pressure-induced ischemic ulceration, and infection leading to amputation, if preventive measures are not taken. Limbs at risk are insensitive to a 10-g monofilament test [Smieja M, Hunt DL, Edelman D, et al. Clinical examination for the detection of protective sensation in the feet of diabetic patients. International Cooperative Group for Clinical Examination Research. *J Gen Intern Med* 1999;14:418–424]. In severe forms, muscle wasting and Charcot joints occur. *Autonomic neuropathy* frequently involves the stomach with gastroparesis and delayed gastric emptying which may make control of blood sugars very difficult. Sudomotor injury contributes to skin fragility and ulceration. Impotence is common and colon and bladder dysfunction not rare. The sensorimotor and autonomic neuropathies are delayed or prevented by tight control of blood glucose. *Diabetic amyotrophy or polyradiculopathy* is an acute, painful, inflammatory or ischemic injury to one or more spinal roots. Patients present with severe back, chest, abdominal or proximal leg pain, and progressive weakness, and may have bowel and bladder dysfunction. It is usually acute in onset and asymmetric. Recovery is expected over months in most people. Isolated *cranial nerve palsies,* especially CN-III, -IV, and -VI are not uncommon and often mistaken for much more serious intracranial pathology. The pupil is spared in CN-III lesions. Diabetic amyotrophy and cranial nerve lesions are not clearly related to the duration of diabetes or degree of blood sugar control.

S KEY SYNDROME

▼ **Median Neuropathy: Carpal Tunnel Syndrome:** *Pathophysiology:* The median nerve is compressed in the carpal tunnel under the flexor retinaculum of the wrist by fibrosis of the tendon sheaths, trauma, arthritis, or soft-tissue swelling. Symptoms include numbness and tingling of the hand in a variable distribution, often the entire volar surface of the hand. Signs include decreased sensation on the volar surface of the thumb, index, middle and radial half of the ring finger. With advanced disease there is atrophy of the thenar eminence and weakness of thumb abduction and opposition. On examination, increased paresthesia and pain may be elicited with flexion of wrists (Phalen sign), or tapping the median nerve in the carpal tunnel (Tinel sign).

✓ *CLINICAL OCCURRENCE:* Causes include repetitive use injury, diabetes mellitus, multiple myeloma, amyloidosis, a congenitally small carpal tunnel, and rheumatoid arthritis.

Disorders of Language and Speech

● KEY SIGN

◤ **Disorders of Speech: Dysarthria, Dysphonia, Ataxia, and Apraxia:** Alterations of speech may be considered in several categories.

ARTICULATION: DYSARTHRIA: Articulation is the production of sounds and their combinations into syllables. Disorders of the brain produce *dysarthria;* specific dysarthrias are identified by the types of sounds which are improperly formed (see Chapter 7, page 226). *Dyslalia* is impaired articulation from non-neurologic structural defects or hearing loss.

VOICE: DYSPHONIA: This concerns phonation, resonation, pitch, quality, and volume. *Dysphonia* is the disturbance in pitch, quality, and volume. *Hypernasality* and *hyponasality* refer to nasal resonance.

RHYTHM: ATAXIA: This deals with the timing and sequence of syllables. Irregular, slow speech with pauses and bursts of sounds is called *scanning speech* and indicates a cerebellar disorder, for example, multiple sclerosis. Faltering or interruptions in speech are termed *stuttering;* this is frequently inherited or may be a developmental disorder.

SOUND SELECTION: APRAXIA: This is the inability to properly and consistently program a correct sequence of sounds, especially consonants. Have the patient repeat the word "artillery" five times; each sound is formed correctly, but they are misplaced and no two attempts may be alike. The problem is evident with writing as well as speech.

S KEY SYNDROME

Disorders of Language: Aphasias: Language is the symbolic representation and interpretation of meaning in voice sounds and written symbols (*symbolization*). It is a far more complex activity than speech, requiring extensive central interconnectivity. Language is evaluated during history-taking and with the Mini-Mental State Exam (MMSE). Six domains are assessed: (a) speech expression, both spontaneous and automatic sequences (e.g., singing, nursery rhymes, and cursing); (b) naming; (c) speech comprehension; (d) repetition; (e) reading; and (f) writing [Damasio AR. Aphasia. *N Engl J Med* 1992;326: 531–539].

APHASIAS: *Pathophysiology:* Language is instantiated in the dominant hemisphere, which is the left hemisphere in >99% of right- and left-handed people. Damage to specific language-processing areas produces distinct aphasias. An acquired inability to use language correctly is termed *aphasia* and indicates acquired disease of the brain. Congenital or developmental disorders of language are called *dysphasias*.

BROCA APHASIA: *Pathophysiology:* There is damage to the Broca area of the left frontal lobe. The speech is nonfluent, often leaving out pronouns, prepositions, and the like; reading and writing are also affected. Patients are aware of their difficulty and become frustrated. They appear to know what they want to say. Speech comprehension is relatively spared for simple communication.

WERNICKE APHASIA: Speech is fluent but words are jumbled and substituted, obscuring all meaning (*paraphasia*). Writing is similarly affected. Reading and verbal comprehension are poor. The patient is unaware of their deficit and may become angry when not understood.

GLOBAL APHASIA: This is a combination of Broca and Wernicke aphasia.

OTHER APHASIAS: See neurology texts for discussion of conduction, anomic, transcortical, and subcortical aphasias.

S KEY SYNDROME

Disorders of Language: Alexia and Agraphia: *Alexia* is the inability to read. *Dyslexia* is an impairment of reading ability. *Agraphia* is the inability to write.

Syndromes of Impaired Mentation

S KEY SYNDROME

Delirium: See Chapter 15, page 890 for the full discussion of delirium.

S KEY SYNDROME

Hepatic Encephalopathy: *Pathophysiology:* Severe hepatocellular dysfunction and/or portal hypertension with portal-systemic shunting allows accumulation of toxic metabolites leading to cerebral dysfunction. This presents four features—only the last two are distinctive: (a) altered mental state varying from slight loss of memory to confusion, slurred speech, sedation, and coma; (b) asterixis, also present in cerebrovascular disease, uremia, and severe pulmonary insufficiency; (c) signs of abnormal liver function such as jaundice, palmar erythema, spider angiomata, hepatomegaly, and ascites; and (d) fetor hepaticus, smelling something like old wine, acetone, or new-mown hay; if present, it is distinctive of hepatic coma.

S KEY SYNDROME

▼ **Wernicke-Korsakoff Syndrome:** *Pathophysiology:* Thiamine deficiency is common in alcoholism and symptoms may occur when administration of glucose causes acute thiamine deficiency (Wernicke encephalopathy) leading to chronic brain injury (Korsakoff syndrome). Wernicke syndrome presents with confusion, nystagmus, ataxia, ophthalmoplegia, impaired memory, and decreased attention. It is essential to recognize and treat the patient immediately with parenteral thiamine. Korsakoff syndrome is an irreversible chronic encephalopathy with antegrade and retrograde amnesia and confabulation.

S KEY SYNDROME

▼ **Dementia:** Dementia is a decline in cognitive function sufficient to impair function. It includes memory loss (recent more than remote; i.e., loss of orientation) and at least one of the following: aphasia, apraxia, agnosia, or abnormal executive function. It is chronic and usually progressive, although the rate of progression is quite variable. Personality changes and loss of normal social inhibitions are late findings in most cases. Dementia is easily missed early in its course if not specifically sought in patients at risk. There are no early physical findings, the release signs being late manifestations of advanced disease. Screening with the Mini-Mental State Exam (MMSE) and clock drawing task are useful. Medical illness can present as dementia so it is essential to exclude reversible medical conditions such as hypothyroidism, other endocrinopathies, medication side effects, and vitamin B_{12} deficiency. There are many causes of dementia, but Alzheimer disease is most common [Karlawish JHT, Clark CM. Diagnostic evaluation of elderly patients with mild memory problems. *Ann Intern Med* 2003;138:411–419].

✓ *DEMENTIA—CLINICAL OCCURRENCE:* *Congenital* Familial Alzheimer disease, adrenoleukodystrophy, Huntington disease, lipopolysaccharidoses, Wilson disease, mitochondrial disease, porphyria, Down syndrome (trisomy 21); *Endocrine* hypothyroidism, Addison disease, Cushing syndrome, hyper- and hypoparathyroidism; *Idiopathic* Alzheimer disease, Pick disease, Lewy body disease, progressive supranuclear palsy, frontotemporal dementias; *Inflammatory/Immune* vasculitis, subacute sclerosing panencephalitis, sarcoidosis; *Infectious* HIV infection, syphilis, prion disease (Creutzfeldt-Jacob disease [CJD], bovine spongiform encephalopathy [vCJD], others), progressive multifocal leukoencephalopathy (papovavirus), Whipple disease, postencephalitis; *Metabolic/Toxic* chronic alcoholism, vitamin B_{12}, thiamine, and nicotinic acid deficiency, uremia, liver failure, aluminum toxicity (dialysis dementia), postanoxia, drug intoxication; *Mechanical/Trauma* acute and chronic head trauma, normal pressure hydrocephalus, chronic subdural hematoma; *Neoplastic* paraneoplastic limbic encephalitis, brain tumors, and metastatic cancer; *Neurologic* nonconvulsive seizures, Parkinson disease; *Psychosocial* depression (pseudodementia), schizophrenia; *Vascular* vascular dementias (multiinfarct, Binswanger disease).

ALZHEIMER DISEASE: *Pathophysiology:* Neurofibrillatory tangles and plaques with extracellular deposition of amyloid precursor protein accumulate in the brain. The cause is partly genetic and possibly partly environmental. Slowly progressive dementia usually begins in the seventh or eighth decade of life; it may occur at younger ages, especially in the hereditary syndromes. The identical syndrome occurs uniformly in patients with trisomy 21 (Down syndrome) at an earlier age, usually in the fourth decade of life. The mental deterioration begins insidiously with memory loss, depression, anxiety, suspicion, and later amnesia, agnosia, aphasia, shuffling gait, and rigidity. The diagnosis is clinical, after excluding treatable forms of dementia. Imaging reveals diffuse atrophy of the cerebral cortex with symmetrical enlargement of the lateral and third ventricles. DDX: If severe psychiatric symptoms are present (e.g., hallucinations, psychosis), consider Lewy body disease. If the dementia is rapidly progressive, consider Creutzfeldt-Jacob disease (CJD) or variant CJD (vCJD, bovine spongiform encephalopathy).

S KEY SYNDROME

▼ **Psychosis:** See Chapter 15, page 896.

Other Syndromes

S KEY SYNDROME

▼ **Leg Discomfort Relieved by Walking: Restless Legs Syndrome (Ekbom Syndrome):** The patient complains of leg discomfort at rest, often prior to sleep. The sensation may be aching, drawing, pulling, prickling, restlessness, formication, or completely nondescript. Always bilateral, the sensations are relieved by walking or massage. There are no pertinent physical findings. The cause is unknown, but has been reported with iron and folate deficiency and uremia. Familial forms occur. Many patients also have periodic limb movements of sleep. Most patients obtain some relief with dopamine agonists [Earley CJ. Restless legs syndrome. *N Engl J Med* 2003;348:2103–2109].

S KEY SYNDROME

▼ **Horner Syndrome:** A lesion of the cervical sympathetic chain produces the following signs on the ipsilateral side: (a) partial ptosis of the upper eyelid and some elevation of the lower lid ("inverse ptosis"), (b) constriction of the pupil, miosis, accompanied by pupil dilation or delay after a light reflex, and (c) absence of sweating on the forehead and face of the affected side (see Fig. 14-20A, page 848). If damage to the sympathetics occurs early in life, pigmentation of the iris may be affected; for example, the affected iris may remain blue when the other changes to brown if the patient is brown-eyed. Horner syndrome occurs with ipsilateral mediastinal tumor and has been reported with spontaneous pneumothorax and brainstem stroke.

S KEY SYNDROME

Complex Regional Pain Syndrome (CRPS): Reflex Sympathetic Dystrophy, Causalgia: See Chapter 4, page 97.

Repeated Bell Palsy: Melkersson Syndrome: This is a triad of scrotal tongue (lingua plicata) with repeated attacks of Bell palsy and painless, nonpitting, facial edema. The cause is unknown.

S KEY SYNDROME

► **Death:** Death is an obvious fact of life. Most adults can make a reasonably accurate diagnosis of death, but occasional cases prove too complicated for the laypersons' abilities. One of the horror stories in medical history is a probably apocryphal episode in the life of Vesalius. In 1564, during the height of his European fame as an anatomist, he was appointed physician to Philip II of Spain. He is said to have conducted an autopsy in Madrid on a young nobleman who had been his patient. According to the custom of the time, this was carried out before a large crowd of citizens. When the thorax of the body was opened, the heart was seen to be beating, and the anatomist was compelled to leave Spain hastily. Such experiences have made it necessary to have a physician or other trained person pronounce the death of a patient.

Biological death is the cessation of function of all bodily tissues. In the process of dying, tissues and organ functions deteriorate at varying rates, so a precise end point is difficult to define. For ordinary purposes, it is conclusive to recognize the irreversible cessation of circulatory, respiratory, brain, or brainstem functions. This is partially assessed by unconsciousness and absence of the "vital signs" (cardiac activity, respirations, and maintained body temperature), but these indicators have proved inadequate in victims of cold water drowning, for example, when unconsciousness, apnea, and imperceptible heartbeat are still compatible with resuscitation and full recovery. Different criteria are also required for patients receiving mechanical respiration and cardiac pacing.

DEATH EXAMINATION (FOR MOST PATIENTS): Examine for evidence of heart contraction by palpating for pulsations in the carotid arteries and auscultating the precordium for heart sounds. An ECG will determine if cardiac electrical activity is present in the absence of mechanical contraction. Search for respiratory activity by placing the diaphragm of your stethoscope over the patient's mouth while listening for breath sounds. Also, hold a cold mirror at the nostrils and mouth to detect a deposit of water vapor. Neurologic function is assessed by several tests: call to the patient to test responsiveness; retract the eyelids to observe the pupillary reaction to light (fixed dilated pupils are seen with death and some drug intoxications); rotate the head from side to side with the lids retracted to observe whether the eyes remain fixed in their orbits or move in conjugate (doll's eyes), indicating an intact brainstem; perform ice water caloric stimulation if there are no eye movements; press the sternum and squeeze the Achilles tendons to look for a response to deep pain; lift and let fall the limbs to test for muscle tone; check for gag and corneal reflexes [Wijdicks EFM. The diagnosis of brain death. *N Engl J Med* 2001; 344:1215–1221].

▶ SUPPLEMENTARY DEATH EXAMINATION (ESPECIALLY FOR NEAR-DROWNING AND PATIENTS WITH MECHANICAL VENTILATORS AND PACEMAKERS): Victims of cold water immersion drowning experience rapid total body cooling (severe hypothermia) and may meet all the preceding criteria of death yet still be capable of resuscitation with excellent neurologic function after immersion of up to 1 hour. A reasonable practical guideline is that such patients are not dead until they are warm and dead. Other patients needing special consideration are those sustained by mechanical ventilation and pacemakers who fail to meet the cardiac and respiratory criteria for death, but who may be dead by irreversible loss of brain function. The clinician should always seek consultation from a neurologist in these complicated, atypical clinical situations.

Psychiatric and social disorders are common in medical settings. They are associated with an increased risk for nonpsychiatric illness and frequently confound the evaluation of patients presenting with nonspecific complaints. The student of medicine at all levels should read more specialized texts that deal with psychiatric illness and seek formal psychiatric consultation whenever doubt exists concerning psychiatric diagnosis. It is imperative to recognize that the presence of a psychiatric diagnosis in no way decreases the probability of serious organic disease in a patient with appropriate signs or symptoms. The challenge is to render appropriate diagnosis and therapy for all coexistent psychiatric and nonpsychiatric illnesses simultaneously, not sequentially. Delay in the diagnosis of organic disease in patients with psychiatric illness is all too common and should caution the clinician to take extra care in their evaluation.

The distinction between what we classify as neurologic versus psychiatric illness is a function of our understanding of brain physiology and pathophysiology. The distinction often rests on the presence of identifiable structural, genetic, physiological, or biochemical disorders in the neurologic category and their absence in psychiatric disease. Many psychiatric syndromes show genetic predispositions and respond to medications that alter brain function. Functional imaging studies are increasingly identifying localized abnormalities of brain function in some psychiatric disorders. For the practitioner, it is sufficient to recognize that the disorders we classify as psychiatric, although representing disorders of brain function, will be recognized by their clinical signs with abnormalities of thought, mood, affect, and behavior rather than specific tests of brain structure and clinical laboratory testing.

Social behavioral disorders and violence are also common problems in our society. To properly evaluate and care for patients, clinicians must be knowledgeable about the social situation of their patient. Social factors lead to patients presenting with a wide variety of complaints both physical and psychiatric. A complete social and psychiatric history with attention to current safety, a history of abuse (physical, sexual, emotional, financial), and the resources available to the patients for their care is essential in the evaluation of all patients.

This chapter does not provide a complete diagnostic approach to psychiatric illness. Rather, our purpose is to alert the clinician to the common psychiatric syndromes likely to be encountered in clinical practice and to provide some guidance to their recognition. The *Diagnostic and Statistical Manual of Mental Disorders (DSM-IV)*, published by the American Psychiatric Association, is a particularly valuable resource with which all practitioners should become familiar [American Psychiatric Association. *Diagnostic and Statistical Manual of Mental Disorders*. 4th ed. Washington, DC, American Psychiatric Association, 1994]. In addition to diagnostic criteria, the manual provides an overview of the epidemiology and presentation of mental disorders.

Section 1   THE MENTAL STATUS AND PSYCHIATRIC EVALUATION

THE MENTAL STATUS EVALUATION

Psychiatric diagnosis is based upon the patient interview and the exclusion of medical illness by appropriate history, physical examination, and, if needed, a selection of laboratory tests. The psychiatric interview requires time, patience, and experience. A wide variety of screening questionnaires are available to assist the clinician in the evaluation of psychological symptoms. Useful screening tools include the Mini-Mental State Exam (MMSE, page 827), clock drawing test, Beck Depression Inventory, Hamilton Depression Scale, and the Prime MD instruments [Spitzer RL, Williams JBW, Kroenke K, et al. Utility of a new procedure for diagnosing mental disorders in primary care: The Prime-MD 1000 study. *JAMA* 1994;272:1749–1756]. Overreliance upon these tools is not encouraged, but they can assist in the evaluation and selection of patients for referral.

The psychiatric evaluation addresses several dimensions of mental processes that are briefly discussed below.

- **Level of Consciousness.** See page 861. Patients are described as alert, lethargic, stuporous, or in coma. These are arbitrary categories and the patient's mental status may fluctuate. Though patients with mental illness may be lethargic from medications or intoxications, all patients who are less than fully alert should be assumed to have an organic neurologic disorder until such has been excluded.
- **Orientation**. This has three dimensions: person, place, and time. Does the patient know who he and others in the room are? Does he know their name and roles? Does he know where he is, the place, city, state, country? Does he know the year, season, day, and date?
- **Attention**. This is the ability to stay on task and follow the course of a conversation and interview, avoid distractions and focus on tasks. Attention deficits are the hallmark of delirium and should alert the clinician to the possibility of a metabolic disorder. Decreased attention is too frequently attributed to a lack of cooperativeness when, in fact, the patient is unable to cooperate. Tests of serial 7s, serial 3s (subtract 3 sequentially starting at 20), and attempting to spell "world" backwards are tests of attention. Always consider the patient's level of education in interpreting these tasks.

- **Memory**. This is the ability to register and retain material from previous experience. Memory is a complex phenomenon. It is usefully classified as immediate recall (registration), short- and long-term memory. Immediate recall is the ability to register items presented. Short-term memory is the ability to recall the registered items within 5–10 minutes. Long-term memory is the ability to recall events from the more distant past from days to years. Specific tests of immediate recall and short-term memory are included in the MMSE. Short-term and long-term memory are evaluated while taking the history.
- **Thought**. Thought has several dimensions. The *content* of thought is what the patient is thinking about. Is it appropriate to his situation and a reasonable perception of the world? The *sequence* of thoughts is also important. How are they linked one to the next? Can the patient digress and get back to the original point? The *logic* a person uses to connect events and explanations should be evaluated. What is the nature of cause and effect in his life? What are the reasons he gives for seeking care? *Insight* is the ability to look at one's self and situation with comprehension and understanding. Lack of insight into the nature or consequences of behaviors or thoughts is an important clue to mental illness. *Judgment* is the ability to make reasonable assessments of the external world and choices between alternative actions. How are decisions made? How does the patient evaluate alternatives? How are potential benefits and risks considered?
- **Perception**. This is global term for the way in which a person perceives the world through the senses. Distortions of perception can be symptoms of either neurologic or psychiatric disease. *Hallucinations* are sensory experiences perceived only by the patient, not by an observer. They may be auditory, visual, tactile, gustatory, or olfactory. Auditory hallucinations are particularly common in psychosis whereas visual hallucinations are more common in delirium. Gustatory and olfactory hallucinations are common in partial seizure disorders (temporal lobe epilepsy). *Illusions* are the incorrect perception of objects seen by both the patient and the observer. These are particularly common with sensory impairment such as visual loss. *Structural perception* is the ability to place objects and shapes in relation to one another. It can be tested by having the patient copy interlocked pentagons (MMSE) or perform the clock drawing.
- **Intellect**. Intellect is generally held to be an innate brain faculty, though it is difficult to separate deficits of intellect from deficits of education. The practitioner must know the patient's *educational and literacy level* in order to properly evaluate intellect. Culture greatly influences tests of intellect and it is hazardous to make assessments across cultures. Begin by having the patient demonstrate his ability to read and write. There are several dimensions of intellect. What is his *information* level? Does he know about important local, national or international events? What are his sources of information? *Calculations,* the ability to manipulate numbers, is tested by simple and gradually more complex arithmetic tasks. *Abstraction* is the ability to see general principles in concrete statements. Abstractions are tested by asking the patient to interpret proverbs, for example, "peo-

ple in glass houses shouldn't throw stones" = "don't criticize others for things you have probably done yourself." Interpretation at the simplest level, for example, "they would break the windows" is indicative of concrete thinking and a deficit in abstract thinking. Remember that proverbs are culturally bound and may not be recognizable to people from different cultural backgrounds. *Reasoning* is the ability to solve problems involving simple logical sequences. *Language* is tested in the interview and by having the patient follow both written and verbal instructions, and write a sentence (MMSE). Assess the patient's vocabulary and the complexity of the patient's spoken language.

- **Mood**. Mood is the sustained affective state of the patient. It is more like the tidal flow of emotion than the waves of affect. Mood is classified as normal, depressed or elevated. Mood should be assessed by asking the patient how his mood has been over the last 2 weeks. Other questions used to evaluate mood include questions regarding how the patient feels about his life, the patient's thoughts of the future, the patient's confidence in his abilities, and the patient's hopes, and the intensity of these feelings. If depression is suspected, it is mandatory to inquire about suicidal thoughts or plans. Depressed patients may show blunted affect with little range.
- **Affect**. This is the more transient state of emotion, which varies from minute to minute and day to day, depending upon the setting and types of social and personal interactions in which a person is engaged. Affect is the clinician's assessment of emotion and is assessed by facial expression, tone, and modulation of voice and specific questions about how the patient feels. Affect is also measured by considering intensity and range of expression. Affective states include happy, sad, angry, fearful, worried, and wary.
- **Appearance and Behavior.** Close observation of the patient during the interview will provide important information. How is the patient dressed and groomed? How is the patient's personal hygiene? Does the patient make and sustain eye contact? Does the patient answer questions promptly and fully? Are there areas of questioning that the patient avoids or tries to deflect? What is the patient's body language? Is the patient fidgeting or unusually still? What is the patient's tone of voice, volume, and speech rhythm?

Psychiatric Symptoms and Signs

This chapter discusses symptoms and signs together because in psychiatric illness, the symptoms and signs manifest together as the patient's behaviors and the patient's perception and description of those behaviors.

Abnormal Perceptions

We perceive the world through our senses which we take as reliable and valid measures of the external environment. Sensory perceptions are distorted as a result of injury to the sensory organs or pathways, from abnormal processing of the sensory perceptions or from false perceptions arising within the brain. Abnormal perceptions arising from primary injury to the sensory organs and their pathways are often negative (loss of perception) or represent an exaggeration or distortion of the normal sensory signal (e.g., tinnitus, paresthesia, hyperalgesia, allodynia). Abnormal perceptions arising in the processing centers and cortex are more often complex.

KEY SYMPTOM
Hallucinations: Hallucinations are abnormal sensory perceptions (auditory, visual, olfactory, or gustatory) that the patient may or may not recognize as unreal. They arise without external cues. Auditory hallucinations are common in schizophrenia, whereas visual hallucinations are more typical of delirium. Olfactory and gustatory hallucinations are common with partial seizures.

KEY SYMPTOM
Confusion: Delirium: See page 890.

KEY SYMPTOM
Abnormal Sleep Perceptions: Parasomnias:
These are disorders of perception or behavior associated with the sleeping state. The most common parasomnias are nightmares and sleep terrors. Auditory hallucinations occurring upon falling asleep and awakening are common, and do not indicate pathology in the absence of other hypnagogic symptoms.

Abnormal Affect and Mood

Feelings are the way we react emotionally to the perceptions and events of our lives. Normally we have a range of feelings throughout the day and the intensity of our feelings may vary over time, from periods or relative intensity to periods of less intensity. Abnormal extremes of feelings, either in degree or duration, may indicate psychiatric disorders.

KEY SYMPTOM
Change in Behavior and Mood: Any significant change in a person's behavior should raise the possibility of underlying medical or psychiatric illness. Changes in school or job performance and withdrawal from social activities should raise concerns about disorders of mood, thought or substance abuse.

ELEVATED AFFECT AND MOOD: Elevation of mood is a normal transient response to positive events. With abnormal elevations of mood patients experience grandiosity or inflated self-esteem, elation, lack of a need for sleep, racing thoughts ("flight of ideas"), loquaciousness, hyperexcitability, agitation, and increased risk taking in pleasurable activities (physical, sexual, financial). When persistent and associated with changes in sleep pattern it may be indicative of *hypomania;* when grandiose and irrational it is indicative of *mania.*

DEPRESSED AFFECT AND MOOD: *Depressed affect* is a transient normal response to negative events and feelings. *Depression of mood* is accompanied by the loss of interest in activities or pleasure, anorexia, weight loss, insomnia or somnolence, psychomotor agitation or retardation, fatigue, inappropriate guilt and/or a sense of worthlessness, loss of the ability to concentrate, thoughts of death and suicidal ideation. When persistent for more than 2 weeks and accompanied by changes in sleep, eating, and behavior, it may indicate an episode of *major depression. Dysthymia* is a persistent, usually lifelong form of mildly depressed affect, not meeting criteria for a major depression.

ANXIETY: This is a state of apprehension or fear accompanied by increased sympathetic nervous system activity. It is a normal response to threats, either physical or psychological, which resolves with resolution of the threat. It is abnormal when the feeling occurs or persists in the absence of real danger.

PHOBIAS: These are irrational fears of situations, events or objects that produce uncontrollable fear and anxiety in the patient. They are pathological when they lead to alterations in social or psychological function.

ANHEDONIA: This is an absence of pleasure from normally emotionally rewarding activities including eating, sexual stimulation, social activities, and personal or business success. It is characteristic of depression.

DEPERSONALIZATION: This is a feeling of being outside the body, an observer of yourself and surroundings. It is accompanied by a loss of affective connection with the people and events in one's environment. It is normal during highly stressful, traumatic events, but abnormal in other situations, especially if persistent or recurrent. Depersonalization may occur with anxiety disorders.

Abnormal Thinking

Thinking is the process by which we connect and explain events to ourselves and others. It is a relational activity of great complexity. Thought disorders may be manifest by verbal symptoms expressed by the patient or by abnormal behaviors resulting from the disordered thoughts.

KEY SYMPTOM

Paranoia: This is a feeling of being systematically threatened or persecuted by a person, persons, or organizations. It is pathological when the paranoia results from a fixed delusion and leads to alterations in activities. Paranoia may be a relatively mild personality trait or a manifestation of psychosis.

KEY SYMPTOM

Disordered Thinking: Thinking is usually logical and linked to an explicit rational system of cause and effect. The train of thought connecting each sequential idea is either apparent to an observer or readily explained by the patient and comprehensible to the observer. Disordered thinking is unconnected from thought to thought or connected by irrational or incomprehensible explanations. It is a sign of schizophrenia.

KEY SYMPTOM
Delusions: Delusions are unreal perceptions of the causal relations between perceptions, events and people. They have their basis in real sensory perceptions and occurrences, but the linkage between the real people or events are illusory. Delusions are often described as fixed, false beliefs, and are pathological when they continue to be believed despite strong, otherwise persuasive, evidence to the contrary. Delusions are characteristic of schizophrenia, manic psychosis, and delirium.

KEY SYMPTOM
Obsessions: Obsessions are recurrent, intrusive thoughts or fears that the person is unable to suppress or control despite recognizing that they are unreasonable. When disruptive of function they indicate obsessive-compulsive disorder.

KEY SYMPTOM
Compulsions: Compulsive activities are repetitive stereotypic behaviors that the patient feels compelled to perform in order to reduce distress or fear of an unavoidable outcome should they not be done. When disruptive of function they indicate obsessive-compulsive disorder.

Abnormal Memory

KEY SIGN
Amnesia: Amnesia is a loss of memory. It can be retrograde for events of the past, or antegrade, the inability to form new memories. It can be either global or selective for particular events or domains of memory. It is indicative of brain injury or psychological disorder.

Abnormal Behaviors

How we behave, our actions in private and public, is the result of how we feel, how we think, and how we perceive the constraints and rewards of the social environment. Behavior is culturally bound such that behaviors appropriate in one culture or setting may be quite inappropriate in another. Normative evaluations of thought, feelings, and private behavior are problematic at best; however, public behaviors are reasonably and readily subject to normative evaluation. Behaviors which are consistently abnormal or unacceptable are indicative of personality or psychiatric disorders.

KEY SYMPTOM
Suicidal Behavior: Expressed suicidal ideation, threats, gestures, and attempts are progressively more serious signs of a potentially life-threatening situation. All such behaviors should be taken seriously. The patient's safety is the first concern; identification and treat-

ment of the underlying problems should be undertaken either primarily or with referral.

KEY SIGN

Stereotypic Behaviors: Activities, movements, or vocalizations that are stereotypically repeated without appropriate precipitants or explanation suggest either tics, compulsions, or possibly complex partial seizures.

KEY SIGN

Catatonia: Catatonic patients exhibit a profound retardation in motor activity, retaining postures, expressing negativism, and repeating the phrases or motions of other persons (echolalia, echopraxia). It is indicative of psychotic states.

KEY SYMPTOM

Abnormal Sexual Feelings and Behaviors: Paraphilias: Paraphilias are abnormal and/or unusually intense feelings of sexual arousal toward inappropriate sexual objects such as children, animals, or nonhuman objects, or the need for inappropriate behaviors such as sadism or masochism during sexual activity. Paraphilic thoughts are not necessarily abnormal, but when acted upon, especially with nonconsenting partners or children, they are indicative of psychiatric illness.

KEY SIGN

Abnormal Eating Behaviors: Bulimia: Bulimia is alternating binge eating and purging with either induced vomiting or other cathartic activity. When the pattern is sustained and secretive it is indicative of a major eating disorder.

KEY SYMPTOM

Abnormal Eating Behaviors: Anorexia: See *Psychiatric Syndromes: Anorexia Nervosa and Bulimia Nervosa*, page 894.

KEY SYMPTOM

Abnormal Sleep Behaviors: Dyssomnias: These include difficulty getting to or maintaining sleep (*insomnia*), abnormal daytime sleepiness or sudden sleep onset (*narcolepsy*), sleep-disorder breathing (obstructive or central sleep apnea, and other disorders of the circadian sleep cycle (e.g., jet lag). The system review should always include questions about sleep quality and disruption. Abnormal sleep patterns may result from or lead to psychiatric disorders. Terminal insomnia is associated with major depression, while initial insomnia characterizes atypical depressive disorder [Schenek CH, Mahowald MW, Sack RL. Assessment and management of insomnia. *JAMA* 2003;289:2475–2479].

ABNORMAL SLEEP BEHAVIORS: SLEEP WALKING: This is classified as a parasomnia, like sleep terrors and nightmares. The patient may perform complex activities while asleep and awakens with no recollection. Hypnotic drugs are associated with an increased risk of sleep-walking behaviors related to the induction of antegrade amnesia.

ABNORMAL SLEEP BEHAVIORS: PERIODIC LEG MOVEMENTS OF SLEEP: Frequent leg movements during sleep are associated with arousals in obstructive and central sleep apneas. They can be quite disturbing to the bed partner, but the patient is unaware of the activity, other than finding the partner absent or the bedding disrupted. When the patient complains of an inability to hold the legs still on going to bed, consider restless legs syndrome (Chapter 14, page 878).

Psychiatric Syndromes

The disorders in this section are presented to help the clinician recognize them for the purposes of treatment or referral to a psychiatrist. Indications for psychiatric consultation or referral include suicidal or homicidal ideation, psychotic symptoms, severe anxiety or depression, mania, dissociative symptoms, and failure to respond to therapy.

To facilitate research, the American Psychiatric Association developed criteria for the diagnosis and classification of mental disorders. These have proved reliable and have improved the diagnosis and therapy of these problems. Practitioners should have a copy of its manual, the *Diagnostic and Statistical Manual (DSM-IV-TR)*, for assistance in your practice [American Psychiatric Association. *Diagnostic and Statistical Manual of Mental Disorders*. 4th ed. Washington, DC, American Psychiatric Association, 1994].

Multiaxial Assessment

The *DSM-IV* uses a multiaxial assessment method that provides a systematic approach to the description of each patient's disorders. Every practitioner should be familiar with this system.

Axis I: Clinical Disorders; Other Conditions That May be a Focus of Clinical Attention.
These are the major psychiatric and behavior syndromes addressed in the *DSM-IV*. If more than one disorder is present, the principle disorder or reason for the current visit is listed first.

Axis II: Personality Disorders; Mental Retardation
These are listed separately from Axis I disorders because they may coexist and complicate the diagnosis and management of Axis I problems.

Axis III: General Medical Conditions.
Here are listed medical conditions, by system, which may be important in the understanding and management of the Axis I and II disorders.

Axis IV: Psychosocial and Environmental Problems.

Problems in the social environment of the patient which influence the diagnosis, management or prognosis of the Axis I, II, and III problems are enumerated here.

Axis V: Global Assessment of Functioning.

The practitioner's assessment of the patient's global level of function is recorded using the Global Assessment of Functioning (GAF) Scale, a 0–100 scale descriptive of the degree of function and impairment as a consequence of the psychiatric (Axis I and II) disorders. The full scale is available in the *DSM-IV* at page 32.

The publications *Prime MD* (Roerig/Pfizer, New York) and *Symptom-Driven Diagnostic System for Primary Care* (Pharmacia-Upjohn, Kalamazoo, Michigan) are screening questionnaires based on diagnostic criteria for anxiety, mood, somatoform, eating disorders, and alcohol abuse. There are few, if any, specific signs or laboratory findings of psychiatric disease, so diagnosis depends principally upon an experienced observer obtaining a complete history from the patient and a collateral informant. The reader is encouraged to review specialized publications in the field.

Acute and Subacute Confusion

S KEY SYNDROME

Delirium: Acute Brain Syndrome, Acute Confusional State, Metabolic Encephalopathy:
Pathophysiology: Metabolic abnormalities (including prescription and nonprescription drugs), pain, restraints, or sleep deprivation impair cognitive function, particularly attention, judgment, and perception. This is actually a metabolic encephalopathy, but is discussed here because it is frequently confused with a primary psychiatric disorder, especially by examiners who have not known the patient in their premorbid state. This is a symptom complex characterized by fluctuations of mental status, progressive loss of orientation, confusion, and a high risk for long-term disability. Persons at highest risk are the elderly, especially those on multiple medications at the time of hospitalization. The chief features are *decreased attentiveness* (distractibility, loss of train of thought), *alteration of consciousness* (from hypervigilance and agitation to lethargy or coma), *disorientation* (for time and place), *illusions* (misinterpreted sensory impressions), *hallucinations* (mostly visual), *wandering and fragmented thoughts, delusions, recent memory loss,* and *affective changes.* The patient may be restless, or picking at the bedclothes. Myoclonus may be present. Some forms of delirium, for example, alcohol withdrawal, produce prominent autonomic dysfunction with fever, tachycardia, and hypertension (*delirium tremens*).

✓ *DELIRIUM—CLINICAL OCCURRENCE:* Common causes of delirium include drugs (e.g., sedatives, tranquilizers, alcohol, steroids, salicylates, digitalis, alkaloids), liver disease, uremia, hypoxia, hypoventilation, congestive heart failure, electrolyte abnormalities, urinary retention, fever, and infection. In hospitalized patients, sensory deficits, restraints, Foley catheters and invasive procedures are associated with an increased incidence of delirium.

Anxiety Disorders

S KEY SYNDROME

Generalized Anxiety Disorder: *Pathophysiology:* Anxiety is an experienced emotional state caused by activity in the deep cortical structures of the limbic system. In addition to the subjective feelings, anxiety triggers stress responses via the autonomic nervous system, which are felt by the patient and may heighten the sense of anxiety. Most persons experience some anxiety in response to stress, but excessive or continuous unfocused anxiety may be so debilitating as to require therapy. The causes of anxiety may be real, potential, or imagined. Autonomically mediated symptoms and signs include palpitations, tachycardia, tremor, chest pain, hyperventilation with paresthesias and dizziness, faintness, fatigue, diaphoresis, nausea, vomiting, diarrhea, and abdominal distress. The Hamilton Anxiety Rating Scale can be used to assess the severity of the symptoms. Significant impairment of social, occupational, or other important functioning is required for diagnosis.

S KEY SYNDROME

Anxiety Disorder: Panic Attack: Sudden intense fear or discomfort occurs often without an evident external cue. Symptoms include palpitations, sweating, tremor, shortness of breath, choking, chest pain, nausea, faintness or dizziness, paresthesias, and/or flushing accompanied by overwhelming cognitive turmoil, as in fear of dying, losing control, or "going crazy." Symptoms peak within 10 minutes and rarely last more than 30 minutes, leaving the patient feeling exhausted.

S KEY SYNDROME

Anxiety Disorder: Panic Disorder: This is the condition of recurrent panic attacks accompanied by an ongoing apprehension of recurrent attacks, worry about the prognostic implications of the attacks (their physical and psychologic meaning), or significant changes in behaviors as a result of the attacks.

KEY SYMPTOM

Anxiety Disorder: Agoraphobia: The agora was the marketplace in ancient Greece; hence the term agoraphobia, which implies a fear of crowding. This is a persistent fear of certain situations which might cause embarrassment or discomfort without escape, or which might precipitate a panic attack. These are often social situations involving groups of people, particularly within confined surroundings such as classrooms, churches, and stores. Agoraphobia commonly accompanies panic disorder.

Anxiety Disorder: Social Phobia: These patients have a compelling desire to avoid social contact, fearing embarrassment or humiliation.

Anxiety Disorder: Specific Phobias: Phobia may develop for almost any specific type of event or interaction. To qualify as a phobia, the anxiety must be consistently produced by the exposure, the fear must be excessive and unreasonable and recognized as such by the patient who then alters her usual patterns of behavior in order to avoid the situation, leading to social disruption or extreme distress.

S KEY SYNDROME

Anxiety Disorder: Acute and Posttraumatic Stress Disorders: Persons experiencing an event involving threatened or actual injury or death to themselves or others may develop significant anxiety either soon afterwards in an acute stress disorder or later with recurrences in a posttraumatic stress disorder. Flashbacks, depersonalization, denial, avoidance of stimuli that induce the memories, and enhanced arousal are manifestations of stress disorders [Yehuda R. Post-traumatic stress disorder. *N Engl J Med* 2002;346: 108–114].

S KEY SYNDROME

Anxiety   Disorder: Obsessive-Compulsive Disorder: Obsessive thoughts and compulsive behaviors occur in any combination. The patient recognizes the unreasonableness of a connection between the behavior and the feared event or outcome. The obsessive and compulsive behaviors, such as handwashing, door locking, and cleaning or arranging of possessions, consume more than 1 hour a day and interfere with social functioning.

Disorders of Mood

Mood is the sustained affective state of the patient. Mood can be depressed or elevated, or can cycle between depression and elevation. It is important to ascertain both the *amplitude* of the swings (the severity of the depression or elevation) and the *rate of cycling* between the states. Depressed and elevated moods are part of normal life. Grieving for a lost spouse or loved one may last for several months, but does not globally impair function.

S KEY SYNDROME

Disorders of Mood: Dysthymia: This is a chronic state of mildly depressed mood that is persistent, but not sufficiently severe to meet the criteria for major depression. Unlike depression, which is episodic, dysthymia is more chronic; a trait rather than a state.

S KEY SYNDROME

Disorders of Mood: Depression: See page 886. Depression is a sustained lowering of mood every day for at least 2 weeks in the absence of an obvious or appropriate precipitating event. Depression accompanies many serious medical illnesses or the medications prescribed for their treatment, which must be excluded as the cause before a diagnosis of major depression can be made [William JW, Noel

PH, Cordes JA, et al. The rational clinical examination. Is this patient clinically depressed? *JAMA* 2002;287:1160–1170].

S KEY SYNDROME

Disorders of Mood: Hypomania, Mania, Bipolar Disorder and Mixed Episodes: See page 885. Mania is characterized by episodes of abnormally elevated mood lasting for at least 1 week. Hypomania is less extreme and functionally successful, as opposed to the destructive consequences of mania. Mania or depression may occur alone (unipolar), or the patient may cycle between mania and depression sequentially over weeks, months, or years (bipolar), or within a single day (mixed episode).

S KEY SYNDROME

Suicide: Suicide attempt is a common and frequently fatal manifestation of psychiatric illness. Persons at highest risk include older men and adolescents, those with a specific plan, those with the intent to use firearms in their possession, and those with previous aborted attempts. All threats of suicide and expressions of suicidal ideation or intent should be taken seriously and immediate psychiatric consultation should be obtained. The practitioner's first obligation is to ensure the safety of the patient pending psychiatric evaluation.

Personality Disorders

S KEY SYNDROME

Abnormal Behaviors and Personality Disorders: Personality is a global description of how we think, feel, and interact with the world around us. Acceptable feeling and behaviors are culturally determined. Personality disorders are defined as persistent (rather than episodic) lifelong patterns of maladaptive feelings, thoughts, and behaviors. Patients have two or more of the following: *abnormal cognition*, that is, how they perceive other people, actions, and themselves; *abnormal feelings* about themselves, people, and events either in type, intensity, or duration; *difficulty functioning* with other people socially, educationally, or occupationally; *difficulty with impulse control*, leading to inappropriate behaviors. The personality traits are consistent over time, regardless of changes in the social surroundings, and produce significant stress and disruption of their lives. Underlying medical disorders and substance abuse must be excluded before the diagnosis can be made. Examples include narcissism, borderline, antisocial, histrionic, dependent, avoidant, and obsessive-compulsive personality disorders.

S KEY SYNDROME

Somatoform and Related Disorders: Hysteria, Hypochondriasis, Briquet Syndrome: Patients with these disorders have many symptoms without identifiable pathology to account for them. They have usually visited several physicians, who "can't seem to find out what's wrong with me." The diagnosis should not be made until organic causes for the complaints are excluded by thorough examination. Patients have often had many extensive evaluations so, absent serious abnormalities on the screening physical and laboratory examinations, the clinician should always obtain complete records of all previous workups before initiating expensive or invasive evaluations [McCahill ME. Somatoform and related disorders: Delivery of diagnosis as the first step. *Am Fam Physician* 1995;52:193–203].

SOMATOFORM DISORDERS: SOMATIZATION DISORDER: This disorder, which is much more common in women, begins before the age of 30 years and leads to frequent medical visits for evaluation and treatment of symptoms to such a degree that social, school, and job performances are impaired. Diagnostic criteria include pain in at least four different sites, two or more nonpainful gastrointestinal symptoms, at least one sexual or reproductive symptom without pain, and one pseudoneurologic symptom. The symptoms cannot be those expected of a general medical illness or a result of medications or abuse of alcohol or illicit drugs. Unlike in factitious disorder, the patient is not intentionally injuring herself or fabricating the symptoms [Barsky AJ, Borus JF. Functional somatic syndromes. *Ann Intern Med* 1999;130(11):910–921].

SOMATOFORM DISORDERS: HYPOCHONDRIASIS: Hypochondriac patients persist in expressing the fear of a serious illness despite the reassurance of concerned physicians who have searched thoroughly for clinical evidence of organic disease and found none [Barsky AJ. Clinical practice. The patient with hypochondriasis. *N Engl J Med* 2001;345:1395–1399].

S KEY SYNDROME
Factitious Disorders: In these disorders, patients consciously and intentionally produce symptoms and/or signs of disease to gratify psychological needs.

FACTITIOUS DISORDERS: MUNCHAUSEN SYNDROME: Munchausen syndrome is dramatic or dangerous behavior resulting in frequent hospitalizations for presumed severe illness. The most common symptoms and signs simulated by persons engaged in factitious behavior are bleeding from the urinary or gastrointestinal tract, diarrhea, fever, seizures, and hypoglycemia.

FACTITIOUS DISORDERS: MALINGERING: This represents intentionally deceptive behavior in which persons claim to have symptoms or signs of disease that will benefit them in some way, for example, obtaining narcotics for pain relief or financial support for disability.

S KEY SYNDROME
Eating Disorders: Marked changes in food selection and abnormal eating behaviors can indicate either organic disease or psychiatric disease.

ANOREXIA NERVOSA: Anorexia nervosa is most common in adolescent and young women with an overwhelming concern about body image and weight. It is accompanied by a distortion of the perceived body image—the patient seeing an overweight person where observers see normal body form or even emaciation. The patients may be obsessed with food, preparing meals for others but not eating themselves. Excessive exercise may accompany the anorexia as a means of achieving the desired body image. Appetite is severely suppressed or absent. Patients become severely malnourished with retardation of secondary sexual maturation, absent menses, and osteoporosis. Patients are at high risk for death from complications of malnutrition. Early recognition and intensive treatment is essential.

BULIMIA NERVOSA: Bulimia is recurrent, secretive, binge eating. The patient feels unable to control the compulsive eating and resorts to induced vomiting, purging with laxatives, and/or abuse of diuretics to avoid weight gain. Clues include erosion of tooth enamel from acid emesis, abrasions on the roof of the mouth and callus on the backs of the fingers from induced vomiting, and electrolyte disorders from use of laxatives and diuretics. Nutritional deficiencies and malnutrition are uncommon.

S KEY SYNDROME

Chronic Alcoholism: This is a compulsive behavioral disorder of imbibing ethyl alcohol repeatedly in biologically damaging quantities and repeatedly creating circumstances that are physically damaging and socially degrading to the drinker and others. It is a common ailment. Positive responses to the CAGE questions should raise the index of suspicion for chronic alcoholism. CAGE is an acronym helping the physician to recall questions that focus on *cutting* down, *annoyance* by criticism, *guilty* feeling, and *eye* openers (early morning drinks). The diagnosis is assured when behaviors that do damage to the drinker's health and reputation occur repeatedly. Such behavior is socially stigmatized; the patient is often reluctant to reveal it to the physician and may use all sorts of subterfuges and untruths to conceal it. To circumvent this and uncover the facts, the clinician must be persistent and gain the patient's confidence. Often, the questioning must be oblique instead of blunt. Details are sought that are pertinent to the diagnosis but not recognizable to the patient as being associated with alcoholism. A history of previous treatment for alcoholism, injury without explanation, unexplained seizures ("rum fits"), job loss, and arrests for driving under the influence are important. Physical signs consistent with chronic alcoholism include vascular spiders on the skin, hepatomegaly, wristdrop, peripheral sensorimotor neuropathy, cerebellar ataxia, and alcohol or aldehyde on the breath [Kitchens JM. The rational clinical examination. Does this patient have an alcohol problem? *JAMA* 1994;272: 1782–1787].

S KEY SYNDROME

Abnormal Impulsive Behaviors: Impulse Control Disorders: This group of disorders includes repetitive behaviors that range from the relatively minor (hair twisting and pulling:

trichotillomania), to the socially disruptive (compulsive gambling, explosive disorder) to the criminal (kleptomania, pyromania). Repetitive impulsive socially disruptive behaviors may be the result of psychiatric disorders, epilepsy, or tics (Tourette syndrome).

S KEY SYNDROME

Abnormal Behaviors: Adjustment Disorders: Sudden, especially unwanted, disruptions of the social environment can produce profound changes in mood and behavior. Failure to adjust in a reasonable period of time with restoration of normal mood or persistent maladaptive or self-destructive behaviors is indicative of an adjustment disorder with or without accompanying anxiety or depression. Common events requiring adjustment are termination of an intimate relationship, divorce, changing schools or communities, loss of employment, getting married, and becoming a parent.

S KEY SYNDROME

Abnormal Behaviors: Prolonged Grieving: Grieving the loss of a loved one is a normal event, an adjustment to a new type of life. The form and pattern of appropriate grieving is both individually and culturally determined. Normal grieving is a gradual process resolving the acute loss with a developing new appreciation for the lost person. With this resolution comes a restoration of a sense of purpose and the ability to find joy in life. Grieving associated with social withdrawal and depression disrupting normal activities and relationships and persisting for more than 2 months may indicate transition from the normal grief process to a psychiatric disorder.

Thought Disorders

S KEY SYNDROME

Schizophrenia and Other Psychoses: As the prototypical psychosis, schizophrenia is now considered to comprise a group of diseases that are probably etiologically distinct. Primary psychotic disorders occur in adolescence or young adult life. Onset of psychotic symptoms at older ages should raise concern about organic brain disease, drug intoxication or withdrawal, or psychosis complicating major depressive or bipolar disease. Schizophrenia involves problems in thinking, affect, socializing, action, language, and perception. *Positive symptoms* represent an exaggeration or distortion of normal functions, including delusions and hallucinations, especially auditory. *Negative symptoms* reveal loss of normal functions such as affective flattening, alogia, anhedonia, and avolition. *Disorganizational symptoms* include disorganized speech or behavior and short or absent attention span. Several subtypes are recognized. *Catatonic* patients exhibit a profound change in motor activity, retaining postures, expressing negativism, and repeating the phrases or motions of other persons (echolalia, echopraxia). *Paranoid* patients are preoccupied with at least one systematized delusion or auditory hallucination related to a single subject. *Disorganized* schizophrenic patients are disorganized in their speech and behavior and display a superficial or inappropriate affect.

Other Disorders

Other major categories of psychiatric syndromes which we do not have space to present inclusively include substance-related disorders, disorders usually first diagnosed in infancy, childhood or adolescence (including mental retardation, learning disorders, autism, attention-deficit and disruptive behavioral disorders, and tic disorders), dissociative disorders, sexual and gender identity disorders, eating disorders, sleep disorders, impulse-control disorders, adjustment disorders, personality disorders, relational problems (e.g., parent to child, siblings), and problems related to abuse or neglect. The reader should consult the *DSM-IV* for detailed discussion of these diagnoses.

Section 2   THE SOCIAL EVALUATION

Evaluation of Social Function and Risk

Health status is strongly correlated with socioeconomic standing. Among the factors known to correlate with health status are family income, community of residence, education, social connectedness (the number and strength of interpersonal relationships), marital status, and employment status. In addition to any role the social environment plays in the incidence of ill health, it often places significant limitations on the ability of an individual and family to cope with the financial and social demands of illness. The result is a vicious spiral of unmet needs.

Evaluation of the patient's social environment should be part of a global patient assessment. The clinician should inquire about marital status, living arrangements, financial limitations and concerns, health insurance, education, literacy (do not assume that several years of elementary and secondary education equates to being able to read or write), interpersonal relationships and personal support system, use of community social support systems, and sense of personal safety and security. It is important to inquire about the availability of heat in the winter and air conditioning in the summer for the elderly and chronically ill near the poverty level.

When questions arise or problems are identified, consultation with your local social service agencies is strongly advised. They are often able to assist patients with medications, transportation, and a wide variety of other services. **Identification of abuse or neglect is especially im-**

portant and the caregiver is required to report to the appropriate social agency children (younger than age 18 years) or elders (older than
age 64 years) who may be victims of abuse or neglect. The first prior-
ity in this situation is securing the safety of the patient, which may require hospitalization.

A description of a complete social evaluation is beyond the scope of
this text. Axis IV of the *DSM-IV* lists the following specific areas of psychosocial and environmental problems. This list is an excellent organizational scheme for identification and classification of these problems:

1. Problems with primary support group.
2. Problems related to the social environment.
3. Educational problems.
4. Occupational problems.
5. Housing problems.
6. Economic problems.
7. Problems with access to health care services.
8. Problems related to interaction with the legal system/crime.
9. Other psychosocial and environmental problems.

Common Social Syndromes and Problems

S KEY SYNDROME
Illiteracy: Inability to read and/or write is not uncommon. The
patient is often embarrassed by the problem and will not volunteer this
information. Learn to inquire tactfully and nonjudgmentally about the
patient's educational and literacy skills. Illiteracy should be suspected
when poor adherence to therapy plans and follow-up is identified.

S KEY SYNDROME
Homelessness: Homeless persons are at high risk for medical illness and abuse, and have high rates of serious psychiatric illness.

S KEY SYNDROME
Abuse and Neglect: Abuse is common and can affect
persons of any age and either sex. Child and elder abuse affects both
males and females, while women are much more commonly affected in
midlife. Abuse can be physical, sexual, emotional, or financial. The examiner should first inquire whether the patients have ever felt unsafe
in a relationship, then whether they have concerns about their current
safety, and last whether they wish help in dealing with the current problems. The safety of the patient, not the identification of a perpetrator, is
the first and most important goal of the interview. Remember that re-
porting of both child and elder abuse and neglect are mandatory.

S KEY SYNDROME

▼ **Isolation:** Social isolation is common, especially in the elderly, in those with impaired motor or communication skills, and in those with financial limitations. Isolation makes dealing with chronic illness more difficult and may increase the rate of cognitive decline in the elderly.

S KEY SYNDROME

▼ **Institutionalization:** A significant proportion of our society spends time living in various institutional settings from the relatively benign, such as boarding schools, to the punitive, such as prisons. Other institutional settings that may impact on health status are nursing homes and homes for the developmentally disabled. It is important to know the stresses and limitations each of these environments places on our patients.

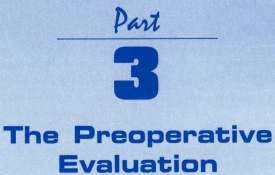

Part

3

The Preoperative Evaluation

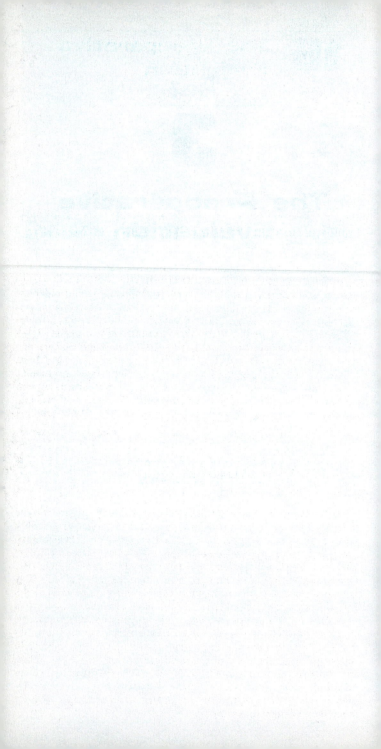

16 The Preoperative Evaluation

Introduction to Preoperative Screening

The goal of preoperative screening is to estimate the patient's risks and to minimize perioperative complications without unnecessarily delaying surgery or causing undue morbidity or cost. To appropriately counsel the surgeon and patient, your history, physical examination, and other studies should assess the risks for myocardial infarction, arrhythmias, heart failure, endocarditis, stroke, pulmonary insufficiency, venous thrombosis and pulmonary embolism, hemorrhage, diabetic acidosis, renal or hepatic failure, and, in the immunocompromised host, infection. When needed, you must make recommendations to minimize these risks by specific preoperative evaluations or treatments or with specific perioperative management strategies. Clinicians must balance the risks of proceeding directly to surgery against the risks of delaying a necessary procedure.

The History

First, determine the type and urgency of the proposed surgery and the patient's age and functional capacity. Ask if your patient can climb a flight of stairs or walk 2 blocks without symptoms. Patients who have symptoms with activities of less than four metabolic equivalents (METs) have poor functional capacity and have increased perioperative risk. One MET is defined as the energy expenditure for sitting quietly. This is equivalent to an oxygen consumption for the average adult of 3.5 mL/kg body weight per minute. Activities that correlate with 4–5 METs of activity include mopping floors, cleaning windows, painting walls, pushing a power lawnmower, raking leaves, weeding a garden, or walking up 1 flight of stairs. Walking 4 miles (6.4 km) per hour or cycling 10 miles (16 km) per hour on level ground constitutes 5–6 METs of activity. The ability to accomplish these activities without symptoms correlates with moderate or greater functional capacity and a lower perioperative risk. If the patient cannot perform these activities without symptoms, what are the symptoms?

Find out if complications have occurred with previous operations. Then focus the history and physical examination upon the specific areas of concern as outlined below.

Assessment of Cardiovascular and Pulmonary Risk from History

The most frequent cause of non-surgical perioperative morbidity and mortality is acute myocardial infarction. The patient's current history is the best method of risk assessment.

Ischemic Heart Disease

Does your patient have angina? If so, how frequent are the episodes of chest pain? Are they progressing in frequency? Do they occur at rest? Have they become less responsive to medication? Is there a history or ECG evidence of myocardial infarction? Has the patient had prior cardiac evaluations (stress tests or coronary angiography), coronary angioplasty, or bypass? If so, when, where, and what was found?

Heart Failure and Pulmonary Disease

Are there symptoms of congestive heart failure or pulmonary abnormality now or in the past, such as exertional dyspnea, orthopnea, paroxysmal nocturnal dyspnea, cough, or peripheral edema? If so, are these symptoms stable? Have there been prior estimates of cardiopulmonary function, such as cardiac catheterization, echocardiography, or pulmonary function tests? If so, when, and what were the results?

Dysrhythmias and Pacemakers

Has your patient experienced palpitations, syncope, or other symptoms of arrhythmias, or have arrhythmias been documented on prior ECGs or ambulatory monitoring? Specifically, is there high-grade atrioventricular block, symptomatic ventricular arrhythmias, especially those associated with structural heart disease, or supraventricular tachycardias at uncontrolled rates. Does the patient have an electronic pacemaker? If so, what is the type and model? When was it implanted, and when was it last checked?

Valvular and Congenital Heart Disease

Are there cardiac shunts or valvular abnormalities that require endocarditis prophylaxis? If these abnormalities are present, when was the last echocardiographic evaluation done, and what was the result? Is there evidence for severe valvular heart disease (e.g., aortic stenosis) that might require cardiac surgical intervention before proceeding with noncardiac surgery?

Cerebrovascular Disease

Have there been symptoms or a history of vascular insufficiency to the brain (transient ischemic attacks or stroke) or extremities (claudication)? If so, when, and what prior evaluations or interventions have been performed?

Venous Thromboembolism

Is there a history of deep venous thrombosis or pulmonary embolism? Have there been symptoms of hemoptysis, edema of the extremities, or pleuritic chest pains that might suggest these diagnoses? Have there been venous Doppler studies of the legs or studies of thrombophilia, for example, measurement of factor V Leiden mutation, lupus anticoagulant, antithrombin III, protein C or S?

Assessment of Bleeding Risk from History

A negative history assures you that the patient is not at increased risk for bleeding. If concerns arise from the history, a laboratory evaluation may be indicated.

Personal and Familial Coagulation Disorders

Did excessive hemorrhage occur with previous dental extractions, surgery, or childbirth? Is there a family history of excessive bleeding in these circumstances?

Platelet and Vessel Disorders

Does the patient experience gingival bleeding, epistaxis, menorrhagia, hematuria, melena, or excessive bleeding or bruising at venipuncture sites or from minor cuts? Has the patient noticed petechiae, spontaneous bruising, or bruises larger than a silver dollar with minor trauma?

Transfusion History

Has the patient ever had a blood transfusion or received procoagulant factor replacement at surgery?

Assessment of Metabolic Risk: Diabetes, Renal and Hepatic Insufficiency

Metabolic abnormalities are assessed so that they can be controlled preoperatively and managed through the perioperative period.

Diabetes

Are there symptoms of polyuria, polydipsia, polyphagia, or weight loss, or a history of diabetes mellitus? If the patient is known to have diabetes, what has been the recent blood sugar control? Does the patient use insulin? If so, what types, schedule, and doses? Does the patient use oral hypoglycemic agents? If so, which medications, schedules, and doses?

Hypoglycemia and Glucose Intolerance

Was there hypoglycemia, hyperglycemia, or acidosis with past surgeries, gestation, or infections?

Kidney Disease

Is there a history of renal insufficiency? If so, has the patient required dialysis in the past? What is the current state of their renal disease?

Liver Disease

Is there a history of hepatic insufficiency? If so, what is the current state of their liver disease? What is their albumin and prothrombin time/INR (international normalized ratio)?

Family History

Is there a family history of adverse reaction to anesthesia (for instance, malignant hyperthermia), deep venous thrombosis or pulmonary embolism, bleeding problems, diabetes mellitus, elevated cholesterol, hypertension, or heart disease?

Medications

Most chronic medications can be continued through the perioperative period. The exceptions are aspirin, warfarin, and nonsteroidal antiinflammatory drugs (NSAIDs) for certain procedures, and hypoglycemic agents whose dose should be reduced or held on the morning of surgery. All unnecessary medications should be discontinued. Avoid altering a chronic medication program just prior to surgery. The goal is to manage the medications and the medical problems through the perioperative period.

Beta-blockers have been shown to reduce cardiovascular complications in patients undergoing high risk surgery. If the patient is taking a beta-blocker, it should always be continued throughout the perioperative period.

Cardiovascular Drugs

Is the patient taking cardiac, antiarrhythmic or antihypertensive medications (e.g., adrenergic blocking drugs, a digitalis preparation, vasodilators including nitrates)?

Drugs Affecting Hemostasis

Is the patient taking any drugs that would affect hemostasis or increase the risk for thromboembolism, for example, NSAIDs, antiplatelet agents (including aspirin), warfarin, oral contraceptives, estrogens?

Pulmonary Mediations

Does the patient use bronchodilators for asthma or obstructive lung disease? If so, which medications and how often are they used?

Corticosteroids

Has the patient received corticosteroids in the last 12 months? If so, when, how much, for what reason, and for how long? Steroid-induced adrenal suppression may persist for up to a year after even relatively short courses of corticosteroids in doses above 10 mg/d. If this has occurred, coverage with stress doses of steroids starting just before surgery and continuing for 48–72 hours is advised.

Insulin and Hypoglycemics

Does the patient use insulin or other medications for diabetes mellitus? If so, what is the type of insulin, the schedule of administration, and the degree of control of the blood sugar?

Allergies and Drug Intolerances

Has the patient had an adverse reaction to any substance, including medications and radiology contrast materials? If so, describe the adverse reaction.

Personal Habits

Knowledge of a patient's habits will help you be alert for problems in the perioperative period such as drug or alcohol withdrawal.

Substance Use and Abuse

Has the patient been using alcohol or illicit or addicting drugs? If so, which drugs and when was the last time they were used? Drug withdrawal should be anticipated in the postoperative period if addicting drugs, including alcohol, were used recently.

Tobacco

Does the patient smoke? If so, how many cigarettes daily? Quitting smoking for at least 8 weeks prior to surgery is optimal.

Mechanical and Positioning Risks

Musculoskeletal Conditions

Does the patient have rheumatoid arthritis? Cervical spine instability can cause serious or fatal injury at the time of endotracheal intubation. Does the patient require particular care in positioning to avoid excessive pressure on deformed limbs? Has the patient been treated with corticosteroids (see page 906)?

The Physical Examination

Direct the physical examination at identifying active medical problems in key organ systems that could increase the risk of surgery or change the perioperative management.

Vital Signs

Obtain vital signs, including blood pressure, heart rate and regularity of rhythm, rate and ease of respiration, and temperature. Systolic blood pressure >180 mmHg, diastolic pressure ≥110 mmHg, or hypotension with clinical evidence of hypoperfusion or shock should be stabilized before proceeding to non-urgent surgery.

Heart Exam

Look for significant heart murmurs, gallop rhythms, evidence of ventricular overactivity, abnormalities of the jugular pulse and peripheral edema.

Vascular Exam

Examine for carotid, abdominal, and femoral bruits.

Lung Exam

Examine the lungs for crackles, wheezes, decreased breath sounds, prolonged expiratory phase, and effusions.

Skin Signs of Hemostatic Disorder

Examine for integrity of the skin, evidence of venous stasis in the lower extremities, petechiae, and unusual bruises.

Mental Status

Assess the patient's mental status. This is especially important in the elderly patient because cognitive dysfunction, which is easily missed without specific testing, greatly increases the risk for postoperative delirium [Inouye SK, Charpentier PA. Precipitating factors for delirium in hospitalized elderly persons. *JAMA* 1996;275:852–857].

Laboratory Tests

Based on the results of the history and physical examination, select the appropriate laboratory studies for confirmation and quantification of abnormalities. Routine laboratory tests are not useful unless there is a specific medical indication.

Electrocardiogram

Current evidence indicates that an ECG is not indicated for asymptomatic subjects undergoing low-risk procedures. Such low-risk procedures include endoscopic procedures, superficial procedures, transurethral prostate resection, cataract surgery, and breast surgery.

Obtain a 12-lead resting ECG for all patients with a recent episode of chest pain or ischemic equivalent (e.g., shortness of breath), patients with diabetes, and for intermediate or high-risk patients scheduled for intermediate or high-risk procedures.

Many, but not all, agree that an ECG should be obtained on all patients with prior coronary revascularization procedures, patients with prior hospitalization for heart disease, and on asymptomatic male patients older than 45 years of age or females patients older than 55 years of age with two or more risk factors for atherosclerosis.

Myocardial Perfusion Imaging

If the patient has known or suspected active coronary artery disease *and* an intermediate risk of perioperative cardiac complications, an intermediate-risk surgery, or poor functional capacity, *or* is to undergo a high-risk surgical procedure (aortic and other major vascular procedures or surgery with anticipated prolonged operative times associated with large fluid shifts and/or blood loss), consider further risk stratification using pharmacologic stress echocardiography or radioisotope myocardial perfusion imaging. *Intermediate-risk patients* have two or more of the following: mild stable angina pectoris (Canadian class I or II), insulin-treated diabetes mellitus, pathological Q waves on the ECG, a history of myocardial infarction or congestive heart failure, and/or renal insufficiency (creatinine ≥2.0). Some clinicians also include advanced age in this list. The need for surgery is not an independent indication for invasive coronary diagnostic or therapeutic procedures.

Chest X-Ray

A chest x-ray is indicated for all patients with respiratory symptoms, suspected congestive heart failure, valvular heart disease, or cardiac shunts.

Pulmonary Function Tests

If you identify severe pulmonary disease *and* the patient is undergoing a thoracic or upper abdominal procedure (higher risk for pulmonary complications), obtain pulmonary function tests with measurement of arterial blood gas. These will assist in the perioperative management of the patient.

Serum Chemistries

Serum chemistries are not required for low-risk procedures. For intermediate- and high-risk procedures, in the presence of diabetes mellitus, cardiac or renal disease, or when surgery is anticipated to be prolonged or associated with significant blood loss, obtain blood urea nitrogen (BUN), serum creatinine, blood glucose, and a complete blood cell count (CBC). Serum electrolytes, or at least potassium, should be included for patients with hypertension or for those taking medications likely to alter electrolyte balance.

Coagulation Studies

Obtain coagulation studies only for patients with a personal or family history suggesting a bleeding diathesis or thrombophilia.

All the above studies should be obtained for patients with poor or unstable general medical conditions.

Summative Risk Assessment

The purpose of the preoperative assessment is to estimate the risk for serious medical morbidity and death so that the surgeon and patient can make reasonable choices regarding the timing and risks of the planned surgical procedure. It is not the task of the medical consultant to either stop a planned surgical procedure or "clear" a patient for surgery. The consultant's task is to provide a sound risk assessment to the patient and surgeon. Avoid the common medical vernacular of "surgical clearance." The final decision of whether to operate, and when, is to be made by the patient and surgeon after reflection on the medical risk attendant to the surgery.

The major nonsurgical cause of perioperative mortality is myocardial infarction. Beginning with Goldman in 1977, a series of articles and guidelines have been published to assist the clinician in estimating the risk for cardiovascular complications in patients undergoing major surgery. These risk indices have been tested and refined over the years. A review of this literature is beyond the scope of this text; readers are encouraged to review the January 2003 issue of *Medical Clinics of North America* for a complete discussion of these topics [Cohn SL (ed). Preoperative medical consultation. *Med Clin North Am* 2003;1:1–289. This is a collection of 15 essays on preoperative and perioperative care].

One of the most recent and well-validated indices is that of Lee et al., the Revised Cardiac Risk Index [Lee TH, Marcantonio ER, Mangione CM, et al. Derivation and prospective validation of a simple index for prediction of cardiac risk of major noncardiac surgery. *Circulation* 1999; 100:1043–1049]. They identify six independent risk factors for cardiac complications: high-risk surgery, a known history of ischemic heart disease, congestive heart failure (current or by history), cerebrovascular disease, insulin-treated diabetes, and a creatinine ≥2.0. The risk for complications if 0 or 1 risk factor was present was <1.0%; for 2 risk factors, 1.3%; for 3 risk factors, 4%; and for ≥3 risk factors, 9%. This is a simple and easy to use index, but the clinician still must combine this with an assessment of the significant noncardiac risks.

Beta-blockers should be considered for all patients with coronary artery disease undergoing high risk procedures [Cohn SL, Goldman L. Preoperative risk evaluation and perioperative management of patients with coronary artery disease. *Med Clin North Am* 2003;87:111–136], absent any absolute contraindications. Their benefit in other patient groups or with lower risk procedures is unclear.

BIBLIOGRAPHY AND ADDITIONAL READING

1. ACC/AHA Task Force Report. Guideline update for perioperative cardiovascular evaluation for noncardiac surgery. *Circulation* 2002; 105:1257–1268, or *J Am Coll Cardiol* 2002;39:542–553.
2. Kajani AS, Taubert KA, Wilson W, et al. Prevention of bacterial endocarditis: Recommendations by the American Heart Association. *JAMA* 1997;277:1794–1801.

3. Palda VA, Desky AS (Clinical Efficacy Assessment Subcommittee of the American College of Physicians). Guidelines for assessing and managing the perioperative risk from coronary artery disease associated with major noncardiac surgery. *Ann Intern Med* 1997;127:309–312, and 313–328.
4. Smetana GW. Preoperative pulmonary evaluation. *N Engl J Med* 1999; 340:937–944.
5. Velanovich V. Preoperative laboratory evaluation. *J Am Coll Surg* 1996;183:79–87.
6. Goldmann DR, Brown FH, Guarnieri DM (eds). *Perioperative Medicine: The Medical Care of the Surgical Patient.* 2nd ed. New York, McGraw-Hill, 1994.

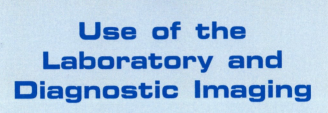

Part

4

Use of the Laboratory and Diagnostic Imaging

Where is the wisdom we have lost in knowledge?
Where is the knowledge we have lost in information?

T.S. Eliot
Choruses from "The Rock"

17 Principles of Diagnostic Testing

Diagnostic accuracy has been greatly enhanced by the sensitive and specific tests available in modern clinical laboratories and the rapid advances in clinical imaging. However, it is essential to recognize that proper use of the laboratory and imaging modalities is dependent upon accurate clinical hypotheses generated by the clinician at the bedside. Laboratory tests and diagnostic imaging can provide reliable and valid answers to well-conceived clinical questions, but they are also liable to overinterpretation and can be quite misleading if not interpreted in the clinical context as answers to particular questions. Beyond a few screening tests, these studies should be used to test physiologic and diagnostic hypotheses generated during the history and physical examination. The laboratory and the radiology suite are not the places to go looking for ideas; they are the place to test your ideas. If you are unable to generate testable hypotheses after the history, physical exam, and screening tests, it will be more useful to seek consultation than to begin an undirected series of laboratory and radiologic studies.

A full discussion of the proper use of diagnostic tests is beyond the scope of this text. The reader is referred to the reading list at the end of this chapter. *Clinical Epidemiology: The Essentials* by Fletcher et al. is especially valuable. The reader is advised to read this text and incorporate the principles of clinical epidemiology into your everyday practice.

Principles of Laboratory Testing

Laboratory testing is principally done for two reasons: (a) to obtain information that cannot be determined clinically, but which is often important in forming hypotheses; and (b) to test hypotheses.

Tests in the first category are those commonly described as "routine" testing and include serum electrolytes, blood urea nitrogen (BUN), creatinine, complete blood counts, urinalysis, and, less commonly, transaminases and erythrocyte sedimentation rate or C-reactive protein. Some, or all, of these tests are performed in patients with significant illness in order to help the clinician identify significant abnormalities in major organ function or laboratory signs of inflammation or infection.

Tests in the second category are innumerable, and more are being developed as you read this. They are used to identify specific abnormalities and diseases. The diagnostic performance of these tests is highly dependent upon the patient population tested. Tests in this category are most useful when the diagnosis in question is in the mid-range of probability on the basis of your clinical assessment—that is, the probability for the disease being present is roughly between 20 and 80%.

To understand why this is so, it is necessary to understand the measures of test performance and how interpretation is dependent on both the diagnostic criteria for a disease or condition and the pretest probability that the disease is present.

Principles of Testing for Disease

Disease Present or Absent

The first question is how do we determine who has the disease and who does not? This is done with an independent test or set of criteria accepted as establishing "the diagnosis." The assumption is that a disease is either present or absent. Although this may seem obvious for diseases such as cancer or an infection where a tissue biopsy or culture are the diagnostic standards, most biologic measurements are continuous variables, not either/or determinations; it is often difficult to say whether rheumatoid arthritis is present or not, or which level of creatinine determines renal failure.

Most diseases have variable clinical severity; hence the diagnostic standard used to establish the disease can be either very inclusive (sensitive) or more exclusive (specific). A good example is the American Rheumatologic Association (ARA) criteria for the diagnosis of rheumatic syndromes. These criteria were developed because no laboratory tests of sufficient accuracy are available to identify these patients. The goal was to identify persons eligible for inclusion in research studies of the specific diseases. Hence, the criteria for diagnosis of these syndromes is set to be quite specific; that is to say, that patients meeting the criteria are very likely to have the syndrome. However, it cannot be concluded that patients not meeting the criteria, who have many of the features and no other explanation, do not have the syndrome.

Test Positive or Negative

The definition of normal for continuous variables is a statistical determination (see the discussion of cholesterol in Chapter 18 for an exception). At what point "abnormal" becomes an illness or disease is a judgment based upon the desire to identify those with disease (*true positives*), but not include a significant portion of patients without the disease (*false positives*). Furthermore, most tests are not positive in all the patients with a given disease, so there will be patients with the disease who are missed by the test (*false negatives*). Finally, we want to be sure that a very high proportion of patients who don't have the disease, have a negative test (*true negatives*).

The decision of what cutpoint constitutes an abnormal test is determined by comparing the distribution of the test results in patients with

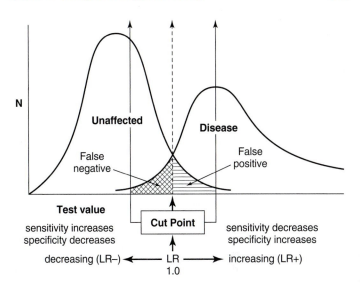

Fig. 17-1 Interpretation of Test Results. *A population of unaffected patients is compared with a population of diseased patients. The cut point for determining normal-abnormal is the value with the best compromise between sensitivity and specificity. Likelihood ratios can be calculated for test values above and below the usual cut point.*

the disease (determined as above) and in those without the disease (Fig. 17-1). When the two populations overlap in part of their range, a cutpoint is chosen to minimize the misallocation of patients (false positives and false negatives).

Note, however, that much of the information is lost in looking at tests of continuous variables as positive or negative: very abnormal tests are more likely to be associated with disease than mildly abnormal tests. As we discuss below, likelihood ratios are a good way to capture this information for making diagnostic decisions.

Probability and Odds

Probability is a ratio or proportion of one part of a population to the population as a whole. A racehorse that wins 1 race in 20 has a probability of winning of 0.05 (1/20 = 0.05).

Odds are the ratio of two probabilities. Because most events are uncommon (otherwise we wouldn't need to make all these calculations), odds are customarily expressed as the odds against an event. For our horse the probability of losing is 0.95 while the probability of winning is 0.05., that is, the odds are 19:1 that it will lose.

Odds and probabilities can be derived from one another:

$$\text{Odds} = \text{Probability}/(1 - \text{Probability})$$
$$\text{Probability} = \text{Odds}/(1 + \text{Odds})$$

Pretest Probability

We have generated a set of hypotheses at the bedside and have formulated a differential diagnosis (see Chapter 1). An essential part of the differential diagnosis process is to make a conscious assessment of the probability for the patient to have each disease in the differential diagnosis. If we were to see 100 patients exactly like the patient before us—same age, sex, comorbidities, presenting symptoms and physical signs—how many would have each condition? This estimate is the *pretest probability*. Expressed as odds (the probability of having the disease over the probability of not having the disease) this known as the *prior odds*.

2 × 2 Tables

Tests can be systematically evaluated in a 2-cell × 2-cell table whose parameters are whether the disease is present or absent and whether the test is positive or negative (Fig. 17-2) by predetermined criteria. The four cells, conventionally labeled *a, b, c,* and *d,* represent the true positive tests (disease present and test positive), the false-positives tests (disease absent, but test positive), the false-negative tests (disease present, but test negative), and the true negative tests (disease absent and test negative), respectively.

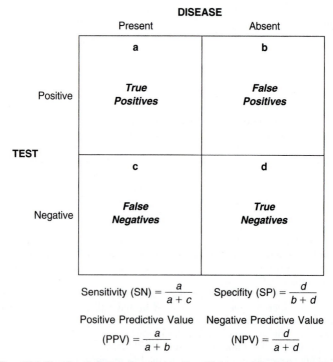

Fig. 17-2 The 2 × 2 Table: Sensitivity, Specificity, and Positive and Negative Predictive Values.

Prevalence of Disease

What additional information is in the table? We can see in the first column all the patients who have the disease $(a + c)$ and in the second column all the patients who are free of disease $(b + d)$. The ratio of the first column to the sum of the two columns is the *prevalence* of disease in the group of patients who generated the data in the table: *prevalence = $(a + c)/(a + b + c + d)$*.

To know how to interpret this prevalence, we need to know how the patients were selected for inclusion in each column. If this was a randomly selected, population-based sample, then the prevalence is that of the disease in the population, often a useful number. On the other hand, the investigators may have selected a group of patients with the disease and another group known not to have the disease in a predetermined ratio or by some nonrandom method. If this is the case, the "prevalence" is essentially meaningless for understanding disease prevalence in any useful clinical sense.

Aids in the Selection and Interpretation of Tests

Sensitivity (Sn)

Sensitivity is the number of patients with the disease who have a positive test, divided by the total number with the disease: *sensitivity = $a/(a + c)$*, a probability. *With highly sensitive tests, the vast majority of patients with the disease have a positive test (very few false negatives).* Tests with high sensitivity (>0.95) are most useful when negative, thereby making the diagnosis less likely. Note that the sensitivity of a test, because it is calculated only in those with the disease, is independent of the prevalence of the disease. Sensitivity can be increased by changing the cutoff for defining a positive test to a less abnormal value (see Fig. 17-1).

Because sensitivity is independent of prevalence, it is susceptible to overinterpretation when disease prevalence is very low (see *Example 1* below). In this case, the false-positive tests (b) may significantly out number the true positives (a).

Sensitive tests are used when you do not wish to miss a serious disease because of the consequences of a delayed diagnosis. A negative result makes the disease unlikely and helps to reassure the patient and clinician, and serves to narrow the diagnostic possibilities. A positive test needs to be confirmed with more specific tests before a diagnosis can be established.

Specificity (Sp)

Specificity is the proportion of patients without the disease who have a negative test: *specificity = $d/(b + d)$*, a probability. *With highly specific tests, the vast majority of patients without the disease have negative tests (very few false positives).* However, the test may also be negative in those with the disease. Note that patients with the disease do not enter into the determination of specificity; it, like sensitivity, is independent of the disease prevalence. Specificity can also be improved by changing the cutpoint for defining abnormal to a more abnormal value (see Fig. 17-1).

Because specificity is independent of prevalence, it is susceptible to overinterpretation when disease prevalence (pretest probability) is high (see *Example 4* below). In this case, the false-negative tests (c) may significantly out number the true negatives (d).

Highly specific tests are used to confirm a diagnosis. This is especially important when the consequences of the diagnosis are serious for the patient, either for prognosis or therapy.

Setting Your Positive/Negative Cutpoint

For most diagnostic tests, the clinical laboratory supplies a reference range (see Chapter 18). This range is determined by testing hundreds of samples of unselected patients, patients with the disease, and patients known to not have the disease. From this data, graphs such as Fig. 17-1 can be generated. The data are analyzed to determine the statistical best fit for distinguishing the diseased from the nondiseased populations.

For many clinical tests, such as treadmill exercise tests, interpretation of imaging studies, and application of diagnostic tests, the clinician must decide, based upon the clinical scenario and the type of diagnostic question being asked (screening, case finding, hypothesis testing) what cutpoint will best serve to answer the question. Consultation with specialists in laboratory medicine and with experts in the diseases in your differential diagnosis can assist you in determining what should be regarded as a positive or negative test in each specific clinical situation.

Predictive Values

When we do a test, we are not really interested in the test (sensitivity and specificity), but in how it can help us in understanding our patient's problem: does the presence of a positive test predict that the patient has the disease (*positive predictive value*) and does a negative test predict the absence of the disease (*negative predictive value*). Predictive values are calculated from 2×2 tables (see Fig. 17-2). As we shall see, the predictive values for a test are dependent upon the population which was used to generate the data in the 2×2 table; different populations have different disease prevalence. To generate meaningful predictive values, the patients generating the data must be chosen randomly from a clinical population that is relevant to your question and patient.

POSITIVE PREDICTIVE VALUE (PPV). The PPV is calculated from our 2×2 table. It is the proportion of patients with a positive test who have the disease: $PPV = a/(a + b)$, a probability. Tests with a high PPV have few false-positive tests, therefore a positive test supports the diagnosis. Note, however, that if the disease is rare in the population (therefore $(b + d) >> (a + c)$, the test will have to be extremely specific (low false positives, b) for the true positives to be greater than the false positives (see examples). Therefore, when the pretest probability of disease is low (low prevalence), even seemingly good tests (sensitivity, specificity) may perform badly for predicting the presence of disease.

NEGATIVE PREDICTIVE VALUE (NPV). The NPV is the proportion of patients with a negative test who do not have the disease: $NPV = d/(c + d)$, a probability. Tests with a high negative predictive value have few false negatives, therefore a negative test argues against the disease. When the condition is very likely in the population to begin with, a negative test may not be very helpful; that is, the NPV may be low and the disease may be present despite a negative test.

Consequently, to use the PPV and NPV, the clinician must know, or have a good estimate of, the prevalence of the condition being tested for in the clinician's population. Most clinicians do not have this data readily available. What we do have is our clinical estimate of the probability of disease that we have generated from our history and physical examination in generating our differential diagnosis.

Likelihood Ratios (LR)

Another way of expressing the usefulness of a test is in *likelihood ratios (LR)*. A *positive likelihood ratio (LR+)* is the ratio of the probability of a *positive* test in people with the disease (the sensitivity) to the probability of a *positive* test in people without the disease: $LR+ = [a/(a + c)] \div [b/(b + d)]$. A *negative likelihood ratio (LR−)* is the probability of a *negative* test in patients with the disease divided by the probability of a *negative* test in people without the disease (the specificity): $LR− = [(c/a + c)] \div [d/(b + d)]$ (Fig. 17-3). Likelihood ratios, the ratio of two probabilities, *are odds*.

Likelihood ratios show how well a result more abnormal (LR+) or less abnormal (LR−) than a given value for the test (the cutpoint for "test positive" in the 2×2 table) discriminates between those with and without the disease. They are a function of the defined parameters of the test and are independent of the prevalence of the disease (see the examples). Likelihood ratios contain all the sensitivity and specificity information *and* express the relationship between sensitivity and specificity for positive and negative results.

A big advantage of likelihood ratios is that they can be calculated for a range of test values, rather than the single normal/abnormal cutpoint used for sensitivity and specificity. Thus, likelihood ratios allow us to use all the information, rather than the limited information in a single normal/abnormal cutpoint.

As the LR+ becomes larger, the likelihood of the disease increases; as the LR− approaches zero, the disease becomes much less likely. Generally speaking, LR between 0.5 and 2.0 are not useful and those <0.5 but >0.2 or >2.0 but <5.0 are suggestive but not conclusive. Values of LR+ >5 argue strongly for the disease whereas LR− <0.2 argue strongly against the disease.

Posttest Probability

Likelihood ratios include information from each cell of the 2×2 table; they are not susceptible to the errors that occur in the application of pre-

DISEASE

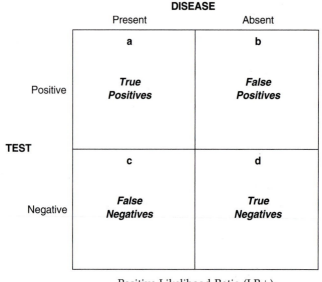

Positive Likelihood Ratio (LR+)
LR+ = [a/(a + c)] ÷ [b/(b + d)]

Negative Likelihood Ratio (LR−)
LR− = [c/(a + c)] ÷ [d/(b + d)]

Fig. 17-3 Positive and Negative Likelihood Ratios.

dictive values to conditions of low and high prevalence, respectively, as discussed above. This makes them much more useful diagnostically.

Because likelihood ratios are a ratio of probabilities, they are an expression of odds. We can use them to derive a new probability for the disease based upon the test result. Because this new probability is determined after the test is done, it is the *posttest probability* (PP). To calculate the posttest probability, convert the pretest probability to pretest odds and then multiply by the LR to get the posttest odds *(posterior odds)*. Then, convert the posttest odds back to the posttest probability (see example 1). The posttest probability can be calculated for both a positive test and a negative test.

Clinicians should learn to think in terms of the likelihood ratio for the parameter ranges of the tests they use. This is the implicit reasoning that experienced and efficient clinicians use in selecting and interpreting their laboratory tests. It is useful to make this process explicit. This allows us to actually do the calculations in the occasional situation where it will be useful, but also helps us to understand and dissect our decision making processes and to avoid misinterpretation of the significance of either normal or abnormal laboratory results [Barry HC, Ebell MH. Test characteristics and decision rules. *Endocrinol Metab Clin North Am* 1997;26:45–65].

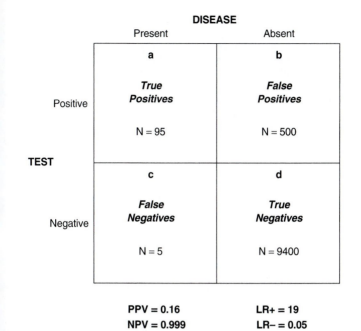

DISEASE

	Present	Absent
Positive	**a** *True Positives* N = 95	**b** *False Positives* N = 500
Negative	**c** *False Negatives* N = 5	**d** *True Negatives* N = 9400

TEST

PPV = 0.16   **LR+ = 19**
NPV = 0.999   **LR− = 0.05**

Fig. 17-4 Example 1: Disease Prevalence 1%. *The test has a sensitivity of 0.95 and a specificity of 0.95.*

Examples

Four examples of clinical testing scenarios are given, each with different estimated disease prevalence. For each example the test is assumed to have 95% sensitivity and 95% specificity. These examples should help you to understand the concepts discussed above.

Example 1: Disease Prevalence 1% (Fig. 17-4)

Of 10,000 patients, only 100 have the disease (99:1 odds against). False positives are five times more likely to be found than true positives. The calculations will only be shown for this example.

Calculation of Positive and Negative Predictive Values:

$$\text{PPV} = \frac{a}{a+b} = \frac{95}{95+500} = .16$$

$$\text{NPV} = \frac{d}{c+d} = \frac{9400}{5+9400} = .999$$

Calculation of Positive and Negative Likelihood Ratios:

$$\text{LR+} = [a/(a+c)] \div [b/(b+d)] = [95/(95+5)]$$
$$\div [500/(500+9400)] = 19$$

$$\text{LR−} = [c/(a+c)] \div [d/(b+d)] = [5/(95+5)]$$
$$\div [9400/(500+9400)] = 0.05$$

The PPV is better than the baseline risk (0.01), but is still quite low, so a positive test doesn't even make the diagnosis very probable. The NPV is 0.999 (1 in 10,000), which sounds good, but is actually not much better than the already low baseline risk of 0.01 (1 in 100).

Has this highly sensitive and specific test helped you in this situation? Not much. Although the odds of disease are much higher with a positive test (from 99:1 to 16:1), still most positive tests are false positives and further evaluation is necessary.

This example is typical of a screening situation for an uncommon disease in an asymptomatic population. The test has to be very sensitive and very specific to be useful. An example of such a test is HIV testing in pregnant women, but most clinical tests have neither the sensitivity nor specificity required to be effective when disease prevalence is low.

Example 2: Disease Prevalence 10% (Fig. 17-5)

Of 1000 patients, 100 have the disease (9:1 odds against).

    PPV = 0.65   LR+ = 19
    NPV = 0.999   LR− = 0.05

In this scenario, 65% of the patients with a positive test have the disease; a definite improvement over 10% at baseline. A positive test is

DISEASE

		Present	Absent
		a	**b**
Positive		*True Positives*	*False Positives*
		N = 95	N = 45
TEST		**c**	**d**
Negative		*False Negatives*	*True Negatives*
		N = 5	N = 855

PPV = 0.65   LR+ = 19
NPV = 0.999   LR− = 0.05

Fig. 17-5 Example 2: Disease Prevalence 10%. The test has a sensitivity of 0.95 and a specificity of 0.95.

twice as likely to be a true positive as a false positive. The NPV is quite low, so a negative test is helpful for reducing the likelihood of disease.

Are either the positive or negative results likely to be diagnostically sufficient? A negative test is useful to reduce the posttest probability of disease below any reasonable clinical threshold. A positive test will need to be followed with more specific testing to confirm the diagnosis (raise the probability of disease above the level needed for clinical certainty). This is especially true for any disease with an adverse prognosis or for which therapies are potentially toxic.

This scenario is representative of a case finding strategy in an at risk population. A test with 95% sensitivity and specificity could be used to separate the population into a low-risk pool and a high-risk pool, the latter to undergo further testing.

Example 3: Disease Prevalence 50% (Fig. 17-6)

You have worked up a patient and your clinical impression is that the patient has a 50% chance (1:1 odds) of having the disease (disease prevalence of 0.5). You construct a 2 × 2 table with what you know.

PPV = 0.95   LR+ = 19
NPV = 0.95   LR− = 0.05

DISEASE

		Present	Absent
TEST	Positive	**a** **True Positives** N = 95	**b** **False Positives** N = 5
	Negative	**c** **False Negatives** N = 5	**d** **True Negatives** N = 95

PPV = 0.95   LR+ = 19
NPV = 0.95   LR− = 0.05

Fig. 17-6 Example 3: Disease Prevalence 50%. For these examples the test has a sensitivity of 0.95 and a specificity of 0.95.

The PPV and NPV are both significant improvements over the baseline risk of 0.5. There are relatively few false positives or false negatives.

Does the test help you in this clinical situation? The test is clinically useful regardless of the result. Both a positive and a negative test make substantial changes in the disease probability, and both probably exceed the level of certainty required in most clinical situations.

This example is representative of the situation in which laboratory testing is most useful—true uncertainty, with even odds for and against the disease. Selecting tests with good likelihood ratios in this setting will have a profound impact on your diagnostic process.

Example 4: Disease Prevalence 90% (Fig. 17-7)

You have worked up a patient and your clinical impression is that the patient has a 90% chance (9:1 odds in favor) of having the disease (disease prevalence of 0.9). You construct a 2 × 2 table with what you know.

PPV = 0.95   LR+ = 19
NPV = 0.73   LR− = 0.05

It is quite likely the patient has the disease based upon your clinical assessment. A positive test (PPV) only minimally improves your accu-

	DISEASE	
	Present	Absent
Positive	**a** *True Positives* N = 855	**b** *False Positives* N = 5
Negative	**c** *False Negatives* N = 45	**d** *True Negatives* N = 95

TEST

PPV = 0.95   LR+ = 19
NPV = 0.73   LR− = 0.05

Fig. 17-7 Example 4: Disease Prevalence 90%. *The test has a sensitivity of 0.95 and a specificity of 0.95.*

racy. A negative test (NPV) reduces the probability, but it is still the most likely diagnosis, and one-third of those with a negative test will be misclassified (false negatives).

Has the test helped you in reaching your predetermined levels of certainty required to either diagnose the disease or exclude it from further consideration? No, a positive result adds nothing and a negative result is likely to be an error.

This scenario is representative of a situation when too high a level of certainty is expected for the clinical situation. Neither a positive or negative test is helpful.

COMMENT. Note that the test has excellent likelihood ratios, and the likelihood ratios are the same regardless of the prevalence of disease. Like sensitivity and specificity, likelihood ratios are a function of the value of the test chosen as the cutpoint. This confirms that the likelihood ratio tells how well a positive and negative test discriminate the population into higher and lower risk groups. However, the interpretation and usefulness of the test still depends upon the baseline probability of disease (pretest probability): a 20 times improvement in very long odds is still long odds (999:1 to 49:1), and a 20 times decrease in very short odds is still an almost even proposition (1:24 to 20:24).

The reader is encouraged to construct their own examples and vary the prevalence of disease and the sensitivity and specificity of the test in order to familiarize themselves with these concepts. The formal calculations are rarely done in clinical practice, but the principles and concepts are used every day by skilled clinicians in deciding how to evaluate their differential diagnoses.

As demonstrated in Example 3, diagnostic testing is most useful when true uncertainty exists with nearly even odds for and against the condition. The purpose of forming a probabilistic differential diagnosis is to identify the conditions which are truly uncertain (approximately even odds) where testing can improve your probability assessment. When clinical probability estimates are either very high or very low, further testing is not useful.

Most physical findings do not have likelihood ratios of sufficient magnitude to be used as a clinical test for the diagnosis [McGee S. *Evidence-Based Physical Diagnosis.* Philadelphia, WB Saunders, 2001]. Many laboratory tests do, however, have likelihood ratios that allow accurate diagnostic discrimination. Remember that the history and physical exam are primarily for hypothesis generation; the laboratory is usually the best place to test your specific hypotheses.

2 × 2 Tables Revisited: Caveat Emptor

If you plan to use the sensitivity, specificity or likelihood ratios generated from a 2 × 2 table, it is necessary to understand the methods used for selection of the test sample that produced the data. Each of these parameters is dependent upon the inclusion criteria for the categories disease-present and disease-absent, and the method for identifying the population(s) that were tested.

Severity of Disease

Most diseases have a broad spectrum of severity that is generally reflected in the amount of aberration in the tests characteristic of the disease: more-severe disease, more abnormal tests; less-severe disease, less abnormal or even normal test results. As can be seen from Fig. 17-1 and the preceding discussion, if the investigators choose to define the presence of disease as those with more-severe disease (cutpoint moved to the right), the test will appear more specific and less sensitive, and the positive likelihood ratio will improve, while the negative likelihood ratio becomes less useful. If they choose an inclusive definition to reflect the broad range of those with the disease (cutpoint moved to the left), the test will be more sensitive and less specific, and the negative likelihood ratio will improve, while the positive likelihood ratio becomes less useful. In addition, if the 2×2 table was constructed using patients with unusually severe disease (as may be seen in an academic referral practice), the sensitivity and specificity calculated may be inappropriately high if applied to a more representative population of patients.

Sampling

Broadly speaking there are three methods of identifying patients to generate data for a 2×2 table.

By far the easiest method is to take patients from a known diseased group (e.g., patients with known lupus attending a rheumatology clinic) and another group of patients from a nondiseased population (e.g., blood donors) and apply the test (e.g., an antinuclear antibody test) to both groups. This will generate a 2×2 table weighted to more-severe disease because the patients are already diagnosed and attending a clinic (see *Severity of Disease* above). The apparent prevalence is not a real population prevalence; it is an a priori choice of the investigators as to how many people they want in each group. Tests evaluated by this method often appear very good when you calculate the sensitivity, specificity, and likelihood ratios. Because the population of the table is really two independent populations, the PPV and NPV have no meaning. The clinical usefulness of information generated by this sampling method is marginal at best when the clinician attempts to apply the test parameters to an unselected population.

The second, far more difficult, method is to select a population of patients that represent the community at large (e.g., a random sample of adults), perform the test on all of them, and also evaluate *all* of them by the gold-standard criteria for the disease. When diseases have a low prevalence in the population (e.g., systemic lupus erythematosus), huge numbers of patients would need very thorough evaluations at tremendous expense to identify enough cases to produce any meaningful data. Hence, this method is only applied to the evaluation of screening tests proposed for large populations (e.g., fecal occult blood testing for colon cancer). This method also doesn't generate clinically useful data for the clinician outside of the screening paradigm.

The most clinically useful information is generated by selecting patients from a population that presents with the challenge faced by the physician: patients who might have the disease based upon history and physical exam (an intermediate pretest probability, near even odds). A consecutive series of such patients is identified and the test and diagnostic gold standard are applied to *all*. The data generated in this way is far more useful to the clinician when faced with a diagnostic challenge. The test parameters (likelihood ratios, sensitivity, and specificity), the prevalence of disease, and the PPV and NPV are much more likely to be applicable to clinical decision making. The clinician still must assess whether the gender, ethnic mix, ages, and comorbidities of the test population are representative of their patient population.

Rule In; Rule Out

The phrases "rule in" and "rule out" are commonplace in the clinical vernacular, but are discouraged.

Some diagnoses can be *confirmed* by specific pathologic tests (e.g., neoplasms, vasculitis), by laboratory tests (e.g., HIV infection, myocardial injury, sickle cell disease), and by microbiologic tests (e.g., cultures and polymerase chain reaction [PCR] identification of specific organisms).

It is impossible, short of necropsy, to "rule out" a diagnosis. When tests with highly negative likelihood ratios are negative in patients with intermediate or low pretest probability for the disease, the *probability* of the disease becomes very small, but never zero. In each clinical case, we empirically set a clinical level of certainty required to confirm a diagnosis, as we discussed in Chapter 1. We also determine a level of certainty needed to effectively exclude a diagnosis from consideration. This will depend upon the patient, the clinical scenario, and the risk associated with drawing a false-negative conclusion. When we have assured ourselves that the diagnosis is less probable than our threshold, we can say it is excluded clinically, but it is never "ruled out."

Furthermore, many clinical conditions, especially syndromes (e.g., rheumatoid arthritis), have no gold-standard diagnostic test or exclusion criteria.

Summary

The skilled clinician uses a patient's history and physical examination to generate pathophysiologic and diagnostic hypotheses. A differential diagnosis includes those diseases with the highest estimated probability of being present *in this patient*, and less likely diseases associated with severe morbidity if not promptly diagnosed. An explicit estimation of the probability for each is made. Tests are selected for which the result (positive, negative, or a specific value or finding) will generate a posttest probability (applying the likelihood ratios) of a clinically significant high or low level. On the basis of the first round of test results and repeat examination of the patient, a refined differential diagnosis is generated and a second round of tests may be ordered. This process is repeated until the posttest probability for the diagnosis exceeds the threshold required by the clinical situation. At that point, a working diagnosis is established.

Principles of Diagnostic Imaging

Imaging techniques include standard radiography and computed axial tomography (CT) using x-rays with or without contrast, magnetic resonance imaging (MRI), ultrasonography (including Doppler flow measurements), and radioisotope imaging (standard nuclear medicine and positron emission tomography [PET]). The amount of information contained in an imaging study is enormous, especially with CT and MRI technologies. This increase in information may be essential for the care of patients, or it may be a distraction in the diagnostic process. Imaging techniques are rapidly evolving, so it is essential to work closely with your radiologist to select the appropriate imaging studies to answer your questions.

Static images reveal the structure of the body; the questions they are able to answer are anatomic, not physiologic questions. Images tell us where anatomy is altered and suggest how it is altered. Images cannot make pathologic, microbiologic or physiologic diagnoses. Be sure your radiologist describes the images and the anatomic abnormalities using descriptive language, rather than conclusions. Radiologists cannot diagnose granulomas, tuberculosis, cancer or infection. They can describe lesions with characteristics suggestive of these diagnoses.

Dynamic imaging allows accurate evaluation of the mechanical properties of certain organs, such as blood flow in arteries and veins and heart muscle and valve function. They also allow reasonably good estimates of intravascular pressure gradients from the Bernoulli equation, which relates flow to the pressure gradient across areas of restricted flow.

As with all tests you order, beyond the most standard laboratory evaluation discussed above, each imaging study must be ordered to answer a specific question. Ordering imaging studies without a hypothesis or specific question, is a bad practice and often leads to the identification of incidental findings (anatomic variants, degenerative conditions, benign neoplasms, cysts, and hemangiomas) that distract the attention of the clinician, even when they have no plausible bearing on the patient's presenting complaints. It is easy to begin evaluating the imaging studies (and the laboratory abnormalities) rather than the patient.

The conclusions drawn from an imaging study need to be drawn by the clinicians who are familiar with the patient. You want the diagnostic and physiologic hypotheses of the radiologists, but only after you have their descriptions. Again, an easily made mistake is to let the imaging specialist begin to direct the evaluation, often of incidental findings or clinically irrelevant questions. Clinically important questions relevant to the presenting problem should be the drivers of the imaging evaluation. Incidental findings can be followed up, if needed, at a later time.

It is extremely uncommon for incidental findings to have major significance for the patient.

ADDITIONAL READING

1. Fletcher RH, Fletcher SW, Wagner EH. *Clinical Epidemiology: The Essentials*. 3rd ed. Baltimore, MD, Williams & Wilkins, 1996.
2. McGee S. *Evidence-Based Physical Diagnosis*. Philadelphia, WB Saunders, 2001.

This chapter discusses the normal and pathologic values for commonly ordered tests of the blood (cells and chemistries), urine, cerebrospinal fluid, and other serous fluids. The tests discussed here are those in common use for helping to formulate physiologic and diagnostic hypotheses. There are many more tests used in the diagnosis of a specific disease. These tests are highly specific, but may not be sensitive. They are a useful means for confirming an hypothesis, but should not be used until a narrow differential diagnosis has been established. These more specific tests are not discussed here.

Laboratory tests are ordered by the clinician for one of four reasons:

1. **Screening:** A small number of tests have been demonstrated to find "silent" disease in the patient who has no symptoms or signs or specific risk factors for the disease. Common examples include testing for hemochromatosis with iron studies and for hypercholesterolemia.
2. **Case finding:** Some tests are used to find disease in specific clinical populations at risk, even if signs or symptoms are not present. They differ from screening tests because they are not used in the general population. An example is testing the bone density of elderly women for osteoporosis.
3. **Diagnosis:** This is the use of tests to assist in making (or excluding) a diagnosis suggested by the symptoms and signs in patients. See the discussion in Chapter 17 for a summary of the proper approach to diagnostic testing.
4. **Monitoring:** Tests are often used to monitor the progress of disease, response to therapy, or concentration of medication.

Many laboratory tests are used for more than one, or even for all, of these reasons, depending on the clinical situation. For example, blood glucose is used to screen for diabetes mellitus, to identify cases amongst obese patients with a family history of diabetes who are at high risk for diabetes, to confirm the diagnosis, and to monitor treatment in patients found to have the disease.

The decision as to which tests, if any, should be obtained routinely can be debated interminably. Certainly, the prevalence of the disease in the population of which your patient is a member should affect the selection [HC Sox: Probability theory in the use of diagnostic tests. *Ann Intern Med* 1986;104:60–66]. In addition to assisting in the diagnosis, quantitative test results help to grade the severity of the physiologic abnormalities and provide objective verification for the purposes of documentation. Tests and their usefulness continually change, so the clinician must keep abreast of current indications and uses for tests available in his clinical laboratory. Consultation with the pathologist in charge of the clinical laboratory is often useful when questions arise.

The reference ranges are presented for purposes of illustration only. Because each clinical laboratory determines its own reference ranges, those we have listed are not intended to be definitive.

Many organizations, including the American Medical Association, have supported the proposal of the American National Metric Council to convert units of measurement to Système International (SI) d'Unités units. Citing what they perceive to be good reasons, US physicians and staffs of laboratories and hospitals have been reluctant to convert to SI units introduced in the mid-1980s. Indeed, excellent medical journals have chosen to use conventional (or both) units rather than to insist on conformity. For the non-American reader's convenience, we have included values with SI units in parentheses following the conventional units. (Most of the laboratory reference values were adopted from *Harrison's Principles of Internal Medicine*, 15th ed., Appendix A [*Harrison's Principles of Internal Medicine*, 15th ed. New York, McGraw-Hill, 2001].

Each test is followed by lists of diseases and disorders in which abnormal values occur. The lists of associated diseases, syndromes, and conditions highlight the more prevalent causes of the abnormalities and some important rarer diseases. The lists are not inclusive of all possibilities, but should be used as a guide for your thinking.

Consult textbooks of laboratory medicine for more complete discussions.

Blood Chemistries

ALBUMIN.   See *Proteins*, page 948.

ALKALINE PHOSPHATASE, SERUM.   *Pathophysiology:* This includes a number of cellular enzymes that hydrolyze phosphate esters. They are named from their optimum activity in alkaline media. High concentrations of the enzymes occur in the blood during periods of rapid growth, either physiologic or pathologic, and from cellular injury. The enzymes are normally plentiful in hepatic parenchyma, osteoblasts, intestinal mucosa, placental cells, and renal epithelium. Abnormally rapid growth or cell destruction will augment the blood concentration of these enzymes.

Normal Alkaline Phosphatase: 30–120 U/L (SI Units: 0.5–2.0 nkat/L). It is high in newborns, declining until puberty and then rising every decade after 60 years of age.

Increased Alkaline Phosphatase. This is usually associated with disorders of bone, liver or the biliary tract. *CLINICAL OCCURRENCE: Technical Error* dehydration of blood specimen; *Endocrine* hyperparathyroidism (osteitis fibrosa cystica), acromegaly, hyperthyroidism (effect on bone), subacute thyroiditis, last half of pregnancy; *Idiopathic* Paget disease, benign transient hyperphosphatasemia; *Infectious* liver infections (hepatitis, abscesses, parasitic infestations and infectious mononucleosis), chronic osteomyelitis; *Inflammatory/Immune* primary biliary cirrhosis, sarcoidosis; *Mechanical/Trauma* healing fractures, common bile duct obstruction from stone or carcinoma, intrahepatic cholestasis, passive congestion of the liver; *Metabolic/Toxic* osteomalacia, rickets, drug reactions (intrahepatic cholestasis), chlorpropamide, ergosterol, sometimes intravenous injection of albumin, pernicious anemia, hyperphosphatasia, dehydration, rapid loss of weight; *Neoplastic* osteoblastic bone tumors, metastatic carcinoma in bone, myeloma, liver metastases, cholangiocarcinoma; *Neurologic* cerebral damage; *Psychosocial* abuse with skeletal trauma; *Vascular* myocardial, renal, and sometimes pulmonary infarction.

Decreased Alkaline Phosphatase. *CLINICAL OCCURRENCE: Technical Errors* use of oxalate in blood collection; *Endocrine* hypothyroidism; *Idiopathic* osteoporosis; *Inflammatory/Immune* celiac disease; *Metabolic/Toxic* vitamin D toxicity, scurvy (vitamin C deficiency), milk-alkali syndrome, pernicious anemia/B_{12} deficiency.

ANION GAP, SERUM. *Pathophysiology:* The anion gap is the difference between the concentrations of measured cations and the measured anions in the blood, measured in milliequivalents per liter, mEq/L: $AG = [Na^+] - ([Cl^-] + [HCO_3^-])$. The anion gap accounts for phosphates, sulfates, amino acids, and albumin.

Normal Anion Gap: 12 ± 2.

Increased Anion Gap. An increased anion gap indicates the accumulation of organic acids and the presence of an *anion gap metabolic acidosis*. *CLINICAL OCCURRENCE:* Ketoacidosis (diabetes, alcoholism, starvation), intoxication with salicylates, methanol or ethylene glycol, lactic acidosis, or renal failure.

Decreased Anion Gap. This occurs uncommonly and suggests the accumulation of positively charged proteins in the blood. *CLINICAL OCCURRENCE:* Multiple myeloma.

ALANINE AMINOTRANSFERASE, SERUM: ALT. *Pathophysiology:* This enzyme occurs mostly in hepatocytes with smaller quantities in skeletal and heart muscle. It is released into the circulation when cells are damaged or necrotic.

Normal Concentration: 0–35 U/L (SI units: 0–0.58 μkat/L).

Increased ALT. Increased ALT usually indicates damage to the liver, although severe damage to skeletal muscle can produce significant elevations. *CLINICAL OCCURRENCE: Infectious* viral hepatitis, infectious mononucleosis, liver abscess; *Mechanical/Trauma* passive liver congestion, extrahepatic biliary obstruction; *Metabolic/Toxic* drug-induced liver disease, alcohol; *Neoplastic* hepatocellular carcinoma, liver metastases.

ASPARTATE AMINOTRANSFERASE, SERUM: AST. *Pathophysiology:* This enzyme is concentrated mostly in the cells of the heart, liver, muscle, and kidney; lesser amounts are in pancreas, spleen, lung, brain, and erythrocytes. Tissue injury releases the enzyme into the extracellular fluids, but not necessarily in amounts proportionate to the injury.

Normal AST: 9–40 U/L.

Increased AST. This usually reflects damage to the liver, the muscles, including the heart, and, less commonly, to other organs. It usually rises in concert with the ALT. When the AST is ≥2.0 times the ALT, alcohol abuse with cirrhosis or alcoholic hepatitis should be suspected. *CLINICAL OCCURRENCE: Technical Error* false-positive from opiates and erythromycin, dehydration of blood specimen; *Congenital* muscular dystrophy; *Endocrine* diabetes mellitus; *Idiopathic* Paget disease, cholecystitis; *Infectious* viral hepatitis, pulmonary infections; *Inflammatory/Immune* hemolytic diseases, polymyositis, pancreatitis, regional ileitis, ulcerative colitis; *Mechanical/Trauma* severe exercise, clonic and tonic seizures, crushing or burning or necrosis of muscle, inflammation from intramuscular injections, rhabdomyolysis, peptic ulcer, extrahepatic biliary obstruction; *Metabolic/Toxic* hepatic necrosis and drug-induced hepatitis, uremia, myoglobinemia, pernicious anemia, drugs (salicylates, alcohol), dehydration; *Neoplastic* bone metastasis, myeloma; *Neurologic; Psychosocial; Vascular* myocardial, renal and cerebral infarction.

Decreased AST. *CLINICAL OCCURRENCE: Endocrine* pregnancy; *Metabolic/Toxic* chronic dialysis, uremia, pyridoxine deficiency, ketoacidosis, beriberi, severe liver disease.

BICARBONATE, TOTAL SERUM (HCO_3^-, CO_2 CONTENT). *Pathophysiology:* Bicarbonate (HCO_3^-) is formed in the kidney by carbonic anhydrase and diffused through the body fluids as ionized bicarbonate in association with sodium. Bicarbonate is the major buffer consumed when protons (H^+) are produced by the metabolism of amino acids or the increased production or ingestion of organic acids. It accumulates to buffer the acidosis of hypoventilation (increased $PaCO_2$). In respiratory alkalosis with a low $PaCO_2$, the kidney excretes bicarbonate to maintain the blood pH and the bicarbonate concentration falls.

Normal Serum Bicarbonate: 22–26 mEq/L (SI: 22–26 mmol/L).

Increased Bicarbonate.   This indicates a *metabolic alkalosis*, either primary or secondary to a respiratory acidosis. *CLINICAL OCCURRENCE: Endocrine* hyperaldosteronism, Cushing disease, severe hypothyroidism;   *Metabolic/Toxic* primary metabolic alkalosis (diarrhea, gastric suction, nausea, and vomiting), diuretics (especially loop diuretics), hypercapnia;   *Psychosocial*   bulimia, purging.

Decreased Bicarbonate.   A decreased bicarbonate concentration indicates the presence of a *metabolic acidosis*. These are further classified by the anion gap, see page 935. *CLINICAL OCCURRENCE: Endocrine* Addison   disease;   *Metabolic/Toxic* hypocapnia   from hyperventilation, metabolic acidosis, for example, renal failure, ketoacidosis (diabetic, alcoholic, starvation), lactic acidosis, salicylate intoxication, methanol or ethylene glycol intoxication, renal tubular acidosis.

BILIRUBIN, TOTAL SERUM. *Pathophysiology:* See *Jaundice, page 539.* Unconjugated bilirubin is insoluble in water until conjugated in the liver with glucuronic acid. Four-fifths or more is derived from the catabolism of the heme from aging erythrocytes. The water-soluble conjugated bilirubin is normally excreted in the bile. It is bound to the plasma proteins; when the level exceeds 0.4 mg/dL, the water-soluble form appears in the urine.

Normal Serum Bilirubin: 0.3–1.0 mg/dL (SI Units: 5.1–17 μmol/L).

Increased Bilirubin: Hyperbilirubinemia.   Increased bilirubin indicates an increased breakdown of red blood cells or failure of hepatic excretion. *CLINICAL OCCURRENCE: Congenital* Dubin-Johnson disease, Gilbert syndrome;   *Idiopathic* acute cholecystitis; *Infectious* viral hepatitis, infectious mononucleosis;   *Inflammatory/ Immune* hemolysis;   *Mechanical/Trauma* common bile duct obstruction, hemolysis;   *Metabolic/Toxic* drug-induced hepatitis, alcoholic hepatitis, cirrhosis, or any cause;   *Vascular* pulmonary infarction, gastrointestinal bleeding, hematoma.

Unconjugated Hyperbilirubinemia.   This is caused by hemolysis, ineffective erythropoiesis, decreased hepatic uptake of unconjugated bilirubin (Gilbert syndrome), or impaired hepatic conjugation (neonatal jaundice, drugs or Crigler-Najjar syndrome).

Conjugated Hyperbilirubinemia.   Because the liver is able to conjugate bilirubin, the problem is either hepatocyte excretion (Dubin-Johnson syndrome, Rotor syndrome), intrahepatic cholestasis (hepatitis, drugs, granulomatous disease), or bile duct obstruction.

Decreased Bilirubin: Hypobilirubinemia.   Nonhemolytic anemias and hypoalbuminemia.

BLOOD UREA NITROGEN, SERUM: BUN.   *Pathophysiology:*   Molecular weight 60. Urea is synthesized in the liver from ammonia derived from the metabolism of protein in the body and gut. It is filtered and reabsorbed by the kidney; reabsorption is inversely related to the rate of urine flow.

Normal Serum Blood Urea Nitrogen (BUN):   10–20mg/dL (SI Units: 3.6–7.1 mmol/L).

Increased BUN.   An increase indicates decreased glomerular filtration and/or increased tubular reabsorption, or increased production in the gut from ingested protein or blood. *CLINICAL OCCURRENCE: Prerenal*   hypotension, hemorrhage, dehydration (vomiting, diarrhea, excessive sweating), Addison disease, hyperthyroidism, heart failure, sepsis, upper gastrointestinal hemorrhage, increased protein ingestion;   *Renal*   any cause of acute or chronic renal insufficiency; *Postrenal*   obstruction of the ureters, bladder, or urethra.

Decreased BUN.   *CLINICAL OCCURRENCE:* Low-protein diets, muscle wasting, starvation, cirrhosis, cachexia, high urine flow.

BUN:Creatinine Ratio Greater than 10:1.   This indicates relatively preserved glomerular filtration with either increased urea production or decreased urine flow. *CLINICAL OCCURRENCE:* Excessive protein intake, blood in the gut, excessive tissue destruction (cachexia, burns, fever, corticosteroid therapy); postrenal obstruction, inadequate renal circulation (heart failure, dehydration, shock).

BUN:Creatinine Ratio Less than 10:1.   This indicates decreased urea production. *CLINICAL OCCURRENCE:* Low protein intake, multiple dialyses, severe diarrhea or vomiting, hepatic insufficiency.

B-TYPE   NATRURETIC   PEPTIDE.   *Pathophysiology:* Heart failure is accompanied by increased wall tension in the ventricles and atria because of dilation. Natruretic peptides types A and B are released into the circulation in congestive heart failure.

Normal Concentration: <50 pg/mL.

INCREASED B-TYPE NATRURETIC PEPTIDE.   This test is used to identify patients with dyspnea and pulmonary infiltrates who have heart failure from those with primary pulmonary disorders [Maisel AS, Krishnaswamy P, Nowak RM, et al. Rapid measurement of B-type natriuretic peptide in the emergency diagnosis of heart failure. *N Engl J Med* 2002;347:161–167].

CALCIUM, SERUM (CA²⁺). *Pathophysiology:* Approximately 99% of the body calcium is in the form of insoluble phosphate and carbonate bound to the collagen matrix of the bones. It is in equilibrium with a small amount in the extracellular fluid. The amount varies with the rate of absorption of Ca^{2+} from the small intestine and the resorption rate in the kidney. Calcium is present in the three forms: *ionized* or *free* Ca^{2+} that is physiologically active; *protein-bound* or *nondiffusible* Ca^{2+}, most of which is loosely bound to plasma albumin; and *complexed* or *complex-bound* Ca^{2+}, which forms relatively soluble fractions complexed with carbonates, citrates, or phosphates. *Parathormone (PTH)* accelerates release of Ca^{2+} and PO_4^{3-} from bone with increased excretion of urinary PO_4^{3-}. PTH stimulates conversion of vitamin D to its active 1,25-$(OH)_2$ form by the kidney. *Calcitonin* inhibits bone resorption and decreases serum Ca^{2+} and Ca^{2+} in the extracellular fluids.

Normal Serum Calcium: 9.0–10.5 mg/dL (SI Units: 2.2–2.6 mmol/L).

Increased Calcium: Hypercalcemia. Hypercalcemia indicates increased bone breakdown, decreased renal excretion and/or vitamin D intoxication. *CLINICAL OCCURRENCE: Endocrine* hyperthyroidism, hypothyroidism, primary hyperparathyroidism, Cushing disease, Addison disease; *Idiopathic* osteoporosis, Paget disease; *Inflammatory/Immune* sarcoidosis; *Mechanical/Trauma* immobilization; *Metabolic/Toxic* vitamin D intoxication, milk–alkali syndrome, hyperproteinemia (sarcoidosis, multiple myeloma), drugs (thiazide diuretics), poisons (berylliosis); *Neoplastic* tumor metastatic to bone, lymphoma, multiple myeloma, leukemia.

Decreased Calcium: Hypocalcemia. A low serum calcium can be caused by decreased binding proteins, vitamin D deficiency or resistance, precipitation of calcium phosphate salts or calcium soaps, or PTH deficiency. *CLINICAL OCCURRENCE: Endocrine* hypoparathyroidism (postthyroidectomy, idiopathic or pseudohypoparathyroidism), hypothyroidism, late pregnancy; *Inflammatory/Immune* acute pancreatitis with fat necrosis; *Metabolic/Toxic* renal insufficiency, excessive fluid intake, malabsorption of calcium and vitamin D or dietary vitamin D deficiency (osteomalacia and rickets), hypoproteinemia (cachexia, nephrosis, celiac disease, cystic fibrosis of the pancreas), drugs (antacids), corticosteroids.

CHLORIDE, SERUM (CL⁻). *Pathophysiology:* This is the principal anion in the extracellular fluid. By contrast, in the cellular fluid the chief anions are phosphate and sulfate. The quantity of Cl^- is usually proportionate to Na^+ (see discussion of anion gap, page 935).

Normal Serum Chloride: 98–106 mEq/L (SI Units: 98–106 mmol/L).

TABLE 18-1

	Total Cholesterol		Triglycerides	
	mg/dL	SI, mmol/L	mg/dL	SI, mmol/L
Desirable	<200	<5.2	<150	<1.69
Borderline High	200–239	5.20–6.18	150–199	1.69–2.25
High	≥240	≥6.21	≥200	≥2.26

Increased Chloride: Hyperchloremia. *CLINICAL OCCURRENCE: Technical Error* bromide in blood gives false test for Cl⁻; *Endocrine* hyperparathyroidism, diabetes mellitus, diabetes insipidus; *Metabolic/Toxic* renal tubular acidosis, acute renal failure, respiratory alkalosis, nonanion gap metabolic acidosis, drugs (Diamox, ammonium salts, salicylates), dehydration.

Decreased Chloride: Hypochloremia. The chloride concentration is low when organic acids accumulate in anion gap metabolic acidosis or bicarbonate replaces chloride in metabolic alkalosis. *CLINICAL OCCURRENCE: Endocrine* diabetic ketoacidosis, Addison disease, primary aldosteronism; *Mechanical/Trauma* congestive cardiac failure, pyloric obstruction; *Metabolic/Toxic* anion gap metabolic acidosis, metabolic alkalosis, pulmonary emphysema, excessive sweating, diarrhea, malabsorption, drugs (diuretics).

CHOLESTEROL, SERUM. *Pathophysiology:* As a lipid, cholesterol is insoluble in water. It is carried in the circulation in association with lipoprotein. The low-density lipoproteins (LDLs) have the highest concentration of cholesterol. Cholesterol comes from the diet and is synthesized by the liver. Cholesterol is essential to every cell; it is a precursor to adrenal steroids, gonadal steroids, and bile salts. Elevated cholesterol, particularly LDL cholesterol, is associated with accelerated atherogenesis. In contrast, elevated high-density lipoprotein (HDL) cholesterol is protective.

TABLE 18-2

	LDL Cholesterol	
	mg/dL	SI, mmol/L
Optimal	<100	<2.59
Desirable	<130	<3.36
Borderline High	130–159	3.36–4.11
High	160–189	4.14–4.89
Very High	≥190	>4.91

TABLE 18-3

	HDL Cholesterol	
	mg/dL	SI, mmol/L
High	≥60	≥1.55
Low	≤39	≤1.01

Normal Concentrations: See Tables 18-1, 18-2 and 18-3. *It is of particular note, that cholesterol and triglycerides are the only serum chemistries reported as socially determined "desirable" and "undesirable" levels, rather than normally distributed population-based ranges, that is, normal.*

Increased Cholesterol: Hypercholesterolemia. *CLINICAL OCCURRENCE: Congenital* familial hypercholesterolemia and combined hyperlipidemia; *Endocrine* hypothyroidism, diabetes mellitus; *Inflammatory/Immune* chronic nephritis, amyloidosis, systemic lupus erythematosus (SLE), polyarteritis; *Mechanical/Trauma* biliary obstruction (gallstone, carcinoma, cholangiolitic cirrhosis); *Metabolic/Toxic* obesity, metabolic syndrome, nephrotic syndrome, maldigestion and malabsorption, cirrhosis, lipodystrophy, alcohol; *Vascular* renal vein thrombosis.

Decreased Cholesterol: Hypocholesterolemia. *CLINICAL OCCURRENCE: Congenital* Tangier disease; *Infectious* chronic infections; *Inflammatory/Immune* cirrhosis, severe hepatitis; *Metabolic/Toxic* malnutrition, alcohol, starvation, uremia, steatorrhea, pernicious anemia, drugs (lipid-lowering agents, cortisone, adrenocorticotropic hormone [ACTH]).

C-REACTIVE PROTEIN (CRP). *Pathophysiology:* This is an acute-phase reactant that has a short half-life, so it rises rapidly (within 4–6 hours) of the onset of inflammation or tissue injury, and declines relatively rapidly (T½ 5–7 hours) when resolution occurs.

Normal CRP: Consult local labs.

Elevated CRP. CRP rises with any acute or chronic inflammation, infection or tissue damage. Levels tend to correlate with the erythrocyte sedimentation rate (ESR), see page 957, but respond more rapidly to changes in the patient's status. Higher levels within the normal range measured by the highly sensitive CRP are associated with an increased risk for coronary artery disease. The mechanism is unknown.

CREATINE KINASE (CK), SERUM. *Pathophysiology:* This enzyme catalyzes the transfer of high-energy phosphate between creatine and phosphocreatine, and between adenosine diphosphate

(ADP) and adenosine triphosphate (ATP). Principal concentrations are found in cardiac and skeletal muscle and in the brain. Erythrocytes lack this enzyme, so autolyzed serum specimens are acceptable for testing.

Normal CK: **Males: 25–90 mU/mL (SI Units: 0.42–1.50 μkat/L); females: 10–70 mU/mL (SI Units: 0.17–1.17 μkat/L).**

Increased Creatine Kinase. Increased CK suggests muscle or brain damage. The isoenzyme pattern (CK-MB from cardiac muscle, CK-BB from brain) can indicate the likely source. *CLINICAL OCCURRENCE: Congenital:* progressive muscular dystrophy; *Endocrine:* hypothyroidism, last few weeks of pregnancy; *Infectious:* pyomyositis; *Inflammatory/Immune:* polymyositis, dermatomyositis, inclusion-body myositis, pancreatitis; *Mechanical/Trauma:* severe exercise, muscle spasms, clonic and tonic seizures, muscle trauma (crush syndrome, postoperatively for about 5 days), electroshock for defibrillation, muscle necrosis and atrophy, intramuscular injections for 48 hours, dissecting aneurysm; *Metabolic/Toxic* megaloblastic anemia, drugs (salicylates, alcohol) *Vascular* myocardial and cerebral infarction.

Decreased Creatine Kinase. *CLINICAL OCCURRENCE: Technical Error* drug interference; *Endocrine* early pregnancy; *Inflammatory/Immune* pancreatitis; *Metabolic/Toxic* decreased muscle mass.

CREATININE, SERUM. *Pathophysiology:* This is an organic acid resulting from the metabolism of creatine in the muscles. It is distributed throughout the body water. Creatine is formed in the liver and pancreas from arginine and glycine; it is taken up by muscle tissue and converted to creatine phosphate, catalyzed by the enzyme CPK. The creatine decomposes to creatinine at a rate of 1 or 2% per day. The amount of creatinine produced increases with muscle mass and decreases with muscle wasting. Creatinine is cleared from the blood by the glomerular filtration (75%) and tubular secretion (25%), without reabsorption. The rate of urinary creatinine excretion is an indicator of glomerular filtration.

Normal Serum Creatinine: **<1.5 mg/dL (SI Units: <133 μmol/L).**

Increased Creatinine. Elevated creatinine indicates a decrease in renal function, particularly glomerular filtration from prerenal, renal, or postrenal causes. Because creatinine is dependent upon muscle mass, decreased renal function may be masked in patients with decreasing muscle mass, especially in women and the elderly. *CLINICAL OCCURRENCE: Technical Error* drug interference with the assay (cephalosporins, ketones); *Endocrine* acromegaly; *Idiopathic* renal insufficiency of any cause; *Mechanical/Trauma* burns, crush injury; *Metabolic/Toxic* increased muscle mass, ingestion of roast beef with excess of creatinine, excessive intake of protein, dehydration, ureterocolostomy with urinary resorption, medications (cimetidine, probenecid, trimethoprim);   *Vascular*   inadequate blood flow to the kidneys, renal failure, heart failure.

Decreased Creatinine.   *CLINICAL OCCURRENCE:* Cachexia, decreased muscle mass, and increased glomerular filtration (e.g., the osmotic diuresis of early diabetes) will decrease the creatinine from baseline.

FERRITIN, SERUM.   *Pathophysiology:*   As the major iron-storage protein in the body, it reflects iron stored in the reticuloendothelial system. Ferritin is an acute-phase reactant and is, therefore, best interpreted with a test of the acute-phase reaction such as the C-reactive protein or erythrocyte sedimentation rate (ESR).

Normal Ferritin: Females: 10–200 ng/mL (SI 10–200 μg/L); males: 15–400 ng/mL (SI Units: 15–400 μg/L).

Increased Serum Ferritin.   *CLINICAL OCCURRENCE:* Increased body iron stores (from transfusion hemosiderosis, anemias of chronic disease, leukemias, Hodgkin disease), excess dietary iron, transfusion hemosiderosis, hemochromatosis (usually >400 ng/dL, often >1000 ng/dL), inflammation, infection, or cancer.

Decreased Serum Ferritin.   *CLINICAL OCCURRENCE:* Iron deficiency.

GLUCOSE, SERUM.   *Pathophysiology:*   This is a six-carbon monosaccharide, a primary energy source for metabolism. The serum level remains fairly constant during fasting; there is a moderate rise after the ingestion of food. Hepatocytes convert other carbohydrates to glucose. Surpluses of glucose are converted to glycogen in the liver and muscle, or form fat that is deposited throughout the body, predominately in adipocytes. Glucose uptake by the liver, muscle, and adipocytes is insulin dependent. After an average meal, the normal person has a blood sugar rise to approximately 180 mg/dL serum; this returns to normal fasting levels within 2 hours. Higher blood glucose levels result from excessively rapid absorption or impaired peripheral disposition, usually related to insulin insufficiency or resistance. When the blood concentration of glucose becomes high, the tubular reabsorption threshold is exceeded and glucose is excreted in the urine (*glycosuria*). The normal renal threshold occurs at a serum glucose of 160–190 mg/dL. This may be higher in a damaged kidney.

Normal Serum Glucose: 75–110 mg/dL (SI Units: 4.2–6.4 mmol/L).

Diagnostic Criteria for Diabetes.

1. A fasting glucose of ≥126 mg/dL (SI Units: ≥7.0 mmol/L); or
2. Symptoms of diabetes plus a random glucose of ≥200 mg/dL (SI Units: ≥11.1 mmol/dL); or
3. A plasma glucose ≥200 mg/dL (SI Units: ≥11.1 mmol/L) 2 hours following a 75-g oral glucose load.

The abnormal test must be confirmed on another day.

Diagnostic of Impaired Fasting Glucose (IFG).   A fasting glucose of 110–126 mg/dL (SI Units: 6.1–7.0 mmol/L).

Diagnostic of Impaired Glucose Tolerance (GT).   A blood glucose of 140–199 mg/dL (SI Units: 7.8–11.0 mmol/L) 2 hours after a 75-g oral glucose load.

Increased Glucose: Hyperglycemia.   Hyperglycemia indicates insulin resistance from the metabolic syndrome, diabetes or release of stress-associated hormones (epinephrine, cortisol, growth hormone). *CLINICAL OCCURRENCE: Endocrine*   diabetes mellitus, impaired glucose tolerance, acromegaly, hyperthyroidism, Cushing disease, increased adrenalin, adrenocorticotropic hormone (ACTH), pheochromocytoma, pregnancy, toxemia of pregnancy;   *Infectious*   any acute severe infection, for example, pneumonia;   *Inflammatory/Immune* systemic inflammatory response syndrome (SIRS), regional enteritis, ulcerative colitis;   *Metabolic/Toxic*   drugs (corticosteroids, diazoxide, epinephrine), poisoning (streptozotocin);   *Neurologic*   Wernicke syndrome, subarachnoid hemorrhage, hypothalamic lesions, convulsions;   *Vascular*   myocardial infarction, pulmonary embolism, hemorrhage.

Decreased Glucose: Hypoglycemia.   Inability to maintain a normal blood glucose indicates excessive insulin secretion or administration, or severely impaired hepatic gluconeogenesis. *CLINICAL OCCURRENCE: Congenital*   galactosuria, maple syrup urine disease, hepatic glycogenoses;   *Endocrine*   hypopituitarism, hypothalamic lesions, hypothyroidism, Addison disease;   *Infectious*   sepsis;   *Inflammatory/Immune*   pancreatitis;   *Mechanical/Trauma*   postgastrectomy dumping syndrome, gastroenterostomy;   *Metabolic/Toxic*   insulin administration, oral hypoglycemics, glycogen deficiency, hepatitis, cirrhosis, malnutrition;   *Neoplastic*   insulinoma, some sarcomas.

HEMOGLOBIN A_{1C}:   GLYCOHEMOGLOBIN. *Pathophysiology:*   Glycosylation of cellular and extracellular proteins occurs at a rate dependent upon the ambient plasma glucose concentration. Hemoglobin is glycosylated in this manner and the amount of glycosylated hemoglobin is an accurate measure of the average blood sugar over the average life of the circulating erythrocytes, approximately 6 weeks. Measurement of one glycosylated form of hemoglobin, hemoglobin A_{1c}, is used to estimate the average blood sugar as a determinate of diabetes control.

Normal Hemoglobin A_{1c}:   3.8–6.4% (SI Units: 0.038–0.064).

IRON, SERUM (FE^{2+}).   *Pathophysiology:*   The body contains about 3–4 g of iron. It is a component of hemoglobin, the cytochromes, and other cellular metalloproteins. Approximately 1 mg of iron is absorbed and excreted each day. Most of the iron circulates in erythrocyte hemoglobin (1.0 mg/1.0 mL packed erythrocytes), with the rest bound to ferritin in stores (approximately 1.0 g), in myoglobin, and with a small fraction incorporated into respiratory enzymes and other sites. Iron is absorbed in the duodenum by a complex pathway regulated at the level of the enterocyte; most ingested iron is not absorbed, or is sloughed in the enterocytes, never entering the plasma. Absorbed iron is bound to transferrin. Iron is cleared from the plasma with a half-time of 60–120 minutes, and 80–90% is incorporated into new circulating erythrocytes over the subsequent 2 weeks. The serum concentration of iron decreases by 50–100 μg/dL with the diurnal acceleration of erythropoiesis in the afternoon, so the time of day the specimen is drawn and its relationship to meals should be known. Iron deficiency is a very common disorder.

Normal Serum Iron: 50–100 μg/dL (SI Units: 9–27 μmol/L).

Increased Serum Iron: Hyperferremia. An increase in serum iron may be seen following a high-iron meal, or with hemochromatosis and liver disease. *CLINICAL OCCURRENCE: Congenital* hemochromatosis, thalassemia; *Inflammatory/Immune* acute hepatic necrosis, aplastic anemia, hemolytic anemia; *Metabolic/Toxic* excessive absorption (iron therapy, dietary excess), cirrhosis, pernicious anemia.

Decreased Serum Iron: Hypoferremia. Low serum iron results from inadequate dietary intake, excessive blood loss (both with increased iron-binding capacity), or chronic inflammation (decreased iron-binding capacity). *CLINICAL OCCURRENCE: Endocrine* iron loss to the fetus during gestation; *Infectious* tuberculosis, osteomyelitis, hookworm; *Inflammatory/Immune* celiac disease, rheumatoid arthritis, systemic lupus erythematosus (SLE); *Mechanical/ Trauma* intravascular hemolysis with hemoglobinuria (paroxysmal nocturnal hemoglobinuria, march hemoglobinuria, prosthetic heart valves); *Metabolic/Toxic* iron deficiency, repeated phlebotomy, diminished absorption (decreased ingestion, celiac disease, pica, postgastrectomy); *Neoplastic* gastrointestinal cancers, loss of transferrin in nephrotic syndrome; *Psychosocial* poverty; *Vascular* intrapulmonary hemorrhage (e.g., idiopathic pulmonary hemosiderosis), chronic bleeding (e.g., menorrhagia, hematuria, peptic ulcer disease, gastritis, polyps, ulcerative colitis, colon carcinoma).

IRON-BINDING CAPACITY (TIBC), SERUM TOTAL.   The TIBC mainly reflects transferrin and, with the serum iron, helps to distinguish iron deficiency anemias from the anemia of chronic inflammation.

Normal Iron-Binding Capacity: 250–370 μg/dL (SI Units: 45–66 μmol/L).

Increased Iron-Binding Capacity. This generally reflects a response to iron deficiency. *CLINICAL OCCURRENCE:* Iron deficiency, acute or chronic blood loss, hepatitis, late pregnancy.

Decreased Iron-Binding Capacity. Transferrin falls with chronic inflammation. *CLINICAL OCCURRENCE:* Anemias of chronic disorders (infections, inflammations, and cancer), thalassemia, cirrhosis, nephrotic syndrome.

LACTIC DEHYDROGENASE (LDH), SERUM. *Pathophysiology:* This enzyme catalyzes the oxidation of lactate to pyruvate reversibly. It is found in all tissues, so an elevation of the blood level is a nonspecific indicator of tissue damage.

Normal LDH: **100–190 U/L (SI Units: 1.7–3.2 μkat/L).**

Increased LDH. Elevations of LDH suggest injury to the muscles, liver, hemolysis, or rapid cell division as in lymphomas. *CLINICAL OCCURRENCE: Congenital* muscular dystrophy in 10% of cases, progressive muscular dystrophy, myotonic dystrophy (but creatine phosphokinase [CPK] is more specific for muscle than LDH); *Endocrine* hypothyroidism; *Infectious* hepatitis with jaundice, infectious mononucleosis; *Inflammatory/Immune* polymyositis in 25% of cases, dermatomyositis, hemolytic anemias; *Mechanical/Trauma* cardiovascular surgery, common bile duct obstruction, intestinal obstruction; *Metabolic/Toxic* muscle necrosis, celiac disease, untreated pernicious anemia, alcohol; *Neoplastic* 50% of cases of lymphoma and leukemia; *Vascular* acute myocardial infarction, pulmonary embolism or infarction.

Decreased LDH.   *CLINICAL OCCURRENCE:* Irradiation, ingestion of clofibrate.

PHOSPHATE, SERUM INORGANIC. *Pathophysiology:* This term includes the inorganic phosphorus of ionized HPO_4^{2-} and H_2PO_4 in equilibrium in the serum; only 10–20% is protein bound. Phosphorus is necessary for synthesizing nucleotides, phospholipids, and the high-energy adenosine triphosphate (ATP). Phosphates are excreted by the kidney; parathormone (PTH) increases phosphate excretion. When the energy demands are great for glycolysis, the serum inorganic P is decreased.

Normal Phosphate: **3.0–4.5 mg/dL (SI Units: 1.0–1.4 mmol/L).**

Increased Phosphate: Hyperphosphatemia. *CLINICAL OCCURRENCE: Congenital* Fanconi disease; *Endocrine* acromegaly, hyperparathyroidism; *Idiopathic* Paget disease; *Infectious* sepsis; *Inflammatory/Immune* sarcoidosis; *Mechanical/Trauma* healing fractures, crush injury, high intestinal obstruction; *Metabolic/Toxic* acute and chronic renal failure, vitamin D deficiency (rickets, osteomalacia), muscle necrosis, milk–alkali syndrome, respiratory alkalosis, excess of vitamin D; *Neoplastic* multiple myelomas, osteolytic metastases, myelocytic leukemia.

Decreased Phosphate: Hypophosphatemia. *CLINICAL OCCURRENCE: Congenital* primary hypophosphatemia; *Endocrine* hyperparathyroidism, diabetes mellitus; *Metabolic/Toxic* renal tubular defects (Fanconi syndrome), anorexia, vomiting, diarrhea, lack of vitamin D, in refeeding after starvation, malnutrition, gout, ketoacidosis, respiratory alkalosis, hypokalemia, hypomagnesemia, primary hypophosphatemia, drugs (intravenous glucose, anabolic steroids, androgens, epinephrine, glucagon, insulin, salicylates, phosphorus-binding antacids, diuretic drugs, alcohol).

POTASSIUM, SERUM [K$^+$]. *Pathophysiology:* This is the predominant cation in the intracellular fluid, while sodium predominates in the extracellular fluids. Approximately 90% of the exchangeable K$^+$ is within the cells; less than 1% is in the normal serum. Small shifts of K$^+$ from the cells causes relatively large changes in the smaller serum [K$^+$]. Intracellular acidosis causes an extracellular shift of K$^+$. Plasma [K$^+$] is tightly regulated by the kidney; hyperkalemia leads to aldosterone secretion and potassium excretion. Changes in serum concentration of K$^+$ produce profound effects on nerve excitation, muscle contraction, and in cardiac conduction. Because the concentration of K$^+$ in the erythrocytes is about 18 times as great as that in the serum, hemolysis occurring during sample collection falsely elevates the serum K$^+$.

Normal Potassium: 3.5–5.0 mEq/L (SI Units: 3.5–5.0 mmol/L).

Increased Potassium: Hyperkalemia. (*Note*: high levels of serum K$^+$ pose great danger of producing cardiac arrest.) *CLINICAL OCCURRENCE: Technical Error* hemolysis in performing venipuncture or intentional clotting in collecting blood specimens, especially with thrombocytosis; *Congenital* hyperkalemic periodic paralysis; *Endocrine* primary and secondary hypoaldosteronism, adrenal insufficiency (Addison disease, adrenal hemorrhage); *Mechanical/Trauma* rhabdomyolysis, crush injury, hemolyzed transfused blood, urinary obstruction; *Metabolic/Toxic* acute and chronic renal failure, acidosis (metabolic or respiratory), muscle necrosis, drugs (amiloride, spironolactone, triamterene, angiotensin-converting enzyme inhibitors), foods (fruit juices, soft drinks, oranges, peaches, bananas, tomatoes, high-protein diet), dehydration; *Neurologic* status epilepticus; *Vascular* gastrointestinal hemorrhage, hemorrhage into tissues.

Decreased Potassium: Hypokalemia. This is almost always associated with depletion of in total body K$^+$. *CLINICAL OCCURRENCE: Endocrine* diabetes mellitus, Cushing syndrome, hyperaldosteronism; *Mechanical/Trauma* ureterosigmoidostomy with urinary reabsorption, adynamic ileus; *Metabolic/Toxic* vomiting, gastric suction, postgastrectomy dumping syndrome, gastric atony, laxative abuse, polyuria, renal injury, salt-losing nephritis, metabolic alkalosis (from diuresis, primary aldosteronism, pseudoaldosteronism), metabolic acidosis (from renal tubular acidosis, diuresis phase of tubular necrosis, chronic pyelonephritis, diuresis after release of urinary obstruction), malabsorption and malnutrition, drugs (diuretics, estrogens, salicylates, corticosteroids) *Neoplastic* aldosteronoma, villous adenoma, colonic cancer, Zollinger-Ellison syndrome.

PROTEIN, TOTAL SERUM. *Pathophysiology:* Most serum proteins are synthesized in the liver (albumin and others) or by mature plasma cells (immunoglobulins). Increases or decreases in serum proteins represent a balance between synthesis and protein catabolism or loss into third spaces or in the urine. This is the total of the serum albumin and the serum globulins; the fibrinogen was discarded in the clot that separated from the plasma to form the serum specimen. The quantity of the total serum protein, minus the albumin fraction, gives an estimate of the serum globulins.

Normal Total Protein: 5.5–8.0 g/dL (SI Units: 55–80 g/L).

Increased Total Protein: Hyperproteinemia. This represents increased concentration of normal proteins, or excessive production of immunoglobulins. *CLINICAL OCCURRENCE:* Water depletion, multiple myeloma, macroglobulinemia, and sarcoidosis.

Decreased Total Protein: Hypoproteinemia. This is caused by decreased synthesis, increased catabolism because of malnutrition, or loss into third spaces or into the urine in nephrotic syndrome. *CLINICAL OCCURRENCE:* Congestive cardiac failure, ulcerative colitis, nephrotic syndrome, chronic glomerulonephritis, cirrhosis, viral hepatitis, burns, malnutrition.

PROTEIN: ALBUMIN, SERUM. *Pathophysiology:* Molecular weight about 65,000. Normally, albumin comprises more than half the total serum protein. Because its molecular weight is low compared to that of the globulins (between 44,000 and 435,000), its smaller molecules exert 80% of osmotic pressure of the plasma. In addition, (a) serum albumin serves as a protein store for the body that can be used when a deficit develops; (b) it serves as a solvent for fatty acids and bile salts; and (c) it serves as a transport vehicle by loosely binding hormones, amino acids, drugs, and metals.

Normal Albumin: 3.5–5.5 g/dL (SI Units: 35–55 g/L).

Increased Albumin: Hyperalbuminemia. No significant correlation with diseases.

Decreased Albumin: Hypoalbuminemia. *CLINICAL OCCURRENCE: Congenital* analbuminemia; *Endocrine* diabetes mellitus;

Infectious viral hepatitis; *Inflammatory/Immune* ulcerative colitis, protein-losing enteropathies, chronic glomerulonephritis, lupus erythematosus, polyarteritis, rheumatoid arthritis, rheumatic fever; *Mechanical/Trauma* peptic ulcer; *Metabolic/Toxic* congestive cardiac failure, cirrhosis, nephrotic syndrome, malnutrition, drugs (estrogens); *Neoplastic* multiple myeloma, Hodgkin disease, lymphocytic leukemia, macroglobulinemia.

PROTEIN: GLOBULINS, SERUM. The difference between the values for total serum protein and for serum albumin is referred to as the *serum globulin fraction* of the serum protein. When the globulin level is increased, fractionation of the globulins is indicated to identify each component. This is accomplished by *serum protein electrophoresis*.

SERUM PROTEIN ELECTROPHORESIS (SPEP). The proteins are separated by electrophoresis; the proteins migrate, each at its own rate, dependent on its charge and molecular weight. A serum specimen contains proteins that separate into several *zones* according to their mobility. The proteins are named for the zone in which they are found (named with Greek lowercase letters): *alpha 0* (for albumin), *alpha 1* (α_1), *alpha 2* (α_2), *beta* (β), *gamma* (γ), and *phi* (ϕ) (for fibrinogen).

PROTEIN: ALPHA-1 (α_1)-GLOBULINS. Alpha-1-globulins include α_1-antitrypsin, oromucil, and some cortisol-binding globulin.

Increased α_1-Globulins. Hodgkin disease, peptic ulcer, ulcerative colitis, cirrhosis, metastatic carcinoma, protein-losing enteropathy.

Decreased α_1-Globulins. Viral hepatitis.

PROTEIN: ALPHA-2 (α_2)-GLOBULINS. Alpha-2-globulins include macroglobulins, haptoglobin, HS glycoprotein, ceruloplasmin, and some immunoglobulins.

Increased α_2-Globulins. Hodgkin disease, peptic ulcer, ulcerative colitis, cirrhosis, nephrotic syndrome, chronic glomerulonephritis, systemic lupus erythematosus, polyarteritis nodosa, rheumatoid arthritis, metastatic carcinoma, protein-losing enteropathies.

Decreased α_2-Globulins. Cirrhosis, viral hepatitis.

PROTEIN: BETA (β)-GLOBULINS. Beta-globulins include transferrin, hemopexin, and some immunoglobulins.

Increased β-Globulins. Rheumatoid arthritis, rheumatic fever, analbuminemia.

Decreased β-Globulins.   Nephrotic syndrome, lymphocytic leukemia, metastatic carcinoma.

PROTEIN: GAMMA (γ)-GLOBULINS.   Gamma globulins are predominately immunoglobulins of the IgG class. Increases in gamma globulins can be (a) *monoclonal*, arising from a clonal proliferation of plasma cells or lymphocytes, or (b) *polyclonal*, as part of an inflammatory response. Polyclonal gamma globulins produce a *broad-based pattern* in the gamma zone, indicating the presence of proteins from many cell lines.

Increased Polyclonal γ-Globulins.   Cirrhosis, myelocytic leukemia, lupus erythematosus, rheumatoid arthritis, analbuminemia.

Decreased Polyclonal γ-Globulins.   Nephrotic syndrome, lymphocytic leukemia, common variable immunodeficiency, hypogammaglobulinemia, protein-losing enteropathies.

PROTEIN: IMMUNOGLOBULIN IgG.   *Pathophysiology:*   Molecular weight 160,000. This is the smallest molecule of the immunoglobulins and the only one that can pass the placental membrane; consequently, it serves as a protection for the newborn until the child's own immunoglobulins can be generated. IgG is synthesized after IgM in response to a new antigen. IgG producing plasma cells are the major humoral effector of chronic inflammation.

Normal IgG: 800–1500 mg/dL (SI Units: 8.0–15.00 g/L).

Increased IgG.   *CLINICAL OCCURRENCE: Infectious*   pulmonary tuberculosis, hepatitis, osteomyelitis;   *Inflammatory/Immune* systemic lupus erythematosus, rheumatoid arthritis, vasculitis;   *Metabolic/Toxic*   cirrhosis;   *Neoplastic*   myeloma, monoclonal gammopathy of undetermined significance (MGUS).

Decreased IgG.   *CLINICAL OCCURRENCE: Congenital*   lymphoid aplasia, agammaglobulinemia;   *Inflammatory/Immune*   common variable immunodeficiency, nephrotic syndrome;   *Neoplastic*   heavy-chain disease, IgA myeloma, macroglobulinemia, chronic lymphocytic leukemia.

PROTEIN: IMMUNOGLOBULIN IgA.   *Pathophysiology:*   Molecular weight 170,000. This globulin is especially involved in the protection against viral infections. It has an *excretory form* with a molecular weight of 400,000, found in colostrum, saliva, tears, bronchial secretions, gastrointestinal secretions, and nasal discharges. It has a special action against viruses of influenza, poliomyelitis, adenoviral diseases, and rhinoviruses.

Normal IgA: 90–325 mg/dL (SI Units: 0.90–3.2 g/L).

Increased IgA. *CLINICAL OCCURRENCE:* *Congenital* Wiskott-Aldrich syndrome; *Inflammatory/Immune* systemic lupus erythematosus, rheumatoid arthritis, sarcoidosis; *Metabolic/Toxic* cirrhosis; *Neoplastic* IgA myeloma.

Decreased IgA. *CLINICAL OCCURRENCE:* *Congenital* absent in some people, hereditary telangiectasia, lymphoid aplasia; *Inflammatory/Immune* nephrotic syndrome, Still disease, systemic lupus erythematosus, common variable immunodeficiency, agammaglobulinemia; *Metabolic/Toxic* cirrhosis; *Neoplastic* heavy-chain disease, acute lymphocytic leukemia, chronic lymphocytic leukemia, chronic myelocytic leukemia.

PROTEIN: IMMUNOGLOBULIN IgM. *Pathophysiology:* Molecular weight 900,000. This is the largest of the immunoglobulins. It is formed during a primary antibody response. The rheumatoid factor and the isoantibodies anti-A and anti-B belong mostly to this class.

Normal IgM: 45–150 mg/dL (SI Units: 0.45–1.5 g/L).

Increased IgM. *CLINICAL OCCURRENCE:* *Infectious* hepatitis, trypanosomiasis; *Inflammatory/Immune* biliary cirrhosis, rheumatoid arthritis, systemic lupus erythematosus; *Neoplastic* macroglobulinemia.

PROTEIN: IMMUNOGLOBULIN IgD. *Pathophysiology:* Molecular weight 185,000. There is no known specific activity for this protein.

Normal IgD: 0–8 mg/dL (SI Units: 0–0.08 g/L).

Increased IgD. Chronic infections, IgD myeloma.

PROTEIN: IMMUNOGLOBULIN IgE. *Pathophysiology:* Molecular weight 200,000. IgE binds to mast cells in body tissue. Specific antigen (allergen) binding to mast cell IgE causes degranulation of the mast cell and an allergic response. This protein is involved in allergic and atopic reactions.

Normal IgE: <0.025 mg/dL (SI Units: <0.00025 g/L).

Increased IgE. Extrinsic asthma (60% of cases), hay fever (30% of cases), atopic eczema, parasitic infestations, IgE myeloma.

PROTEIN: MONOCLONAL GAMMA GLOBULINS. *Pathophysiology:* These are recognized in the serum protein electrophoresis (SPEP) by a *sharp and narrow* spike (M-spike) in the gamma region. An M-spike indicates homogeneous proteins from a single cell line. The exact nature of the immunoglobulin is determined by immunoelectrophoresis. They are characterized by the proliferation of one or, rarely, more of the five human immunoglobulins normally present in human serum: IgG, IgA, IgM, IgD, and IgE. Each contains a specific heavy chain (H chain) coupled to one of two types of *light chains* (L chains). The heavy chains are named with lowercase Greek letters, corresponding to the capital letters designating immunoglobulin type: IgA (α), IgG (γ), IgM (μ), IgD (δ), IgE (ϵ). The light chains are called kappa (κ) and lambda (λ). The five immunoglobulins can be identified by *immunofixation electrophoresis*. In this procedure, after electrophoresis, specific antibodies are used to identify the H and L chains.

Monoclonal Immunoglobulin *CLINICAL OCCURRENCE:* Multiple myeloma, macroglobulinemia, malignant lymphoma, amyloidosis, monoclonal gammopathy of undetermined significance.

SODIUM, SERUM (NA⁺). *Pathophysiology:* Molecular weight 23. This is the predominant cation in the extracellular fluid. Together with Cl^- it makes a major contribution to the osmotic pressure of the plasma. Loss of Na^+ is frequently accompanied by an equivalent amount of water (as an isotonic solution), so normal levels of serum Na^+ do not exclude total body loss of Na^+. Assessment of total body Na^+ status is done by assessing extracellular volume. To maintain extracellular volume, the kidney retains sodium, and with it, enough water to maintain normal osmolarity. Because water moves between the intracellular and extracellular compartments to maintain iso-osmolarity between the two, an increase or decrease in the $[Na^+]$ represents an inverse change in the total body water, that is, an increased serum Na^+ indicates a water deficit and a decreased serum Na^+ indicates water excess.

Normal Sodium: 136–145 mEq/L (136–145 mmol/L).

Increased Serum Sodium: Hypernatremia. This always indicates a *relative total body water deficit*, regardless of the extracellular volume status [Adrogué HJ, Madias NE. Hypernatremia. *N Engl J Med* 2000;342:1493–1499]. *CLINICAL OCCURRENCE: Endocrine* diabetes insipidus, diabetes mellitus, hyperparathyroidism, hyperaldosteronism; *Metabolic/Toxic* water loss greater than Na loss (vomiting, sweating, hyperpnea, diarrhea), drugs (corticosteroids, diuretics), diuretic phase of acute tubular necrosis, diuresis after relief of urinary obstruction, excessive sodium intake, hypercalcemia, hypokalemic nephropathy; *Neurologic* thalamic lesions.

Decreased Serum Sodium: Hyponatremia. This always indicates a *relative total body water excess*, from excess water ingestion or inability of the kidney to excrete a sufficiently dilute urine, regardless of the extracellular volume status [Adrogué HJ, Madia NE. Hyponatremia. *N Engl J Med* 2000;342:1581–1589]. *CLINICAL OCCURRENCE: Technical Error* spuriously normal serum osmolality (hyperlipidemia, hyperglycemia); *Endocrine* Addison disease; *Infectious* pneumonia, meningitis, brain abscess (all cause syndrome of inappropriate antidiuretic hormone [SIADH] secretion); *Metabolic/Toxic* congestive cardiac failure, salt-losing nephropathy, cirrhosis with ascites, fluid and electrolyte loss with replacement by hypotonic fluids, for example, water (vomiting, sweating, diarrhea, diuresis), malnutrition, SIADH secretion; *Neoplastic* antidiuretic hormone (ADH)-secreting tumors, especially lung cancers; *Psychosocial* anorexia nervosa, psychogenic polydipsia.

TRIGLYCERIDES. *Pathophysiology:* Triglycerides are absorbed from the gut following ingestion of a fatty meal. They are transported in chylomicrons to the adipose tissue where they are deposited by the action of lipoprotein lipase, leading to the formation of less triglyceride enriched very low density and intermediate density lipoproteins (VLDL and IDL, respectively). Triglycerides are the major form of energy storage. They are broken down to free fatty acids which are a highly efficient cellular energy source.

Normal Triglycerides: See Table 18-1, page 940.

Increased Triglycerides: Hypertriglyceridemia: *CLINICAL OCCURRENCE:* *Cogenital* lipoprotein lipase deficiency, familial combined hyperlipidemia; familial hypertriglyceridemia, dysbetalipomotanemia; *Endocrine* diabetes, hypothyroidism; *Metabolic/ Toxic* alcohol ingestion, high fat diets, metabolic syndrome, drugs (oral contraceptives).

UREA NITROGEN. See *Blood Urea Nitrogen*, page 938.

URIC ACID, SERUM. *Pathophysiology:* Molecular weight 169. Uric acid is the end product of purine metabolism. Normally uric acid is produced at the rate of 10 mg/kg per day in a healthy adult. The body pool is about 1200 mg, distributed in the body water. Increased nucleic acid breakdown results in increased uric acid production. Uric acid leaves the body through renal excretion and by bacterial catabolism of uric acid in the gut. Renal excretion of uric acid is increased by expansion of body fluids (by salt or osmotic diuresis). Excretion of uric acid is decreased by dehydration and diuretics.

Normal Uric Acid: Males: 2.5–8.0 mg/dL (SI Units: 150–480 μmol/L); Females: 1.5–6.0 mg/dL (SI Units: 90–360 μmol/L).

Increased Uric Acid: Hyperuricemia. *Note: High values for uric acid are among the most common abnormalities encountered in routine testing. This probably accounts for the much-too-frequent diagnosis of gout. The serum uric acid is elevated in only two-thirds of the cases of gouty arthritis, but the same elevation is noted in 25% of the cases of acute nongouty arthritis, and in 25% of relatives of gouty patients. CLINICAL OCCURRENCE: Congenital* polycystic kidneys, sickle cell anemia, Wilson disease, Fanconi disease, von Gierke disease, Down syndrome, certain normal *populations* (Blackfoot and Pima Indians, Filipinos, New Zealand Maoris); *Endocrine* hypothyroidism, hypoparathyroidism, primary hyperparathyroidism, toxemia of pregnancy; *Infectious* resolving pneumonia; *Inflammatory/Immune* psoriasis, hemolytic anemias, sarcoidosis; *Metabolic/Toxic* renal failure, drugs (diuretics, small doses of salicylates), high-protein low-calorie diet, high-purine diet (sweetbreads, liver), starvation, gout, relatives of gouty patients, poisons (acute alcoholism, lead poisoning, berylliosis); *Neoplastic* leukemia, multiple myeloma, polycythemia vera, lymphoma, other disseminated cancers.

Decreased Uric Acid: Hypouricemia. *CLINICAL OCCURRENCE:* *Congenital* xanthinuria, Fanconi syndrome, Wilson disease, healthy adults with Dalmatian-dog mutation (isolated defect in tubular transport of uric acid); *Endocrine* acromegaly; *Inflammatory/Immune* celiac disease; *Metabolic/Toxic* drugs (uricosuric medication, allopurinol, adrenocorticotropic hormone [ACTH], glyceryl guaiacolate, x-ray contrast media); *Neoplastic* carcinomas, Hodgkin disease.

Hematologic Data

Blood Cells

BLOOD FILM EXAMINATION. A blood film provides the physician with an opportunity to immediately evaluate clues from the history and physical examination and to confirm results of automated blood analyzers. Here, we give examples of information that can be obtained; the reader is encouraged to consult standard textbooks of hematology for comprehensive treatment of these subjects. Appreciate that cellular morphology may vary depending on the preparation technique, stain, and location you examine on the blood smear. Select an area where the erythrocytes are close but do not touch each other.

Erythrocyte Morphology. Evaluate color, size, shape, and contents.

Macrocytes reticulocytosis, liver disease, megaloblastic anemia.

Hypochromic Microcytes defects in hemoglobin synthesis (iron deficiency, thalassemias, sickle cell disease, and other hemoglobinopathies).

Spherocytes hereditary spherocytosis, immune hemolysis.

Schistocytes microangiopathic hemolytic anemias (disseminated intravascular coagulation, thrombotic thrombocytopenic purpura, vasculitis, thrombotic microangiopathy, prosthetic heart valves, malignant hypertension, scleroderma renal crisis).

Teardrops (Dacryocytes) marrow damage, for example, extramedullary hemopoiesis, myelophthisic anemia.

Erythroblasts extramedullary hemopoiesis, myelophthisic anemia, severe hemolytic anemia, erythroleukemia.

Howell-Jolly Bodies postsplenectomy, megaloblastic anemia.

Basophilic Stippling lead poisoning, hemolytic disease.

Malaria, Babesia, and Bartonella parasites.

Leukocyte Morphology. Confirm the automated differential leukocyte count.

Toxic Granulation of Neutrophils and Metamyelocytes bacterial infections.

Giant Cytoplasmic Granules Chediak-Higashi syndrome.

Bilobed Neutrophils hereditary Pelger-Huet anomaly or pseudo–Pelger-Huet anomaly in acute leukemia.

Hypersegmented Neutrophils nuclear maturation defect, for example, pernicious anemia, vitamin deficiency, folate deficiency, myeloproliferative diseases.

Neutrophil Inclusions granulocytic ehrlichiosis.

Myeloblasts, Promyelocytes, Myelocytes depending on the number and appearance of immature cells, consider acute myeloblastic leukemia, acute promyelocytic leukemia, chronic myelocytic leukemia, myelofibrosis, polycythemia vera.

Atypical Lymphocytes viral infections, especially Ebstein-Barr virus (acute infectious mononucleosis) and cytomegalovirus (CMV).

Large Granular Lymphocytes natural killer cells of T-gamma lymphoproliferative disease.

Lymphoblasts acute lymphoblastic leukemia, prolymphocytic leukemia, malignant lymphoma, chronic lymphocytic leukemia, infectious mononucleosis.

Monocyte Inclusions monocytic ehrlichiosis.

Plasma Cells multiple myeloma.

Platelet Morphology. Confirm the automated platelet count. In oil immersion fields at 1000 magnification, where the erythrocytes are close but not touching, the number of platelets in an average field $\times$ 15 is approximately equal to the platelet count per mm^3. Scan the sides of the smear for clumps of platelets that may have been counted inaccurately by instrument.

Megathrombocytes   platelets greater than 2 μm in diameter may be increased in conditions of accelerated platelet production compensating for increased destruction (e.g., idiopathic thrombocytopenic purpura [ITP]), B_{12} deficiency, folate deficiency, myeloproliferative diseases, Bernard-Soulier syndrome.

ERYTHROCYTE MEASUREMENTS: COUNTS, HEMOGLOBIN CONTENT, AND HEMATOCRIT.
The volume of erythrocytes in the blood is determined by the hematocrit expressed as a percent of the blood volume occupied by erythrocytes in a centrifuged specimen. The hemoglobin measures the grams of hemoglobin per deciliter of whole blood. The total number of erythrocytes per mm^3 is counted by machine or a hemocytometer.

Normal Values: Hematocrit: males, 42–52%; females, 37–48%; hemoglobin: males, 13–18 g/dL; females, 12–16 g/dL; erythrocyte count: 4.15–4.90 $\times$ 10^6 per mm^3.

ERYTHROCYTIC INDICES.   These values are all calculated from the red blood cell (RBC) counts, hemoglobin content, and hematocrit.

Normal Values: Mean corpuscular hemoglobin (MCH): 28–33 pg/cell; mean corpuscular volume (MCV): 86–98 fL; mean corpuscular hemoglobin concentration (MCHC): 32–36 g/dL.

High RBC Count: Erythrocytosis. This usually represents intravascular and extracellular fluid volume loss, chronic hypoxia, iatrogenic or endogenous erythropoietin excess, or polycythemia vera. *CLINICAL OCCURRENCE: Endocrine* diabetic acidosis, third to ninth month of pregnancy and to third week postpartum, ruptured ectopic pregnancy; *Inflammatory/Immune* chronic obstructive and restrictive lung disease with hypoxia; *Mechanical/Trauma* burns (contracted plasma volume), high-altitude hypoxia; *Metabolic/Toxic* contracted plasma volume (dehydration, diarrhea, burns, shock), carboxyhemoglobinemia, sulfhemoglobinemia, secondary polycythemia, drugs (erythropoietin, androgens, diuretics); *Neoplastic* polycythemia vera, renal cyst or carcinoma; *Vascular* venous-arterial shunt (right-to-left shunt).

Low RBC Counts: Anemia. See also Chapter 5, page 116. Anemia results from decreased RBC production, hemorrhage, increased RBC destruction (hemolysis), dilution or sequestration in hypersplenism. *CLINICAL OCCURRENCE: Congenital* thalassemia; *Idiopathic* bone marrow failure; *Inflammatory/Immune* hemolysis; *Mechanical/Trauma* hemolysis or bleeding; *Metabolic/Toxic* renal failure, oliguria, macrocytic anemia (pernicious anemia/vitamin B_{12} deficiency), folate deficiency, myelodysplasia, normocytic normochromic anemias (hemolysis, chronic disease, infections, renal failure, liver disease), microcytic hypochromic anemias (Fe deficiency, pyridoxine-responsive anemia, hemoglobinopathies); *Neoplastic* refractory anemia; *Vascular* congestive cardiac failure, acute hemorrhage.

RETICULOCYTE COUNTS. *Pathophysiology:* Reticulocytes are immature erythrocytes released from the bone marrow into the blood. The retained ribosomal RNA is revealed as basophilic stippling with supravital stain. It disappears within 24–48 hours. Values are expressed as a percent of erythrocytes or as an absolute number. Increased absolute numbers of reticulocytes reflect accelerated erythropoiesis.

Normal Reticulocytes: 0.5–1.8%; 29–87 × 10^9/L.

Increased Reticulocytes: Accelerated Erythropoiesis.   *Note*: There must be adequate iron, folate, and protein. Causes are hemorrhage or hemolysis, response to erythropoietin from tissue hypoxia or from its therapeutic administration, and response to therapy of nutrient deprivation (iron, folate, protein).

Decreased Reticulocytes: Decreased Erythropoiesis.   *Nutrient deprivation* (iron deficiency, pernicious anemia/B$_{12}$ deficiency, folate deficiency, starvation), *anemia of chronic disease* (inflammation, infection, cancer) and *bone marrow failure* (alcohol abuse, idiosyncratic drug reactions, cancer chemotherapy, total body irradiation, aplastic anemia, leukemia, lymphoma, multiple myeloma, and other cancers invading bone marrow).

ERYTHROCYTE SEDIMENTATION RATE (ESR). *Pathophysiology:* Erythrocytes sediment as a result of gravity. Increased proteins in the blood (especially fibrinogen, other acute-phase reactants, and immunoglobulins) decrease the repulsive force between erythrocytes allowing aggregation of larger clumps of cells (seen on the smear as rouleaux formation), which accelerates the rate of sedimentation.

Normal ESR: Males 1–17 mm/h; females, 0–25 mm/h.

Increased ESR.   This is a very nonspecific finding indicating increased inflammation associated with infection, inflammatory diseases, and some cancers. ***CLINICAL OCCURRENCE:*** *Endocrine* hyperthyroidism, hypothyroidism, normal pregnancy from third month to termination plus 3 weeks postpartum, menstruation; *Infectious* many, but especially tuberculosis, endocarditis, osteomyelitis, and pelvic inflammation; *Inflammatory/Immune* rheumatoid arthritis, systemic lupus erythematosus, polymyalgia rheumatica, giant cell arteritis, vasculitis; *Metabolic/Toxic* hyperglobulinemia, hypoalbuminemia, dextran or polyvinyl plasma substitutes; *Neoplastic* many cancers; *Vascular* vasculitis.

LEUKOCYTES, TOTAL COUNT: WHITE BLOOD CELL COUNT (WBC). This cellular compartment of the blood contains the neutrophils, eosinophils, basophils, lymphocytes, and monocytes.

Normal WBC: 4.3–10.8 × 10³/mm³.

Normal Neutrophil Count: 45–74% of total.

Increase in All Cellular Elements of the Blood (Erythrocytes, Leukocytes, Platelets): Pancytosis. *CLINICAL OCCURRENCE:* *Metabolic/Toxic* dehydration; *Neoplastic* polycythemia vera, the myeloproliferative syndromes.

Decrease in All Cellular Elements of the Blood (Erythrocytes, Leukocytes, Platelets): Pancytopenia. *CLINICAL OCCURRENCE:* *Idiopathic* marrow failure (aplastic anemia), paroxysmal nocturnal hemoglobinuria; *Infectious* bacterial (tuberculosis); viral (hepatitis); *Inflammatory/Immune* systemic lupus erythematosus; *Mechanical/Trauma* irradiation; *Metabolic/Toxic* pernicious anemia or folate deficiency, drugs (cancer chemotherapy, chloramphenicol), poisons (benzene); *Neoplastic* multiple myeloma, carcinomatous invasion, lymphoma, myelodysplasia, acute leukemia, myelofibrosis.

Increased Neutrophils: Leukocytosis, Neutrophilia. Leukocytosis usually represents a response to tissue injury or invasion by pathologic organisms. Always inspect the peripheral smear to detect band forms and toxic granulation. *CLINICAL OCCURRENCE: Endocrine* eclampsia; *Idiopathic* leukemoid reactions; *Infectious* acute pyogenic infections including pneumonia, meningitis, pyelonephritis, pelvic inflammatory disease, deep abscesses, endocarditis; *Inflammatory/Immune* acute necrotizing vasculitis; *Mechanical/ Trauma* burns, acute hemolysis; *Metabolic/Toxic* exercise, uremia, diabetic acidosis, gout, drugs (granulocyte colony-stimulating factor [G-CSF], granulocyte-macrophage colony-stimulating factor [GM-CSF], epinephrine, corticosteroids, lithium carbonate, parenteral foreign proteins, vaccines), poisons (venoms, mercury, black widow spider venom); *Neoplastic* myeloproliferative diseases (polycythemia vera, chronic myelocytic leukemia, myelofibrosis, idiopathic thrombocythemia); *Neurologic* seizures *Vascular* tissue necrosis, myocardial infarction, acute hemorrhage.

Decreased Neutrophils: Leukopenia or Neutropenia. *CLINICAL OCCURRENCE: Congenital* Gaucher disease; *Idiopathic* bone marrow failure (aplastic anemia), cyclic neutropenia; *Infectious* viral (infectious mononucleosis, hepatitis, HIV, influenza, rubeola, psittacosis), bacterial (streptococcal, staphylococcal diseases, sepsis, tularemia, brucellosis, tuberculosis), rickettsial disease (scrub typhus, sandfly fever); protozoa (malaria, kala-azar); *Inflammatory/Immune* hypersplenism, Felty syndrome, autoimmune neutropenia, systemic lupus erythematosus; *Mechanical/Trauma* portal hypertension; *Metabolic/Toxic* uremia, pernicious anemia/B_{12} deficiency, folate deficiency, cirrhosis, cachexia, drugs and therapy (cancer chemotherapy, sulfonamides, antibiotics, analgesics, antidepressants, arsenicals, antithyroid drugs, X-radiation), poisons (benzene); *Neoplastic* aleukemic leukemia, acute myeloblastic leukemia.

EOSINOPHIL COUNTS. *Pathophysiology:* Eosinophils are important in the defense against multicellular parasite infections.

Normal Eosinophil Count: 0%–7% of white blood cells (WBCs).

Increased Eosinophils: Eosinophilia. *CLINICAL OCCURRENCE:* *Idiopathic* Loeffler endocarditis, hypereosinophilic syndrome; *Infectious* scarlet fever, parasitic infestations (e.g., trichinosis, echinococcosis); *Inflammatory/Immune* asthma, hay fever, urticaria, drug reactions, erythema multiforme, pemphigus, dermatitis herpetiformis, eosinophilic gastroenteritis, ulcerative colitis, regional enteritis, polyarteritis nodosa, sarcoidosis pernicious anemia, eosinophilic fasciitis; *Mechanical/Trauma* postsplenectomy, black widow spider bite; *Metabolic/Toxic* poisons (phosphorus); *Neoplastic* metastatic carcinoma to bone, chronic myelocytic leukemia, polycythemia vera, Hodgkin disease; *Vascular* vasculitis (polyarteritis nodosa).

Decreased Eosinophils: Eosinopenia. Bone Marrow failure, adrenal insufficiency (Addison disease).

BASOPHIL COUNTS. *Pathophysiology:* The function of basophils is uncertain. They are similar to tissue mast cells.

Normal Basophil Count: 0–2.0% of white blood cells (WBCs).

Increased Basophils: Basophilia. *CLINICAL OCCURRENCE:* *Endocrine* hypothyroidism (myxedema); *Infectious* varicella, variola; *Inflammatory/Immune* chronic hemolytic anemias; *Mechanical/Trauma* postsplenectomy; *Metabolic/Toxic* nephrotic syndrome; *Neoplastic* chronic myelocytic leukemia, polycythemia vera, myeloid metaplasia, Hodgkin disease.

Decreased Basophils. *CLINICAL OCCURRENCE: Endocrine* hyperthyroidism, pregnancy; *Idiopathic* bone marrow failure, aplastic anemia; *Metabolic/Toxic* drugs (chemotherapy, glucocorticoids).

LYMPHOCYTE COUNTS. *Pathophysiology:* Most circulating lymphocytes are T cells, which traffic continuously between the blood, the tissues, and the lymph nodes until they become activated by exposure to specific antigen on antigen-presenting cells.

Normal Lymphocyte Count: 16–45% of white blood cells (WBCs).

Increased Lymphocytes: Lymphocytosis. *CLINICAL OCCUR-RENCE: Infectious* infectious mononucleosis, tuberculosis, viral pneumonia, infectious hepatitis, cholera, rubella, brucellosis, systemic syphilis, toxoplasmosis, pertussis; *Neoplastic* lymphocytic leukemia, malignant lymphoma.

Decreased Lymphocytes: Lymphopenia. *CLINICAL OCCUR-RENCE: Idiopathic* idiopathic lymphopenia; *Infectious* acute infections (viral, HIV), chronic HIV; *Metabolic/Toxic* drugs (corticosteroids, irradiation therapy, cancer chemotherapy); *Neoplastic* carcinoma, lymphoma.

MONOCYTE COUNTS. *Pathophysiology:* Monocytes circulate in the blood and then enter the tissue and terminally differentiate into tissue macrophages, which are important antigen-presenting cells.

Normal Monocyte Count: 4–10% of white blood cells (WBCs).

Increased Monocytes: Monocytosis. *CLINICAL OCCURRENCE: Congenital* Gaucher disease; *Infectious* protozoal (malaria, kala-azar, trypanosomiasis), rickettsial (Rocky Mountain spotted fever, typhus), bacterial (subacute bacterial endocarditis, tuberculosis, brucellosis, syphilis); *Inflammatory/Immune* ulcerative colitis, regional enteritis, systemic lupus erythematosus, sarcoidosis; *Neoplastic* monocytic leukemia, myeloid metaplasia, recovery from agranulocytosis.

PLATELET COUNTS (THROMBOCYTES). *Pathophysiology:* Platelets are primarily responsible for initial hemostasis by aggregation at the sites of endothelial damage. The platelet plug is then stabilized by fibrin deposition from activated coagulation.

Normal Platelet Count: 130,000–400,000/mm^3.

Increased Platelet Count: Thrombocytosis or Thrombocythemia. Platelets respond like an acute-phase reactant to tissue injury and many acute infections. *CLINICAL OCCURRENCE: Infectious* acute infections; *Inflammatory/Immune* rheumatoid arthritis; *Mechanical/Trauma* burns, postsplenectomy; *Metabolic/Toxic* exercise, cirrhosis, iron deficiency; *Neoplastic* myeloproliferative diseases (polycythemia vera, essential thrombocythemia, myelocytic leukemia); *Vascular* hemorrhage.

Decreased Platelet Count: Thrombocytopenia. *CLINICAL OCCURRENCE: Congenital* May-Hegglin anomaly, Gaucher disease, Kasabach-Merritt syndrome; *Idiopathic* aplastic anemia, marrow failure; *Infectious* subacute bacterial endocarditis, sepsis, AIDS, typhus; *Inflammatory/Immune* autoimmune thrombocytopenic purpura (ITP), hemolytic uremic syndrome (HUS), acquired hemolytic anemia, thrombotic thrombocytopenic purpura (TTP), disseminated intravascular coagulation (DIC); *Mechanical/Trauma* hypersplenism (congestive splenomegaly, sarcoidosis, splenomegaly, Felty syndrome), massive blood transfusions, irradiation, heat stroke; *Metabolic/Toxic* uremia, pernicious anemia, folate deficiency, drugs (cancer chemotherapy, chloramphenicol, heparin induced thrombocytopenia, tranquilizers, antipyretics, heavy metals), poisons (benzol, snake bite, insect bites); *Neoplastic* polycythemia vera, myelocytic leukemia.

Coagulation

NORMAL COAGULATION. *Pathophysiology:* Coagulation is a complex process involving many different blood proteins, platelets, calcium, and tissue factors. There is a constant balance between initiation of coagulation and coagulation inhibitors designed to protect against inappropriate coagulation while directing clot formation to the sites of vessel injury. Two major tests of the coagulation pathways are commonly used.

PROTHROMBIN TIME (PT). The PT is standardized by the International Normalized Ratio (INR), which adjusts the raw clotting time for the International Sensitivity Index (ISI) of the particular thromboplastin in use. It tests factors VII, V, X, thrombin (II), and fibrinogen (I). The PT/INR is particularly sensitive to decreases in the vitamin K-dependent coagulation factors (II, VII, IX and X).

Normal PT: 11–15 seconds (this is highly dependent upon the thromboplastin used).

Normal INR: 1.0–1.2.

Prolonged PT/INR: Deficiencies in factors I, II, V, VII, or X, liver disease, disseminated intravascular coagulation, vitamin K deficiency, steatorrhea, idiopathic, hemodilution, Warfarin administration, greatly decreased or abnormal fibrinogen. *Technical Error* incomplete filling of the Vacutainer tube during the blood draw.

ACTIVATED PARTIAL THROMBOPLASTIN TIME (APTT). The PTT assesses the intrinsic pathway of coagulation which uses factors XII, XI, IX, VIII, V, X, II and I.

Normal aPTT: 22–39 seconds.

Prolonged PTT. Deficiency of *any of the* clotting factors—I, II, V, VIII, IX, X, XI, or XII; disseminated intravascular coagulation, heparin, lupus erythematosus (lupus anticoagulant), antiphospholipid syndrome, and antibody-mediated inhibitors of clotting factor activity.

FIBRINOGEN.   *Pathophysiology:*   The conversion of fibrinogen to fibrin by thrombin is the final pathway in clot formation. Abnormal fibrinogen levels indicate decreased synthesis or, more commonly, increased consumption because of diffuse activation of clotting.

Normal Fibrinogen: 200–400 mg/dL.

Increased Fibrinogen.   Fibrinogen is an acute-phase reactant that increases during menstruation and pregnancy, infections, inflammation and hyperthyroidism.

Decreased Fibrinogen.   Congenital afibrinogenemia, disseminated intravascular coagulation (DIC), hemodilution, fibrinolysis.

Urinalysis

Considerable information can be rapidly obtained from examination of the urine. Optimally, urine is collected as a midstream specimen from the first morning voiding and is examined within 30 minutes. This tests renal-concentrating ability and permits identification of casts before they disintegrate. As with the peripheral smear, experience is required for interpretation. The clinician should establish the habit of examining the urine personally, especially in challenging cases.

COLOR.   Either clear or cloudy (from precipitated normally excreted urates, phosphates, or sulfates), the urine is usually yellow to amber. Other colors provide clues to the presence of abnormal substances for which chemical tests should be performed.

Abnormal-Colored Urine.   *Dark yellow to green* (bilirubin); *red to black* (erythrocytes, hemoglobin, myoglobin); *purple to brown* on standing in the sunlight from porphyrins.

ACIDITY.   Normally the urine is acid, and the urine pH can reach 5.0 with an acid load. High urine pH suggests either an alkali load or inability to fully acidify the urine by excreting H^+ in the distal tubule. Interpretation of the urine pH requires an assessment of the serum or plasma acid–base status. Monitoring of urinary pH helps physicians attempting to alkalinize or acidify the urine to enhance the solubility and excretion of certain substances and drugs.

Normal Range of pH: 4.6–6.0.

Increased Urine pH. Infection with urea-splitting organisms (e.g., *Proteus*), systemic alkalosis, renal tubular acidosis, carbonic anhydrase inhibitors.

SPECIFIC GRAVITY. An index of weight per unit volume, the specific gravity measures the kidney's ability to concentrate urine in response to the secretion of antidiuretic hormone (ADH), and to dilute the urine with a water load. Fasting during 8 hours of sleep should produce a first morning specimen with a specific gravity exceeding 1.018.

Normal Urine Specific Gravity Range: 1.003–1.030, achieved with forced water-drinking and fasting, respectively.

Increased Urine Specific Gravity. Fasting and dehydration, glycosuria, proteinuria, radiographic contrast media.

Decreased Urine Specific Gravity. Compulsive water drinking, diabetes insipidus.

Fixed Specific Gravity: Isosthenuria (1.010). This suggests inability to concentrate or dilute the urine, indicating damage to the renal medulla. *CLINICAL OCCURRENCE:* Severe renal parenchymal damage from many causes, for example, gout, prolonged potassium deficiency, hypercalcemia, myeloma kidney, sickle cell disease.

PROTEINURIA. *Pathophysiology:* Normally, only the smallest protein molecules can pass the filtration barrier of the glomerulus, and most of these are reabsorbed by the tubules. Glomerular disease produces measurable proteinuria by allowing filtration of more and larger molecules than normal. Because of its low molecular weight, increased albumin in the urine is an early sign of glomerular injury. Tubular injury limits reabsorption of filtered proteins.

Normal Urine Protein: 5–15 mg/dL; males: 0–60 mg/d; females: 0–90 mg/d.

Elevated Urine Protein. *CLINICAL OCCURRENCE: Mild Elevations* Pyelonephritis, fever, benign orthostatic proteinuria, idiopathic focal glomerulonephritis. *Severe Proteinuria* Nephrotic syndrome is defined as >3.5 g/d of proteinuria. Glomerulonephritis, diabetes mellitus, systemic lupus erythematosus, renal vein thrombosis, amyloidosis, and other causes of nephrotic syndrome.

GLUCOSE. *Pathophysiology:* Glucose is normally filtered in the glomerulus and completely reabsorbed, mostly in the proximal tubule. Glucose in randomly collected fresh urine specimens is normally undetectable. When the serum glucose rises above 200 mg/dL, the filtered load will exceed the capacity for tubular reabsorption and glucose will appear in the urine. Dipsticks, impregnated with glucose oxidase and an indicator color, provide a convenient, rapid and semiquantitative estimate for the patient and physician.

Normal Glucose Excretion: 3–25 mg/dL; 50–300 mg/d.

Increased Urine Glucose: Glucosuria. *CLINICAL OCCURRENCE:* Hyperglycemia in diabetes mellitus; infrequently with renal abnormalities, including acute tubular damage, hereditary renal glycosuria, and proximal tubular dysfunction as in the Fanconi syndrome.

KETONES. *Pathophysiology:* Ketones are the products of fatty acid metabolism. Increased ketones in the urine indicate that cellular metabolism is dependent upon fatty acids rather than glucose for energy. Progressively diminished glucose utilization in uncontrolled diabetes mellitus leads to lipolysis with increasing plasma and urinary concentrations of acetoacetic acid, beta-hydroxybutyric acid, and ketones.

Increased Urinary Ketones: Ketonuria. *CLINICAL OCCURRENCE:* Diabetic acidosis, fasting, starvation, alcoholic ketoacidosis, isopropyl alcohol intoxication (the clue is an obtunded patient with normal glucose and acid–base status and urine tests positive for ketones).

URINARY SEDIMENT. *Pathophysiology:* Normally erythrocytes, leukocytes, hyaline casts, and crystals (urate, phosphate, oxalate) are found in the sediment of a fresh specimen collected after a night's fast.

PROCEDURE FOR EXAMINING THE URINARY SEDIMENT. Centrifuge 10 mL of urine in a conical tube for 5 minutes, decant the supernatant, flick the tube to disperse formed elements in the remaining drop, and place it on a slide under a cover slip to be examined with the high-power objective of a microscope (hpf). Abnormal numbers of cells and casts or any bacteria reveal the presence of disease.

Erythrocytes: Hematuria. *Normal: 0–5 red blood cells (RBCs)/hpf. CLINICAL OCCURRENCE: Microscopic hematuria* may occur with fever and exercise and many lesions of the urinary tract from the glomerulus to the urethral meatus [Cohen RA, Brown RS. Microscopic Hematuria. NEJM 2003;348:2330–2338]. Causes of *gross hematuria* include coagulation defects, renal papillary necrosis, renal infarction, sickle cell disease, glomerulonephritis, Goodpasture syndrome, stone or carcinoma of the kidney, hemorrhagic cystitis, stone or carcinoma of the bladder, and prostatitis.

Leukocytes: Pyuria. *Normal: 0–10 white blood cells (WBCs)/hpf. CLINICAL OCCURRENCE:* In addition to neutrophils excreted into the urine from the same anatomic sites as erythrocytes, leukocytes from vaginal exudates frequently contaminate routine specimens collected from women. When pyuria exceeding 10 WBCs/hpf is present in an uncontaminated specimen, a site of infection or inflammation in the urinary tract or kidney should be sought.

Casts. Occasional *hyalin casts*, arising from the normal renal tubular secretion of mucoproteins, are seen in fresh concentrated specimens. Finding many broad, fine, or coarse *granular casts* (composed of serum proteins like albumin, IgG, transferrin, haptoglobin) in urine containing excessive protein indicates renal parenchymal disease. *Red cell casts* generally indicate glomerular disease with RBCs passing the damaged glomeruli in large quantities. The urine of patients with the nephrotic syndrome, who exhibit glomerular proteinuria and hyperlipoproteinuria, contains *fatty casts*, casts with *doubly refractile fat bodies*, and *Maltese crosses* when examined in polarized light. *Red cell casts*, containing 10 to 50 distinct erythrocytes and doubly refractile fat bodies, indicate glomerular disease (glomerulonephritis). *White cell and/or renal tubular epithelial cell casts* are found in the urinary sediment of patients with pyelonephritis, polyarteritis, exudative glomerulonephritis, and renal infarction. *Bacteria* accompanying white cell casts indicate urinary tract infection. Broad orange or brown *hematin casts* occur in acute tubular injury and chronic renal failure.

Cerebrospinal Fluid (CSF)

The brain and spinal cord are surrounded by, and suspended in, a clear, colorless fluid. Patients with acute CNS symptoms often require testing of the fluid. Below are found the most commonly ordered tests, their reference ranges, and the more frequent causes of abnormality.

PROTEIN. **Normal CSF Protein: 20–50 mg/dL (SI Units: 0.5–2.0 g/L).**

Increased CSF Protein. Traumatic tap, infection, hemorrhage, metabolic and demyelinating disorders.

Decreased CSF Protein. Young children, CSF leakage, water intoxication, CSF removal, hyperthyroidism.

GLUCOSE. **Normal CSF Glucose: 40–70 mg/dL (SI Units: 2.2–3/9 mmol/L).**

Elevated CSF Glucose. Hyperglycemia.

Decreased CSF Glucose. Hypoglycemia, infection (especially bacterial or mycobacterial), meningeal malignancy.

CELL COUNT AND DIFFERENTIAL. **Normal CSF Cell Count: Adult, 0–5 mononuclear cells per microliter; neonates, 0–30 mononuclear cells per microliter.**

Increased CSF Leukocytes. *Mononuclear cells* increase in infection of the CNS (viral and early bacterial meningitis, meningoencephalitis, or abscess), neurologic disorders, and hematologic malignancies. *Neutrophils* increase in bacterial infection, hemorrhage, and meningeal malignancy. *Eosinophils* increase in shunt, parasitic infection, and allergic reactions.

Serous Body Fluids

Normally, a very small amount of fluid resides in the pleural, pericardial and peritoneal spaces. Any clinically detectable accumulation of fluid (effusion or ascites) in the cavity is caused by a pathologic condition. Effusions should be examined microscopically to determine the distribution (differential count) of cells and to detect malignant cells. Cell counts are useful in peritoneal fluid (below), but are somewhat less helpful in pleural fluid. Increased inflammatory cells have indications similar to those in other locations: *Neutrophils* (infection, neoplasm, leukemia); *lymphocytes* (infection, infarction, lymphoma, leukemia, neoplasm, rheumatologic serositis); *eosinophils* (air in cavity, infection, infarction, neoplasm, rheumatologic disease, congestive heart failure). Microbiologic examination, stains, and culture are indicated in exudates; cytologic examination will identify abnormal/malignant cells. Effusions are generally classified as *transudate* (low protein) or *exudate* (high protein).

Transudates. Transudates, commonly bilateral in the pleural cavities, are secondary to heart failure or medical conditions that cause a low serum albumin, for example, cirrhosis or nephrotic syndrome. Clear and pale, straw-colored fluids are usually transudates, and additional information is rarely provided by testing beyond that required to confirm that the fluid is a transudate. The few cells found in transudates are mesothelial cells and mononuclear cells (lymphocytes and monocytes) with very few neutrophils.

Exudates. Exudates are more frequently unilateral in the pleural cavities and secondary to localized disorders such as infection or neoplasm. Exudates can be cloudy from cellular increases (leukocytes), red or pink from hemorrhage (or trauma), green white from purulence, or milky from increased lipid.

PLEURAL EFFUSION. See page 397. Tests frequently useful in pleural effusions include gross appearance, fluid/serum protein ratios (<0.5 = transudate; >0.5 = exudate), fluid/serum lactate dehydrogenase (LDH) ratios (<0.6 = transudate; >0.6 = exudate), fluid/serum cholesterol ratio (<0.3 = transudate; >0.3 = exudate), morphologic exam (hematology and cytology), and pH (<7.20 with white blood cell count [WBC] $>1000/mm^3$ and low glucose suggests empyema). *Note*: If the protein and LDH ratios are equivocal, the cholesterol ratios may help identify transudate/exudate. Transudates rarely benefit from further testing. Cell counts are rarely useful.

PERITONEAL EFFUSION: ASCITES. See page 542.
Tests frequently useful in peritoneal effusion include gross appearance,
serum/ascites albumin concentration gradient, cell count and differential, cytology and cultures for bacteria and mycobacteria.

Serum/Ascites Albumin Gradient. Subtracting peritoneal albumin
from simultaneously determined serum albumin determines the
serum/ascites albumin gradient. Values <1.1 indicate an exudate (bacterial peritonitis, neoplasm, nephrotic syndrome, pancreatitis, vasculitis); values >1.1 indicate a transudate (portal hypertension
caused by cirrhosis, hepatic vein thrombosis, portal vein thrombosis,
congestive heart failure). *Note*: Protein and lactate dehydrogenase
(LDH) ratios described above for pleural fluid are not reliable in peritoneal fluid to separate transudates from exudates.

White Blood Cell Counts. Detection of spontaneous bacterial peritonitis in patients with transudative ascites is important. Neutrophil
counts of >250/mm^3 indicate infection and the need for treatment
and long-term prophylaxis. High leukocyte counts (>500/mm^3),
mostly mononuclear cells, are also seen in malignancy.

ADDITIONAL READING

1. RH Fletcher, SW Fletcher, EH Wagner: *Clinical Epidemiology*. 3rd ed.
   Baltimore, MD, Williams & Wilkins, 1996.
2. DS Young, EJ Huth: *SI Units for Clinical Measurement*. Philadelphia,
   American College of Physicians, 1998.
3. Black ER, Bordley DR, Tape TG, Panzer RJ (eds): *Diagnostic Strategies
   for Common Medical Problems*. 2nd ed. Philadelphia, American College
   of Physicians, 1999.

Index

Note: Page numbers followed by f indicate figures; those followed by t indicate tables.

Knee (*Cont.*)
  loose body in, 761–762
  motions and deviations of, 686, 686*f*
  movement of, 826
  pain in
    anterior, 761
    examination for, 705–707, 706*f*
    post-traumatic, 760–761, 761*f*, 762–764
  palpation of, 703–704
  superficial anatomy of, 683–687, 685*f*, 686*f*
  swelling of, 757–760, 758*f*, 759*f*
Knee extension, lack of, 846*f*, 847
Knee jerk, 810–811, 810*f*
Knee ligaments, examination of, 704–705, 705*f*
Knee signs, 757–764, 758*f*, 759*f*, 761*f*
Knock-knee, 686*f*, 757
Kocher test, 314
Koebner phenomena, 171
KOH preparation, 135
Koilonychia, 153, 153*f*
Koplik spots, 290, 290*f*
Korotkoff sounds, 82–83
Korsakoff syndrome, 877
KP (keratitic precipitates), 318
Krönig isthmus, 357, 357*f*, 358
Kussmaul breathing, 80–81
Kussmaul sign, 440
Kyphoscoliosis, 720
Kyphosis, 380–381, 380*f*
  thoracic, 719*f*, 720

Labial corners, inflamed, 288, 288*f*
Labial deformity, 287
Labial enlargement, 287
Labial frenulum, 202
Labial inflammation, 288, 288*f*
Labial pigmentation, due to intestinal polyposis, 288*f*, 289
Labial scaling lesion, 289
Labial scarring, 288*f*, 289
Labial ulcer, 288–289
Labial vesicles, 287
Labia majora
  anatomy of, 624, 626*f*
  swelling of, 634

Labia minora, anatomy of, 624, 626*f*
Labioinguinal hernia, 634
Laboratory examination, 5
Laboratory results, in medical record, 32
Laboratory test(s), 933–967
  aids in selection and interpretation of, 919–922, 922*f*
  of blood chemistries, 934–954
  of cerebrospinal fluid, 965–966
  for hematologic data, 954–962
  preoperative, 908–909
  reasons for, 933–934
  selection of, 11
  of serous body fluids, 966–967
  for urinalysis, 962–965
Laboratory testing
  for disease present or absent, 916
  examples of, 923–927, 923*f*–926*f*
  likelihood ratios in, 921, 922*f*
  posttest probability in, 921–922
  predictive values in, 918*f*, 920–921
  pretest probability in, 918
  for prevalence of disease, 919
  principles of, 915–930
  probability and odds in, 917
  reasons for, 915–916
  routine, 915
  rule in and rule out in, 929
  sampling in, 928–929
  sensitivity of, 918*f*, 919
  setting cutpoint in, 916–917, 917*f*, 920
  severity of disease in, 928
  specificity of, 918*f*, 919–920
  test positive or negative in, 916–917, 917*f*
  2×2 tables in, 918, 918*f*, 927
Labyrinth, 193, 195
Labyrinthine disorder, 246
Labyrinthine hydrops, 322, 323–324
Labyrinthine tests, 210–211, 211*f*
Labyrinthitis, acute, 323
Laceration, of scrotum, 665
Lachman test, 704–705, 705*f*
Lacrimal duct, 198
  inflammation of, 251*f*, 252

Vasomotor rhinitis, 324–325